# Place-of-Service Codes for Professional Claims

Listed below are place-of-service codes and descriptions. These codes should be used on professional claims to specify the entity where service(s) were rendered. Check with individual payers (eg, Medicare, Medicaid, other private insurance) for reimbursement policies regarding these codes. If you would like to comment on a code(s) or description(s), please send your request to posinfo@cms.hhs.gov.

| Place of Service Code(s) | Place of Service Name | Place of Service Description |
|---|---|---|
| 01 | Pharmacy | A facility or location where drugs and other medically related items and services are sold, dispensed, or otherwise provided directly to patients. (effective 10/1/05) |
| 02 | Unassigned | N/A |
| 03 | School | A facility whose primary purpose is education. |
| 04 | Homeless shelter | A facility or location whose primary purpose is to provide temporary housing to homeless individuals (eg, emergency shelters, individual or family shelters). |
| 05 | Indian Health Service freestanding facility | A facility or location, owned and operated by the Indian Health Service, which provides diagnostic, therapeutic (surgical and nonsurgical), and rehabilitation services to American Indians and Alaska Natives who do not require hospitalization. |
| 06 | Indian Health Service provider-based facility | A facility or location, owned and operated by the Indian Health Service, which provides diagnostic, therapeutic (surgical and nonsurgical), and rehabilitation services rendered by, or under the supervision of, physicians to American Indians and Alaska Natives admitted as inpatients or outpatients. |
| 07 | Tribal 638 freestanding facility | A facility or location owned and operated by a federally recognized American Indian or Alaska Native tribe or tribal organization under a 638 agreement which provides diagnostic, therapeutic (surgical and nonsurgical), and rehabilitation services to tribal members who do not require hospitalization. |
| 08 | Tribal 638 provider-based facility | A facility or location owned and operated by a federally recognized American Indian or Alaska Native tribe or tribal organization under a 638 agreement which provides diagnostic, therapeutic (surgical and nonsurgical), and rehabilitation services to tribal members admitted as inpatients or outpatients. |
| 09 | Prison-Correctional facility | A prison, jail, reformatory, work farm, detention center, or any other similar facility maintained by either Federal, State, or local authorities for the purpose of confinement or rehabilitation of adult or juvenile criminal offenders. |
| 10 | Unassigned | N/A |
| 11 | Office | Location, other than a hospital, skilled nursing facility (SNF), military treatment facility, community health center, State or local public health clinic, or intermediate care facility (ICF), where the health professional routinely provides health examinations, diagnosis, and treatment of illness or injury on an ambulatory basis. |
| 12 | Home | Location, other than a hospital or other facility, where the patient receives care in a private residence. |
| 13 | Assisted living facility | Congregate residential facility with self-contained living units providing assessment of each resident's needs and on-site support 24 hours a day, seven days a week, with the capacity to deliver or arrange for services including some health care and other services. |
| 14 | Group home | A residence, with shared living areas, where clients receive supervision and other services such as social and/or behavioral services, custodial service, and minimal services (eg, medication administration) (effective 4/1/04) |
| 15 | Mobile unit | A facility or unit that moves from place to place and is equipped to provide preventive, screening, diagnostic, and/or treatment services. |
| 16 | Temporary lodging | A short term accommodation such as a hotel, camp ground, hostel, cruise ship, or resort where the patient receives care, and which is not identified by any other POS code. |
| 17 | Walk-in retail health clinic | A walk-in health clinic, other than an office, urgent care facility, pharmacy, or independent clinic, and which is not described by any other Place of Service code, that is located within a retail operation and provides on an ambulatory basis, preventive and primary care services. (This code is available for use immediately with a final effective date of May 1, 2010.) |
| 18-19 | Unassigned | N/A |
| 20 | Urgent care facility | Location, distinct from a hospital emergency department, an office, or a clinic, whose purpose is to diagnose and treat illness or injury for unscheduled, ambulatory patients seeking immediate medical attention. |
| 21 | Inpatient hospital | A facility, other than psychiatric, which primarily provides diagnostic, therapeutic (both surgical and nonsurgical), and rehabilitation services by, or under, the supervision of physicians to patients admitted for a variety of medical conditions. |
| 22 | Outpatient hospital | A portion of a hospital that provides diagnostic, therapeutic (both surgical and nonsurgical), and rehabilitation services to sick or injured persons who do not require hospitalization or institutionalization. |
| 23 | Emergency Room—hospital | A portion of a hospital where emergency diagnosis and treatment of illness or injury is provided. |
| 24 | Ambulatory surgical center | A freestanding facility, other than a physician's office, where surgical and diagnostic services are provided on an ambulatory basis. |
| 25 | Birthing center | A facility, other than a hospital's maternity facilities or a physician's office, which provides a setting for labor, delivery, and immediate postpartum care as well as immediate care of newborn infants. |
| 26 | Military treatment facility | A medical facility operated by one or more of the Uniformed Services. Military treatment facility (MTF) also refers to certain former US Public Health Service (USPHS) facilities now designated as Uniformed Service Treatment Facilities (USTF). |
| 27-30 | Unassigned | N/A |

| 31 | Skilled nursing facility | A facility that primarily provides inpatient skilled nursing care and related services to patients who require medical, nursing, or rehabilitative services but does not provide the level of care or treatment available in a hospital. |
|---|---|---|
| 32 | Nursing facility | A facility that primarily provides to residents skilled nursing care and related services for the rehabilitation of injured, disabled, or sick persons, or, on a regular basis, health-related care services above the level of custodial care to other than mentally retarded individuals. |
| 33 | Custodial care facility | A facility that provides room, board, and other personal assistance services, generally on a long-term basis, and does not include a medical component. |
| 34 | Hospice | A facility, other than a patient's home, in which palliative and supportive care for terminally ill patients and their families are provided. |
| 35-40 | Unassigned | N/A |
| 41 | Ambulance—land | A land vehicle specifically designed, equipped, and staffed for lifesaving and transporting the sick or injured. |
| 42 | Ambulance—air or water | An air or water vehicle specifically designed, equipped, and staffed for lifesaving and transporting the sick or injured. |
| 43-48 | Unassigned | N/A |
| 49 | Independent clinic | A location, not part of a hospital and not described by any other Place of Service code, that is organized and operated to provide preventive, diagnostic, therapeutic, rehabilitative, or palliative services to outpatients only. (effective 10/1/03) |
| 50 | Federally qualified health center | A facility located in a medically underserved area that provides Medicare beneficiaries preventive primary medical care under the general direction of a physician. |
| 51 | Inpatient psychiatric facility | A facility that provides inpatient psychiatric services for the diagnosis and treatment of mental illness on a 24-hour basis, by or under the supervision of a physician. |
| 52 | Psychiatric facility— partial hospitalization | A facility for the diagnosis and treatment of mental illness that provides a planned therapeutic program for patients who do not require full-time hospitalization but who need broader programs than are possible from outpatient visits to a hospital-based or hospital-affiliated facility. |
| 53 | Community mental health center | A facility that provides the following services: outpatient services, including specialized outpatient services for children, the elderly, individuals who are chronically ill, and residents of the CMHC's community mental health area who have been discharged from inpatient treatment at a mental health facility; 24-hour a day emergency care services; day treatment, other partial hospitalization services, or psychosocial rehabilitation services; screening for patients being considered for admission to State mental health facilities to determine the appropriateness of such admission; and consultation and education services. |
| 54 | Intermediate care facility/mentally retarded | A facility that primarily provides health-related care and services above the level of custodial care to mentally retarded individuals but does not provide the level of care or treatment available in a hospital or SNF. |
| 55 | Residential substance abuse treatment facility | A facility which provides treatment for substance (alcohol and drug) abuse to live-in residents who do not require acute medical care. Services include individual and group therapy and counseling, family counseling, laboratory tests, drugs and supplies, psychological testing, and room and board. |
| 56 | Psychiatric residential treatment center | A facility or distinct part of a facility for psychiatric care which provides a total 24-hour therapeutically planned and professionally staffed group living and learning environment. |
| 57 | Nonresidential substance abuse treatment facility | A location that provides treatment for substance (alcohol and drug) abuse on an ambulatory basis. Services include individual and group therapy and counseling, family counseling, laboratory tests, drugs and supplies, and psychological testing. |
| 58-59 | Unassigned | N/A |
| 60 | Mass immunization center | A location where providers administer pneumococcal pneumonia and influenza virus vaccinations and submit these services as electronic media claims or paper claims or by using the roster billing method. This generally takes place in a mass immunization setting, such as a public health center, pharmacy, or mall but may include a physician office setting. |
| 61 | Comprehensive inpatient rehabilitation facility | A facility that provides comprehensive rehabilitation services under the supervision of a physician to inpatients with physical disabilities. Services include physical therapy, occupational therapy, speech pathology, social or psychological services, and orthotics and prosthetics services. |
| 62 | Comprehensive outpatient rehabilitation facility | A facility that provides comprehensive rehabilitation services under the supervision of a physician to outpatients with physical disabilities. Services include physical therapy, occupational therapy, and speech pathology services. |
| 63-64 | Unassigned | N/A |
| 65 | End-stage renal disease treatment facility | A facility, other than a hospital, that provides dialysis treatment, maintenance, and/or training to patients or caregivers on an ambulatory or home-care basis. |
| 66-70 | Unassigned | N/A |
| 71 | Public health clinic | A facility maintained by either State or local health departments that provides ambulatory primary medical care under the general direction of a physician. |
| 72 | Rural health clinic | A certified facility located in a rural, medically underserved area that provides ambulatory primary medical care under the general direction of a physician. |
| 73-80 | Unassigned | N/A |
| 81 | Independent laboratory | A laboratory certified to perform diagnostic and/or clinical tests independent of an institution or a physician's office. |
| 82-98 | Unassigned | N/A |
| 99 | Other place of service | Other place of service not identified above. |

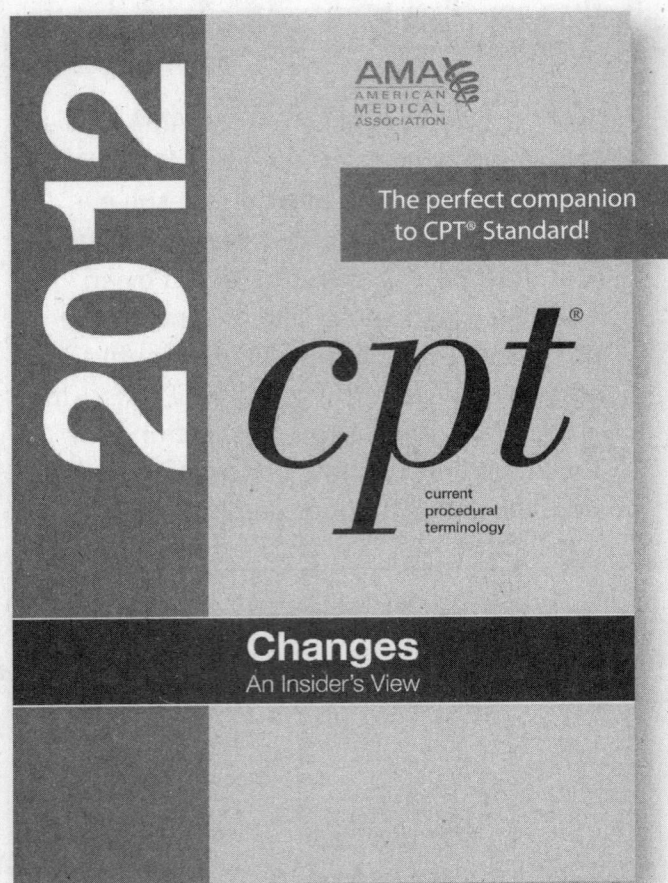

current procedural terminology

# *cpt*®
## 2012

# Standard Edition

Michelle Abraham, MHA
Jay T. Ahlman
Caryn Anderson, RHIT
Angela J. Boudreau
Judy Connelly
Desiree D. Evans, AAS
Rejina L. Glenn
Gloria Green, BA

DeHandro Hayden, BS
Grace M. Kotowicz, RN, BS
Elizabeth Lumakovska, MPA, RHIT
Janette Meggs, RHIA
Marie L. Mindeman, BA, RHIT
Karen E. O'Hara, BS, CCS-P
Mary R. O'Heron, RHIA
Danielle Pavloski, BS, RHIT, CCS-P

Marjorie C. Rallins, DPM
Dan Reyes
Desiree Rozell, MPA
Lianne Stancik, RHIT
Peggy Thompson, MS, RHIA, CCS
Susan Tracy, MA, RHIT
Ada Walker, CCA
Arletrice Watkins, MHA, RHIA

AMA
AMERICAN MEDICAL
ASSOCIATION

Standard ISBN: 978-1-60359-567-4
ISSN: 0276-8283

# Foreword

*Current Procedural Terminology* (CPT®), Fourth Edition, is a listing of descriptive terms and identifying codes for reporting medical services and procedures performed by physicians. The purpose of the terminology is to provide a uniform language that will accurately describe medical, surgical, and diagnostic services, and will thereby provide an effective means for reliable nationwide communication among physicians, patients, and third parties. *CPT 2012* is the most recent revision of a work that first appeared in 1966.

CPT descriptive terms and identifying codes currently serve a wide variety of important functions in the field of medical nomenclature. The CPT code set is useful for administrative management purposes such as claims processing and for the development of guidelines for medical care review. The uniform language is also applicable to medical education and outcomes, health services, and quality research by providing a useful basis for local, regional, and national utilization comparisons. The CPT code set is the most widely accepted nomenclature for the reporting of physician procedures and services under government and private health insurance programs. In 2000, the CPT code set was designated by the Department of Health and Human Services as the national coding standard for physician and other health care professional services and procedures under the Health Insurance Portability and Accountability Act (HIPAA). This means that for all financial and administrative health care transactions sent electronically, the CPT code set will need to be used.

The changes that appear in this revision have been prepared by the CPT Editorial Panel with the assistance of physicians representing all specialties of medicine, and with important contributions from many third-party payers and governmental agencies.

The American Medical Association trusts that this revision will continue the usefulness of its predecessors in identifying, describing, and coding medical, surgical, and diagnostic services.

# Acknowledgments

Publication of the annual CPT codebook represents many challenges and opportunities. From reconciling the many differences of opinion about the best way to describe a procedure, to the last details on placement of a semicolon, many individuals and organizations devote their energies and expertise to the preparation of this revision.

The editorial staff wishes to express sincere thanks to the many national medical specialty societies, health insurance organizations and agencies, and individual physicians and other health professionals who have made contributions.

Thanks are due to Robert A. Musacchio, PhD, Sr VP, American Medical Association; Claudia Bonnell, Blue Cross and Blue Shield Association; Nelly Leon-Chisen, American Hospital Association; Terry Leone, America's Health Insurance Plans; and Sue Bowman, RHIA, American Health Information Management Association, for their invaluable assistance in enhancing the CPT code set.

For their assistance in development of the CPT Category II codes:

Jeffrey Cozzens, MD
Ronald A. Gabel, MD
Darryl T. Gray, MD, ScD
Sam J. W. Romeo, MD, MBA

We recognize the following people for efforts in working with the Physician Consortium for Performance Improvement® (PCPI™) and other quality measurement organizations:

Mark Antman, DDS, MBA
Katherine Ast, MSW, LCSW
Heidi Bossley, MSN, MBA
Christopher D. Carlucci, MBA
Kendra Hanley, MS
Diedra D. Joseph, MPH
Karen S. Kmetik, PhD
Stephanie Moncada, MS
Marjorie C. Rallins, DPM
Kimberly Smuk, BS, RHIA
Beth Tapper, MA
Samantha Tierney, MPH
Jennifer Trajkovski, MJ, RHIT

# AMA CPT Editorial Panel

*Chair*
William T. Thorwarth, Jr, MD, FACR*

*Vice-Chair*
Peter A. Hollmann, MD*

Albert E. Bothe, Jr, MD, FACS
Kenneth P. Brin, MD, PhD, FACC
Boyd R. Buser, DO, FACOFP
Patrick J. Cafferty, MPAS, PA-C*
Jeffrey W. Cozzens, MD, FACS
Frank J. Dubeck, Jr, MD, FACP
Richard Duszak, Jr, MD, FACR*
David A. Ellington, MD
Ronald A. Gabel, MD†
M. Bradford Henley, MD, MBA
Andrea H. McGuire, MD, MBA
Victor L. Lewis, MD†
Antonio E. Puente, PhD
Kenneth B. Simon, MD, MBA*
Mark S. Synovec, MD, MBA

*Secretary*
Marie L. Mindeman, BA, RHIT

*Member of the CPT Executive Committee
†New Panel Member April 2010
‡New Advisors

# AMA CPT Advisory Committee

*Academy of Pharmaceutical Physicians and Investigators*
Grant P. Bagley, MD
*American Academy of Allergy, Asthma and Immunology*
Donald W. Aaronson, MD, JD, MPH
*American Academy of Child & Adolescent Psychiatry*
David I. Berland, MD
*American Academy of Dermatology*
Dirk M. Elston, MD
Alexander Miller, MD‡
*American Academy of Disability Evaluating Physicians*
Douglas W. Martin, MD, FAADEP, FACOEM‡
*American Academy of Family Physicians*
Robert J. Carr, Jr, MD
Gretchen M. Dickson, MD, MBA‡
*American Academy of Neurology*
Marc R. Nuwer, MD, PhD
Bruce H. Cohen, MD, FAAN‡
*American Academy of Ophthalmology*
Michael X. Repka, MD
*American Academy of Orthopaedic Surgeons*
Richard J. Friedman, MD, FACSC
*American Academy of Otolaryngic Allergy*
Paul T. Fass, MD, FACS
Bryan D. Leatherman, MD‡
*American Academy of Otolaryngology Head and Neck Surgery*
Bradley F. Marple, MD, FAAOA‡
Brendan C. Stack, Jr, MD, FACS, FACE‡
*American Academy of Pain Medicine*
Eduardo M. Fraifeld, MD
Lee T. Snook, Jr, MD, FACP, DABPM‡
*American Academy of Pediatrics*
Richard A. Molteni, MD
Julia M. Pillsbury, DO, FAAO, FACOP‡
*American Academy of Physical Medicine and Rehabilitation*
Francis P. Lagattuta, MD

*American Academy of Sleep Medicine*
Samuel A. Fleishman, MD
Amy J. Aronsky, DO, FAAP, FACOP‡
*American Association for Clinical Chemistry*
Robert L. Murray, JD, PhD
*American Association for Thoracic Surgery*
Kirk R. Kanter, MD
Stephen J. Lahey, MD‡
*American Association of Clinical Endocrinologists*
Eric A. Orzeck, MD, FACP, FACE
*American Association of Neurological Surgeons*
R. Patrick Jacob, MD
*American Association of Neuromuscular and Electrodiagnostic Medicine*
Andrea J. Boon, MD
*American Association of Public Health Physicians*
Arvind K. Goyal, MD, MPH, FAAFP, FACPM
*American Clinical Neurophysiology Society*
Marc R. Nuwer, MD, PhD
*American College of Allergy, Asthma and Immunology*
Gary N. Gross, MD
*American College of Cardiology*
Robert N. Piana, MD, FACC
Patricio A. Frais, MD, FACC‡
*American College of Chest Physicians*
Steve G. Peters, MD
Michael E. Nelson, MD, FCCP‡
*American College of Emergency Physicians*
Kenneth L. DeHart, MD, FACEP
*American College of Gastroenterology*
Daniel C. DeMarco, MD, FACG
*American College of Medical Genetics*
David B. Flannery, MD
*American College of Medical Quality*
Joel Grossman, MD
*American College of Mohs Surgery*
David B. Pharis, MD, PC‡
*American College of Nuclear Medicine*
Scott C. Bartley, MD‡
*American College of Occupational and Environmental Medicine*
Lee S. Glass, MD, JD‡
*American College of Physicians*
R. Scott Hanson, MD, MPH
Jeannine Z. Engel, MD, FACP‡
*American College of Preventive Medicine*
Ryung Suh, MD, MPP, MBA, MPH
*American College of Radiation Oncology*
Andy W. Su, MD‡
Paul E. Wallner, DO, FACR, FAOCR, FASTRO, FACRO‡
*American College of Radiology*
Daniel Picus, MD, FACR, RCC
*American College of Rheumatology*
Gerald M. Eisenberg, MD, FACP, FACR‡
Robert J. Lloyd, MD, FACR
*American College of Surgeons*
Linda M. Barney, MD, FACS
Mark T. Savarise, MD, FACS‡
*American Congress of Obstetricians and Gynecologists*
Jordan G. Pritzker, MD, MBA, FACOG
Jon K. Hathaway, MD, PhD‡
*American Dental Association*
Anthony M. Spina, DDS, MD
Joseph F. Piecuch, DMD, MD‡
*American Gastroenterological Association*
Joel V. Brill, MD, AGAF, FASGE, FACG, CHCQM

American Geriatric Society
Robert A. Zorowitz, MD, MBA, FACP, AGSF, CMD
American Institute of Ultrasound in Medicine
Harvey L. Nisenbaum, MD
American Medical Directors Association
Dennis L. Stone, MD, MBA
American Orthopaedic Association
Blair C. Filler, MD
American Orthopaedic Foot and Ankle Society
Walter J. Pedowitz, MD
David I. Pedowitz, MD‡
American Osteopathic Association
Judith A. O'Connell, DO, FAAO
American Psychiatric Association
David K. Nace, MD
American Roentgen Ray Society
Mark D. Alson, MD
American Society for Aesthetic Plastic Surgery, Inc.
Paul R. Weiss, MD
American Society for Clinical Pathology
Lee H. Hilborne, MD, MPH, FASCP
American Society for Dermatologic Surgery
Murad Alam, MD
Jeremy S. Bordeaux, MD, MPH‡
American Society for Gastrointestinal Endoscopy
Glenn D. Littenberg, MD, FACP
Christopher Y. Kim, MD, MBA, FACG, FASGE, AGAF, FACP‡
American Society for Radiation Oncology
David C. Beyer, MD, FACR, FACRO, FASTRO‡
American Society for Reproductive Medicine
John T. Queenan, Jr, MD, FACOG
American Society for Surgery of the Hand
Daniel J. Nagle, MD
American Society of Abdominal Surgeons
Louis F. Alfano, Jr, MD
American Society of Anesthesiologists
Doug G. Merrill, MD, MBA
Peter A. Goldzweig, DO‡
American Society of Cataract and Refractive Surgery
Stephen S. Lane, MD
American Society of Clinical Oncology
William C. Penley, MD
American Society of Colon and Rectal Surgeons
James I. Merlino, MD
American Society of Cytopathology
Carol A. Filomena, MD‡
American Society of General Surgeons
Charles Drueck, III, MD, FACS
American Society of Hematology
Samuel M. Silver, MD, PhD, FACP, FAHA
American Society of Interventional Pain Physicians
Frank J. E. Falco, MD‡
American Society of Neuroradiology
Jacqueline A. Bello, MD, FACR‡
C. Douglas Phillips, MD, FACR
American Society of Ophthalmic Plastic and Reconstructive Surgery
L. Neal Freeman, MD, MBA, CCS-P, FACS
American Society of Plastic Surgeons
Raymond V. Janevicius, MD
American Thoracic Society
Stephen P. Hoffmann, MD
Kathrin Nicolacakis, MD‡
American Urological Association
Jeffrey A. Dann, MD, MBA
Ronald P. Kaufman, Jr, MD, FACS‡

Association of University Radiologists
Robert K. Zeman, MD, FACR
College of American Pathologists
Michael D. McEachin, MD
Congress of Neurological Surgeons
Joseph S. Cheng, MD
Heart Rhythm Society
Amit J. Shanker, MD‡
Kevin R. Wheelen, MD‡
Infectious Disease Society of America
Steven K. Schmitt, MD
International Spinal Intervention Society
Scott I. Horn, DO
Claire Tibiletti, MD‡
National Association of Medical Examiners
Paul A. Raslavicus, MD, MHA, CPE
North American Spine Society
William Mitchell, MD
David R. O'Brien, Jr, MD‡
Radiological Society of North America
Timothy A. Crummy, MD
Renal Physicians Association
Chester A. Amedia, Jr, MD, FACP‡
Richard J. Hamburger, MD
Society for Investigative Dermatology
Stephen P. Stone, MD
Society for Vascular Surgery
Sean Roddy, MD, FACS
Society of American Gastrointestinal Endoscopic Surgeons
Michael B. Edye, MD‡
Society of Critical Care Medicine
George A. Sample, MD, FCCP
Society of Interventional Radiology
Katharine L. Krol, MD
Donald F. Denny, Jr, MD‡
Society of Nuclear Medicine
Gary L. Dillehay, MD, FACNP, FACR‡
Society of Thoracic Surgeons
Francis C. Nichols, III, MD
Jeffrey P. Jacobs, MD, FACS, FACC, FCCP‡
The Endocrine Society
Richard A. Guthrie, MD
The Triological Society
Richard W. Waguespack, MD, FACS
United States and Canadian Academy of Pathology
David S. Wilkinson, MD, PhD

# AMA Health Care Professionals Advisory Committee (HCPAC)

William T. Thorwarth, Jr, MD, FACR, Co-Chair
AMA CPT Editorial Panel
Patrick J. Cafferty, MPAS, PA-C, Co-Chair
AMA CPT Editorial Panel
American Academy of Physician Assistants
Terry E. Carlisle, PA-C, MPAS
American Association of Naturopathic Physicians
Wendell B. Milliman, ND
Eva Miller, ND‡
American Association for Respiratory Care
Susan Rinaldo-Gallo, Med, RRT
American Chiropractic Association
Craig S. Little, DC, FACO

# Contents

## Radiology Guidelines (Including Nuclear Medicine and Diagnostic Ultrasound)

# Introduction

*Current Procedural Terminology* (CPT®), Fourth Edition, is a set of codes, descriptions, and guidelines intended to describe procedures and services performed by physicians and other health care providers. Each procedure or service is identified with a five-digit code. The use of CPT codes simplifies the reporting of services.

Inclusion of a descriptor and its associated five-digit code number in the CPT codebook is based on whether the procedure is consistent with contemporary medical practice and is performed by many practitioners in clinical practice in multiple locations. Inclusion in the CPT codebook does not represent endorsement by the American Medical Association (AMA) of any particular diagnostic or therapeutic procedure. Inclusion or exclusion of a procedure does not imply any health insurance coverage or reimbursement policy.

The CPT code set is published annually in the late summer or early fall as both electronic data files and books. The release of CPT data files on the Internet typically precedes the book by several weeks. In any case, January 1 is the effective date for use of the update of the CPT code set. The interval between the release of the update and the effective date is considered the implementation period and is intended to allow physicians and other providers, payers, and vendors to incorporate CPT changes into their systems. The exceptions to this schedule of release and effective dates are CPT Category III and vaccine product codes, which are released twice a year on January 1 or July 1 with effective dates for use six months later, and CPT Category II codes. Changes to the CPT code set are meant to be applied prospectively from the effective date.

The main body of the Category I section is listed in six sections. Each section is divided into subsections with anatomic, procedural, condition, or descriptor subheadings. The procedures and services with their identifying codes are presented in numeric order with one exception—the entire **Evaluation and Management** section (99201-99499) appears at the beginning of the listed procedures. These items are used by most physicians in reporting a significant portion of their services.

## Section Numbers and Their Sequences

**Evaluation and Management** . . . . . . . . . . . . 99201-99499
**Anesthesiology** . . . . . . . . . . . . 00100-01999, 99100-99140
**Surgery** . . . . . . . . . . . . . . . . . . . . . . . . . . . . . . 10021-69990
**Radiology (Including Nuclear Medicine
    and Diagnostic Ultrasound)** . . . . . . . . . 70010-79999
**Pathology and Laboratory** . . . . . . . . . . . . . . 80048-89356
**Medicine (except
    Anesthesiology)** . . . . . . . 90281-99199, 99500-99602

The first and last code numbers and the subsection name of the items appear at the top margin of most pages (eg, "11010-11306 Surgery/Integumentary System"). The continuous pagination of the CPT codebook is found on the lower margin of each page along with explanation of any code symbols that are found on that page.

## Instructions for Use of the CPT Codebook

Select the name of the procedure or service that accurately identifies the service performed. Do not select a CPT code that merely approximates the service provided. If no such specific code exists, then report the service using the appropriate unlisted procedure or service code. In surgery, it may be an operation; in medicine, a diagnostic or therapeutic procedure; in radiology, a radiograph. Other additional procedures performed or pertinent special services are also listed. When necessary, any modifying or extenuating circumstances are added. Any service or procedure should be adequately documented in the medical record.

It is important to recognize that the listing of a service or procedure and its code number in a specific section of this book does not restrict its use to a specific specialty group. Any procedure or service in any section of this book may be used to designate the services rendered by any qualified physician or other qualified health care professional or entity (eg, hospital, clinical laboratory, home health agency).

A "physician or other qualified healthcare professional" is an individual who is qualified by education, training, licensure/regulation (when applicable), and facility privileging (when applicable) who performs a professional service within his/her scope of practice and independently reports that professional service. These professionals are distinct from "clinical staff". A clinical staff member is a person who works under the supervision of a physician or other qualified healthcare professional and who is allowed by law, regulation and facility policy to perform or assist in the performance of a specified professional service, but who does not individually report that professional service. Other policies may also affect who may report specific services.

Instructions, typically included as parenthetical notes, with selected codes indicate that a code should not be reported with another code or codes. These instructions are intended to prevent errors of significant probability and are not all inclusive. For example, the code with such instructions may be a component of another code and therefore it would be incorrect to report both codes even when the component service is performed. These instructions are not intended as a listing of all possible code combinations that should not be reported, nor to indicate all possible code combinations that are appropriately reported. When reporting codes for services provided, it is important to assure the accuracy and quality of coding through verification of the intent of the code by use of the related guidelines, parenthetical instructions, and coding resources, including *CPT Assistant* and other publications resulting from collaborative efforts of the American Medical Association with the medical specialty societies (ie, *Clinical Examples in Radiology*).

## Format of the Terminology

The CPT code set has been developed as stand-alone descriptions of medical procedures. However, some of the procedures in the CPT codebook are not printed in their entirety but refer back to a common portion of the procedure listed in a preceding entry. This is evident when an entry is followed by one or more indentations. This is done in an effort to conserve space.

*Example*

**25100**    Arthrotomy, wrist joint; with biopsy

**25105**        with synovectomy

Note that the common part of code 25100 (the part before the semicolon) should be considered part of code 25105. Therefore, the full procedure represented by code 25105 should read:

**25105**    Arthrotomy, wrist joint; with synovectomy

## Requests to Update the CPT Nomenclature

The effectiveness of the CPT nomenclature depends on constant updating to reflect changes in medical practice. This can only be accomplished through the interest and timely suggestions of practicing physicians, medical specialty societies, state medical associations, and other organizations and agencies. Accordingly, the AMA welcomes correspondence, inquiries, and suggestions concerning old and new procedures, as well as other matters such as codes and indices.

To submit a suggestion to add, delete, or revise codes contained in the CPT codebook, please contact:

CPT Editorial Research & Development
American Medical Association
515 North State Street
Chicago, Illinois 60654

Coding change request forms are available at the AMA's CPT Web site: www.ama-assn.org/ama/pub/category/3866.html.

All proposed changes of the CPT codebook will be considered by the CPT Editorial Panel with consultation of appropriate medical specialty societies.

## Guidelines

Specific guidelines are presented at the beginning of each of the sections. These guidelines define items that are necessary to appropriately interpret and report the procedures and services contained in that section. For example, in the **Medicine** section, specific instructions are provided for handling unlisted services or procedures, special reports, and supplies and materials provided. Guidelines also provide explanations regarding terms that apply only to a particular section. For instance, **Radiology Guidelines** provide a definition of the unique term, "radiological supervision and interpretation." While in **Anesthesia,** a discussion of reporting time is included.

## Add-on Codes

Some of the listed procedures are commonly carried out in addition to the primary procedure performed. These additional or supplemental procedures are designated as add-on codes with the ✚ symbol and they are listed in **Appendix D** of the CPT codebook. Add-on codes in *CPT 2012* can be

readily identified by specific descriptor nomenclature that includes phrases such as "each additional" or "(List separately in addition to primary procedure)."

The add-on code concept in *CPT 2012* applies only to add-on procedures or services performed by the same physician. Add-on codes describe additional intra-service work associated with the primary procedure, eg, additional digit(s), lesion(s), neurorrhaphy(s), vertebral segment(s), tendon(s), joint(s).

Add-on codes are always performed in addition to the primary service or procedure and must never be reported as a stand-alone code. All add-on codes found in the CPT codebook are exempt from the multiple procedure concept (see the modifier 51 definition in **Appendix A**).

## Modifiers

A modifier provides the means to report or indicate that a service or procedure that has been performed has been altered by some specific circumstance but not changed in its definition or code. Modifiers also enable health care professionals to effectively respond to payment policy requirements established by other entities. The judicious application of modifiers obviates the necessity for separate procedure listings that may describe the modifying circumstance. Modifiers may be used to indicate to the recipient of a report that:

- A service or procedure had both a professional and technical component.
- A service or procedure was performed by more than one physician and/or in more than one location.
- A service or procedure was increased or reduced.
- Only part of a service was performed.
- An adjunctive service was performed.
- A bilateral procedure was performed.
- A service or procedure was provided more than once.
- Unusual events occurred.

*Example*

A physician providing diagnostic or therapeutic radiology services, ultrasound, or nuclear medicine services in a hospital would add modifier 26 to report the professional component.

73090 with modifier 26 = Professional component only for an X-ray of the forearm

*Example*

Two surgeons may be required to manage a specific surgical problem. When two surgeons work together as primary surgeons performing distinct part(s) of a procedure, each surgeon should report his/her distinct operative work by adding modifier 62 to the procedure code and any associated code(s) for that procedure as long as both surgeons continue to work together as primary surgeons. Each surgeon should report the co-surgery once using the same procedure code. Modifier 62 would be applicable. For instance, a neurological surgeon and an otolaryngologist are working as co-surgeons in performing transphenoidal excision of a pituitary neoplasm.

The first surgeon would report:

61548 62 = Hypophysectomy or excision of pituitary tumor, transnasal or transseptal approach, nonstereotactic + two surgeons modifier

AND the second surgeon would report:

61548 62 = Hypophysectomy or excision of pituitary tumor, transnasal or transseptal approach, nonstereotactic + two surgeons modifier

If additional procedure(s) (including add-on procedure[s]) are performed during the same surgical session, separate code(s) may also be reported with modifier 62 added. It should be noted that if a co-surgeon acts as an assistant in the performance of additional procedure(s) during the same surgical session, those services may be reported using separate procedure code(s) with modifier 80 or modifier 82 added, as appropriate. A complete listing of modifiers is found in **Appendix A.**

## Place of Service and Facility Reporting

Some codes have specified places of service (eg, evaluation and management codes are specific to a setting). Other services and procedures may have instructions specific to the place of service (eg, therapeutic, prophylactic, and diagnostic injections and infusions). The CPT code set is designated for reporting physician and qualified health care professional services. It is also the designated code set for reporting services by organizational or facility providers (eg, hospitals) in specific circumstances. Facilities are entities that may report services in addition to the physician or qualified health care professional for the same service. For example, a physician may report a procedure performed in the outpatient department of the hospital and the hospital may report the same procedure. The CPT code set uses the term *facility* to describe such providers and the term *nonfacility* to describe services where no facility reporting may occur. Services provided in the home by an agency are facility services. Services provided in the home by a physician or qualified health care professional who is not a representative of the agency are nonfacility services.

## Unlisted Procedure or Service

It is recognized that there may be services or procedures performed by physicians or other qualified health care professionals that are not found in the CPT code set. Therefore, a number of specific code numbers have been designated for reporting unlisted procedures. When an unlisted procedure number is used, the service or procedure should be described (see specific section guidelines). Each of these unlisted procedural code numbers (with the appropriate accompanying topical entry) relates to a specific section of the book and is presented in the guidelines of that section.

In some cases alternative coding and procedural nomenclature as contained in other code sets may allow appropriate reporting of a more specific code. CPT references to use an unlisted procedure code do not preclude the reporting of an appropriate code that may be found in other code sets.

## Results, Testing, Interpretation, and Report

Results are the technical component of a service. Testing leads to results; results lead to interpretation. Reports are the work product of the interpretation of test results. Certain procedures or services described in CPT involve a technical component (eg, tests) which produce "results" (eg, data, images, slides). For clinical use, some of these results require interpretation. Some CPT descriptors specifically require interpretation and reporting to report that code.

## Special Report

A service that is rarely provided, unusual, variable, or new may require a special report. Pertinent information should include an adequate definition or description of the nature, extent, and need for the procedure and the time, effort, and equipment necessary to provide the service.

## Time

The CPT code set contains many codes with a time basis for code selection. The following standards shall apply to time measurement, unless there are code or code-range–specific instructions in guidelines, parenthetical instructions, or code descriptors to the contrary. Time is the face-to-face time with the patient. Phrases such as "interpretation and report" in the code descriptor are not intended to indicate in all cases that report writing is part of the reported time. A unit of time is attained when the mid-point is passed. For example, an hour is attained when 31 minutes have elapsed (more than midway between zero and sixty minutes). A second hour is attained when a total of 91 minutes have elapsed. When codes are ranked in sequential typical times and the actual time is between two typical times, the code with the typical time closest to the actual time is used. See also the Evaluation and Management (E/M) Services Guidelines. When another service is performed concurrently with a time based service, the time associated with the concurrent service should not be included in the time used for reporting the time-based service. Some services measured in units other than days extend across calendar dates. When this occurs a continuous service does not reset and create a first hour. However, any disruption in the service does create a new initial service. For example, if intravenous hydration (96360, 96361) is given from 11 PM to 2 AM 96360 would be reported once and 96361 twice. However, if instead of a continuous infusion, a medication was given by intravenous push at 10 PM and 2 AM, as the service was not continuous, both administrations would be reported as initial (96374). For continuous services that last beyond midnight, use the date in which the service began and report the total units of time provided continuously.

## Code Symbols

A summary listing of additions, deletions, and revisions applicable to the CPT codebook is found in **Appendix B.** New procedure numbers added to the CPT codebook are identified throughout the text with the symbol ● placed before the code number. In instances where a code revision has resulted in a substantially altered procedure descriptor, the symbol ▲ is placed before the code number. The symbols ► ◄ are used to indicate new and revised text other than the procedure descriptors. These symbols indicate CPT Editorial Panel actions. The symbol ○ is used to indicate reinstated/recycled code. The AMA reserves the right to correct typographical errors and make stylistic improvements.

CPT add-on codes are annotated by the symbol ✚ and are listed in **Appendix D.** The symbol ⊘ is used to identify codes that are exempt from the use of modifier 51 but have not been designated as CPT add-on procedures or services. A list of codes exempt from modifier 51 usage is included in **Appendix E.** The symbol ⊙ is used to identify codes that include moderate sedation (see **Appendix G**). The symbol ∕ is used to identify codes for vaccines that are pending FDA approval (see **Appendix K**). The symbol # is used to identify codes that are listed out of numerical sequence (see **Appendix N**).

Resequenced codes that are not placed numerically are identified with the # symbol, and a reference placed numerically (eg, Code is out of numerical sequence. See…) as a navigational alert to direct the user to the location of the out-of-sequence code (see Appendix N). Resequencing is utilized to allow placement of related concepts in appropriate locations within the families of codes regardless of the availability of numbers for sequential numerical placement.

## Alphabetical Reference Index

This codebook features an expanded alphabetical index that includes listings by procedure and anatomic site. Procedures and services commonly known by their eponyms or other designations are also included.

## *CPT 2012* in Electronic Formats

*CPT 2012* procedure codes and descriptions are available on CD-ROM as data files and electronic software. Data files are available in ASCII and EBCDIC formats and can be imported into any billing and claims reporting software that accepts a text (.TXT) file format. *CPT 2012 Electronic Professional* software, with *Netter's Atlas of Human Anatomy for CPT Coding*, provides access to the entire *CPT 2012 Professional Edition* codebook on your desktop. Easy-to-use and fully searchable, this invaluable software contains all of the favorite *CPT Professional* features plus CPT codes and quick linking access between CPT codes, guidelines, modifiers, appendices, index, and more. For more information call (800) 621-8335 or visit *www.amabookstore.com*.

## References to AMA Resources

The symbols ➋ and ➋ appear after many codes throughout this codebook and indicate that the AMA has published reference material regarding that particular code.

The symbol ➋ refers to the *CPT Assistant* monthly newsletter and *CPT Changes: An Insider's View*, an annual book with all of the coding changes for the current year. The symbol ➋ refers to the quarterly newsletter *Clinical Examples in Radiology*.

### Example

**36598**    Contrast injection(s) for radiologic evaluation of existing central venous access device, including fluoroscopy, image documentation and report
➋ *CPT Changes: An Insider's View* 2006
➋ *Clinical Examples in Radiology* Winter 2006:15

(For placement of centrally inserted non-tunneled central venous catheter, without subcutaneous port or pump, age 5 years or older, use 36556)

In this example, the green reference symbol indicates that in the 2006 edition of *CPT Changes: An Insider's View* material is available that may assist in understanding the application of the code. The red reference symbol indicates that the 2006 issue of *Clinical Examples in Radiology* (page 15) should be consulted.

Subscriptions to *CPT Assistant* and *Clinical Examples in Radiology* can be purchased by calling the AMA's Unified Service Center at (800) 621-8335. Individual back issues are available for purchase and immediate download at *www.amabookstore.com*.

An archive software product with every issue of *CPT Assistant* is also available. *CPT Assistant Archives 1990-2011* provides convenient access to 20 years of *CPT Assistant* newsletter articles on your desktop. Search past issues of the AMA's authoritative coding newsletter by keyword, phrase, CPT code number, newsletter issue, article index, or codebook table of contents. This product offers simple search capabilities and a complete historical CPT code list from 1990-2011 that references when a code was added, deleted, and/or revised. Call (800) 621-8335 or visit *www.amabookstore.com* for more information.

Current and past editions of *CPT Changes: An Insider's View* can be purchased by calling the AMA's Unified Service Center at (800) 621-8335 or visiting *www.amabookstore.com*.

Additionally, an archives software product with all content from past and present editions of *CPT Changes: An Insider's View* is available. *CPT Changes Archives 2000-2011* provides access to current and historical CPT code and guideline changes on your computer desktop. Search by keyword, phrase, CPT code number, edition, and CPT codebook table of contents. For more information, call (800) 621-8335 or visit *www.amabookstore.com*.

# Illustrated Anatomical and Procedural Review

It is essential that coders have a thorough understanding of medical terminology and anatomy to code accurately. The following section reviewing the basics of vocabulary and anatomy can be used as a quick reference to help you with your coding. It is not intended as a replacement for up-to-date medical dictionaries and anatomy texts, which are essential tools for accurate coding.

## Prefixes, Suffixes, and Roots

Although medical terminology may seem complex, many medical terms can be broken into component parts, which makes them easier to understand. Many of these terms are derived from Latin or Greek words, but some include the names of physicians.

Prefixes are word parts that appear at the beginning of a word and modify its meaning; suffixes are found at the end of words. By learning what various prefixes and suffixes mean, it is possible to decipher the meaning of a word quickly. The following lists are a quick reference for some common prefixes and suffixes.

## Numbers

| Prefix | Meaning | Example |
|---|---|---|
| mono-, uni- | one | monocyte, unilateral |
| bi- | two | bilateral |
| tri- | three | triad |
| quadr- | four | quadriplegia |
| hex-, sex- | six | hexose |
| diplo- | double | diplopia |

## Surgical Procedures

| Suffix | Meaning | Example |
|---|---|---|
| -centesis | puncture a cavity to remove fluid | amniocentesis |
| -ectomy | surgical removal (excision) | appendectomy |
| -ostomy | a new permanent opening | colostomy |
| -otomy | cutting into (incision) | tracheotomy |
| -orrhaphy | surgical repair/suture | herniorrhaphy |
| -opexy | surgical fixation | nephropexy |
| -oplasty | surgical repair | rhinoplasty |
| -otripsy | crushing, destroying | lithotripsy |

## Conditions

| Prefix | Meaning | Example |
|---|---|---|
| ambi- | both | ambidextrous |
| aniso- | unequal | anisocoria |
| dys- | bad, painful, difficult | dysphoria |
| eu- | good, normal | euthanasia |
| hetero- | different | heterogeneous |
| homo- | same | homogeneous |
| hyper- | excessive, above | hypergastric |
| hypo- | deficient, below | hypogastric |
| iso- | equal, same | isotonic |
| mal- | bad, poor | malaise |
| megalo- | large | megalocardia |

| Suffix | Meaning | Example |
|---|---|---|
| -algia | pain | neuralgia |
| -asthenia | weakness | myasthenia |
| -emia | blood | anemia |
| -iasis | condition of | amebiasis |
| -itis | inflammation | appendicitis |
| -lysis | destruction, break down | hemolysis |
| -lytic | destroy, break down | hemolytic |
| -oid | like | lipoid |
| -oma | tumor | carcinoma |
| -opathy | disease of | arthropathy |
| -orrhagia | hemorrhage | menorrhagia |
| -orrhea | flow or discharge | amenorrhea |
| -osis | abnormal condition of | tuberculosis |
| -paresis | weakness | hemiparesis |
| -plasia | growth | hyperplasia |
| -plegia | paralysis | paraplegia |
| -pnea | breathing | apnea |

## Directions and Positions

| Prefix | Meaning | Example |
| --- | --- | --- |
| ab- | away from | abduction |
| ad- | toward | adduction |
| ecto, exo- | outside | ectopic, exocrine |
| endo- | within | endoscope |
| epi- | upon | epigastric |
| infra- | below, under | infrastructure |
| ipsi- | same | ipsilateral |
| meso- | middle | mesopexy |
| meta- | after, beyond, transformation | metastasis |
| peri- | surrounding | pericardium |
| retro- | behind, back | retroversion |
| trans- | across, through | transvaginal |

| Word | Meaning |
| --- | --- |
| anterior or ventral | at or near the front surface of the body |
| posterior or dorsal | at or near the back surface of the body |
| superior | above |
| inferior | below |
| lateral | side |
| distal | farthest from center |
| proximal | nearest to center |
| medial | middle |
| supine | face up or palm up |
| prone | face down or palm down |
| sagittal | vertical body plane, divides the body into equal right and left sides |
| transverse | horizontal body plane, divides the body into top and bottom sections |
| coronal | vertical body plane, divides the body into front and back sections |

# Additional References

For best coding results, you will need to use other reference materials in addition to your coding books. These references include a medical dictionary and one or more anatomy books that can be purchased from the American Medical Association by calling 800 621-8335.

## Medical Dictionaries

*Stedman's CPT® Dictionary, 2nd ed.*
Chicago, IL: American Medical Association, 2009.
OP300609

*Merriam-Webster's Medical Desk Dictionary.*
Springfield, Mass: Merriam Webster.
OP941493

*Stedman's Medical Dictionary.* 27th ed.
Baltimore, Md: Williams & Wilkins; 2000.
OP982900

## Anatomy References

Kirschner, CG. *Netter's Atlas of Human Anatomy for CPT® Coding, 2nd ed.*
Chicago, Ill: American Medical Association; 2005.
OP490609

Kirschner, CG. *Netter's Atlas of Human Anatomy for CPT® and ICD-9-CM Coding Series: Musculoskeletal.*
Chicago, Ill: American Medical Association
OP492206

Netter, FH. *Atlas of Human Anatomy.* 3rd ed.
East Hanover, NJ: Novartis; 2003.
OP936798

# Lists of Illustrations

To further aid coders in properly assigning CPT codes, the codebook contains a number of anatomical and procedural illustrations.

## Anatomical Illustrations

## Figure 1A
### Body Planes — 3/4 View

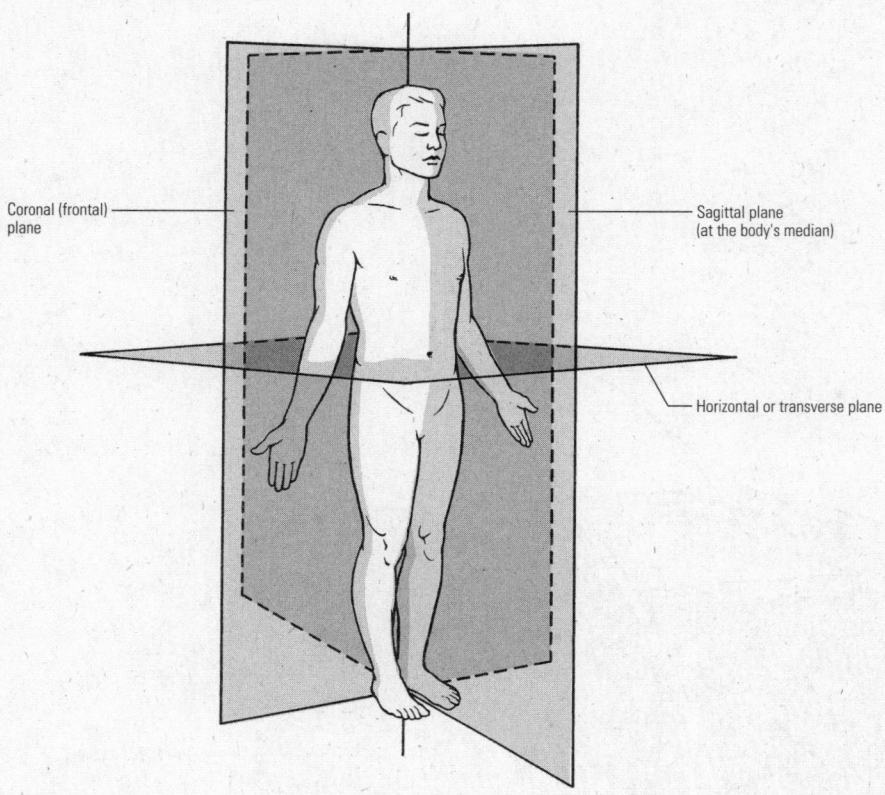

Coronal (frontal) plane

Sagittal plane (at the body's median)

Horizontal or transverse plane

## Figure 1B
### Body Aspects — Side View

Superior (cranial) aspect

Posterior aspect

Anterior aspect

Dorsal surface of hand

Palmar surface of hand

Dorsal surface of foot

Plantar surface of foot

Inferior aspect

## Figure 1C
### Body Planes — Front View

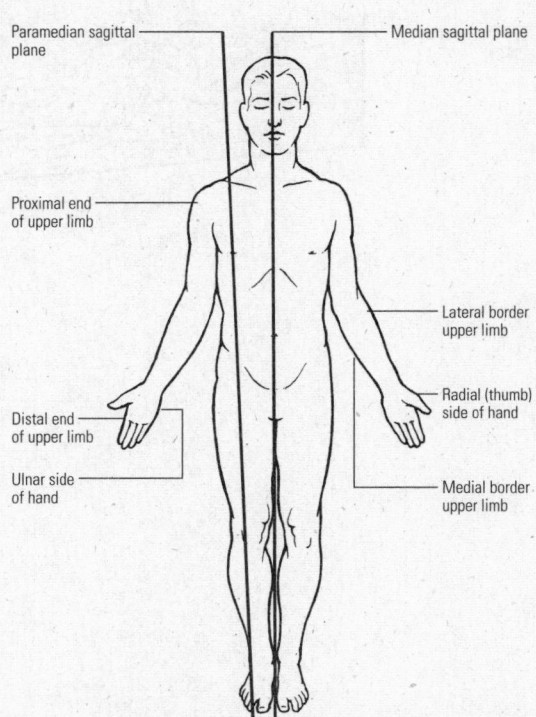

Paramedian sagittal plane

Median sagittal plane

Proximal end of upper limb

Lateral border upper limb

Radial (thumb) side of hand

Distal end of upper limb

Ulnar side of hand

Medial border upper limb

## Figure 2
## Structure of Skin

Hair shaft

Hair root

Epidermis

Dermis

Subcutaneous tissue

Sebaceous gland

Nerve endings

Hair bulb

Sweat gland

Cutaneous nerve

Blood vessels

Figure 3
**Skeletal System**

Skull
Maxilla
Mandible
Cervical vertebra
First rib
Scapula
Sternum

Clavicle
Humerus

Lumbar vertebra
Ilium
Sacrum
Pubis
Ischium

Radius
Ulna
Carpals
Metacarpals
Phalanges

Femur

Patella
Tibia
Fibula

Tarsals
Metatarsals
Phalanges

Figure 4
## Skull

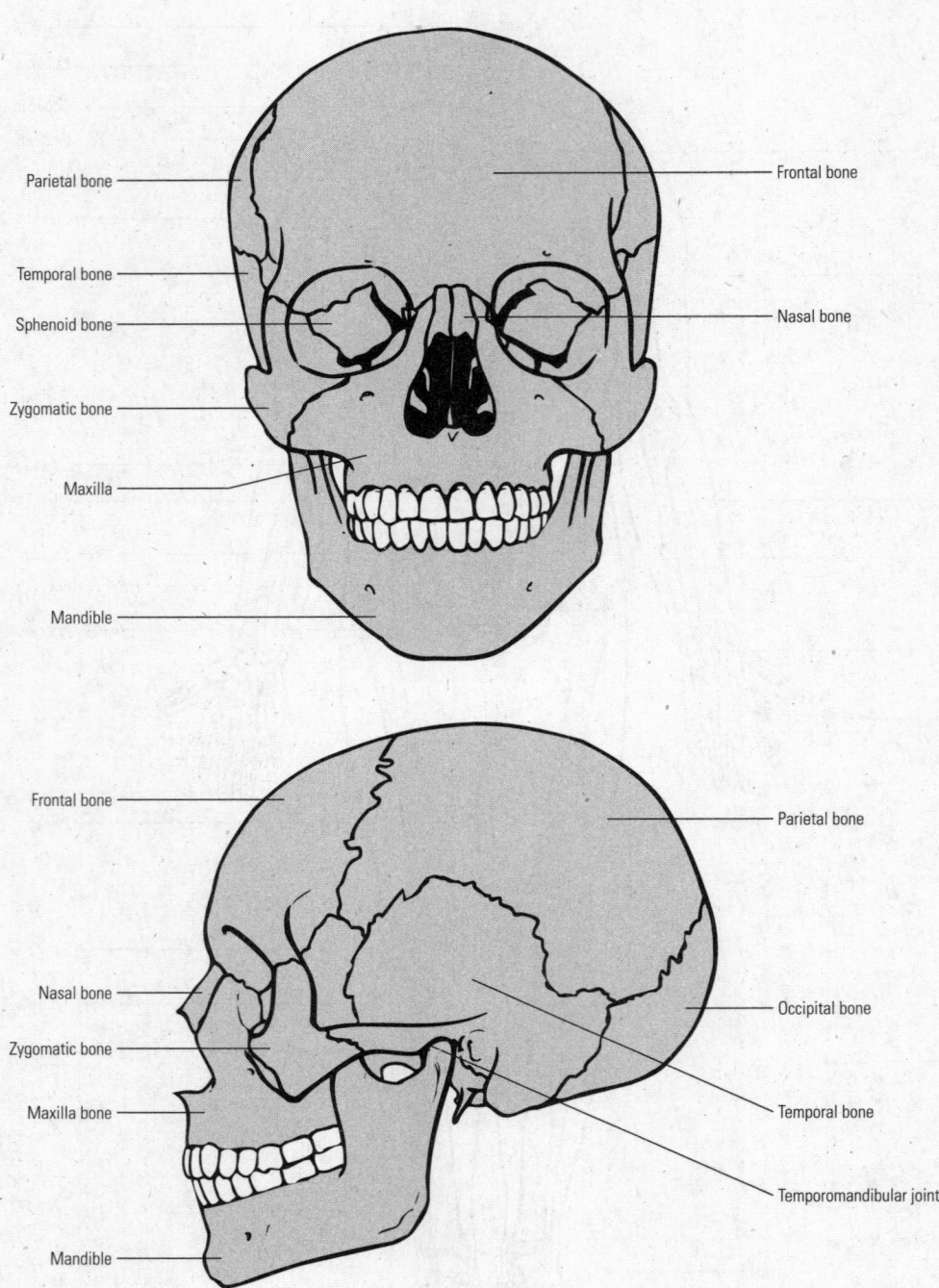

Parietal bone
Frontal bone
Temporal bone
Nasal bone
Sphenoid bone
Zygomatic bone
Maxilla
Mandible

Frontal bone
Parietal bone
Nasal bone
Occipital bone
Zygomatic bone
Maxilla bone
Temporal bone
Mandible
Temporomandibular joint

Figure 5A
**Muscular System — Front**

Sternocleidomastoid m.
Omohyoid m.
Sternohyoid m.
Trapezius m.
Deltoid m.
Pectoralis major m.
Latissimus dorsi m.
Serratas anterior m.
Oblique external m.
Rectus abdominus m.

Biceps m.
Brachialus m.
Brachioradialus m.
Pronator teres m.
Flexor carpi radialus m.
Palmaris longus m.
Flexor digitorum superficialus m.
Flexor carpi ulnaris m.

Pectineus m.
Adductor longus m.
Adductor magnus m.
Gracilis m.
Sartorius m.
Rectus femoris m.
Vastus medialis m. ⎤
Vastus lateralis m. ⎦ — Quadriceps

Peroneus longus m.
Tibialis anterior m.
Gastrocnemius m.
Extensor digitorum longus m.
Soleus m.

Figure 5B
**Muscular System — Back**

Trapezius m.
Deltoid m.
Infraspinatus m.
Teres minor m.
Teres major m.
Triceps m.
Latissimus dorsi m.
Anconeus m.
Extensor carpi radialis longus m.
Flexor carpi ulnaris m.
Extensor carpi radialis brevis m.
Extensor digitorum m.
Extensor carpi ulnaris m.
Abductor pollicis longus m.
Extensor pollicis brevis m.

Gluteus medius m.
Gluteus maximus m.
Adductor magnus m.
Biceps femoris m.
Semitendinosus m.
Gracilis m.
Semimembranosus m.
Vastus lateralis m.
Sartorius m.
Gastrocnemius m.
Peroneus longus m.
Flexor hallicis longus m.

Figure 6A
# Thoracic Vertebra—Superior View

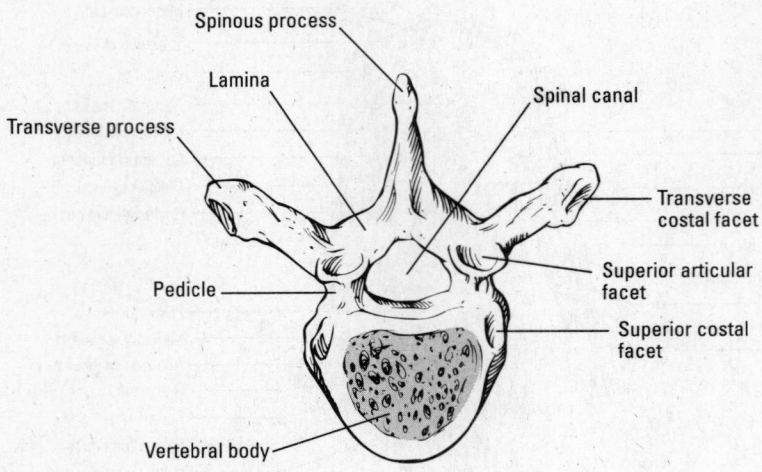

Spinous process

Lamina

Transverse process

Spinal canal

Transverse costal facet

Superior articular facet

Superior costal facet

Pedicle

Vertebral body

Figure 6B
# Lumbar Vertebra—Superior View

Spinous process

Lamina

Superior articular process

Mamillary process

Spinal canal

Pedicle

Transverse process

Vertebral body

Figure 7
# Lumbar Vertebrae—Lateral View

Pedicle

Superior articular process

Transverse process

Spinous process

Vertebral body

Inferior articular process

Intervertebral discs

Inferior vertebral notch

Intervertebral foramen

Superior vertebral notch

L1

L2

L3

L4

L5

Figure 8
## Bones, Muscles, and Tendons of Hand

Phalanges

Metacarpal bones

Carpal bones

Ulna

Radius

Transmetacarpal ligament

Lumbrical muscles

Tendons of flexor digitorum superficialis muscle

Abductor digiti minimi muscle

Flexor digiti minimi brevis muscle

Opponens digiti minimi muscle

Fibrous digital sheath, cruciform part

Fibrous digital sheath, annular part

Adductor pollicis muscle

Flexor pollicis brevis muscle

Abductor pollicis brevis muscle

Opponens pollicis muscle

Flexor retinaculum sheath

Figure 9
## Bones and Muscles of Foot

Phalanges

Metatarsal bones

Tarsal bones

Talus

Calcaneus

Tendon of flexor hallucis longus muscle

Flexor hallucis brevis muscle

Abductor hallucis muscle

Lumbrical muscles

Flexor digitorum brevis muscle

Flexor digiti minimi brevis muscle

Abductor digiti minimi muscle

Figure 10
**Paranasal Sinuses**

Frontal

Ethmoid

Sphenoid

Maxillary

Figure 11
**Respiratory System**

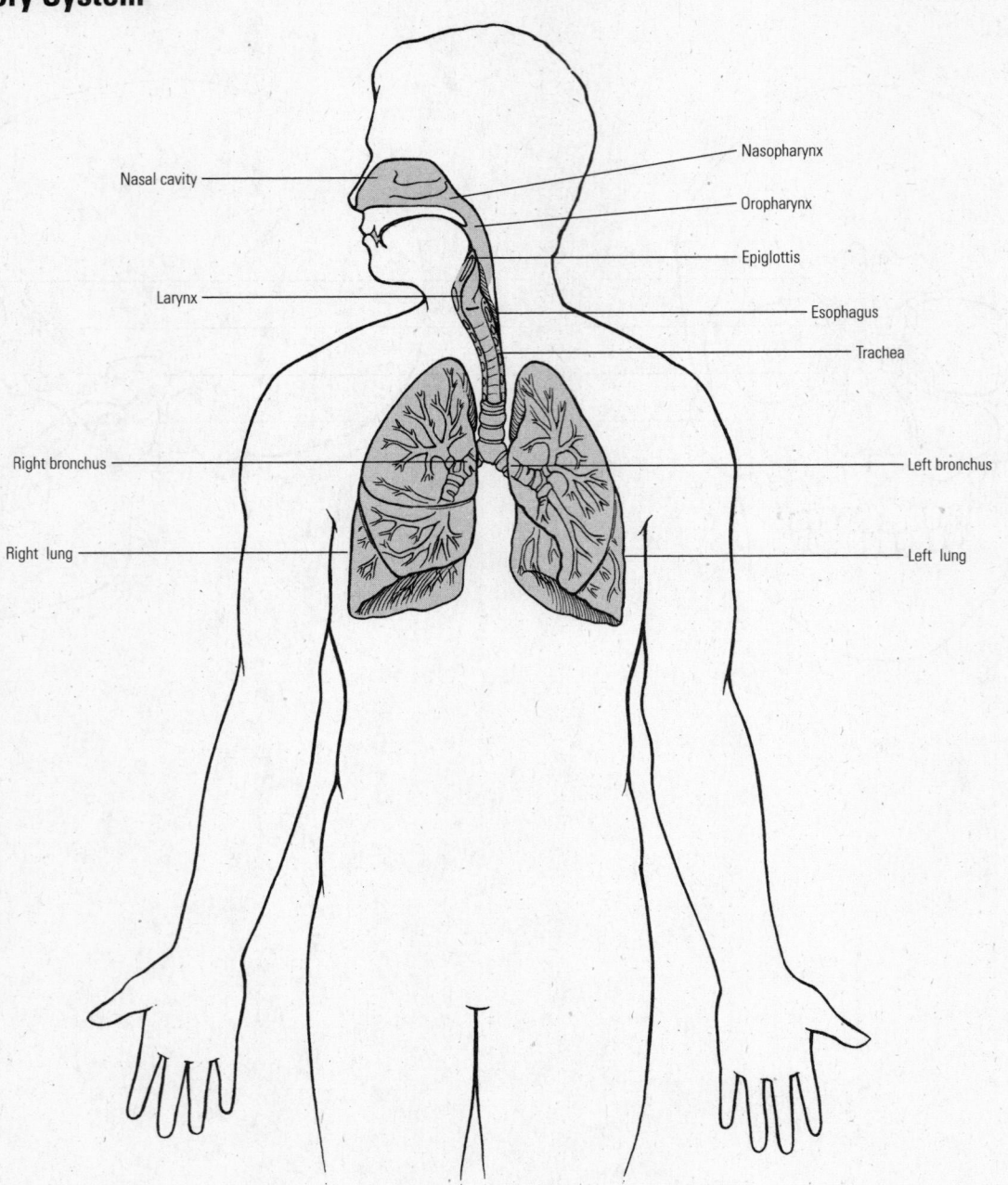

Nasal cavity

Nasopharynx

Oropharynx

Epiglottis

Larynx

Esophagus

Trachea

Right bronchus

Left bronchus

Right lung

Left lung

Figure 12
# Circulatory System — Arteries

Superficial temporal a.
Posterior auricular a.
Common carotid a.
Subclavian a.
Brachiocephalic trunk
Axillary a.
Deep brachial a.
Brachial a.
Aorta
Radial a.
Interosseous a.
Ulnar a.
Deep palmar arch
Superficial palmar arch
Descending genicular a.

External carotid a.
Internal carotid a.
Vertebral a.
Aorta and arch
Pulmonary a.
Cardiac a.
Thoracic aorta
Celiac trunk
Superior mesenteric a.
Renal a.
Gonadal a.
Inferior mesenteric a.
Common iliac a.
External iliac a.
Internal iliac a.
Deep femoral a.
Femoral a.
Popliteal a.
Anterior tibial a.
Peroneal a.
Posterior tibial a.

Figure 13
# Cardiac Anatomy

Superior vena cava
Right pulmonary artery
Pulmonary valve
Location of sinoatrial node
Location of atrioventricular node
Right atrium
Tricuspid valve
Right ventricle
Inferior vena cava

Aorta
Pulmonary artery
Left atrium
Aortic valve
Mitral valve
Left ventricle
Ventricular septum
Descending thoracic aorta

Figure 14
## Circulatory System — Veins

Superficial temporal v.

Facial v.

Internal jugular v.

External jugular v.

Subclavian v.

Brachiocephalic v.

Axillary v.

Brachial v.

Cephalic v.

Basilic v.

Median cubital v.

Medial antebrachial v.

Superficial venous palmar arch

Small saphenous v.

Superior vena cava

Hepatic v.

Renal v.

Gonadal v.

Inferior vena cava

Common iliac v.

Internal iliac v.

External iliac v.

Deep femoral v.

Femoral v.

Great saphenous v.

Popliteal v.

Anterior tibial v.

Posterior tibial v.

Dorsal venous arch

Figure 15
**Lymphatic System**

Cervical lymph nodes

Right lymphatic duct

Thoracic lymph nodes

Axillary lymph nodes

Supratrochlear lymph nodes

Mesenteric lymph nodes

Iliac lymph nodes

Inguinal lymph nodes

Left lymphatic duct

Heart

Thoracic duct

Spleen

Cisterna chyli

Lumbar lymph nodes

Popliteal lymph nodes

Figure 16
**Digestive System**

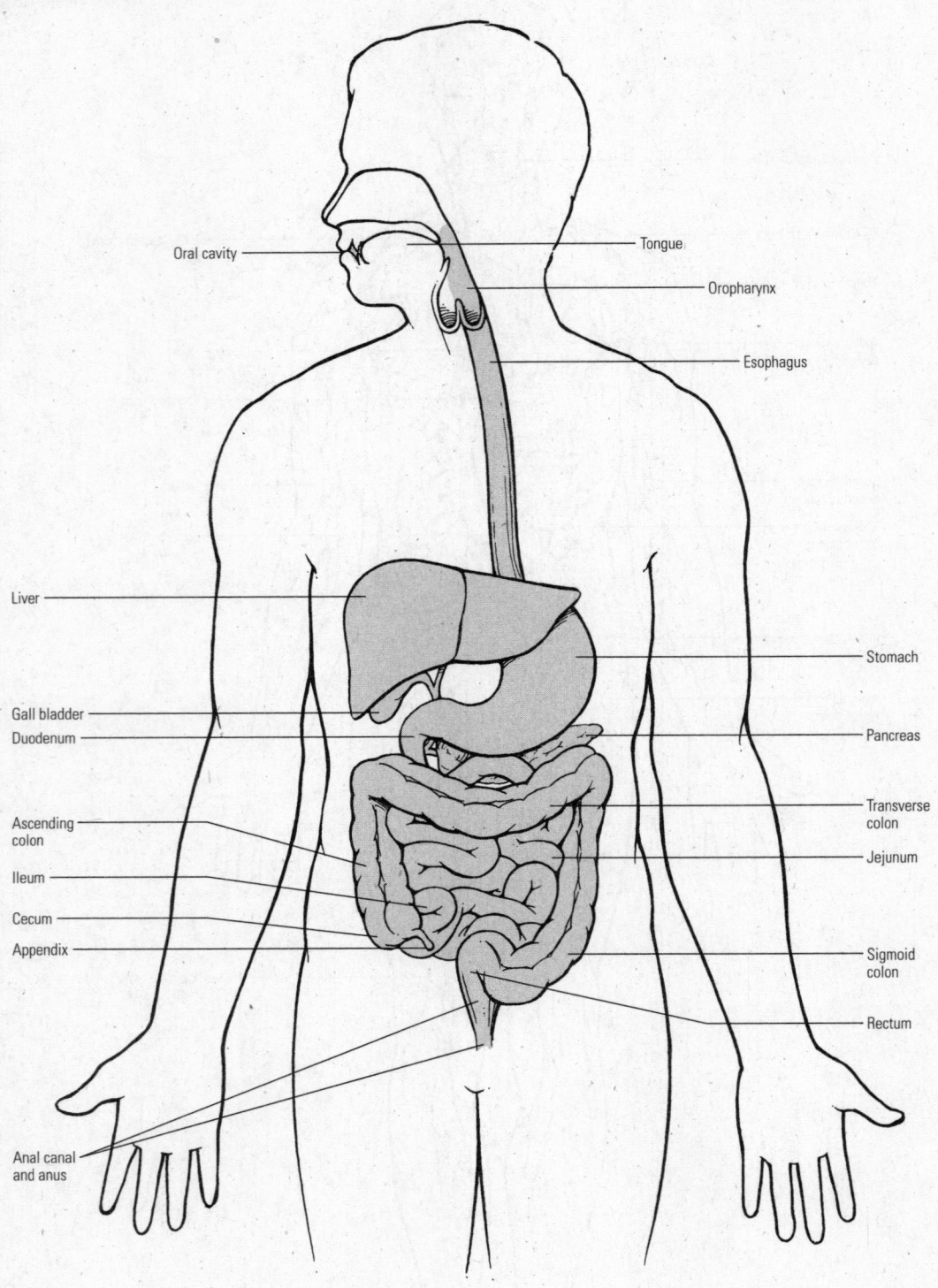

Oral cavity

Tongue

Oropharynx

Esophagus

Liver

Stomach

Gall bladder

Duodenum

Pancreas

Transverse colon

Ascending colon

Jejunum

Ileum

Cecum

Appendix

Sigmoid colon

Rectum

Anal canal and anus

Figure 17
**Urinary System**

Right kidney

Left kidney

Ureters

Urinary bladder

Urethra (empties through
penis or in front
of vagina)

Figure 18
## Male Genital System

Deferent duct

Urinary bladder
and cavity

Corpus
cavernosa

Corpus
spongiosum

Penis

Glans penis

Prepuce

Seminal
vesicle

Ejaculatory
duct

Prostate
gland

Spermatic cord
and deferent duct

Epididymus

Testes

Scrotum

Figure 19
**Female Genital System**

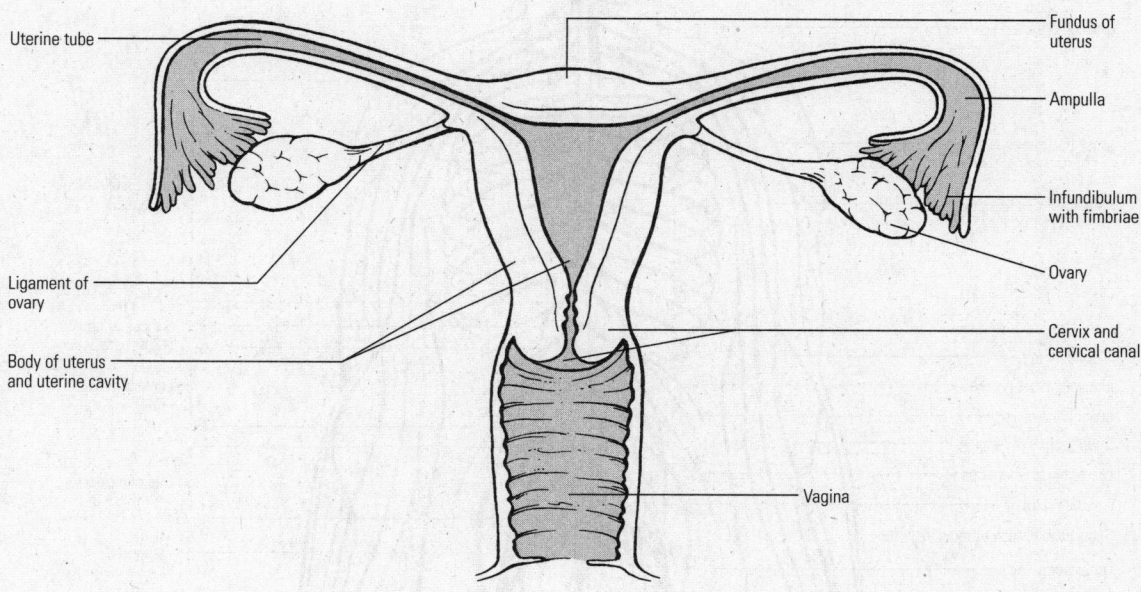

Uterine tube

Fundus of uterus

Ampulla

Infundibulum with fimbriae

Ovary

Ligament of ovary

Body of uterus and uterine cavity

Cervix and cervical canal

Vagina

Figure 20
**Nervous System**

Brain

Cerebellum

Spinal cord

Brachial plexus

Musculocutaneous n.

Radial n.

Intercostal nerves
(with ribs)

Subcostal nerve
(12th thoracic)

Lumbar plexus

Median n.

Iliohypogastric n.

Ilioinguinal n.

Deep branch of radial n.

Lat. femoral cutaneous n.

Genitofemoral n.

Superficial branch of radial n.

Obturator n.

Sacral plexus

Femoral n.

Pudendal n.

Sciatic n.

Ulnar n.

Muscular branches
of femoral n.

Saphenous n.

Common peroneal n.

Tibial n.

Deep peroneal n.

Superficial peroneal n.

Figure 21A
**Brain Anatomy**

Figure 21B
**Sagittal Section of Brain and Brain Stem**

Figure 22
**Eye Anatomy**

Transverse (horizontal) section of eyeball

Figure 23
**Ear**

Figure 24
# Endocrine System

Hypothalamus

Pineal body

Pituitary

Parathyroids

Thyroid gland

Thymus gland

Adrenal glands

Pancreas

Ovaries

Testes

# Evaluation and Management (E/M) Services Guidelines

In addition to the information presented in the Introduction, several other items unique to this section are defined or identified here.

## Classification of Evaluation and Management (E/M) Services

The E/M section is divided into broad categories such as office visits, hospital visits, and consultations. Most of the categories are further divided into two or more subcategories of E/M services. For example, there are two subcategories of office visits (new patient and established patient) and there are two subcategories of hospital visits (initial and subsequent). The subcategories of E/M services are further classified into levels of E/M services that are identified by specific codes. This classification is important because the nature of physician work varies by type of service, place of service, and the patient's status.

The basic format of the levels of E/M services is the same for most categories. First, a unique code number is listed. Second, the place and/or type of service is specified, eg, office consultation. Third, the content of the service is defined, eg, comprehensive history and comprehensive examination. (See "Levels of E/M Services," page 2, for details on the content of E/M services.) Fourth, the nature of the presenting problem(s) usually associated with a given level is described. Fifth, the time typically required to provide the service is specified. (A detailed discussion of time is provided on page 3.)

## Definitions of Commonly Used Terms

Certain key words and phrases are used throughout the E/M section. The following definitions are intended to reduce the potential for differing interpretations and to increase the consistency of reporting by physicians in differing specialties. E/M services may also be reported by other qualified health care professionals who are authorized to perform such services within the scope of their practice.

## New and Established Patient

▶Solely for the purposes of distinguishing between new and established patients, **professional services** are those face-to-face services rendered by a physician and reported by a specific CPT code(s). A new patient is one who has not received any professional services from the physician or another physician of the **exact** same specialty **and subspecialty** who belongs to the same group practice, within the past three years.◀

▶An established patient is one who has received professional services from the physician or another physician of the **exact** same specialty **and subspecialty** who belongs to the same group practice, within the past three years. See Decision Tree.◀

In the instance where a physician is on call for or covering for another physician, the patient's encounter will be classified as it would have been by the physician who is not available.

No distinction is made between new and established patients in the emergency department. E/M services in the emergency department category may be reported for any new or established patient who presents for treatment in the emergency department.

▶The decision tree on page 7 is provided to aid in determining whether to report the E/M service provided as a new or an established patient encounter. ◀

## Chief Complaint

A chief complaint is a concise statement describing the symptom, problem, condition, diagnosis, or other factor that is the reason for the encounter, usually stated in the patient's words.

## Concurrent Care and Transfer of Care

Concurrent care is the provision of similar services (eg, hospital visits) to the same patient by more than one physician on the same day. When concurrent care is provided, no special reporting is required. Transfer of care is the process whereby a physician who is providing management for some or all of a patient's problems relinquishes this responsibility to another physician who explicitly agrees to accept this responsibility and who, from the initial encounter, is not providing consultative services. The physician transferring care is then no longer providing care for these problems though he or she may continue providing care for other conditions when appropriate. Consultation codes should not be reported by the physician who has agreed to accept transfer of care before an initial evaluation but are appropriate to report if the decision to accept transfer of care cannot be made until after the initial consultation evaluation, regardless of site of service.

## Counseling

Counseling is a discussion with a patient and/or family concerning one or more of the following areas:

- Diagnostic results, impressions, and/or recommended diagnostic studies
- Prognosis
- Risks and benefits of management (treatment) options
- Instructions for management (treatment) and/or follow-up
- Importance of compliance with chosen management (treatment) options
- Risk factor reduction
- Patient and family education

(For psychotherapy, see 90804-90857)

## Family History

A review of medical events in the patient's family that includes significant information about:

- The health status or cause of death of parents, siblings, and children
- Specific diseases related to problems identified in the Chief Complaint or History of the Present Illness, and/or System Review
- Diseases of family members that may be hereditary or place the patient at risk

## History of Present Illness

A chronological description of the development of the patient's present illness from the first sign and/or symptom to the present. This includes a description of location, quality, severity, timing, context, modifying factors, and associated signs and symptoms significantly related to the presenting problem(s).

## Levels of E/M Services

Within each category or subcategory of E/M service, there are three to five levels of E/M services available for reporting purposes. Levels of E/M services are **not** interchangeable among the different categories or subcategories of service. For example, the first level of E/M services in the subcategory of office visit, new patient, does not have the same definition as the first level of E/M services in the subcategory of office visit, established patient.

The levels of E/M services include examinations, evaluations, treatments, conferences with or concerning patients, preventive pediatric and adult health supervision, and similar medical services, such as the determination of the need and/or location for appropriate care. Medical screening includes the history, examination, and medical decision-making required to determine the need and/or location for appropriate care and treatment of the patient (eg, office and other outpatient setting, emergency department, nursing facility). The levels of E/M services encompass the wide variations in skill, effort, time, responsibility, and medical knowledge required for the prevention or diagnosis and treatment of illness or injury and the promotion of optimal health. Each level of E/M services may be used by all physicians.

The descriptors for the levels of E/M services recognize seven components, six of which are used in defining the levels of E/M services. These components are:

- History
- Examination
- Medical decision making
- Counseling
- Coordination of care
- Nature of presenting problem
- Time

The first three of these components (history, examination, and medical decision making) are considered the **key** components in selecting a level of E/M services. (See "Determine the Extent of History Obtained," page 5.)

The next three components (counseling, coordination of care, and the nature of the presenting problem) are considered **contributory** factors in the majority of encounters. Although the first two of these contributory factors are important E/M services, it is not required that these services be provided at every patient encounter.

Coordination of care with other providers or agencies without a patient encounter on that day is reported using the case management codes.

The final component, time, is discussed in detail on page 3.

Any specifically identifiable procedure (ie, identified with a specific CPT code) performed on or subsequent to the date of initial or subsequent E/M services should be reported separately.

The actual performance and/or interpretation of diagnostic tests/studies ordered during a patient encounter are not included in the levels of E/M services. Physician performance of diagnostic tests/studies for which specific CPT codes are available may be reported separately, in addition to the appropriate E/M code. The physician's interpretation of the results of diagnostic tests/ studies (ie, professional component) with preparation of a separate distinctly identifiable signed written report may also be reported separately, using the appropriate CPT code with modifier 26 appended.

The physician may need to indicate that on the day a procedure or service identified by a CPT code was performed, the patient's condition required a significant separately identifiable E/M service above and beyond other services provided or beyond the usual preservice and postservice care associated with the procedure that was performed. The E/M service may be caused or prompted by the symptoms or condition for which the procedure and/or service was provided. This circumstance may be reported by adding modifier 25 to the appropriate level of E/M service. As such, different diagnoses are not required for reporting of the procedure and the E/M services on the same date.

## Nature of Presenting Problem

A presenting problem is a disease, condition, illness, injury, symptom, sign, finding, complaint, or other reason for encounter, with or without a diagnosis being established at the time of the encounter. The E/M codes recognize five types of presenting problems that are defined as follows:

*Minimal:* A problem that may not require the presence of the physician, but service is provided under the physician's supervision.

*Self-limited or minor:* A problem that runs a definite and prescribed course, is transient in nature, and is not likely to permanently alter health status OR has a good prognosis with management/compliance.

*Low severity:* A problem where the risk of morbidity without treatment is low; there is little to no risk of mortality without treatment; full recovery without functional impairment is expected.

*Moderate severity:* A problem where the risk of morbidity without treatment is moderate; there is moderate risk of mortality without treatment; uncertain prognosis OR increased probability of prolonged functional impairment.

*High severity:* A problem where the risk of morbidity without treatment is high to extreme; there is a moderate to high risk of mortality without treatment OR high probability of severe, prolonged functional impairment.

## Past History

A review of the patient's past experiences with illnesses, injuries, and treatments that includes significant information about:

- Prior major illnesses and injuries
- Prior operations
- Prior hospitalizations
- Current medications

- Allergies (eg, drug, food)
- Age appropriate immunization status
- Age appropriate feeding/dietary status

## Social History

An age appropriate review of past and current activities that includes significant information about:

- Marital status and/or living arrangements
- Current employment
- Occupational history
- Use of drugs, alcohol, and tobacco
- Level of education
- Sexual history
- Other relevant social factors

## System Review (Review of Systems)

An inventory of body systems obtained through a series of questions seeking to identify signs and/or symptoms that the patient may be experiencing or has experienced. For the purposes of the CPT codebook the following elements of a system review have been identified:

- Constitutional symptoms (fever, weight loss, etc)
- Eyes
- Ears, nose, mouth, throat
- Cardiovascular
- Respiratory
- Gastrointestinal
- Genitourinary
- Musculoskeletal
- Integumentary (skin and/or breast)
- Neurological
- Psychiatric
- Endocrine
- Hematologic/lymphatic
- Allergic/immunologic

The review of systems helps define the problem, clarify the differential diagnosis, identify needed testing, or serves as baseline data on other systems that might be affected by any possible management options.

## Time

The inclusion of time in the definitions of levels of E/M services has been implicit in prior editions of the CPT codebook. The inclusion of time as an explicit factor beginning in *CPT 1992* is done to assist physicians in selecting the most appropriate level of E/M services. It should be recognized that the specific times expressed in the visit code descriptors are averages and, therefore, represent a range of times that may be higher or lower depending on actual clinical circumstances.

Time is **not** a descriptive component for the emergency department levels of E/M services because emergency department services are typically provided on a variable intensity basis, often involving multiple encounters with several patients over an extended period of time. Therefore, it is often difficult for physicians to provide accurate estimates of the time spent face-to-face with the patient.

Studies to establish levels of E/M services employed surveys of practicing physicians to obtain data on the amount of time and work associated with typical E/M services. Since "work" is not easily quantifiable, the codes must rely on other objective, verifiable measures that correlate with physicians' estimates of their "work." It has been demonstrated that physicians' estimations of **intraservice** time (as explained on the next page), both within and across specialties, is a variable that is predictive of the "work" of E/M services. This same research has shown there is a strong relationship between intraservice time and total time for E/M services. Intraservice time, rather than total time, was chosen for inclusion with the codes because of its relative ease of measurement and because of its direct correlation with measurements of the total amount of time and work associated with typical E/M services.

Intraservice times are defined as **face-to-face** time for office and other outpatient visits and as **unit/floor** time for hospital and other inpatient visits. This distinction is necessary because most of the work of typical office visits takes place during the face-to-face time with the patient, while most of the work of typical hospital visits takes place during the time spent on the patient's floor or unit. When prolonged time occurs in either the office or the inpatient areas, the appropriate add-on code should be reported.

*Face-to-face time (office and other outpatient visits and office consultations):* For coding purposes, face-to-face time for these services is defined as only that time that the physician spends face-to-face with the patient and/or family. This includes the time in which the physician performs such tasks as obtaining a history, performing an examination, and counseling the patient.

Physicians also spend time doing work before or after the face-to-face time with the patient, performing such tasks as reviewing records and tests, arranging for further services, and communicating further with other professionals and the patient through written reports and telephone contact.

This **non-face-to-face** time for office services—also called pre- and postencounter time—is not included in the time component described in the E/M codes. However, the pre- and post-non-face-to-face work associated with an encounter was included in calculating the total work of typical services in physician surveys.

Thus, the face-to-face time associated with the services described by any E/M code is a valid proxy for the total work done before, during, and after the visit.

*Unit/floor time (hospital observation services, inpatient hospital care, initial inpatient hospital consultations, nursing facility):* For reporting purposes, intraservice time for these services is defined as unit/floor time, which includes the time that the physician is present on the patient's hospital unit and at the bedside rendering services for that patient. This includes the time in which the physician establishes and/or reviews the patient's chart, examines the patient, writes notes, and communicates with other professionals and the patient's family.

In the hospital, pre- and post-time includes time spent off the patient's floor performing such tasks as reviewing pathology and radiology findings in another part of the hospital.

This pre- and postvisit time is not included in the time component described in these codes. However, the pre- and postwork performed during the time spent off the floor or unit was included in calculating the total work of typical services in physician surveys.

Thus, the unit/floor time associated with the services described by any code is a valid proxy for the total work done before, during, and after the visit.

# Unlisted Service

An E/M service may be provided that is not listed in this section of the CPT codebook. When reporting such a service, the appropriate unlisted code may be used to indicate the service, identifying it by "Special Report," as discussed in the following paragraph. The "Unlisted Services" and accompanying codes for the E/M section are as follows:

**99429**   **Unlisted preventive** medicine service

**99499**   **Unlisted evaluation and management** service

# Special Report

An unlisted service or one that is unusual, variable, or new may require a special report demonstrating the medical appropriateness of the service. Pertinent information should include an adequate definition or description of the nature, extent, and need for the procedure and the time, effort, and equipment necessary to provide the service. Additional items that may be included are complexity of symptoms, final diagnosis, pertinent physical findings, diagnostic and therapeutic procedures, concurrent problems, and follow-up care.

# Clinical Examples

Clinical examples of the codes for E/M services are provided to assist physicians in understanding the meaning of the descriptors and selecting the correct code. The clinical examples are listed in Appendix C. Each example was developed by physicians in the specialties shown.

The same problem, when seen by physicians in different specialties, may involve different amounts of work. Therefore, the appropriate level of encounter should be reported using the descriptors rather than the examples.

The examples have been tested for validity and approved by the CPT Editorial Panel. Physicians were given the examples and asked to assign a code or assess the amount of time and work involved. Only examples that were rated consistently have been included in Appendix C.

# Instructions for Selecting a Level of E/M Service

## Review the Reporting Instructions for the Selected Category or Subcategory

Most of the categories and many of the subcategories of service have special guidelines or instructions unique to that category or subcategory. Where these are indicated, eg, "Inpatient Hospital Care," special instructions will be presented preceding the levels of E/M services.

## Review the Level of E/M Service Descriptors and Examples in the Selected Category or Subcategory

The descriptors for the levels of E/M services recognize seven components, six of which are used in defining the levels of E/M services. These components are:

- History
- Examination
- Medical decision making
- Counseling
- Coordination of care
- Nature of presenting problem
- Time

The first three of these components (ie, history, examination, and medical decision making) should be considered the **key** components in selecting the level of E/M services. An exception to this rule is in the case of visits that consist predominantly of counseling or coordination of care (see numbered paragraph 3, page 6).

The nature of the presenting problem and time are provided in some levels to assist the physician in determining the appropriate level of E/M service.

## Determine the Extent of History Obtained

The extent of the history is dependent upon clinical judgment and on the nature of the presenting problem(s). The levels of E/M services recognize four types of history that are defined as follows:

*Problem focused:* Chief complaint; brief history of present illness or problem.

*Expanded problem focused:* Chief complaint; brief history of present illness; problem pertinent system review.

*Detailed:* Chief complaint; extended history of present illness; problem pertinent system review extended to include a review of a limited number of additional systems; **pertinent** past, family, and/or social history **directly related to the patient's problems.**

*Comprehensive:* Chief complaint; extended history of present illness; review of systems that is directly related to the problem(s) identified in the history of the present illness plus a review of all additional body systems; **complete** past, family, and social history.

The comprehensive history obtained as part of the preventive medicine E/M service is not problem-oriented and does not involve a chief complaint or present illness. It does, however, include a comprehensive system review and comprehensive or interval past, family, and social history as well as a comprehensive assessment/history of pertinent risk factors.

## Determine the Extent of Examination Performed

The extent of the examination performed is dependent on clinical judgment and on the nature of the presenting problem(s). The levels of E/M services recognize four types of examination that are defined as follows:

*Problem focused:* A limited examination of the affected body area or organ system.

*Expanded problem focused:* A limited examination of the affected body area or organ system and other symptomatic or related organ system(s).

*Detailed:* An extended examination of the affected body area(s) and other symptomatic or related organ system(s).

*Comprehensive:* A general multisystem examination or a complete examination of a single organ system. **Note:** The comprehensive examination performed as part of the preventive medicine E/M service is multisystem, but its extent is based on age and risk factors identified.

For the purposes of these CPT definitions, the following body areas are recognized:

- Head, including the face
- Neck
- Chest, including breasts and axilla
- Abdomen
- Genitalia, groin, buttocks
- Back
- Each extremity

For the purposes of these CPT definitions, the following organ systems are recognized:

- Eyes
- Ears, nose, mouth, and throat
- Cardiovascular
- Respiratory
- Gastrointestinal
- Genitourinary
- Musculoskeletal
- Skin
- Neurologic
- Psychiatric
- Hematologic/lymphatic/immunologic

## Determine the Complexity of Medical Decision Making

Medical decision making refers to the complexity of establishing a diagnosis and/or selecting a management option as measured by:

- The number of possible diagnoses and/or the number of management options that must be considered
- The amount and/or complexity of medical records, diagnostic tests, and/or other information that must be obtained, reviewed, and analyzed
- The risk of significant complications, morbidity, and/or mortality, as well as comorbidities, associated with the patient's presenting problem(s), the diagnostic procedure(s), and/or the possible management options

Four types of medical decision making are recognized: straightforward, low complexity, moderate complexity, and high complexity. To qualify for a given type of decision making, two of the three elements in Table 1 must be met or exceeded.

Comorbidities/underlying diseases, in and of themselves, are not considered in selecting a level of E/M services *unless* their presence significantly increases the complexity of the medical decision making.

## Select the Appropriate Level of E/M Services Based on the Following

1. For the following categories/subcategories, **all of the key components,** ie, history, examination, and medical decision making, must meet or exceed the stated requirements to qualify for a particular level of E/M service: office, new patient; hospital observation services; initial hospital care; office consultations; initial inpatient consultations; emergency department services; initial nursing facility care; domiciliary care, new patient; and home, new patient.

2. For the following categories/subcategories, **two of the three key components** (ie, history, examination, and medical decision making) must meet or exceed the stated requirements to qualify for a particular level of E/M services: office, established patient; subsequent hospital care; subsequent nursing facility care; domiciliary care, established patient; and home, established patient.

3. When counseling and/or coordination of care dominates (more than 50%) the physician/patient and/or family encounter (face-to-face time in the office or other outpatient setting or floor/unit time in the hospital or nursing facility), then **time** shall be considered the key or controlling factor to qualify for a particular level of E/M services. This includes time spent with parties who have assumed responsibility for the care of the patient or decision making whether or not they are family members (eg, foster parents, person acting in loco parentis, legal guardian). The extent of counseling and/or coordination of care must be documented in the medical record.

Table 1
**Complexity of Medical Decision Making**

| Number of Diagnoses or Management Options | Amount and/or Complexity of Data to be Reviewed | Risk of Complications and/or Morbidity or Mortality | Type of Decision Making |
|---|---|---|---|
| minimal | minimal or none | minimal | **straightforward** |
| limited | limited | low | **low complexity** |
| multiple | moderate | moderate | **moderate complexity** |
| extensive | extensive | high | **high complexity** |

# Decision Tree for New vs Established Patients

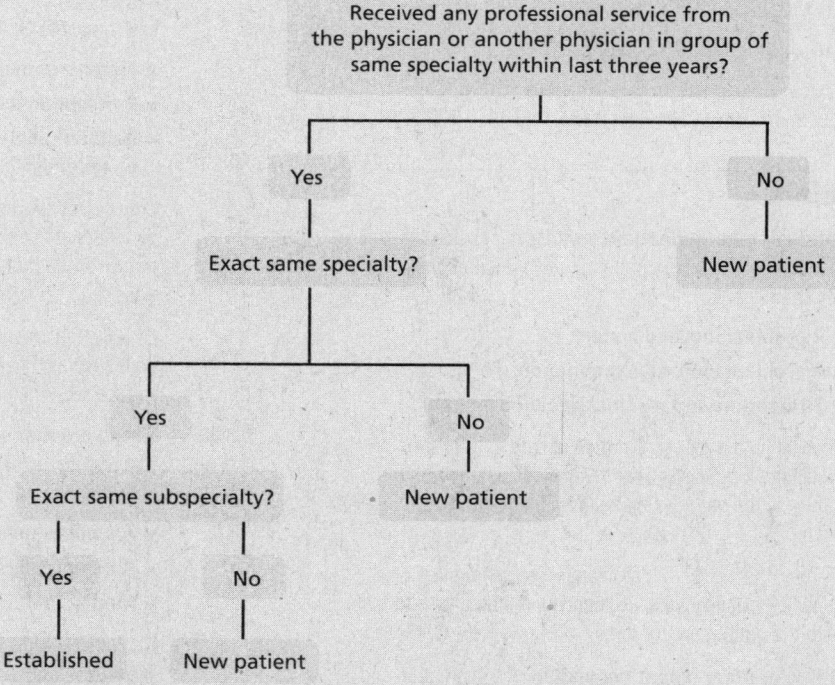

Received any professional service from the physician or another physician in group of same specialty within last three years?

Yes

No

Exact same specialty?

New patient

Yes

No

Exact same subspecialty?

New patient

Yes

No

Established

New patient

# Evaluation and Management

## Office or Other Outpatient Services

The following codes are used to report evaluation and management services provided in the physician's office or in an outpatient or other ambulatory facility. A patient is considered an outpatient until inpatient admission to a health care facility occurs.

To report services provided to a patient who is admitted to a hospital or nursing facility in the course of an encounter in the office or other ambulatory facility, see the notes for initial hospital inpatient care (page 11) or initial nursing facility care (page 19).

For services provided by physicians in the emergency department, see 99281-99285.

For observation care, see 99217-99226.

For observation or inpatient care services (including admission and discharge services), see 99234-99236.

### New Patient

**99201**  **Office or other outpatient visit** for the evaluation and management of a new patient, which requires these 3 key components:

- **A problem focused history;**
- **A problem focused examination;**
- **Straightforward medical decision making.**

Counseling and/or coordination of care with other providers or agencies are provided consistent with the nature of the problem(s) and the patient's and/or family's needs.

Usually, the presenting problem(s) are self limited or minor. Physicians typically spend 10 minutes face-to-face with the patient and/or family.

**99202**  **Office or other outpatient visit** for the evaluation and management of a new patient, which requires these 3 key components:

- **An expanded problem focused history;**
- **An expanded problem focused examination;**
- **Straightforward medical decision making.**

Counseling and/or coordination of care with other providers or agencies are provided consistent with the nature of the problem(s) and the patient's and/or family's needs.

Usually, the presenting problem(s) are of low to moderate severity. Physicians typically spend 20 minutes face-to-face with the patient and/or family.

**99203**  **Office or other outpatient visit** for the evaluation and management of a new patient, which requires these 3 key components:

- **A detailed history;**
- **A detailed examination;**
- **Medical decision making of low complexity.**

Counseling and/or coordination of care with other providers or agencies are provided consistent with the nature of the problem(s) and the patient's and/or family's needs.

Usually, the presenting problem(s) are of moderate severity. Physicians typically spend 30 minutes face-to-face with the patient and/or family.

**99204**  **Office or other outpatient visit** for the evaluation and management of a new patient, which requires these 3 key components:

- **A comprehensive history;**
- **A comprehensive examination;**
- **Medical decision making of moderate complexity.**

Counseling and/or coordination of care with other providers or agencies are provided consistent with the nature of the problem(s) and the patient's and/or family's needs.

Usually, the presenting problem(s) are of moderate to high severity. Physicians typically spend 45 minutes face-to-face with the patient and/or family.

**99205**  **Office or other outpatient visit** for the evaluation and management of a new patient, which requires these 3 key components:

- **A comprehensive history;**
- **A comprehensive examination;**
- **Medical decision making of high complexity.**

Counseling and/or coordination of care with other providers or agencies are provided consistent with the nature of the problem(s) and the patient's and/or family's needs.

Usually, the presenting problem(s) are of moderate to high severity. Physicians typically spend 60 minutes face-to-face with the patient and/or family.

### Established Patient

**99211**  **Office or other outpatient visit** for the evaluation and management of an established patient, that may not require the presence of a physician. Usually, the presenting problem(s) are minimal. Typically, 5 minutes are spent performing or supervising these services.

**99212**    **Office or other outpatient visit** for the evaluation and management of an established patient, which requires at least 2 of these 3 key components:

- **A problem focused history;**
- **A problem focused examination;**
- **Straightforward medical decision making.**

Counseling and/or coordination of care with other providers or agencies are provided consistent with the nature of the problem(s) and the patient's and/or family's needs.

Usually, the presenting problem(s) are self limited or minor. Physicians typically spend 10 minutes face-to-face with the patient and/or family.

**99213**    **Office or other outpatient visit** for the evaluation and management of an established patient, which requires at least 2 of these 3 key components:

- **An expanded problem focused history;**
- **An expanded problem focused examination;**
- **Medical decision making of low complexity.**

Counseling and coordination of care with other providers or agencies are provided consistent with the nature of the problem(s) and the patient's and/or family's needs.

Usually, the presenting problem(s) are of low to moderate severity. Physicians typically spend 15 minutes face-to-face with the patient and/or family.

**99214**    **Office or other outpatient visit** for the evaluation and management of an established patient, which requires at least 2 of these 3 key components:

- **A detailed history;**
- **A detailed examination;**
- **Medical decision making of moderate complexity.**

Counseling and/or coordination of care with other providers or agencies are provided consistent with the nature of the problem(s) and the patient's and/or family's needs.

Usually, the presenting problem(s) are of moderate to high severity. Physicians typically spend 25 minutes face-to-face with the patient and/or family.

**99215**    **Office or other outpatient visit** for the evaluation and management of an established patient, which requires at least 2 of these 3 key components:

- **A comprehensive history;**
- **A comprehensive examination;**
- **Medical decision making of high complexity.**

Counseling and/or coordination of care with other providers or agencies are provided consistent with the nature of the problem(s) and the patient's and/or family's needs.

Usually, the presenting problem(s) are of moderate to high severity. Physicians typically spend 40 minutes face-to-face with the patient and/or family.

# Hospital Observation Services

The following codes are used to report evaluation and management services provided to patients designated/admitted as "observation status" in a hospital. It is not necessary that the patient be located in an observation area designated by the hospital.

If such an area does exist in a hospital (as a separate unit in the hospital, in the emergency department, etc.), these codes are to be utilized if the patient is placed in such an area.

For definitions of key components and commonly used terms, please see **Evaluation and Management Services Guidelines.**

## Observation Care Discharge Services

Observation care discharge of a patient from "observation status" includes final examination of the patient, discussion of the hospital stay, instructions for continuing care, and preparation of discharge records. For observation or inpatient hospital care including the admission and discharge of the patient on the same date, see codes 99234-99236 as appropriate.

**99217**    **Observation care discharge** day management (This code is to be utilized by the physician to report all services provided to a patient on discharge from "observation status" if the discharge is on other than the initial date of "observation status." To report services to a patient designated as "observation status" or "inpatient status" and discharged on the same date, use the codes for Observation or Inpatient Care Services [including Admission and Discharge Services, 99234-99236 as appropriate.])

# Initial Observation Care

## New or Established Patient

The following codes are used to report the encounter(s) by the supervising physician with the patient when designated as "observation status." This refers to the initiation of observation status, supervision of the care plan for observation and performance of periodic reassessments. For observation encounters by other physicians, see Office or Other Outpatient Consultation codes (99241-99245) or subsequent observation care codes (99224-99226) as appropriate.

To report services provided to a patient who is admitted to the hospital after receiving hospital observation care services on the same date, see the notes for initial hospital inpatient care (page 11). For observation care services on other than the initial or discharge date, see subsequent observation services codes (99224-99226). For a patient admitted to the hospital on a date subsequent to the date of observation status, the hospital admission would be reported with the appropriate Initial Hospital Care code (99221-99223). For a patient admitted and discharged from observation or inpatient status on the same date, the services should be reported with codes 99234-99236 as appropriate. Do not report observation discharge (99217) in conjunction with a hospital admission.

When "observation status" is initiated in the course of an encounter in another site of service (eg, hospital emergency department, physician's office, nursing facility) all evaluation and management services provided by the supervising physician in conjunction with initiating "observation status" are considered part of the initial observation care when performed on the same date. The observation care level of service reported by the supervising physician should include the services related to initiating "observation status" provided in the other sites of service as well as in the observation setting.

Evaluation and management services on the same date provided in sites that are related to initiating "observation status" should **not** be reported separately.

These codes may not be utilized for post-operative recovery if the procedure is considered part of the surgical "package." These codes apply to all evaluation and management services that are provided on the same date of initiating "observation status."

▲ **99218** **Initial observation care,** per day, for the evaluation and management of a patient which requires these 3 key components:

- **A detailed or comprehensive history;**
- **A detailed or comprehensive examination; and**
- **Medical decision making that is straightforward or of low complexity.**

Counseling and/or coordination of care with other providers or agencies are provided consistent with the nature of the problem(s) and the patient's and/or family's needs.

Usually, the problem(s) requiring admission to "observation status" are of low severity. Physicians typically spend 30 minutes at the bedside and on the patient's hospital floor or unit.

▲ **99219** **Initial observation care,** per day, for the evaluation and management of a patient, which requires these 3 key components:

- **A comprehensive history;**
- **A comprehensive examination; and**
- **Medical decision making of moderate complexity.**

Counseling and/or coordination of care with other providers or agencies are provided consistent with the nature of the problem(s) and the patient's and/or family's needs.

Usually, the problem(s) requiring admission to "observation status" are of moderate severity. Physicians typically spend 50 minutes at the bedside and on the patient's hospital floor or unit.

▲ **99220** **Initial observation care,** per day, for the evaluation and management of a patient, which requires these 3 key components:

- **A comprehensive history;**
- **A comprehensive examination; and**
- **Medical decision making of high complexity.**

Counseling and/or coordination of care with other providers or agencies are provided consistent with the nature of the problem(s) and the patient's and/or family's needs.

Usually, the problem(s) requiring admission to "observation status" are of high severity. Physicians typically spend 70 minutes at the bedside and on the patient's hospital floor or unit.

## Subsequent Observation Care

All levels of subsequent observation care include reviewing the medical record and reviewing the results of diagnostic studies and changes in the patient's status (ie, changes in history, physical condition, and response to management) since the last assessment by the physician.

\# **99224** **Subsequent observation care,** per day, for the evaluation and management of a patient, which requires at least 2 of these 3 key components:

- **Problem focused interval history;**
- **Problem focused examination;**
- **Medical decision making that is straightforward or of low complexity.**

Counseling and/or coordination of care with other providers or agencies are provided consistent with the nature of the problem(s) and the patient's and/or family's needs.

Usually, the patient is stable, recovering, or improving. Physicians typically spend 15 minutes at the bedside and on the patient's hospital floor or unit.

\# **99225** **Subsequent observation care,** per day, for the evaluation and management of a patient, which requires at least 2 of these 3 key components:

- **An expanded problem focused interval history;**
- **An expanded problem focused examination;**
- **Medical decision making of moderate complexity.**

Counseling and/or coordination of care with other providers or agencies are provided consistent with the nature of the problem(s) and the patient's and/or family's needs.

Usually, the patient is responding inadequately to therapy or has developed a minor complication. Physicians typically spend 25 minutes at the bedside and on the patient's hospital floor or unit.

**# 99226**    **Subsequent observation care,** per day, for the evaluation and management of a patient, which requires at least 2 of these 3 key components:

- **A detailed interval history;**
- **A detailed examination;**
- **Medical decision making of high complexity.**

Counseling and/or coordination of care with other providers or agencies are provided consistent with the nature of the problem(s) and the patient's and/or family's needs.

Usually, the patient is unstable or has developed a significant complication or a significant new problem. Physicians typically spend 35 minutes at the bedside and on the patient's hospital floor or unit.

# Hospital Inpatient Services

The following codes are used to report evaluation and management services provided to hospital inpatients. Hospital inpatient services include those services provided to patients in a "partial hospital" setting. These codes are to be used to report these partial hospitalization services. See also psychiatry notes in the full text of the CPT codebook.

For definitions of key components and commonly used terms, please see **Evaluation and Management Services Guidelines.** For Hospital Observation Services, see 99218-99220, 99224-99226. For a patient admitted and discharged from observation or inpatient status on the same date, the services should be reported with codes 99234-99236 as appropriate.

## Initial Hospital Care

### New or Established Patient

The following codes are used to report the first hospital inpatient encounter with the patient by the admitting physician.

For initial inpatient encounters by physicians other than the admitting physician, see initial inpatient consultation codes (99251-99255) or subsequent hospital care codes (99231-99233) as appropriate.

For admission services for the neonate (28 days of age or younger) requiring intensive observation, frequent interventions, and other intensive care services, see 99477.

When the patient is admitted to the hospital as an inpatient in the course of an encounter in another site of service (eg, hospital emergency department, observation status in a hospital, physician's office, nursing facility) all evaluation and management services provided by that physician in conjunction with that admission are considered part of the initial hospital care when performed on the same date as the admission. The inpatient care level of service reported by the admitting physician should include the services related to the admission he/she provided in the other sites of service as well as in the inpatient setting.

Evaluation and management services on the same date provided in sites that are related to the admission "observation status" should **not** be reported separately. For a patient admitted and discharged from observation or inpatient status on the same date, the services should be reported with codes 99234-99236 as appropriate.

**99221**    **Initial hospital care,** per day, for the evaluation and management of a patient, which requires these 3 key components:

- **A detailed or comprehensive history;**
- **A detailed or comprehensive examination; and**
- **Medical decision making that is straightforward or of low complexity.**

Counseling and/or coordination of care with other providers or agencies are provided consistent with the nature of the problem(s) and the patient's and/or family's needs.

Usually, the problem(s) requiring admission are of low severity. Physicians typically spend 30 minutes at the bedside and on the patient's hospital floor or unit.

**99222**    **Initial hospital care,** per day, for the evaluation and management of a patient, which requires these 3 key components:

- **A comprehensive history;**
- **A comprehensive examination; and**
- **Medical decision making of moderate complexity.**

Counseling and/or coordination of care with other providers or agencies are provided consistent with the nature of the problem(s) and the patient's and/or family's needs.

Usually, the problem(s) requiring admission are of moderate severity. Physicians typically spend 50 minutes at the bedside and on the patient's hospital floor or unit.

**99223**    **Initial hospital care,** per day, for the evaluation and management of a patient, which requires these 3 key components:

- **A comprehensive history;**
- **A comprehensive examination; and**
- **Medical decision making of high complexity.**

Counseling and/or coordination of care with other providers or agencies are provided consistent with the nature of the problem(s) and the patient's and/or family's needs.

**Evaluation and Management**

Usually, the problem(s) requiring admission are of high severity. Physicians typically spend 70 minutes at the bedside and on the patient's hospital floor or unit.

**99224**  Code 99224 is out of numerical sequence. See 99224-99226

**99225**  Code 99225 is out of numerical sequence. See 99224-99226

**99226**  Code 99226 is out of numerical sequence. See 99224-99226

# Subsequent Hospital Care

All levels of subsequent hospital care include reviewing the medical record and reviewing the results of diagnostic studies and changes in the patient's status (ie, changes in history, physical condition and response to management) since the last assessment by the physician.

**99231**  **Subsequent hospital care,** per day, for the evaluation and management of a patient, which requires at least 2 of these 3 key components:

- **A problem focused interval history;**
- **A problem focused examination;**
- **Medical decision making that is straightforward or of low complexity.**

Counseling and/or coordination of care with other providers or agencies are provided consistent with the nature of the problem(s) and the patient's and/or family's needs.

Usually, the patient is stable, recovering or improving. Physicians typically spend 15 minutes at the bedside and on the patient's hospital floor or unit.

**99232**  **Subsequent hospital care,** per day, for the evaluation and management of a patient, which requires at least 2 of these 3 key components:

- **An expanded problem focused interval history;**
- **An expanded problem focused examination;**
- **Medical decision making of moderate complexity.**

Counseling and/or coordination of care with other providers or agencies are provided consistent with the nature of the problem(s) and the patient's and/or family's needs.

Usually, the patient is responding inadequately to therapy or has developed a minor complication. Physicians typically spend 25 minutes at the bedside and on the patient's hospital floor or unit.

**99233**  **Subsequent hospital care,** per day, for the evaluation and management of a patient, which requires at least 2 of these 3 key components:

- **A detailed interval history;**
- **A detailed examination;**
- **Medical decision making of high complexity.**

Counseling and/or coordination of care with other providers or agencies are provided consistent with the nature of the problem(s) and the patient's and/or family's needs.

Usually, the patient is unstable or has developed a significant complication or a significant new problem. Physicians typically spend 35 minutes at the bedside and on the patient's hospital floor or unit.

# Observation or Inpatient Care Services (Including Admission and Discharge Services)

The following codes are used to report observation or inpatient hospital care services provided to patients admitted and discharged on the same date of service. When a patient is admitted to the hospital from observation status on the same date, the physician should report only the initial hospital care code. The initial hospital care code reported by the admitting physician should include the services related to the observation status services he/she provided on the same date of inpatient admission.

When "observation status" is initiated in the course of an encounter in another site of service (eg, hospital emergency department, physician's office, nursing facility) all evaluation and management services provided by the supervising physician in conjunction with initiating "observation status" are considered part of the initial observation care when performed on the same date. The observation care level of service should include the services related to initiating "observation status" provided in the other sites of service as well as in the observation setting when provided by the same physician.

For patients admitted to observation or inpatient care and discharged on a different date, see codes 99218-99220, 99224-99226, 99217, or 99221-99223, 99238 and 99239.

**99234**  **Observation or inpatient hospital care,** for the evaluation and management of a patient including admission and discharge on the same date, which requires these 3 key components:

- **A detailed or comprehensive history;**
- **A detailed or comprehensive examination; and**
- **Medical decision making that is straightforward or of low complexity.**

Counseling and/or coordination of care with other providers or agencies are provided consistent with the nature of the problem(s) and the patient's and/or family's needs.

Usually the presenting problem(s) requiring admission are of low severity.

**99235**  **Observation or inpatient hospital care,** for the evaluation and management of a patient including admission and discharge on the same date, which requires these 3 key components:

■ **A comprehensive history;**

■ **A comprehensive examination; and**

■ **Medical decision making of moderate complexity.**

Counseling and/or coordination of care with other providers or agencies are provided consistent with the nature of the problem(s) and the patient's and/or family's needs.

Usually the presenting problem(s) requiring admission are of moderate severity.

**99236**  **Observation or inpatient hospital care,** for the evaluation and management of a patient including admission and discharge on the same date, which requires these 3 key components:

■ **A comprehensive history;**

■ **A comprehensive examination; and**

■ **Medical decision making of high complexity.**

Counseling and/or coordination of care with other providers or agencies are provided consistent with the nature of the problem(s) and the patient's and/or family's needs.

Usually the presenting problem(s) requiring admission are of high severity.

## Hospital Discharge Services

The hospital discharge day management codes are to be used to report the total duration of time spent by a physician for final hospital discharge of a patient. The codes include, as appropriate, final examination of the patient, discussion of the hospital stay, even if the time spent by the physician on that date is not continuous, instructions for continuing care to all relevant caregivers, and preparation of discharge records, prescriptions and referral forms. For a patient admitted and discharged from observation or inpatient status on the same date, the services should be reported with codes 99234-99236 as appropriate.

**99238**  **Hospital discharge day management**; 30 minutes or less

**99239**  more than 30 minutes

(These codes are to be utilized by the physician to report all services provided to a patient on the date of discharge, if other than the initial date of inpatient status. To report services to a patient who is admitted as an inpatient and discharged on the same date, see codes 99234-99236 for observation or inpatient hospital care including the admission and discharge of the patient on the same date. To report concurrent care services provided by a physician[s] other than the attending physician, use subsequent hospital care codes [99231-99233] on the day of discharge.)

(For Observation Care Discharge, use 99217)

(For observation or inpatient hospital care including the admission and discharge of the patient on the same date, see 99234-99236)

(For Nursing Facility Care Discharge, see 99315, 99316)

(For discharge services provided to newborns admitted and discharged on the same date, use 99463)

## Consultations

A consultation is a type of evaluation and management service provided by a physician at the request of another physician or appropriate source to either recommend care for a specific condition or problem or to determine whether to accept responsibility for ongoing management of the patient's entire care or for the care of a specific condition or problem.

A physician consultant may initiate diagnostic and/or therapeutic services at the same or subsequent visit.

A "consultation" initiated by a patient and/or family, and not requested by a physician or other appropriate source (eg, physician assistant, nurse practitioner, doctor of chiropractic, physical therapist, occupational therapist, speech-language pathologist, psychologist, social worker, lawyer, or insurance company), is not reported using the consultation codes but may be reported using the office visit, home service, or domiciliary/rest home care codes as appropriate.

The written or verbal request for consult may be made by a physician or other appropriate source and documented in the patient's medical record by either the consulting or requesting physician or appropriate source. The consultant's opinion and any services that were ordered or performed must also be documented in the patient's medical record and communicated by written report to the requesting physician or other appropriate source.

If a consultation is mandated (eg, by a third-party payer) modifier 32 should also be reported.

Any specifically identifiable procedure (ie, identified with a specific CPT code) performed on or subsequent to the date of the initial consultation should be reported separately.

If subsequent to the completion of a consultation the consultant assumes responsibility for management of a portion or all of the patient's condition(s), the appropriate **Evaluation and Management** services code for the site of service should be reported. In the hospital or nursing facility setting, the consulting physician should use the appropriate inpatient consultation code for the initial encounter and then subsequent hospital or nursing facility care codes. In the office setting, the physician should use the appropriate office or other outpatient consultation codes and then the established patient office or other outpatient services codes.

**Evaluation and Management**

To report services provided to a patient who is admitted to a hospital or nursing facility in the course of an encounter in the office or other ambulatory facility, see the notes for Initial Hospital Inpatient Care (page 11) or Initial Nursing Facility Care (page 19).

For definitions of key components and commonly used terms, please see **Evaluation and Management Services Guidelines.**

# Office or Other Outpatient Consultations

## New or Established Patient

The following codes are used to report consultations provided in the physician's office or in an outpatient or other ambulatory facility, including hospital observation services, home services, domiciliary, rest home, or emergency department (see the preceding consultation definition above). Follow-up visits in the consultant's office or other outpatient facility that are initiated by the physician consultant or patient are reported using the appropriate codes for established patients, office visits (99211-99215), domiciliary, rest home (99334-99337), or home (99347-99350). If an additional request for an opinion or advice regarding the same or a new problem is received from another physician or other appropriate source and documented in the medical record, the office consultation codes may be used again. Services that constitute transfer of care (ie, are provided for the management of the patient's entire care or for the care of a specific condition or problem) are reported with the appropriate new or established patient codes for office or other outpatient visits, domiciliary, rest home services, or home services.

**99241**    **Office consultation** for a new or established patient, which requires these 3 key components:

- A problem focused history;
- A problem focused examination; and
- Straightforward medical decision making.

Counseling and/or coordination of care with other providers or agencies are provided consistent with the nature of the problem(s) and the patient's and/or family's needs.

Usually, the presenting problem(s) are self limited or minor. Physicians typically spend 15 minutes face-to-face with the patient and/or family.

**99242**    **Office consultation** for a new or established patient, which requires these 3 key components:

- An expanded problem focused history;
- An expanded problem focused examination; and
- Straightforward medical decision making.

Counseling and/or coordination of care with other providers or agencies are provided consistent with the nature of the problem(s) and the patient's and/or family's needs.

Usually, the presenting problem(s) are of low severity. Physicians typically spend 30 minutes face-to-face with the patient and/or family.

**99243**    **Office consultation** for a new or established patient, which requires these 3 key components:

- A detailed history;
- A detailed examination; and
- Medical decision making of low complexity.

Counseling and/or coordination of care with other providers or agencies are provided consistent with the nature of the problem(s) and the patient's and/or family's needs.

Usually, the presenting problem(s) are of moderate severity. Physicians typically spend 40 minutes face-to-face with the patient and/or family.

**99244**    **Office consultation** for a new or established patient, which requires these 3 key components:

- A comprehensive history;
- A comprehensive examination; and
- Medical decision making of moderate complexity.

Counseling and/or coordination of care with other providers or agencies are provided consistent with the nature of the problem(s) and the patient's and/or family's needs.

Usually, the presenting problem(s) are of moderate to high severity. Physicians typically spend 60 minutes face-to-face with the patient and/or family.

**99245**    **Office consultation** for a new or established patient, which requires these 3 key components:

- A comprehensive history;
- A comprehensive examination; and
- Medical decision making of high complexity.

Counseling and/or coordination of care with other providers or agencies are provided consistent with the nature of the problem(s) and the patient's and/or family's needs.

Usually, the presenting problem(s) are of moderate to high severity. Physicians typically spend 80 minutes face-to-face with the patient and/or family.

# Inpatient Consultations

## New or Established Patient

The following codes are used to report physician consultations provided to hospital inpatients, residents of nursing facilities, or patients in a partial hospital setting. Only one consultation should be reported by a consultant per admission. Subsequent services during the same admission are reported using subsequent hospital care codes (99231-99233) or subsequent nursing facility care codes (99307-99310), including services to complete the initial consultation, monitor progress, revise recommendations, or address a new problem. Use subsequent hospital care codes (99231-99233) or subsequent nursing facility care codes (99307-99310) to report transfer of care services (see page 4, Concurrent Care and Transfer of Care definitions).

When an inpatient consultation is performed on a date that a patient is admitted to a hospital or nursing facility, all evaluation and management services provided by the consultant related to the admission are reported with the inpatient consultation service code (99251-99255). If a patient is admitted after an outpatient consultation (office, emergency department, etc), and the patient is not seen on the unit on the date of admission, only report the outpatient consultation code (99241-99245). If the patient is seen by the consultant on the unit on the date of admission, report all evaluation and management services provided by the consultant related to the admission with either the inpatient consultation code (99251-99255) or with the initial inpatient admission service code (99221-99223). Do not report both an outpatient consultation and inpatient consultation for services related to the same inpatient stay. When transfer of care services are provided on a date subsequent to the outpatient consultation, use the subsequent hospital care codes (99231-99233) or subsequent nursing facility care codes (99307-99310).

**99251** **Inpatient consultation** for a new or established patient, which requires these 3 key components:

- **A problem focused history;**
- **A problem focused examination; and**
- **Straightforward medical decision making.**

Counseling and/or coordination of care with other providers or agencies are provided consistent with the nature of the problem(s) and the patient's and/or family's needs.

Usually, the presenting problem(s) are self limited or minor. Physicians typically spend 20 minutes at the bedside and on the patient's hospital floor or unit.

**99252** **Inpatient consultation** for a new or established patient, which requires these 3 key components:

- **An expanded problem focused history;**
- **An expanded problem focused examination; and**
- **Straightforward medical decision making.**

Counseling and/or coordination of care with other providers or agencies are provided consistent with the nature of the problem(s) and the patient's and/or family's needs.

Usually, the presenting problem(s) are of low severity. Physicians typically spend 40 minutes at the bedside and on the patient's hospital floor or unit.

**99253** **Inpatient consultation** for a new or established patient, which requires these 3 key components:

- **A detailed history;**
- **A detailed examination; and**
- **Medical decision making of low complexity.**

Counseling and/or coordination of care with other providers or agencies are provided consistent with the nature of the problem(s) and the patient's and/or family's needs.

Usually, the presenting problem(s) are of moderate severity. Physicians typically spend 55 minutes at the bedside and on the patient's hospital floor or unit.

**99254** **Inpatient consultation** for a new or established patient, which requires these 3 key components:

- **A comprehensive history;**
- **A comprehensive examination; and**
- **Medical decision making of moderate complexity.**

Counseling and/or coordination of care with other providers or agencies are provided consistent with the nature of the problem(s) and the patient's and/or family's needs.

Usually, the presenting problem(s) are of moderate to high severity. Physicians typically spend 80 minutes at the bedside and on the patient's hospital floor or unit.

**99255** **Inpatient consultation** for a new or established patient, which requires these 3 key components:

- **A comprehensive history;**
- **A comprehensive examination; and**
- **Medical decision making of high complexity.**

Counseling and/or coordination of care with other providers or agencies are provided consistent with the nature of the problem(s) and the patient's and/or family's needs.

Usually, the presenting problem(s) are of moderate to high severity. Physicians typically spend 110 minutes at the bedside and on the patient's hospital floor or unit.

Evaluation and Management

**Evaluation and Management**

# Emergency Department Services

## New or Established Patient

The following codes are used to report evaluation and management services provided in the emergency department. No distinction is made between new and established patients in the emergency department.

An emergency department is defined as an organized hospital-based facility for the provision of unscheduled episodic services to patients who present for immediate medical attention. The facility must be available 24 hours a day.

For critical care services provided in the emergency department, see Critical Care notes and 99291, 99292.

For evaluation and management services provided to a patient in an observation area of a hospital, see 99217-99220.

For observation or inpatient care services (including admission and discharge services), see 99234-99236.

**99281**    **Emergency department visit** for the evaluation and management of a patient, which requires these 3 key components:

- **A problem focused history;**
- **A problem focused examination; and**
- **Straightforward medical decision making.**

Counseling and/or coordination of care with other providers or agencies are provided consistent with the nature of the problem(s) and the patient's and/or family's needs.

Usually, the presenting problem(s) are self limited or minor.

**99282**    **Emergency department visit** for the evaluation and management of a patient, which requires these 3 key components:

- **An expanded problem focused history;**
- **An expanded problem focused examination; and**
- **Medical decision making of low complexity.**

Counseling and/or coordination of care with other providers or agencies are provided consistent with the nature of the problem(s) and the patient's and/or family's needs.

Usually, the presenting problem(s) are of low to moderate severity.

**99283**    **Emergency department visit** for the evaluation and management of a patient, which requires these 3 key components:

- **An expanded problem focused history;**
- **An expanded problem focused examination; and**
- **Medical decision making of moderate complexity.**

Counseling and/or coordination of care with other providers or agencies are provided consistent with the nature of the problem(s) and the patient's and/or family's needs.

Usually, the presenting problem(s) are of moderate severity.

**99284**    **Emergency department visit** for the evaluation and management of a patient, which requires these 3 key components:

- **A detailed history;**
- **A detailed examination; and**
- **Medical decision making of moderate complexity.**

Counseling and/or coordination of care with other providers or agencies are provided consistent with the nature of the problem(s) and the patient's and/or family's needs.

Usually, the presenting problem(s) are of high severity, and require urgent evaluation by the physician but do not pose an immediate significant threat to life or physiologic function.

**99285**    **Emergency department visit** for the evaluation and management of a patient, which requires these 3 key components within the constraints imposed by the urgency of the patient's clinical condition and/or mental status:

- **A comprehensive history;**
- **A comprehensive examination; and**
- **Medical decision making of high complexity.**

Counseling and/or coordination of care with other providers or agencies are provided consistent with the nature of the problem(s) and the patient's and/or family's needs.

Usually, the presenting problem(s) are of high severity and pose an immediate significant threat to life or physiologic function.

## Other Emergency Services

In physician directed emergency care, advanced life support, the physician is located in a hospital emergency or critical care department, and is in two-way voice communication with ambulance or rescue personnel outside the hospital. The physician directs the performance of necessary medical procedures, including but not limited to: telemetry of cardiac rhythm; cardiac and/or pulmonary resuscitation; endotracheal or esophageal obturator airway intubation; administration of intravenous fluids and/or administration of intramuscular, intratracheal or subcutaneous drugs; and/or electrical conversion of arrhythmia.

**99288**    **Physician direction of** emergency medical systems (EMS) emergency care, advanced life support

     (99289 has been deleted. To report, use 99466)

     (99290 has been deleted. To report, use 99467)

## Critical Care Services

Critical care is the direct delivery by a physician(s) of medical care for a critically ill or critically injured patient. A critical illness or injury acutely impairs one or more vital organ systems such that there is a high probability of imminent or life threatening deterioration in the patient's condition. Critical care involves high complexity decision making to assess, manipulate, and support vital system function(s) to treat single or multiple vital organ system failure and/or to prevent further life threatening deterioration of the patient's condition. Examples of vital organ system failure include, but are not limited to: central nervous system failure, circulatory failure, shock, renal, hepatic, metabolic, and/or respiratory failure. Although critical care typically requires interpretation of multiple physiologic parameters and/or application of advanced technology(s), critical care may be provided in life threatening situations when these elements are not present. Critical care may be provided on multiple days, even if no changes are made in the treatment rendered to the patient, provided that the patient's condition continues to require the level of physician attention described above.

Providing medical care to a critically ill, injured, or post-operative patient qualifies as a critical care service only if both the illness or injury and the treatment being provided meet the above requirements. Critical care is usually, but not always, given in a critical care area, such as the coronary care unit, intensive care unit, pediatric intensive care unit, respiratory care unit, or the emergency care facility.

Inpatient critical care services provided to infants 29 days through 71 months of age are reported with pediatric critical care codes 99471-99476. The pediatric critical care codes are reported as long as the infant/young child qualifies for critical care services during the hospital stay through 71 months of age. Inpatient critical care services provided to neonates (28 days of age or younger) are reported with the neonatal critical care codes 99468 and 99469. The neonatal critical care codes are reported as long as the neonate qualifies for critical care services during the hospital stay through the 28th postnatal day. The reporting of the pediatric and neonatal critical care services is not based on time or the type of unit (eg, pediatric or neonatal critical care unit) and it is not dependent upon the type of provider delivering the care. To report critical care services provided in the outpatient setting (eg, emergency department or office), for neonates and pediatric patients up through 71 months of age, see the critical care codes 99291, 99292. If the same physician provides critical care services for a neonatal or pediatric patient in both the outpatient and inpatient settings on the same day, report only the appropriate neonatal or pediatric critical care code 99468-99472 for all critical care services provided on that day. Also report 99291-99292 for neonatal or pediatric critical care services provided by the physician providing critical care at one facility but transferring the patient to another facility. Critical care services provided by a second physician of a different specialty not reporting a per day neonatal or pediatric critical care code can be reported with codes 99291-99292. For additional instructions on reporting these services, see the Neonatal and Pediatric Critical Care section and codes 99468-99476.

Services for a patient who is not critically ill but happens to be in a critical care unit are reported using other appropriate E/M codes.

Critical care and other E/M services may be provided to the same patient on the same date by the same physician.

For reporting by professionals, the following services are included in critical care when performed during the critical period by the physician(s) providing critical care: the interpretation of cardiac output measurements (93561, 93562), chest X-rays (71010, 71015, 71020), pulse oximetry (94760, 94761, 94762), blood gases, and information data stored in computers (eg, ECGs, blood pressures, hematologic data [99090]); gastric intubation (43752, 43753); temporary transcutaneous pacing (92953); ventilatory management (94002-94004, 94660, 94662); and vascular access procedures (36000, 36410, 36415, 36591, 36600). Any services performed that are not included in this listing should be reported separately. Facilities may report the above services separately.

Codes 99291, 99292 should be reported for the physician's attendance during the transport of critically ill or critically injured patients older than 24 months of age to or from a facility or hospital. For physician transport services of critically ill or critically injured pediatric patients 24 months of age or younger, see 99466, 99467.

The critical care codes 99291 and 99292 are used to report the total duration of time spent by a physician providing critical care services to a critically ill or critically injured patient, even if the time spent by the physician on that date is not continuous. For any given period of time spent providing critical care services, the physician must devote his or her full attention to the patient and, therefore, cannot provide services to any other patient during the same period of time.

Time spent with the individual patient should be recorded in the patient's record. The time that can be reported as critical care is the time spent engaged in work directly related to the individual patient's care whether that time was spent at the immediate bedside or elsewhere on the floor or unit. For example, time spent on the unit or at the nursing station on the floor reviewing test results or imaging studies, discussing the critically ill patient's care with other medical staff or documenting critical care services in the medical record would be reported as critical care, even though it does not occur at the bedside. Also, when the patient is unable or lacks capacity to participate in discussions, time spent on the floor or unit with family members or surrogate decision makers obtaining a medical history, reviewing the patient's condition or prognosis, or discussing treatment or limitation(s) of treatment may be reported as critical care, provided that the conversation bears directly on the management of the patient.

Time spent in activities that occur outside of the unit or off the floor (eg, telephone calls whether taken at home, in the office, or elsewhere in the hospital) may not be reported as critical care since the physician is not immediately available to the patient. Time spent in activities that do not directly contribute to the treatment of the patient may not be reported as critical care, even if they are performed in the critical care unit (eg, participation in administrative meetings or telephone calls to discuss other patients). Time spent performing separately reportable procedures or services should not be included in the time reported as critical care time. No physician may report remote real-time interactive video-conferenced critical care services (0188T, 0189T) for the period in which any physician reports 99291-99292.

Code 99291 is used to report the first 30-74 minutes of critical care on a given date. It should be used only once per date even if the time spent by the physician is not continuous on that date. Critical care of less than 30 minutes total duration on a given date should be reported with the appropriate E/M code.

Code 99292 is used to report additional block(s) of time, of up to 30 minutes each beyond the first 74 minutes. (See the following table.)

The following examples illustrate the correct reporting of critical care services:

| Total Duration of Critical Care | Codes |
|---|---|
| less than 30 minutes | appropriate E/M codes |
| 30-74 minutes (30 minutes - 1 hr. 14 min.) | 99291 X 1 |
| 75-104 minutes (1 hr. 15 min. - 1 hr. 44 min.) | 99291 X 1 AND 99292 X 1 |
| 105-134 minutes (1 hr. 45 min. - 2 hr. 14 min.) | 99291 X 1 AND 99292 X 2 |
| 135-164 minutes (2 hr. 15 min. - 2 hr. 44 min.) | 99291 X 1 AND 99292 X 3 |
| 165-194 minutes (2 hr. 45 min. - 3 hr. 14 min.) | 99291 X 1 AND 99292 X 4 |
| 195 minutes or longer (3 hr. 15 min. - etc.) | 99291 and 99292 as appropriate (see illustrated reporting examples above) |

**99291** **Critical care, evaluation and management** of the critically ill or critically injured patient; first 30-74 minutes

+ **99292** each additional 30 minutes (List separately in addition to code for primary service)

(Use 99292 in conjunction with 99291)

(99293 has been deleted. To report, use 99471)

(99294 has been deleted. To report, use 99472)

(99295 has been deleted. To report, use 99468)

(99296 has been deleted. To report, use 99469)

(99298 has been deleted. To report, use 99478)

(99299 has been deleted. To report, use 99479)

(99300 has been deleted. To report, use 99480)

# Nursing Facility Services

The following codes are used to report evaluation and management services to patients in nursing facilities (formerly called skilled nursing facilities [SNFs], intermediate care facilities [ICFs], or long-term care facilities [LTCFs]).

These codes should also be used to report evaluation and management services provided to a patient in a psychiatric residential treatment center (a facility or a distinct part of a facility for psychiatric care, which provides a 24-hour therapeutically planned and professionally staffed group living and learning environment). If procedures such as medical psychotherapy are provided in addition to evaluation and management services, these should be reported in addition to the evaluation and management services provided.

Nursing facilities that provide convalescent, rehabilitative, or long term care are required to conduct comprehensive, accurate, standardized, and reproducible assessments of each resident's functional capacity using a Resident Assessment Instrument (RAI). All RAIs include the Minimum Data Set (MDS), Resident Assessment Protocols (RAPs), and utilization guidelines. The MDS is the primary screening and assessment tool; the RAPs trigger the identification of potential problems and provide guidelines for follow-up assessments.

Physicians have a central role in assuring that all residents receive thorough assessments and that medical plans of care are instituted or revised to enhance or maintain the residents' physical and psychosocial functioning. This role includes providing input in the development of the MDS and a multi-disciplinary plan of care, as required by regulations pertaining to the care of nursing facility residents.

Two major subcategories of nursing facility services are recognized: Initial Nursing Facility Care and Subsequent Nursing Facility Care. Both subcategories apply to new or established patients.

For definitions of key components and commonly used terms, please see **Evaluation and Management Services Guidelines.**

> (For care plan oversight services provided to nursing facility residents, see 99379-99380)

# Initial Nursing Facility Care

## New or Established Patient

When the patient is admitted to the nursing facility in the course of an encounter in another site of service (eg, hospital emergency department, physician's office), all evaluation and management services provided by that physician in conjunction with that admission are considered part of the initial nursing facility care when performed on the same date as the admission or readmission. The nursing facility care level of service reported by the admitting physician should include the services related to the admission he/she provided in the other sites of service as well as in the nursing facility setting.

Hospital discharge or observation discharge services performed on the same date of nursing facility admission or readmission may be reported separately. For a patient discharged from inpatient status on the same date of

nursing facility admission or readmission, the hospital discharge services should be reported with codes 99238, 99239 as appropriate. For a patient discharged from observation status on the same date of nursing facility admission or readmission, the observation care discharge services should be reported with code 99217. For a patient admitted and discharged from observation or inpatient status on the same date, see codes 99234-99236.

(For nursing facility care discharge, see 99315, 99316)

**99304**    Initial nursing facility care, per day, for the evaluation and management of a patient, which requires these 3 key components:

- **A detailed or comprehensive history;**
- **A detailed or comprehensive examination; and**
- **Medical decision making that is straightforward or of low complexity.**

Counseling and/or coordination of care with other providers or agencies are provided consistent with the nature of the problem(s) and the patient's and/or family's needs.

Usually, the problem(s) requiring admission are of low severity. Physicians typically spend 25 minutes at the bedside and on the patient's facility floor or unit.

**99305**    Initial nursing facility care, per day, for the evaluation and management of a patient, which requires these 3 key components:

- **A comprehensive history;**
- **A comprehensive examination; and**
- **Medical decision making of moderate complexity.**

Counseling and/or coordination of care with other providers or agencies are provided consistent with the nature of the problem(s) and the patient's and/or family's needs.

Usually, the problem(s) requiring admission are of moderate severity. Physicians typically spend 35 minutes at the bedside and on the patient's facility floor or unit.

**99306**    Initial nursing facility care, per day, for the evaluation and management of a patient, which requires these 3 key components:

- **A comprehensive history;**
- **A comprehensive examination; and**
- **Medical decision making of high complexity.**

Counseling and/or coordination of care with other providers or agencies are provided consistent with the nature of the problem(s) and the patient's and/or family's needs.

Usually, the problem(s) requiring admission are of high severity. Physicians typically spend 45 minutes at the bedside and on the patient's facility floor or unit.

**Evaluation and Management**

# Subsequent Nursing Facility Care

All levels of subsequent nursing facility care include reviewing the medical record and reviewing the results of diagnostic studies and changes in the patient's status (ie, changes in history, physical condition, and response to management) since the last assessment by the physician.

**99307**    Subsequent nursing facility care, per day, for the evaluation and management of a patient, which requires at least 2 of these 3 key components:

- **A problem focused interval history;**
- **A problem focused examination;**
- **Straightforward medical decision making.**

Counseling and/or coordination of care with other providers or agencies are provided consistent with the nature of the problem(s) and the patient's and/or family's needs.

Usually, the patient is stable, recovering, or improving. Physicians typically spend 10 minutes at the bedside and on the patient's facility floor or unit.

**99308**    Subsequent nursing facility care, per day, for the evaluation and management of a patient, which requires at least 2 of these 3 key components:

- **An expanded problem focused interval history;**
- **An expanded problem focused examination;**
- **Medical decision making of low complexity.**

Counseling and/or coordination of care with other providers or agencies are provided consistent with the nature of the problem(s) and the patient's and/or family's needs.

Usually, the patient is responding inadequately to therapy or has developed a minor complication. Physicians typically spend 15 minutes at the bedside and on the patient's facility floor or unit.

**99309**    Subsequent nursing facility care, per day, for the evaluation and management of a patient, which requires at least 2 of these 3 key components:

- **A detailed interval history;**
- **A detailed examination;**
- **Medical decision making of moderate complexity.**

Counseling and/or coordination of care with other providers or agencies are provided consistent with the nature of the problem(s) and the patient's and/or family's needs.

Usually, the patient has developed a significant complication or a significant new problem. Physicians typically spend 25 minutes at the bedside and on the patient's facility floor or unit.

**99310**    Subsequent nursing facility care, per day, for the evaluation and management of a patient, which requires at least 2 of these 3 key components:

- **A comprehensive interval history;**
- **A comprehensive examination;**
- **Medical decision making of high complexity.**

Counseling and/or coordination of care with other providers or agencies are provided consistent with the nature of the problem(s) and the patient's and/or family's needs.

The patient may be unstable or may have developed a significant new problem requiring immediate physician attention. Physicians typically spend 35 minutes at the bedside and on the patient's facility floor or unit.

# Nursing Facility Discharge Services

The nursing facility discharge day management codes are to be used to report the total duration of time spent by a physician for the final nursing facility discharge of a patient. The codes include, as appropriate, final examination of the patient, discussion of the nursing facility stay, even if the time spent by the physician on that date is not continuous. Instructions are given for continuing care to all relevant caregivers, and preparation of discharge records, prescriptions and referral forms.

**99315**    Nursing facility discharge day management; 30 minutes or less

**99316**        more than 30 minutes

# Other Nursing Facility Services

**99318**    Evaluation and management of a patient involving an annual nursing facility assessment, which requires these 3 key components:

- **A detailed interval history;**
- **A comprehensive examination; and**
- **Medical decision making that is of low to moderate complexity.**

Counseling and/or coordination of care with other providers or agencies are provided consistent with the nature of the problem(s) and the patient's and/or family's needs.

Usually, the patient is stable, recovering, or improving. Physicians typically spend 30 minutes at the bedside and on the patient's facility floor or unit.

(Do not report 99318 on the same date of service as nursing facility services codes 99304-99316)

# Domiciliary, Rest Home (eg, Boarding Home), or Custodial Care Services

The following codes are used to report evaluation and management services in a facility which provides room, board and other personal assistance services, generally on a long-term basis. They also are used to report evaluation and management services in an assisted living facility.

The facility's services do not include a medical component.

For definitions of key components and commonly used terms, please see **Evaluation and Management Services Guidelines**.

> (For care plan oversight services provided to a patient in a domiciliary facility under the care of a home health agency, see 99374-99375)

> (For care plan oversight services provided to a patient in a domiciliary facility under the individual supervision of a physician, see 99339, 99340)

## New Patient

99324    Domiciliary or rest home visit for the evaluation and management of a new patient, which requires these 3 key components:

- **A problem focused history;**
- **A problem focused examination; and**
- **Straightforward medical decision making.**

Counseling and/or coordination of care with other providers or agencies are provided consistent with the nature of the problem(s) and the patient's and/or family's needs.

Usually, the presenting problem(s) are of low severity. Physicians typically spend 20 minutes with the patient and/or family or caregiver.

99325    Domiciliary or rest home visit for the evaluation and management of a new patient, which requires these 3 key components:

- **An expanded problem focused history;**
- **An expanded problem focused examination; and**
- **Medical decision making of low complexity.**

Counseling and/or coordination of care with other providers or agencies are provided consistent with the nature of the problem(s) and the patient's and/or family's needs.

Usually, the presenting problem(s) are of moderate severity. Physicians typically spend 30 minutes with the patient and/or family or caregiver.

99326    Domiciliary or rest home visit for the evaluation and management of a new patient, which requires these 3 key components:

- **A detailed history;**
- **A detailed examination; and**
- **Medical decision making of moderate complexity.**

Counseling and/or coordination of care with other providers or agencies are provided consistent with the nature of the problem(s) and the patient's and/or family's needs.

Usually, the presenting problem(s) are of moderate to high severity. Physicians typically spend 45 minutes with the patient and/or family or caregiver.

99327    Domiciliary or rest home visit for the evaluation and management of a new patient, which requires these 3 key components:

- **A comprehensive history;**
- **A comprehensive examination; and**
- **Medical decision making of moderate complexity.**

Counseling and/or coordination of care with other providers or agencies are provided consistent with the nature of the problem(s) and the patient's and/or family's needs.

Usually, the presenting problem(s) are of high severity. Physicians typically spend 60 minutes with the patient and/or family or caregiver.

99328    Domiciliary or rest home visit for the evaluation and management of a new patient, which requires these 3 key components:

- **A comprehensive history;**
- **A comprehensive examination; and**
- **Medical decision making of high complexity.**

Counseling and/or coordination of care with other providers or agencies are provided consistent with the nature of the problem(s) and the patient's and/or family's needs.

Usually, the patient is unstable or has developed a significant new problem requiring immediate physician attention. Physicians typically spend 75 minutes with the patient and/or family or caregiver.

## Established Patient

99334    Domiciliary or rest home visit for the evaluation and management of an established patient, which requires at least 2 of these 3 key components:

- **A problem focused interval history;**
- **A problem focused examination;**
- **Straightforward medical decision making.**

**Evaluation and Management**

Counseling and/or coordination of care with other providers or agencies are provided consistent with the nature of the problem(s) and the patient's and/or family's needs.

Usually, the presenting problem(s) are self-limited or minor. Physicians typically spend 15 minutes with the patient and/or family or caregiver.

**99335** Domiciliary or rest home visit for the evaluation and management of an established patient, which requires at least 2 of these 3 key components:

- **An expanded problem focused interval history;**
- **An expanded problem focused examination;**
- **Medical decision making of low complexity.**

Counseling and/or coordination of care with other providers or agencies are provided consistent with the nature of the problem(s) and the patient's and/or family's needs.

Usually, the presenting problem(s) are of low to moderate severity. Physicians typically spend 25 minutes with the patient and/or family or caregiver.

**99336** Domiciliary or rest home visit for the evaluation and management of an established patient, which requires at least 2 of these 3 key components:

- **A detailed interval history;**
- **A detailed examination;**
- **Medical decision making of moderate complexity.**

Counseling and/or coordination of care with other providers or agencies are provided consistent with the nature of the problem(s) and the patient's and/or family's needs.

Usually, the presenting problem(s) are of moderate to high severity. Physicians typically spend 40 minutes with the patient and/or family or caregiver.

**99337** Domiciliary or rest home visit for the evaluation and management of an established patient, which requires at least 2 of these 3 key components:

- **A comprehensive interval history;**
- **A comprehensive examination;**
- **Medical decision making of moderate to high complexity.**

Counseling and/or coordination of care with other providers or agencies are provided consistent with the nature of the problem(s) and the patient's and/or family's needs.

Usually, the presenting problem(s) are of moderate to high severity. The patient may be unstable or may have developed a significant new problem requiring immediate physician attention. Physicians typically spend 60 minutes with the patient and/or family or caregiver.

# Domiciliary, Rest Home (eg, Assisted Living Facility), or Home Care Plan Oversight Services

(For instructions on the use of 99339, 99340, see introductory notes for 99374-99380)

(For care plan oversight services for patients under the care of a home health agency, hospice, or nursing facility, see 99374-99380)

(Do not report 99339, 99340 for time reported with 98966-98969, 99441-99444)

**99339** Individual physician supervision of a patient (patient not present) in home, domiciliary or rest home (eg, assisted living facility) requiring complex and multidisciplinary care modalities involving regular physician development and/or revision of care plans, review of subsequent reports of patient status, review of related laboratory and other studies, communication (including telephone calls) for purposes of assessment or care decisions with health care professional(s), family member(s), surrogate decision maker(s) (eg, legal guardian) and/or key caregiver(s) involved in patient's care, integration of new information into the medical treatment plan and/or adjustment of medical therapy, within a calendar month; 15-29 minutes

**99340**        30 minutes or more

(Do not report 99339, 99340 for patients under the care of a home health agency, enrolled in a hospice program, or for nursing facility residents)

# Home Services

The following codes are used to report evaluation and management services provided in a private residence.

For definitions of key components and commonly used terms, please see **Evaluation and Management Services Guidelines.**

(For care plan oversight services provided to a patient in the home under the care of a home health agency, see 99374-99375)

(For care plan oversight services provided to a patient in the home under the individual supervision of a physician, see 99339, 99340)

## New Patient

**99341** **Home visit** for the evaluation and management of a new patient, which requires these 3 key components:

- **A problem focused history;**
- **A problem focused examination; and**
- **Straightforward medical decision making.**

Counseling and/or coordination of care with other providers or agencies are provided consistent with the nature of the problem(s) and the patient's and/or family's needs.

Usually, the presenting problem(s) are of low severity. Physicians typically spend 20 minutes face-to-face with the patient and/or family.

**99342**    **Home visit** for the evaluation and management of a new patient, which requires these 3 key components:

- **An expanded problem focused history;**
- **An expanded problem focused examination; and**
- **Medical decision making of low complexity.**

Counseling and/or coordination of care with other providers or agencies are provided consistent with the nature of the problem(s) and the patient's and/or family's needs.

Usually, the presenting problem(s) are of moderate severity. Physicians typically spend 30 minutes face-to-face with the patient and/or family.

**99343**    **Home visit** for the evaluation and management of a new patient, which requires these 3 key components:

- **A detailed history;**
- **A detailed examination; and**
- **Medical decision making of moderate complexity.**

Counseling and/or coordination of care with other providers or agencies are provided consistent with the nature of the problem(s) and the patient's and/or family's needs.

Usually, the presenting problem(s) are of moderate to high severity. Physicians typically spend 45 minutes face-to-face with the patient and/or family.

**99344**    **Home visit** for the evaluation and management of a new patient, which requires these 3 key components:

- **A comprehensive history;**
- **A comprehensive examination; and**
- **Medical decision making of moderate complexity.**

Counseling and/or coordination of care with other providers or agencies are provided consistent with the nature of the problem(s) and the patient's and/or family's needs.

Usually, the presenting problem(s) are of high severity. Physicians typically spend 60 minutes face-to-face with the patient and/or family.

**99345**    **Home visit** for the evaluation and management of a new patient, which requires these 3 key components:

- **A comprehensive history;**
- **A comprehensive examination; and**
- **Medical decision making of high complexity.**

Counseling and/or coordination of care with other providers or agencies are provided consistent with the nature of the problem(s) and the patient's and/or family's needs.

Usually, the patient is unstable or has developed a significant new problem requiring immediate physician attention. Physicians typically spend 75 minutes face-to-face with the patient and/or family.

## Established Patient

**99347**    **Home visit** for the evaluation and management of an established patient, which requires at least 2 of these 3 key components:

- **A problem focused interval history;**
- **A problem focused examination;**
- **Straightforward medical decision making.**

Counseling and/or coordination of care with other providers or agencies are provided consistent with the nature of the problem(s) and the patient's and/or family's needs.

Usually, the presenting problem(s) are self limited or minor. Physicians typically spend 15 minutes face-to-face with the patient and/or family.

**99348**    **Home visit** for the evaluation and management of an established patient, which requires at least 2 of these 3 key components:

- **An expanded problem focused interval history;**
- **An expanded problem focused examination;**
- **Medical decision making of low complexity.**

Counseling and/or coordination of care with other providers or agencies are provided consistent with the nature of the problem(s) and the patient's and/or family's needs.

Usually, the presenting problem(s) are of low to moderate severity. Physicians typically spend 25 minutes face-to-face with the patient and/or family.

**99349**    **Home visit** for the evaluation and management of an established patient, which requires at least 2 of these 3 key components:

- **A detailed interval history;**
- **A detailed examination;**
- **Medical decision making of moderate complexity.**

Counseling and/or coordination of care with other providers or agencies are provided consistent with the nature of the problem(s) and the patient's and/or family's needs.

Usually, the presenting problem(s) are moderate to high severity. Physicians typically spend 40 minutes face-to-face with the patient and/or family.

**99350**   **Home visit** for the evaluation and management of an established patient, which requires at least 2 of these 3 key components:

- **A comprehensive interval history;**
- **A comprehensive examination;**
- **Medical decision making of moderate to high complexity.**

Counseling and/or coordination of care with other providers or agencies are provided consistent with the nature of the problem(s) and the patient's and/or family's needs.

Usually, the presenting problem(s) are of moderate to high severity. The patient may be unstable or may have developed a significant new problem requiring immediate physician attention. Physicians typically spend 60 minutes face-to-face with the patient and/or family.

# Prolonged Services

## ►Prolonged Service With Direct Patient Contact◄

►Codes 99354-99357 are used when a physician or other qualified health care professional provides prolonged service involving direct patient contact that is provided beyond the usual service in either the inpatient or outpatient setting. Direct patient contact is face-to-face and includes additional non-face-to-face services on the patient's floor or unit in the hospital or nursing facility during the same session. This service is reported in addition to the designated evaluation and management services at any level and any other services provided at the same session as evaluation and management services. Appropriate codes should be selected for supplies provided or procedures performed in the care of the patient during this period.

Codes 99354-99355 are used to report the total duration of face-to-face time spent by a physician or other qualified health care professional on a given date providing prolonged service in the office or other outpatient setting, even if the time spent by the physician or other qualified health care professional on that date is not continuous. Codes 99356-99357 are used to report the total duration of time spent by a physician or other qualified health care professional at the bedside and on the patient's floor or unit, in the hospital or nursing facility on a given date providing prolonged service to a patient, even if the time spent by the physician or other qualified health care professional on that date is not continuous.◄

Code 99354 or 99356 is used to report the first hour of prolonged service on a given date, depending on the place of service.

►Either code should be used only once per date, even if the time spent by the physician or other qualified health care professional is not continuous on that date. Prolonged service of less than 30 minutes total duration on a given date is not separately reported because the work involved is included in the total work of the evaluation and management codes.◄

Code 99355 or 99357 is used to report each additional 30 minutes beyond the first hour, depending on the place of service. Either code may also be used to report the final 15-30 minutes of prolonged service on a given date. Prolonged service of less than 15 minutes beyond the first hour or less than 15 minutes beyond the final 30 minutes is not reported separately.

The use of the time based add-on codes requires that the primary evaluation and management service have a typical or specified time published in the CPT codebook.

►The following examples illustrate the correct reporting of prolonged physician or other qualified health care professional service with direct patient contact in the office setting:◄

| Total Duration of Prolonged Services | Code(s) |
|---|---|
| less than 30 minutes | Not reported separately |
| 30-74 minutes (30 minutes - 1 hr. 14 min.) | 99354 X 1 |
| 75-104 minutes (1 hr. 15 min. - 1 hr. 44 min.) | 99354 X 1 AND 99355 X 1 |
| 105 or more (1 hr. 45 min. or more) | 99354 X 1 AND 99355 X 2 or more for each additional 30 minutes. |

**+▲ 99354**   Prolonged service in the office or other outpatient setting requiring direct patient contact beyond the usual service; first hour (List separately in addition to code for office or other outpatient **Evaluation and Management** service)

(Use 99354 in conjunction with 99201-99215, 99241-99245, 99324-99337, 99341-99350, 90809, 90815)

**+▲ 99355**   each additional 30 minutes (List separately in addition to code for prolonged service)

(Use 99355 in conjunction with 99354)

**+▲ 99356**   Prolonged service in the inpatient or observation setting, requiring unit/floor time beyond the usual service; first hour (List separately in addition to code for inpatient **Evaluation and Management** service)

►(Use 99356 in conjunction with 99218-99220, 99221-99233, 99251-99255, 99304-99310, 90822, 90829)◄

**+▲ 99357**   each additional 30 minutes (List separately in addition to code for prolonged service)

(Use 99357 in conjunction with 99356)

Evaluation and Management

## ►Prolonged Service Without Direct Patient Contact◄

►Codes 99358 and 99359 are used when a prolonged service is provided that is neither face-to-face time in the office or outpatient setting, nor additional unit/floor time in the hospital or nursing facility setting during the same session of an evaluation and management service and is beyond the usual physician or other qualified health care professional service time.

This service is to be reported in relation to other physician or other qualified health care professional services, including evaluation and management services at any level. This prolonged service may be reported on a different date than the primary service to which it is related. For example, extensive record review may relate to a previous evaluation and management service performed earlier and commences upon receipt of past records. However, it must relate to a service or patient where (face-to-face) patient care has occurred or will occur and relate to ongoing patient management. A typical time for the primary service need not be established within the CPT code set.◄

►Codes 99358 and 99359 are used to report the total duration of non-face-to-face time spent by a physician or other qualified health care professional on a given date providing prolonged service, even if the time spent by the physician or other qualified health care professional on that date is not continuous. Code 99358 is used to report the first hour of prolonged service on a given date regardless of the place of service. It should be used only once per date.◄

Prolonged service of less than 30 minutes total duration on a given date is not separately reported.

Code 99359 is used to report each additional 30 minutes beyond the first hour regardless of the place of service. It may also be used to report the final 15 to 30 minutes of prolonged service on a given date.

Prolonged service of less than 15 minutes beyond the first hour or less than 15 minutes beyond the final 30 minutes is not reported separately.

Do not report 99358-99359 for time spent in medical team conferences, on-line medical evaluations, care plan oversight services, anticoagulation management, or other non-face-to-face services that have more specific codes and no upper time limit in the CPT code set. Codes 99358-99359 may be reported when related to other non-face-to-face services codes that have a published maximum time (eg, telephone services).

▲ **99358**     **Prolonged evaluation and management service**
before and/or after direct patient care; first hour

+▲ **99359**     each additional 30 minutes (List separately in addition to code for prolonged service)

(Use 99359 in conjunction with 99358)

## Physician Standby Services

Code 99360 is used to report physician standby services that are requested by another physician and that involve prolonged physician attendance without direct (face-to-face) patient contact. The physician may not be providing care or services to other patients during this period. This code is not used to report time spent proctoring another physician. It is also not used if the period of standby ends with the performance of a procedure, subject to a surgical package by the physician who was on standby.

Code 99360 is used to report the total duration of time spent by a physician on a given date on standby. Standby service of less than 30 minutes total duration on a given date is not reported separately.

Second and subsequent periods of standby beyond the first 30 minutes may be reported only if a full 30 minutes of standby was provided for each unit of service reported.

**99360**     **Physician standby service,** requiring prolonged physician attendance, each 30 minutes (eg, operative standby, standby for frozen section, for cesarean/high risk delivery, for monitoring EEG)

(For hospital mandated on call services, see 99026, 99027)

(99360 may be reported in addition to 99460, 99465 as appropriate)

(Do not report 99360 in conjunction with 99464)

# Case Management Services

Case management is a process in which a physician or another qualified health care professional is responsible for direct care of a patient and, additionally, for coordinating, managing access to, initiating, and/or supervising other health care services needed by the patient.

## Anticoagulant Management

Anticoagulant services are intended to describe the outpatient management of warfarin therapy, including ordering, review, and interpretation of International Normalized Ratio (INR) testing, communication with patient, and dosage adjustments as appropriate.

When reporting these services, the work of anticoagulant management may not be used as a basis for reporting an evaluation and management (E/M) service or care plan oversight time during the reporting period. Do not report these services with 98966-98969, 99441-99444 when telephone or on-line services address anticoagulation with warfarin management. If a significant, separately identifiable E/M service is performed, report the appropriate E/M service code using modifier 25.

These services are outpatient services only. When anticoagulation therapy is initiated or continued in the inpatient or observation setting, a new period begins after discharge and is reported with 99364. Do not report 99363-99364 with 99217-99239, 99291-99292, 99304-99318, 99471-99480 or other code(s) for physician review, interpretation, and patient management of home INR testing for a patient with mechanical heart valve(s).

Any period less than 60 continuous outpatient days is not reported. If less than the specified minimum number of services per period are performed, do not report the anticoagulant management services (99363-99364).

**99363**    Anticoagulant management for an outpatient taking warfarin, physician review and interpretation of International Normalized Ratio (INR) testing, patient instructions, dosage adjustment (as needed), and ordering of additional tests; initial 90 days of therapy (must include a minimum of 8 INR measurements)

**99364**    each subsequent 90 days of therapy (must include a minimum of 3 INR measurements)

# Medical Team Conferences

Medical team conferences include face-to-face participation by a minimum of three qualified health care professionals from different specialties or disciplines (each of whom provide direct care to the patient), with or without the presence of the patient, family member(s), community agencies, surrogate decision maker(s) (eg, legal guardian), and/or caregiver(s). The participants are actively involved in the development, revision, coordination, and implementation of health care services needed by the patient. Reporting participants shall have performed face-to-face evaluations or treatments of the patient, independent of any team conference, within the previous 60 days.

Physicians may report their time spent in a team conference with the patient and/or family present using evaluation and management (E/M) codes (and time as the key controlling factor for code selection when counseling and/or coordination of care dominates the service). These introductory guidelines do not apply to services reported using E/M codes (see E/M services guidelines). However, the physician must be directly involved with the patient, providing face-to-face services outside of the conference visit with other providers or agencies.

Reporting participants shall document their participation in the team conference as well as their contributed information and subsequent treatment recommendations.

No more than one individual from the same specialty may report 99366-99368 at the same encounter.

Individuals should not report 99366-99368 when their participation in the medical team conference is part of a facility or organizational service contractually provided by the organizational or facility provider.

The team conference starts at the beginning of the review of an individual patient and ends at the conclusion of the review. Time related to record keeping and report generation is not reported. The reporting participant shall be present for all time reported. The time reported is not limited to the time that the participant is communicating to the other team members or patient and/or family. Time reported for medical team conferences may not be used in the determination of time for other services such as care plan oversight (99374-99380), home, domiciliary, or rest home care plan oversight (99339-99340), prolonged services (99354-99359), psychotherapy, or any E/M service. For team conferences where the patient is present for any part of the duration of the conference, nonphysician qualified health care professionals report the team conference face-to-face code 99366.

# Medical Team Conference, Direct (Face-to-Face) Contact With Patient and/or Family

**99366**    **Medical team conference** with interdisciplinary team of health care professionals, face-to-face with patient and/or family, 30 minutes or more, participation by nonphysician qualified health care professional

(Team conference services of less than 30 minutes duration are not reported separately)

(For team conference services by a physician with patient and/or family present, see Evaluation and Management services)

# Medical Team Conference, Without Direct (Face-to-Face) Contact With Patient and/or Family

**99367**    **Medical team conference** with interdisciplinary team of health care professionals, patient and/or family not present, 30 minutes or more; participation by physician

**99368**    participation by nonphysician qualified health care professional

(Team conference services of less than 30 minutes duration are not reported separately)

# Care Plan Oversight Services

Care plan oversight services are reported separately from codes for office/outpatient, hospital, home, nursing facility or domiciliary, or non-face-to-face services. The complexity and approximate physician time of the care plan oversight services provided within a 30-day period determine code selection. Only one physician may report services for a given period of time, to reflect that physician's sole or predominant supervisory role with a particular patient. These codes should not be reported for supervision of patients in nursing facilities or under the care of home health agencies unless they require recurrent supervision of therapy.

The work involved in providing very low intensity or infrequent supervision services is included in the pre- and post-encounter work for home, office/outpatient and nursing facility or domiciliary visit codes.

> (For care plan oversight services of patients in the home, domiciliary, or rest home (eg, assisted living facility) under the individual supervision of a physician, see 99339, 99340)

> (Do not report 99374-99380 for time reported with 98966-98969, 99441-99444)

**99374**    **Physician supervision** of a patient under care of home health agency (patient not present) in home, domiciliary or equivalent environment (eg, Alzheimer's facility) requiring complex and multidisciplinary care modalities involving regular physician development and/or revision of care plans, review of subsequent reports of patient status, review of related laboratory and other studies, communication (including telephone calls) for purposes of assessment or care decisions with health care professional(s), family member(s), surrogate decision maker(s) (eg, legal guardian) and/or key caregiver(s) involved in patient's care, integration of new information into the medical treatment plan and/or adjustment of medical therapy, within a calendar month; 15-29 minutes

**99375**    30 minutes or more

**99377**    **Physician supervision** of a hospice patient (patient not present) requiring complex and multidisciplinary care modalities involving regular physician development and/or revision of care plans, review of subsequent reports of patient status, review of related laboratory and other studies, communication (including telephone calls) for purposes of assessment or care decisions with health care professional(s), family member(s), surrogate decision maker(s) (eg, legal guardian) and/or key caregiver(s) involved in patient's care, integration of new information into the medical treatment plan and/or adjustment of medical therapy, within a calendar month; 15-29 minutes

**99378**    30 minutes or more

**99379**    **Physician supervision** of a nursing facility patient (patient not present) requiring complex and multidisciplinary care modalities involving regular physician development and/or revision of care plans, review of subsequent reports of patient status, review of related laboratory and other studies, communication (including telephone calls) for purposes of assessment or care decisions with health care professional(s), family member(s), surrogate decision maker(s) (eg, legal guardian) and/or key caregiver(s) involved in patient's care, integration of new information into the medical treatment plan and/or adjustment of medical therapy, within a calendar month; 15-29 minutes

**99380**    30 minutes or more

# Preventive Medicine Services

The following codes are used to report the preventive medicine evaluation and management of infants, children, adolescents, and adults.

The extent and focus of the services will largely depend on the age of the patient.

If an abnormality is encountered or a preexisting problem is addressed in the process of performing this preventive medicine evaluation and management service, and if the problem or abnormality is significant enough to require additional work to perform the key components of a problem-oriented E/M service, then the appropriate Office/Outpatient code 99201-99215 should also be reported. Modifier 25 should be added to the Office/Outpatient code to indicate that a significant, separately identifiable evaluation and management service was provided by the same physician on the same day as the preventive medicine service. The appropriate preventive medicine service is additionally reported.

An insignificant or trivial problem/abnormality that is encountered in the process of performing the preventive medicine evaluation and management service and which does not require additional work and the performance of the key components of a problem-oriented E/M service should not be reported.

The "comprehensive" nature of the Preventive Medicine Services codes 99381-99397 reflects an age and gender appropriate history/exam and is **not** synonymous with the "comprehensive" examination required in Evaluation and Management codes 99201-99350.

Codes 99381-99397 include counseling/anticipatory guidance/risk factor reduction interventions which are provided at the time of the initial or periodic comprehensive preventive medicine examination. (Refer to codes 99401-99412 for reporting those counseling/anticipatory guidance/risk factor reduction interventions that are provided at an encounter separate from the preventive medicine examination.)

Vaccine/toxoid products, immunization administrations, ancillary studies involving laboratory, radiology, other procedures, or screening tests (eg, vision, hearing, developmental) identified with a specific CPT code are reported separately. For immunization administration and vaccine risk/benefit counseling, see 90460, 90461, 90471-90474. For vaccine/toxoid products, see 90476-90749.

**Evaluation and Management**

## New Patient

**99381**  **Initial comprehensive preventive medicine** evaluation and management of an individual including an age and gender appropriate history, examination, counseling/anticipatory guidance/risk factor reduction interventions, and the ordering of laboratory/diagnostic procedures, new patient; infant (age younger than 1 year)

**99382**  early childhood (age 1 through 4 years)

**99383**  late childhood (age 5 through 11 years)

**99384**  adolescent (age 12 through 17 years)

**99385**  18-39 years

**99386**  40-64 years

**99387**  65 years and older

## Established Patient

**99391**  **Periodic comprehensive preventive medicine** reevaluation and management of an individual including an age and gender appropriate history, examination, counseling/anticipatory guidance/risk factor reduction interventions, and the ordering of laboratory/diagnostic procedures, established patient; infant (age younger than 1 year)

**99392**  early childhood (age 1 through 4 years)

**99393**  late childhood (age 5 through 11 years)

**99394**  adolescent (age 12 through 17 years)

**99395**  18-39 years

**99396**  40-64 years

**99397**  65 years and older

# Counseling Risk Factor Reduction and Behavior Change Intervention

## New or Established Patient

These codes are used to report services provided face-to-face by a physician or other qualified health care professional for the purpose of promoting health and preventing illness or injury. They are distinct from evaluation and management (E/M) services that may be reported separately when performed. Risk factor reduction services are used for persons without a specific illness for which the counseling might otherwise be used as part of treatment.

Preventive medicine counseling and risk factor reduction interventions will vary with age and should address such issues as family problems, diet and exercise, substance use, sexual practices, injury prevention, dental health, and diagnostic and laboratory test results available at the time of the encounter.

Behavior change interventions are for persons who have a behavior that is often considered an illness itself, such as tobacco use and addiction, substance abuse/misuse, or obesity. Behavior change services may be reported when performed as part of the treatment of condition(s) related to or potentially exacerbated by the behavior or when performed to change the harmful behavior that has not yet resulted in illness. Any E/M services reported on the same day must be distinct, and time spent providing these services may not be used as a basis for the E/M code selection. Behavior change services involve specific validated interventions of assessing readiness for change and barriers to change, advising a change in behavior, assisting by providing specific suggested actions and motivational counseling, and arranging for services and follow-up.

For counseling groups of patients with symptoms or established illness, use 99078.

Health and Behavior Assessment/Intervention services (96150-96155) should not be reported on the same day.

### Preventive Medicine, Individual Counseling

**99401**  **Preventive medicine counseling** and/or risk factor reduction intervention(s) provided to an individual (separate procedure); approximately 15 minutes

**99402**  approximately 30 minutes

**99403**  approximately 45 minutes

**99404**  approximately 60 minutes

### Behavior Change Interventions, Individual

**99406**  Smoking and tobacco use cessation counseling visit; intermediate, greater than 3 minutes up to 10 minutes

**99407**  intensive, greater than 10 minutes

(Do not report 99407 in conjunction with 99406)

**99408**  Alcohol and/or substance (other than tobacco) abuse structured screening (eg, AUDIT, DAST), and brief intervention (SBI) services; 15 to 30 minutes

(Do not report services of less than 15 minutes with 99408)

**99409**  greater than 30 minutes

(Do not report 99409 in conjunction with 99408)

(Do not report 99408, 99409 in conjunction with 99420)

(Use 99408, 99409 only for initial screening and brief intervention)

### Preventive Medicine, Group Counseling

**99411**    **Preventive medicine counseling** and/or risk factor reduction intervention(s) provided to individuals in a group setting (separate procedure); approximately 30 minutes

**99412**        approximately 60 minutes

## Other Preventive Medicine Services

**99420**    **Administration and interpretation** of health risk assessment instrument (eg, health hazard appraisal)

**99429**    **Unlisted preventive** medicine service

(99431 has been deleted. To report, use 99460)

(99432 has been deleted. To report, use 99461)

(99433 has been deleted. To report, use 99462)

(99435 has been deleted. To report, use 99463)

(99436 has been deleted. To report, use 99464)

(99440 has been deleted. To report, use 99465)

# Non-Face-to-Face Physician Services

## Telephone Services

Telephone services are non-face-to-face evaluation and management (E/M) services provided by a physician to a patient using the telephone. These codes are used to report episodes of care by the physician initiated by an established patient or guardian of an established patient. If the telephone service ends with a decision to see the patient within 24 hours or next available urgent visit appointment, the code is not reported; rather the encounter is considered part of the preservice work of the subsequent E/M service, procedure, and visit. Likewise if the telephone call refers to an E/M service performed and reported by the physician within the previous seven days (either physician requested or unsolicited patient follow-up) or within the postoperative period of the previously completed procedure, then the service(s) are considered part of that previous E/M service or procedure. (Do not report 99441-99443 if reporting 99441-99444 performed in the previous seven days.)

(For telephone services provided by a qualified nonphysician health care professional, see 98966-98968)

**99441**    Telephone evaluation and management service provided by a physician to an established patient, parent, or guardian not originating from a related E/M service provided within the previous 7 days nor leading to an E/M service or procedure within the next 24 hours or soonest available appointment; 5-10 minutes of medical discussion

**99442**      11-20 minutes of medical discussion

**99443**      21-30 minutes of medical discussion

(Do not report 99441-99443 when using 99339-99340, 99374-99380 for the same call[s])

(Do not report 99441-99443 for anticoagulation management when reporting 99363-99364)

## On-Line Medical Evaluation

An on-line electronic medical evaluation is a non-face-to-face evaluation and management (E/M) service by a physician to a patient using Internet resources in response to a patient's on-line inquiry. Reportable services involve the physician's personal timely response to the patient's inquiry and must involve permanent storage (electronic or hard copy) of the encounter. This service is reported only once for the same episode of care during a seven-day period, although multiple physicians could report their exchange with the same patient. If the on-line medical evaluation refers to an E/M service previously performed and reported by the physician within the previous seven days (either physician requested or unsolicited patient follow-up) or within the postoperative period of the previously completed procedure, then the service(s) are considered covered by the previous E/M service or procedure. A reportable service encompasses the sum of communication (eg, related telephone calls, prescription provision, laboratory orders) pertaining to the on-line patient encounter.

(For an on-line medical evaluation provided by a qualified nonphysician health care professional, use 98969)

**99444**    Online evaluation and management service provided by a physician to an established patient, guardian, or health care provider not originating from a related E/M service provided within the previous 7 days, using the Internet or similar electronic communications network

(Do not report 99444 when using 99339-99340, 99374-99380 for the same communication[s])

(Do not report 99444 for anticoagulation management when reporting 99363, 99364)

# Special Evaluation and Management Services

The following codes are used to report evaluations performed to establish baseline information prior to life or disability insurance certificates being issued. This service is performed in the office or other setting, and applies to both new and established patients. When using these codes, no active management of the problem(s) is undertaken during the encounter.

**Evaluation and Management** (sidebar)

If other evaluation and management services and/or procedures are performed on the same date, the appropriate E/M or procedure code(s) should be reported in addition to these codes.

## Basic Life and/or Disability Evaluation Services

**99450**    **Basic life** and/or disability examination that includes:

- **Measurement of height, weight, and blood pressure;**
- **Completion of a medical history following a life insurance pro forma;**
- **Collection of blood sample and/or urinalysis complying with "chain of custody" protocols; and**
- **Completion of necessary documentation/ certificates.**

## Work Related or Medical Disability Evaluation Services

**99455**    **Work related** or medical disability examination by the treating physician that includes:

- **Completion of a medical history commensurate with the patient's condition;**
- **Performance of an examination commensurate with the patient's condition;**
- **Formulation of a diagnosis, assessment of capabilities and stability, and calculation of impairment;**
- **Development of future medical treatment plan; and**
- **Completion of necessary documentation/ certificates and report.**

**99456**    **Work related** or medical disability examination by other than the treating physician that includes:

- **Completion of a medical history commensurate with the patient's condition;**
- **Performance of an examination commensurate with the patient's condition;**
- **Formulation of a diagnosis, assessment of capabilities and stability, and calculation of impairment;**
- **Development of future medical treatment plan; and**
- **Completion of necessary documentation/ certificates and report.**

(Do not report 99455, 99456 in conjunction with 99080 for the completion of Workman's Compensation forms)

# Newborn Care Services

The following codes are used to report the services provided to newborns (birth through the first 28 days) in several different settings. Use of the normal newborn codes is limited to the initial care of the newborn in the first days after birth prior to home discharge.

Evaluation and Management (E/M) services for the newborn include maternal and/or fetal and newborn history, newborn physical examination(s), ordering of diagnostic tests and treatments, meetings with the family, and documentation in the medical record.

When delivery room attendance services (99464) or delivery room resuscitation services (99465) are required, report these in addition to normal newborn services Evaluation and Management codes.

For E/M services provided to newborns who are other than normal, see codes for hospital inpatient services (99221-99233) and neonatal intensive and critical care services (99466-99469, 99477-99480). When normal newborn services are provided by the same physician on the same date that the newborn later becomes ill and receives additional intensive or critical care services, report the appropriate E/M code with modifier 25 for these services in addition to the normal newborn code.

Procedures (eg, 54150, newborn circumcision) are not included with the normal newborn codes, and when performed, should be reported in addition to the newborn services.

When newborns are seen in follow-up after the date of discharge in the office or outpatient setting, see 99201-99215, 99381, 99391 as appropriate.

**99460**    Initial hospital or birthing center care, per day, for evaluation and management of normal newborn infant

**99461**    Initial care, per day, for evaluation and management of normal newborn infant seen in other than hospital or birthing center

**99462**    Subsequent hospital care, per day, for evaluation and management of normal newborn

**99463**    Initial hospital or birthing center care, per day, for evaluation and management of normal newborn infant admitted and discharged on the same date

(For newborn hospital discharge services provided on a date subsequent to the admission date, see 99238, 99239)

## Delivery/Birthing Room Attendance and Resuscitation Services

**99464**    Attendance at delivery (when requested by the delivering physician) and initial stabilization of newborn

(99464 may be reported in conjunction with 99460, 99468, 99477)

(Do not report 99464 in conjunction with 99465)

**99465**   Delivery/birthing room resuscitation, provision of positive pressure ventilation and/or chest compressions in the presence of acute inadequate ventilation and/or cardiac output

(99465 may be reported in conjunction with 99460, 99468, 99477)

(Do not report 99465 in conjunction with 99464)

(Procedures that are performed as a necessary part of the resuscitation [eg, intubation, vascular lines] are reported separately in addition to 99465. In order to report these procedures, they must be performed as a necessary component of the resuscitation and not as a convenience before admission to the neonatal intensive care unit)

# Inpatient Neonatal Intensive Care Services and Pediatric and Neonatal Critical Care Services

## Pediatric Critical Care Patient Transport

The following codes (99466, 99467) are used to report the physical attendance and direct face-to-face care by a physician during the interfacility transport of a critically ill or critically injured pediatric patient 24 months of age or younger. For the purpose of reporting codes 99466 and 99467, face-to-face care begins when the physician assumes primary responsibility of the pediatric patient at the referring hospital/facility, and ends when the receiving hospital/facility accepts responsibility for the pediatric patient's care. Only the time the physician spends in direct face-to-face contact with the patient during the transport should be reported. Pediatric patient transport services involving less than 30 minutes of face-to-face physician care should not be reported using codes 99466, 99467. Procedure(s) or service(s) performed by other members of the transporting team may not be reported by the supervising physician.

For the definition of the critically injured pediatric patient, see the **Neonatal and Pediatric Critical Care Services** section.

The direction of emergency care to transporting staff by a physician located in a hospital or other facility by two-way communication is not considered direct face-to-face care and should not be reported with 99466, 99467. Physician-directed emergency care through outside voice communication to transporting staff personnel is reported with 99288.

Emergency department services (99281-99285), initial hospital care (99221-99223), critical care (99291, 99292), initial date neonatal intensive (99477) or critical care (99468) are only reported after the patient has been

admitted to the emergency department, the inpatient floor, or the critical care unit of the receiving facility. If inpatient critical care services are reported in the referring facility prior to transfer to the receiving hospital, use the critical care codes (99291, 99292).

The following services are included when performed during the pediatric patient transport by the physician providing critical care and may not be reported separately: routine monitoring evaluations (eg, heart rate, respiratory rate, blood pressure, and pulse oximetry), the interpretation of cardiac output measurements (93562), chest X-rays (71010, 71015, 71020), pulse oximetry (94760, 94761, 94762), blood gases and information data stored in computers (eg, ECGs, blood pressures, hematologic data) (99090), gastric intubation (43752, 43753), temporary transcutaneous pacing (92953), ventilatory management (94002, 94003, 94660, 94662) and vascular access procedures (36000, 36400, 36405, 36406, 36415, 36591, 36600). Any services performed which are not listed above should be reported separately.

Code 99466 is used to report the first 30 to 74 minutes of direct face-to-face time with the transport pediatric patient and should be reported only once on a given date. Code 99467 is used to report each additional 30 minutes provided on a given date. Face-to-face services of less than 30 minutes should not be reported with these codes.

►(For total body cooling of neonates, see 0260T, 0261T)◄

**99466**   **Critical care** services delivered by a physician, face-to-face, during an interfacility transport of critically ill or critically injured pediatric patient, 24 months of age or younger; first 30-74 minutes of hands-on care during transport

**+ 99467**        each additional 30 minutes (List separately in addition to code for primary service)

(Use 99467 in conjunction with 99466)

(Critical care of less than 30 minutes total duration should be reported with the appropriate E/M code)

## Inpatient Neonatal and Pediatric Critical Care

The same definitions for critical care services apply for the adult, child, and neonate.

Codes 99468, 99469 are used to report services provided by a physician directing the inpatient care of a critically ill neonate or infant 28 days of age or younger. They represent care starting with the date of admission (99468) and subsequent day(s) (99469) that the neonate remains critical. These codes may be reported only by a single physician and only once per day, per patient.

The initial day neonatal critical care code (99468) can be used in addition to 99464 or 99465 as appropriate, when the physician is present for the delivery (99464) or resuscitation (99465) is required. Other procedures performed as a necessary part of the resuscitation (eg, endotracheal intubation [31500]) are also reported separately when performed as part of the pre-admission delivery room care. In order to report these procedures separately, they must be performed as a necessary component of the resuscitation and not simply as a convenience before admission to the neonatal intensive care unit.

Codes 99471-99476 are used to report services provided by a physician directing the inpatient care of a critically ill infant or young child from 29 days of postnatal age through five years of age. They represent care starting with the date of admission (99471, 99475) and subsequent day(s) (99472, 99476) the infant or child remains critical. These codes may be reported only by a single physician and only once per day, per patient in a given setting. Service for the critically ill or critically injured child older than five years of age would be reported with critical care codes (99291, 99292).

▶The pediatric and neonatal critical care codes include those procedures listed for the critical care codes (99291, 99292). In addition, the following procedures are also included (and are not separately reported by professionals, but may be reported by facilities) in the pediatric and neonatal critical care service codes (99468-99472, 99475, 99476) and the intensive care services codes (99477-99480):◀

▶Any services performed that are not included in these listings may be reported separately. Facilities may report the included services separately.◀

Invasive or non-invasive electronic monitoring of vital signs

Vascular access procedures

    Peripheral vessel catheterization (36000)

    Other arterial catheters (36140, 36620)

    Umbilical venous catheters (36510)

    Central vessel catheterization (36555)

    Vascular access procedures (36400, 36405, 36406)

    Vascular punctures (36420, 36600)

    Umbilical arterial catheters (36660)

Airway and ventilation management

    Endotracheal intubation (31500)

    Ventilatory management (94002-94004)

    Bedside pulmonary function testing (94375)

    Surfactant administration (94610)

    Continuous positive airway pressure (CPAP) (94660)

Monitoring or interpretation of blood gases or oxygen saturation (94760-94762)

▶Car Seat Evaluation (94780-94781)◀

Transfusion of blood components (36430, 36440)

Oral or nasogastric tube placement (43752)

Suprapubic bladder aspiration (51100)

Bladder catheterization (51701, 51702)

Lumbar puncture (62270)

Any services performed which are not listed above may be reported separately.

When a neonate or infant is not critically ill but requires intensive observation, frequent interventions, and other intensive care services, the Continuing Intensive Care Services codes (99477-99480) should be used to report these services.

To report critical care services provided in the outpatient setting (eg, emergency department or office) for neonates and pediatric patients of any age, see the Critical Care codes 99291, 99292. If the same physician provides critical care services for a neonatal or pediatric patient in both the outpatient and inpatient settings on the same day, report only the appropriate Neonatal or Pediatric Critical Care codes 99468-99476 for all critical care services provided on that day. Critical care services provided by a second physician of a different specialty not reporting a per-day neonatal or pediatric critical care code can be reported with 99291, 99292.

When critical care services are provided to neonates or pediatric patients less than five years of age at two separate institutions by a physician from a different group on the same date of service, the physician from the referring institution should report their critical care services with the critical care codes (99291, 99292) and the receiving institution should report the appropriate global admission code (99468, 99471, 99475, 99476) for the same date of service.

Critical care services to a pediatric patient six years of age or older are reported with the critical care codes 99291, 99292.

Critical care services to a neonate or pediatric patient provided in an outpatient environment are reported with the critical care codes 99291, 99292.

Critical care services provided by a second physician of a different specialty not reporting a 24-hour global code can be reported with the critical care codes 99291, 99292.

▶When the critically ill neonate or pediatric patient improves and is transferred to a lower level of care, the transferring physician does not report a per day critical care service. Subsequent Hospital Care (99231-99233) or Critical Care Services (99291-99292) is reported, as appropriate based upon the condition of the neonate or child. The receiving physician reports a Subsequent Intensive Care (99478-99480) or Subsequent Hospital Care (99231-99233), as appropriate based upon the condition of the neonate or child.◀

No physician may report remote real-time videoconferenced critical care (0188T, 0189T) when neonatal or pediatric intensive or critical care services (99468-99476) are reported.

**99468**    **Initial inpatient neonatal critical care,** per day, for the evaluation and management of a critically ill neonate, 28 days of age or younger

**99469**    **Subsequent inpatient neonatal critical care,** per day, for the evaluation and management of a critically ill neonate, 28 days of age or younger

**99471**    **Initial inpatient pediatric critical care,** per day, for the evaluation and management of a critically ill infant or young child, 29 days through 24 months of age

**99472**    **Subsequent inpatient pediatric critical care,** per day, for the evaluation and management of a critically ill infant or young child, 29 days through 24 months of age

**99475**    **Initial inpatient pediatric critical care,** per day, for the evaluation and  management of a critically ill infant or young child, 2 through 5 years of age

**99476**    **Subsequent inpatient pediatric critical care,** per day, for the evaluation and management of a critically ill infant or young child, 2 through 5 years of age

## Initial and Continuing Intensive Care Services

Code 99477 represents the initial day of inpatient care for the child who is not critically ill but requires intensive observation, frequent interventions, and other intensive care services. Codes 99478-99480 are used to report subsequent day services provided by a physician directing the continuing intensive care of the low birth weight (LBW 1500-2500 grams) present body weight infant, very low birth weight (VLBW less than 1500 grams) present body weight infant, or normal (2501-5000 grams) present body weight newborn who does not meet the definition of critically ill but continues to require intensive observation, frequent interventions, and other intensive care services. These services are for infants and neonates who are not critically ill but continue to require intensive cardiac and respiratory monitoring, continuous and/or frequent vital sign monitoring, heat maintenance, enteral and/or parenteral nutritional adjustments, laboratory and oxygen monitoring, and constant observation by the health care team under direct physician supervision. Codes 99477-99480 may be reported by only one physician and only once per day, per patient. These codes include the same procedures that are outlined in the **Pediatric Critical Care Services** section and these services should not be separately reported.

►When the neonate or infant improves after the initial day and is transferred to a lower level of care, the transferring physician does not report a per day intensive care service, Subsequent Hospital Care (99231-99233) is reported. When the neonate or infant becomes critically ill on a day when Initial or Subsequent Intensive Care Services have been performed and is transferred to a critical care level of care performed by a different physician, the transferring physician reports either the Critical Care Services performed (99291-99292) or the Intensive Care Service performed, but not both. The

receiving physician reports Subsequent Inpatient Neonatal or Pediatric Critical Care (99469, 99472).◄

For the subsequent care of the sick neonate younger than 28 days of age but more than 5000 grams who does not require intensive or critical care services, use codes 99231-99233.

**99477**    **Initial hospital care,** per day, for the evaluation and management of the neonate, 28 days of age or younger, who requires intensive observation, frequent interventions, and other intensive care services

(For the initiation of inpatient care of the normal newborn, use 99460)

(For the initiation of care of the critically ill neonate, use 99468)

(For initiation of inpatient hospital care of the ill neonate not requiring intensive observation, frequent interventions, and other intensive care services, see 99221-99223)

**99478**    **Subsequent intensive care,** per day, for the evaluation and management of the recovering very low birth weight infant (present body weight less than 1500 grams)

**99479**    **Subsequent intensive care,** per day, for the evaluation and management of the recovering low birth weight infant (present body weight of 1500-2500 grams)

**99480**    **Subsequent intensive care,** per day, for the evaluation and management of the recovering infant (present body weight of 2501-5000 grams)

## Other Evaluation and Management Services

**99499**    **Unlisted evaluation and management** service

---

# Notes

# Anesthesia Guidelines

Services involving administration of anesthesia are reported by the use of the anesthesia five-digit procedure code (00100-01999) plus modifier codes (defined under "Anesthesia Modifiers" later in these Guidelines).

The reporting of anesthesia services is appropriate by or under the responsible supervision of a physician. These services may include but are not limited to general, regional, supplementation of local anesthesia, or other supportive services in order to afford the patient the anesthesia care deemed optimal by the anesthesiologist during any procedure. These services include the usual preoperative and postoperative visits, the anesthesia care during the procedure, the administration of fluids and/or blood and the usual monitoring services (eg, ECG, temperature, blood pressure, oximetry, capnography, and mass spectrometry). Unusual forms of monitoring (eg, intra-arterial, central venous, and Swan-Ganz) are not included.

Items used by all physicians in reporting their services are presented in the **Introduction.** Some of the commonalities are repeated in this section for the convenience of those physicians referring to this section on **Anesthesia.** Other definitions and items unique to anesthesia are also listed.

To report moderate (conscious) sedation provided by a physician also performing the service for which conscious sedation is being provided, see codes 99143-99145.

For the procedures listed in Appendix G, when a second physician other than the health care professional performing the diagnostic or therapeutic services provides moderate (conscious) sedation in the facility setting (eg, hospital, outpatient hospital/ambulatory surgery center, skilled nursing facility), the second physician reports the associated moderate sedation procedure/service 99148-99150; when these services are performed by the second physician in the nonfacility setting (eg, physician office, freestanding imaging center), codes 99148-99150 would not be reported. Moderate sedation does not include minimal sedation (anxiolysis), deep sedation, or monitored anesthesia care (00100-01999).

To report regional or general anesthesia provided by a physician also performing the services for which the anesthesia is being provided, see modifier 47 in Appendix A.

## Time Reporting

Time for anesthesia procedures may be reported as is customary in the local area. Anesthesia time begins when the anesthesiologist begins to prepare the patient for the induction of anesthesia in the operating room (or in an equivalent area) and ends when the anesthesiologist is no longer in personal attendance, that is, when the patient may be safely placed under postoperative supervision.

## Physician's Services

Physician's services rendered in the office, home, or hospital; consultation; and other medical services are listed in the section titled **Evaluation and Management Services** (99201-99499 series) found on page 1. "Special Services and Reporting" (99000-99091 series) are listed in the **Medicine** section.

## Materials Supplied by Physician

Supplies and materials provided by the physician (eg, sterile trays, drugs) over and above those usually included with the office visit or other services rendered may be listed separately. Drugs, tray supplies, and materials provided should be listed and identified with 99070 or the appropriate supply code.

## Separate or Multiple Procedures

When multiple surgical procedures are performed during a single anesthetic administration, the anesthesia code representing the most complex procedure is reported. The time reported is the combined total for all procedures.

## Special Report

A service that is rarely provided, unusual, variable, or new may require a special report. Pertinent information should include an adequate definition or description of the nature, extent, and need for the procedure and the time, effort, and equipment necessary to provide the service.

# Anesthesia Modifiers

All anesthesia services are reported by use of the anesthesia five-digit procedure code (00100-01999) plus the addition of a physical status modifier. The use of other optional modifiers may be appropriate.

## Physical Status Modifiers

Physical Status modifiers are represented by the initial letter 'P' followed by a single digit from 1 to 6 as defined in the following list:

**P1:** A normal healthy patient

**P2:** A patient with mild systemic disease

**P3:** A patient with severe systemic disease

**P4:** A patient with severe systemic disease that is a constant threat to life

**P5:** A moribund patient who is not expected to survive without the operation

**P6:** A declared brain-dead patient whose organs are being removed for donor purposes

These six levels are consistent with the American Society of Anesthesiologists (ASA) ranking of patient physical status. Physical status is included in the CPT codebook to distinguish among various levels of complexity of the anesthesia service provided.

Example: 00100-P1

# Qualifying Circumstances

More than one qualifying circumstance may be selected.

Many anesthesia services are provided under particularly difficult circumstances, depending on factors such as extraordinary condition of patient, notable operative conditions, and/or unusual risk factors. This section includes a list of important qualifying circumstances that significantly affect the character of the anesthesia service provided. These procedures would not be reported alone but would be reported as additional procedure numbers qualifying an anesthesia procedure or service.

**+ 99100**  Anesthesia for patient of extreme age, younger than 1 year and older than 70 (List separately in addition to code for primary anesthesia procedure)

(For procedure performed on infants younger than 1 year of age at time of surgery, see 00326, 00561, 00834, 00836)

**+ 99116**  Anesthesia complicated by utilization of total body hypothermia (List separately in addition to code for primary anesthesia procedure)

**+ 99135**  Anesthesia complicated by utilization of controlled hypotension (List separately in addition to code for primary anesthesia procedure)

**+ 99140**  Anesthesia complicated by emergency conditions (specify) (List separately in addition to code for primary anesthesia procedure)

(An emergency is defined as existing when delay in treatment of the patient would lead to a significant increase in the threat to life or body part.)

# Anesthesia

## Head

**00100**    Anesthesia for procedures on salivary glands, including biopsy

**00102**    Anesthesia for procedures involving plastic repair of cleft lip

**00103**    Anesthesia for reconstructive procedures of eyelid (eg, blepharoplasty, ptosis surgery)

**00104**    Anesthesia for electroconvulsive therapy

**00120**    Anesthesia for procedures on external, middle, and inner ear including biopsy; not otherwise specified

**00124**        otoscopy

**00126**        tympanotomy

**00140**    Anesthesia for procedures on eye; not otherwise specified

**00142**        lens surgery

**00144**        corneal transplant

**00145**        vitreoretinal surgery

**00147**        iridectomy

**00148**        ophthalmoscopy

**00160**    Anesthesia for procedures on nose and accessory sinuses; not otherwise specified

**00162**        radical surgery

**00164**        biopsy, soft tissue

**00170**    Anesthesia for intraoral procedures, including biopsy; not otherwise specified

**00172**        repair of cleft palate

**00174**        excision of retropharyngeal tumor

**00176**        radical surgery

**00190**    Anesthesia for procedures on facial bones or skull; not otherwise specified

**00192**        radical surgery (including prognathism)

**00210**    Anesthesia for intracranial procedures; not otherwise specified

**00211**        craniotomy or craniectomy for evacuation of hematoma

**00212**        subdural taps

**00214**        burr holes, including ventriculography

**00215**        cranioplasty or elevation of depressed skull fracture, extradural (simple or compound)

**00216**        vascular procedures

**00218**        procedures in sitting position

**00220**        cerebrospinal fluid shunting procedures

**00222**        electrocoagulation of intracranial nerve

## Neck

**00300**    Anesthesia for all procedures on the integumentary system, muscles and nerves of head, neck, and posterior trunk, not otherwise specified

**00320**    Anesthesia for all procedures on esophagus, thyroid, larynx, trachea and lymphatic system of neck; not otherwise specified, age 1 year or older

**00322**        needle biopsy of thyroid

         (For procedures on cervical spine and cord, see 00600, 00604, 00670)

**00326**    Anesthesia for all procedures on the larynx and trachea in children younger than 1 year of age

         (Do not report 00326 in conjunction with 99100)

**00350**    Anesthesia for procedures on major vessels of neck; not otherwise specified

**00352**        simple ligation

         (For arteriography, use 01916)

## Thorax (Chest Wall and Shoulder Girdle)

**00400**    Anesthesia for procedures on the integumentary system on the extremities, anterior trunk and perineum; not otherwise specified

**00402**        reconstructive procedures on breast (eg, reduction or augmentation mammoplasty, muscle flaps)

**00404**        radical or modified radical procedures on breast

**00406**        radical or modified radical procedures on breast with internal mammary node dissection

**00410**        electrical conversion of arrhythmias

**00450**    Anesthesia for procedures on clavicle and scapula; not otherwise specified

**00452**        radical surgery

**00454**        biopsy of clavicle

**00470**    Anesthesia for partial rib resection; not otherwise specified

**00472**        thoracoplasty (any type)

**00474**        radical procedures (eg, pectus excavatum)

**Anesthesia**

# Intrathoracic

00500    Anesthesia for all procedures on esophagus

00520    Anesthesia for closed chest procedures; (including bronchoscopy) not otherwise specified

00522        needle biopsy of pleura

00524        pneumocentesis

00528        mediastinoscopy and diagnostic thoracoscopy not utilizing 1 lung ventilation

(For tracheobronchial reconstruction, use 00539)

00529        mediastinoscopy and diagnostic thoracoscopy utilizing 1 lung ventilation

00530    Anesthesia for permanent transvenous pacemaker insertion

00532    Anesthesia for access to central venous circulation

00534    Anesthesia for transvenous insertion or replacement of pacing cardioverter-defibrillator

(For transthoracic approach, use 00560)

00537    Anesthesia for cardiac electrophysiologic procedures including radiofrequency ablation

00539    Anesthesia for tracheobronchial reconstruction

00540    Anesthesia for thoracotomy procedures involving lungs, pleura, diaphragm, and mediastinum (including surgical thoracoscopy); not otherwise specified

00541        utilizing 1 lung ventilation

(For thoracic spine and cord anesthesia procedures via an anterior transthoracic approach, see 00625-00626)

00542        decortication

00546        pulmonary resection with thoracoplasty

00548        intrathoracic procedures on the trachea and bronchi

00550    Anesthesia for sternal debridement

00560    Anesthesia for procedures on heart, pericardial sac, and great vessels of chest; without pump oxygenator

00561        with pump oxygenator, younger than 1 year of age

(Do not report 00561 in conjunction with 99100, 99116, and 99135)

00562        with pump oxygenator, age 1 year or older, for all non-coronary bypass procedures (eg, valve procedures) or for re-operation for coronary bypass more than 1 month after original operation

00563        with pump oxygenator with hypothermic circulatory arrest

00566    Anesthesia for direct coronary artery bypass grafting; without pump oxygenator

00567        with pump oxygenator

00580    Anesthesia for heart transplant or heart/lung transplant

# Spine and Spinal Cord

00600    Anesthesia for procedures on cervical spine and cord; not otherwise specified

(For percutaneous image-guided spine and spinal cord anesthesia procedures, see 01935, 01936)

00604        procedures with patient in the sitting position

00620    Anesthesia for procedures on thoracic spine and cord; not otherwise specified

00622        thoracolumbar sympathectomy

00625    Anesthesia for procedures on the thoracic spine and cord, via an anterior transthoracic approach; not utilizing 1 lung ventilation

00626        utilizing 1 lung ventilation

(For anesthesia for thoracotomy procedures other than spinal, see 00540-00541)

00630    Anesthesia for procedures in lumbar region; not otherwise specified

00632        lumbar sympathectomy

00634        chemonucleolysis

00635        diagnostic or therapeutic lumbar puncture

00640    Anesthesia for manipulation of the spine or for closed procedures on the cervical, thoracic or lumbar spine

00670    Anesthesia for extensive spine and spinal cord procedures (eg, spinal instrumentation or vascular procedures)

# Upper Abdomen

00700    Anesthesia for procedures on upper anterior abdominal wall; not otherwise specified

00702        percutaneous liver biopsy

00730    Anesthesia for procedures on upper posterior abdominal wall

00740    Anesthesia for upper gastrointestinal endoscopic procedures, endoscope introduced proximal to duodenum

00750    Anesthesia for hernia repairs in upper abdomen; not otherwise specified

00752        lumbar and ventral (incisional) hernias and/or wound dehiscence

00754        omphalocele

00756        transabdominal repair of diaphragmatic hernia

00770    Anesthesia for all procedures on major abdominal blood vessels

00790    Anesthesia for intraperitoneal procedures in upper abdomen including laparoscopy; not otherwise specified

00792        partial hepatectomy or management of liver hemorrhage (excluding liver biopsy)

| | |
|---|---|
| 00794 | pancreatectomy, partial or total (eg, Whipple procedure) |
| 00796 | liver transplant (recipient) |
| | (For harvesting of liver, use 01990) |
| 00797 | gastric restrictive procedure for morbid obesity |

## Lower Abdomen

| | |
|---|---|
| 00800 | Anesthesia for procedures on lower anterior abdominal wall; not otherwise specified |
| 00802 | panniculectomy |
| 00810 | Anesthesia for lower intestinal endoscopic procedures, endoscope introduced distal to duodenum |
| 00820 | Anesthesia for procedures on lower posterior abdominal wall |
| 00830 | Anesthesia for hernia repairs in lower abdomen; not otherwise specified |
| 00832 | ventral and incisional hernias |
| | (For hernia repairs in the infant 1 year of age or younger, see 00834, 00836) |
| 00834 | Anesthesia for hernia repairs in the lower abdomen not otherwise specified, younger than 1 year of age |
| | (Do not report 00834 in conjunction with 99100) |
| 00836 | Anesthesia for hernia repairs in the lower abdomen not otherwise specified, infants younger than 37 weeks gestational age at birth and younger than 50 weeks gestational age at time of surgery |
| | (Do not report 00836 in conjunction with 99100) |
| 00840 | Anesthesia for intraperitoneal procedures in lower abdomen including laparoscopy; not otherwise specified |
| 00842 | amniocentesis |
| 00844 | abdominoperineal resection |
| 00846 | radical hysterectomy |
| 00848 | pelvic exenteration |
| 00851 | tubal ligation/transection |
| 00860 | Anesthesia for extraperitoneal procedures in lower abdomen, including urinary tract; not otherwise specified |
| 00862 | renal procedures, including upper one-third of ureter, or donor nephrectomy |
| 00864 | total cystectomy |
| 00865 | radical prostatectomy (suprapubic, retropubic) |
| 00866 | adrenalectomy |
| 00868 | renal transplant (recipient) |
| | (For donor nephrectomy, use 00862) |
| | (For harvesting kidney from brain-dead patient, use 01990) |

| | |
|---|---|
| 00870 | cystolithotomy |
| 00872 | Anesthesia for lithotripsy, extracorporeal shock wave; with water bath |
| 00873 | without water bath |
| 00880 | Anesthesia for procedures on major lower abdominal vessels; not otherwise specified |
| 00882 | inferior vena cava ligation |

## Perineum

| | |
|---|---|
| | (For perineal procedures on integumentary system, muscles and nerves, see 00300, 00400) |
| 00902 | Anesthesia for; anorectal procedure |
| 00904 | radical perineal procedure |
| 00906 | vulvectomy |
| 00908 | perineal prostatectomy |
| 00910 | Anesthesia for transurethral procedures (including urethrocystoscopy); not otherwise specified |
| 00912 | transurethral resection of bladder tumor(s) |
| 00914 | transurethral resection of prostate |
| 00916 | post-transurethral resection bleeding |
| 00918 | with fragmentation, manipulation and/or removal of ureteral calculus |
| 00920 | Anesthesia for procedures on male genitalia (including open urethral procedures); not otherwise specified |
| 00921 | vasectomy, unilateral or bilateral |
| 00922 | seminal vesicles |
| 00924 | undescended testis, unilateral or bilateral |
| 00926 | radical orchiectomy, inguinal |
| 00928 | radical orchiectomy, abdominal |
| 00930 | orchiopexy, unilateral or bilateral |
| 00932 | complete amputation of penis |
| 00934 | radical amputation of penis with bilateral inguinal lymphadenectomy |
| 00936 | radical amputation of penis with bilateral inguinal and iliac lymphadenectomy |
| 00938 | insertion of penile prosthesis (perineal approach) |
| 00940 | Anesthesia for vaginal procedures (including biopsy of labia, vagina, cervix or endometrium); not otherwise specified |
| 00942 | colpotomy, vaginectomy, colporrhaphy, and open urethral procedures |
| 00944 | vaginal hysterectomy |
| 00948 | cervical cerclage |
| 00950 | culdoscopy |

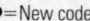

Anesthesia

**Anesthesia**

00952        hysteroscopy and/or hysterosalpingography

# Pelvis (Except Hip)

01112    Anesthesia for bone marrow aspiration and/or biopsy, anterior or posterior iliac crest

01120    Anesthesia for procedures on bony pelvis

01130    Anesthesia for body cast application or revision

01140    Anesthesia for interpelviabdominal (hindquarter) amputation

01150    Anesthesia for radical procedures for tumor of pelvis, except hindquarter amputation

01160    Anesthesia for closed procedures involving symphysis pubis or sacroiliac joint

01170    Anesthesia for open procedures involving symphysis pubis or sacroiliac joint

01173    Anesthesia for open repair of fracture disruption of pelvis or column fracture involving acetabulum

01180    Anesthesia for obturator neurectomy; extrapelvic

01190        intrapelvic

# Upper Leg (Except Knee)

01200    Anesthesia for all closed procedures involving hip joint

01202    Anesthesia for arthroscopic procedures of hip joint

01210    Anesthesia for open procedures involving hip joint; not otherwise specified

01212        hip disarticulation

01214        total hip arthroplasty

01215        revision of total hip arthroplasty

01220    Anesthesia for all closed procedures involving upper two-thirds of femur

01230    Anesthesia for open procedures involving upper two-thirds of femur; not otherwise specified

01232        amputation

01234        radical resection

01250    Anesthesia for all procedures on nerves, muscles, tendons, fascia, and bursae of upper leg

01260    Anesthesia for all procedures involving veins of upper leg, including exploration

01270    Anesthesia for procedures involving arteries of upper leg, including bypass graft; not otherwise specified

01272        femoral artery ligation

01274        femoral artery embolectomy

# Knee and Popliteal Area

01320    Anesthesia for all procedures on nerves, muscles, tendons, fascia, and bursae of knee and/or popliteal area

01340    Anesthesia for all closed procedures on lower one-third of femur

01360    Anesthesia for all open procedures on lower one-third of femur

01380    Anesthesia for all closed procedures on knee joint

01382    Anesthesia for diagnostic arthroscopic procedures of knee joint

01390    Anesthesia for all closed procedures on upper ends of tibia, fibula, and/or patella

01392    Anesthesia for all open procedures on upper ends of tibia, fibula, and/or patella

01400    Anesthesia for open or surgical arthroscopic procedures on knee joint; not otherwise specified

01402        total knee arthroplasty

01404        disarticulation at knee

01420    Anesthesia for all cast applications, removal, or repair involving knee joint

01430    Anesthesia for procedures on veins of knee and popliteal area; not otherwise specified

01432        arteriovenous fistula

01440    Anesthesia for procedures on arteries of knee and popliteal area; not otherwise specified

01442        popliteal thromboendarterectomy, with or without patch graft

01444        popliteal excision and graft or repair for occlusion or aneurysm

# Lower Leg (Below Knee, Includes Ankle and Foot)

01462    Anesthesia for all closed procedures on lower leg, ankle, and foot

01464    Anesthesia for arthroscopic procedures of ankle and/or foot

01470    Anesthesia for procedures on nerves, muscles, tendons, and fascia of lower leg, ankle, and foot; not otherwise specified

01472        repair of ruptured Achilles tendon, with or without graft

01474        gastrocnemius recession (eg, Strayer procedure)

01480    Anesthesia for open procedures on bones of lower leg, ankle, and foot; not otherwise specified

01482        radical resection (including below knee amputation)

01484        osteotomy or osteoplasty of tibia and/or fibula

**01486**      total ankle replacement

**01490**      Anesthesia for lower leg cast application, removal, or repair

**01500**      Anesthesia for procedures on arteries of lower leg, including bypass graft; not otherwise specified

**01502**      embolectomy, direct or with catheter

**01520**      Anesthesia for procedures on veins of lower leg; not otherwise specified

**01522**      venous thrombectomy, direct or with catheter

# Shoulder and Axilla

Includes humeral head and neck, sternoclavicular joint, acromioclavicular joint, and shoulder joint.

**01610**      Anesthesia for all procedures on nerves, muscles, tendons, fascia, and bursae of shoulder and axilla

**01620**      Anesthesia for all closed procedures on humeral head and neck, sternoclavicular joint, acromioclavicular joint, and shoulder joint

**01622**      Anesthesia for diagnostic arthroscopic procedures of shoulder joint

**01630**      Anesthesia for open or surgical arthroscopic procedures on humeral head and neck, sternoclavicular joint, acromioclavicular joint, and shoulder joint; not otherwise specified

         (01632 has been deleted. To report, see 01630, 01638)

**01634**      shoulder disarticulation

**01636**      interthoracoscapular (forequarter) amputation

**01638**      total shoulder replacement

**01650**      Anesthesia for procedures on arteries of shoulder and axilla; not otherwise specified

**01652**      axillary-brachial aneurysm

**01654**      bypass graft

**01656**      axillary-femoral bypass graft

**01670**      Anesthesia for all procedures on veins of shoulder and axilla

**01680**      Anesthesia for shoulder cast application, removal or repair; not otherwise specified

**01682**      shoulder spica

# Upper Arm and Elbow

**01710**      Anesthesia for procedures on nerves, muscles, tendons, fascia, and bursae of upper arm and elbow; not otherwise specified

**01712**      tenotomy, elbow to shoulder, open

**01714**      tenoplasty, elbow to shoulder

**01716**      tenodesis, rupture of long tendon of biceps

**01730**      Anesthesia for all closed procedures on humerus and elbow

**01732**      Anesthesia for diagnostic arthroscopic procedures of elbow joint

**01740**      Anesthesia for open or surgical arthroscopic procedures of the elbow; not otherwise specified

**01742**      osteotomy of humerus

**01744**      repair of nonunion or malunion of humerus

**01756**      radical procedures

**01758**      excision of cyst or tumor of humerus

**01760**      total elbow replacement

**01770**      Anesthesia for procedures on arteries of upper arm and elbow; not otherwise specified

**01772**      embolectomy

**01780**      Anesthesia for procedures on veins of upper arm and elbow; not otherwise specified

**01782**      phleborrhaphy

# Forearm, Wrist, and Hand

**01810**      Anesthesia for all procedures on nerves, muscles, tendons, fascia, and bursae of forearm, wrist, and hand

**01820**      Anesthesia for all closed procedures on radius, ulna, wrist, or hand bones

**01829**      Anesthesia for diagnostic arthroscopic procedures on the wrist

**01830**      Anesthesia for open or surgical arthroscopic/endoscopic procedures on distal radius, distal ulna, wrist, or hand joints; not otherwise specified

**01832**      total wrist replacement

**01840**      Anesthesia for procedures on arteries of forearm, wrist, and hand; not otherwise specified

**01842**      embolectomy

**01844**      Anesthesia for vascular shunt, or shunt revision, any type (eg, dialysis)

**01850**      Anesthesia for procedures on veins of forearm, wrist, and hand; not otherwise specified

**01852**      phleborrhaphy

**01860**      Anesthesia for forearm, wrist, or hand cast application, removal, or repair

# Radiological Procedures

**01916**      Anesthesia for diagnostic arteriography/venography

         (Do not report 01916 in conjunction with therapeutic codes 01924-01926, 01930-01933)

Anesthesia

**Anesthesia**

01920    Anesthesia for cardiac catheterization including coronary angiography and ventriculography (not to include Swan-Ganz catheter)

01922    Anesthesia for non-invasive imaging or radiation therapy

01924    Anesthesia for therapeutic interventional radiological procedures involving the arterial system; not otherwise specified

01925         carotid or coronary

01926         intracranial, intracardiac, or aortic

01930    Anesthesia for therapeutic interventional radiological procedures involving the venous/lymphatic system (not to include access to the central circulation); not otherwise specified

01931         intrahepatic or portal circulation (eg, transvenous intrahepatic portosystemic shunt[s] [TIPS])

01932         intrathoracic or jugular

01933         intracranial

01935    Anesthesia for percutaneous image guided procedures on the spine and spinal cord; diagnostic

01936         therapeutic

# Burn Excisions or Debridement

01951    Anesthesia for second- and third-degree burn excision or debridement with or without skin grafting, any site, for total body surface area (TBSA) treated during anesthesia and surgery; less than 4% total body surface area

01952         between 4% and 9% of total body surface area

+ 01953       each additional 9% total body surface area or part thereof (List separately in addition to code for primary procedure)

         (Use 01953 in conjunction with 01952)

# Obstetric

01958    Anesthesia for external cephalic version procedure

01960    Anesthesia for vaginal delivery only

01961    Anesthesia for cesarean delivery only

01962    Anesthesia for urgent hysterectomy following delivery

01963    Anesthesia for cesarean hysterectomy without any labor analgesia/anesthesia care

01965    Anesthesia for incomplete or missed abortion procedures

01966    Anesthesia for induced abortion procedures

01967    Neuraxial labor analgesia/anesthesia for planned vaginal delivery (this includes any repeat subarachnoid needle placement and drug injection and/or any necessary replacement of an epidural catheter during labor)

+ 01968    Anesthesia for cesarean delivery following neuraxial labor analgesia/anesthesia (List separately in addition to code for primary procedure performed)

         (Use 01968 in conjunction with 01967)

+ 01969    Anesthesia for cesarean hysterectomy following neuraxial labor analgesia/anesthesia (List separately in addition to code for primary procedure performed)

         (Use 01969 in conjunction with 01967)

# Other Procedures

01990    Physiological support for harvesting of organ(s) from brain-dead patient

01991    Anesthesia for diagnostic or therapeutic nerve blocks and injections (when block or injection is performed by a different provider); other than the prone position

01992         prone position

         (Do not report 01991 or 01992 in conjunction with 99143-99150)

         (When regional intravenous administration of local anesthetic agent or other medication in the upper or lower extremity is used as the anesthetic for a surgical procedure, report the appropriate anesthesia code. To report a Bier block for pain management, use 64999)

         (For intra-arterial or intravenous therapy for pain management, see 96373, 96374)

01996    Daily hospital management of epidural or subarachnoid continuous drug administration

         (Report code 01996 for daily hospital management of continuous epidural or subarachnoid drug administration performed after insertion of an epidural or subarachnoid catheter)

01999    Unlisted anesthesia procedure(s)

# Surgery Guidelines

Items used by all physicians in reporting their services are presented in the **Introduction.** Some of the commonalities are repeated here for the convenience of those physicians referring to this section on **Surgery.** Other definitions and items unique to Surgery are also listed.

## Physicians' Services

Physicians' services rendered in the office, home, or hospital, consultations, and other medical services are listed in the section entitled **Evaluation and Management Services** (99201-99499) found in the front of the book, beginning on page 8. "Special Services and Reports" (99000 series) is presented in the **Medicine** section.

## CPT Surgical Package Definition

The services provided by the physician to any patient by their very nature are variable. The CPT codes that represent a readily identifiable surgical procedure thereby include, on a procedure-by-procedure basis, a variety of services. In defining the specific services "included" in a given CPT surgical code, the following services are always included in addition to the operation per se:

- Local infiltration, metacarpal/metatarsal/digital block or topical anesthesia
- Subsequent to the decision for surgery, one related Evaluation and Management (E/M) encounter on the date immediately prior to or on the date of procedure (including history and physical)
- Immediate postoperative care, including dictating operative notes, talking with the family and other physicians
- Writing orders
- Evaluating the patient in the postanesthesia recovery area
- Typical postoperative follow-up care

## Follow-Up Care for Diagnostic Procedures

Follow-up care for diagnostic procedures (eg, endoscopy, arthroscopy, injection procedures for radiography) includes only that care related to recovery from the diagnostic procedure itself. Care of the condition for which the diagnostic procedure was performed or of other concomitant conditions is not included and may be listed separately.

## Follow-Up Care for Therapeutic Surgical Procedures

Follow-up care for therapeutic surgical procedures includes only that care which is usually a part of the surgical service. Complications, exacerbations, recurrence, or the presence of other diseases or injuries requiring additional services should be separately reported.

## Materials Supplied by Physician

Supplies and materials provided by the physician (eg, sterile trays/drugs), over and above those usually included with the procedure(s) rendered are reported separately. List drugs, trays, supplies, and materials provided. Identify as 99070 or specific supply code.

## Reporting More Than One Procedure/Service

When a physician performs more than one procedure/service on the same date, same session or during a post-operative period (subject to the "surgical package" concept), several CPT modifiers may apply (see Appendix A for definition).

## Separate Procedure

Some of the procedures or services listed in the CPT codebook that are commonly carried out as an integral component of a total service or procedure have been identified by the inclusion of the term "separate procedure." The codes designated as "separate procedure" should not be reported in addition to the code for the total procedure or service of which it is considered an integral component.

However, when a procedure or service that is designated as a "separate procedure" is carried out independently or considered to be unrelated or distinct from other procedures/services provided at that time, it may be reported by itself, or in addition to other procedures/services by appending modifier 59 to the specific "separate procedure" code to indicate that the procedure is not considered to be a component of another procedure, but is a distinct, independent procedure. This may represent a different session, different procedure or surgery, different site or organ system, separate incision/excision, separate lesion, or separate injury (or area of injury in extensive injuries).

# Unlisted Service or Procedure

A service or procedure may be provided that is not listed in this edition of the CPT codebook. When reporting such a service, the appropriate "Unlisted Procedure" code may be used to indicate the service, identifying it by "Special Report" as discussed in the section below. The "Unlisted Procedures" and accompanying codes for **Surgery** are as follows:

| | |
|---|---|
| 15999 | Unlisted procedure, excision pressure ulcer |
| 17999 | Unlisted procedure, skin, mucous membrane and subcutaneous tissue |
| 19499 | Unlisted procedure, breast |
| 20999 | Unlisted procedure, musculoskeletal system, general |
| 21089 | Unlisted maxillofacial prosthetic procedure |
| 21299 | Unlisted craniofacial and maxillofacial procedure |
| 21499 | Unlisted musculoskeletal procedure, head |
| 21899 | Unlisted procedure, neck or thorax |
| 22899 | Unlisted procedure, spine |
| 22999 | Unlisted procedure, abdomen, musculoskeletal system |
| 23929 | Unlisted procedure, shoulder |
| 24999 | Unlisted procedure, humerus or elbow |
| 25999 | Unlisted procedure, forearm or wrist |
| 26989 | Unlisted procedure, hands or fingers |
| 27299 | Unlisted procedure, pelvis or hip joint |
| 27599 | Unlisted procedure, femur or knee |
| 27899 | Unlisted procedure, leg or ankle |
| 28899 | Unlisted procedure, foot or toes |
| 29799 | Unlisted procedure, casting or strapping |
| 29999 | Unlisted procedure, arthroscopy |
| 30999 | Unlisted procedure, nose |
| 31299 | Unlisted procedure, accessory sinuses |
| 31599 | Unlisted procedure, larynx |
| 31899 | Unlisted procedure, trachea, bronchi |
| 32999 | Unlisted procedure, lungs and pleura |
| 33999 | Unlisted procedure, cardiac surgery |
| 36299 | Unlisted procedure, vascular injection |

| | |
|---|---|
| 37501 | Unlisted vascular endoscopy procedure |
| 37799 | Unlisted procedure, vascular surgery |
| 38129 | Unlisted laparoscopy procedure, spleen |
| 38589 | Unlisted laparoscopy procedure, lymphatic system |
| 38999 | Unlisted procedure, hemic or lymphatic system |
| 39499 | Unlisted procedure, mediastinum |
| 39599 | Unlisted procedure, diaphragm |
| 40799 | Unlisted procedure, lips |
| 40899 | Unlisted procedure, vestibule of mouth |
| 41599 | Unlisted procedure, tongue, floor of mouth |
| 41899 | Unlisted procedure, dentoalveolar structures |
| 42299 | Unlisted procedure, palate, uvula |
| 42699 | Unlisted procedure, salivary glands or ducts |
| 42999 | Unlisted procedure, pharynx, adenoids, or tonsils |
| 43289 | Unlisted laparoscopy procedure, esophagus |
| 43499 | Unlisted procedure, esophagus |
| 43659 | Unlisted laparoscopy procedure, stomach |
| 43999 | Unlisted procedure, stomach |
| 44238 | Unlisted laparoscopy procedure, intestine (except rectum) |
| 44799 | Unlisted procedure, intestine |
| 44899 | Unlisted procedure, Meckel's diverticulum and the mesentery |
| 44979 | Unlisted laparoscopy procedure, appendix |
| 45499 | Unlisted laparoscopy procedure, rectum |
| 45999 | Unlisted procedure, rectum |
| 46999 | Unlisted procedure, anus |
| 47379 | Unlisted laparoscopic procedure, liver |
| 47399 | Unlisted procedure, liver |
| 47579 | Unlisted laparoscopy procedure, biliary tract |
| 47999 | Unlisted procedure, biliary tract |
| 48999 | Unlisted procedure, pancreas |
| 49329 | Unlisted laparoscopy procedure, abdomen, peritoneum and omentum |
| 49659 | Unlisted laparoscopy procedure, hernioplasty, herniorrhaphy, herniotomy |
| 49999 | Unlisted procedure, abdomen, peritoneum and omentum |
| 50549 | Unlisted laparoscopy procedure, renal |
| 50949 | Unlisted laparoscopy procedure, ureter |
| 51999 | Unlisted laparoscopy procedure, bladder |
| 53899 | Unlisted procedure, urinary system |
| 54699 | Unlisted laparoscopy procedure, testis |
| 55559 | Unlisted laparoscopy procedure, spermatic cord |

⊙=Moderate sedation  ✚=Add-on code  ✗=FDA approval pending  #=Resequenced code  ○=Recycled/reinstated code

| 55899 | Unlisted procedure, male genital system |
|---|---|
| 58578 | Unlisted laparoscopy procedure, uterus |
| 58579 | Unlisted hysteroscopy procedure, uterus |
| 58679 | Unlisted laparoscopy procedure, oviduct, ovary |
| 58999 | Unlisted procedure, female genital system (nonobstetrical) |
| 59897 | Unlisted fetal invasive procedure, including ultrasound guidance, when performed |
| 59898 | Unlisted laparoscopy procedure, maternity care and delivery |
| 59899 | Unlisted procedure, maternity care and delivery |
| 60659 | Unlisted laparoscopy procedure, endocrine system |
| 60699 | Unlisted procedure, endocrine system |
| 64999 | Unlisted procedure, nervous system |
| 66999 | Unlisted procedure, anterior segment of eye |
| 67299 | Unlisted procedure, posterior segment |
| 67399 | Unlisted procedure, ocular muscle |
| 67599 | Unlisted procedure, orbit |
| 67999 | Unlisted procedure, eyelids |
| 68399 | Unlisted procedure, conjunctiva |
| 68899 | Unlisted procedure, lacrimal system |
| 69399 | Unlisted procedure, external ear |
| 69799 | Unlisted procedure, middle ear |
| 69949 | Unlisted procedure, inner ear |
| 69979 | Unlisted procedure, temporal bone, middle fossa approach |

# Special Report

A service that is rarely provided, unusual, variable, or new may require a special report. Pertinent information should include an adequate definition or description of the nature, extent, and need for the procedure, and the time, effort, and equipment necessary to provide the service.

# Surgical Destruction

Surgical destruction is a part of a surgical procedure and different methods of destruction are not ordinarily listed separately unless the technique substantially alters the standard management of a problem or condition. Exceptions under special circumstances are provided for by separate code numbers.

# Surgery

## General

**10021** Fine needle aspiration; without imaging guidance

**10022** with imaging guidance

(For placement of percutaneous localization clip during breast biopsy, use 19295)

(For radiological supervision and interpretation, see 76942, 77002, 77012, 77021)

(For percutaneous needle biopsy other than fine needle aspiration, see 20206 for muscle, 32400 for pleura, 32405 for lung or mediastinum, 42400 for salivary gland, 47000 for liver, 48102 for pancreas, 49180 for abdominal or retroperitoneal mass, 50200 for kidney, 54500 for testis, 54800 for epididymis, 60100 for thyroid, 62267 for nucleus pulposus, intervertebral disc, or paravertebral tissue, 62269 for spinal cord)

(For evaluation of fine needle aspirate, see 88172, 88173)

## Integumentary System

### Skin, Subcutaneous, and Accessory Structures

#### Incision and Drainage

(For excision, see 11400, et seq)

**10040** Acne surgery (eg, marsupialization, opening or removal of multiple milia, comedones, cysts, pustules)

**10060** Incision and drainage of abscess (eg, carbuncle, suppurative hidradenitis, cutaneous or subcutaneous abscess, cyst, furuncle, or paronychia); simple or single

**10061** complicated or multiple

**10080** Incision and drainage of pilonidal cyst; simple

**10081** complicated

(For excision of pilonidal cyst, see 11770-11772)

**10120** Incision and removal of foreign body, subcutaneous tissues; simple

**10121** complicated

(To report wound exploration due to penetrating trauma without laparotomy or thoracotomy, see 20100-20103, as appropriate)

(To report debridement associated with open fracture(s) and/or dislocation(s), use 11010-11012, as appropriate)

**10140** Incision and drainage of hematoma, seroma or fluid collection

(If imaging guidance is performed, see 76942, 77012, 77021)

**10160** Puncture aspiration of abscess, hematoma, bulla, or cyst

(If imaging guidance is performed, see 76942, 77012, 77021)

**10180** Incision and drainage, complex, postoperative wound infection

(For secondary closure of surgical wound, see 12020, 12021, 13160)

## Debridement

▶Wound debridements (11042-11047) are reported by depth of tissue that is removed and by surface area of the wound. These services may be reported for injuries, infections, wounds and chronic ulcers. When performing debridement of a single wound, report depth using the deepest level of tissue removed. In multiple wounds, sum the surface area of those wounds that are at the same depth, but do not combine sums from different depths. For example: When bone is debrided from a 4 sq cm heel ulcer and from a 10 sq cm ischial ulcer, report the work with a single code, 11044. When subcutaneous tissue is debrided from a 16 sq cm dehisced abdominal wound and a 10 sq cm thigh wound, report the work with 11042 for the first 20 sq cm and 11045 for the second 6 sq cm. If all four wounds were debrided on the same day, use modifier 59 with either 11042, or 11044 as appropriate.◀

(For dermabrasions, see 15780-15783)

(For nail debridement, see 11720-11721)

(For burn(s), see 16000-16035)

(For pressure ulcers, see 15920-15999)

**11000** Debridement of extensive eczematous or infected skin; up to 10% of body surface

(For abdominal wall or genitalia debridement for necrotizing soft tissue infection, see 11004-11006)

**+ 11001** each additional 10% of the body surface, or part thereof (List separately in addition to code for primary procedure)

(Use 11001 in conjunction with 11000)

**11004** Debridement of skin, subcutaneous tissue, muscle and fascia for necrotizing soft tissue infection; external genitalia and perineum

**11005** abdominal wall, with or without fascial closure

**11006**     external genitalia, perineum and abdominal wall, with or without fascial closure

(If orchiectomy is performed, use 54520)

(If testicular transplantation is performed, use 54680)

**+ 11008**   Removal of prosthetic material or mesh, abdominal wall for infection (eg, for chronic or recurrent mesh infection or necrotizing soft tissue infection) (List separately in addition to code for primary procedure)

(Use 11008 in conjunction with 10180, 11004-11006)

(Do not report 11008 in conjunction with 11000-11001, 11010-11044)

(Report skin grafts or flaps separately when performed for closure at the same session as 11004-11008)

(When insertion of mesh is used for closure, use 49568)

**11010**   Debridement including removal of foreign material at the site of an open fracture and/or an open dislocation (eg, excisional debridement); skin and subcutaneous tissues

**11011**     skin, subcutaneous tissue, muscle fascia, and muscle

**11012**     skin, subcutaneous tissue, muscle fascia, muscle, and bone

(11040, 11041 have been deleted)

(For debridement of skin, ie, epidermis and/or dermis only, see 97597, 97598)

(For active wound care management, see 97597, 97598)

(For debridement of burn wounds, see 16020-16030)

**11042**   Debridement, subcutaneous tissue (includes epidermis and dermis, if performed); first 20 sq cm or less

(For debridement of skin [ie, epidermis and/or dermis only], see 97597, 97598)

**#+ 11045**     each additional 20 sq cm, or part thereof (List separately in addition to code for primary procedure)

(Use 11045 in conjunction with 11042)

**11043**   Debridement, muscle and/or fascia (includes epidermis, dermis, and subcutaneous tissue, if performed); first 20 sq cm or less

**#+ 11046**     each additional 20 sq cm, or part thereof (List separately in addition to code for primary procedure)

(Use 11046 in conjunction with 11043)

**11044**   Debridement, bone (includes epidermis, dermis, subcutaneous tissue, muscle and/or fascia, if performed); first 20 sq cm or less

**11045**   Code is out of numerical sequence. See 11000-11047

**11046**   Code is out of numerical sequence. See 11000-11047

**#+ 11047**     each additional 20 sq cm, or part thereof (List separately in addition to code for primary procedure)

(Do not report 11042-11047 in conjunction with 97597-97602 for the same wound)

(Use 11047 in conjunction with 11044)

## Paring or Cutting

(To report destruction, see 17000-17004)

**11055**   Paring or cutting of benign hyperkeratotic lesion (eg, corn or callus); single lesion

**11056**     2 to 4 lesions

**11057**     more than 4 lesions

## Biopsy

During certain surgical procedures in the integumentary system, such as excision, destruction, or shave removals, the removed tissue is often submitted for pathologic examination. The obtaining of tissue for pathology during the course of these procedures is a routine component of such procedures. This obtaining of tissue is not considered a separate biopsy procedure and is not separately reported. The use of a biopsy procedure code (eg, 11100, 11101) indicates that the procedure to obtain tissue for pathologic examination was performed independently, or was unrelated or distinct from other procedures/services provided at that time. Such biopsies are not considered components of other procedures when performed on different lesions or different sites on the same date, and are to be reported separately.

(For biopsy of conjunctiva, use 68100; eyelid, use 67810)

**11100**   Biopsy of skin, subcutaneous tissue and/or mucous membrane (including simple closure), unless otherwise listed; single lesion

**+ 11101**     each separate/additional lesion (List separately in addition to code for primary procedure)

(Use 11101 in conjunction with 11100)

## Removal of Skin Tags

Removal by scissoring or any sharp method, ligature strangulation, electrosurgical destruction or combination of treatment modalities, including chemical destruction or electrocauterization of wound, with or without local anesthesia.

**11200**   Removal of skin tags, multiple fibrocutaneous tags, any area; up to and including 15 lesions

**+ 11201**     each additional 10 lesions, or part thereof (List separately in addition to code for primary procedure)

(Use 11201 in conjunction with 11200)

## Shaving of Epidermal or Dermal Lesions

Shaving is the sharp removal by transverse incision or horizontal slicing to remove epidermal and dermal lesions without a full-thickness dermal excision. This includes local anesthesia, chemical or electrocauterization of the wound. The wound does not require suture closure.

**11300** Shaving of epidermal or dermal lesion, single lesion, trunk, arms or legs; lesion diameter 0.5 cm or less

**11301** lesion diameter 0.6 to 1.0 cm

**11302** lesion diameter 1.1 to 2.0 cm

**11303** lesion diameter over 2.0 cm

**11305** Shaving of epidermal or dermal lesion, single lesion, scalp, neck, hands, feet, genitalia; lesion diameter 0.5 cm or less

**11306** lesion diameter 0.6 to 1.0 cm

**11307** lesion diameter 1.1 to 2.0 cm

**11308** lesion diameter over 2.0 cm

**11310** Shaving of epidermal or dermal lesion, single lesion, face, ears, eyelids, nose, lips, mucous membrane; lesion diameter 0.5 cm or less

**11311** lesion diameter 0.6 to 1.0 cm

**11312** lesion diameter 1.1 to 2.0 cm

**11313** lesion diameter over 2.0 cm

## Excision—Benign Lesions

Excision (including simple closure) of benign lesions of skin (eg, neoplasm, cicatricial, fibrous, inflammatory, congenital, cystic lesions), includes local anesthesia. See appropriate size and area below. For shave removal, see 11300 et seq, and for electrosurgical and other methods see 17000 et seq.

Excision is defined as full-thickness (through the dermis) removal of a lesion, including margins, and includes simple (non-layered) closure when performed. Report separately each benign lesion excised. Code selection is determined by measuring the greatest clinical diameter of the apparent lesion plus that margin required for complete excision (lesion diameter plus the most narrow margins required equals the excised diameter). The margins refer to the most narrow margin required to adequately excise the lesion, based on the physician's judgment. The measurement of lesion plus margin is made prior to excision. The excised diameter is the same whether the surgical defect is repaired in a linear fashion, or reconstructed (eg, with a skin graft).

The closure of defects created by incision, excision, or trauma may require intermediate or complex closure. Repair by intermediate or complex closure should be reported separately. For excision of benign lesions requiring more than simple closure, ie, requiring

intermediate or complex closure, report 11400-11446 in addition to appropriate intermediate (12031-12057) or complex closure (13100-13153) codes. For reconstructive closure, see 15002-15261, 15570-15770. For excision performed in conjunction with adjacent tissue transfer, report only the adjacent tissue transfer code (14000-14302). Excision of lesion (11400-11446) is not separately reportable with adjacent tissue transfer. See page 50 for the definition of *intermediate* or *complex* closure.

**11400** Excision, benign lesion including margins, except skin tag (unless listed elsewhere), trunk, arms or legs; excised diameter 0.5 cm or less

**11401** excised diameter 0.6 to 1.0 cm

**11402** excised diameter 1.1 to 2.0 cm

**11403** excised diameter 2.1 to 3.0 cm

**11404** excised diameter 3.1 to 4.0 cm

**11406** excised diameter over 4.0 cm

(For unusual or complicated excision, add modifier 22)

**11420** Excision, benign lesion including margins, except skin tag (unless listed elsewhere), scalp, neck, hands, feet, genitalia; excised diameter 0.5 cm or less

**11421** excised diameter 0.6 to 1.0 cm

**11422** excised diameter 1.1 to 2.0 cm

**11423** excised diameter 2.1 to 3.0 cm

**11424** excised diameter 3.1 to 4.0 cm

**11426** excised diameter over 4.0 cm

(For unusual or complicated excision, add modifier 22)

**11440** Excision, other benign lesion including margins, except skin tag (unless listed elsewhere), face, ears, eyelids, nose, lips, mucous membrane; excised diameter 0.5 cm or less

**11441** excised diameter 0.6 to 1.0 cm

**11442** excised diameter 1.1 to 2.0 cm

**11443** excised diameter 2.1 to 3.0 cm

**11444** excised diameter 3.1 to 4.0 cm

**11446** excised diameter over 4.0 cm

(For unusual or complicated excision, add modifier 22)

(For eyelids involving more than skin, see also 67800 et seq)

**11450** Excision of skin and subcutaneous tissue for hidradenitis, axillary; with simple or intermediate repair

**11451** with complex repair

**11462** Excision of skin and subcutaneous tissue for hidradenitis, inguinal; with simple or intermediate repair

**11463** with complex repair

**11470** Excision of skin and subcutaneous tissue for hidradenitis, perianal, perineal, or umbilical; with simple or intermediate repair

**11471** with complex repair

(When skin graft or flap is used for closure, use appropriate procedure code in addition)

(For bilateral procedure, add modifier 50)

## Excision—Malignant Lesions

Excision (including simple closure) of malignant lesions of skin (eg, basal cell carcinoma, squamous cell carcinoma, melanoma) includes local anesthesia. (See appropriate size and body area below.) For destruction of malignant lesions of skin, see destruction codes 17260-17286.

Excision is defined as full-thickness (through the dermis) removal of a lesion including margins, and includes simple (non-layered) closure when performed. Report separately each malignant lesion excised. Code selection is determined by measuring the greatest clinical diameter of the apparent lesion plus that margin required for complete excision (lesion diameter plus the most narrow margins required equals the excised diameter). The margins refer to the most narrow margin required to adequately excise the lesion, based on the physician's judgment. The measurement of lesion plus margin is made prior to excision. The excised diameter is the same whether the surgical defect is repaired in a linear fashion, or reconstructed (eg, with a skin graft).

The closure of defects created by incision, excision, or trauma may require intermediate or complex closure. Repair by intermediate or complex closure should be reported separately. For excision of malignant lesions requiring more than simple closure, ie, requiring intermediate or complex closure, report 11600-11646 in addition to appropriate intermediate (12031-12057) or complex closure (13100-13153) codes. For reconstructive closure, see 15002-15261, 15570-15770. For excision performed in conjunction with adjacent tissue transfer, report only the adjacent tissue transfer code (14000-14302). Excision of lesion (11600-11646) is not separately reportable with adjacent tissue transfer. See page 50 for the definition of *intermediate* or *complex* closure.

When frozen section pathology shows the margins of excision were not adequate, an additional excision may be necessary for complete tumor removal. Use only one code to report the additional excision and re-excision(s) based on the final widest excised diameter required for complete tumor removal at the same operative session. To report a re-excision procedure performed to widen margins at a subsequent operative session, see codes 11600-11646, as appropriate. Append modifier 58 if the re-excision procedure is performed during the postoperative period of the primary excision procedure.

**11600** Excision, malignant lesion including margins, trunk, arms, or legs; excised diameter 0.5 cm or less

**11601** excised diameter 0.6 to 1.0 cm

**11602** excised diameter 1.1 to 2.0 cm

**11603** excised diameter 2.1 to 3.0 cm

**11604** excised diameter 3.1 to 4.0 cm

**11606** excised diameter over 4.0 cm

**11620** Excision, malignant lesion including margins, scalp, neck, hands, feet, genitalia; excised diameter 0.5 cm or less

**11621** excised diameter 0.6 to 1.0 cm

**11622** excised diameter 1.1 to 2.0 cm

**11623** excised diameter 2.1 to 3.0 cm

**11624** excised diameter 3.1 to 4.0 cm

**11626** excised diameter over 4.0 cm

**11640** Excision, malignant lesion including margins, face, ears, eyelids, nose, lips; excised diameter 0.5 cm or less

**11641** excised diameter 0.6 to 1.0 cm

**11642** excised diameter 1.1 to 2.0 cm

**11643** excised diameter 2.1 to 3.0 cm

**11644** excised diameter 3.1 to 4.0 cm

**11646** excised diameter over 4.0 cm

(For eyelids involving more than skin, see also 67800 et seq)

## Nails

(For drainage of paronychia or onychia, see 10060, 10061)

**11719** Trimming of nondystrophic nails, any number

**11720** Debridement of nail(s) by any method(s); 1 to 5

**11721** 6 or more

**11730** Avulsion of nail plate, partial or complete, simple; single

**+ 11732** each additional nail plate (List separately in addition to code for primary procedure)

(Use 11732 in conjunction with 11730)

**11740** Evacuation of subungual hematoma

**11750** Excision of nail and nail matrix, partial or complete (eg, ingrown or deformed nail), for permanent removal;

**11752** with amputation of tuft of distal phalanx

(For skin graft, if used, use 15050)

**11755** Biopsy of nail unit (eg, plate, bed, matrix, hyponychium, proximal and lateral nail folds) (separate procedure)

**11760** Repair of nail bed

**11762** Reconstruction of nail bed with graft

**11765** Wedge excision of skin of nail fold (eg, for ingrown toenail)

Surgery: Integumentary System

# Pilonidal Cyst

**11770**   Excision of pilonidal cyst or sinus; simple

**11771**        extensive

**11772**        complicated

(For incision of pilonidal cyst, see 10080, 10081)

# Introduction

**11900**   Injection, intralesional; up to and including 7 lesions

**11901**        more than 7 lesions

(11900, 11901 are not to be used for preoperative local anesthetic injection)

(For veins, see 36470, 36471)

(For intralesional chemotherapy administration, see 96405, 96406)

**11920**   Tattooing, intradermal introduction of insoluble opaque pigments to correct color defects of skin, including micropigmentation; 6.0 sq cm or less

**11921**        6.1 to 20.0 sq cm

**+ 11922**      each additional 20.0 sq cm, or part thereof (List separately in addition to code for primary procedure)

(Use 11922 in conjunction with 11921)

**11950**   Subcutaneous injection of filling material (eg, collagen); 1 cc or less

**11951**        1.1 to 5.0 cc

**11952**        5.1 to 10.0 cc

**11954**        over 10.0 cc

**11960**   Insertion of tissue expander(s) for other than breast, including subsequent expansion

(For breast reconstruction with tissue expander(s), use 19357)

**11970**   Replacement of tissue expander with permanent prosthesis

**11971**   Removal of tissue expander(s) without insertion of prosthesis

►(11975 has been deleted. To report insertion of non-biodegradable drug delivery implant for contraception, use 11981)◄

**11976**   Removal, implantable contraceptive capsules

►(11977 has been deleted. To report removal of implantable contraceptive capsules with subsequent insertion of non-biodegradable drug delivery implant, use 11976 and 11981)◄

**11980**   Subcutaneous hormone pellet implantation (implantation of estradiol and/or testosterone pellets beneath the skin)

**11981**   Insertion, non-biodegradable drug delivery implant

**11982**   Removal, non-biodegradable drug delivery implant

**11983**   Removal with reinsertion, non-biodegradable drug delivery implant

# Repair (Closure)

Use the codes in this section to designate wound closure utilizing sutures, staples, or tissue adhesives (eg, 2-cyanoacrylate), either singly or in combination with each other, or in combination with adhesive strips. Wound closure utilizing adhesive strips as the sole repair material should be coded using the appropriate E/M code.

### Definitions

The repair of wounds may be classified as Simple, Intermediate, or Complex.

***Simple repair*** is used when the wound is superficial; eg, involving primarily epidermis or dermis, or subcutaneous tissues without significant involvement of deeper structures, and requires simple one layer closure. This includes local anesthesia and chemical or electrocauterization of wounds not closed.

***Intermediate repair*** includes the repair of wounds that, in addition to the above, require layered closure of one or more of the deeper layers of subcutaneous tissue and superficial (non-muscle) fascia, in addition to the skin (epidermal and dermal) closure. Single-layer closure of heavily contaminated wounds that have required extensive cleaning or removal of particulate matter also constitutes intermediate repair.

***Complex repair*** includes the repair of wounds requiring more than layered closure, viz., scar revision, debridement (eg, traumatic lacerations or avulsions), extensive undermining, stents or retention sutures. Necessary preparation includes creation of a limited defect for repairs or the debridement of complicated lacerations or avulsions. Complex repair does not include excision of benign (11400-11446) or malignant (11600-11646) lesions, excisional preparation of a wound bed (15002-15005) or debridement of an open fracture or open dislocation.

Instructions for listing services at time of wound repair:

1. The repaired wound(s) should be measured and recorded in centimeters, whether curved, angular, or stellate.

2. When multiple wounds are repaired, add together the lengths of those in the same classification (see above) and from all anatomic sites that are grouped together into the same code descriptor. For example, add together the lengths of intermediate repairs to the trunk and extremities. Do not add lengths of repairs from different groupings of anatomic sites (eg, face and extremities). Also, do not add together lengths of different classifications (eg, intermediate and complex repairs).

▶When more than one classification of wounds is repaired, list the more complicated as the primary procedure and the less complicated as the secondary procedure, using modifier 59.◀

3. Decontamination and/or debridement: Debridement is considered a separate procedure only when gross contamination requires prolonged cleansing, when appreciable amounts of devitalized or contaminated tissue are removed, or when debridement is carried out separately without immediate primary closure.

(For extensive debridement of soft tissue and/or bone, not associated with open fracture(s) and/or dislocation(s) resulting from penetrating and/or blunt trauma, see 11042-11047.)

(For extensive debridement of subcutaneous tissue, muscle fascia, muscle, and/or bone associated with open fracture(s) and/or dislocation(s), see 11010-11012.)

▶4. Involvement of nerves, blood vessels and tendons: Report under appropriate system (Nervous, Cardiovascular, Musculoskeletal) for repair of these structures. The repair of these associated wounds is included in the primary procedure unless it qualifies as a complex repair, in which case modifier 59 applies.◀

Simple ligation of vessels in an open wound is considered as part of any wound closure.

Simple "exploration" of nerves, blood vessels or tendons exposed in an open wound is also considered part of the essential treatment of the wound and is not a separate procedure unless appreciable dissection is required. If the wound requires enlargement, extension of dissection (to determine penetration), debridement, removal of foreign body(s), ligation or coagulation of minor subcutaneous and/or muscular blood vessel(s) of the subcutaneous tissue, muscle fascia, and/or muscle, not requiring thoracotomy or laparotomy, use codes 20100-20103, as appropriate.

## Repair—Simple

Sum of lengths of repairs for each group of anatomic sites.

| 12001 | Simple repair of superficial wounds of scalp, neck, axillae, external genitalia, trunk and/or extremities (including hands and feet); 2.5 cm or less |
|---|---|
| 12002 | 2.6 cm to 7.5 cm |
| 12004 | 7.6 cm to 12.5 cm |
| 12005 | 12.6 cm to 20.0 cm |
| 12006 | 20.1 cm to 30.0 cm |
| 12007 | over 30.0 cm |
| 12011 | Simple repair of superficial wounds of face, ears, eyelids, nose, lips and/or mucous membranes; 2.5 cm or less |
| 12013 | 2.6 cm to 5.0 cm |
| 12014 | 5.1 cm to 7.5 cm |

| 12015 | 7.6 cm to 12.5 cm |
|---|---|
| 12016 | 12.6 cm to 20.0 cm |
| 12017 | 20.1 cm to 30.0 cm |
| 12018 | over 30.0 cm |
| 12020 | Treatment of superficial wound dehiscence; simple closure |
| 12021 | with packing |

(For extensive or complicated secondary wound closure, use 13160)

## Repair—Intermediate

Sum of lengths of repairs for each group of anatomic sites.

| 12031 | Repair, intermediate, wounds of scalp, axillae, trunk and/or extremities (excluding hands and feet); 2.5 cm or less |
|---|---|
| 12032 | 2.6 cm to 7.5 cm |
| 12034 | 7.6 cm to 12.5 cm |
| 12035 | 12.6 cm to 20.0 cm |
| 12036 | 20.1 cm to 30.0 cm |
| 12037 | over 30.0 cm |
| 12041 | Repair, intermediate, wounds of neck, hands, feet and/or external genitalia; 2.5 cm or less |
| 12042 | 2.6 cm to 7.5 cm |
| 12044 | 7.6 cm to 12.5 cm |
| 12045 | 12.6 cm to 20.0 cm |
| 12046 | 20.1 cm to 30.0 cm |
| 12047 | over 30.0 cm |
| 12051 | Repair, intermediate, wounds of face, ears, eyelids, nose, lips and/or mucous membranes; 2.5 cm or less |
| 12052 | 2.6 cm to 5.0 cm |
| 12053 | 5.1 cm to 7.5 cm |
| 12054 | 7.6 cm to 12.5 cm |
| 12055 | 12.6 cm to 20.0 cm |
| 12056 | 20.1 cm to 30.0 cm |
| 12057 | over 30.0 cm |

## Repair—Complex

Reconstructive procedures, complicated wound closure.

Sum of lengths of repairs for each group of anatomic sites.

(For full thickness repair of lip or eyelid, see respective anatomical subsections)

| 13100 | Repair, complex, trunk; 1.1 cm to 2.5 cm |
|---|---|

(For 1.0 cm or less, see simple or intermediate repairs)

Surgery: Integumentary System

| | |
|---|---|
| 13101 | 2.6 cm to 7.5 cm |
| + 13102 | each additional 5 cm or less (List separately in addition to code for primary procedure) |
| | (Use 13102 in conjunction with 13101) |
| 13120 | Repair, complex, scalp, arms, and/or legs; 1.1 cm to 2.5 cm |
| | (For 1.0 cm or less, see simple or intermediate repairs) |
| 13121 | 2.6 cm to 7.5 cm |
| + 13122 | each additional 5 cm or less (List separately in addition to code for primary procedure) |
| | (Use 13122 in conjunction with 13121) |
| 13131 | Repair, complex, forehead, cheeks, chin, mouth, neck, axillae, genitalia, hands and/or feet; 1.1 cm to 2.5 cm |
| | (For 1.0 cm or less, see simple or intermediate repairs) |
| 13132 | 2.6 cm to 7.5 cm |
| + 13133 | each additional 5 cm or less (List separately in addition to code for primary procedure) |
| | (Use 13133 in conjunction with 13132) |
| 13150 | Repair, complex, eyelids, nose, ears and/or lips; 1.0 cm or less |
| | (See also 40650-40654, 67961-67975) |
| 13151 | 1.1 cm to 2.5 cm |
| 13152 | 2.6 cm to 7.5 cm |
| + 13153 | each additional 5 cm or less (List separately in addition to code for primary procedure) |
| | (Use 13153 in conjunction with 13152) |
| 13160 | Secondary closure of surgical wound or dehiscence, extensive or complicated |
| | (For packing or simple secondary wound closure, see 12020, 12021) |

## Adjacent Tissue Transfer or Rearrangement

For full thickness repair of lip or eyelid, see respective anatomical subsections.

Codes 14000-14302 are used for excision (including lesion) and/or repair by adjacent tissue transfer or rearrangement (eg, Z-plasty, W-plasty, V-Y plasty, rotation flap, random island flap, advancement flap). When applied in repairing lacerations, the procedures listed must be performed by the surgeon to accomplish the repair. They do not apply to direct closure or rearrangement of traumatic wounds incidentally resulting in these configurations. Undermining alone of adjacent tissues to achieve closure, without additional incisions, does not constitute adjacent tissue transfer, see complex repair codes 13100-13160. The excision of a benign lesion (11400-11446) or a malignant lesion (11600-

11646) is not separately reportable with codes 14000-14302.

Skin graft necessary to close secondary defect is considered an additional procedure. For purposes of code selection, the term "defect" includes the primary and secondary defects. The primary defect resulting from the excision and the secondary defect resulting from flap design to perform the reconstruction are measured together to determine the code.

| | |
|---|---|
| 14000 | Adjacent tissue transfer or rearrangement, trunk; defect 10 sq cm or less |
| 14001 | defect 10.1 sq cm to 30.0 sq cm |
| 14020 | Adjacent tissue transfer or rearrangement, scalp, arms and/or legs; defect 10 sq cm or less |
| 14021 | defect 10.1 sq cm to 30.0 sq cm |
| 14040 | Adjacent tissue transfer or rearrangement, forehead, cheeks, chin, mouth, neck, axillae, genitalia, hands and/or feet; defect 10 sq cm or less |
| 14041 | defect 10.1 sq cm to 30.0 sq cm |
| 14060 | Adjacent tissue transfer or rearrangement, eyelids, nose, ears and/or lips; defect 10 sq cm or less |
| 14061 | defect 10.1 sq cm to 30.0 sq cm |
| | (For eyelid, full thickness, see 67961 et seq) |
| | (14300 has been deleted. To report, see 14301, 14302) |
| 14301 | Adjacent tissue transfer or rearrangement, any area; defect 30.1 sq cm to 60.0 sq cm |
| + 14302 | each additional 30.0 sq cm, or part thereof (List separately in addition to code for primary procedure) |
| | (Use 14302 in conjunction with 14301) |
| 14350 | Filleted finger or toe flap, including preparation of recipient site |

## ▶Skin Replacement Surgery◀

▶Skin replacement surgery consists of *surgical preparation* and topical placement of an *autograft* (including tissue cultured autograft) or *skin substitute graft* (ie, homograft, allograft, xenograft). The graft is anchored using the provider's choice of fixation. When services are performed in the office, routine dressing supplies are not reported separately.

The following definition should be applied to those codes that reference "100 sq cm or 1% of body area of infants and children" when determining the involvement of body size: The measurement of 100 sq cm is applicable to adults and children 10 years of age and older; and percentages of body surface area apply to infants and children younger than 10 years of age. The measurements apply to the size of the recipient area.

Procedures involving wrist and/or ankle are reported with codes that include arm or leg in the descriptor.

When a primary procedure requires a skin substitute or skin autograft for definitive skin closure (eg, orbitectomy, radical mastectomy, deep tumor removal), use 15100-15278 in conjunction with primary procedure.

For biological implant for soft tissue reinforcement, use 15777 in conjunction with primary procedure.

The supply of skin substitute graft(s) should be reported separately in conjunction with 15271-15278.◄

### ►Definitions◄

►Surgical preparation codes 15002-15005 for skin replacement surgery describe the initial services related to preparing a clean and viable wound surface for placement of an autograft, flap, skin substitute graft or for negative pressure wound therapy. In some cases, closure may be possible using adjacent tissue transfer (14000-14061) or complex repair (13100-13153). In all cases, appreciable nonviable tissue is removed to treat a burn, traumatic wound or a necrotizing infection. The clean wound bed may also be created by incisional release of a scar contracture resulting in a surface defect from separation of tissues. The intent is to heal the wound by primary intention, or by the use of negative pressure wound therapy. Patient conditions may require the closure or application of graft, flap, or skin substitute to be delayed, but in all cases the intent is to include these treatments or negative pressure wound therapy to heal the wound. Do not report 15002-15005 for removal of nonviable tissue/debris in a chronic wound (eg, venous or diabetic) when the wound is left to heal by secondary intention. See active wound management codes (97597, 97598) and debridement codes (11042-11047) for this service. For necrotizing soft tissue infections in specific anatomic locations, see 11004-11008.

Select the appropriate code from 15002-15005 based upon location and size of the resultant defect. For multiple wounds, sum the surface area of all wounds from all anatomic sites that are grouped together into the same code descriptor. For example, sum the surface area of all wounds on the trunk and arms. Do not sum wounds from different groupings of anatomic sites (eg, face and arms). Use 15002 or 15004, as appropriate, for excisions and incisional releases resulting in wounds up to and including 100 sq cm of surface area. Use 15003 or 15005 for each additional 100 sq cm or part thereof. For example: Surgical preparation of a 20 sq cm wound on the right hand and a 15 sq cm wound on the left hand would be reported with a single code, 15004. Surgical preparation of a 75 sq cm wound on the right thigh and a 75 sq cm wound on the left thigh would be reported with 15002 for the first 100 sq cm and 15003 for the second 50 sq cm. If all four wounds required surgical preparation on the same day, use modifier 59 with 15002, and 15004.

*Autografts/tissue cultured autografts* include the harvest and/or application of an autologous skin graft. Repair of donor site requiring skin graft or local flaps is reported

separately. Removal of current graft and/or simple cleansing of the wound is included, when performed. Do not report 97602. Debridement is considered a separate procedure only when gross contamination requires prolonged cleansing, when appreciable amounts of devitalized or contaminated tissue are removed, or when debridement is carried out separately without immediate primary closure.

Select the appropriate code from 15040-15261 based upon type of autograft and location and size of the defect. The measurements apply to the size of the recipient area. For multiple wounds, sum the surface area of all wounds from all anatomic sites that are grouped together into the same code descriptor. For example, sum the surface area of all wounds on the trunk and arms. Do not sum wounds from different groupings of anatomic sites (eg, face and arms).

*Skin substitute grafts* include non-autologous human skin (dermal or epidermal, cellular and acellular) grafts (eg, homograft, allograft), non-human skin substitute grafts (ie, xenograft), and biological products that form a sheet scaffolding for skin growth. These codes are not to be reported for application of non-graft wound dressings (eg, gel, ointment, foam, liquid) or injected skin substitutes. Removal of current graft and/or simple cleansing of the wound is included, when performed. Do not report 97602. Debridement is considered a separate procedure only when gross contamination requires prolonged cleansing, when appreciable amounts of devitalized or contaminated tissue are removed, or when debridement is carried out separately without immediate primary closure.

Select the appropriate code from 15271-15278 based upon location and size of the defect. For multiple wounds, sum the surface area of all wounds from all anatomic sites that are grouped together into the same code descriptor. For example, sum the surface area of all wounds on the trunk and arms. Do not sum wounds from different groupings of anatomic sites (eg, face and arms).◄

### ►Surgical Preparation◄

**15002**   Surgical preparation or creation of recipient site by excision of open wounds, burn eschar, or scar (including subcutaneous tissues), or incisional release of scar contracture, trunk, arms, legs; first 100 sq cm or 1% of body area of infants and children

(For linear scar revision, see 13100-13153)

**+ 15003**   each additional 100 sq cm, or part ~~~~ additional 1% of body ~~~~ (List separately in ~~~~ procedure)

(Use 15003 in conjuncti~~~~

54

**Surgery: Integumentary System**

**15004** Surgical preparation or creation of recipient site by excision of open wounds, burn eschar, or scar (including subcutaneous tissues), or incisional release of scar contracture, face, scalp, eyelids, mouth, neck, ears, orbits, genitalia, hands, feet and/or multiple digits; first 100 sq cm or 1% of body area of infants and children

+ **15005** each additional 100 sq cm, or part thereof, or each additional 1% of body area of infants and children (List separately in addition to code for primary procedure)

(Use 15005 in conjunction with 15004)

## *Autografts/Tissue Cultured Autograft*

**15040** Harvest of skin for tissue cultured skin autograft, 100 sq cm or less

**15050** Pinch graft, single or multiple, to cover small ulcer, tip of digit, or other minimal open area (except on face), up to defect size 2 cm diameter

**15100** Split-thickness autograft, trunk, arms, legs; first 100 sq cm or less, or 1% of body area of infants and children (except 15050)

+ **15101** each additional 100 sq cm, or each additional 1% of body area of infants and children, or part thereof (List separately in addition to code for primary procedure)

(Use 15101 in conjunction with 15100)

**15110** Epidermal autograft, trunk, arms, legs; first 100 sq cm or less, or 1% of body area of infants and children

+ **15111** each additional 100 sq cm, or each additional 1% of body area of infants and children, or part thereof (List separately in addition to code for primary procedure)

(Use 15111 in conjunction with 15110)

**15115** Epidermal autograft, face, scalp, eyelids, mouth, neck, ears, orbits, genitalia, hands, feet, and/or multiple digits; first 100 sq cm or less, or 1% of body area of infants and children

+ **15116** each additional 100 sq cm, or each additional 1% of body area of infants and children, or part thereof (List separately in addition to code for primary procedure)

(Use 15116 in conjunction with 15115)

**15120** Split-thickness autograft, face, scalp, eyelids, mouth, neck, ears, orbits, genitalia, hands, feet, and/or multiple digits; first 100 sq cm or less, or 1% of body area of infants and children (except 15050)

+ **15121** each additional 100 sq cm, or each additional 1% of body area of infants and children, or part thereof (List separately in addition to code for primary procedure)

(Use 15121 in conjunction with 15120)

►(For eyelids, see also 67961-67975)◄

**15130** Dermal autograft, trunk, arms, legs; first 100 sq cm or less, or 1% of body area of infants and children

+ **15131** each additional 100 sq cm, or each additional 1% of body area of infants and children, or part thereof (List separately in addition to code for primary procedure)

(Use 15131 in conjunction with 15130)

**15135** Dermal autograft, face, scalp, eyelids, mouth, neck, ears, orbits, genitalia, hands, feet, and/or multiple digits; first 100 sq cm or less, or 1% of body area of infants and children

+ **15136** each additional 100 sq cm, or each additional 1% of body area of infants and children, or part thereof (List separately in addition to code for primary procedure)

(Use 15136 in conjunction with 15135)

▲ **15150** Tissue cultured skin autograft, trunk, arms, legs; first 25 sq cm or less

+▲ **15151** additional 1 sq cm to 75 sq cm (List separately in addition to code for primary procedure)

(Do not report 15151 more than once per session)

(Use 15151 in conjunction with 15150)

+▲ **15152** each additional 100 sq cm, or each additional 1% of body area of infants and children, or part thereof (List separately in addition to code for primary procedure)

(Use 15152 in conjunction with 15151)

▲ **15155** Tissue cultured skin autograft, face, scalp, eyelids, mouth, neck, ears, orbits, genitalia, hands, feet, and/or multiple digits; first 25 sq cm or less

+▲ **15156** additional 1 sq cm to 75 sq cm (List separately in addition to code for primary procedure)

(Do not report 15156 more than once per session)

(Use 15156 in conjunction with 15155)

+▲ **15157** each additional 100 sq cm, or each additional 1% of body area of infants and children, or part thereof (List separately in addition to code for primary procedure)

(Use 15157 in conjunction with 15156)

►(15170-15176 have been deleted. To report, see 15271-15278)◄

**15200** Full thickness graft, free, including direct closure of donor site, trunk; 20 sq cm or less

+ **15201** each additional 20 sq cm, or part thereof (List separately in addition to code for primary procedure)

(Use 15201 in conjunction with 15200)

**15220** Full thickness graft, free, including direct closure of donor site, scalp, arms, and/or legs; 20 sq cm or less

+ **15221** each additional 20 sq cm, or part thereof (List separately in addition to code for primary procedure)

(Use 15221 in conjunction with 15220)

**15240** Full thickness graft, free, including direct closure of donor site, forehead, cheeks, chin, mouth, neck, axillae, genitalia, hands, and/or feet; 20 sq cm or less

(For finger tip graft, use 15050)

(For repair of syndactyly, fingers, see 26560-26562)

**+ 15241**      each additional 20 sq cm, or part thereof (List separately in addition to code for primary procedure)

(Use 15241 in conjunction with 15240)

**15260**      Full thickness graft, free, including direct closure of donor site, nose, ears, eyelids, and/or lips; 20 sq cm or less

**+ 15261**      each additional 20 sq cm, or part thereof (List separately in addition to code for primary procedure)

(Use 15261 in conjunction with 15260)

►(For eyelids, see also 67961-67975)◄

►(Repair of donor site requiring skin graft or local flaps is considered a separate procedure)◄

### ►*Skin Substitute Grafts*◄

►The supply of skin substitute graft(s) should be reported separately in conjunction with 15271-15278. For biologic implant for soft tissue reinforcement, use 15777 in conjunction with code for primary procedure.◄

**● 15271**      Application of skin substitute graft to trunk, arms, legs, total wound surface area up to 100 sq cm; first 25 sq cm or less wound surface area

**+● 15272**      each additional 25 sq cm wound surface area, or part thereof (List separately in addition to code for primary procedure)

►(Use 15272 in conjunction with 15271)◄

►(For total wound surface area greater than or equal to 100 sq cm, see 15273, 15274)◄

►(Do not report 15271, 15272 in conjunction with 15273, 15274)◄

**● 15273**      Application of skin substitute graft to trunk, arms, legs, total wound surface area greater than or equal to 100 sq cm; first 100 sq cm wound surface area, or 1% of body area of infants and children

**+● 15274**      each additional 100 sq cm wound surface area, or part thereof, or each additional 1% of body area of infants and children, or part thereof (List separately in addition to code for primary procedure)

►(Use 15274 in conjunction with 15273)◄

►(For total wound surface area up to 100 sq cm, see 15271, 15272)◄

**● 15275**      Application of skin substitute graft to face, scalp, eyelids, mouth, neck, ears, orbits, genitalia, hands, feet, and/or multiple digits, total wound surface area up to 100 sq cm; first 25 sq cm or less wound surface area

**+● 15276**      each additional 25 sq cm wound surface area, or part thereof (List separately in addition to code for primary procedure)

►(Use 15276 in conjunction with 15275)◄

►(For total wound surface area greater than or equal to 100 sq cm, see 15277, 15278)◄

►(Do not report 15275, 15276 in conjunction with 15277, 15278)◄

**● 15277**      Application of skin substitute graft to face, scalp, eyelids, mouth, neck, ears, orbits, genitalia, hands, feet, and/or multiple digits, total wound surface area greater than or equal to 100 sq cm; first 100 sq cm wound surface area, or 1% of body area of infants and children

**+● 15278**      each additional 100 sq cm wound surface area, or part thereof, or each additional 1% of body area of infants and children, or part thereof (List separately in addition to code for primary procedure)

►(Use 15278 in conjunction with 15277)◄

►(For total wound surface area up to 100 sq cm, see 15275, 15276)◄

►(Do not report 15271-15278 in conjunction with 97602)◄

►(15300, 15301 have been deleted. To report, see 15271-15274)◄

►(15320, 15321 have been deleted. To report, see 15275-15278)◄

►(15330, 15331 have been deleted. To report, see 15271-15274)◄

►(15335, 15336 have been deleted. To report, see 15275-15278)◄

►(15340, 15341 have been deleted. To report, see 15271-15278)◄

►(15360, 15361 have been deleted. To report, see 15271-15274)◄

►(15365, 15366 have been deleted. To report, see 15275-15278)◄

►(15400, 15401 have been deleted. To report, see 15271-15274)◄

►(15420, 15421 have been deleted. To report, see 15275-15278)◄

►(15430, 15431 have been deleted. To report, see 15271-15278)◄

## Flaps (Skin and/or Deep Tissues)

The regions listed refer to the recipient area (not the donor site) when a flap is being attached in a transfer or to a final site.

The regions listed refer to a donor site when a tube is formed for later transfer or when a "delay" of [...] prior to the transfer. Codes 1573[...] by donor site of the muscle, [...] fasciocutaneous flap.

▲=Revised code   ●=New code   ►◄=Contains new or revised text   ⊘=Modifier 51 exempt

**Surgery: Integumentary System**

Codes 15570-15738 do not include extensive immobilization (eg, large plaster casts and other immobilizing devices are considered additional separate procedures).

A repair of a donor site requiring a skin graft or local flaps is considered an additional separate procedure.

> (For microvascular flaps, see 15756-15758)
>
> (For flaps without inclusion of a vascular pedicle, see 15570-15576)
>
> (For adjacent tissue transfer flaps, see 14000-14302)

**15570** Formation of direct or tubed pedicle, with or without transfer; trunk

**15572** scalp, arms, or legs

**15574** forehead, cheeks, chin, mouth, neck, axillae, genitalia, hands or feet

**15576** eyelids, nose, ears, lips, or intraoral

**15600** Delay of flap or sectioning of flap (division and inset); at trunk

**15610** at scalp, arms, or legs

**15620** at forehead, cheeks, chin, neck, axillae, genitalia, hands, or feet

**15630** at eyelids, nose, ears, or lips

**15650** Transfer, intermediate, of any pedicle flap (eg, abdomen to wrist, Walking tube), any location

> (For eyelids, nose, ears, or lips, see also anatomical area)
>
> (For revision, defatting or rearranging of transferred pedicle flap or skin graft, see 13100-14302)

**15731** Forehead flap with preservation of vascular pedicle (eg, axial pattern flap, paramedian forehead flap)

> (For muscle, myocutaneous, or fasciocutaneous flap of the head or neck, use 15732)

**15732** Muscle, myocutaneous, or fasciocutaneous flap; head and neck (eg, temporalis, masseter muscle, sternocleidomastoid, levator scapulae)

> (For forehead flap with preservation of vascular pedicle, use 15731)

**15734** trunk

**15736** upper extremity

**15738** lower extremity

## Other Flaps and Grafts

Code 15740 describes a cutaneous flap, transposed into a nearby but not immediately adjacent defect, with a pedicle that incorporates an axial vessel into its design. The flap is typically transferred through a tunnel underneath the skin and sutured into its new position. The donor site is closed directly.

Neurovascular pedicle procedures are reported with 15750. This code includes not only skin but also a functional motor or sensory nerve(s). The flap serves to reinnervate a damaged portion of the body dependent on touch or movement (eg, thumb).

Repair of donor site requiring skin graft or local flaps should be reported as an additional procedure.

**15740** Flap; island pedicle

**15750** neurovascular pedicle

> (For random island flaps, V-Y subcutaneous flaps and other flaps from adjacent areas, see 14000-14302)

**15756** Free muscle or myocutaneous flap with microvascular anastomosis

> (Do not report code 69990 in addition to code 15756)

**15757** Free skin flap with microvascular anastomosis

> (Do not report code 69990 in addition to code 15757)

**15758** Free fascial flap with microvascular anastomosis

> (Do not report code 69990 in addition to code 15758)

**15760** Graft; composite (eg, full thickness of external ear or nasal ala), including primary closure, donor area

**15770** derma-fat-fascia

**15775** Punch graft for hair transplant; 1 to 15 punch grafts

**15776** more than 15 punch grafts

> (For strip transplant, use 15220)

+● **15777** Implantation of biologic implant (eg, acellular dermal matrix) for soft tissue reinforcement (eg, breast, trunk) (List separately in addition to code for primary procedure)

> ►(For bilateral breast procedure, report 15777 with modifier 50)◄
>
> ►(For implantation of mesh or other prosthesis for open incisional or ventral hernia repair, use 49568 in conjunction with 49560-49566)◄
>
> ►(For insertion of mesh or other prosthesis for closure of a necrotizing soft tissue infection wound, use 49568 in conjunction with 11004-11006)◄
>
> ►(For topical application of skin substitute graft to a wound surface, see 15271-15278)◄
>
> ►(For repair of anorectal fistula with plug (eg, porcine small intestine submucosa [SIS]), use 46707)◄
>
> ►(For insertion of mesh or other prosthesis for repair of pelvic floor defect, use 57267)◄
>
> ►(The supply of biologic implant should be reported separately in conjunction with 15777)◄

## Other Procedures

**15780**    Dermabrasion; total face (eg, for acne scarring, fine wrinkling, rhytids, general keratosis)

**15781**        segmental, face

**15782**        regional, other than face

**15783**        superficial, any site (eg, tattoo removal)

**15786**    Abrasion; single lesion (eg, keratosis, scar)

**+ 15787**        each additional 4 lesions or less (List separately in addition to code for primary procedure)

(Use 15787 in conjunction with 15786)

**15788**    Chemical peel, facial; epidermal

**15789**        dermal

**15792**    Chemical peel, nonfacial; epidermal

**15793**        dermal

**15819**    Cervicoplasty

**15820**    Blepharoplasty, lower eyelid;

**15821**        with extensive herniated fat pad

**15822**    Blepharoplasty, upper eyelid;

**15823**        with excessive skin weighting down lid

(For bilateral blepharoplasty, add modifier 50)

**15824**    Rhytidectomy; forehead

(For repair of brow ptosis, use 67900)

**15825**        neck with platysmal tightening (platysmal flap, P-flap)

**15826**        glabellar frown lines

**15828**        cheek, chin, and neck

**15829**        superficial musculoaponeurotic system (SMAS) flap

(For bilateral rhytidectomy, add modifier 50)

**15830**    Excision, excessive skin and subcutaneous tissue (includes lipectomy); abdomen, infraumbilical panniculectomy

(Do not report 15830 in conjunction with 12031-12037, 13100-13102, 14000, 14001, 14302)

**15832**        thigh

**15833**        leg

**15834**        hip

**15835**        buttock

**15836**        arm

**15837**        forearm or hand

**15838**        submental fat pad

**15839**        other area

(For bilateral procedure, add modifier 50)

**15840**    Graft for facial nerve paralysis; free fascia graft (including obtaining fascia)

(For bilateral procedure, add modifier 50)

**15841**        free muscle graft (including obtaining graft)

**15842**        free muscle flap by microsurgical technique

(Do not report code 69990 in addition to code 15842)

**15845**        regional muscle transfer

(For intravenous fluorescein examination of blood flow in graft or flap, use 15860)

(For nerve transfers, decompression, or repair, see 64831-64876, 64905, 64907, 69720, 69725, 69740, 69745, 69955)

**+ 15847**    Excision, excessive skin and subcutaneous tissue (includes lipectomy), abdomen (eg, abdominoplasty) (includes umbilical transposition and fascial plication) (List separately in addition to code for primary procedure)

(Use 15847 in conjunction with 15830)

(For abdominal wall hernia repair, see 49491-49587)

(To report other abdominoplasty, use 17999)

**15850**    Removal of sutures under anesthesia (other than local), same surgeon

**15851**    Removal of sutures under anesthesia (other than local), other surgeon

**15852**    Dressing change (for other than burns) under anesthesia (other than local)

**15860**    Intravenous injection of agent (eg, fluorescein) to test vascular flow in flap or graft

**15876**    Suction assisted lipectomy; head and neck

**15877**        trunk

**15878**        upper extremity

**15879**        lower extremity

## Pressure Ulcers (Decubitus Ulcers)

**15920**    Excision, coccygeal pressure ulcer, with coccygectomy; with primary suture

**15922**        with flap closure

**15931**    Excision, sacral pressure ulcer, with primary suture;

**15933**        with ostectomy

**15934**    Excision, sacral pressure ulcer, with skin flap closure;

**15935**        with ostectomy

**15936**    Excision, sacral pressure ulcer, in prepar... or myocutaneous flap or skin...

**15937**        with ostectomy

(For repair of defect using
use code(s) 15734 and/or 1...
15937. For repair of defect u...
codes 15100 and/or 15101 in...

**15940** Excision, ischial pressure ulcer, with primary suture;

**15941** with ostectomy (ischiectomy)

**15944** Excision, ischial pressure ulcer, with skin flap closure;

**15945** with ostectomy

**15946** Excision, ischial pressure ulcer, with ostectomy, in preparation for muscle or myocutaneous flap or skin graft closure

(For repair of defect using muscle or myocutaneous flap, use code(s) 15734 and/or 15738 in addition to 15946. For repair of defect using split skin graft, use codes 15100 and/or 15101 in addition to 15946)

**15950** Excision, trochanteric pressure ulcer, with primary suture;

**15951** with ostectomy

**15952** Excision, trochanteric pressure ulcer, with skin flap closure;

**15953** with ostectomy

**15956** Excision, trochanteric pressure ulcer, in preparation for muscle or myocutaneous flap or skin graft closure;

**15958** with ostectomy

(For repair of defect using muscle or myocutaneous flap, use code(s) 15734 and/or 15738 in addition to 15956, 15958. For repair of defect using split skin graft, use codes 15100 and/or 15101 in addition to 15956, 15958)

**15999** Unlisted procedure, excision pressure ulcer

(For free skin graft to close ulcer or donor site, see 15002 et seq)

## Burns, Local Treatment

▶Procedures 16000-16036 refer to local treatment of burned surface only. Codes 16020-16030 include the application of materials (eg, dressings) not described in codes 15100-15278.◀

List percentage of body surface involved and depth of burn.

For necessary related medical services (eg, hospital visits, detention) in management of burned patients, see appropriate services in **Evaluation and Management** and **Medicine** sections.

For the application of skin grafts or skin substitutes, see codes 15100-15650.

**16000** Initial treatment, first degree burn, when no more than local treatment is required

**16020** Dressings and/or debridement of partial-thickness burns, initial or subsequent; small (less than 5% total body surface area)

**16025** medium (eg, whole face or whole extremity, or 5% to 10% total body surface area)

**16030** large (eg, more than 1 extremity, or greater than 10% total body surface area)

**16035** Escharotomy; initial incision

**+ 16036** each additional incision (List separately in addition to code for primary procedure)

(Use 16036 in conjunction with 16035)

(For debridement, curettement of burn wound, see 16020-16030)

## Destruction

*Destruction* means the ablation of benign, premalignant or malignant tissues by any method, with or without curettement, including local anesthesia, and not usually requiring closure.

Any method includes electrosurgery, cryosurgery, laser and chemical treatment. Lesions include condylomata, papillomata, molluscum contagiosum, herpetic lesions, warts (ie, common, plantar, flat), milia, or other benign, premalignant (eg, actinic keratoses), or malignant lesions.

(For destruction of lesion(s) in specific anatomic sites, see 40820, 46900-46917, 46924, 54050-54057, 54065, 56501, 56515, 57061, 57065, 67850, 68135)

(For laser treatment for inflammatory skin disease, see 96920-96922)

(For paring or cutting of benign hyperkeratotic lesions (eg, corns or calluses), see 11055-11057)

(For sharp removal or electrosurgical destruction of skin tags and fibrocutaneous tags, see 11200, 11201)

(For cryotherapy of acne, use 17340)

(For initiation or follow-up care of topical chemotherapy (eg, 5-FU or similar agents), see appropriate office visits)

(For shaving of epidermal or dermal lesions, see 11300-11313)

## Destruction, Benign or Premalignant Lesions

**17000** Destruction (eg, laser surgery, electrosurgery, cryosurgery, chemosurgery, surgical curettement), premalignant lesions (eg, actinic keratoses); first lesion

**+ 17003** second through 14 lesions, each (List separately in addition to code for first lesion)

(Use 17003 in conjunction with 17000)

(For destruction of common or plantar warts, see 17110, 17111)

⊘ **17004** Destruction (eg, laser surgery, electrosurgery, cryosurgery, chemosurgery, surgical curettement), premalignant lesions (eg, actinic keratoses), 15 or more lesions

(Do not report 17004 in conjunction with 17000-17003)

**17106** Destruction of cutaneous vascular proliferative lesions (eg, laser technique); less than 10 sq cm

| | |
|---|---|
| **17107** | 10.0 to 50.0 sq cm |
| **17108** | over 50.0 sq cm |
| **17110** | Destruction (eg, laser surgery, electrosurgery, cryosurgery, chemosurgery, surgical curettement), of benign lesions other than skin tags or cutaneous vascular proliferative lesions; up to 14 lesions |
| **17111** | 15 or more lesions |
| **17250** | Chemical cauterization of granulation tissue (proud flesh, sinus or fistula) |

(17250 is not to be used with removal or excision codes for the same lesion)

## Destruction, Malignant Lesions, Any Method

| | |
|---|---|
| **17260** | Destruction, malignant lesion (eg, laser surgery, electrosurgery, cryosurgery, chemosurgery, surgical curettement), trunk, arms or legs; lesion diameter 0.5 cm or less |
| **17261** | lesion diameter 0.6 to 1.0 cm |
| **17262** | lesion diameter 1.1 to 2.0 cm |
| **17263** | lesion diameter 2.1 to 3.0 cm |
| **17264** | lesion diameter 3.1 to 4.0 cm |
| **17266** | lesion diameter over 4.0 cm |
| **17270** | Destruction, malignant lesion (eg, laser surgery, electrosurgery, cryosurgery, chemosurgery, surgical curettement), scalp, neck, hands, feet, genitalia; lesion diameter 0.5 cm or less |
| **17271** | lesion diameter 0.6 to 1.0 cm |
| **17272** | lesion diameter 1.1 to 2.0 cm |
| **17273** | lesion diameter 2.1 to 3.0 cm |
| **17274** | lesion diameter 3.1 to 4.0 cm |
| **17276** | lesion diameter over 4.0 cm |
| **17280** | Destruction, malignant lesion (eg, laser surgery, electrosurgery, cryosurgery, chemosurgery, surgical curettement), face, ears, eyelids, nose, lips, mucous membrane; lesion diameter 0.5 cm or less |
| **17281** | lesion diameter 0.6 to 1.0 cm |
| **17282** | lesion diameter 1.1 to 2.0 cm |
| **17283** | lesion diameter 2.1 to 3.0 cm |
| **17284** | lesion diameter 3.1 to 4.0 cm |
| **17286** | lesion diameter over 4.0 cm |

## Mohs Micrographic Surgery

Mohs micrographic surgery is a technique for the removal of complex or ill-defined skin cancer with histologic examination of 100% of the surgical margins. It requires a single physician to act in two integrated but separate and distinct capacities: surgeon and pathologist. If either of these responsibilities is delegated to another physician who reports the services separately, these codes should not be reported. The Mohs surgeon removes the tumor tissue and maps and divides the tumor specimen into pieces, and each piece is embedded into an individual tissue block for histopathologic examination. Thus a tissue block in Mohs surgery is defined as an individual tissue piece embedded in a mounting medium for sectioning.

If repair is performed, use separate repair, flap, or graft codes. If a biopsy of a suspected skin cancer is performed on the same day as Mohs surgery because there was no prior pathology confirmation of a diagnosis, then report diagnostic skin biopsy (11100, 11101) and frozen section pathology (88331) with modifier 59 to distinguish from the subsequent definitive surgical procedure of Mohs surgery.

(If additional special pathology procedures, stains or immunostains are required, use 88311-88314, 88342)

(Do not report 88314 in conjunction with 17311-17315 for routine frozen section stain (eg, hematoxylin and eosin, toluidine blue) performed during Mohs surgery. When a nonroutine histochemical stain on frozen tissue is utilized, report 88314 with modifier 59)

(Do not report 88302-88309 on the same specimen as part of the Mohs surgery)

| | |
|---|---|
| **17311** | Mohs micrographic technique, including removal of all gross tumor, surgical excision of tissue specimens, mapping, color coding of specimens, microscopic examination of specimens by the surgeon, and histopathologic preparation including routine stain(s) (eg, hematoxylin and eosin, toluidine blue), head, neck, hands, feet, genitalia, or any location with surgery directly involving muscle, cartilage, bone, tendon, major nerves, or vessels; first stage, up to 5 tissue blocks |
| **+ 17312** | each additional stage after the first stage, up to 5 tissue blocks (List separately in addition to code for primary procedure) |

(Use 17312 in conjunction with 17311)

| | |
|---|---|
| **17313** | Mohs micrographic technique, including removal of all gross tumor, surgical excision of tissue specimens, mapping, color coding of specimens, microscopic examination of specimens by the surgeon, and histopathologic preparation including routi~~ne~~ hematoxylin and eosin, toluidine ~~blue~~ or legs; first stage, up t~~o~~ |
| **+ 17314** | each additional stage tissue blocks (List sepa~~rately~~ primary procedure) |

(Use 17314 in conjunction wi~~th~~

▲=Revised code    ●=New code    ►◄=Contains new or revised text    ⊘=Modifier 51 exempt

American M~~edical~~

**+ 17315** Mohs micrographic technique, including removal of all gross tumor, surgical excision of tissue specimens, mapping, color coding of specimens, microscopic examination of specimens by the surgeon, and histopathologic preparation including routine stain(s) (eg, hematoxylin and eosin, toluidine blue), each additional block after the first 5 tissue blocks, any stage (List separately in addition to code for primary procedure)

(Use 17315 in conjunction with 17311-17314)

## Other Procedures

**17340** Cryotherapy ($CO_2$ slush, liquid $N_2$) for acne

**17360** Chemical exfoliation for acne (eg, acne paste, acid)

**17380** Electrolysis epilation, each 30 minutes

(For actinotherapy, use 96900)

**17999** Unlisted procedure, skin, mucous membrane and subcutaneous tissue

# Breast

## Incision

**19000** Puncture aspiration of cyst of breast;

**+ 19001** each additional cyst (List separately in addition to code for primary procedure)

(Use 19001 in conjunction with 19000)

(If imaging guidance is performed, see 76942, 77021, 77031, 77032)

**19020** Mastotomy with exploration or drainage of abscess, deep

**19030** Injection procedure only for mammary ductogram or galactogram

(For radiological supervision and interpretation, see 77053, 77054)

## Excision

Excisional breast surgery includes certain biopsy procedures, the removal of cysts or other benign or malignant tumors or lesions, and the surgical treatment of breast and chest wall malignancies. Biopsy procedures may be percutaneous or open, and they involve the removal of differing amounts of tissue for diagnosis.

Breast biopsies are reported using codes 19100-19103. The open excision of breast lesions (eg, lesions of the breast ducts, cysts, benign or malignant tumors), without specific attention to adequate surgical margins, with or without the preoperative placement of radiological markers, is reported using codes 19110-19126. Partial mastectomy procedures (eg, lumpectomy, tylectomy, quadrantectomy, or segmentectomy) describe open excisions of breast tissue with specific attention to adequate surgical margins.

Partial mastectomy procedures are reported using codes 19301 or 19302 as appropriate. Documentation for partial mastectomy procedures includes attention to the removal of adequate surgical margins surrounding the breast mass or lesion.

Total mastectomy procedures include simple mastectomy, complete mastectomy, subcutaneous mastectomy, modified radical mastectomy, radical mastectomy, and more extended procedures (eg, Urban type operation). Total mastectomy procedures are reported using codes 19303-19307 as appropriate.

Excisions or resections of chest wall tumors including ribs, with or without reconstruction, with or without mediastinal lymphadenectomy, are reported using codes 19260, 19271, or 19272. Codes 19260-19272 are not restricted to breast tumors and are used to report resections of chest wall tumors originating from any chest wall component. (For excision of lung or pleura, see 32310 et seq)

(To report bilateral procedure, report modifier 50 with the procedure code)

**19100** Biopsy of breast; percutaneous, needle core, not using imaging guidance (separate procedure)

(For fine needle aspiration, use 10021)

(For image guided breast biopsy, see 19102, 19103, 10022)

**19101** open, incisional

**19102** percutaneous, needle core, using imaging guidance

(For placement of percutaneous localization clip, use 19295)

**19103** percutaneous, automated vacuum assisted or rotating biopsy device, using imaging guidance

(For imaging guidance performed in conjunction with 19102, 19103, see 76942, 77012, 77021, 77031, 77032)

(For placement of percutaneous localization clip, use 19295)

**19105** Ablation, cryosurgical, of fibroadenoma, including ultrasound guidance, each fibroadenoma

(Do not report 19105 in conjunction with 76940, 76942)

(For adjacent lesions treated with 1 cryoprobe insertion, report once)

**19110** Nipple exploration, with or without excision of a solitary lactiferous duct or a papilloma lactiferous duct

**19112** Excision of lactiferous duct fistula

**19120** Excision of cyst, fibroadenoma, or other benign or malignant tumor, aberrant breast tissue, duct lesion, nipple or areolar lesion (except 19300), open, male or female, 1 or more lesions

**19125** Excision of breast lesion identified by preoperative placement of radiological marker, open; single lesion

Surgery: Integumentary System

**+ 19126**     each additional lesion separately identified by a preoperative radiological marker (List separately in addition to code for primary procedure)

(Use 19126 in conjunction with 19125)

**19260**     Excision of chest wall tumor including ribs

**19271**     Excision of chest wall tumor involving ribs, with plastic reconstruction; without mediastinal lymphadenectomy

**19272**     with mediastinal lymphadenectomy

(Do not report 19260, 19271, 19272 in conjunction with 32100, 32422, 32503, 32504, 32551)

## Introduction

**19290**     Preoperative placement of needle localization wire, breast;

**+ 19291**     each additional lesion (List separately in addition to code for primary procedure)

(Use 19291 in conjunction with 19290)

(For radiological supervision and interpretation, see 76942, 77031, 77032)

**+ 19295**     Image guided placement, metallic localization clip, percutaneous, during breast biopsy/aspiration (List separately in addition to code for primary procedure)

(Use 19295 in conjunction with 10022, 19102, 19103)

**19296**     Placement of radiotherapy afterloading expandable catheter (single or multichannel) into the breast for interstitial radioelement application following partial mastectomy, includes imaging guidance; on date separate from partial mastectomy

**+ 19297**     concurrent with partial mastectomy (List separately in addition to code for primary procedure)

(Use 19297 in conjunction with 19301 or 19302)

**⊙ 19298**     Placement of radiotherapy afterloading brachytherapy catheters (multiple tube and button type) into the breast for interstitial radioelement application following (at the time of or subsequent to) partial mastectomy, includes imaging guidance

## Mastectomy Procedures

**19300**     Mastectomy for gynecomastia

**19301**     Mastectomy, partial (eg, lumpectomy, tylectomy, quadrantectomy, segmentectomy);

**19302**     with axillary lymphadenectomy

(For placement of radiotherapy afterloading balloon/brachytherapy catheters, see 19296-19298)

**19303**     Mastectomy, simple, complete

(For immediate or delayed insertion of implant, see 19340, 19342)

(For gynecomastia, use 19300)

**19304**     Mastectomy, subcutaneous

(For immediate or delayed insertion of implant, see 19340, 19342)

**19305**     Mastectomy, radical, including pectoral muscles, axillary lymph nodes

(For immediate or delayed insertion of implant, see 19340, 19342)

**19306**     Mastectomy, radical, including pectoral muscles, axillary and internal mammary lymph nodes (Urban type operation)

(For immediate or delayed insertion of implant, see 19340, 19342)

**19307**     Mastectomy, modified radical, including axillary lymph nodes, with or without pectoralis minor muscle, but excluding pectoralis major muscle

(For immediate or delayed insertion of implant, see 19340, 19342)

## Repair and/or Reconstruction

(To report bilateral procedure, report modifier 50 with the procedure code)

▶(For biologic implant for soft tissue reinforcement, use 15777 in conjunction with primary procedure)◀

**19316**     Mastopexy

**19318**     Reduction mammaplasty

**19324**     Mammaplasty, augmentation; without prosthetic implant

**19325**     with prosthetic implant

(For flap or graft, use also appropriate number)

**19328**     Removal of intact mammary implant

**19330**     Removal of mammary implant material

**19340**     Immediate insertion of breast prosthesis following mastopexy, mastectomy or in reconstruction

**19342**     Delayed insertion of breast prosthesis following mastopexy, mastectomy or in reconstruction

(For supply of implant, use 99070)

(For preparation of custom breast implant, use 19396)

**19350**     Nipple/areola reconstruction

**19355**     Correction of inverted nipples

**19357**     Breast reconstruction, immediate or delayed, with tissue expander, including subsequent expansion

**19361**     Breast reconstruction with latissimus dorsi flap, without prosthetic implant

(For insertion of prosthesis, use

**Surgery: Integumentary System**

**19364** Breast reconstruction with free flap

(Do not report code 69990 in addition to code 19364)

(19364 includes harvesting of the flap, microvascular transfer, closure of the donor site, and inset shaping the flap into a breast)

**19366** Breast reconstruction with other technique

(For operating microscope, use 69990)

(For insertion of prosthesis, use also 19340 or 19342)

**19367** Breast reconstruction with transverse rectus abdominis myocutaneous flap (TRAM), single pedicle, including closure of donor site;

**19368** with microvascular anastomosis (supercharging)

(Do not report code 69990 in addition to code 19368)

**19369** Breast reconstruction with transverse rectus abdominis myocutaneous flap (TRAM), double pedicle, including closure of donor site

**19370** Open periprosthetic capsulotomy, breast

**19371** Periprosthetic capsulectomy, breast

**19380** Revision of reconstructed breast

**19396** Preparation of moulage for custom breast implant

# Other Procedures

**19499** Unlisted procedure, breast

# Musculoskeletal System

Cast and strapping procedures appear at the end of this section.

The services listed below include the application and removal of the first cast or traction device only. Subsequent replacement of cast and/or traction device may require an additional listing.

**Definitions**

The terms "closed treatment," "open treatment," and "percutaneous skeletal fixation" have been carefully chosen to accurately reflect current orthopaedic procedural treatments.

*Closed treatment* specifically means that the fracture site is not surgically opened (exposed to the external environment and directly visualized). This terminology is used to describe procedures that treat fractures by three methods: (1) without manipulation; (2) with manipulation; or (3) with or without traction.

*Open treatment* is used when the fractured bone is either: (1) surgically opened (exposed to the external environment) and the fracture (bone ends) visualized and internal fixation may be used; or (2) the fractured bone is opened remote from the fracture site in order to insert an intramedullary nail across the fracture site (the fracture site is not opened and visualized).

*Percutaneous skeletal fixation* describes fracture treatment which is neither open nor closed. In this procedure, the fracture fragments are not visualized, but fixation (eg, pins) is placed across the fracture site, usually under X-ray imaging.

The type of fracture (eg, open, compound, closed) does not have any coding correlation with the type of treatment (eg, closed, open, or percutaneous) provided.

The codes for treatment of fractures and joint injuries (dislocations) are categorized by the type of manipulation (reduction) and stabilization (fixation or immobilization). These codes can apply to either open (compound) or closed fractures or joint injuries.

Skeletal traction is the application of a force (distracting or traction force) to a limb segment through a wire, pin, screw, or clamp that is attached (eg, penetrates) to bone.

Skin traction is the application of a force (longitudinal) to a limb using felt or strapping applied directly to skin only.

External fixation is the usage of skeletal pins plus an attaching mechanism/device used for temporary or definitive treatment of acute or chronic bony deformity.

Codes for obtaining autogenous bone grafts, cartilage, tendon, fascia lata grafts or other tissues through separate incisions are to be used only when the graft is not already listed as part of the basic procedure.

Re-reduction of a fracture and/or dislocation performed by the primary physician may be identified by the addition of the modifier 76 to the usual procedure number to indicate "Repeat Procedure or Service by Same Physician." (See Appendix A guidelines.)

Codes for external fixation are to be used only when external fixation is not already listed as part of the basic procedure.

All codes for suction irrigation have been deleted. To report, list only the primary surgical procedure performed (eg, sequestrectomy, deep incision).

*Manipulation* is used throughout the musculoskeletal fracture and dislocation subsections to specifically mean the attempted reduction or restoration of a fracture or joint dislocation to its normal anatomic alignment by the application of manually applied forces.

*Excision of subcutaneous soft tissue tumors* (including simple or intermediate repair) involves the simple or marginal resection of tumors confined to subcutaneous tissue below the skin but above the deep fascia. These tumors are usually benign and are resected without removing a significant amount of surrounding normal tissue. Code selection is based on the location and size of the tumor. Code selection is determined by measuring the greatest diameter of the tumor plus that margin required for complete excision of the tumor. The margins refer to the most narrow margin required to adequately excise the tumor, based on the physician's judgment. The measurement of the tumor plus margin is made at the time of the excision. Appreciable vessel exploration and/or neuroplasty should be reported separately. Extensive undermining or other techniques to close a defect created by skin excision may require a complex repair which should be reported separately. Dissection or elevation of tissue planes to permit resection of the tumor is included in the excision.

*Excision of fascial or subfascial soft tissue tumors* (including simple or intermediate repair) involves the resection of tumors confined to the tissue within or below the deep fascia, but not involving the bone. These tumors are usually benign, are often intramuscular, and are resected without removing a significant amount of surrounding normal tissue. Code selection is based on size and location of the tumor. Code selection is determined by measuring the greatest diameter of the tumor plus that margin required for complete excision of the tumor. The margins refer to the most narrow margin required to adequately excise the tumor, based on the physician's judgment. The measurement of the tumor plus margin is made at the time of the excision. Appreciable vessel exploration and/or neuroplasty be reported separately. Extensive undermin techniques to close a defect created require a complex repair which s separately. Dissection or elevation permit resection of the tumor is inc

Surgery: Musculoskeletal System

**Surgery: Musculoskeletal System**

Digital (ie, fingers and toes) subfascial tumors are defined as those tumors involving the tendons, tendon sheaths, or joints of the digit. Tumors which simply abut but do not breach the tendon, tendon sheath, or joint capsule are considered subcutaneous soft tissue tumors.

*Radical resection of soft tissue tumors* (including simple or intermediate repair) involves the resection of the tumor with wide margins of normal tissue. Appreciable vessel exploration and/or neuroplasty repair or reconstruction (eg, adjacent tissue transfer[s], flap[s]) should be reported separately. Extensive undermining or other techniques to close a defect created by skin excision may require a complex repair which should be reported separately. Dissection or elevation of tissue planes to permit resection of the tumor is included in the excision. Although these tumors may be confined to a specific layer (eg, subcutaneous, subfascial), radical resection may involve removal of tissue from one or more layers. Radical resection of soft tissue tumors is most commonly used for malignant tumors or very aggressive benign tumors. Code selection is based on size and location of the tumor. Code selection is determined by measuring the greatest diameter of the tumor plus that margin required for complete excision of the tumor. The margins refer to the most narrow margin required to adequately excise the tumor, based on the physician's judgment. The measurement of the tumor plus margin is made at the time of the excision. For radical resection of tumors of cutaneous origin, (eg, melanoma) see 11600-11646.

*Radical resection of bone tumors* (including simple or intermediate repair) involves the resection of the tumor with wide margins of normal tissue. Appreciable vessel exploration and/or neuroplasty and complex bone repair or reconstruction (eg, adjacent tissue transfer[s], flap[s]) should be reported separately. Extensive undermining or other techniques to close a defect created by skin excision may require a complex repair which should be reported separately. Dissection or elevation of tissue planes to permit resection of the tumor is included in the excision. It may require removal of the entire bone if tumor growth is extensive (eg, clavicle). Radical resection of bone tumors is usually performed for malignant tumors or very aggressive benign tumors. If surrounding soft tissue is removed during these procedures, the radical resection of soft tissue tumor codes should not be reported separately. Code selection is based solely on the location of the tumor, **not** on the size of the tumor or whether the tumor is benign or malignant, primary or metastatic.

# General

## Incision

(20000 has been deleted)

(For incision and drainage procedures, cutaneous/subcutaneous, see 10060, 10061)

| | |
|---|---|
| 20005 | Incision and drainage of soft tissue abscess, subfascial (ie, involves the soft tissue below the deep fascia) |

## Wound Exploration—Trauma (eg, Penetrating Gunshot, Stab Wound)

20100-20103 relate to wound(s) resulting from penetrating trauma. These codes describe surgical exploration and enlargement of the wound, extension of dissection (to determine penetration), debridement, removal of foreign body(s), ligation or coagulation of minor subcutaneous and/or muscular blood vessel(s), of the subcutaneous tissue, muscle fascia, and/or muscle, not requiring thoracotomy or laparotomy. If a repair is done to major structure(s) or major blood vessel(s) requiring thoracotomy or laparotomy, then those specific code(s) would supersede the use of codes 20100-20103. To report simple, intermediate, or complex repair of wound(s) that do not require enlargement of the wound, extension of dissection, etc, as stated above, use specific Repair code(s) in the **Integumentary System** section.

| | |
|---|---|
| 20100 | Exploration of penetrating wound (separate procedure); neck |
| 20101 | chest |
| 20102 | abdomen/flank/back |
| 20103 | extremity |

## Excision

| | |
|---|---|
| 20150 | Excision of epiphyseal bar, with or without autogenous soft tissue graft obtained through same fascial incision |
| | (For aspiration of bone marrow, use 38220) |
| 20200 | Biopsy, muscle; superficial |
| 20205 | deep |
| 20206 | Biopsy, muscle, percutaneous needle |
| | (If imaging guidance is performed, see 76942, 77012, 77021) |
| | (For fine needle aspiration, use 10021 or 10022) |
| | (For evaluation of fine needle aspirate, see 88172-88173) |
| | (For excision of muscle tumor, deep, see specific anatomic section) |
| 20220 | Biopsy, bone, trocar, or needle; superficial (eg, ilium, sternum, spinous process, ribs) |
| 20225 | deep (eg, vertebral body, femur) |
| | (For bone marrow biopsy, use 38221) |
| | (For radiologic supervision and interpretation, see 77002, 77012, 77021) |
| 20240 | Biopsy, bone, open; superficial (eg, ilium, sternum, spinous process, ribs, trochanter of femur) |
| 20245 | deep (eg, humerus, ischium, femur) |

**20250**    Biopsy, vertebral body, open; thoracic

**20251**         lumbar or cervical

         (For sequestrectomy, osteomyelitis or drainage of bone abscess, see anatomical area)

## Introduction or Removal

         (For injection procedure for arthrography, see anatomical area)

**20500**    Injection of sinus tract; therapeutic (separate procedure)

**20501**         diagnostic (sinogram)

         (For radiological supervision and interpretation, use 76080)

         (For contrast injection[s] and radiological assessment of gastrostomy, duodenostomy, jejunostomy, gastro-jejunostomy, or cecostomy [or other colonic] tube including fluoroscopic imaging guidance, use 49465)

**20520**    Removal of foreign body in muscle or tendon sheath; simple

**20525**         deep or complicated

**20526**    Injection, therapeutic (eg, local anesthetic, corticosteroid), carpal tunnel

● **20527**    Injection, enzyme (eg, collagenase), palmar fascial cord (ie, Dupuytren's contracture)

         ►(For manipulation of palmar fascial cord (ie, Dupuytren's cord) post enzyme injection (eg, collagenase), use 26341)◄

**20550**    Injection(s); single tendon sheath, or ligament, aponeurosis (eg, plantar "fascia")

         (For injection of Morton's neuroma, see 64455, 64632)

**20551**         single tendon origin/insertion

         (Do not report 20550, 20551 in conjunction with 0232T)

         (For injection(s) of platelet rich plasma, use 0232T)

**20552**    Injection(s); single or multiple trigger point(s), 1 or 2 muscle(s)

**20553**         single or multiple trigger point(s), 3 or more muscle(s)

         (If imaging guidance is performed, see 76942, 77002, 77021)

**20555**    Placement of needles or catheters into muscle and/or soft tissue for subsequent interstitial radioelement application (at the time of or subsequent to the procedure)

         (For placement of devices into the breast for interstitial radioelement application, see 19296-19298)

         (For placement of needles, catheters, or devices into muscle or soft tissue of the head and neck, for interstitial radioelement application, use 41019)

         (For placement of needles or catheters for interstitial radioelement application into prostate, use 55875)

         (For placement of needles or catheters into the pelvic organs or genitalia [except prostate] for interstitial radioelement application, use 55920)

         (For interstitial radioelement application, see 77776-77778, 77785-77787)

         (For imaging guidance, see 76942, 77002, 77012, 77021)

**20600**    Arthrocentesis, aspiration and/or injection; small joint or bursa (eg, fingers, toes)

**20605**         intermediate joint or bursa (eg, temporomandibular, acromioclavicular, wrist, elbow or ankle, olecranon bursa)

**20610**         major joint or bursa (eg, shoulder, hip, knee joint, subacromial bursa)

         (If imaging guidance is performed, see 76942, 77002, 77012, 77021)

**20612**    Aspiration and/or injection of ganglion cyst(s) any location

         (To report multiple ganglion cyst aspirations/injections, use 20612 and append modifier 59)

**20615**    Aspiration and injection for treatment of bone cyst

**20650**    Insertion of wire or pin with application of skeletal traction, including removal (separate procedure)

**20660**    Application of cranial tongs, caliper, or stereotactic frame, including removal (separate procedure)

**20661**    Application of halo, including removal; cranial

**20662**         pelvic

**20663**         femoral

**20664**    Application of halo, including removal, cranial, 6 or more pins placed, for thin skull osteology (eg, pediatric patients, hydrocephalus, osteogenesis imperfecta)

**20665**    Removal of tongs or halo applied by another physician

**20670**    Removal of implant; superficial (eg, buried wire, pin or rod) (separate procedure)

**20680**         deep (eg, buried wire, pin, screw, metal band, nail, rod or plate)

**20690**    Application of a uniplane (pins or wires in 1 plane), unilateral, external fixation system

**20692**    Application of a multiplane (pins or wires in more than 1 plane), unilateral, external fixation system (eg, Ilizarov, Monticelli type)

**20693**    Adjustment or revision of external fixation system requiring anesthesia (eg, new pin[s] or wire[s] and/or new ring[s] or bar[s])

**20694**    Removal, under anesthesia, of external fixation system

---

▲ =Revised code   ● =New code   ► ◄ =Contains new or revised text   ⊘ =Modifier 51 exempt          American Medic

**20696**   Application of multiplane (pins or wires in more than 1 plane), unilateral, external fixation with stereotactic computer-assisted adjustment (eg, spatial frame), including imaging; initial and subsequent alignment(s), assessment(s), and computation(s) of adjustment schedule(s)

(Do not report 20696 in conjunction with 20692, 20697)

⊘ **20697**      exchange (ie, removal and replacement) of strut, each

(Do not report 20697 in conjunction with 20692, 20696)

## Replantation

**20802**   Replantation, arm (includes surgical neck of humerus through elbow joint), complete amputation

(To report replantation of incomplete arm amputation, see specific code[s] for repair of bone[s], ligament[s], tendon[s], nerve[s], or blood vessel[s] with modifier 52)

**20805**   Replantation, forearm (includes radius and ulna to radial carpal joint), complete amputation

(To report replantation of incomplete forearm amputation, see specific code[s] for repair of bone[s], ligament[s], tendon[s], nerve[s], or blood vessel[s] with modifier 52)

**20808**   Replantation, hand (includes hand through metacarpophalangeal joints), complete amputation

(To report replantation of incomplete hand amputation, see specific code[s] for repair of bone[s], ligament[s], tendon[s], nerve[s], or blood vessel[s] with modifier 52)

**20816**   Replantation, digit, excluding thumb (includes metacarpophalangeal joint to insertion of flexor sublimis tendon), complete amputation

(To report replantation of incomplete digit amputation, excluding thumb, see specific code[s] for repair of bone[s], ligament[s], tendon[s], nerve[s], or blood vessel[s] with modifier 52)

**20822**   Replantation, digit, excluding thumb (includes distal tip to sublimis tendon insertion), complete amputation

(To report replantation of incomplete digit amputation, excluding thumb, see specific code[s] for repair of bone[s], ligament[s], tendon[s], nerve[s], or blood vessel[s] with modifier 52)

**20824**   Replantation, thumb (includes carpometacarpal joint to MP joint), complete amputation

(To report replantation of incomplete thumb amputation, see specific code[s] for repair of bone[s], ligament[s], tendon[s], nerve[s], or blood vessel[s] with modifier 52)

**20827**   Replantation, thumb (includes distal tip to MP joint), complete amputation

(To report replantation of incomplete thumb amputation, see specific code[s] for repair of bone[s], ligament[s], tendon[s], nerve[s], or blood vessel[s] with modifier 52)

(To report replantation of complete leg amputation, see specific code[s] for repair of bone[s], ligament[s], tendon[s], nerve[s], or blood vessel[s] with modifier 52)

(To report replantation of incomplete leg amputation, see specific code[s] for repair of bone[s], ligament[s], tendon[s], nerve[s], or blood vessel[s] with modifier 52)

**20838**   Replantation, foot, complete amputation

(To report replantation of incomplete foot amputation, see specific code[s] for repair of bone[s], ligament[s], tendon[s], nerve[s], or blood vessel[s] with modifier 52)

## Grafts (or Implants)

Codes for obtaining autogenous bone, cartilage, tendon, fascia lata grafts, or other tissues through separate skin/fascial incisions should be reported separately unless the code descriptor references the harvesting of the graft or implant (eg, includes obtaining graft).

Do not append modifier 62 to bone graft codes 20900-20938.

(For spinal surgery bone graft[s] see codes 20930-20938)

**20900**   Bone graft, any donor area; minor or small (eg, dowel or button)

**20902**      major or large

**20910**   Cartilage graft; costochondral

**20912**      nasal septum

(For ear cartilage, use 21235)

**20920**   Fascia lata graft; by stripper

**20922**      by incision and area exposure, complex or sheet

**20924**   Tendon graft, from a distance (eg, palmaris, toe extensor, plantaris)

**20926**   Tissue grafts, other (eg, paratenon, fat, dermis)

(For injection(s) of platelet rich plasma, use 0232T)

+ **20930**   Allograft, morselized, or placement of osteopromotive material, for spine surgery only (List separately in addition to code for primary procedure)

(Use 20930 in conjunction with 22319, 22532, 22533, 22548-22558, 22590-22612, 22630, 22800-22812, 0195T, 0196T)

+ **20931**   Allograft, structural, for spine surgery only (List separately in addition to code for primary procedure)

(Use 20931 in conjunction with 22319, 22532-22533, 22548-22558, 22590-22612, 22630, 22800-22812)

+ **20936**   Autograft for spine surgery only (includes harvesting the graft); local (eg, ribs, spinous process, or laminar fragments) obtained from same incision (List separately in addition to code for primary procedure)

(Use 20936 in conjunction with 22319, 22532, 22533, 22548-22558, 22590-22612, 22630, 22800-22812, 0195T, 0196T)

---

⊙ =Moderate sedation    ✚ =Add-on code    ✗ =FDA approval pending    # =Resequenced code    ⊘ =Recycled/reinstated code

**+ 20937**     morselized (through separate skin or fascial incision) (List separately in addition to code for primary procedure)

     (Use 20937 in conjunction with 22319, 22532, 22533, 22548-22558, 22590-22612, 22630, 22800-22812, 0195T, 0196T)

**+ 20938**     structural, bicortical or tricortical (through separate skin or fascial incision) (List separately in addition to code for primary procedure)

     (Use 20938 in conjunction with 22319, 22532, 22533, 22548-22558, 22590-22612, 22630, 22800-22812)

     (For needle aspiration of bone marrow for the purpose of bone grafting, use 38220)

## Other Procedures

**20950**     Monitoring of interstitial fluid pressure (includes insertion of device, eg, wick catheter technique, needle manometer technique) in detection of muscle compartment syndrome

**20955**     Bone graft with microvascular anastomosis; fibula

**20956**     iliac crest

**20957**     metatarsal

**20962**     other than fibula, iliac crest, or metatarsal

     (Do not report code 69990 in addition to codes 20955-20962)

**20969**     Free osteocutaneous flap with microvascular anastomosis; other than iliac crest, metatarsal, or great toe

**20970**     iliac crest

**20972**     metatarsal

**20973**     great toe with web space

     (Do not report code 69990 in addition to codes 20969-20973)

     (For great toe, wrap-around procedure, use 26551)

⃠ **20974**     Electrical stimulation to aid bone healing; noninvasive (nonoperative)

⃠ **20975**     invasive (operative)

**20979**     Low intensity ultrasound stimulation to aid bone healing, noninvasive (nonoperative)

⊙ **20982**     Ablation, bone tumor(s) (eg, osteoid osteoma, metastasis) radiofrequency, percutaneous, including computed tomographic guidance

     (Do not report 20982 in conjunction with 77013)

**+ 20985**     Computer-assisted surgical navigational procedure for musculoskeletal procedures, image-less (List separately in addition to code for primary procedure)

     (Do not report 20985 in conjunction with 61781-61783)

     (20986, 20987 have been deleted)

     (For computer-assisted navigational procedures with image guidance based on pre-operative and intraoperatively obtained images, see 0054T, 0055T)

**20999**     Unlisted procedure, musculoskeletal system, general

# Head

Skull, facial bones, and temporomandibular joint.

## Incision

     (For incision and drainage of superficial abscess and hematoma, see 10060, 10061)

     (For incision and drainage of soft tissue abscess, use 20005)

     (For removal of embedded foreign body from dentoalveolar structure, see 41805, 41806)

**21010**     Arthrotomy, temporomandibular joint

     (To report bilateral procedure, report 21010 with modifier 50)

## Excision

**21011**     Excision, tumor, soft tissue of face or scalp, subcutaneous; less than 2 cm

**21012**     2 cm or greater

**21013**     Excision, tumor, soft tissue of face and scalp, subfascial (eg, subgaleal, intramuscular); less than 2 cm

**21014**     2 cm or greater

**21015**     Radical resection of tumor (eg, malignant neoplasm), soft tissue of face or scalp; less than 2 cm

     (To report excision of skull tumor for osteomyelitis, use 61501)

**21016**     2 cm or greater

**21025**     Excision of bone (eg, for osteomyelitis or bone abscess); mandible

**21026**     facial bone(s)

**21029**     Removal by contouring of benign tumor of facial bone (eg, fibrous dysplasia)

**21030**     Excision of benign tumor or cyst of maxilla or zygoma by enucleation and curettage

**21031**     Excision of torus mandibularis

**21032**     Excision of maxillary torus palatinus

**21034**     Excision of malignant tumor of maxilla or zygoma

**21040**     Excision of benign tumor or cyst of mandible, by enucleation and/or curettage

     (For enucleation and/or curettage of benign cysts or tumors of mandible not requiring osteotomy

     (For excision of benign tumor or cyst requiring osteotomy, see 21046-2

**Surgery: Musculoskeletal System**

21044    Excision of malignant tumor of mandible;

21045      radical resection

(For bone graft, use 21215)

21046    Excision of benign tumor or cyst of mandible; requiring intra-oral osteotomy (eg, locally aggressive or destructive lesion(s))

21047      requiring extra-oral osteotomy and partial mandibulectomy (eg, locally aggressive or destructive lesion(s))

21048    Excision of benign tumor or cyst of maxilla; requiring intra-oral osteotomy (eg, locally aggressive or destructive lesion(s))

21049      requiring extra-oral osteotomy and partial maxillectomy (eg, locally aggressive or destructive lesion(s))

21050    Condylectomy, temporomandibular joint (separate procedure)

(For bilateral procedures, report 21050 with modifier 50)

21060    Meniscectomy, partial or complete, temporomandibular joint (separate procedure)

(For bilateral procedures, report 21060 with modifier 50)

21070    Coronoidectomy (separate procedure)

(For bilateral procedures, report 21070 with modifier 50)

## Manipulation

21073    Manipulation of temporomandibular joint(s) (TMJ), therapeutic, requiring an anesthesia service (ie, general or monitored anesthesia care)

(For TMJ manipulation without an anesthesia service [ie, general or monitored anesthesia care], see 97140, 98925-98929, 98943)

(For closed treatment of temporomandibular dislocation, see 21480, 21485)

## Head Prosthesis

Codes 21076-21089 describe professional services for the rehabilitation of patients with oral, facial, or other anatomical deficiencies by means of prostheses such as an artificial eye, ear, or nose or intraoral obturator to close a cleft. Codes 21076-21089 should only be used when the physician actually designs and prepares the prosthesis (ie, not prepared by an outside laboratory).

(For application or removal of caliper or tongs, see 20660, 20665)

21076    Impression and custom preparation; surgical obturator prosthesis

21077      orbital prosthesis

21079      interim obturator prosthesis

21080      definitive obturator prosthesis

21081      mandibular resection prosthesis

21082      palatal augmentation prosthesis

21083      palatal lift prosthesis

21084      speech aid prosthesis

21085      oral surgical splint

21086      auricular prosthesis

21087      nasal prosthesis

21088      facial prosthesis

### Other Procedures

21089    Unlisted maxillofacial prosthetic procedure

## Introduction or Removal

21100    Application of halo type appliance for maxillofacial fixation, includes removal (separate procedure)

21110    Application of interdental fixation device for conditions other than fracture or dislocation, includes removal

(For removal of interdental fixation by another physician, see 20670-20680)

21116    Injection procedure for temporomandibular joint arthrography

(For radiological supervision and interpretation, use 70332. Do not report 77002 in conjunction with 70332)

## Repair, Revision, and/or Reconstruction

(For cranioplasty, see 21179, 21180 and 62116, 62120, 62140-62147)

21120    Genioplasty; augmentation (autograft, allograft, prosthetic material)

21121      sliding osteotomy, single piece

21122      sliding osteotomies, 2 or more osteotomies (eg, wedge excision or bone wedge reversal for asymmetrical chin)

21123      sliding, augmentation with interpositional bone grafts (includes obtaining autografts)

21125    Augmentation, mandibular body or angle; prosthetic material

21127      with bone graft, onlay or interpositional (includes obtaining autograft)

21137    Reduction forehead; contouring only

21138      contouring and application of prosthetic material or bone graft (includes obtaining autograft)

21139      contouring and setback of anterior frontal sinus wall

21141    Reconstruction midface, LeFort I; single piece, segment movement in any direction (eg, for Long Face Syndrome), without bone graft

   ⊙=Moderate sedation    ✚=Add-on code    ∕=FDA approval pending    #=Resequenced code    ○=Recycled/reinstated code

**21142**   2 pieces, segment movement in any direction, without bone graft

**21143**   3 or more pieces, segment movement in any direction, without bone graft

**21145**   single piece, segment movement in any direction, requiring bone grafts (includes obtaining autografts)

**21146**   2 pieces, segment movement in any direction, requiring bone grafts (includes obtaining autografts) (eg, ungrafted unilateral alveolar cleft)

**21147**   3 or more pieces, segment movement in any direction, requiring bone grafts (includes obtaining autografts) (eg, ungrafted bilateral alveolar cleft or multiple osteotomies)

**21150**   Reconstruction midface, LeFort II; anterior intrusion (eg, Treacher-Collins Syndrome)

**21151**   any direction, requiring bone grafts (includes obtaining autografts)

**21154**   Reconstruction midface, LeFort III (extracranial), any type, requiring bone grafts (includes obtaining autografts); without LeFort I

**21155**   with LeFort I

**21159**   Reconstruction midface, LeFort III (extra and intracranial) with forehead advancement (eg, mono bloc), requiring bone grafts (includes obtaining autografts); without LeFort I

**21160**   with LeFort I

**21172**   Reconstruction superior-lateral orbital rim and lower forehead, advancement or alteration, with or without grafts (includes obtaining autografts)

(For frontal or parietal craniotomy performed for craniosynostosis, use 61556)

**21175**   Reconstruction, bifrontal, superior-lateral orbital rims and lower forehead, advancement or alteration (eg, plagiocephaly, trigonocephaly, brachycephaly), with or without grafts (includes obtaining autografts)

(For bifrontal craniotomy performed for craniosynostosis, use 61557)

**21179**   Reconstruction, entire or majority of forehead and/or supraorbital rims; with grafts (allograft or prosthetic material)

**21180**   with autograft (includes obtaining grafts)

(For extensive craniectomy for multiple suture craniosynostosis, use only 61558 or 61559)

**21181**   Reconstruction by contouring of benign tumor of cranial bones (eg, fibrous dysplasia), extracranial

**21182**   Reconstruction of orbital walls, rims, forehead, nasoethmoid complex following intra- and extracranial excision of benign tumor of cranial bone (eg, fibrous dysplasia), with multiple autografts (includes obtaining grafts); total area of bone grafting less than 40 sq cm

**21183**   total area of bone grafting greater than 40 sq cm but less than 80 sq cm

**21184**   total area of bone grafting greater than 80 sq cm

(For excision of benign tumor of cranial bones, see 61563, 61564)

**21188**   Reconstruction midface, osteotomies (other than LeFort type) and bone grafts (includes obtaining autografts)

**21193**   Reconstruction of mandibular rami, horizontal, vertical, C, or L osteotomy; without bone graft

**21194**   with bone graft (includes obtaining graft)

**21195**   Reconstruction of mandibular rami and/or body, sagittal split; without internal rigid fixation

**21196**   with internal rigid fixation

**21198**   Osteotomy, mandible, segmental;

**21199**   with genioglossus advancement

(To report total osteotomy of the maxilla, see 21141-21160)

**21206**   Osteotomy, maxilla, segmental (eg, Wassmund or Schuchard)

**21208**   Osteoplasty, facial bones; augmentation (autograft, allograft, or prosthetic implant)

**21209**   reduction

**21210**   Graft, bone; nasal, maxillary or malar areas (includes obtaining graft)

(For cleft palate repair, see 42200-42225)

**21215**   mandible (includes obtaining graft)

**21230**   Graft; rib cartilage, autogenous, to face, chin, nose or ear (includes obtaining graft)

**21235**   ear cartilage, autogenous, to nose or ear (includes obtaining graft)

(To report graft augmentation of facial bones, use 21208)

**21240**   Arthroplasty, temporomandibular joint, with or without autograft (includes obtaining graft)

**21242**   Arthroplasty, temporomandibular joint, with allograft

**21243**   Arthroplasty, temporomandibular joint, with prosthetic joint replacement

**21244**   Reconstruction of mandible, extraoral, with transosteal bone plate (eg, mandibular staple bone plate)

**21245**   Reconstruction of mandible or maxilla, subperiosteal implant; partial

**21246**   complete

**21247**   Reconstruction of mandibular condyle with bone and cartilage autografts (includes obtaining grafts) (eg, for hemifacial microsomia)

**21248**   Reconstruction of mandible or maxilla, endosteal (eg, blade, cylinder); partial

**Surgery: Musculoskeletal System**

**Surgery: Musculoskeletal System**

**21249** complete

(To report midface reconstruction, see 21141-21160)

**21255** Reconstruction of zygomatic arch and glenoid fossa with bone and cartilage (includes obtaining autografts)

**21256** Reconstruction of orbit with osteotomies (extracranial) and with bone grafts (includes obtaining autografts) (eg, micro-ophthalmia)

**21260** Periorbital osteotomies for orbital hypertelorism, with bone grafts; extracranial approach

**21261** combined intra- and extracranial approach

**21263** with forehead advancement

**21267** Orbital repositioning, periorbital osteotomies, unilateral, with bone grafts; extracranial approach

**21268** combined intra- and extracranial approach

**21270** Malar augmentation, prosthetic material

(For malar augmentation with bone graft, use 21210)

**21275** Secondary revision of orbitocraniofacial reconstruction

**21280** Medial canthopexy (separate procedure)

(For medial canthoplasty, use 67950)

**21282** Lateral canthopexy

**21295** Reduction of masseter muscle and bone (eg, for treatment of benign masseteric hypertrophy); extraoral approach

**21296** intraoral approach

## Other Procedures

**21299** Unlisted craniofacial and maxillofacial procedure

## Fracture and/or Dislocation

(For operative repair of skull fracture, see 62000-62010)

(To report closed treatment of skull fracture, use the appropriate Evaluation and Management code)

**21310** Closed treatment of nasal bone fracture without manipulation

**21315** Closed treatment of nasal bone fracture; without stabilization

**21320** with stabilization

**21325** Open treatment of nasal fracture; uncomplicated

**21330** complicated, with internal and/or external skeletal fixation

**21335** with concomitant open treatment of fractured septum

**21336** Open treatment of nasal septal fracture, with or without stabilization

**21337** Closed treatment of nasal septal fracture, with or without stabilization

**21338** Open treatment of nasoethmoid fracture; without external fixation

**21339** with external fixation

**21340** Percutaneous treatment of nasoethmoid complex fracture, with splint, wire or headcap fixation, including repair of canthal ligaments and/or the nasolacrimal apparatus

**21343** Open treatment of depressed frontal sinus fracture

**21344** Open treatment of complicated (eg, comminuted or involving posterior wall) frontal sinus fracture, via coronal or multiple approaches

**21345** Closed treatment of nasomaxillary complex fracture (LeFort II type), with interdental wire fixation or fixation of denture or splint

**21346** Open treatment of nasomaxillary complex fracture (LeFort II type); with wiring and/or local fixation

**21347** requiring multiple open approaches

**21348** with bone grafting (includes obtaining graft)

**21355** Percutaneous treatment of fracture of malar area, including zygomatic arch and malar tripod, with manipulation

**21356** Open treatment of depressed zygomatic arch fracture (eg, Gillies approach)

**21360** Open treatment of depressed malar fracture, including zygomatic arch and malar tripod

**21365** Open treatment of complicated (eg, comminuted or involving cranial nerve foramina) fracture(s) of malar area, including zygomatic arch and malar tripod; with internal fixation and multiple surgical approaches

**21366** with bone grafting (includes obtaining graft)

**21385** Open treatment of orbital floor blowout fracture; transantral approach (Caldwell-Luc type operation)

**21386** periorbital approach

**21387** combined approach

**21390** periorbital approach, with alloplastic or other implant

**21395** periorbital approach with bone graft (includes obtaining graft)

**21400** Closed treatment of fracture of orbit, except blowout; without manipulation

**21401** with manipulation

**21406** Open treatment of fracture of orbit, except blowout; without implant

**21407** with implant

**21408** with bone grafting (includes obtaining graft)

**21421** Closed treatment of palatal or maxillary fracture (LeFort I type), with interdental wire fixation or fixation of denture or splint

**21422** Open treatment of palatal or maxillary fracture (LeFort I type);

**21423**        complicated (comminuted or involving cranial nerve foramina), multiple approaches

**21431**    Closed treatment of craniofacial separation (LeFort III type) using interdental wire fixation of denture or splint

**21432**    Open treatment of craniofacial separation (LeFort III type); with wiring and/or internal fixation

**21433**        complicated (eg, comminuted or involving cranial nerve foramina), multiple surgical approaches

**21435**        complicated, utilizing internal and/or external fixation techniques (eg, head cap, halo device, and/or intermaxillary fixation)

(For removal of internal or external fixation device, use 20670)

**21436**        complicated, multiple surgical approaches, internal fixation, with bone grafting (includes obtaining graft)

**21440**    Closed treatment of mandibular or maxillary alveolar ridge fracture (separate procedure)

**21445**    Open treatment of mandibular or maxillary alveolar ridge fracture (separate procedure)

**21450**    Closed treatment of mandibular fracture; without manipulation

**21451**        with manipulation

**21452**    Percutaneous treatment of mandibular fracture, with external fixation

**21453**    Closed treatment of mandibular fracture with interdental fixation

**21454**    Open treatment of mandibular fracture with external fixation

**21461**    Open treatment of mandibular fracture; without interdental fixation

**21462**        with interdental fixation

**21465**    Open treatment of mandibular condylar fracture

**21470**    Open treatment of complicated mandibular fracture by multiple surgical approaches including internal fixation, interdental fixation, and/or wiring of dentures or splints

**21480**    Closed treatment of temporomandibular dislocation; initial or subsequent

**21485**        complicated (eg, recurrent requiring intermaxillary fixation or splinting), initial or subsequent

**21490**    Open treatment of temporomandibular dislocation

(For interdental wire fixation, use 21497)

**21495**    Open treatment of hyoid fracture

(For laryngoplasty with open reduction of fracture, use 31584)

(To report treatment of closed fracture of larynx, use the applicable Evaluation and Management codes)

**21497**    Interdental wiring, for condition other than fracture

## Other Procedures

**21499**    Unlisted musculoskeletal procedure, head

(For unlisted craniofacial or maxillofacial procedure, use 21299)

# Neck (Soft Tissues) and Thorax

(For cervical spine and back, see 21920 et seq)

(For injection of fracture site or trigger point, use 20550)

## Incision

(For incision and drainage of abscess or hematoma, superficial, see 10060, 10140)

**21501**    Incision and drainage, deep abscess or hematoma, soft tissues of neck or thorax;

(For posterior spine subfascial incision and drainage, see 22010-22015)

**21502**        with partial rib ostectomy

**21510**    Incision, deep, with opening of bone cortex (eg, for osteomyelitis or bone abscess), thorax

## Excision

(For bone biopsy, see 20220-20251)

**21550**    Biopsy, soft tissue of neck or thorax

(For needle biopsy of soft tissue, use 20206)

**21552**    Code is out of numerical sequence. See 21550-21632

**21554**    Code is out of numerical sequence. See 21550-21632

**21555**    Excision, tumor, soft tissue of neck or anterior thorax, subcutaneous; less than 3 cm

**# 21552**        3 cm or greater

**21556**    Excision, tumor, soft tissue of neck or anterior thorax, subfascial (eg, intramuscular); less than 5 cm

**# 21554**        5 cm or greater

**21557**    Radical resection of tumor (eg, malignant neoplasm), soft tissue of neck or anterior thorax; less than 5 cm

**21558**        5 cm or greater

**21600**    Excision of rib, partial

(For radical resection of chest wall and rib cage for tumor, use 19260)

(For radical debridement of chest wall and rib cage for injury, see 11044, 11047)

**21610**    Costotransversectomy (separate procedure)

**21615**    Excision first and/or cervical rib;

**21616**        with sympathectomy

**21620**    Ostectomy of sternum, partial

**Surgery: Musculoskeletal System**

**21627** Sternal debridement

(For debridement and closure, use 21750)

**21630** Radical resection of sternum;

**21632** with mediastinal lymphadenectomy

## Repair, Revision, and/or Reconstruction

(For superficial wound, see **Integumentary System** section under Repair—Simple)

**21685** Hyoid myotomy and suspension

**21700** Division of scalenus anticus; without resection of cervical rib

**21705** with resection of cervical rib

**21720** Division of sternocleidomastoid for torticollis, open operation; without cast application

(For transection of spinal accessory and cervical nerves, see 63191, 64722)

**21725** with cast application

**21740** Reconstructive repair of pectus excavatum or carinatum; open

**21742** minimally invasive approach (Nuss procedure), without thoracoscopy

**21743** minimally invasive approach (Nuss procedure), with thoracoscopy

**21750** Closure of median sternotomy separation with or without debridement (separate procedure)

## Fracture and/or Dislocation

**21800** Closed treatment of rib fracture, uncomplicated, each

**21805** Open treatment of rib fracture without fixation, each

**21810** Treatment of rib fracture requiring external fixation (flail chest)

**21820** Closed treatment of sternum fracture

**21825** Open treatment of sternum fracture with or without skeletal fixation

(For sternoclavicular dislocation, see 23520-23532)

## Other Procedures

**21899** Unlisted procedure, neck or thorax

# Back and Flank

## Excision

**21920** Biopsy, soft tissue of back or flank; superficial

**21925** deep

(For needle biopsy of soft tissue, use 20206)

**21930** Excision, tumor, soft tissue of back or flank, subcutaneous; less than 3 cm

**21931** 3 cm or greater

**21932** Excision, tumor, soft tissue of back or flank, subfascial (eg, intramuscular); less than 5 cm

**21933** 5 cm or greater

**21935** Radical resection of tumor (eg, malignant neoplasm), soft tissue of back or flank; less than 5 cm

**21936** 5 cm or greater

# Spine (Vertebral Column)

Cervical, thoracic, and lumbar spine.

Within the spine section, bone grafting procedures are reported separately and in addition to arthrodesis. For bone grafts in other Musculoskeletal sections, see specific code(s) descriptor(s) and/or accompanying guidelines.

To report bone grafts performed after arthrodesis, see 20930-20938. Do not append modifier 62 to bone graft codes 20900-20938.

*Example:*

Posterior arthrodesis of L5-S1 for degenerative disc disease utilizing morselized autogenous iliac bone graft harvested through a separate fascial incision.

Report as 22612 and 20937.

Within the spine section, instrumentation is reported separately and in addition to arthrodesis. To report instrumentation procedures performed with definitive vertebral procedure(s), see 22840-22855. Instrumentation procedure codes 22840-22848 and 22851 are reported in addition to the definitive procedure(s). Modifier 62 may not be appended to the definitive or add-on spinal instrumentation procedure code(s) 22840-22848 and 22850-22852.

*Example:*

Posterior arthrodesis of L4-S1, utilizing morselized autogenous iliac bone graft harvested through separate fascial incision, and pedicle screw fixation.

Report as 22612, 22614, 22842, and 20937.

Vertebral procedures are sometimes followed by arthrodesis and in addition may include bone grafts and instrumentation.

When arthrodesis is performed in addition to another procedure, the arthrodesis should be reported in addition to the original procedure with modifier 51 (multiple procedures). Examples are after osteotomy, fracture care, vertebral corpectomy, and laminectomy. Bone grafts and instrumentation are never performed without arthrodesis.

*Example:*

Treatment of a burst fracture of L2 by corpectomy followed by arthrodesis of L1-L3, utilizing anterior instrumentation L1-L3 and structural allograft.

Report as 63090, 22558-51, 22585, 22845, and 20931.

When two surgeons work together as primary surgeons performing distinct part(s) of a single reportable procedure, each surgeon should report his/her distinct operative work by appending modifier 62 to the single definitive procedure code. If additional procedure(s) (including add-on procedure[s]) are performed during the same surgical session, separate code(s) may be reported by each co-surgeon, with modifier 62 appended (see Appendix A).

*Example:*

A 42-year-old male with a history of posttraumatic degenerative disc disease at L3-4 and L4-5 (internal disc disruption) underwent surgical repair. Surgeon A performed an anterior exposure of the spine with mobilization of the great vessels. Surgeon B performed anterior (minimal) discectomy and fusion at L3-4 and L4-5 using anterior interbody technique.

Report surgeon A: 22558 append modifier 62, 22585 append modifier 62

Report surgeon B: 22558 append modifier 62, 22585 append modifier 62, 20931

(Do not append modifier 62 to bone graft code 20931)

(For injection procedure for myelography, use 62284)

(For injection procedure for discography, see 62290, 62291)

(For injection procedure, chemonucleolysis, single or multiple levels, use 62292)

►(For injection procedure for facet joints, see 64490-64495, 64633-64636)◄

(For needle or trocar biopsy, see 20220-20225)

## Incision

**22010**    Incision and drainage, open, of deep abscess (subfascial), posterior spine; cervical, thoracic, or cervicothoracic

**22015**        lumbar, sacral, or lumbosacral

(Do not report 22015 in conjunction with 22010)

(Do not report 22015 in conjunction with instrumentation removal, 10180, 22850, 22852)

(For incision and drainage of abscess or hematoma, superficial, see 10060, 10140)

## Excision

For the following codes, when two surgeons work together as primary surgeons performing distinct part(s) of partial vertebral body excision, each surgeon should report his/her distinct operative work by appending modifier 62 to the procedure code. In this situation, modifier 62 may be appended to the procedure code(s) 22100-22102, 22110-22114 and, as appropriate, to the

associated additional vertebral segment add-on code(s) 22103, 22116 as long as both surgeons continue to work together as primary surgeons.

(For bone biopsy, see 20220-20251)

(To report soft tissue biopsy of back or flank, see 21920-21925)

(For needle biopsy of soft tissue, use 20206)

(To report excision of soft tissue tumor of back or flank, use 21930)

**22100**    Partial excision of posterior vertebral component (eg, spinous process, lamina or facet) for intrinsic bony lesion, single vertebral segment; cervical

**22101**        thoracic

**22102**        lumbar

(For insertion of posterior spinous process distraction devices, see 0171T, 0172T)

**+ 22103**        each additional segment (List separately in addition to code for primary procedure)

(Use 22103 in conjunction with 22100, 22101, 22102)

**22110**    Partial excision of vertebral body, for intrinsic bony lesion, without decompression of spinal cord or nerve root(s), single vertebral segment; cervical

**22112**        thoracic

**22114**        lumbar

**+ 22116**        each additional vertebral segment (List separately in addition to code for primary procedure)

(Use 22116 in conjunction with 22110, 22112, 22114)

(For complete or near complete resection of vertebral body, see vertebral corpectomy, 63081-63091)

(For spinal reconstruction with bone graft (autograft, allograft) and/or methylmethacrylate of cervical vertebral body, use 63081 and 22554 and 20931 or 20938)

(For spinal reconstruction with bone graft (autograft, allograft) and/or methylmethacrylate of thoracic vertebral body, use 63085 or 63087 and 22556 and 20931 or 20938)

(For spinal reconstruction with bone graft (autograft, allograft) and/or methylmethacrylate of lumbar vertebral body, use 63087 or 63090 and 22558 and 20931 or 20938)

(For spinal reconstruction following vertebral body resection, use 63082 or 63086 or 63088 or 63091, and 22585)

(For harvest of bone autograft for vertebral reconstruction, see 20931 or 20938)

(For cervical spinal reconstruction with prosthetic replacement of resected vertebral bodies, see codes 63081 and 22554 and 20931 or 20938 and 22851)

(For thoracic spinal reconstruction with prosthetic replacement of resected vertebral bodies, see 63085 or 63087 and 22556 and 20931 or 20938 and 22851)

(For lumbar spinal reconstruction with prosthetic replacement of resected vertebral bodies, see codes 63087 or 63090 and 22558, and 20931 or 20938 and 22851)

(For osteotomy of spine, see 22210-22226)

## Osteotomy

To report arthrodesis, see codes 22590-22632. (Report in addition to code[s] for the definitive procedure with modifier 51.)

To report instrumentation procedures, see 22840-22855. (Report in addition to code[s] for the definitive procedure[s].) Do not append modifier 62 to spinal instrumentation codes 22840-22848 and 22850-22852.

To report bone graft procedures, see 20930-20938. (Report in addition to code[s] for the definitive procedure[s].) Do not append modifier 62 to bone graft codes 20900-20938.

For the following codes, when two surgeons work together as primary surgeons performing distinct part(s) of an anterior spine osteotomy, each surgeon should report his/her distinct operative work by appending modifier 62 to the procedure code. In this situation, modifier 62 may be appended to the procedure code(s) 22210-22214, 22220-22224 and, as appropriate, to associated additional segment add-on code(s) 22216, 22226 as long as both surgeons continue to work together as primary surgeons.

Spinal osteotomy procedures are reported when a portion(s) of the vertebral segment(s) is cut and removed in preparation for re-aligning the spine as part of a spinal deformity correction. For excision of an intrinsic lesion of the vertebra without deformity correction, see 22100-22116. For decompression of the spinal cord and/or nerve roots, see 63001-63308.

The three columns are defined as anterior (anterior two-thirds of the vertebral body), middle (posterior third of the vertebral body and the pedicle), and posterior (articular facets, lamina, and spinous process).

**22206** Osteotomy of spine, posterior or posterolateral approach, 3 columns, 1 vertebral segment (eg, pedicle/vertebral body subtraction); thoracic

(Do not report 22206 in conjunction with 22207)

**22207** lumbar

(Do not report 22207 in conjunction with 22206)

**+ 22208** each additional vertebral segment (List separately in addition to code for primary procedure)

(Use 22208 in conjunction with 22206, 22207)

(Do not report 22206, 22207, 22208 in conjunction with 22210-22226, 22830, 63001-63048, 63055-63066, 63075-63091, 63101-63103, when performed at the same level)

**22210** Osteotomy of spine, posterior or posterolateral approach, 1 vertebral segment; cervical

**22212** thoracic

**22214** lumbar

**+ 22216** each additional vertebral segment (List separately in addition to primary procedure)

(Use 22216 in conjunction with 22210, 22212, 22214)

**22220** Osteotomy of spine, including discectomy, anterior approach, single vertebral segment; cervical

**22222** thoracic

**22224** lumbar

**+ 22226** each additional vertebral segment (List separately in addition to code for primary procedure)

(Use 22226 in conjunction with 22220, 22222, 22224)

(For vertebral corpectomy, see 63081-63091)

## Fracture and/or Dislocation

To report arthrodesis, see codes 22590-22632. (Report in addition to code[s] for the definitive procedure with modifier 51.)

To report instrumentation procedures, see 22840-22855. (Report in addition to code[s] for the definitive procedure[s].) Do not append modifier 62 to spinal instrumentation codes 22840-22848 and 22850-22852.

To report bone graft procedures, see 20930-20938. (Report in addition to code[s] for the definitive procedure[s].) Do not append modifier 62 to bone graft codes 20900-20938.

For the following codes, when two surgeons work together as primary surgeons performing distinct part(s) of open fracture and/or dislocation procedure(s), each surgeon should report his/her distinct operative work by appending modifier 62 to the procedure code. In this situation, modifier 62 may be appended to the procedure code(s) 22318-22327 and, as appropriate, the associated additional fracture vertebrae or dislocated segment add-on code 22328 as long as both surgeons continue to work together as primary surgeons.

**22305** Closed treatment of vertebral process fracture(s)

**22310** Closed treatment of vertebral body fracture(s), without manipulation, requiring and including casting or bracing

**22315** Closed treatment of vertebral fracture(s) and/or dislocation(s) requiring casting or bracing, with and including casting and/or bracing by manipulation or traction

(For spinal subluxation, use 97140)

**22318** Open treatment and/or reduction of odontoid fracture(s) and or dislocation(s) (including os odontoideum), anterior approach, including placement of internal fixation; without grafting

| 22319 | with grafting |
|---|---|

**22325** Open treatment and/or reduction of vertebral fracture(s) and/or dislocation(s), posterior approach, 1 fractured vertebra or dislocated segment; lumbar

**22326** cervical

**22327** thoracic

**+ 22328** each additional fractured vertebra or dislocated segment (List separately in addition to code for primary procedure)

(Use 22328 in conjunction with 22325-22327)

(For treatment of vertebral fracture by the anterior approach, see corpectomy 63081-63091, and appropriate arthrodesis, bone graft and instrument codes)

(For decompression of spine following fracture, see 63001-63091; for arthrodesis of spine following fracture, see 22548-22632)

## Manipulation

(For spinal manipulation without anesthesia, use 97140)

**22505** Manipulation of spine requiring anesthesia, any region

## Vertebral Body, Embolization or Injection

⊙▲ **22520** Percutaneous vertebroplasty (bone biopsy included when performed), 1 vertebral body, unilateral or bilateral injection; thoracic

⊙▲ **22521** lumbar

+▲ **22522** each additional thoracic or lumbar vertebral body (List separately in addition to code for primary procedure)

►(Do not report 22520-22522 in conjunction with 20225, 22310-22315, 22325, 22327 when performed at the same level as 22520-22522)◄

(Use 22522 in conjunction with 22520, 22521 as appropriate)

(For radiological supervision and interpretation, see 72291, 72292)

**22523** Percutaneous vertebral augmentation, including cavity creation (fracture reduction and bone biopsy included when performed) using mechanical device, 1 vertebral body, unilateral or bilateral cannulation (eg, kyphoplasty); thoracic

**22524** lumbar

+ **22525** each additional thoracic or lumbar vertebral body (List separately in addition to code for primary procedure)

►(Do not report 22523-22525 in conjunction with 20225, 22310-22315, 22325, 22327 when performed at the same level as 22523-22525)◄

(Use 22525 in conjunction with 22523, 22524)

(For radiological supervision and interpretation, see 72291, 72292)

⊙ **22526** Percutaneous intradiscal electrothermal annuloplasty, unilateral or bilateral including fluoroscopic guidance; single level

⊙+ **22527** 1 or more additional levels (List separately in addition to code for primary procedure)

(Use 22527 in conjunction with 22526)

(Do not report codes 22526, 22527 in conjunction with 77002, 77003)

(For percutaneous intradiscal annuloplasty using method other than electrothermal, use 22899)

## Arthrodesis

Arthrodesis may be performed in the absence of other procedures and therefore when it is combined with another definitive procedure (eg, osteotomy, fracture care, vertebral corpectomy or laminectomy), modifier 51 is appropriate. However, arthrodesis codes 22585, 22614, and 22632 are considered add-on procedure codes and should not be used with modifier 51.

To report instrumentation procedures, see 22840-22855. (Codes 22840-22848, 22851 are reported in conjunction with code[s] for the definitive procedure[s]. When instrumentation reinsertion or removal is reported in conjunction with other definitive procedures including arthrodesis, decompression, and exploration of fusion, append modifier 51 to 22849, 22850, 22852, and 22855.) To report exploration of fusion, use 22830. (When exploration is reported in conjunction with other definitive procedures, including arthrodesis and decompression, append modifier 51 to 22830.) Do not append modifier 62 to spinal instrumentation codes 22840-22848 and 22850-22852.

To report bone graft procedures, see 20930-20938. (Report in addition to code[s] for the definitive procedure[s].) Do not append modifier 62 to bone graft codes 20900-20938.

### Lateral Extracavitary Approach Technique

**22532** Arthrodesis, lateral extracavitary technique, including minimal discectomy to prepare interspace (other than for decompression); thoracic

**22533** lumbar

+ **22534** thoracic or lumbar, each additional vertebral segment (List separately in addition to code for primary procedure)

(Use 22534 in conjunction with 22532 and 22533)

## Anterior or Anterolateral Approach Technique

Procedure codes 22554-22558 are for SINGLE interspace; for additional interspaces, use 22585. A vertebral interspace is the non-bony compartment between two adjacent vertebral bodies, which contains the intervertebral disc, and includes the nucleus pulposus, annulus fibrosus, and two cartilagenous endplates.

For the following codes, when two surgeons work together as primary surgeons performing distinct part(s) of an anterior interbody arthrodesis, each surgeon should report his/her distinct operative work by appending modifier 62 to the procedure code. In this situation, modifier 62 may be appended to the procedure code(s) 22548-22558 and, as appropriate, to the associated additional interspace add-on code 22585 as long as both surgeons continue to work together as primary surgeons.

**22548** Arthrodesis, anterior transoral or extraoral technique, clivus-C1-C2 (atlas-axis), with or without excision of odontoid process

(For intervertebral disc excision by laminotomy or laminectomy, see 63020-63042)

**22551** Arthrodesis, anterior interbody, including disc space preparation, discectomy, osteophytectomy and decompression of spinal cord and/or nerve roots; cervical below C2;

**+ 22552** cervical below C2, each additional interspace (List separately in addition to code for separate procedure)

(Use 22552 in conjunction with 22551)

**22554** Arthrodesis, anterior interbody technique, including minimal discectomy to prepare interspace (other than for decompression); cervical below C2

(Do not report 22554 in conjunction with 63075, even if performed by separate providers. To report anterior cervical discectomy and interbody fusion at the same level during the same session, use 22551)

**22556** thoracic

**22558** lumbar

**+ 22585** each additional interspace (List separately in addition to code for primary procedure)

(Use 22585 in conjunction with 22554, 22556, 22558)

(Do not report 22585 in conjunction with 63075, even if performed by separate providers. To report anterior cervical discectomy and interbody fusion at the same level during the same session, use 22552)

## Posterior, Posterolateral or Lateral Transverse Process Technique

To report instrumentation procedures, see 22840-22855. (Report in addition to code[s] for the definitive procedure[s].) Do not append modifier 62 to spinal instrumentation codes 22840-22848 and 22850-22852.

To report bone graft procedures, see 20930-20938. (Report in addition to code[s] for the definitive procedure[s].) Do not append modifier 62 to bone graft codes 20900-20938.

A vertebral segment describes the basic constituent part into which the spine may be divided. It represents a single complete vertebral bone with its associated articular processes and laminae. A vertebral interspace is the non-bony compartment between two adjacent vertebral bodies which contains the intervertebral disc, and includes the nucleus pulposus, annulus fibrosus, and two cartilagenous endplates.

**22590** Arthrodesis, posterior technique, craniocervical (occiput-C2)

**22595** Arthrodesis, posterior technique, atlas-axis (C1-C2)

**22600** Arthrodesis, posterior or posterolateral technique, single level; cervical below C2 segment

▲ **22610** thoracic (with lateral transverse technique, when performed)

▲ **22612** lumbar (with lateral transverse technique, when performed)

►(Do not report 22612 in conjunction with 22630 for the same interspace and segment, use 22633)◄

**+ 22614** each additional vertebral segment (List separately in addition to code for primary procedure)

►Use 22614 in conjunction with 22600, 22610, 22612, 22630 or 22633 when performed at a different level. When performing a posterior or posterolateral technique for fusion/arthrodesis at an additional level, use 22614. When performing a posterior interbody fusion arthrodesis at an additional level, use 22632. When performing a combined posterior or posterolateral technique with posterior interbody arthrodesis at an additional level, use 22634)◄

►(For facet joint fusion, see 0219T-0222T)◄

(For placement of a posterior intrafacet implant, see 0219T-0222T)

**22630** Arthrodesis, posterior interbody technique, including laminectomy and/or discectomy to prepare interspace (other than for decompression), single interspace; lumbar

►(Do not report 22630 in conjunction with 22612 for the same interspace and segment, use 22633)◄

**+ 22632**    each additional interspace (List separately in addition to code for primary procedure)

▶(Use 22632 in conjunction with 22612, 22630, or 22633 when performed at a different level. When performing a posterior interbody fusion arthrodesis at an additional level, use 22632. When performing a posterior or posterolateral technique for fusion/arthrodesis at an additional level, use 22614. When performing a combined posterior or posterolateral technique with posterior interbody arthrodesis at an additional level, use 22634)◀

**● 22633**    Arthrodesis, combined posterior or posterolateral technique with posterior interbody technique including laminectomy and/or discectomy sufficient to prepare interspace (other than for decompression), single interspace and segment; lumbar

▶(Do not report with 22612 or 22630 at the same level)◀

**+● 22634**    each additional interspace and segment (List separately in addition to code for primary procedure)

▶(Use 22634 in conjunction with 22633)◀

## Spine Deformity (eg, Scoliosis, Kyphosis)

To report instrumentation procedures, see 22840-22855. (Report in addition to code[s] for the definitive procedure[s].) Do not append modifier 62 to spinal instrumentation codes 22840-22848 and 22850-22852.

To report bone graft procedures, see 20930-20938. (Report in addition to code[s] for the definitive procedure[s].) Do not append modifier 62 to bone graft codes 20900-20938.

A vertebral segment describes the basic constituent part into which the spine may be divided. It represents a single complete vertebral bone with its associated articular processes and laminae.

For the following codes, when two surgeons work together as primary surgeons performing distinct part(s) of an arthrodesis for spinal deformity, each surgeon should report his/her distinct operative work by appending modifier 62 to the procedure code. In this situation, modifier 62 may be appended to procedure code(s) 22800-22819 as long as both surgeons continue to work together as primary surgeons.

**22800**    Arthrodesis, posterior, for spinal deformity, with or without cast; up to 6 vertebral segments

**22802**    7 to 12 vertebral segments

**22804**    13 or more vertebral segments

**22808**    Arthrodesis, anterior, for spinal deformity, with or without cast; 2 to 3 vertebral segments

**22810**    4 to 7 vertebral segments

**22812**    8 or more vertebral segments

**22818**    Kyphectomy, circumferential exposure of spine and resection of vertebral segment(s) (including body and posterior elements); single or 2 segments

**22819**    3 or more segments

(To report arthrodesis, see 22800-22804 and add modifier 51)

## Exploration

To report instrumentation procedures, see 22840-22855. (Codes 22840-22848 and 22851 are reported in conjunction with code[s] for the definitive procedure[s]. When instrumentation reinsertion or removal is reported in conjunction with other definitive procedures including arthrodesis, decompression, and exploration of fusion, append modifier 51 to 22849, 22850, 22852 and 22855.) Code 22849 should not be reported with 22850, 22852, and 22855 at the same spinal levels. To report exploration of fusion, see 22830. (When exploration is reported in conjunction with other definitive procedures, including arthrodesis and decompression, append modifier 51 to 22830.)

(To report bone graft procedures, see 20930-20938)

**22830**    Exploration of spinal fusion

## Spinal Instrumentation

Segmental instrumentation is defined as fixation at each end of the construct and at least one additional interposed bony attachment.

Non-segmental instrumentation is defined as fixation at each end of the construct and may span several vertebral segments without attachment to the intervening segments.

Insertion of spinal instrumentation is reported separately and in addition to arthrodesis. Instrumentation procedure codes 22840-22848 and 22851 are reported in addition to the definitive procedure(s). Do not append modifier 62 to spinal instrumentation codes 22840-22848 and 22850-22852.

To report bone graft procedures, see 20930-20938. (Report in addition to code[s] for definitive procedure[s].) Do not append modifier 62 to bone graft codes 20900-20938.

A vertebral segment describes the basic constituent part into which the spine may be divided. It represents a single complete vertebral bone with its associated articular processes and laminae. A vertebral interspace is the non-bony compartment between two adjacent vertebral bodies, which contains the intervertebral disc, and includes the nucleus pulposus, annulus fibrosus, and two cartilagenous endplates.

**Surgery: Musculoskeletal System**

►Codes 22849, 22850, 22852, and 22855 are subject to modifier 51 if reported with other definitive procedure(s), including arthrodesis, decompression, and exploration of fusion. Code 22849 should not be reported in conjunction with 22850, 22852, and 22855 at the same spinal levels. Only the appropriate insertion code (22840-22848) should be reported when previously placed spinal instrumentation is being removed or revised during the same session where new instrumentation is inserted at levels including all or part of the previously instrumented segments. Do not report the reinsertion (22849) or removal (22850, 22852, 22855) procedures in addition to the insertion of the new instrumentation (22840-22848).◄

+ **22840**   Posterior non-segmental instrumentation (eg, Harrington rod technique, pedicle fixation across 1 interspace, atlantoaxial transarticular screw fixation, sublaminar wiring at C1, facet screw fixation) (List separately in addition to code for primary procedure)

(Use 22840 in conjunction with 22100-22102, 22110-22114, 22206, 22207, 22210-22214, 22220-22224, 22305-22327, 22532, 22533, 22548-22558, 22590-22612, 22630, 22800-22812, 63001-63030, 63040-63042, 63045-63047, 63050-63056, 63064, 63075, 63077, 63081, 63085, 63087, 63090, 63101, 63102, 63170-63290, 63300-63307)

(For insertion of posterior spinous process distraction devices, see 0171T, 0172T)

+ **22841**   Internal spinal fixation by wiring of spinous processes (List separately in addition to code for primary procedure)

(Use 22841 in conjunction with 22100-22102, 22110-22114, 22206, 22207, 22210-22214, 22220-22224, 22305-22327, 22532, 22533, 22548-22558, 22590-22612, 22630, 22800-22812, 63001-63030, 63040-63042, 63045-63047, 63050-63056, 63064, 63075, 63077, 63081, 63085, 63087, 63090, 63101, 63102, 63170-63290, 63300-63307)

+ **22842**   Posterior segmental instrumentation (eg, pedicle fixation, dual rods with multiple hooks and sublaminar wires); 3 to 6 vertebral segments (List separately in addition to code for primary procedure)

(Use 22842 in conjunction with 22100-22102, 22110-22114, 22206, 22207, 22210-22214, 22220-22224, 22305-22327, 22532, 22533, 22548-22558, 22590-22612, 22630, 22800-22812, 63001-63030, 63040-63042, 63045-63047, 63050-63056, 63064, 63075, 63077, 63081, 63085, 63087, 63090, 63101, 63102, 63170-63290, 63300-63307)

+ **22843**   7 to 12 vertebral segments (List separately in addition to code for primary procedure)

(Use 22843 in conjunction with 22100-22102, 22110-22114, 22206, 22207, 22210-22214, 22220-22224, 22305-22327, 22532, 22533, 22548-22558, 22590-22612, 22630, 22800-22812, 63001-63030, 63040-63042, 63045-63047, 63050-63056, 63064, 63075, 63077, 63081, 63085, 63087, 63090, 63101, 63102, 63170-63290, 63300-63307)

+ **22844**   13 or more vertebral segments (List separately in addition to code for primary procedure)

(Use 22844 in conjunction with 22100-22102, 22110-22114, 22206, 22207, 22210-22214, 22220-22224, 22305-22327, 22532, 22533, 22548-22558, 22590-22612, 22630, 22800-22812, 63001-63030, 63040-63042, 63045-63047, 63050-63056, 63064, 63075, 63077, 63081, 63085, 63087, 63090, 63101, 63102, 63170-63290, 63300-63307)

+ **22845**   Anterior instrumentation; 2 to 3 vertebral segments (List separately in addition to code for primary procedure)

(Use 22845 in conjunction with 22100-22102, 22110-22114, 22206, 22207, 22210-22214, 22220-22224, 22305-22327, 22532, 22533, 22548-22558, 22590-22612, 22630, 22800-22812, 63001-63030, 63040-63042, 63045-63047, 63050-63056, 63064, 63075, 63077, 63081, 63085, 63087, 63090, 63101, 63102, 63170-63290, 63300-63307)

+ **22846**   4 to 7 vertebral segments (List separately in addition to code for primary procedure)

(Use 22846 in conjunction with 22100-22102, 22110-22114, 22206, 22207, 22210-22214, 22220-22224, 22305-22327, 22532, 22533, 22548-22558, 22590-22612, 22630, 22800-22812, 63001-63030, 63040-63042, 63045-63047, 63050-63056, 63064, 63075, 63077, 63081, 63085, 63087, 63090, 63101, 63102, 63170-63290, 63300-63307)

+ **22847**   8 or more vertebral segments (List separately in addition to code for primary procedure)

(Use 22847 in conjunction with 22100-22102, 22110-22114, 22206, 22207, 22210-22214, 22220-22224, 22305-22327, 22532, 22533, 22548-22558, 22590-22612, 22630, 22800-22812, 63001-63030, 63040-63042, 63045-63047, 63050-63056, 63064, 63075, 63077, 63081, 63085, 63087, 63090, 63101, 63102, 63170-63290, 63300-63307)

+ **22848**   Pelvic fixation (attachment of caudal end of instrumentation to pelvic bony structures) other than sacrum (List separately in addition to code for primary procedure)

(Use 22848 in conjunction with 22100-22102, 22110-22114, 22206, 22207, 22210-22214, 22220-22224, 22305-22327, 22532, 22533, 22548-22558, 22590-22612, 22630, 22800-22812, 63001-63030, 63040-63042, 63045-63047, 63050-63056, 63064, 63075, 63077, 63081, 63085, 63087, 63090, 63101, 63102, 63170-63290, 63300-63307)

**22849**   Reinsertion of spinal fixation device

**22850**   Removal of posterior nonsegmental instrumentation (eg, Harrington rod)

+ **22851**   Application of intervertebral biomechanical device(s) (eg, synthetic cage(s), methylmethacrylate) to vertebral defect or interspace (List separately in addition to code for primary procedure)

(Use 22851 in conjunction with 22100-22102, 22110-22114, 22206, 22207, 22210-22214, 22220-22224, 22305-22327, 22532, 22533, 22548-22558, 22590-22612, 22630, 22800-22812, 63001-63030, 63040-63042, 63045-63047, 63050-63056, 63064, 63075, 63077, 63081, 63085, 63087, 63090, 63101, 63102, 63170-63290, 63300-63307)

(For application of an intervertebral bone device/graft, see 20930-20938)

(For insertion of posterior spinous process distraction devices, see 0171T, 0172T)

**22852**  Removal of posterior segmental instrumentation

**22855**  Removal of anterior instrumentation

**22856**  Total disc arthroplasty (artificial disc), anterior approach, including discectomy with end plate preparation (includes osteophytectomy for nerve root or spinal cord decompression and microdissection), single interspace, cervical

(Do not report 22856 in conjunction with 22554, 22845, 22851, 63075 when performed at the same level)

(Do not report 22856 in conjunction with 69990)

(For additional interspace cervical total disc arthroplasty, use 0092T)

**22857**  Total disc arthroplasty (artificial disc), anterior approach, including discectomy to prepare interspace (other than for decompression), single interspace, lumbar

(Do not report 22857 in conjunction with 22558, 22845, 22851, 49010 when performed at the same level)

(For additional interspace, use Category III code 0163T)

**22861**  Revision including replacement of total disc arthroplasty (artificial disc), anterior approach, single interspace; cervical

(Do not report 22861 in conjunction with 22845, 22851, 22864, 63075 when performed at the same level)

(Do not report 22861 in conjunction with 69990)

(For additional interspace revision of cervical total disc arthroplasty, use 0098T)

**22862**      lumbar

(Do not report 22862 in conjunction with 22558, 22845, 22851, 22865, 49010 when performed at the same level)

(For additional interspace, use Category III code 0165T)

**22864**  Removal of total disc arthroplasty (artificial disc), anterior approach, single interspace; cervical

(Do not report 22864 in conjunction with 22861, 69990)

(For additional interspace removal of cervical total disc arthroplasty, use 0095T)

**22865**      lumbar

(Do not report 22865 in conjunction with 49010)

(For additional interspace, see Category III code 0164T)

(22856-22865 include fluoroscopy when performed)

(For decompression, see 63001-63048)

## Other Procedures

**22899**  Unlisted procedure, spine

# Abdomen

## Excision

**22900**  Excision, tumor, soft tissue of abdominal wall, subfascial (eg, intramuscular); less than 5 cm

**22901**      5 cm or greater

**22902**  Excision, tumor, soft tissue of abdominal wall, subcutaneous; less than 3 cm

**22903**      3 cm or greater

**22904**  Radical resection of tumor (eg, malignant neoplasm), soft tissue of abdominal wall; less than 5 cm

**22905**      5 cm or greater

## Other Procedures

**22999**  Unlisted procedure, abdomen, musculoskeletal system

# Shoulder

The area known as the shoulder is made up of the clavicle, scapula, humerus head and neck, sterno-clavicular joint, acromioclavicular joint, and shoulder joint.

## Incision

**23000**  Removal of subdeltoid calcareous deposits, open

(For arthroscopic removal of bursal deposits, use 29999)

**23020**  Capsular contracture release (eg, Sever type procedure)

(For incision and drainage procedures, superficial, see 10040-10160)

**23030**  Incision and drainage, shoulder area; deep abscess or hematoma

**23031**      infected bursa

**23035**  Incision, bone cortex (eg, osteomyelitis or bone abscess), shoulder area

**23040**  Arthrotomy, glenohumeral joint, including exploration, drainage, or removal of foreign body

**23044**  Arthrotomy, acromioclavicular, sternoclavicular joint, including exploration, drainage, or removal of foreign body

## Excision

**23065**  Biopsy, soft tissue of shoulder area; superficial

**23066**      deep

(For needle biopsy of soft tissue, use 20206)

**23071**  Code is out of numerical sequence. See 23065-23220

**23073**  Code is out of numerical sequence. See 23065-23220

**Surgery: Musculoskeletal System**

**23075** Excision, tumor, soft tissue of shoulder area, subcutaneous; less than 3 cm

# **23071** 3 cm or greater

**23076** Excision, tumor, soft tissue of shoulder area, subfascial (eg, intramuscular); less than 5 cm

# **23073** 5 cm or greater

**23077** Radical resection of tumor (eg, malignant neoplasm), soft tissue of shoulder area; less than 5 cm

**23078** 5 cm or greater

**23100** Arthrotomy, glenohumeral joint, including biopsy

**23101** Arthrotomy, acromioclavicular joint or sternoclavicular joint, including biopsy and/or excision of torn cartilage

**23105** Arthrotomy; glenohumeral joint, with synovectomy, with or without biopsy

**23106** sternoclavicular joint, with synovectomy, with or without biopsy

**23107** Arthrotomy, glenohumeral joint, with joint exploration, with or without removal of loose or foreign body

**23120** Claviculectomy; partial

(For arthroscopic procedure, use 29824)

**23125** total

**23130** Acromioplasty or acromionectomy, partial, with or without coracoacromial ligament release

**23140** Excision or curettage of bone cyst or benign tumor of clavicle or scapula;

**23145** with autograft (includes obtaining graft)

**23146** with allograft

**23150** Excision or curettage of bone cyst or benign tumor of proximal humerus;

**23155** with autograft (includes obtaining graft)

**23156** with allograft

**23170** Sequestrectomy (eg, for osteomyelitis or bone abscess), clavicle

**23172** Sequestrectomy (eg, for osteomyelitis or bone abscess), scapula

**23174** Sequestrectomy (eg, for osteomyelitis or bone abscess), humeral head to surgical neck

**23180** Partial excision (craterization, saucerization, or diaphysectomy) bone (eg, osteomyelitis), clavicle

**23182** Partial excision (craterization, saucerization, or diaphysectomy) bone (eg, osteomyelitis), scapula

**23184** Partial excision (craterization, saucerization, or diaphysectomy) bone (eg, osteomyelitis), proximal humerus

**23190** Ostectomy of scapula, partial (eg, superior medial angle)

**23195** Resection, humeral head

(For replacement with implant, use 23470)

**23200** Radical resection of tumor; clavicle

**23210** scapula

**23220** Radical resection of tumor, proximal humerus

(23221, 23222 have been deleted)

## Introduction or Removal

(For arthrocentesis or needling of bursa, use 20610)

(For K-wire or pin insertion or removal, see 20650, 20670, 20680)

**23330** Removal of foreign body, shoulder; subcutaneous

**23331** deep (eg, Neer hemiarthroplasty removal)

**23332** complicated (eg, total shoulder)

**23350** Injection procedure for shoulder arthrography or enhanced CT/MRI shoulder arthrography

(For radiographic arthrography, radiological supervision and interpretation, use 73040. Fluoroscopy [77002] is inclusive of radiographic arthrography)

(When fluoroscopic guided injection is performed for enhanced CT arthrography, use 23350, 77002, and 73201 or 73202)

(When fluoroscopic guided injection is performed for enhanced MR arthrography, use 23350, 77002, and 73222 or 73223)

(For enhanced CT or enhanced MRI arthrography, use 77002 and either 73201, 73202, 73222, or 73223)

(To report biopsy of the shoulder and joint, see 29805-29826)

## Repair, Revision, and/or Reconstruction

**23395** Muscle transfer, any type, shoulder or upper arm; single

**23397** multiple

**23400** Scapulopexy (eg, Sprengels deformity or for paralysis)

**23405** Tenotomy, shoulder area; single tendon

**23406** multiple tendons through same incision

**23410** Repair of ruptured musculotendinous cuff (eg, rotator cuff) open; acute

**23412** chronic

(For arthroscopic procedure, use 29827)

**23415** Coracoacromial ligament release, with or without acromioplasty

(For arthroscopic procedure, use 29826)

**23420** Reconstruction of complete shoulder (rotator) cuff avulsion, chronic (includes acromioplasty)

**23430** Tenodesis of long tendon of biceps

(For arthroscopic biceps tenodesis, use 29828)

**23440** Resection or transplantation of long tendon of biceps

**23450** Capsulorrhaphy, anterior; Putti-Platt procedure or Magnuson type operation

(To report arthroscopic thermal capsulorrhaphy, use 29999)

**23455** with labral repair (eg, Bankart procedure)

(For arthroscopic procedure, use 29806)

**23460** Capsulorrhaphy, anterior, any type; with bone block

**23462** with coracoid process transfer

(To report open thermal capsulorrhaphy, use 23929)

**23465** Capsulorrhaphy, glenohumeral joint, posterior, with or without bone block

(For sternoclavicular and acromioclavicular reconstruction, see 23530, 23550)

**23466** Capsulorrhaphy, glenohumeral joint, any type multi-directional instability

**23470** Arthroplasty, glenohumeral joint; hemiarthroplasty

**23472** total shoulder (glenoid and proximal humeral replacement (eg, total shoulder))

(For removal of total shoulder implants, see 23331, 23332)

(For osteotomy, proximal humerus, use 24400)

**23480** Osteotomy, clavicle, with or without internal fixation;

**23485** with bone graft for nonunion or malunion (includes obtaining graft and/or necessary fixation)

**23490** Prophylactic treatment (nailing, pinning, plating or wiring) with or without methylmethacrylate; clavicle

**23491** proximal humerus

## Fracture and/or Dislocation

**23500** Closed treatment of clavicular fracture; without manipulation

**23505** with manipulation

**23515** Open treatment of clavicular fracture, includes internal fixation, when performed

**23520** Closed treatment of sternoclavicular dislocation; without manipulation

**23525** with manipulation

**23530** Open treatment of sternoclavicular dislocation, acute or chronic;

**23532** with fascial graft (includes obtaining graft)

**23540** Closed treatment of acromioclavicular dislocation; without manipulation

**23545** with manipulation

**23550** Open treatment of acromioclavicular dislocation, acute or chronic;

**23552** with fascial graft (includes obtaining graft)

**23570** Closed treatment of scapular fracture; without manipulation

**23575** with manipulation, with or without skeletal traction (with or without shoulder joint involvement)

**23585** Open treatment of scapular fracture (body, glenoid or acromion) includes internal fixation, when performed

**23600** Closed treatment of proximal humeral (surgical or anatomical neck) fracture; without manipulation

**23605** with manipulation, with or without skeletal traction

**23615** Open treatment of proximal humeral (surgical or anatomical neck) fracture, includes internal fixation, when performed, includes repair of tuberosity(s), when performed;

**23616** with proximal humeral prosthetic replacement

**23620** Closed treatment of greater humeral tuberosity fracture; without manipulation

**23625** with manipulation

**23630** Open treatment of greater humeral tuberosity fracture, includes internal fixation, when performed

**23650** Closed treatment of shoulder dislocation, with manipulation; without anesthesia

**23655** requiring anesthesia

**23660** Open treatment of acute shoulder dislocation

(Repairs for recurrent dislocations, see 23450-23466)

**23665** Closed treatment of shoulder dislocation, with fracture of greater humeral tuberosity, with manipulation

**23670** Open treatment of shoulder dislocation, with fracture of greater humeral tuberosity, includes internal fixation, when performed

**23675** Closed treatment of shoulder dislocation, with surgical or anatomical neck fracture, with manipulation

**23680** Open treatment of shoulder dislocation, with surgical or anatomical neck fracture, includes internal fixation, when performed

## Manipulation

**23700** Manipulation under anesthesia, shoulder joint, including application of fixation apparatus (dislocation excluded)

## Arthrodesis

**23800** Arthrodesis, glenohumeral joint;

**23802** with autogenous graft (includes obtaining graft)

## Amputation

**23900** Interthoracoscapular amputation (forequarter)

**23920** Disarticulation of shoulder;

**23921** secondary closure or scar revision

## Other Procedures

**23929**  Unlisted procedure, shoulder

# Humerus (Upper Arm) and Elbow

The elbow area includes the head and neck of the radius and olecranon process.

## Incision

(For incision and drainage procedures, superficial, see 10040-10160)

**23930**  Incision and drainage, upper arm or elbow area; deep abscess or hematoma

**23931**  bursa

**23935**  Incision, deep, with opening of bone cortex (eg, for osteomyelitis or bone abscess), humerus or elbow

**24000**  Arthrotomy, elbow, including exploration, drainage, or removal of foreign body

**24006**  Arthrotomy of the elbow, with capsular excision for capsular release (separate procedure)

## Excision

**24065**  Biopsy, soft tissue of upper arm or elbow area; superficial

**24066**  deep (subfascial or intramuscular)

(For needle biopsy of soft tissue, use 20206)

**24071**  Code is out of numerical sequence. See 24065-54155

**24073**  Code is out of numerical sequence. See 24065-24155

**24075**  Excision, tumor, soft tissue of upper arm or elbow area, subcutaneous; less than 3 cm

**# 24071**  3 cm or greater

**24076**  Excision, tumor, soft tissue of upper arm or elbow area, subfascial (eg, intramuscular); less than 5 cm

**# 24073**  5 cm or greater

**24077**  Radical resection of tumor (eg, malignant neoplasm), soft tissue of upper arm or elbow area; less than 5 cm

**24079**  5 cm or greater

**24100**  Arthrotomy, elbow; with synovial biopsy only

**24101**  with joint exploration, with or without biopsy, with or without removal of loose or foreign body

**24102**  with synovectomy

**24105**  Excision, olecranon bursa

**24110**  Excision or curettage of bone cyst or benign tumor, humerus;

**24115**  with autograft (includes obtaining graft)

**24116**  with allograft

**24120**  Excision or curettage of bone cyst or benign tumor of head or neck of radius or olecranon process;

**24125**  with autograft (includes obtaining graft)

**24126**  with allograft

**24130**  Excision, radial head

(For replacement with implant, use 24366)

**24134**  Sequestrectomy (eg, for osteomyelitis or bone abscess), shaft or distal humerus

**24136**  Sequestrectomy (eg, for osteomyelitis or bone abscess), radial head or neck

**24138**  Sequestrectomy (eg, for osteomyelitis or bone abscess), olecranon process

**24140**  Partial excision (craterization, saucerization, or diaphysectomy) bone (eg, osteomyelitis), humerus

**24145**  Partial excision (craterization, saucerization, or diaphysectomy) bone (eg, osteomyelitis), radial head or neck

**24147**  Partial excision (craterization, saucerization, or diaphysectomy) bone (eg, osteomyelitis), olecranon process

**24149**  Radical resection of capsule, soft tissue, and heterotopic bone, elbow, with contracture release (separate procedure)

(For capsular and soft tissue release only, use 24006)

**24150**  Radical resection of tumor, shaft or distal humerus

(24151 has been deleted)

**24152**  Radical resection of tumor, radial head or neck

(24153 has been deleted)

**24155**  Resection of elbow joint (arthrectomy)

## Introduction or Removal

(For K-wire or pin insertion or removal, see 20650, 20670, 20680)

(For arthrocentesis or needling of bursa or joint, use 20605)

**24160**  Implant removal; elbow joint

**24164**  radial head

**24200**  Removal of foreign body, upper arm or elbow area; subcutaneous

**24201**  deep (subfascial or intramuscular)

**24220**  Injection procedure for elbow arthrography

(For radiological supervision and interpretation, use 73085. Do not report 77002 in conjunction with 73085)

(For injection for tennis elbow, use 20550)

## Repair, Revision, and/or Reconstruction

**24300**  Manipulation, elbow, under anesthesia

(For application of external fixation, see 20690 or 20692)

**24301**    Muscle or tendon transfer, any type, upper arm or elbow, single (excluding 24320-24331)

**24305**    Tendon lengthening, upper arm or elbow, each tendon

**24310**    Tenotomy, open, elbow to shoulder, each tendon

**24320**    Tenoplasty, with muscle transfer, with or without free graft, elbow to shoulder, single (Seddon-Brookes type procedure)

**24330**    Flexor-plasty, elbow (eg, Steindler type advancement);

**24331**       with extensor advancement

**24332**    Tenolysis, triceps

**24340**    Tenodesis of biceps tendon at elbow (separate procedure)

**24341**    Repair, tendon or muscle, upper arm or elbow, each tendon or muscle, primary or secondary (excludes rotator cuff)

**24342**    Reinsertion of ruptured biceps or triceps tendon, distal, with or without tendon graft

**24343**    Repair lateral collateral ligament, elbow, with local tissue

**24344**    Reconstruction lateral collateral ligament, elbow, with tendon graft (includes harvesting of graft)

**24345**    Repair medial collateral ligament, elbow, with local tissue

**24346**    Reconstruction medial collateral ligament, elbow, with tendon graft (includes harvesting of graft)

**24357**    Tenotomy, elbow, lateral or medial (eg, epicondylitis, tennis elbow, golfer's elbow); percutaneous

**24358**       debridement, soft tissue and/or bone, open

**24359**       debridement, soft tissue and/or bone, open with tendon repair or reattachment

       (Do not report 24357-24359 in conjunction with 29837, 29838)

**24360**    Arthroplasty, elbow; with membrane (eg, fascial)

**24361**       with distal humeral prosthetic replacement

**24362**       with implant and fascia lata ligament reconstruction

**24363**       with distal humerus and proximal ulnar prosthetic replacement (eg, total elbow)

**24365**    Arthroplasty, radial head;

**24366**       with implant

**24400**    Osteotomy, humerus, with or without internal fixation

**24410**    Multiple osteotomies with realignment on intramedullary rod, humeral shaft (Sofield type procedure)

**24420**    Osteoplasty, humerus (eg, shortening or lengthening) (excluding 64876)

**24430**    Repair of nonunion or malunion, humerus; without graft (eg, compression technique)

**24435**       with iliac or other autograft (includes obtaining graft)

       (For proximal radius and/or ulna, see 25400-25420)

**24470**    Hemiepiphyseal arrest (eg, cubitus varus or valgus, distal humerus)

**24495**    Decompression fasciotomy, forearm, with brachial artery exploration

**24498**    Prophylactic treatment (nailing, pinning, plating or wiring), with or without methylmethacrylate, humeral shaft

# Fracture and/or Dislocation

**24500**    Closed treatment of humeral shaft fracture; without manipulation

**24505**       with manipulation, with or without skeletal traction

**24515**    Open treatment of humeral shaft fracture with plate/screws, with or without cerclage

**24516**    Treatment of humeral shaft fracture, with insertion of intramedullary implant, with or without cerclage and/or locking screws

**24530**    Closed treatment of supracondylar or transcondylar humeral fracture, with or without intercondylar extension; without manipulation

**24535**       with manipulation, with or without skin or skeletal traction

**24538**    Percutaneous skeletal fixation of supracondylar or transcondylar humeral fracture, with or without intercondylar extension

**24545**    Open treatment of humeral supracondylar or transcondylar fracture, includes internal fixation, when performed; without intercondylar extension

**24546**       with intercondylar extension

**24560**    Closed treatment of humeral epicondylar fracture, medial or lateral; without manipulation

**24565**       with manipulation

**24566**    Percutaneous skeletal fixation of humeral epicondylar fracture, medial or lateral, with manipulation

**24575**    Open treatment of humeral epicondylar fracture, medial or lateral, includes internal fixation, when performed

**24576**    Closed treatment of humeral condylar fracture, medial or lateral; without manipulation

**24577**       with manipulation

**24579**    Open treatment of humeral condylar fracture, medial or lateral, includes internal fixation, when performed

       (To report closed treatment of fractures without manipulation, see 24530, 24560, 24576, 24650, 24670)

       (To report closed treatment of fractures with manipulation, see 24535, 24565, 24577, 24675)

**24582**    Percutaneous skeletal fixation of humeral condylar fracture, medial or lateral, with manipulation

**24586**    Open treatment of periarticular fracture and/or dislocation of the elbow (fracture distal humerus and proximal ulna and/or proximal radius);

**24587**      with implant arthroplasty

(See also 24361)

**24600**   Treatment of closed elbow dislocation; without anesthesia

**24605**      requiring anesthesia

**24615**   Open treatment of acute or chronic elbow dislocation

**24620**   Closed treatment of Monteggia type of fracture dislocation at elbow (fracture proximal end of ulna with dislocation of radial head), with manipulation

**24635**   Open treatment of Monteggia type of fracture dislocation at elbow (fracture proximal end of ulna with dislocation of radial head), includes internal fixation, when performed

**24640**   Closed treatment of radial head subluxation in child, nursemaid elbow, with manipulation

**24650**   Closed treatment of radial head or neck fracture; without manipulation

**24655**      with manipulation

**24665**   Open treatment of radial head or neck fracture, includes internal fixation or radial head excision, when performed;

**24666**      with radial head prosthetic replacement

**24670**   Closed treatment of ulnar fracture, proximal end (eg, olecranon or coronoid process[es]); without manipulation

**24675**      with manipulation

**24685**   Open treatment of ulnar fracture, proximal end (eg, olecranon or coronoid process[es]), includes internal fixation, when performed

(Do not report 24685 in conjunction with 24100-24102)

## Arthrodesis

**24800**   Arthrodesis, elbow joint; local

**24802**      with autogenous graft (includes obtaining graft)

## Amputation

**24900**   Amputation, arm through humerus; with primary closure

**24920**      open, circular (guillotine)

**24925**      secondary closure or scar revision

**24930**      re-amputation

**24931**      with implant

**24935**   Stump elongation, upper extremity

**24940**   Cineplasty, upper extremity, complete procedure

## Other Procedures

**24999**   Unlisted procedure, humerus or elbow

# Forearm and Wrist

Radius, ulna, carpal bones, and joints.

## Incision

**25000**   Incision, extensor tendon sheath, wrist (eg, deQuervains disease)

(For decompression median nerve or for carpal tunnel syndrome, use 64721)

**25001**   Incision, flexor tendon sheath, wrist (eg, flexor carpi radialis)

**25020**   Decompression fasciotomy, forearm and/or wrist, flexor OR extensor compartment; without debridement of nonviable muscle and/or nerve

**25023**      with debridement of nonviable muscle and/or nerve

(For decompression fasciotomy with brachial artery exploration, use 24495)

(For incision and drainage procedures, superficial, see 10060-10160)

(For debridement, see also 11000-11044)

**25024**   Decompression fasciotomy, forearm and/or wrist, flexor AND extensor compartment; without debridement of nonviable muscle and/or nerve

**25025**      with debridement of nonviable muscle and/or nerve

**25028**   Incision and drainage, forearm and/or wrist; deep abscess or hematoma

**25031**      bursa

**25035**   Incision, deep, bone cortex, forearm and/or wrist (eg, osteomyelitis or bone abscess)

**25040**   Arthrotomy, radiocarpal or midcarpal joint, with exploration, drainage, or removal of foreign body

## Excision

**25065**   Biopsy, soft tissue of forearm and/or wrist; superficial

**25066**      deep (subfascial or intramuscular)

(For needle biopsy of soft tissue, use 20206)

**25071**   Code is out of numerical sequence. See 25065-25240

**25073**   Code is out of numerical sequence. See 25065-25240

**25075**   Excision, tumor, soft tissue of forearm and/or wrist area, subcutaneous; less than 3 cm

**# 25071**      3 cm or greater

**25076**   Excision, tumor, soft tissue of forearm and/or wrist area, subfascial (eg, intramuscular); less than 3 cm

**# 25073**      3 cm or greater

**25077**   Radical resection of tumor (eg, malignant neoplasm), soft tissue of forearm and/or wrist area; less than 3 cm

**25078**      3 cm or greater

**25085**   Capsulotomy, wrist (eg, contracture)

**25100**   Arthrotomy, wrist joint; with biopsy

**25101**        with joint exploration, with or without biopsy, with or without removal of loose or foreign body

**25105**        with synovectomy

**25107**   Arthrotomy, distal radioulnar joint including repair of triangular cartilage, complex

**25109**   Excision of tendon, forearm and/or wrist, flexor or extensor, each

**25110**   Excision, lesion of tendon sheath, forearm and/or wrist

**25111**   Excision of ganglion, wrist (dorsal or volar); primary

**25112**        recurrent

        (For hand or finger, use 26160)

**25115**   Radical excision of bursa, synovia of wrist, or forearm tendon sheaths (eg, tenosynovitis, fungus, Tbc, or other granulomas, rheumatoid arthritis); flexors

**25116**        extensors, with or without transposition of dorsal retinaculum

        (For finger synovectomies, use 26145)

**25118**   Synovectomy, extensor tendon sheath, wrist, single compartment;

**25119**        with resection of distal ulna

**25120**   Excision or curettage of bone cyst or benign tumor of radius or ulna (excluding head or neck of radius and olecranon process);

        (For head or neck of radius or olecranon process, see 24120-24126)

**25125**        with autograft (includes obtaining graft)

**25126**        with allograft

**25130**   Excision or curettage of bone cyst or benign tumor of carpal bones;

**25135**        with autograft (includes obtaining graft)

**25136**        with allograft

**25145**   Sequestrectomy (eg, for osteomyelitis or bone abscess), forearm and/or wrist

**25150**   Partial excision (craterization, saucerization, or diaphysectomy) of bone (eg, for osteomyelitis); ulna

**25151**        radius

        (For head or neck of radius or olecranon process, see 24145, 24147)

**25170**   Radical resection of tumor, radius or ulna

**25210**   Carpectomy; 1 bone

        (For carpectomy with implant, see 25441-25445)

**25215**        all bones of proximal row

**25230**   Radial styloidectomy (separate procedure)

**25240**   Excision distal ulna partial or complete (eg, Darrach type or matched resection)

        (For implant replacement, distal ulna, use 25442)

        (For obtaining fascia for interposition, see 20920, 20922)

## Introduction or Removal

        (For K-wire, pin or rod insertion or removal, see 20650, 20670, 20680)

**25246**   Injection procedure for wrist arthrography

        (For radiological supervision and interpretation, use 73115. Do not report 77002 in conjunction with 73115)

        (For foreign body removal, superficial use 20520)

**25248**   Exploration with removal of deep foreign body, forearm or wrist

**25250**   Removal of wrist prosthesis; (separate procedure)

**25251**        complicated, including total wrist

**25259**   Manipulation, wrist, under anesthesia

        (For application of external fixation, see 20690 or 20692)

## Repair, Revision, and/or Reconstruction

**25260**   Repair, tendon or muscle, flexor, forearm and/or wrist; primary, single, each tendon or muscle

**25263**        secondary, single, each tendon or muscle

**25265**        secondary, with free graft (includes obtaining graft), each tendon or muscle

**25270**   Repair, tendon or muscle, extensor, forearm and/or wrist; primary, single, each tendon or muscle

**25272**        secondary, single, each tendon or muscle

**25274**        secondary, with free graft (includes obtaining graft), each tendon or muscle

**25275**   Repair, tendon sheath, extensor, forearm and/or wrist, with free graft (includes obtaining graft) (eg, for extensor carpi ulnaris subluxation)

**25280**   Lengthening or shortening of flexor or extensor tendon, forearm and/or wrist, single, each tendon

**25290**   Tenotomy, open, flexor or extensor tendon, forearm and/or wrist, single, each tendon

**25295**   Tenolysis, flexor or extensor tendon, forearm and/or wrist, single, each tendon

**25300**   Tenodesis at wrist; flexors of fingers

**25301**        extensors of fingers

**25310**   Tendon transplantation or transfer, flexor or extensor, forearm and/or wrist, single; each tendon

**25312**        with tendon graft(s) (includes obtaining graft), each tendon

**25315**   Flexor origin slide (eg, for cerebral palsy, Volkmann contracture), forearm and/or wrist;

**Surgery: Musculoskeletal System**

| | |
|---|---|
| 25316 | with tendon(s) transfer |
| 25320 | Capsulorrhaphy or reconstruction, wrist, open (eg, capsulodesis, ligament repair, tendon transfer or graft) (includes synovectomy, capsulotomy and open reduction) for carpal instability |
| 25332 | Arthroplasty, wrist, with or without interposition, with or without external or internal fixation |
| | (For obtaining fascia for interposition, see 20920, 20922) |
| | (For prosthetic replacement arthroplasty, see 25441-25446) |
| 25335 | Centralization of wrist on ulna (eg, radial club hand) |
| 25337 | Reconstruction for stabilization of unstable distal ulna or distal radioulnar joint, secondary by soft tissue stabilization (eg, tendon transfer, tendon graft or weave, or tenodesis) with or without open reduction of distal radioulnar joint |
| | (For harvesting of fascia lata graft, see 20920, 20922) |
| 25350 | Osteotomy, radius; distal third |
| 25355 | middle or proximal third |
| 25360 | Osteotomy; ulna |
| 25365 | radius AND ulna |
| 25370 | Multiple osteotomies, with realignment on intramedullary rod (Sofield type procedure); radius OR ulna |
| 25375 | radius AND ulna |
| 25390 | Osteoplasty, radius OR ulna; shortening |
| 25391 | lengthening with autograft |
| 25392 | Osteoplasty, radius AND ulna; shortening (excluding 64876) |
| 25393 | lengthening with autograft |
| 25394 | Osteoplasty, carpal bone, shortening |
| 25400 | Repair of nonunion or malunion, radius OR ulna; without graft (eg, compression technique) |
| 25405 | with autograft (includes obtaining graft) |
| 25415 | Repair of nonunion or malunion, radius AND ulna; without graft (eg, compression technique) |
| 25420 | with autograft (includes obtaining graft) |
| 25425 | Repair of defect with autograft; radius OR ulna |
| 25426 | radius AND ulna |
| 25430 | Insertion of vascular pedicle into carpal bone (eg, Hori procedure) |
| 25431 | Repair of nonunion of carpal bone (excluding carpal scaphoid (navicular)) (includes obtaining graft and necessary fixation), each bone |
| 25440 | Repair of nonunion, scaphoid carpal (navicular) bone, with or without radial styloidectomy (includes obtaining graft and necessary fixation) |
| 25441 | Arthroplasty with prosthetic replacement; distal radius |

| | |
|---|---|
| 25442 | distal ulna |
| 25443 | scaphoid carpal (navicular) |
| 25444 | lunate |
| 25445 | trapezium |
| 25446 | distal radius and partial or entire carpus (total wrist) |
| 25447 | Arthroplasty, interposition, intercarpal or carpometacarpal joints |
| | (For wrist arthroplasty, use 25332) |
| 25449 | Revision of arthroplasty, including removal of implant, wrist joint |
| 25450 | Epiphyseal arrest by epiphysiodesis or stapling; distal radius OR ulna |
| 25455 | distal radius AND ulna |
| 25490 | Prophylactic treatment (nailing, pinning, plating or wiring) with or without methylmethacrylate; radius |
| 25491 | ulna |
| 25492 | radius AND ulna |

## Fracture and/or Dislocation

(For application of external fixation in addition to internal fixation, use 20690 and the appropriate internal fixation code)

| | |
|---|---|
| 25500 | Closed treatment of radial shaft fracture; without manipulation |
| 25505 | with manipulation |
| 25515 | Open treatment of radial shaft fracture, includes internal fixation, when performed |
| 25520 | Closed treatment of radial shaft fracture and closed treatment of dislocation of distal radioulnar joint (Galeazzi fracture/dislocation) |
| 25525 | Open treatment of radial shaft fracture, includes internal fixation, when performed, and closed treatment of distal radioulnar joint dislocation (Galeazzi fracture/dislocation), includes percutaneous skeletal fixation, when performed |
| 25526 | Open treatment of radial shaft fracture, includes internal fixation, when performed, and open treatment of distal radioulnar joint dislocation (Galeazzi fracture/dislocation), includes internal fixation, when performed, includes repair of triangular fibrocartilage complex |
| 25530 | Closed treatment of ulnar shaft fracture; without manipulation |
| 25535 | with manipulation |
| 25545 | Open treatment of ulnar shaft fracture, includes internal fixation, when performed |
| 25560 | Closed treatment of radial and ulnar shaft fractures; without manipulation |
| 25565 | with manipulation |

**25574**   Open treatment of radial AND ulnar shaft fractures, with internal fixation, when performed; of radius OR ulna

**25575**       of radius AND ulna

**25600**   Closed treatment of distal radial fracture (eg, Colles or Smith type) or epiphyseal separation, includes closed treatment of fracture of ulnar styloid, when performed; without manipulation

**25605**       with manipulation

           (Do not report 25600, 25605 in conjunction with 25650)

**25606**   Percutaneous skeletal fixation of distal radial fracture or epiphyseal separation

           (Do not report 25606 in conjunction with 25650)

           (For percutaneous treatment of ulnar styloid fracture, use 25651)

           (For open treatment of ulnar styloid fracture, use 25652)

**25607**   Open treatment of distal radial extra-articular fracture or epiphyseal separation, with internal fixation

           (Do not report 25607 in conjunction with 25650)

           (For percutaneous treatment of ulnar styloid fracture, use 25651)

           (For open treatment of ulnar styloid fracture, use 25652)

**25608**   Open treatment of distal radial intra-articular fracture or epiphyseal separation; with internal fixation of 2 fragments

           (Do not report 25608 in conjunction with 25609)

**25609**       with internal fixation of 3 or more fragments

           (Do not report 25608, 25609 in conjunction with 25650)

           (For percutaneous treatment of ulnar styloid fracture, use 25651)

           (For open treatment of ulnar styloid fracture, use 25652)

**25622**   Closed treatment of carpal scaphoid (navicular) fracture; without manipulation

**25624**       with manipulation

**25628**   Open treatment of carpal scaphoid (navicular) fracture, includes internal fixation, when performed

**25630**   Closed treatment of carpal bone fracture (excluding carpal scaphoid [navicular]); without manipulation, each bone

**25635**       with manipulation, each bone

**25645**   Open treatment of carpal bone fracture (other than carpal scaphoid [navicular]), each bone

**25650**   Closed treatment of ulnar styloid fracture

           (Do not report 25650 in conjunction with 25600, 25605, 25607-25609)

**25651**   Percutaneous skeletal fixation of ulnar styloid fracture

**25652**   Open treatment of ulnar styloid fracture

**25660**   Closed treatment of radiocarpal or intercarpal dislocation, 1 or more bones, with manipulation

**25670**   Open treatment of radiocarpal or intercarpal dislocation, 1 or more bones

**25671**   Percutaneous skeletal fixation of distal radioulnar dislocation

**25675**   Closed treatment of distal radioulnar dislocation with manipulation

**25676**   Open treatment of distal radioulnar dislocation, acute or chronic

**25680**   Closed treatment of trans-scaphoperilunar type of fracture dislocation, with manipulation

**25685**   Open treatment of trans-scaphoperilunar type of fracture dislocation

**25690**   Closed treatment of lunate dislocation, with manipulation

**25695**   Open treatment of lunate dislocation

## Arthrodesis

**25800**   Arthrodesis, wrist; complete, without bone graft (includes radiocarpal and/or intercarpal and/or carpometacarpal joints)

**25805**       with sliding graft

**25810**       with iliac or other autograft (includes obtaining graft)

**25820**   Arthrodesis, wrist; limited, without bone graft (eg, intercarpal or radiocarpal)

**25825**       with autograft (includes obtaining graft)

**25830**   Arthrodesis, distal radioulnar joint with segmental resection of ulna, with or without bone graft (eg, Sauve-Kapandji procedure)

## Amputation

**25900**   Amputation, forearm, through radius and ulna;

**25905**       open, circular (guillotine)

**25907**       secondary closure or scar revision

**25909**       re-amputation

**25915**   Krukenberg procedure

**25920**   Disarticulation through wrist;

**25922**       secondary closure or scar revision

**25924**       re-amputation

**25927**   Transmetacarpal amputation;

**25929**       secondary closure or scar revision

**25931**       re-amputation

## Other Procedures

**25999**   Unlisted procedure, forearm or wrist

# Hand and Fingers

## Incision

**26010**    Drainage of finger abscess; simple

**26011**        complicated (eg, felon)

**26020**    Drainage of tendon sheath, digit and/or palm, each

**26025**    Drainage of palmar bursa; single, bursa

**26030**        multiple bursa

**26034**    Incision, bone cortex, hand or finger (eg, osteomyelitis or bone abscess)

**26035**    Decompression fingers and/or hand, injection injury (eg, grease gun)

**26037**    Decompressive fasciotomy, hand (excludes 26035)

(For injection injury, use 26035)

**26040**    Fasciotomy, palmar (eg, Dupuytren's contracture); percutaneous

**26045**        open, partial

▶(For palmar fasciotomy by enzyme injection (eg, collagenase), see 20527, 26341)◀

(For fasciectomy, see 26121-26125)

**26055**    Tendon sheath incision (eg, for trigger finger)

**26060**    Tenotomy, percutaneous, single, each digit

**26070**    Arthrotomy, with exploration, drainage, or removal of loose or foreign body; carpometacarpal joint

**26075**        metacarpophalangeal joint, each

**26080**        interphalangeal joint, each

## Excision

**26100**    Arthrotomy with biopsy; carpometacarpal joint, each

**26105**        metacarpophalangeal joint, each

**26110**        interphalangeal joint, each

**26111**    Code is out of numerical sequence. See 26100-26262

**26113**    Code is out of numerical sequence. See 26100-26262

**26115**    Excision, tumor or vascular malformation, soft tissue of hand or finger, subcutaneous; less than 1.5 cm

**# 26111**        1.5 cm or greater

**26116**    Excision, tumor, soft tissue, or vascular malformation, of hand or finger, subfascial (eg, intramuscular); less than 1.5 cm

**# 26113**        1.5 cm or greater

**26117**    Radical resection of tumor (eg, malignant neoplasm), soft tissue of hand or finger; less than 3 cm

**26118**        3 cm or greater

**26121**    Fasciectomy, palm only, with or without Z-plasty, other local tissue rearrangement, or skin grafting (includes obtaining graft)

**26123**    Fasciectomy, partial palmar with release of single digit including proximal interphalangeal joint, with or without Z-plasty, other local tissue rearrangement, or skin grafting (includes obtaining graft);

**+ 26125**        each additional digit (List separately in addition to code for primary procedure)

(Use 26125 in conjunction with 26123)

▶(For palmar fasciotomy by enzyme injection (eg, collagenase), see 20527, 26341)◀

(For fasciotomy, see 26040, 26045)

**26130**    Synovectomy, carpometacarpal joint

**26135**    Synovectomy, metacarpophalangeal joint including intrinsic release and extensor hood reconstruction, each digit

**26140**    Synovectomy, proximal interphalangeal joint, including extensor reconstruction, each interphalangeal joint

**26145**    Synovectomy, tendon sheath, radical (tenosynovectomy), flexor tendon, palm and/or finger, each tendon

(For tendon sheath synovectomies at wrist, see 25115, 25116)

**26160**    Excision of lesion of tendon sheath or joint capsule (eg, cyst, mucous cyst, or ganglion), hand or finger

(For wrist ganglion, see 25111, 25112)

(For trigger digit, use 26055)

**26170**    Excision of tendon, palm, flexor or extensor, single, each tendon

(Do not report 26170 in conjunction with 26390, 26415)

**26180**    Excision of tendon, finger, flexor or extensor, each tendon

(Do not report 26180 in conjunction with 26390, 26415)

**26185**    Sesamoidectomy, thumb or finger (separate procedure)

**26200**    Excision or curettage of bone cyst or benign tumor of metacarpal;

**26205**        with autograft (includes obtaining graft)

**26210**    Excision or curettage of bone cyst or benign tumor of proximal, middle, or distal phalanx of finger;

**26215**        with autograft (includes obtaining graft)

**26230**    Partial excision (craterization, saucerization, or diaphysectomy) bone (eg, osteomyelitis); metacarpal

**26235**        proximal or middle phalanx of finger

**26236**        distal phalanx of finger

**26250**    Radical resection of tumor, metacarpal

(26255 has been deleted)

26260 Radical resection of tumor, proximal or middle phalanx of finger

(26261 has been deleted)

26262 Radical resection of tumor, distal phalanx of finger

## Introduction or Removal

26320 Removal of implant from finger or hand

(For removal of foreign body in hand or finger, see 20520, 20525)

## Repair, Revision, and/or Reconstruction

26340 Manipulation, finger joint, under anesthesia, each joint

(For application of external fixation, see 20690 or 20692)

● 26341 Manipulation, palmar fascial cord (ie, Dupuytren's cord), post enzyme injection (eg, collagenase), single cord

▶(For enzyme injection (eg, collagenase), palmar fascial cord (eg, Dupuytren's contracture), use 20527)◀

▶(Report custom orthotic fabrication/application separately)◀

26350 Repair or advancement, flexor tendon, not in zone 2 digital flexor tendon sheath (eg, no man's land); primary or secondary without free graft, each tendon

26352 secondary with free graft (includes obtaining graft), each tendon

26356 Repair or advancement, flexor tendon, in zone 2 digital flexor tendon sheath (eg, no man's land); primary, without free graft, each tendon

26357 secondary, without free graft, each tendon

26358 secondary, with free graft (includes obtaining graft), each tendon

26370 Repair or advancement of profundus tendon, with intact superficialis tendon; primary, each tendon

26372 secondary with free graft (includes obtaining graft), each tendon

26373 secondary without free graft, each tendon

26390 Excision flexor tendon, with implantation of synthetic rod for delayed tendon graft, hand or finger, each rod

26392 Removal of synthetic rod and insertion of flexor tendon graft, hand or finger (includes obtaining graft), each rod

26410 Repair, extensor tendon, hand, primary or secondary; without free graft, each tendon

26412 with free graft (includes obtaining graft), each tendon

26415 Excision of extensor tendon, with implantation of synthetic rod for delayed tendon graft, hand or finger, each rod

26416 Removal of synthetic rod and insertion of extensor tendon graft (includes obtaining graft), hand or finger, each rod

26418 Repair, extensor tendon, finger, primary or secondary; without free graft, each tendon

26420 with free graft (includes obtaining graft) each tendon

26426 Repair of extensor tendon, central slip, secondary (eg, boutonniere deformity); using local tissue(s), including lateral band(s), each finger

26428 with free graft (includes obtaining graft), each finger

26432 Closed treatment of distal extensor tendon insertion, with or without percutaneous pinning (eg, mallet finger)

26433 Repair of extensor tendon, distal insertion, primary or secondary; without graft (eg, mallet finger)

26434 with free graft (includes obtaining graft)

(For tenovaginotomy for trigger finger, use 26055)

26437 Realignment of extensor tendon, hand, each tendon

26440 Tenolysis, flexor tendon; palm OR finger, each tendon

26442 palm AND finger, each tendon

26445 Tenolysis, extensor tendon, hand OR finger, each tendon

26449 Tenolysis, complex, extensor tendon, finger, including forearm, each tendon

26450 Tenotomy, flexor, palm, open, each tendon

26455 Tenotomy, flexor, finger, open, each tendon

26460 Tenotomy, extensor, hand or finger, open, each tendon

26471 Tenodesis; of proximal interphalangeal joint, each joint

26474 of distal joint, each joint

26476 Lengthening of tendon, extensor, hand or finger, each tendon

26477 Shortening of tendon, extensor, hand or finger, each tendon

26478 Lengthening of tendon, flexor, hand or finger, each tendon

26479 Shortening of tendon, flexor, hand or finger, each tendon

26480 Transfer or transplant of tendon, carpometacarpal area or dorsum of hand; without free graft, each tendon

26483 with free tendon graft (includes obtaining graft), each tendon

26485 Transfer or transplant of tendon, palmar; without free tendon graft, each tendon

26489 with free tendon graft (includes obtaining graft), each tendon

26490 Opponensplasty; superficialis tendon transfer type, each tendon

26492 tendon transfer with graft (includes obtaining graft), each tendon

26494 hypothenar muscle transfer

26496 other methods

(For thumb fusion in opposition, use 26820)

**Surgery: Musculoskeletal System**

**26497**  Transfer of tendon to restore intrinsic function; ring and small finger

**26498**      all 4 fingers

**26499**  Correction claw finger, other methods

**26500**  Reconstruction of tendon pulley, each tendon; with local tissues (separate procedure)

**26502**      with tendon or fascial graft (includes obtaining graft) (separate procedure)

**26508**  Release of thenar muscle(s) (eg, thumb contracture)

**26510**  Cross intrinsic transfer, each tendon

**26516**  Capsulodesis, metacarpophalangeal joint; single digit

**26517**      2 digits

**26518**      3 or 4 digits

**26520**  Capsulectomy or capsulotomy; metacarpophalangeal joint, each joint

**26525**      interphalangeal joint, each joint

(To report carpometacarpal joint arthroplasty, use 25447)

**26530**  Arthroplasty, metacarpophalangeal joint; each joint

**26531**      with prosthetic implant, each joint

**26535**  Arthroplasty, interphalangeal joint; each joint

**26536**      with prosthetic implant, each joint

**26540**  Repair of collateral ligament, metacarpophalangeal or interphalangeal joint

**26541**  Reconstruction, collateral ligament, metacarpophalangeal joint, single; with tendon or fascial graft (includes obtaining graft)

**26542**      with local tissue (eg, adductor advancement)

**26545**  Reconstruction, collateral ligament, interphalangeal joint, single, including graft, each joint

**26546**  Repair non-union, metacarpal or phalanx (includes obtaining bone graft with or without external or internal fixation)

**26548**  Repair and reconstruction, finger, volar plate, interphalangeal joint

**26550**  Pollicization of a digit

**26551**  Transfer, toe-to-hand with microvascular anastomosis; great toe wrap-around with bone graft

(For great toe with web space, use 20973)

**26553**      other than great toe, single

**26554**      other than great toe, double

(Do not report code 69990 in addition to codes 26551-26554)

**26555**  Transfer, finger to another position without microvascular anastomosis

**26556**  Transfer, free toe joint, with microvascular anastomosis

(Do not report code 69990 in addition to code 26556)

(To report great toe-to-hand transfer, use 20973)

**26560**  Repair of syndactyly (web finger) each web space; with skin flaps

**26561**      with skin flaps and grafts

**26562**      complex (eg, involving bone, nails)

**26565**  Osteotomy; metacarpal, each

**26567**      phalanx of finger, each

**26568**  Osteoplasty, lengthening, metacarpal or phalanx

**26580**  Repair cleft hand

**26587**  Reconstruction of polydactylous digit, soft tissue and bone

(For excision of polydactylous digit, soft tissue only, use 11200)

**26590**  Repair macrodactylia, each digit

**26591**  Repair, intrinsic muscles of hand, each muscle

**26593**  Release, intrinsic muscles of hand, each muscle

**26596**  Excision of constricting ring of finger, with multiple Z-plasties

(To report release of scar contracture or graft repairs see 11042, 14040-14041, or 15120, 15240)

## Fracture and/or Dislocation

**26600**  Closed treatment of metacarpal fracture, single; without manipulation, each bone

**26605**      with manipulation, each bone

**26607**  Closed treatment of metacarpal fracture, with manipulation, with external fixation, each bone

**26608**  Percutaneous skeletal fixation of metacarpal fracture, each bone

**26615**  Open treatment of metacarpal fracture, single, includes internal fixation, when performed, each bone

**26641**  Closed treatment of carpometacarpal dislocation, thumb, with manipulation

**26645**  Closed treatment of carpometacarpal fracture dislocation, thumb (Bennett fracture), with manipulation

**26650**  Percutaneous skeletal fixation of carpometacarpal fracture dislocation, thumb (Bennett fracture), with manipulation

**26665**  Open treatment of carpometacarpal fracture dislocation, thumb (Bennett fracture), includes internal fixation, when performed

**26670**  Closed treatment of carpometacarpal dislocation, other than thumb, with manipulation, each joint; without anesthesia

| | |
|---|---|
| 26675 | requiring anesthesia |
| 26676 | Percutaneous skeletal fixation of carpometacarpal dislocation, other than thumb, with manipulation, each joint |
| 26685 | Open treatment of carpometacarpal dislocation, other than thumb; includes internal fixation, when performed, each joint |
| 26686 | complex, multiple, or delayed reduction |
| 26700 | Closed treatment of metacarpophalangeal dislocation, single, with manipulation; without anesthesia |
| 26705 | requiring anesthesia |
| 26706 | Percutaneous skeletal fixation of metacarpophalangeal dislocation, single, with manipulation |
| 26715 | Open treatment of metacarpophalangeal dislocation, single, includes internal fixation, when performed |
| 26720 | Closed treatment of phalangeal shaft fracture, proximal or middle phalanx, finger or thumb; without manipulation, each |
| 26725 | with manipulation, with or without skin or skeletal traction, each |
| 26727 | Percutaneous skeletal fixation of unstable phalangeal shaft fracture, proximal or middle phalanx, finger or thumb, with manipulation, each |
| 26735 | Open treatment of phalangeal shaft fracture, proximal or middle phalanx, finger or thumb, includes internal fixation, when performed, each |
| 26740 | Closed treatment of articular fracture, involving metacarpophalangeal or interphalangeal joint; without manipulation, each |
| 26742 | with manipulation, each |
| 26746 | Open treatment of articular fracture, involving metacarpophalangeal or interphalangeal joint, includes internal fixation, when performed, each |
| 26750 | Closed treatment of distal phalangeal fracture, finger or thumb; without manipulation, each |
| 26755 | with manipulation, each |
| 26756 | Percutaneous skeletal fixation of distal phalangeal fracture, finger or thumb, each |
| 26765 | Open treatment of distal phalangeal fracture, finger or thumb, includes internal fixation, when performed, each |
| 26770 | Closed treatment of interphalangeal joint dislocation, single, with manipulation; without anesthesia |
| 26775 | requiring anesthesia |
| 26776 | Percutaneous skeletal fixation of interphalangeal joint dislocation, single, with manipulation |
| 26785 | Open treatment of interphalangeal joint dislocation, includes internal fixation, when performed, single |

## Arthrodesis

| | |
|---|---|
| 26820 | Fusion in opposition, thumb, with autogenous graft (includes obtaining graft) |
| 26841 | Arthrodesis, carpometacarpal joint, thumb, with or without internal fixation; |
| 26842 | with autograft (includes obtaining graft) |
| 26843 | Arthrodesis, carpometacarpal joint, digit, other than thumb, each; |
| 26844 | with autograft (includes obtaining graft) |
| 26850 | Arthrodesis, metacarpophalangeal joint, with or without internal fixation; |
| 26852 | with autograft (includes obtaining graft) |
| 26860 | Arthrodesis, interphalangeal joint, with or without internal fixation; |
| + 26861 | each additional interphalangeal joint (List separately in addition to code for primary procedure) |
| | (Use 26861 in conjunction with 26860) |
| 26862 | with autograft (includes obtaining graft) |
| + 26863 | with autograft (includes obtaining graft), each additional joint (List separately in addition to code for primary procedure) |
| | (Use 26863 in conjunction with 26862) |

## Amputation

(For hand through metacarpal bones, use 25927)

| | |
|---|---|
| 26910 | Amputation, metacarpal, with finger or thumb (ray amputation), single, with or without interosseous transfer |
| | (For repositioning, see 26550, 26555) |
| 26951 | Amputation, finger or thumb, primary or secondary, any joint or phalanx, single, including neurectomies; with direct closure |
| 26952 | with local advancement flaps (V-Y, hood) |
| | (For repair of soft tissue defect requiring split or full thickness graft or other pedicle flaps, see 15050-15758) |

## Other Procedures

| | |
|---|---|
| 26989 | Unlisted procedure, hands or fingers |

# Pelvis and Hip Joint

Including head and neck of femur.

## Incision

(For incision and drainage procedures, superficial, see 10040-10160)

| | |
|---|---|
| 26990 | Incision and drainage, pelvis or hip joint area; deep abscess or hematoma |

**26991**    infected bursa

**26992**    Incision, bone cortex, pelvis and/or hip joint (eg, osteomyelitis or bone abscess)

**27000**    Tenotomy, adductor of hip, percutaneous (separate procedure)

**27001**    Tenotomy, adductor of hip, open

(To report bilateral procedure, report 27001 with modifier 50)

**27003**    Tenotomy, adductor, subcutaneous, open, with obturator neurectomy

(To report bilateral procedure, report 27003 with modifier 50)

**27005**    Tenotomy, hip flexor(s), open (separate procedure)

**27006**    Tenotomy, abductors and/or extensor(s) of hip, open (separate procedure)

**27025**    Fasciotomy, hip or thigh, any type

(To report bilateral procedure, report 27025 with modifier 50)

**27027**    Decompression fasciotomy(ies), pelvic (buttock) compartment(s) (eg, gluteus medius-minimus, gluteus maximus, iliopsoas, and/or tensor fascia lata muscle), unilateral

(To report bilateral procedure, report 27027 with modifier 50)

**27030**    Arthrotomy, hip, with drainage (eg, infection)

**27033**    Arthrotomy, hip, including exploration or removal of loose or foreign body

**27035**    Denervation, hip joint, intrapelvic or extrapelvic intra-articular branches of sciatic, femoral, or obturator nerves

(For obturator neurectomy, see 64763, 64766)

**27036**    Capsulectomy or capsulotomy, hip, with or without excision of heterotopic bone, with release of hip flexor muscles (ie, gluteus medius, gluteus minimus, tensor fascia latae, rectus femoris, sartorius, iliopsoas)

## Excision

**27040**    Biopsy, soft tissue of pelvis and hip area; superficial

**27041**    deep, subfascial or intramuscular

(For needle biopsy of soft tissue, use 20206)

**27043**    Code is out of numerical sequence. See 27040-27080

**27045**    Code is out of numerical sequence. See 27040-27080

**27047**    Excision, tumor, soft tissue of pelvis and hip area, subcutaneous; less than 3 cm

**# 27043**    3 cm or greater

**27048**    Excision, tumor, soft tissue of pelvis and hip area, subfascial (eg, intramuscular); less than 5 cm

**# 27045**    5 cm or greater

**27049**    Radical resection of tumor (eg, malignant neoplasm), soft tissue of pelvis and hip area; less than 5 cm

**# 27059**    5 cm or greater

**27050**    Arthrotomy, with biopsy; sacroiliac joint

**27052**    hip joint

**27054**    Arthrotomy with synovectomy, hip joint

**27057**    Decompression fasciotomy(ies), pelvic (buttock) compartment(s) (eg, gluteus medius-minimus, gluteus maximus, iliopsoas, and/or tensor fascia lata muscle) with debridement of nonviable muscle, unilateral

(To report bilateral procedure, report 27057 with modifier 50)

**27059**    Code is out of numerical sequence. See 27040-27080

**27060**    Excision; ischial bursa

**27062**    trochanteric bursa or calcification

(For arthrocentesis or needling of bursa, use 20610)

**27065**    Excision of bone cyst or benign tumor, wing of ilium, symphysis pubis, or greater trochanter of femur; superficial, includes autograft, when performed

**27066**    deep (subfascial), includes autograft, when performed

**27067**    with autograft requiring separate incision

**27070**    Partial excision, wing of ilium, symphysis pubis, or greater trochanter of femur, (craterization, saucerization) (eg, osteomyelitis or bone abscess); superficial

**27071**    deep (subfascial or intramuscular)

**27075**    Radical resection of tumor; wing of ilium, 1 pubic or ischial ramus or symphysis pubis

**27076**    ilium, including acetabulum, both pubic rami, or ischium and acetabulum

**27077**    innominate bone, total

**27078**    ischial tuberosity and greater trochanter of femur

(27079 has been deleted)

**27080**    Coccygectomy, primary

(For pressure (decubitus) ulcer, see 15920, 15922 and 15931-15958)

## Introduction or Removal

**27086**    Removal of foreign body, pelvis or hip; subcutaneous tissue

**27087**    deep (subfascial or intramuscular)

**27090**    Removal of hip prosthesis; (separate procedure)

**27091**    complicated, including total hip prosthesis, methylmethacrylate with or without insertion of spacer

**27093**    Injection procedure for hip arthrography; without anesthesia

(For radiological supervision and interpretation, use 73525. Do not report 77002 in conjunction with 73525)

**27095**     with anesthesia

(For radiological supervision and interpretation, use 73525. Do not report 77002 in conjunction with 73525)

▲ **27096**   Injection procedure for sacroiliac joint, anesthetic/steroid, with image guidance (fluoroscopy or CT) including arthrography when performed

►(27096 is to be used only with CT or fluoroscopic imaging confirmation of intra-articular needle positioning)◄

►(If CT or fluoroscopy imaging is not performed, use 20552)◄

(Code 27096 is a unilateral procedure. For bilateral procedure, use modifier 50)

# Repair, Revision, and/or Reconstruction

**27097**   Release or recession, hamstring, proximal

**27098**   Transfer, adductor to ischium

**27100**   Transfer external oblique muscle to greater trochanter including fascial or tendon extension (graft)

**27105**   Transfer paraspinal muscle to hip (includes fascial or tendon extension graft)

**27110**   Transfer iliopsoas; to greater trochanter of femur

**27111**     to femoral neck

**27120**   Acetabuloplasty; (eg, Whitman, Colonna, Haygroves, or cup type)

**27122**     resection, femoral head (eg, Girdlestone procedure)

**27125**   Hemiarthroplasty, hip, partial (eg, femoral stem prosthesis, bipolar arthroplasty)

(For prosthetic replacement following fracture of the hip, use 27236)

**27130**   Arthroplasty, acetabular and proximal femoral prosthetic replacement (total hip arthroplasty), with or without autograft or allograft

**27132**   Conversion of previous hip surgery to total hip arthroplasty, with or without autograft or allograft

**27134**   Revision of total hip arthroplasty; both components, with or without autograft or allograft

**27137**     acetabular component only, with or without autograft or allograft

**27138**     femoral component only, with or without allograft

**27140**   Osteotomy and transfer of greater trochanter of femur (separate procedure)

**27146**   Osteotomy, iliac, acetabular or innominate bone;

**27147**     with open reduction of hip

**27151**     with femoral osteotomy

**27156**     with femoral osteotomy and with open reduction of hip

**27158**   Osteotomy, pelvis, bilateral (eg, congenital malformation)

**27161**   Osteotomy, femoral neck (separate procedure)

**27165**   Osteotomy, intertrochanteric or subtrochanteric including internal or external fixation and/or cast

**27170**   Bone graft, femoral head, neck, intertrochanteric or subtrochanteric area (includes obtaining bone graft)

**27175**   Treatment of slipped femoral epiphysis; by traction, without reduction

**27176**     by single or multiple pinning, in situ

**27177**   Open treatment of slipped femoral epiphysis; single or multiple pinning or bone graft (includes obtaining graft)

**27178**     closed manipulation with single or multiple pinning

**27179**     osteoplasty of femoral neck (Heyman type procedure)

**27181**     osteotomy and internal fixation

**27185**   Epiphyseal arrest by epiphysiodesis or stapling, greater trochanter of femur

**27187**   Prophylactic treatment (nailing, pinning, plating or wiring) with or without methylmethacrylate, femoral neck and proximal femur

# Fracture and/or Dislocation

**27193**   Closed treatment of pelvic ring fracture, dislocation, diastasis or subluxation; without manipulation

**27194**     with manipulation, requiring more than local anesthesia

**27200**   Closed treatment of coccygeal fracture

**27202**   Open treatment of coccygeal fracture

**27215**   Open treatment of iliac spine(s), tuberosity avulsion, or iliac wing fracture(s), unilateral, for pelvic bone fracture patterns that do not disrupt the pelvic ring, includes internal fixation, when performed

(To report bilateral procedure, report 27215 with modifier 50)

**27216**   Percutaneous skeletal fixation of posterior pelvic bone fracture and/or dislocation, for fracture patterns that disrupt the pelvic ring, unilateral (includes ipsilateral ilium, sacroiliac joint and/or sacrum)

(To report bilateral procedure, report 27216 with modifier 50)

**27217**   Open treatment of anterior pelvic bone fracture and/or dislocation for fracture patterns that disrupt the pelvic ring, unilateral, includes internal fixation, when performed (includes pubic symphysis and/or ipsilateral superior/inferior rami)

(To report bilateral procedure, report 27217 with modifier 50)

**Surgery: Musculoskeletal System**

27218 Open treatment of posterior pelvic bone fracture and/or dislocation, for fracture patterns that disrupt the pelvic ring, unilateral, includes internal fixation, when performed (includes ipsilateral ilium, sacroiliac joint and/or sacrum)

(To report bilateral procedure, report 27218 with modifier 50)

27220 Closed treatment of acetabulum (hip socket) fracture(s); without manipulation

27222 with manipulation, with or without skeletal traction

27226 Open treatment of posterior or anterior acetabular wall fracture, with internal fixation

27227 Open treatment of acetabular fracture(s) involving anterior or posterior (one) column, or a fracture running transversely across the acetabulum, with internal fixation

27228 Open treatment of acetabular fracture(s) involving anterior and posterior (two) columns, includes T-fracture and both column fracture with complete articular detachment, or single column or transverse fracture with associated acetabular wall fracture, with internal fixation

27230 Closed treatment of femoral fracture, proximal end, neck; without manipulation

27232 with manipulation, with or without skeletal traction

27235 Percutaneous skeletal fixation of femoral fracture, proximal end, neck

27236 Open treatment of femoral fracture, proximal end, neck, internal fixation or prosthetic replacement

27238 Closed treatment of intertrochanteric, peritrochanteric, or subtrochanteric femoral fracture; without manipulation

27240 with manipulation, with or without skin or skeletal traction

27244 Treatment of intertrochanteric, peritrochanteric, or subtrochanteric femoral fracture; with plate/screw type implant, with or without cerclage

27245 with intramedullary implant, with or without interlocking screws and/or cerclage

27246 Closed treatment of greater trochanteric fracture, without manipulation

27248 Open treatment of greater trochanteric fracture, includes internal fixation, when performed

27250 Closed treatment of hip dislocation, traumatic; without anesthesia

27252 requiring anesthesia

27253 Open treatment of hip dislocation, traumatic, without internal fixation

27254 Open treatment of hip dislocation, traumatic, with acetabular wall and femoral head fracture, with or without internal or external fixation

(For treatment of acetabular fracture with fixation, see 27226, 27227)

27256 Treatment of spontaneous hip dislocation (developmental, including congenital or pathological), by abduction, splint or traction; without anesthesia, without manipulation

27257 with manipulation, requiring anesthesia

27258 Open treatment of spontaneous hip dislocation (developmental, including congenital or pathological), replacement of femoral head in acetabulum (including tenotomy, etc);

27259 with femoral shaft shortening

27265 Closed treatment of post hip arthroplasty dislocation; without anesthesia

27266 requiring regional or general anesthesia

27267 Closed treatment of femoral fracture, proximal end, head; without manipulation

27268 with manipulation

27269 Open treatment of femoral fracture, proximal end, head, includes internal fixation, when performed

(Do not report 27269 in conjunction with 27033, 27253)

## Manipulation

27275 Manipulation, hip joint, requiring general anesthesia

## Arthrodesis

27280 Arthrodesis, sacroiliac joint (including obtaining graft)

(To report bilateral procedure, report 27280 with modifier 50)

27282 Arthrodesis, symphysis pubis (including obtaining graft)

27284 Arthrodesis, hip joint (including obtaining graft);

27286 with subtrochanteric osteotomy

## Amputation

27290 Interpelviabdominal amputation (hindquarter amputation)

27295 Disarticulation of hip

## Other Procedures

27299 Unlisted procedure, pelvis or hip joint

# Femur (Thigh Region) and Knee Joint

Including tibial plateaus.

## Incision

(For incision and drainage of abscess or hematoma, superficial, see 10040-10160)

27301 Incision and drainage, deep abscess, bursa, or hematoma, thigh or knee region

| | |
|---|---|
| 27303 | Incision, deep, with opening of bone cortex, femur or knee (eg, osteomyelitis or bone abscess) |
| 27305 | Fasciotomy, iliotibial (tenotomy), open |

(For combined Ober-Yount fasciotomy, use 27025)

| | |
|---|---|
| 27306 | Tenotomy, percutaneous, adductor or hamstring; single tendon (separate procedure) |
| 27307 |      multiple tendons |
| 27310 | Arthrotomy, knee, with exploration, drainage, or removal of foreign body (eg, infection) |

## Excision

| | |
|---|---|
| 27323 | Biopsy, soft tissue of thigh or knee area; superficial |
| 27324 |      deep (subfascial or intramuscular) |

(For needle biopsy of soft tissue, use 20206)

| | |
|---|---|
| 27325 | Neurectomy, hamstring muscle |
| 27326 | Neurectomy, popliteal (gastrocnemius) |
| 27327 | Excision, tumor, soft tissue of thigh or knee area, subcutaneous; less than 3 cm |
| # 27337 |      3 cm or greater |
| 27328 | Excision, tumor, soft tissue of thigh or knee area, subfascial (eg, intramuscular); less than 5 cm |
| # 27339 |      5 cm or greater |
| 27329 | Code is out of numerical sequence. See 27323-27365 |
| 27330 | Arthrotomy, knee; with synovial biopsy only |
| 27331 |      including joint exploration, biopsy, or removal of loose or foreign bodies |
| 27332 | Arthrotomy, with excision of semilunar cartilage (meniscectomy) knee; medial OR lateral |
| 27333 |      medial AND lateral |
| 27334 | Arthrotomy, with synovectomy, knee; anterior OR posterior |
| 27335 |      anterior AND posterior including popliteal area |
| 27337 | Code is out of numerical sequence. See 27323-27365 |
| 27339 | Code is out of numerical sequence. See 27323-27365 |
| 27340 | Excision, prepatellar bursa |
| 27345 | Excision of synovial cyst of popliteal space (eg, Baker's cyst) |
| 27347 | Excision of lesion of meniscus or capsule (eg, cyst, ganglion), knee |
| 27350 | Patellectomy or hemipatellectomy |
| 27355 | Excision or curettage of bone cyst or benign tumor of femur; |
| 27356 |      with allograft |
| 27357 |      with autograft (includes obtaining graft) |

| | |
|---|---|
| + 27358 | with internal fixation (List in addition to code for primary procedure) |

(Use 27358 in conjunction with 27355, 27356, or 27357)

| | |
|---|---|
| 27360 | Partial excision (craterization, saucerization, or diaphysectomy) bone, femur, proximal tibia and/or fibula (eg, osteomyelitis or bone abscess) |
| # 27329 | Radical resection of tumor (eg, malignant neoplasm), soft tissue of thigh or knee area; less than 5 cm |
| 27364 |      5 cm or greater |
| 27365 | Radical resection of tumor, femur or knee |

(For radical resection of tumor, soft tissue of thigh or knee area, see 27329, 27364)

## Introduction or Removal

| | |
|---|---|
| 27370 | Injection procedure for knee arthrography |

(For radiological supervision and interpretation, use 73580. Do not report 77002 in conjunction with 73580)

| | |
|---|---|
| 27372 | Removal of foreign body, deep, thigh region or knee area |

(For removal of knee prosthesis including "total knee," use 27488)

(For surgical arthroscopic knee procedures, see 29870-29887)

## Repair, Revision, and/or Reconstruction

| | |
|---|---|
| 27380 | Suture of infrapatellar tendon; primary |
| 27381 |      secondary reconstruction, including fascial or tendon graft |
| 27385 | Suture of quadriceps or hamstring muscle rupture; primary |
| 27386 |      secondary reconstruction, including fascial or tendon graft |
| 27390 | Tenotomy, open, hamstring, knee to hip; single tendon |
| 27391 |      multiple tendons, 1 leg |
| 27392 |      multiple tendons, bilateral |
| 27393 | Lengthening of hamstring tendon; single tendon |
| 27394 |      multiple tendons, 1 leg |
| 27395 |      multiple tendons, bilateral |
| 27396 | Transplant or transfer (with muscle redirection or rerouting), thigh (eg, extensor to flexor); single tendon |
| 27397 |      multiple tendons |
| 27400 | Transfer, tendon or muscle, hamstrings to femur (eg, Egger's type procedure) |
| 27403 | Arthrotomy with meniscus repair, knee |

(For arthroscopic repair, use 29882)

| | |
|---|---|
| 27405 | Repair, primary, torn ligament and/or capsule, knee; collateral |

---

**Surgery: Musculoskeletal System**

27407  cruciate

(For cruciate ligament reconstruction, use 27427)

27409  collateral and cruciate ligaments

(For ligament reconstruction, see 27427-27429)

27412  Autologous chondrocyte implantation, knee

(Do not report 27412 in conjunction with 20926, 27331, 27570)

(For harvesting of chondrocytes, use 29870)

27415  Osteochondral allograft, knee, open

(For arthroscopic implant of osteochondral allograft, use 29867)

(Do not report 27415 in conjunction with 27416)

27416  Osteochondral autograft(s), knee, open (eg, mosaicplasty) (includes harvesting of autograft[s])

(Do not report 27416 in conjunction with 27415, 29870, 29871, 29875, 29884 when performed at the same session and/or 29874, 29877, 29879, 29885-29887 when performed in the same compartment)

(For arthroscopic osteochondral autograft of knee, use 29866)

27418  Anterior tibial tubercleplasty (eg, Maquet type procedure)

27420  Reconstruction of dislocating patella; (eg, Hauser type procedure)

27422  with extensor realignment and/or muscle advancement or release (eg, Campbell, Goldwaite type procedure)

27424  with patellectomy

27425  Lateral retinacular release, open

(For arthroscopic lateral release, use 29873)

27427  Ligamentous reconstruction (augmentation), knee; extra-articular

27428  intra-articular (open)

27429  intra-articular (open) and extra-articular

(For primary repair of ligament(s) performed in conjunction with reconstruction, report 27405, 27407 or 27409 in conjunction with 27427, 27428 or 27429)

27430  Quadricepsplasty (eg, Bennett or Thompson type)

27435  Capsulotomy, posterior capsular release, knee

27437  Arthroplasty, patella; without prosthesis

27438  with prosthesis

27440  Arthroplasty, knee, tibial plateau;

27441  with debridement and partial synovectomy

27442  Arthroplasty, femoral condyles or tibial plateau(s), knee;

27443  with debridement and partial synovectomy

27445  Arthroplasty, knee, hinge prosthesis (eg, Walldius type)

27446  Arthroplasty, knee, condyle and plateau; medial OR lateral compartment

27447  medial AND lateral compartments with or without patella resurfacing (total knee arthroplasty)

(For revision of total knee arthroplasty, use 27487)

(For removal of total knee prosthesis, use 27488)

27448  Osteotomy, femur, shaft or supracondylar; without fixation

(To report bilateral procedure, report 27448 with modifier 50)

27450  with fixation

(To report bilateral procedure, report 27450 with modifier 50)

27454  Osteotomy, multiple, with realignment on intramedullary rod, femoral shaft (eg, Sofield type procedure)

27455  Osteotomy, proximal tibia, including fibular excision or osteotomy (includes correction of genu varus [bowleg] or genu valgus [knock-knee]); before epiphyseal closure

(To report bilateral procedure, report 27455 with modifier 50)

27457  after epiphyseal closure

(To report bilateral procedure, report 27457 with modifier 50)

27465  Osteoplasty, femur; shortening (excluding 64876)

27466  lengthening

27468  combined, lengthening and shortening with femoral segment transfer

27470  Repair, nonunion or malunion, femur, distal to head and neck; without graft (eg, compression technique)

27472  with iliac or other autogenous bone graft (includes obtaining graft)

27475  Arrest, epiphyseal, any method (eg, epiphysiodesis); distal femur

27477  tibia and fibula, proximal

27479  combined distal femur, proximal tibia and fibula

27485  Arrest, hemiepiphyseal, distal femur or proximal tibia or fibula (eg, genu varus or valgus)

27486  Revision of total knee arthroplasty, with or without allograft; 1 component

27487  femoral and entire tibial component

27488  Removal of prosthesis, including total knee prosthesis, methylmethacrylate with or without insertion of spacer, knee

27495  Prophylactic treatment (nailing, pinning, plating, or wiring) with or without methylmethacrylate, femur

27496  Decompression fasciotomy, thigh and/or knee, 1 compartment (flexor or extensor or adductor);

27497  with debridement of nonviable muscle and/or nerve

27498   Decompression fasciotomy, thigh and/or knee, multiple compartments;

27499     with debridement of nonviable muscle and/or nerve

## Fracture and/or Dislocation

(For arthroscopic treatment of intercondylar spine[s] and tuberosity fracture[s] of the knee, see 29850, 29851)

(For arthroscopic treatment of tibial fracture, see 29855, 29856)

27500   Closed treatment of femoral shaft fracture, without manipulation

27501   Closed treatment of supracondylar or transcondylar femoral fracture with or without intercondylar extension, without manipulation

27502   Closed treatment of femoral shaft fracture, with manipulation, with or without skin or skeletal traction

27503   Closed treatment of supracondylar or transcondylar femoral fracture with or without intercondylar extension, with manipulation, with or without skin or skeletal traction

27506   Open treatment of femoral shaft fracture, with or without external fixation, with insertion of intramedullary implant, with or without cerclage and/or locking screws

27507   Open treatment of femoral shaft fracture with plate/screws, with or without cerclage

27508   Closed treatment of femoral fracture, distal end, medial or lateral condyle, without manipulation

27509   Percutaneous skeletal fixation of femoral fracture, distal end, medial or lateral condyle, or supracondylar or transcondylar, with or without intercondylar extension, or distal femoral epiphyseal separation

27510   Closed treatment of femoral fracture, distal end, medial or lateral condyle, with manipulation

27511   Open treatment of femoral supracondylar or transcondylar fracture without intercondylar extension, includes internal fixation, when performed

27513   Open treatment of femoral supracondylar or transcondylar fracture with intercondylar extension, includes internal fixation, when performed

27514   Open treatment of femoral fracture, distal end, medial or lateral condyle, includes internal fixation, when performed

27516   Closed treatment of distal femoral epiphyseal separation; without manipulation

27517     with manipulation, with or without skin or skeletal traction

27519   Open treatment of distal femoral epiphyseal separation, includes internal fixation, when performed

27520   Closed treatment of patellar fracture, without manipulation

27524   Open treatment of patellar fracture, with internal fixation and/or partial or complete patellectomy and soft tissue repair

27530   Closed treatment of tibial fracture, proximal (plateau); without manipulation

27532     with or without manipulation, with skeletal traction

(For arthroscopic treatment, see 29855, 29856)

27535   Open treatment of tibial fracture, proximal (plateau); unicondylar, includes internal fixation, when performed

27536     bicondylar, with or without internal fixation

(For arthroscopic treatment, see 29855, 29856)

27538   Closed treatment of intercondylar spine(s) and/or tuberosity fracture(s) of knee, with or without manipulation

(For arthroscopic treatment, see 29850, 29851)

27540   Open treatment of intercondylar spine(s) and/or tuberosity fracture(s) of the knee, includes internal fixation, when performed

27550   Closed treatment of knee dislocation; without anesthesia

27552     requiring anesthesia

27556   Open treatment of knee dislocation, includes internal fixation, when performed; without primary ligamentous repair or augmentation/reconstruction

27557     with primary ligamentous repair

27558     with primary ligamentous repair, with augmentation/reconstruction

27560   Closed treatment of patellar dislocation; without anesthesia

(For recurrent dislocation, see 27420-27424)

27562     requiring anesthesia

27566   Open treatment of patellar dislocation, with or without partial or total patellectomy

## Manipulation

27570   Manipulation of knee joint under general anesthesia (includes application of traction or other fixation devices)

## Arthrodesis

27580   Arthrodesis, knee, any technique

## Amputation

27590   Amputation, thigh, through femur, any level;

27591     immediate fitting technique including first cast

27592     open, circular (guillotine)

27594     secondary closure or scar revision

27596     re-amputation

27598   Disarticulation at knee

**Surgery: Musculoskeletal System**

## Other Procedures

**27599**   Unlisted procedure, femur or knee

## Leg (Tibia and Fibula) and Ankle Joint

### Incision

**27600**   Decompression fasciotomy, leg; anterior and/or lateral compartments only

**27601**       posterior compartment(s) only

**27602**       anterior and/or lateral, and posterior compartment(s)

(For incision and drainage procedures, superficial, see 10040-10160)

(For decompression fasciotomy with debridement, see 27892-27894)

**27603**   Incision and drainage, leg or ankle; deep abscess or hematoma

**27604**       infected bursa

**27605**   Tenotomy, percutaneous, Achilles tendon (separate procedure); local anesthesia-

**27606**       general anesthesia

**27607**   Incision (eg, osteomyelitis or bone abscess), leg or ankle

**27610**   Arthrotomy, ankle, including exploration, drainage, or removal of foreign body

**27612**   Arthrotomy, posterior capsular release, ankle, with or without Achilles tendon lengthening

(See also 27685)

### Excision

**27613**   Biopsy, soft tissue of leg or ankle area; superficial

**27614**       deep (subfascial or intramuscular)

(For needle biopsy of soft tissue, use 20206)

**27615**   Radical resection of tumor (eg, malignant neoplasm), soft tissue of leg or ankle area; less than 5 cm

**27616**       5 cm or greater

**27618**   Excision, tumor, soft tissue of leg or ankle area, subcutaneous; less than 3 cm

**# 27632**       3 cm or greater

**27619**   Excision, tumor, soft tissue of leg or ankle area, subfascial (eg, intramuscular); less than 5 cm

**# 27634**       5 cm or greater

**27620**   Arthrotomy, ankle, with joint exploration, with or without biopsy, with or without removal of loose or foreign body

**27625**   Arthrotomy, with synovectomy, ankle;

**27626**       including tenosynovectomy

**27630**   Excision of lesion of tendon sheath or capsule (eg, cyst or ganglion), leg and/or ankle

**27632**   Code is out of numerical sequence. See 27613-27647

**27634**   Code is out of numerical sequence. See 27613-27647

**27635**   Excision or curettage of bone cyst or benign tumor, tibia or fibula;

**27637**       with autograft (includes obtaining graft)

**27638**       with allograft

**27640**   Partial excision (craterization, saucerization, or diaphysectomy), bone (eg, osteomyelitis); tibia

(For exostosis excision, use 27635)

**27641**       fibula

(For exostosis excision, use 27635)

**27645**   Radical resection of tumor; tibia

**27646**       fibula

**27647**       talus or calcaneus

### Introduction or Removal

**27648**   Injection procedure for ankle arthrography

(For radiological supervision and interpretation, use 73615. Do not report 77002 in conjunction with 73615)

(For ankle arthroscopy, see 29894-29898)

### Repair, Revision, and/or Reconstruction

**27650**   Repair, primary, open or percutaneous, ruptured Achilles tendon;

**27652**       with graft (includes obtaining graft)

**27654**   Repair, secondary, Achilles tendon, with or without graft

**27656**   Repair, fascial defect of leg

**27658**   Repair, flexor tendon, leg; primary, without graft, each tendon

**27659**       secondary, with or without graft, each tendon

**27664**   Repair, extensor tendon, leg; primary, without graft, each tendon

**27665**       secondary, with or without graft, each tendon

**27675**   Repair, dislocating peroneal tendons; without fibular osteotomy

**27676**       with fibular osteotomy

**27680**   Tenolysis, flexor or extensor tendon, leg and/or ankle; single, each tendon

**27681**       multiple tendons (through separate incision(s))

**27685**   Lengthening or shortening of tendon, leg or ankle; single tendon (separate procedure)

**27686**       multiple tendons (through same incision), each

**27687**   Gastrocnemius recession (eg, Strayer procedure)

(Toe extensors are considered as a group to be a single tendon when transplanted into midfoot)

**27690**   Transfer or transplant of single tendon (with muscle redirection or rerouting); superficial (eg, anterior tibial extensors into midfoot)

**27691**   deep (eg, anterior tibial or posterior tibial through interosseous space, flexor digitorum longus, flexor hallucis longus, or peroneal tendon to midfoot or hindfoot)

**+ 27692**   each additional tendon (List separately in addition to code for primary procedure)

(Use 27692 in conjunction with 27690, 27691)

**27695**   Repair, primary, disrupted ligament, ankle; collateral

**27696**   both collateral ligaments

**27698**   Repair, secondary, disrupted ligament, ankle, collateral (eg, Watson-Jones procedure)

**27700**   Arthroplasty, ankle;

**27702**   with implant (total ankle)

**27703**   revision, total ankle

**27704**   Removal of ankle implant

**27705**   Osteotomy; tibia

**27707**   fibula

**27709**   tibia and fibula

**27712**   multiple, with realignment on intramedullary rod (eg, Sofield type procedure)

(For osteotomy to correct genu varus [bowleg] or genu valgus [knock-knee], see 27455-27457)

**27715**   Osteoplasty, tibia and fibula, lengthening or shortening

**27720**   Repair of nonunion or malunion, tibia; without graft, (eg, compression technique)

**27722**   with sliding graft

**27724**   with iliac or other autograft (includes obtaining graft)

**27725**   by synostosis, with fibula, any method

**27726**   Repair of fibula nonunion and/or malunion with internal fixation

(Do not report 27726 in conjunction with 27707)

**27727**   Repair of congenital pseudarthrosis, tibia

**27730**   Arrest, epiphyseal (epiphysiodesis), open; distal tibia

**27732**   distal fibula

**27734**   distal tibia and fibula

**27740**   Arrest, epiphyseal (epiphysiodesis), any method, combined, proximal and distal tibia and fibula;

**27742**   and distal femur

(For epiphyseal arrest of proximal tibia and fibula, use 27477)

**27745**   Prophylactic treatment (nailing, pinning, plating or wiring) with or without methylmethacrylate, tibia

## Fracture and/or Dislocation

**27750**   Closed treatment of tibial shaft fracture (with or without fibular fracture); without manipulation

**27752**   with manipulation, with or without skeletal traction

**27756**   Percutaneous skeletal fixation of tibial shaft fracture (with or without fibular fracture) (eg, pins or screws)

**27758**   Open treatment of tibial shaft fracture (with or without fibular fracture), with plate/screws, with or without cerclage

**27759**   Treatment of tibial shaft fracture (with or without fibular fracture) by intramedullary implant, with or without interlocking screws and/or cerclage

**27760**   Closed treatment of medial malleolus fracture; without manipulation

**27762**   with manipulation, with or without skin or skeletal traction

**27766**   Open treatment of medial malleolus fracture, includes internal fixation, when performed

**27767**   Closed treatment of posterior malleolus fracture; without manipulation

**27768**   with manipulation

**27769**   Open treatment of posterior malleolus fracture, includes internal fixation, when performed

(Do not report 27767-27769 in conjunction with 27808-27823)

**27780**   Closed treatment of proximal fibula or shaft fracture; without manipulation

**27781**   with manipulation

**27784**   Open treatment of proximal fibula or shaft fracture, includes internal fixation, when performed

**27786**   Closed treatment of distal fibular fracture (lateral malleolus); without manipulation

**27788**   with manipulation

**27792**   Open treatment of distal fibular fracture (lateral malleolus), includes internal fixation, when performed

(For treatment of tibia and fibula shaft fractures, see 27750-27759)

**27808**   Closed treatment of bimalleolar ankle fracture (eg, lateral and medial malleoli, or lateral and posterior malleoli or medial and posterior malleoli); without manipulation

**27810**   with manipulation

**27814**   Open treatment of bimalleolar ankle fracture (eg, lateral and medial malleoli, or lateral and posterior malleoli, or medial and posterior malleoli), includes internal fixation, when performed

**Surgery: Musculoskeletal System**

27816 Closed treatment of trimalleolar ankle fracture; without manipulation

27818  with manipulation

27822 Open treatment of trimalleolar ankle fracture, includes internal fixation, when performed, medial and/or lateral malleolus; without fixation of posterior lip

27823  with fixation of posterior lip

27824 Closed treatment of fracture of weight bearing articular portion of distal tibia (eg, pilon or tibial plafond), with or without anesthesia; without manipulation

27825  with skeletal traction and/or requiring manipulation

27826 Open treatment of fracture of weight bearing articular surface/portion of distal tibia (eg, pilon or tibial plafond), with internal fixation, when performed; of fibula only

27827  of tibia only

27828  of both tibia and fibula

27829 Open treatment of distal tibiofibular joint (syndesmosis) disruption, includes internal fixation, when performed

27830 Closed treatment of proximal tibiofibular joint dislocation; without anesthesia

27831  requiring anesthesia

27832 Open treatment of proximal tibiofibular joint dislocation, includes internal fixation, when performed, or with excision of proximal fibula

27840 Closed treatment of ankle dislocation; without anesthesia

27842  requiring anesthesia, with or without percutaneous skeletal fixation

27846 Open treatment of ankle dislocation, with or without percutaneous skeletal fixation; without repair or internal fixation

27848  with repair or internal or external fixation

(For surgical or diagnostic arthroscopic procedures, see 29894-29898)

## Manipulation

27860 Manipulation of ankle under general anesthesia (includes application of traction or other fixation apparatus)

## Arthrodesis

27870 Arthrodesis, ankle, open

(For arthroscopic ankle arthrodesis, use 29899)

27871 Arthrodesis, tibiofibular joint, proximal or distal

## Amputation

27880 Amputation, leg, through tibia and fibula;

27881  with immediate fitting technique including application of first cast

27882  open, circular (guillotine)

27884  secondary closure or scar revision

27886  re-amputation

27888 Amputation, ankle, through malleoli of tibia and fibula (eg, Syme, Pirogoff type procedures), with plastic closure and resection of nerves

27889 Ankle disarticulation

## Other Procedures

27892 Decompression fasciotomy, leg; anterior and/or lateral compartments only, with debridement of nonviable muscle and/or nerve

(For decompression fasciotomy of the leg without debridement, use 27600)

27893  posterior compartment(s) only, with debridement of nonviable muscle and/or nerve

(For decompression fasciotomy of the leg without debridement, use 27601)

27894  anterior and/or lateral, and posterior compartment(s), with debridement of nonviable muscle and/or nerve

(For decompression fasciotomy of the leg without debridement, use 27602)

27899 Unlisted procedure, leg or ankle

# Foot and Toes

## Incision

(For incision and drainage procedures, superficial, see 10040-10160)

28001 Incision and drainage, bursa, foot

28002 Incision and drainage below fascia, with or without tendon sheath involvement, foot; single bursal space

28003  multiple areas

28005 Incision, bone cortex (eg, osteomyelitis or bone abscess), foot

28008 Fasciotomy, foot and/or toe

(See also 28060, 28062, 28250)

28010 Tenotomy, percutaneous, toe; single tendon

28011  multiple tendons

(For open tenotomy, see 28230-28234)

28020 Arthrotomy, including exploration, drainage, or removal of loose or foreign body; intertarsal or tarsometatarsal joint

28022  metatarsophalangeal joint

28024  interphalangeal joint

28035 Release, tarsal tunnel (posterior tibial nerve decompression)

(For other nerve entrapments, see 64704, 64722)

⊙=Moderate sedation  ✚=Add-on code  ✔=FDA approval pending  #=Resequenced code  ○=Recycled/reinstated code

# Excision

**28039**   Code is out of numerical sequence. See 28043-28175

**28041**   Code is out of numerical sequence. See 28043-28175

**28043**   Excision, tumor, soft tissue of foot or toe, subcutaneous; less than 1.5 cm

**# 28039**      1.5 cm or greater

**28045**   Excision, tumor, soft tissue of foot or toe, subfascial (eg, intramuscular); less than 1.5 cm

**# 28041**      1.5 cm or greater

**28046**   Radical resection of tumor (eg, malignant neoplasm), soft tissue of foot or toe; less than 3 cm

**28047**      3 cm or greater

**28050**   Arthrotomy with biopsy; intertarsal or tarsometatarsal joint

**28052**      metatarsophalangeal joint

**28054**      interphalangeal joint

**28055**   Neurectomy, intrinsic musculature of foot

**28060**   Fasciectomy, plantar fascia; partial (separate procedure)

**28062**      radical (separate procedure)

(For plantar fasciotomy, see 28008, 28250)

**28070**   Synovectomy; intertarsal or tarsometatarsal joint, each

**28072**      metatarsophalangeal joint, each

**28080**   Excision, interdigital (Morton) neuroma, single, each

**28086**   Synovectomy, tendon sheath, foot; flexor

**28088**      extensor

**28090**   Excision of lesion, tendon, tendon sheath, or capsule (including synovectomy) (eg, cyst or ganglion); foot

**28092**      toe(s), each

**28100**   Excision or curettage of bone cyst or benign tumor, talus or calcaneus;

**28102**      with iliac or other autograft (includes obtaining graft)

**28103**      with allograft

**28104**   Excision or curettage of bone cyst or benign tumor, tarsal or metatarsal, except talus or calcaneus;

**28106**      with iliac or other autograft (includes obtaining graft)

**28107**      with allograft

**28108**   Excision or curettage of bone cyst or benign tumor, phalanges of foot

(For ostectomy, partial (eg, hallux valgus, Silver type procedure), use 28290)

**28110**   Ostectomy, partial excision, fifth metatarsal head (bunionette) (separate procedure)

**28111**   Ostectomy, complete excision; first metatarsal head

**28112**      other metatarsal head (second, third or fourth)

**28113**      fifth metatarsal head

**28114**      all metatarsal heads, with partial proximal phalangectomy, excluding first metatarsal (eg, Clayton type procedure)

**28116**   Ostectomy, excision of tarsal coalition

**28118**   Ostectomy, calcaneus;

**28119**      for spur, with or without plantar fascial release

**28120**   Partial excision (craterization, saucerization, sequestrectomy, or diaphysectomy) bone (eg, osteomyelitis or bossing); talus or calcaneus

**28122**      tarsal or metatarsal bone, except talus or calcaneus

(For partial excision of talus or calcaneus, use 28120)

(For cheilectomy for hallux rigidus, use 28289)

**28124**      phalanx of toe

**28126**   Resection, partial or complete, phalangeal base, each toe

**28130**   Talectomy (astragalectomy)

(For calcanectomy, use 28118)

**28140**   Metatarsectomy

**28150**   Phalangectomy, toe, each toe

**28153**   Resection, condyle(s), distal end of phalanx, each toe

**28160**   Hemiphalangectomy or interphalangeal joint excision, toe, proximal end of phalanx, each

**28171**   Radical resection of tumor; tarsal (except talus or calcaneus)

**28173**      metatarsal

**28175**      phalanx of toe

(For talus or calcaneus, use 27647)

# Introduction or Removal

**28190**   Removal of foreign body, foot; subcutaneous

**28192**      deep

**28193**      complicated

# Repair, Revision, and/or Reconstruction

**28200**   Repair, tendon, flexor, foot; primary or secondary, without free graft, each tendon

**28202**      secondary with free graft, each tendon (includes obtaining graft)

**28208**   Repair, tendon, extensor, foot; primary or secondary, each tendon

**28210**      secondary with free graft, each tendon (includes obtaining graft)

**28220**   Tenolysis, flexor, foot; single tendon

**28222**      multiple tendons

**28225**   Tenolysis, extensor, foot; single tendon

**Surgery: Musculoskeletal System**

| | |
|---|---|
| 28226 | multiple tendons |
| 28230 | Tenotomy, open, tendon flexor; foot, single or multiple tendon(s) (separate procedure) |
| 28232 | toe, single tendon (separate procedure) |
| 28234 | Tenotomy, open, extensor, foot or toe, each tendon |
| | (For tendon transfer to midfoot or hindfoot, see 27690, 27691) |
| 28238 | Reconstruction (advancement), posterior tibial tendon with excision of accessory tarsal navicular bone (eg, Kidner type procedure) |
| | (For subcutaneous tenotomy, see 28010, 28011) |
| | (For transfer or transplant of tendon with muscle redirection or rerouting, see 27690-27692) |
| | (For extensor hallucis longus transfer with great toe IP fusion (Jones procedure), use 28760) |
| 28240 | Tenotomy, lengthening, or release, abductor hallucis muscle |
| 28250 | Division of plantar fascia and muscle (eg, Steindler stripping) (separate procedure) |
| 28260 | Capsulotomy, midfoot; medial release only (separate procedure) |
| 28261 | with tendon lengthening |
| 28262 | extensive, including posterior talotibial capsulotomy and tendon(s) lengthening (eg, resistant clubfoot deformity) |
| 28264 | Capsulotomy, midtarsal (eg, Heyman type procedure) |
| 28270 | Capsulotomy; metatarsophalangeal joint, with or without tenorrhaphy, each joint (separate procedure) |
| 28272 | interphalangeal joint, each joint (separate procedure) |
| 28280 | Syndactylization, toes (eg, webbing or Kelikian type procedure) |
| 28285 | Correction, hammertoe (eg, interphalangeal fusion, partial or total phalangectomy) |
| 28286 | Correction, cock-up fifth toe, with plastic skin closure (eg, Ruiz-Mora type procedure) |
| 28288 | Ostectomy, partial, exostectomy or condylectomy, metatarsal head, each metatarsal head |
| 28289 | Hallux rigidus correction with cheilectomy, debridement and capsular release of the first metatarsophalangeal joint |
| 28290 | Correction, hallux valgus (bunion), with or without sesamoidectomy; simple exostectomy (eg, Silver type procedure) |
| 28292 | Keller, McBride, or Mayo type procedure |
| 28293 | resection of joint with implant |
| 28294 | with tendon transplants (eg, Joplin type procedure) |
| 28296 | with metatarsal osteotomy (eg, Mitchell, Chevron, or concentric type procedures) |

| | |
|---|---|
| 28297 | Lapidus-type procedure |
| 28298 | by phalanx osteotomy |
| 28299 | by double osteotomy |
| 28300 | Osteotomy; calcaneus (eg, Dwyer or Chambers type procedure), with or without internal fixation |
| 28302 | talus |
| 28304 | Osteotomy, tarsal bones, other than calcaneus or talus; |
| 28305 | with autograft (includes obtaining graft) (eg, Fowler type) |
| 28306 | Osteotomy, with or without lengthening, shortening or angular correction, metatarsal; first metatarsal |
| 28307 | first metatarsal with autograft (other than first toe) |
| 28308 | other than first metatarsal, each |
| 28309 | multiple (eg, Swanson type cavus foot procedure) |
| 28310 | Osteotomy, shortening, angular or rotational correction; proximal phalanx, first toe (separate procedure) |
| 28312 | other phalanges, any toe |
| 28313 | Reconstruction, angular deformity of toe, soft tissue procedures only (eg, overlapping second toe, fifth toe, curly toes) |
| 28315 | Sesamoidectomy, first toe (separate procedure) |
| 28320 | Repair, nonunion or malunion; tarsal bones |
| 28322 | metatarsal, with or without bone graft (includes obtaining graft) |
| 28340 | Reconstruction, toe, macrodactyly; soft tissue resection |
| 28341 | requiring bone resection |
| 28344 | Reconstruction, toe(s); polydactyly |
| 28345 | syndactyly, with or without skin graft(s), each web |
| 28360 | Reconstruction, cleft foot |

## Fracture and/or Dislocation

| | |
|---|---|
| 28400 | Closed treatment of calcaneal fracture; without manipulation |
| 28405 | with manipulation |
| 28406 | Percutaneous skeletal fixation of calcaneal fracture, with manipulation |
| 28415 | Open treatment of calcaneal fracture, includes internal fixation, when performed; |
| 28420 | with primary iliac or other autogenous bone graft (includes obtaining graft) |
| 28430 | Closed treatment of talus fracture; without manipulation |
| 28435 | with manipulation |
| 28436 | Percutaneous skeletal fixation of talus fracture, with manipulation |
| 28445 | Open treatment of talus fracture, includes internal fixation, when performed |

**28446** Open osteochondral autograft, talus (includes obtaining graft(s))

(Do not report 28446 in conjunction with 27705, 27707)

(For arthroscopic osteochondral talus graft, use 29892)

(For open osteochondral allograft or repairs with industrial grafts, use 28899)

**28450** Treatment of tarsal bone fracture (except talus and calcaneus); without manipulation, each

**28455** with manipulation, each

**28456** Percutaneous skeletal fixation of tarsal bone fracture (except talus and calcaneus), with manipulation, each

**28465** Open treatment of tarsal bone fracture (except talus and calcaneus), includes internal fixation, when performed, each

**28470** Closed treatment of metatarsal fracture; without manipulation, each

**28475** with manipulation, each

**28476** Percutaneous skeletal fixation of metatarsal fracture, with manipulation, each

**28485** Open treatment of metatarsal fracture, includes internal fixation, when performed, each

**28490** Closed treatment of fracture great toe, phalanx or phalanges; without manipulation

**28495** with manipulation

**28496** Percutaneous skeletal fixation of fracture great toe, phalanx or phalanges, with manipulation

**28505** Open treatment of fracture, great toe, phalanx or phalanges, includes internal fixation, when performed

**28510** Closed treatment of fracture, phalanx or phalanges, other than great toe; without manipulation, each

**28515** with manipulation, each

**28525** Open treatment of fracture, phalanx or phalanges, other than great toe, includes internal fixation, when performed, each

**28530** Closed treatment of sesamoid fracture

**28531** Open treatment of sesamoid fracture, with or without internal fixation

**28540** Closed treatment of tarsal bone dislocation, other than talotarsal; without anesthesia

**28545** requiring anesthesia

**28546** Percutaneous skeletal fixation of tarsal bone dislocation, other than talotarsal, with manipulation

**28555** Open treatment of tarsal bone dislocation, includes internal fixation, when performed

**28570** Closed treatment of talotarsal joint dislocation; without anesthesia

**28575** requiring anesthesia

**28576** Percutaneous skeletal fixation of talotarsal joint dislocation, with manipulation

**28585** Open treatment of talotarsal joint dislocation; includes internal fixation, when performed

**28600** Closed treatment of tarsometatarsal joint dislocation; without anesthesia

**28605** requiring anesthesia

**28606** Percutaneous skeletal fixation of tarsometatarsal joint dislocation, with manipulation

**28615** Open treatment of tarsometatarsal joint dislocation, includes internal fixation, when performed

**28630** Closed treatment of metatarsophalangeal joint dislocation; without anesthesia

**28635** requiring anesthesia

**28636** Percutaneous skeletal fixation of metatarsophalangeal joint dislocation, with manipulation

**28645** Open treatment of metatarsophalangeal joint dislocation, includes internal fixation, when performed

**28660** Closed treatment of interphalangeal joint dislocation; without anesthesia

**28665** requiring anesthesia

**28666** Percutaneous skeletal fixation of interphalangeal joint dislocation, with manipulation

**28675** Open treatment of interphalangeal joint dislocation, includes internal fixation, when performed

## Arthrodesis

**28705** Arthrodesis; pantalar

**28715** triple

**28725** subtalar

**28730** Arthrodesis, midtarsal or tarsometatarsal, multiple or transverse;

**28735** with osteotomy (eg, flatfoot correction)

**28737** Arthrodesis, with tendon lengthening and advancement, midtarsal, tarsal navicular-cuneiform (eg, Miller type procedure)

**28740** Arthrodesis, midtarsal or tarsometatarsal, single joint

**28750** Arthrodesis, great toe; metatarsophalangeal joint

**28755** interphalangeal joint

**28760** Arthrodesis, with extensor hallucis longus transfer to first metatarsal neck, great toe, interphalangeal joint (eg, Jones type procedure)

(For hammertoe operation or interphalangeal fusion, use 28285)

## Amputation

**28800**  Amputation, foot; midtarsal (eg, Chopart type procedure)

**28805**  transmetatarsal

**28810**  Amputation, metatarsal, with toe, single

**28820**  Amputation, toe; metatarsophalangeal joint

**28825**  interphalangeal joint

(For amputation of tuft of distal phalanx, use 11752)

## Other Procedures

**28890**  Extracorporeal shock wave, high energy, performed by a physician, requiring anesthesia other than local, including ultrasound guidance, involving the plantar fascia

(For extracorporeal shock wave therapy involving musculoskeletal system not otherwise specified, see Category III codes 0019T, 0101T, 0102T)

**28899**  Unlisted procedure, foot or toes

# Application of Casts and Strapping

The listed procedures apply when the cast application or strapping is a replacement procedure used during or after the period of follow-up care, or when the cast application or strapping is an initial service performed without a restorative treatment or procedure(s) to stabilize or protect a fracture, injury, or dislocation and/or to afford comfort to a patient. Restorative treatment or procedure(s) rendered by another physician following the application of the initial cast/splint/strap may be reported with a treatment of fracture and/or dislocation code.

A physician who applies the initial cast, strap or splint and also assumes all of the subsequent fracture, dislocation, or injury care cannot use the application of casts and strapping codes as an initial service, since the first cast/splint or strap application is included in the treatment of fracture and/or dislocation codes. (See notes under Musculoskeletal System, page 63.) A temporary cast/splint/strap is not considered to be part of the preoperative care, and the use of the modifier 56 is not applicable. Additional evaluation and management services are reportable only if significant identifiable further services are provided at the time of the cast application or strapping.

If cast application or strapping is provided as an initial service (eg, casting of a sprained ankle or knee) in which no other procedure or treatment (eg, surgical repair, reduction of a fracture, or joint dislocation) is performed or is expected to be performed by a physician rendering the initial care only, use the casting, strapping and/or supply code (99070) in addition to an evaluation and management code as appropriate.

Listed procedures include removal of cast or strapping.

(For orthotics management and training, see 97760-97762)

## Body and Upper Extremity

### Casts

**29000**  Application of halo type body cast (see 20661-20663 for insertion)

**29010**  Application of Risser jacket, localizer, body; only

**29015**  including head

**29020**  Application of turnbuckle jacket, body; only

**29025**  including head

**29035**  Application of body cast, shoulder to hips;

**29040**  including head, Minerva type

**29044**  including 1 thigh

**29046**  including both thighs

**29049**  Application, cast; figure-of-eight

**29055**  shoulder spica

**29058**  plaster Velpeau

**29065**  shoulder to hand (long arm)

**29075**  elbow to finger (short arm)

**29085**  hand and lower forearm (gauntlet)

**29086**  finger (eg, contracture)

### Splints

**29105**  Application of long arm splint (shoulder to hand)

**29125**  Application of short arm splint (forearm to hand); static

**29126**  dynamic

**29130**  Application of finger splint; static

**29131**  dynamic

### Strapping—Any Age

**29200**  Strapping; thorax

(29220 has been deleted)

(To report low back strapping, use 29799)

**29240**  shoulder (eg, Velpeau)

**29260**  elbow or wrist

**29280**  hand or finger

## Lower Extremity

### Casts

**29305**  Application of hip spica cast; 1 leg

**29325**  1 and one-half spica or both legs

(For hip spica (body) cast, including thighs only, use 29046)

| | |
|---|---|
| **29345** | Application of long leg cast (thigh to toes); |
| **29355** | walker or ambulatory type |
| **29358** | Application of long leg cast brace |
| **29365** | Application of cylinder cast (thigh to ankle) |
| **29405** | Application of short leg cast (below knee to toes); |
| **29425** | walking or ambulatory type |
| **29435** | Application of patellar tendon bearing (PTB) cast |
| **29440** | Adding walker to previously applied cast |
| **29445** | Application of rigid total contact leg cast |
| **29450** | Application of clubfoot cast with molding or manipulation, long or short leg |

(To report bilateral procedure, use 29450 with modifier 50)

### Splints

| | |
|---|---|
| **29505** | Application of long leg splint (thigh to ankle or toes) |
| **29515** | Application of short leg splint (calf to foot) |

### Strapping—Any Age

| | |
|---|---|
| **29520** | Strapping; hip |
| **29530** | knee |
| **29540** | ankle and/or foot |

►(Do not report 29540 in conjunction with 29581, 29582)◄

| | |
|---|---|
| **29550** | toes |
| **29580** | Unna boot |

►(Do not report 29580 in conjunction with 29581, 29582)◄

▲ **29581** Application of multi-layer compression system; leg (below knee), including ankle and foot

►(Do not report 29581 in conjunction with 29540, 29580, 29582, 36475, 36478, 97140)◄

● **29582** thigh and leg, including ankle and foot, when performed

►(Do not report 29582 in conjunction with 29540, 29580, 29581, 36475, 36478, 97140)◄

● **29583** upper arm and forearm

►(Do not report 29583 in conjunction with 29584, 97140)◄

● **29584** upper arm, forearm, hand, and fingers

►(Do not report 29584 in conjunction with 29583, 97140)◄

| | |
|---|---|
| **29590** | Denis-Browne splint strapping |

## Removal or Repair

Codes for cast removals should be employed only for casts applied by another physician.

| | |
|---|---|
| **29700** | Removal or bivalving; gauntlet, boot or body cast |
| **29705** | full arm or full leg cast |
| **29710** | shoulder or hip spica, Minerva, or Risser jacket, etc. |
| **29715** | turnbuckle jacket |
| **29720** | Repair of spica, body cast or jacket |
| **29730** | Windowing of cast |
| **29740** | Wedging of cast (except clubfoot casts) |
| **29750** | Wedging of clubfoot cast |

(To report bilateral procedure, use 29750 with modifier 50)

## Other Procedures

| | |
|---|---|
| **29799** | Unlisted procedure, casting or strapping |

# Endoscopy/Arthroscopy

Surgical endoscopy/arthroscopy always includes a diagnostic endoscopy/arthroscopy.

When arthroscopy is performed in conjunction with arthrotomy, add modifier 51.

| | |
|---|---|
| **29800** | Arthroscopy, temporomandibular joint, diagnostic, with or without synovial biopsy (separate procedure) |
| **29804** | Arthroscopy, temporomandibular joint, surgical |

(For open procedure, use 21010)

| | |
|---|---|
| **29805** | Arthroscopy, shoulder, diagnostic, with or without synovial biopsy (separate procedure) |

(For open procedure, see 23065-23066, 23100-23101)

| | |
|---|---|
| **29806** | Arthroscopy, shoulder, surgical; capsulorrhaphy |

(For open procedure, see 23450-23466)

(To report thermal capsulorrhaphy, use 29999)

| | |
|---|---|
| **29807** | repair of SLAP lesion |
| **29819** | with removal of loose body or foreign body |

(For open procedure, see 23040-23044, 23107)

| | |
|---|---|
| **29820** | synovectomy, partial |

(For open procedure, see 23105)

| | |
|---|---|
| **29821** | synovectomy, complete |

(For open procedure, see 23105)

| | |
|---|---|
| **29822** | debridement, limited |

(For open procedure, see specific open shoulder procedure performed)

**29823**    debridement, extensive

(For open procedure, see specific open shoulder procedure performed)

**29824**    distal claviculectomy including distal articular surface (Mumford procedure)

(For open procedure, use 23120)

**29825**    with lysis and resection of adhesions, with or without manipulation

(For open procedure, see specific open shoulder procedure performed)

**+▲ 29826**    decompression of subacromial space with partial acromioplasty, with coracoacromial ligament (ie, arch) release, when performed (List separately in addition to code for primary procedure)

(For open procedure, use 23130 or 23415)

►(Use 29826 in conjunction with 29806-29825, 29827, 29828)◄

**29827**    with rotator cuff repair

(For open or mini-open rotator cuff repair, use 23412)

(When arthroscopic subacromial decompression is performed at the same setting, use 29826 and append modifier 51)

(When arthroscopic distal clavicle resection is performed at the same setting, use 29824 and append modifier 51)

**29828**    biceps tenodesis

(Do not report 29828 in conjunction with 29805, 29820, 29822)

(For open biceps tenodesis, use 23430)

**29830**    Arthroscopy, elbow, diagnostic, with or without synovial biopsy (separate procedure)

**29834**    Arthroscopy, elbow, surgical; with removal of loose body or foreign body

**29835**        synovectomy, partial

**29836**        synovectomy, complete

**29837**        debridement, limited

**29838**        debridement, extensive

**29840**    Arthroscopy, wrist, diagnostic, with or without synovial biopsy (separate procedure)

**29843**    Arthroscopy, wrist, surgical; for infection, lavage and drainage

**29844**        synovectomy, partial

**29845**        synovectomy, complete

**29846**        excision and/or repair of triangular fibrocartilage and/or joint debridement

**29847**        internal fixation for fracture or instability

**29848**    Endoscopy, wrist, surgical, with release of transverse carpal ligament

(For open procedure, use 64721)

**29850**    Arthroscopically aided treatment of intercondylar spine(s) and/or tuberosity fracture(s) of the knee, with or without manipulation; without internal or external fixation (includes arthroscopy)

**29851**        with internal or external fixation (includes arthroscopy)

(For bone graft, use 20900, 20902)

**29855**    Arthroscopically aided treatment of tibial fracture, proximal (plateau); unicondylar, includes internal fixation, when performed (includes arthroscopy)

**29856**        bicondylar, includes internal fixation, when performed (includes arthroscopy)

(For bone graft, use 20900, 20902)

**29860**    Arthroscopy, hip, diagnostic with or without synovial biopsy (separate procedure)

**29861**    Arthroscopy, hip, surgical; with removal of loose body or foreign body

**29862**        with debridement/shaving of articular cartilage (chondroplasty), abrasion arthroplasty, and/or resection of labrum

**29863**        with synovectomy

**# 29914**        with femoroplasty (ie, treatment of cam lesion)

**# 29915**        with acetabuloplasty (ie, treatment of pincer lesion)

(Do not report 29914, 29915 in conjunction with 29862, 29863)

**# 29916**        with labral repair

(Do not report 29916 for labral repair secondary to acetabuloplasty or in conjunction with 29862, 29863)

**29866**    Arthroscopy, knee, surgical; osteochondral autograft(s) (eg, mosaicplasty) (includes harvesting of the autograft[s])

(Do not report 29866 in conjunction with 29870, 29871, 29875, 29884 when performed at the same session and/or 29874, 29877, 29879, 29885-29887 when performed in the same compartment)

(For open osteochondral autograft of knee, use 27416)

**29867**        osteochondral allograft (eg, mosaicplasty)

(Do not report 29867 in conjunction with 27570, 29870, 29871, 29875, 29884 when performed at the same session and/or 29874, 29877, 29879, 29885-29887 when performed in the same compartment)

(Do not report 29867 in conjunction with 27415)

*Surgery: Musculoskeletal System*

**29868**      meniscal transplantation (includes arthrotomy for meniscal insertion), medial or lateral

(Do not report 29868 in conjunction with 29870, 29871, 29875, 29880, 29883, 29884 when performed at the same session or 29874, 29877, 29881, 29882 when performed in the same compartment)

**29870**    Arthroscopy, knee, diagnostic, with or without synovial biopsy (separate procedure)

(For open autologous chondrocyte implantation of the knee, use 27412)

**29871**    Arthroscopy, knee, surgical; for infection, lavage and drainage

(For implantation of osteochondral graft for treatment of articular surface defect, see 27412, 27415, 29866, 29867)

**29873**      with lateral release

(For open lateral release, use 27425)

**29874**      for removal of loose body or foreign body (eg, osteochondritis dissecans fragmentation, chondral fragmentation)

**29875**      synovectomy, limited (eg, plica or shelf resection) (separate procedure)

**29876**      synovectomy, major, 2 or more compartments (eg, medial or lateral)

**29877**      debridement/shaving of articular cartilage (chondroplasty)

►(When performed with arthroscopic meniscectomy, see 29880 or 29881)◄

**29879**      abrasion arthroplasty (includes chondroplasty where necessary) or multiple drilling or microfracture

▲ **29880**      with meniscectomy (medial AND lateral, including any meniscal shaving) including debridement/shaving of articular cartilage (chondroplasty), same or separate compartment(s), when performed

▲ **29881**      with meniscectomy (medial OR lateral, including any meniscal shaving) including debridement/shaving of articular cartilage (chondroplasty), same or separate compartment(s), when performed

**29882**      with meniscus repair (medial OR lateral)

**29883**      with meniscus repair (medial AND lateral)

(For meniscal transplantation, medial or lateral, knee, use 29868)

**29884**      with lysis of adhesions, with or without manipulation (separate procedure)

**29885**      drilling for osteochondritis dissecans with bone grafting, with or without internal fixation (including debridement of base of lesion)

**29886**      drilling for intact osteochondritis dissecans lesion

**29887**      drilling for intact osteochondritis dissecans lesion with internal fixation

**29888**    Arthroscopically aided anterior cruciate ligament repair/augmentation or reconstruction

**29889**    Arthroscopically aided posterior cruciate ligament repair/augmentation or reconstruction

(Procedures 29888 and 29889 should not be used with reconstruction procedures 27427-27429)

**29891**    Arthroscopy, ankle, surgical, excision of osteochondral defect of talus and/or tibia, including drilling of the defect

**29892**    Arthroscopically aided repair of large osteochondritis dissecans lesion, talar dome fracture, or tibial plafond fracture, with or without internal fixation (includes arthroscopy)

**29893**    Endoscopic plantar fasciotomy

**29894**    Arthroscopy, ankle (tibiotalar and fibulotalar joints), surgical; with removal of loose body or foreign body

**29895**      synovectomy, partial

**29897**      debridement, limited

**29898**      debridement, extensive

**29899**      with ankle arthrodesis

(For open ankle arthrodesis, use 27870)

**29900**    Arthroscopy, metacarpophalangeal joint, diagnostic, includes synovial biopsy

(Do not report 29900 with 29901, 29902)

**29901**    Arthroscopy, metacarpophalangeal joint, surgical; with debridement

**29902**      with reduction of displaced ulnar collateral ligament (eg, Stenar lesion)

**29904**    Arthroscopy, subtalar joint, surgical; with removal of loose body or foreign body

**29905**      with synovectomy

**29906**      with debridement

**29907**      with subtalar arthrodesis

**29914**    Code 29914 is out of numerical sequence. See 29800-29999

**29915**    Code 29915 is out of numerical sequence. See 29800-29999

**29916**    Code 29916 is out of numerical sequence. See 29800-29999

**29999**    Unlisted procedure, arthroscopy

Surgery: Musculoskeletal System

# Respiratory System

## Nose

**Surgery: Respiratory System**

### Incision

**30000**  Drainage abscess or hematoma, nasal, internal approach

(For external approach, see 10060, 10140)

**30020**  Drainage abscess or hematoma, nasal septum

(For lateral rhinotomy, see specific application (eg, 30118, 30320))

### Excision

**30100**  Biopsy, intranasal

(For biopsy skin of nose, see 11100, 11101)

**30110**  Excision, nasal polyp(s), simple

(30110 would normally be completed in an office setting)

(To report bilateral procedure, use 30110 with modifier 50)

**30115**  Excision, nasal polyp(s), extensive

(30115 would normally require the facilities available in a hospital setting)

(To report bilateral procedure, use 30115 with modifier 50)

**30117**  Excision or destruction (eg, laser), intranasal lesion; internal approach

**30118**  external approach (lateral rhinotomy)

**30120**  Excision or surgical planing of skin of nose for rhinophyma

**30124**  Excision dermoid cyst, nose; simple, skin, subcutaneous

**30125**  complex, under bone or cartilage

**30130**  Excision inferior turbinate, partial or complete, any method

(For excision of superior or middle turbinate, use 30999)

**30140**  Submucous resection inferior turbinate, partial or complete, any method

(Do not report 30130 or 30140 in conjunction with 30801, 30802, 30930)

(For submucous resection of superior or middle turbinate, use 30999)

(For endoscopic resection of concha bullosa of middle turbinate, use 31240)

(For submucous resection of nasal septum, use 30520)

**30150**  Rhinectomy; partial

**30160**  total

(For closure and/or reconstruction, primary or delayed, see **Integumentary System,**13150-13160, 14060-14302, 15120, 15121, 15260, 15261, 15760, 20900-20912)

### Introduction

**30200**  Injection into turbinate(s), therapeutic

**30210**  Displacement therapy (Proetz type)

**30220**  Insertion, nasal septal prosthesis (button)

### Removal of Foreign Body

**30300**  Removal foreign body, intranasal; office type procedure

**30310**  requiring general anesthesia

**30320**  by lateral rhinotomy

### Repair

(For obtaining tissues for graft, see 20900-20926, 21210)

**30400**  Rhinoplasty, primary; lateral and alar cartilages and/or elevation of nasal tip

(For columellar reconstruction, see 13150 et seq)

**30410**  complete, external parts including bony pyramid, lateral and alar cartilages, and/or elevation of nasal tip

**30420**  including major septal repair

**30430**  Rhinoplasty, secondary; minor revision (small amount of nasal tip work)

**30435**  intermediate revision (bony work with osteotomies)

**30450**  major revision (nasal tip work and osteotomies)

**30460**  Rhinoplasty for nasal deformity secondary to congenital cleft lip and/or palate, including columellar lengthening; tip only

**30462**  tip, septum, osteotomies

**30465**  Repair of nasal vestibular stenosis (eg, spreader grafting, lateral nasal wall reconstruction)

(30465 excludes obtaining graft. For graft procedure, see 20900-20926, 21210)

(30465 is used to report a bilateral procedure. For unilateral procedure, use modifier 52)

**30520**  Septoplasty or submucous resection, with or without cartilage scoring, contouring or replacement with graft

(For submucous resection of turbinates, use 30140)

**30540**  Repair choanal atresia; intranasal

**30545**  transpalatine

(Do not report modifier 63 in conjunction with 30540, 30545)

30560　　Lysis intranasal synechia

30580　　Repair fistula; oromaxillary (combine with 31030 if antrotomy is included)

30600　　　　oronasal

30620　　Septal or other intranasal dermatoplasty (does not include obtaining graft)

30630　　Repair nasal septal perforations

## Destruction

30801　　Ablation, soft tissue of inferior turbinates, unilateral or bilateral, any method (eg, electrocautery, radiofrequency ablation, or tissue volume reduction); superficial

　　　　　(For ablation of superior or middle turbinates, use 30999)

30802　　　　intramural (ie, submucosal)

　　　　　(Do not report 30801 in conjunction with 30802)

　　　　　(Do not report 30801, 30802, 30930 in conjunction with 30130 or 30140)

　　　　　(For cautery performed for control of nasal hemorrhage, see 30901-30906)

## Other Procedures

30901　　Control nasal hemorrhage, anterior, simple (limited cautery and/or packing) any method

　　　　　(To report bilateral procedure, use 30901 with modifier 50)

30903　　Control nasal hemorrhage, anterior, complex (extensive cautery and/or packing) any method

　　　　　(To report bilateral procedure, use 30903 with modifier 50)

30905　　Control nasal hemorrhage, posterior, with posterior nasal packs and/or cautery, any method; initial

30906　　　　subsequent

30915　　Ligation arteries; ethmoidal

30920　　　　internal maxillary artery, transantral

　　　　　(For ligation external carotid artery, use 37600)

30930　　Fracture nasal inferior turbinate(s), therapeutic

　　　　　(Do not report 30801, 30802, 30930 in conjunction with 30130 or 30140)

　　　　　(For fracture of superior or middle turbinate(s), use 30999)

30999　　Unlisted procedure, nose

# Accessory Sinuses

## Incision

31000　　Lavage by cannulation; maxillary sinus (antrum puncture or natural ostium)

　　　　　(To report bilateral procedure, use 31000 with modifier 50)

31002　　　　sphenoid sinus

31020　　Sinusotomy, maxillary (antrotomy); intranasal

　　　　　(To report bilateral procedure, use 31020 with modifier 50)

31030　　　　radical (Caldwell-Luc) without removal of antrochoanal polyps

　　　　　(To report bilateral procedure, use 31030 with modifier 50)

31032　　　　radical (Caldwell-Luc) with removal of antrochoanal polyps

　　　　　(To report bilateral procedure, use 31032 with modifier 50)

31040　　Pterygomaxillary fossa surgery, any approach

　　　　　(For transantral ligation of internal maxillary artery, use 30920)

31050　　Sinusotomy, sphenoid, with or without biopsy;

31051　　　　with mucosal stripping or removal of polyp(s)

31070　　Sinusotomy frontal; external, simple (trephine operation)

　　　　　(For frontal intranasal sinusotomy, use 31276)

31075　　　　transorbital, unilateral (for mucocele or osteoma, Lynch type)

31080　　　　obliterative without osteoplastic flap, brow incision (includes ablation)

31081　　　　obliterative, without osteoplastic flap, coronal incision (includes ablation)

31084　　　　obliterative, with osteoplastic flap, brow incision

31085　　　　obliterative, with osteoplastic flap, coronal incision

31086　　　　nonobliterative, with osteoplastic flap, brow incision

31087　　　　nonobliterative, with osteoplastic flap, coronal incision

31090　　Sinusotomy, unilateral, 3 or more paranasal sinuses (frontal, maxillary, ethmoid, sphenoid)

**Surgery: Respiratory System**

# Excision

**31200** Ethmoidectomy; intranasal, anterior

**31201**   intranasal, total

**31205**   extranasal, total

**31225** Maxillectomy; without orbital exenteration

**31230**   with orbital exenteration (en bloc)

(For orbital exenteration only, see 65110 et seq)

(For skin grafts, see 15120 et seq)

# Endoscopy

A surgical sinus endoscopy includes a sinusotomy (when appropriate) and diagnostic endoscopy.

Codes 31295-31297 describe dilation of sinus ostia by displacement of tissue, any method, and include fluoroscopy if performed.

Codes 31233-31297 are used to report unilateral procedures unless otherwise specified.

Codes 31231-31235 for diagnostic evaluation refer to employing a nasal/sinus endoscope to inspect the interior of the nasal cavity and the middle and superior meatus, the turbinates, and the spheno-ethmoid recess. Any time a diagnostic evaluation is performed all these areas would be inspected and a separate code is not reported for each area.

**31231** Nasal endoscopy, diagnostic, unilateral or bilateral (separate procedure)

**31233** Nasal/sinus endoscopy, diagnostic with maxillary sinusoscopy (via inferior meatus or canine fossa puncture)

(Do not report 31233 in conjunction with 31295 when performed on the same sinus)

**31235** Nasal/sinus endoscopy, diagnostic with sphenoid sinusoscopy (via puncture of sphenoidal face or cannulation of ostium)

(Do not report 31235 in conjunction with 31297 when performed on the same sinus)

**31237** Nasal/sinus endoscopy, surgical; with biopsy, polypectomy or debridement (separate procedure)

**31238**   with control of nasal hemorrhage

**31239**   with dacryocystorhinostomy

**31240**   with concha bullosa resection

(For endoscopic osteomeatal complex [OMC] resection with antrostomy and/or anterior ethmoidectomy, with or without removal of polyp[s], use 31254 and 31256)

(For endoscopic osteomeatal complex [OMC] resection with antrostomy, removal of antral mucosal disease, and/or anterior ethmoidectomy, with or without removal of polyp[s], use 31254 and 31267)

(For endoscopic frontal sinus exploration, osteomeatal complex [OMC] resection and/or anterior ethmoidectomy, with or without removal of polyp[s], use 31254 and 31276)

(For endoscopic frontal sinus exploration, osteomeatal complex [OMC] resection, antrostomy, and/or anterior ethmoidectomy, with or without removal of polyp[s], use 31254, 31256, and 31276)

(For endoscopic nasal diagnostic endoscopy, see 31231-31235)

(For endoscopic osteomeatal complex [OMC] resection, frontal sinus exploration, antrostomy, removal of antral mucosal disease, and/or anterior ethmoidectomy, with or without removal of polyp[s], use 31254, 31267, and 31276)

**31254** Nasal/sinus endoscopy, surgical; with ethmoidectomy, partial (anterior)

**31255**   with ethmoidectomy, total (anterior and posterior)

**31256** Nasal/sinus endoscopy, surgical, with maxillary antrostomy;

(For endoscopic anterior and posterior ethmoidectomy [APE] and antrostomy, with or without removal of polyp[s], use 31255 and 31256)

(For endoscopic anterior and posterior ethmoidectomy [APE], antrostomy and removal of antral mucosal disease, with or without removal of polyp[s], use 31255 and 31267)

(For endoscopic anterior and posterior ethmoidectomy [APE], and frontal sinus exploration, with or without removal of polyp[s], use 31255 and 31276)

**31267**   with removal of tissue from maxillary sinus

(Do not report 31256, 31267 in conjunction with 31295 when performed on the same sinus)

(For endoscopic anterior and posterior ethmoidectomy [APE], and frontal sinus exploration and antrostomy, with or without removal of polyp[s], use 31255, 31256, and 31276)

(For endoscopic anterior and posterior ethmoidectomy [APE], frontal sinus exploration, antrostomy, and removal of antral mucosal disease, with or without removal of polyp[s], use 31255, 31267, and 31276)

**31276** Nasal/sinus endoscopy, surgical with frontal sinus exploration, with or without removal of tissue from frontal sinus

(Do not report 31276 in conjunction with 31296 when performed on the same sinus)

(For endoscopic anterior and posterior ethmoidectomy and sphenoidotomy [APS], with or without removal of polyp[s], use 31255, 31287 or 31288)

(For endoscopic anterior and posterior ethmoidectomy and sphenoidotomy [APS], and antrostomy, with or without removal of polyp[s], use 31255, 31256, and 31287 or 31288)

(For endoscopic anterior and posterior ethmoidectomy and sphenoidotomy [APS], antrostomy and removal of antral mucosal disease, with or without removal of polyp[s], use 31255, 31267, and 31287 or 31288)

(For endoscopic anterior and posterior ethmoidectomy and sphenoidotomy [APS], and frontal sinus exploration with or without removal of polyp[s], use 31255, 31287 or 31288, and 31276)

(For endoscopic anterior and posterior ethmoidectomy and sphenoidotomy [APS], with or without removal of polyp[s], with frontal sinus exploration and antrostomy, use 31255, 31256, 31287 or 31288, and 31276)

(For unilateral endoscopy of 2 or more sinuses, see 31231-31235)

(For endoscopic anterior and posterior ethmoidectomy and sphenoidotomy [APS], frontal sinus exploration, antrostomy and removal of antral mucosal disease, with or without removal of polyp[s], see 31255, 31267, 31287 or 31288 and 31276)

**31287**    Nasal/sinus endoscopy, surgical, with sphenoidotomy;

**31288**       with removal of tissue from the sphenoid sinus

(Do not report 31287, 31288 in conjunction with 31297 when performed on the same sinus)

**31290**    Nasal/sinus endoscopy, surgical, with repair of cerebrospinal fluid leak; ethmoid region

**31291**       sphenoid region

**31292**    Nasal/sinus endoscopy, surgical; with medial or inferior orbital wall decompression

**31293**       with medial orbital wall and inferior orbital wall decompression

**31294**       with optic nerve decompression

**31295**    Nasal/sinus endoscopy, surgical; with dilation of maxillary sinus ostium (eg, balloon dilation), transnasal or via canine fossa;

(Do not report 31295 in conjunction with 31233, 31256, 31267 when performed on the same sinus)

**31296**       with dilation of frontal sinus ostium (eg, balloon dilation)

(Do not report 31296 in conjunction with 31276 when performed on the same sinus)

**31297**       with dilation of sphenoid sinus ostium (eg, balloon dilation)

(Do not report 31297 in conjunction with 31235, 31287, 31288 when performed on the same sinus)

## Other Procedures

(For hypophysectomy, transantral or transeptal approach, use 61548)

(For transcranial hypophysectomy, use 61546)

**31299**    Unlisted procedure, accessory sinuses

## Larynx

### Excision

**31300**    Laryngotomy (thyrotomy, laryngofissure); with removal of tumor or laryngocele, cordectomy

**31320**       diagnostic

**31360**    Laryngectomy; total, without radical neck dissection

**31365**       total, with radical neck dissection

**31367**       subtotal supraglottic, without radical neck dissection

**31368**       subtotal supraglottic, with radical neck dissection

**31370**    Partial laryngectomy (hemilaryngectomy); horizontal

**31375**       laterovertical

**31380**       anterovertical

**31382**       antero-latero-vertical

**31390**    Pharyngolaryngectomy, with radical neck dissection; without reconstruction

**31395**       with reconstruction

**31400**    Arytenoidectomy or arytenoidopexy, external approach

(For endoscopic arytenoidectomy, use 31560)

**31420**    Epiglottidectomy

### Introduction

⊘ **31500**    Intubation, endotracheal, emergency procedure

(For injection procedure for segmental bronchography, use 31656)

**31502**    Tracheotomy tube change prior to establishment of fistula tract

### Endoscopy

For endoscopic procedures, code appropriate endoscopy of each anatomic site examined. If using operating microscope, telescope, or both, use the applicable code only once per operative session.

**31505**    Laryngoscopy, indirect; diagnostic (separate procedure)

**31510**       with biopsy

**31511**       with removal of foreign body

**31512**       with removal of lesion

**31513**       with vocal cord injection

**31515**    Laryngoscopy direct, with or without tracheoscopy; for aspiration

**31520**       diagnostic, newborn

(Do not report modifier 63 in conjunction with 31520)

**31525**       diagnostic, except newborn

---

**Surgery: Respiratory System**

**31526**  diagnostic, with operating microscope or telescope

(Do not report code 69990 in addition to code 31526)

**31527**  with insertion of obturator

**31528**  with dilation, initial

**31529**  with dilation, subsequent

**31530**  Laryngoscopy, direct, operative, with foreign body removal;

**31531**  with operating microscope or telescope

(Do not report code 69990 in addition to code 31531)

**31535**  Laryngoscopy, direct, operative, with biopsy;

**31536**  with operating microscope or telescope

(Do not report code 69990 in addition to code 31536)

**31540**  Laryngoscopy, direct, operative, with excision of tumor and/or stripping of vocal cords or epiglottis;

**31541**  with operating microscope or telescope

(Do not report code 69990 in addition to code 31541)

**31545**  Laryngoscopy, direct, operative, with operating microscope or telescope, with submucosal removal of non-neoplastic lesion(s) of vocal cord; reconstruction with local tissue flap(s)

**31546**  reconstruction with graft(s) (includes obtaining autograft)

(Do not report 31546 in addition to 20926 for graft harvest)

(For reconstruction of vocal cord with allograft, use 31599)

(Do not report 31545 or 31546 in conjunction with 31540, 31541, 69990)

**31560**  Laryngoscopy, direct, operative, with arytenoidectomy;

**31561**  with operating microscope or telescope

(Do not report code 69990 in addition to code 31561)

**31570**  Laryngoscopy, direct, with injection into vocal cord(s), therapeutic;

**31571**  with operating microscope or telescope

(Do not report code 69990 in addition to code 31571)

**31575**  Laryngoscopy, flexible fiberoptic; diagnostic

**31576**  with biopsy

**31577**  with removal of foreign body

**31578**  with removal of lesion

(To report flexible fiberoptic endoscopic evaluation of swallowing, see 92612-92613)

(To report flexible fiberoptic endoscopic evaluation with sensory testing, see 92614-92615)

(To report flexible fiberoptic endoscopic evaluation of swallowing with sensory testing, see 92616-92617)

(For flexible fiberoptic laryngoscopy as part of flexible fiberoptic endoscopic evaluation of swallowing and/or laryngeal sensory testing by cine or video recording, see 92612-92617)

**31579**  Laryngoscopy, flexible or rigid fiberoptic, with stroboscopy

## Repair

**31580**  Laryngoplasty; for laryngeal web, 2-stage, with keel insertion and removal

**31582**  for laryngeal stenosis, with graft or core mold, including tracheotomy

**31584**  with open reduction of fracture

**31587**  Laryngoplasty, cricoid split

**31588**  Laryngoplasty, not otherwise specified (eg, for burns, reconstruction after partial laryngectomy)

**31590**  Laryngeal reinnervation by neuromuscular pedicle

## Destruction

**31595**  Section recurrent laryngeal nerve, therapeutic (separate procedure), unilateral

## Other Procedures

**31599**  Unlisted procedure, larynx

# Trachea and Bronchi

## Incision

**31600**  Tracheostomy, planned (separate procedure);

**31601**  younger than 2 years

**31603**  Tracheostomy, emergency procedure; transtracheal

**31605**  cricothyroid membrane

**31610**  Tracheostomy, fenestration procedure with skin flaps

(For endotracheal intubation, use 31500)

(For tracheal aspiration under direct vision, use 31515)

**31611**  Construction of tracheoesophageal fistula and subsequent insertion of an alaryngeal speech prosthesis (eg, voice button, Blom-Singer prosthesis)

**31612**  Tracheal puncture, percutaneous with transtracheal aspiration and/or injection

**31613**  Tracheostoma revision; simple, without flap rotation

**31614**  complex, with flap rotation

# Endoscopy

For endoscopy procedures, code appropriate endoscopy of each anatomic site examined. Surgical bronchoscopy always includes diagnostic bronchoscopy when performed by the same physician. Codes 31622-31646 include fluoroscopic guidance, when performed.

(For tracheoscopy, see laryngoscopy codes 31515-31578)

⊙ **31615**　Tracheobronchoscopy through established tracheostomy incision

⊙+ **31620**　Endobronchial ultrasound (EBUS) during bronchoscopic diagnostic or therapeutic intervention(s) (List separately in addition to code for primary procedure[s])

(Use 31620 in conjunction with 31622-31646)

⊙ **31622**　Bronchoscopy, rigid or flexible, including fluoroscopic guidance, when performed; diagnostic, with cell washing, when performed (separate procedure)

⊙ **31623**　　with brushing or protected brushings

⊙ **31624**　　with bronchial alveolar lavage

⊙ **31625**　　with bronchial or endobronchial biopsy(s), single or multiple sites

⊙ **31626**　　with placement of fiducial markers, single or multiple

(Report supply of device separately)

⊙+ **31627**　　with computer-assisted, image-guided navigation (List separately in addition to code for primary procedure[s])

(31627 includes 3D reconstruction. Do not report 31627 in conjunction with 76376, 76377)

(Use 31627 in conjunction with 31615, 31622-31631, 31635, 31636, 31638-31643)

⊙ **31628**　　with transbronchial lung biopsy(s), single lobe

(31628 should be reported only once regardless of how many transbronchial lung biopsies are performed in a lobe)

(To report transbronchial lung biopsies performed on additional lobe, use 31632)

⊙ **31629**　　with transbronchial needle aspiration biopsy(s), trachea, main stem and/or lobar bronchus(i)

(31629 should be reported only once for upper airway biopsies regardless of how many transbronchial needle aspiration biopsies are performed in the upper airway or in a lobe)

(To report transbronchial needle aspiration biopsies performed on additional lobe(s), use 31633)

**31630**　　with tracheal/bronchial dilation or closed reduction of fracture

**31631**　　with placement of tracheal stent(s) (includes tracheal/bronchial dilation as required)

(For placement of bronchial stent, see 31636, 31637)

(For revision of tracheal/bronchial stent, use 31638)

+ **31632**　　with transbronchial lung biopsy(s), each additional lobe (List separately in addition to code for primary procedure)

(Use 31632 in conjunction with 31628)

(31632 should be reported only once regardless of how many transbronchial lung biopsies are performed in a lobe)

+ **31633**　　with transbronchial needle aspiration biopsy(s), each additional lobe (List separately in addition to code for primary procedure)

(Use 31633 in conjunction with 31629)

(31633 should be reported only once regardless of how many transbronchial needle aspiration biopsies are performed in the trachea or the additional lobe)

⊙ **31634**　　with balloon occlusion, with assessment of air leak, with administration of occlusive substance (eg, fibrin glue), if performed

⊙ **31635**　　with removal of foreign body

(For removal of implanted bronchial valves, see 0251T, 0252T)

**31636**　　with placement of bronchial stent(s) (includes tracheal/bronchial dilation as required), initial bronchus

+ **31637**　　each additional major bronchus stented (List separately in addition to code for primary procedure)

(Use 31637 in conjunction with 31636)

**31638**　　with revision of tracheal or bronchial stent inserted at previous session (includes tracheal/bronchial dilation as required)

**31640**　　with excision of tumor

**31641**　　with destruction of tumor or relief of stenosis by any method other than excision (eg, laser therapy, cryotherapy)

(For bronchoscopic photodynamic therapy, report 31641 in addition to 96570, 96571 as appropriate)

**31643**　　with placement of catheter(s) for intracavitary radioelement application

(For intracavitary radioelement application, see 77761-77763, 77785-77787)

⊙ **31645**　　with therapeutic aspiration of tracheobronchial tree, initial (eg, drainage of lung abscess)

⊙ **31646**　　with therapeutic aspiration of tracheobronchial tree, subsequent

(For catheter aspiration of tracheobronchial tree at bedside, use 31725)

⊙ **31656**　　with injection of contrast material for segmental bronchography (fiberscope only)

(For radiological supervision and interpretation, see 71040, 71060)

Surgery: Respiratory System

# Introduction

(For endotracheal intubation, use 31500)

(For tracheal aspiration under direct vision, see 31515)

**31715**   Transtracheal injection for bronchography

(For radiological supervision and interpretation, see 71040, 71060)

(For prolonged services, see 99354-99360)

**31717**   Catheterization with bronchial brush biopsy

**31720**   Catheter aspiration (separate procedure); nasotracheal

⊙ **31725**      tracheobronchial with fiberscope, bedside

**31730**   Transtracheal (percutaneous) introduction of needle wire dilator/stent or indwelling tube for oxygen therapy

# Excision, Repair

**31750**   Tracheoplasty; cervical

**31755**      tracheopharyngeal fistulization, each stage

**31760**      intrathoracic

**31766**   Carinal reconstruction

**31770**   Bronchoplasty; graft repair

**31775**      excision stenosis and anastomosis

(For lobectomy and bronchoplasty, use 32501)

**31780**   Excision tracheal stenosis and anastomosis; cervical

**31781**      cervicothoracic

**31785**   Excision of tracheal tumor or carcinoma; cervical

**31786**      thoracic

**31800**   Suture of tracheal wound or injury; cervical

**31805**      intrathoracic

**31820**   Surgical closure tracheostomy or fistula; without plastic repair

**31825**      with plastic repair

(For repair tracheoesophageal fistula, see 43305, 43312)

**31830**   Revision of tracheostomy scar

# Other Procedures

**31899**   Unlisted procedure, trachea, bronchi

# Lungs and Pleura

▶Pleural cavity or lung biopsy procedures may be accomplished using a percutaneous, thoracoscopic (Video-Assisted Thoracoscopic Surgery [VATS]), or thoracotomy approach. They involve the removal of differing amounts of tissue for diagnosis. A biopsy may be performed using different techniques such as incision or wedge. Lung resection procedures include diagnostic and therapeutic procedures, including the removal of blebs, bullae, cysts, and benign or malignant tumors or lesions. These procedures may involve the removal of small portions of the lung or even an entire lung. Additionally, lung resection procedures may require the removal of adjacent structures. Both diagnostic lung biopsies and therapeutic lung resections can be performed utilizing a wedge technique. However, a diagnostic biopsy of a lung nodule using a wedge technique requires only that a tissue sample be obtained without particular attention to resection margins. A therapeutic wedge resection requires attention to margins and complete resection even when the wedge resection is ultimately followed by a more extensive resection. In the case of a wedge resection where intraoperative pathology consultation determines that a more extensive resection is required in the same anatomic location, it becomes classified as a diagnostic wedge resection (32507, 32668). When no more extensive resection is required, the same procedure is a therapeutic wedge resection (32505, 32666).

Pleural or lung biopsies or diagnostic wedge resections should be reported using codes 32096, 32097, 32098, 32400, 32405, 32507, 32607, 32608, 32609 or 32668. The open or thoracoscopic (VATS) therapeutic resection of lung mass or nodules via a wedge resection is reported using codes 32505, 32506, 32666, and 32667. More extensive anatomic lung resection procedures, which can be performed with either thoracotomy or thoracoscopic (VATS) approaches, include: segmentectomy, lobectomy, bilobectomy, and pneumonectomy.

When diagnostic biopsy(ies) of the lung are performed, regardless of the approach (ie, open or thoracoscopic [VATS]), or technique (eg, incisional resection, cautery resection, or stapled wedge), and the specimen is sent for intraoperative pathology consultation, and during that same operative session the surgeon uses these results to determine the extent of the necessary surgical resection that includes the anatomical location biopsied, only the most extensive procedure performed (eg, segmentectomy, lobectomy, thoracoscopic [VATS] lobectomy) should be reported.

The therapeutic wedge resection codes (32505, 32506, 32666, or 32667) should not be reported in addition to the more extensive lung procedure (eg, lobectomy) unless the therapeutic wedge resection was performed on a different lobe or on the contralateral lung, whether or not an intraoperative pathology consultation is used to determine the extent of lung resection. When a diagnostic wedge resection is followed by a more extensive procedure in the same anatomical location, report add-on codes 32507 or 32668 with the more extensive procedure(s). When a therapeutic wedge resection (32505, 32506, 32666, or 32667) is performed in a different lobe than the more extensive lung resection (eg, lobectomy), report the therapeutic wedge resection with modifier 59.◀

# Incision

(32000 has been deleted. To report, use 32421)

(32002 has been deleted. To report, use 32422)

(32005 has been deleted. To report, use 32560)

(32019 has been deleted. To report, use 32550)

(32020 has been deleted. To report, use 32551)

►(To report wound exploration due to penetrating trauma without thoracotomy, use 20101)◄

**32035**    Thoracostomy; with rib resection for empyema

**32036**    with open flap drainage for empyema

►(To report wound exploration due to penetrating trauma without thoractomy, use 20101)◄

►(32095 has been deleted. To report, see 32096, 32097, 32098 for thoracotomy with biopsy of the lung or pleura)◄

● **32096**    Thoracotomy, with diagnostic biopsy(ies) of lung infiltrate(s) (eg, wedge, incisional), unilateral

►(Do not report 32096 more than once per lung)◄

►(Do not report 32096 in conjunction with 32440, 32442, 32445, 32488)◄

● **32097**    Thoracotomy, with diagnostic biopsy(ies) of lung nodule(s) or mass(es) (eg, wedge, incisional), unilateral

►(Do not report 32097 more than once per lung)◄

►(Do not report 32097 in conjunction with 32440, 32442, 32445, 32488)◄

● **32098**    Thoracotomy, with biopsy(ies) of pleura

►(To report wound exploration due to penetrating trauma without thoractomy, use 20101)◄

▲ **32100**    Thoracotomy; with exploration

(Do not report 32100 in conjunction with 19260, 19271, 19272, 32503, 32504)

▲ **32110**    with control of traumatic hemorrhage and/or repair of lung tear

▲ **32120**    for postoperative complications

▲ **32124**    with open intrapleural pneumonolysis

▲ **32140**    with cyst(s) removal, includes pleural procedure when performed

▲ **32141**    with resection-plication of bullae, includes any pleural procedure when performed

(For lung volume reduction, use 32491)

▲ **32150**    with removal of intrapleural foreign body or fibrin deposit

▲ **32151**    with removal of intrapulmonary foreign body

▲ **32160**    with cardiac massage

(For segmental or other resections of lung, see 32480-32504)

**32200**    Pneumonostomy; with open drainage of abscess or cyst

⊙ **32201**    with percutaneous drainage of abscess or cyst

(For radiological supervision and interpretation, use 75989)

**32215**    Pleural scarification for repeat pneumothorax

**32220**    Decortication, pulmonary (separate procedure); total

**32225**    partial

# ►Excision/Resection◄

**32310**    Pleurectomy, parietal (separate procedure)

**32320**    Decortication and parietal pleurectomy

**32400**    Biopsy, pleura; percutaneous needle

(If imaging guidance is performed, see 76942, 77002, 77012, 77021)

(For fine needle aspiration, use 10021 or 10022)

►(32402 has been deleted. To report open biopsy of pleura, use 32098)◄

⊙▲ **32405**    Biopsy, lung or mediastinum, percutaneous needle

►(For open biopsy of lung, see 32096, 32097. For open biopsy of mediastinum, see 39000 or 39010. For thoracoscopic [VATS] biopsy of lung, pleura, pericardium or mediastinal space structure, see 32604, 32606, 32607, 32608, 32609)◄

(For radiological supervision and interpretation, see 76942, 77002, 77012, 77021)

(For fine needle aspiration, use 10022)

# Removal

**32420**    Pneumocentesis, puncture of lung for aspiration

**32421**    Thoracentesis, puncture of pleural cavity for aspiration, initial or subsequent

(If imaging guidance is performed, see 76942, 77002, 77012)

**32422**    Thoracentesis with insertion of tube, includes water seal (eg, for pneumothorax), when performed (separate procedure)

(Do not report 32422 in conjunction with 19260, 19271, 19272, 32503, 32504)

(If imaging guidance is performed, see 76942, 77002, 77012)

▲ **32440**    Removal of lung, pneumonectomy;

▲ **32442**    with resection of segment of trachea followed by broncho-tracheal anastomosis (sleeve pneumonectomy)

Surgery: Respiratory System

▲ 32445         extrapleural

(For extrapleural pneumonectomy, with empyemectomy, use 32445 and 32540)

►(If lung resection is performed with chest wall tumor resection, report the appropriate chest wall tumor resection 19260-19272, in addition to lung resection 32440-32445)◄

▲ 32480   Removal of lung, other than pneumonectomy; single lobe (lobectomy)

▲ 32482         2 lobes (bilobectomy)

▲ 32484         single segment (segmentectomy)

(For removal of lung with bronchoplasty, use 32501)

▲ 32486         with circumferential resection of segment of bronchus followed by broncho-bronchial anastomosis (sleeve lobectomy)

▲ 32488         with all remaining lung following previous removal of a portion of lung (completion pneumonectomy)

►(For lobectomy or segmentectomy, with concomitant decortication, use 32320 and the appropriate removal of lung code)◄

▲ 32491         with resection-plication of emphysematous lung(s) (bullous or non-bullous) for lung volume reduction, sternal split or transthoracic approach, includes any pleural procedure, when performed

►(32500 has been deleted. To report open wedge resection of lung see 32505, 32506, 32507)◄

►(If lung resection is performed with chest wall tumor resection, report the appropriate chest wall tumor resection 19260-19272, in addition to lung resection 32480, 32482, 32484, 32486, 32488, 32505, 32506, 32507)◄

+ 32501   Resection and repair of portion of bronchus (bronchoplasty) when performed at time of lobectomy or segmentectomy (List separately in addition to code for primary procedure)

(Use 32501 in conjunction with 32480, 32482, 32484)

(32501 is to be used when a portion of the bronchus to preserved lung is removed and requires plastic closure to preserve function of that preserved lung. It is not to be used for closure for the proximal end of a resected bronchus)

32503   Resection of apical lung tumor (eg, Pancoast tumor), including chest wall resection, rib(s) resection(s), neurovascular dissection, when performed; without chest wall reconstruction(s)

32504         with chest wall reconstruction

(Do not report 32503, 32504 in conjunction with 19260, 19271, 19272, 32100, 32422, 32551)

● 32505   Thoracotomy; with therapeutic wedge resection (eg, mass, nodule), initial

►(Do not report 32505 in conjunction with 32440, 32442, 32445, 32488)◄

+● 32506         with therapeutic wedge resection (eg, mass or nodule), each additional resection, ipsilateral (List separately in addition to code for primary procedure)

►(Report 32506 only in conjunction with 32505)◄

►(If lung resection is performed with chest wall tumor resection, report the appropriate chest wall tumor resection 19260-19272, in addition to lung resection 32480, 32482, 32484, 32486, 32488, 32505, 32506, 32507)◄

+● 32507         with diagnostic wedge resection followed by anatomic lung resection (List separately in addition to code for primary procedure)

►(Report 32507 in conjunction with 32440, 32442, 32445, 32480, 32482, 32484, 32486, 32488, 32503, 32504)◄

32540   Extrapleural enucleation of empyema (empyemectomy)

(For extrapleural enucleation of empyema (empyemectomy) with lobectomy, use 32540 and the appropriate removal of lung code)

## Introduction and Removal

⊙ 32550   Insertion of indwelling tunneled pleural catheter with cuff

(Do not report 32550 in conjunction with 32421, 32422)

(If imaging guidance is performed, use 75989)

⊙ 32551   Tube thoracostomy, includes water seal (eg, for abscess, hemothorax, empyema), when performed (separate procedure)

(Do not report 32551 in conjunction with 19260, 19271, 19272, 32503, 32504)

(If imaging guidance is performed, use 75989)

32552   Removal of indwelling tunneled pleural catheter with cuff

⊙ 32553   Placement of interstitial device(s) for radiation therapy guidance (eg, fiducial markers, dosimeter), percutaneous, intra-thoracic, single or multiple

(Report supply of device separately)

(For imaging guidance, see 76942, 77002, 77012, 77021)

(For percutaneous placement of interstitial device[s] for intra-abdominal, intrapelvic, and/or retroperitoneal radiation therapy guidance, use 49411)

Surgery: Respiratory System

# Destruction

The instillation of a fibrinolytic agent may be performed multiple times per day over the course of several days. Code 32561 should be reported only once on the initial day treatment. Code 32562 should be reported only once on each subsequent day of treatment.

**32560**   Instillation, via chest tube/catheter, agent for pleurodesis (eg, talc for recurrent or persistent pneumothorax)

(For chest tube insertion, use 32551)

**32561**   Instillation(s), via chest tube/catheter, agent for fibrinolysis (eg, fibrinolytic agent for break up of multiloculated effusion); initial day

(For chest tube insertion, use 32551)

**32562**       subsequent day

(For chest tube insertion, use 32551)

## ►Thoracoscopy (Video-assisted thoracic surgery [VATS])◄

►Surgical thoracoscopy (video-assisted thoracic surgery [VATS]) always includes diagnostic thoracoscopy.◄

▲ **32601**   Thoracoscopy, diagnostic (separate procedure); lungs, pericardial sac, mediastinal or pleural space, without biopsy

►(32602 has been deleted. To report lung or pleural space biopsy(ies), see 32607, 32608, 32609)◄

►(32603 has been deleted. To report diagnostic thoracoscopy, pericardial sac, without biopsy use 32601)◄

**32604**       pericardial sac, with biopsy

►(32605 has been deleted. To report diagnostic thoracoscopy within the mediastinal space, use 32601)◄

►(For open pericardial bipsy, use 39010)◄

**32606**       mediastinal space, with biopsy

● **32607**   Thoracoscopy; with diagnostic biopsy(ies) of lung infiltrate(s) (eg, wedge, incisional), unilateral

►(Do not report 32607 more than once per lung)◄

►(Do not report 32607 in conjunction with 32440, 32442, 32445, 32488, 32671)◄

● **32608**       with diagnostic biopsy(ies) of lung nodule(s) or mass(es) (eg, wedge, incisional), unilateral

►(Do not report 32608 more than once per lung)◄

►(Do not report 32608 in conjunction with 32440, 32442, 32445, 32488, 32671)◄

● **32609**       with biopsy(ies) of pleura

**32650**   Thoracoscopy, surgical; with pleurodesis (eg, mechanical or chemical)

**32651**       with partial pulmonary decortication

**32652**       with total pulmonary decortication, including intrapleural pneumonolysis

**32653**       with removal of intrapleural foreign body or fibrin deposit

**32654**       with control of traumatic hemorrhage

▲ **32655**       with resection-plication of bullae, includes any pleural procedure when performed

►(For thoracoscopic [VATS] lung volume reduction surgery, use 32672)◄

**32656**       with parietal pleurectomy

►(32657 has been deleted. To report thoracoscopic [VATS] wedge resection of lung, see 32666, 32667, 32668)◄

**32658**       with removal of clot or foreign body from pericardial sac

**32659**       with creation of pericardial window or partial resection of pericardial sac for drainage

►(32660 has been deleted)◄

**32661**       with excision of pericardial cyst, tumor, or mass

**32662**       with excision of mediastinal cyst, tumor, or mass

▲ **32663**       with lobectomy (single lobe)

►(For thoracoscopic [VATS] segmentectomy, use 32669)◄

**32664**       with thoracic sympathectomy

**32665**       with esophagomyotomy (Heller type)

►(For exploratory thoracoscopy, and exploratory thoracoscopy with biopsy, see 32601-32609)◄

● **32666**       with therapeutic wedge resection (eg, mass, nodule), initial unilateral

►(To report bilateral procedure, report 32666 with modifier 50)◄

►(Do not report 32666, in conjunction with 32440, 32442, 32445, 32488, 32671)◄

+● **32667**       with therapeutic wedge resection (eg, mass or nodule), each additional resection, ipsilateral (List separately in addition to code for primary procedure)

►(Report 32667 only in conjunction with 32666)◄

►(Do not report 32667 in conjunction with 32440, 32442, 32445, 32488, 32671)◄

+● **32668**       with diagnostic wedge resection followed by anatomic lung resection (List separately in addition to code for primary procedure)

►(Report 32668 in conjunction with 32440, 32442, 32445, 32480, 32482, 32484, 32486, 32488, 32503, 32504, 32663, 32669, 32670, 32671)◄

● **32669**       with removal of a single lung segment (segmentectomy)

● **32670**       with removal of two lobes (bilobectomy)

● **32671**       with removal of lung (pneumonectomy)

---

▲=Revised code   ●=New code   ►◄=Contains new or revised text   ⊘=Modifier 51 exempt

**Surgery: Respiratory System**

● **32672**    with resection-plication for emphysematous lung (bullous or non-bullous) for lung volume reduction (LVRS), unilateral includes any pleural procedure, when performed

● **32673**    with resection of thymus, unilateral or bilateral

▶(For open thymectomy see 60520, 60521, 60522)◀

▶(For open excision mediastinal cyst see 39200, for open excision mediastinal tumor use 39220)◀

▶(For exploratory thoracoscopy, and exploratory thoracoscopy with biopsy, see 32601-32609)◀

+● **32674**    with mediastinal and regional lymphadenectomy (List separately in addition to code for primary procedure)

▶(On the right, mediastinal lymph nodes include the paratracheal, subcarinal, paraesophageal, and inferior pulmonary ligament)◀

▶(On the left, mediastinal lymph nodes include the aortopulmonary window, subcarinal, paraesophageal, and inferior pulmonary ligament)◀

▶(Report 32674 in conjunction with 32440, 32442, 32445, 32480, 32482, 32484, 32486, 32488, 32503, 32504, 32505, 32663, 32666, 32667, 32669, 32670, 32671)◀

▶(To report mediastinal and regional lymphadenectomy via thoracotomy, use 38746)◀

## Repair

**32800**    Repair lung hernia through chest wall

**32810**    Closure of chest wall following open flap drainage for empyema (Clagett type procedure)

**32815**    Open closure of major bronchial fistula

**32820**    Major reconstruction, chest wall (posttraumatic)

## Lung Transplantation

Lung allotransplantation involves three distinct components of physician work:

1. *Cadaver donor pneumonectomy(s)*, which include(s) harvesting the allograft and cold preservation of the allograft (perfusing with cold preservation solution and cold maintenance) (use 32850).

2. *Backbench work*:

Preparation of a cadaver donor single lung allograft prior to transplantation, including dissection of the allograft from surrounding soft tissues to prepare the pulmonary venous/atrial cuff, pulmonary artery, and bronchus unilaterally (use 32855).

Preparation of a cadaver donor double lung allograft prior to transplantation, including dissection of the allograft from surrounding soft tissues to prepare the pulmonary venous/atrial cuff, pulmonary artery, and bronchus bilaterally (use 32856).

3. *Recipient lung allotransplantation*, which includes transplantation of a single or double lung allograft and care of the recipient (see 32851-32854).

**32850**    Donor pneumonectomy(s) (including cold preservation), from cadaver donor

**32851**    Lung transplant, single; without cardiopulmonary bypass

**32852**        with cardiopulmonary bypass

**32853**    Lung transplant, double (bilateral sequential or en bloc); without cardiopulmonary bypass

**32854**        with cardiopulmonary bypass

**32855**    Backbench standard preparation of cadaver donor lung allograft prior to transplantation, including dissection of allograft from surrounding soft tissues to prepare pulmonary venous/atrial cuff, pulmonary artery, and bronchus; unilateral

**32856**        bilateral

(For repair or resection procedures on the donor lung, see 32491, 32500, 35216, or 35276)

## Surgical Collapse Therapy; Thoracoplasty

(See also 32503, 32504)

**32900**    Resection of ribs, extrapleural, all stages

**32905**    Thoracoplasty, Schede type or extrapleural (all stages);

**32906**        with closure of bronchopleural fistula

(For open closure of major bronchial fistula, use 32815)

(For resection of first rib for thoracic outlet compression, see 21615, 21616)

**32940**    Pneumonolysis, extraperiosteal, including filling or packing procedures

**32960**    Pneumothorax, therapeutic, intrapleural injection of air

## Other Procedures

**32997**    Total lung lavage (unilateral)

(For bronchoscopic bronchial alveolar lavage, use 31624)

**32998**    Ablation therapy for reduction or eradication of 1 or more pulmonary tumor(s) including pleura or chest wall when involved by tumor extension, percutaneous, radiofrequency, unilateral

(For imaging guidance and monitoring, see 76940, 77013, 77022)

**32999**    Unlisted procedure, lungs and pleura

# Cardiovascular System

Selective vascular catheterizations should be coded to include introduction and all lesser order selective catheterizations used in the approach (eg, the description for a selective right middle cerebral artery catheterization includes the introduction and placement catheterization of the right common and internal carotid arteries).

Additional second and/or third order arterial catheterizations within the same family of arteries supplied by a single first order artery should be expressed by 36218 or 36248. Additional first order or higher catheterizations in vascular families supplied by a first order vessel different from a previously selected and coded family should be separately coded using the conventions described above.

(For monitoring, operation of pump and other nonsurgical services, see 99190-99192, 99291, 99292, 99354-99360)

(For other medical or laboratory related services, see appropriate section)

(For radiological supervision and interpretation, see 75600-75978)

## Heart and Pericardium

### Pericardium

►(For thoracoscopic (VATS) pericardial procedures, see 32601, 32604, 32658, 32659, 32661)◄

⊙ **33010**   Pericardiocentesis; initial

(For radiological supervision and interpretation, use 76930)

⊙ **33011**      subsequent

(For radiological supervision and interpretation, use 76930)

**33015**   Tube pericardiostomy

**33020**   Pericardiotomy for removal of clot or foreign body (primary procedure)

**33025**   Creation of pericardial window or partial resection for drainage

►(For thoracoscopic (VATS) pericardial window, use 32659)◄

**33030**   Pericardiectomy, subtotal or complete; without cardiopulmonary bypass

**33031**      with cardiopulmonary bypass

▲ **33050**   Resection of pericardial cyst or tumor

►(For open pericardial biopsy, use 39010)◄

►(For thoracoscopic (VATS) resection of pericardial cyst, tumor or mass, use 32661)◄

## Cardiac Tumor

**33120**   Excision of intracardiac tumor, resection with cardiopulmonary bypass

**33130**   Resection of external cardiac tumor

## Transmyocardial Revascularization

**33140**   Transmyocardial laser revascularization, by thoracotomy; (separate procedure)

+ **33141**      performed at the time of other open cardiac procedure(s) (List separately in addition to code for primary procedure)

(Use 33141 in conjunction with 33400-33496, 33510-33536, 33542)

## Pacemaker or Pacing Cardioverter-Defibrillator

A pacemaker system includes a pulse generator containing electronics, a battery, and one or more electrodes (leads). Pulse generators are placed in a subcutaneous "pocket" created in either a subclavicular site or underneath the abdominal muscles just below the ribcage. Electrodes may be inserted through a vein (transvenous) or they may be placed on the surface of the heart (epicardial). The epicardial location of electrodes requires a thoracotomy for electrode insertion.

A single chamber pacemaker system includes a pulse generator and one electrode inserted in either the atrium or ventricle. A dual chamber pacemaker system includes a pulse generator and one electrode inserted in the right atrium and one electrode inserted in the right ventricle. In certain circumstances, an additional electrode may be required to achieve pacing of the left ventricle (bi-ventricular pacing). In this event, transvenous (cardiac vein) placement of the electrode should be separately reported using code 33224 or 33225. Epicardial placement of the electrode should be separately reported using 33202-33203.

►Like a pacemaker system, a pacing cardioverter-defibrillator (ICD) system includes a pulse generator and electrodes, although pacing cardioverter-defibrillators may require multiple leads, even when only a single chamber is being paced. A pacing cardioverter-defibrillator system may be inserted in a single chamber (pacing in the ventricle) or in dual chambers (pacing in atrium and ventricle). These devices use a combination of antitachycardia pacing, low-energy cardioversion or defibrillating shocks to treat ventricular tachycardia or ventricular fibrillation.◄

Pacing cardioverter-defibrillator pulse generators may be implanted in a subcutaneous infraclavicular pocket or in an abdominal pocket. Removal of a pacing cardioverter-defibrillator pulse generator requires opening of the existing subcutaneous pocket and disconnection of the pulse generator from its electrode(s). A thoracotomy (or laparotomy in the case of abdominally placed pulse generators) is not required to remove the pulse generator.

The electrodes (leads) of a pacing cardioverter-defibrillator system are positioned in the heart via the venous system (transvenously), in most circumstances. In certain circumstances, an additional electrode may be required to achieve pacing of the left ventricle (bi-ventricular pacing). In this event, transvenous (cardiac vein) placement of the electrode should be separately reported using code 33224 or 33225. Epicardial placement of the electrode should be separately reported using 33202-33203.

▶Electrode positioning on the epicardial surface of the heart requires a thoracotomy, or thoracoscopic placement of the leads. Removal of electrode(s) may first be attempted by transvenous extraction (33234, 33235, or 33244). However, if transvenous extraction is unsuccessful, a thoracotomy may be required to remove the electrodes (33238 or 33243). Use 33212, 33213, 33221, 33230, 33231, 33240 as appropriate in addition to the thoracotomy or endoscopic epicardial lead placement codes (33202 or 33203) to report the insertion of the generator if done by the same physician during the same session.

When the "battery" of a pacemaker or pacing cardioverter-defibrillator is changed, it is actually the pulse generator that is changed. Removal of pacemaker or pacing cardioverter-defibrillator pulse generator only is reported with 33233 or 33241. Removal of a pacemaker or pacing cardioverter-defibrillator pulse generator with insertion of a new pulse generator without any replacement or insertion of a lead(s) is reported with 33227-33229 and 33262-33264. Insertion of a new pulse generator, when existing leads are already in place and when no prior pulse generator is removed, is reported with 33212, 33213, 33221, 33230, 33231, 33240. When a pulse generator insertion involves the insertion or replacement of one or more lead(s), use the system codes 33206-33208 for pacemaker or 33249 for pacing cardioverter-defibrillator. Removal of a pulse generator (33233 or 33241) or extraction of transvenous leads (33234, 33235 or 33244) should be reported separately. An exception involves a pacemaker upgrade from single to dual system which includes removal of pulse generator, replacement of new pulse generator, and insertion of new lead, reported with 33214.

Repositioning of a pacemaker electrode, pacing cardioverter-defibrillator electrode(s), or a left ventricular pacing electrode is reported using 33215 or 33226, as appropriate.

The pacemaker and pacing cardioverter-defibrillator device evaluation codes 93279-93299 may not be reported in conjunction with pulse generator and lead insertion or revision codes 33206-33249. Defibrillator threshold testing (DFT) during pacing cardioverter-defibrillator insertion or replacement may be separately reported using 93640, 93641.

Radiological supervision and interpretation related to the pacemaker or pacing cardioverter-defibrillator procedure is included in 33206-33249. To report fluoroscopic guidance for diagnostic lead evaluation without lead insertion, replacement, or revision procedures, use 76000.

The following definitions apply to 33206-33249.

**Single lead:** a pacemaker or pacing cardioverter-defibrillator with pacing and sensing function in only one chamber of the heart.

**Dual lead:** a pacemaker or pacing cardioverter-defibrillator with pacing and sensing function in only two chambers of the heart.

**Multiple lead:** a pacemaker or pacing cardioverter-defibrillator with pacing and sensing function in three or more chambers of the heart.◀

**33202**    Insertion of epicardial electrode(s); open incision (eg, thoracotomy, median sternotomy, subxiphoid approach)

**33203**       endoscopic approach (eg, thoracoscopy, pericardioscopy)

▶(When epicardial lead placement is performed with insertion of the generator, report 33202, 33203 in conjunction with 33212, 33213, 33221, 33230, 33231, 33240)◀

⊙▲ **33206**   Insertion of new or replacement of permanent pacemaker with transvenous electrode(s); atrial

⊙▲ **33207**       ventricular

⊙▲ **33208**       atrial and ventricular

(Codes 33206-33208 include subcutaneous insertion of the pulse generator and transvenous placement of electrode[s])

▶(For removal and replacement of pacemaker pulse generator and transvenous electrode(s), use 33233 in conjunction with either 33234 or 33235 and 33206-33208)◀

▶(Do not report 33206-33208 in conjunction with 33227-33229)◀

⊙ **33210**   Insertion or replacement of temporary transvenous single chamber cardiac electrode or pacemaker catheter (separate procedure)

⊙ **33211**   Insertion or replacement of temporary transvenous dual chamber pacing electrodes (separate procedure)

⊙▲ **33212**   Insertion of pacemaker pulse generator only; with existing single lead

| ►Transvenous Procedure | System | |
| --- | --- | --- |
| | **Pacemaker** | **Implantable Cardioverter-Defibrillator** |
| Insert transvenous single lead only without pulse generator | 33216 | 33216 |
| Insert transvenous dual leads without pulse generator | 33217 | 33217 |
| Insert transvenous multiple leads without pulse generator | 33217 + 33224 | 33217 + 33224 |
| Initial pulse generator insertion only with existing single lead | 33212 | 33240 |
| Initial pulse generator insertion only with existing dual leads | 33213 | 33230 |
| Initial pulse generator insertion only with existing multiple leads | 33221 | 33231 |
| Initial pulse generator insertion or replacement plus insertion of transvenous single lead | 33206 (atrial) or 33207 (ventricular) | 33249 |
| Initial pulse generator insertion or replacement plus insertion of transvenous dual leads | 33208 | 33249 |
| Initial pulse generator insertion or replacement plus insertion of transvenous multiple leads | 33208 + 33225 | 33249 + 33225 |
| Upgrade single chamber system to dual chamber system | 33214 (includes removal of existing pulse generator) | 33241 + 33249 |
| Removal pulse generator only (without replacement) | 33233 | 33241 |
| Removal pulse generator with replacement pulse generator only single lead system (transvenous) | 33227 | 33262 |
| Removal pulse generator with replacement pulse generator only dual lead system (transvenous) | 33228 | 33263 |
| Removal pulse generator with replacement pulse generator only multiple lead system (transvenous) | 33229 | 33264 |
| Removal transvenous electrode only single lead system | 33234 | 33244 |
| Removal transvenous electrode only dual lead system | 33235 | 33244 |
| Removal and replacement of pulse generator and transvenous electrodes | 33233 + (33234 or 33235) + (33206 or 33207 or 33208) and 33225, when appropriate | 33241 + 33244 + 33249 and 33225, when appropriate◄ |

⊙▲ **33213**     with existing dual leads

#⊙● **33221**     with existing multiple leads

►(Do not report 33212, 33213, 33221 in conjunction with 33233 for removal and replacement of the pacemaker pulse generator. Use 33227-33229, as appropriate, when pulse generator replacement is indicated)◄

►(When epicardial lead placement is performed with insertion of generator, report 33202, 33203 in conjunction with 33212, 33213, 33221)◄

⊙ **33214**     Upgrade of implanted pacemaker system, conversion of single chamber system to dual chamber system (includes removal of previously placed pulse generator, testing of existing lead, insertion of new lead, insertion of new pulse generator)

►(Do not report 33214 in conjunction with 33227-33229)◄

**33215**     Repositioning of previously implanted transvenous pacemaker or pacing cardioverter-defibrillator (right atrial or right ventricular) electrode

⊙ **33216**     Insertion of a single transvenous electrode, permanent pacemaker or cardioverter-defibrillator

⊙ **33217**     Insertion of 2 transvenous electrodes, permanent pacemaker or cardioverter-defibrillator

(Do not report 33216-33217 in conjunction with 33214)

(For insertion or replacement of a cardiac venous system lead, see 33224, 33225)

⊙▲ **33218**     Repair of single transvenous electrode, permanent pacemaker or pacing cardioverter-defibrillator

►(For repair of single permanent pacemaker or pacing cardioverter-defibrillator electrode with replacement of pulse generator, see 33227-33229 or 33262-33264 and 33218)◄

Surgery: Cardiovascular System

**Surgery: Cardiovascular System**

⊙▲ **33220**   Repair of 2 transvenous electrodes for permanent pacemaker or pacing cardioverter-defibrillator

▶(For repair of 2 transvenous electrodes for permanent pacemaker or pacing cardioverter-defibrillator with replacement of pulse generator, use 33220 in conjunction with 33228, 33229, 33263, 33264)◀

**33221**   Code is out of numerical sequence. See 33202-33249

⊙ **33222**   Revision or relocation of skin pocket for pacemaker

⊙ **33223**   Revision of skin pocket for cardioverter-defibrillator

▲ **33224**   Insertion of pacing electrode, cardiac venous system, for left ventricular pacing, with attachment to previously placed pacemaker or pacing cardioverter-defibrillator pulse generator (including revision of pocket, removal, insertion, and/or replacement of existing generator)

(When epicardial electrode placement is performed, report 33224 in conjunction with 33202, 33203)

+▲ **33225**   Insertion of pacing electrode, cardiac venous system, for left ventricular pacing, at time of insertion of pacing cardioverter-defibrillator or pacemaker pulse generator (including upgrade to dual chamber system and pocket revision) (List separately in addition to code for primary procedure)

▶(Use 33225 in conjunction with 33206, 33207, 33208, 33212, 33213, 33214, 33216, 33217, 33221, 33222, 33230, 33231, 33233, 33234, 33235, 33240, 33249)◀

▲ **33226**   Repositioning of previously implanted cardiac venous system (left ventricular) electrode (including removal, insertion and/or replacement of existing generator)

**33227**   Code is out of numerical sequence. See 33202-33249

**33228**   Code is out of numerical sequence. See 33202-33249

**33229**   Code is out of numerical sequence. See 33202-33249

**33230**   Code is out of numerical sequence. See 33202-33249

**33231**   Code is out of numerical sequence. See 33202-33249

⊙▲ **33233**   Removal of permanent pacemaker pulse generator only

#⊙● **33227**   Removal of permanent pacemaker pulse generator with replacement of pacemaker pulse generator; single lead system

#⊙● **33228**      dual lead system

#⊙● **33229**      multiple lead system

▶(Do not report 33227-33229 in conjunction with 33233)◀

▶(For removal and replacement of pacemaker pulse generator and transvenous electrode[s], use 33233 in conjunction with either 33234 or 33235 and 33206-33208)◀

⊙ **33234**   Removal of transvenous pacemaker electrode(s); single lead system, atrial or ventricular

⊙ **33235**      dual lead system

**33236**   Removal of permanent epicardial pacemaker and electrodes by thoracotomy; single lead system, atrial or ventricular

**33237**      dual lead system

**33238**   Removal of permanent transvenous electrode(s) by thoracotomy

⊙▲ **33240**   Insertion of pacing cardioverter-defibrillator pulse generator only; with existing single lead

(Use 33240, as appropriate, in addition to the epicardial lead placement codes to report the insertion of the generator when done by the same physician during the same session)

#⊙● **33230**      with existing dual leads

#⊙● **33231**      with existing multiple leads

▶(Do not report 33230, 33231, 33240 in conjunction with 33241 for removal and replacement of the pacing cardioverter-defibrillator pulse generator. Use 33262-33264, as appropriate, when pulse generator replacement is indicated)◀

▶(When epicardial lead placement is performed with insertion of generator, report 33202, 33203 in conjunction with 33230, 33231, 33240)◀

⊙▲ **33241**   Removal of pacing cardioverter-defibrillator pulse generator only

▶(For removal and replacement of a pacing cardioverter-defibrillator pulse generator and electrode(s), use 33241 in conjunction with either 33243 or 33244 and 33249)◀

#⊙● **33262**   Removal of pacing cardioverter-defibrillator pulse generator with replacement of pacing cardioverter-defibrillator pulse generator; single lead system

#⊙● **33263**      dual lead system

#⊙● **33264**      multiple lead system

▶(Do not report 33262-33264 in conjunction with 33241)◀

▶(For removal of electrode[s] by thoracotomy in conjunction with pulse generator removal or replacement, use 33243 in conjunction with 33241, 33262-33264)◀

▶(For removal of electrode[s] by transvenous extraction in conjunction with pulse generator removal or replacement, use 33244 in conjunction with 33241, 33262-33264)◀

(For repair of implantable cardioverter-defibrillator pulse generator and/or leads, see 33218, 33220)

**33243**   Removal of single or dual chamber pacing cardioverter-defibrillator electrode(s); by thoracotomy

⊙ **33244**      by transvenous extraction

⊙▲ **33249**   Insertion or replacement of permanent pacing cardioverter-defibrillator system with transvenous lead(s), single or dual chamber

▶(For removal and replacement of a pacing cardioverter-defibrillator system [pulse generator and electrodes], report 33241 in conjunction with either 33243 or 33244 and 33249)◀

▶(For insertion of implantable cardioverter-defibrillator lead(s), without thoracotomy, use 33216 or 33217)◀

⊙=Moderate sedation   +=Add-on code   ⊠=FDA approval pending   #=Resequenced code   ○=Recycled/reinstated code

# Electrophysiologic Operative Procedures

This family of codes describes the surgical treatment of supraventricular dysrhythmias. Tissue ablation, disruption, and reconstruction can be accomplished by many methods including surgical incision or through the use of a variety of energy sources (eg, radiofrequency, cryotherapy, microwave, ultrasound, laser). If excision or isolation of the left atrial appendage by any method, including stapling, oversewing, ligation, or plication, is performed in conjunction with any of the atrial tissue ablation and reconstruction (maze) procedures (33254-33259, 33265-33266), it is considered part of the procedure. Codes 33254-33256 are only to be reported when there is no concurrently performed procedure that requires median sternotomy or cardiopulmonary bypass. The appropriate atrial tissue ablation add-on code, 33257, 33258, 33259 should be reported in addition to an open cardiac procedure requiring sternotomy or cardiopulmonary bypass if performed concurrently.

## Definitions

*Limited* operative ablation and reconstruction includes:

Surgical isolation of triggers of supraventricular dysrhythmias by operative ablation that isolates the pulmonary veins or other anatomically defined triggers in the left or right atrium.

*Extensive* operative ablation and reconstruction includes:

1. The services included in "*limited*"

2. Additional ablation of atrial tissue to eliminate sustained supraventricular dysrhythmias. This must include operative ablation that involves either the right atrium, the atrial septum, or left atrium in continuity with the atrioventricular annulus.

## Incision

33250　Operative ablation of supraventricular arrhythmogenic focus or pathway (eg, Wolff-Parkinson-White, atrioventricular node re-entry), tract(s) and/or focus (foci); without cardiopulmonary bypass

(For intraoperative pacing and mapping by a separate provider, use 93631)

33251　　　with cardiopulmonary bypass

33254　Operative tissue ablation and reconstruction of atria, limited (eg, modified maze procedure)

33255　Operative tissue ablation and reconstruction of atria, extensive (eg, maze procedure); without cardiopulmonary bypass

33256　　　with cardiopulmonary bypass

(Do not report 33254-33256 in conjunction with 32100, 32551, 33120, 33130, 33210, 33211, 33400-33507, 33510-33523, 33533-33548, 33600-33853, 33860-33864, 33910-33920)

+ 33257　Operative tissue ablation and reconstruction of atria, performed at the time of other cardiac procedure(s), limited (eg, modified maze procedure) (List separately in addition to code for primary procedure)

(Use 33257 in conjunction with 33120-33130, 33250-33251, 33261, 33300-33335, 33400-33496, 33500-33507, 33510-33516, 33533-33548, 33600-33619, 33641-33697, 33702-33732, 33735-33767, 33770-33814, 33840-33877, 33910-33922, 33925-33926, 33935, 33945, 33975-33980)

+ 33258　Operative tissue ablation and reconstruction of atria, performed at the time of other cardiac procedure(s), extensive (eg, maze procedure), without cardiopulmonary bypass (List separately in addition to code for primary procedure)

(Use 33258 in conjunction with 33130, 33250, 33300, 33310, 33320, 33321, 33330, 33332, 33401, 33414-33417, 33420, 33470-33472, 33501-33503, 33510-33516, 33533-33536, 33690, 33735, 33737, 33800-33813, 33840-33852, 33915, 33925 when the procedure is performed without cardiopulmonary bypass)

+ 33259　Operative tissue ablation and reconstruction of atria, performed at the time of other cardiac procedure(s), extensive (eg, maze procedure), with cardiopulmonary bypass (List separately in addition to code for primary procedure)

(Use 33259 in conjunction with 33120, 33251, 33261, 33305, 33315, 33322, 33335, 33400, 33403-33413, 33422-33468, 33474-33478, 33496, 33500, 33504-33507, 33510-33516, 33533-33548, 33600-33688, 33692-33722, 33730, 33732, 33736, 33750-33767, 33770-33781, 33786-33788, 33814, 33853, 33860-33877, 33910, 33916-33922, 33926, 33935, 33945, 33975-33980 when the procedure is performed with cardiopulmonary bypass)

(Do not report 33257, 33258 and 33259 in conjunction with 32551, 33210, 33211, 33254-33256, 33265, 33266)

33261　Operative ablation of ventricular arrhythmogenic focus with cardiopulmonary bypass

33262　Code is out of numerical sequence. See 33202-33264

33263　Code is out of numerical sequence. See 33202-33264

33264　Code is out of numerical sequence. See 33202-33264

## Endoscopy

33265　Endoscopy, surgical; operative tissue ablation and reconstruction of atria, limited (eg, modified maze procedure), without cardiopulmonary bypass

33266　　　operative tissue ablation and reconstruction of atria, extensive (eg, maze procedure), without cardiopulmonary bypass

(Do not report 33265-33266 in conjunction with 32551, 33210, 33211)

Surgery: Cardiovascular System

## Patient-Activated Event Recorder

**33282**    Implantation of patient-activated cardiac event recorder

(Initial implantation includes programming. For subsequent electronic analysis and/or reprogramming, use 93285, 93291, 93298)

**33284**    Removal of an implantable, patient-activated cardiac event recorder

## Wounds of the Heart and Great Vessels

**33300**    Repair of cardiac wound; without bypass

**33305**      with cardiopulmonary bypass

**33310**    Cardiotomy, exploratory (includes removal of foreign body, atrial or ventricular thrombus); without bypass

**33315**      with cardiopulmonary bypass

(Do not report removal of thrombus [33310-33315] in conjunction with other cardiac procedures unless a separate incision in the heart is required to remove the atrial or ventricular thrombus)

(If removal of thrombus with cardiopulmonary bypass [33315] is reported in conjunction with 33120, 33130, 33420-33430, 33460-33468, 33496, 33542, 33545, 33641-33647, 33670, 33681, 33975-33980 which requires a separate heart incision, report 33315 with modifier 59)

**33320**    Suture repair of aorta or great vessels; without shunt or cardiopulmonary bypass

**33321**      with shunt bypass

**33322**      with cardiopulmonary bypass

**33330**    Insertion of graft, aorta or great vessels; without shunt, or cardiopulmonary bypass

**33332**      with shunt bypass

**33335**      with cardiopulmonary bypass

## Cardiac Valves

(For multiple valve procedures, see 33400-33478 and add modifier 51 to the secondary valve procedure code)

### Aortic Valve

**33400**    Valvuloplasty, aortic valve; open, with cardiopulmonary bypass

**33401**      open, with inflow occlusion

**33403**      using transventricular dilation, with cardiopulmonary bypass

(Do not report modifier 63 in conjunction with 33401, 33403)

**33404**    Construction of apical-aortic conduit

**33405**    Replacement, aortic valve, with cardiopulmonary bypass; with prosthetic valve other than homograft or stentless valve

**33406**      with allograft valve (freehand)

(For aortic valve valvotomy, [commissurotomy] with inflow occlusion, use 33401)

(For aortic valve valvotomy, [commissurotomy] with cardiopulmonary bypass, use 33403)

**33410**      with stentless tissue valve

**33411**    Replacement, aortic valve; with aortic annulus enlargement, noncoronary sinus

**33412**      with transventricular aortic annulus enlargement (Konno procedure)

**33413**      by translocation of autologous pulmonary valve with allograft replacement of pulmonary valve (Ross procedure)

**33414**    Repair of left ventricular outflow tract obstruction by patch enlargement of the outflow tract

**33415**    Resection or incision of subvalvular tissue for discrete subvalvular aortic stenosis

**33416**    Ventriculomyotomy (-myectomy) for idiopathic hypertrophic subaortic stenosis (eg, asymmetric septal hypertrophy)

**33417**    Aortoplasty (gusset) for supravalvular stenosis

### Mitral Valve

**33420**    Valvotomy, mitral valve; closed heart

**33422**      open heart, with cardiopulmonary bypass

**33425**    Valvuloplasty, mitral valve, with cardiopulmonary bypass;

**33426**      with prosthetic ring

**33427**      radical reconstruction, with or without ring

**33430**    Replacement, mitral valve, with cardiopulmonary bypass

### Tricuspid Valve

**33460**    Valvectomy, tricuspid valve, with cardiopulmonary bypass

**33463**    Valvuloplasty, tricuspid valve; without ring insertion

**33464**      with ring insertion

**33465**    Replacement, tricuspid valve, with cardiopulmonary bypass

**33468**    Tricuspid valve repositioning and plication for Ebstein anomaly

### Pulmonary Valve

**33470**    Valvotomy, pulmonary valve, closed heart; transventricular

(Do not report modifier 63 in conjunction with 33470)

**33471**      via pulmonary artery

(To report percutaneous valvuloplasty of pulmonary valve, use 92990)

Surgery: Cardiovascular System

**33472**   Valvotomy, pulmonary valve, open heart; with inflow occlusion

(Do not report modifier 63 in conjunction with 33472)

**33474**      with cardiopulmonary bypass

**33475**   Replacement, pulmonary valve

**33476**   Right ventricular resection for infundibular stenosis, with or without commissurotomy

**33478**   Outflow tract augmentation (gusset), with or without commissurotomy or infundibular resection

(Use 33478 in conjunction with 33768 when a cavopulmonary anastomosis to a second superior vena cava is performed)

## Other Valvular Procedures

**33496**   Repair of non-structural prosthetic valve dysfunction with cardiopulmonary bypass (separate procedure)

(For reoperation, use 33530 in addition to 33496)

## Coronary Artery Anomalies

Basic procedures include endarterectomy or angioplasty.

**33500**   Repair of coronary arteriovenous or arteriocardiac chamber fistula; with cardiopulmonary bypass

**33501**      without cardiopulmonary bypass

**33502**   Repair of anomalous coronary artery from pulmonary artery origin; by ligation

**33503**      by graft, without cardiopulmonary bypass

(Do not report modifier 63 in conjunction with 33502, 33503)

**33504**      by graft, with cardiopulmonary bypass

**33505**      with construction of intrapulmonary artery tunnel (Takeuchi procedure)

**33506**      by translocation from pulmonary artery to aorta

(Do not report modifier 63 in conjunction with 33505, 33506)

**33507**   Repair of anomalous (eg, intramural) aortic origin of coronary artery by unroofing or translocation

## Endoscopy

Surgical vascular endoscopy always includes diagnostic endoscopy.

+ **33508**   Endoscopy, surgical, including video-assisted harvest of vein(s) for coronary artery bypass procedure (List separately in addition to code for primary procedure)

(Use 33508 in conjunction with 33510-33523)

(For open harvest of upper extremity vein procedure, use 35500)

## Venous Grafting Only for Coronary Artery Bypass

The following codes are used to report coronary artery bypass procedures using venous grafts only. These codes should NOT be used to report the performance of coronary artery bypass procedures using arterial grafts and venous grafts during the same procedure. See 33517-33523 and 33533-33536 for reporting combined arterial-venous grafts.

Procurement of the saphenous vein graft is included in the description of the work for 33510-33516 and should not be reported as a separate service or co-surgery. To report harvesting of an upper extremity vein, use 35500 in addition to the bypass procedure. To report harvesting of a femoropopliteal vein segment, report 35572 in addition to the bypass procedure. When surgical assistant performs graft procurement, add modifier 80 to 33510-33516.

**33510**   Coronary artery bypass, vein only; single coronary venous graft

**33511**      2 coronary venous grafts

**33512**      3 coronary venous grafts

**33513**      4 coronary venous grafts

**33514**      5 coronary venous grafts

**33516**      6 or more coronary venous grafts

## Combined Arterial-Venous Grafting for Coronary Bypass

The following codes are used to report coronary artery bypass procedures using venous grafts and arterial grafts during the same procedure. These codes may NOT be used alone.

To report combined arterial-venous grafts it is necessary to report two codes: (1) the appropriate combined arterial-venous graft code (33517-33523); and (2) the appropriate arterial graft code (33533-33536).

Procurement of the saphenous vein graft is included in the description of the work for 33517-33523 and should not be reported as a separate service or co-surgery. Procurement of the artery for grafting is included in the description of the work for 33533-33536 and should not be reported as a separate service or co-surgery, except when an upper extremity artery (eg, radial artery) is procured. To report harvesting of an upper extremity artery, use 35600 in addition to the bypass procedure. To report harvesting of an upper extremity vein, use 35500 in addition to the bypass procedure. To report harvesting of a femoropopliteal vein segment, report 35572 in addition to the bypass procedure. When surgical assistant performs arterial and/or venous graft procurement, add modifier 80 to 33517-33523, 33533-33536, as appropriate.

**Surgery: Cardiovascular System**

+ **33517** Coronary artery bypass, using venous graft(s) and arterial graft(s); single vein graft (List separately in addition to code for primary procedure)

(Use 33517 in conjunction with 33533-33536)

+ **33518** 2 venous grafts (List separately in addition to code for primary procedure)

(Use 33518 in conjunction with 33533-33536)

+ **33519** 3 venous grafts (List separately in addition to code for primary procedure)

(Use 33519 in conjunction with 33533-33536)

+ **33521** 4 venous grafts (List separately in addition to code for primary procedure)

(Use 33521 in conjunction with 33533-33536)

+ **33522** 5 venous grafts (List separately in addition to code for primary procedure)

(Use 33522 in conjunction with 33533-33536)

+ **33523** 6 or more venous grafts (List separately in addition to code for primary procedure)

(Use 33523 in conjunction with 33533-33536)

+ **33530** Reoperation, coronary artery bypass procedure or valve procedure, more than 1 month after original operation (List separately in addition to code for primary procedure)

(Use 33530 in conjunction with 33400-33496; 33510-33536, 33863)

## Arterial Grafting for Coronary Artery Bypass

The following codes are used to report coronary artery bypass procedures using either arterial grafts only or a combination of arterial-venous grafts. The codes include the use of the internal mammary artery, gastroepiploic artery, epigastric artery, radial artery, and arterial conduits procured from other sites.

To report combined arterial-venous grafts it is necessary to report two codes: (1) the appropriate arterial graft code (33533-33536); and (2) the appropriate combined arterial-venous graft code (33517-33523).

Procurement of the artery for grafting is included in the description of the work for 33533-33536 and should not be reported as a separate service or co-surgery, except when an upper extremity artery (eg, radial artery) is procured. To report harvesting of an upper extremity artery, use 35600 in addition to the bypass procedure. To report harvesting of an upper extremity vein, use 35500 in addition to the bypass procedure. To report harvesting of a femoropopliteal vein segment, report 35572 in addition to the bypass procedure. When surgical assistant performs arterial and/or venous graft procurement, add modifier 80 to 33517-33523, 33533-33536, as appropriate.

**33533** Coronary artery bypass, using arterial graft(s); single arterial graft

**33534** 2 coronary arterial grafts

**33535** 3 coronary arterial grafts

**33536** 4 or more coronary arterial grafts

**33542** Myocardial resection (eg, ventricular aneurysmectomy)

**33545** Repair of postinfarction ventricular septal defect, with or without myocardial resection

**33548** Surgical ventricular restoration procedure, includes prosthetic patch, when performed (eg, ventricular remodeling, SVR, SAVER, Dor procedures)

(Do not report 33548 in conjunction with 32551, 33210, 33211, 33310, 33315)

(For Batista procedure or pachopexy, use 33999)

## Coronary Endarterectomy

+ **33572** Coronary endarterectomy, open, any method, of left anterior descending, circumflex, or right coronary artery performed in conjunction with coronary artery bypass graft procedure, each vessel (List separately in addition to primary procedure)

(Use 33572 in conjunction with 33510-33516, 33533-33536)

## Single Ventricle and Other Complex Cardiac Anomalies

**33600** Closure of atrioventricular valve (mitral or tricuspid) by suture or patch

**33602** Closure of semilunar valve (aortic or pulmonary) by suture or patch

**33606** Anastomosis of pulmonary artery to aorta (Damus-Kaye-Stansel procedure)

**33608** Repair of complex cardiac anomaly other than pulmonary atresia with ventricular septal defect by construction or replacement of conduit from right or left ventricle to pulmonary artery

(For repair of pulmonary artery arborization anomalies by unifocalization, see 33925-33926)

**33610** Repair of complex cardiac anomalies (eg, single ventricle with subaortic obstruction) by surgical enlargement of ventricular septal defect

(Do not report modifier 63 in conjunction with 33610)

**33611** Repair of double outlet right ventricle with intraventricular tunnel repair;

(Do not report modifier 63 in conjunction with 33611)

**33612** with repair of right ventricular outflow tract obstruction

**33615**   Repair of complex cardiac anomalies (eg, tricuspid atresia) by closure of atrial septal defect and anastomosis of atria or vena cava to pulmonary artery (simple Fontan procedure)

**33617**   Repair of complex cardiac anomalies (eg, single ventricle) by modified Fontan procedure

(Use 33617 in conjunction with 33768 when a cavopulmonary anastomosis to a second superior vena cava is performed)

**33619**   Repair of single ventricle with aortic outflow obstruction and aortic arch hypoplasia (hypoplastic left heart syndrome) (eg, Norwood procedure)

(Do not report modifier 63 in conjunction with 33619)

**33620**   Application of right and left pulmonary artery bands (eg, hybrid approach stage 1)

(For banding of the main pulmonary artery related to septal defect, use 33690)

**33621**   Transthoracic insertion of catheter for stent placement with catheter removal and closure (eg, hybrid approach stage 1)

(For placement of stent, use 37207)

(Report both 33620, 33621 if performed in same session)

**33622**   Reconstruction of complex cardiac anomaly (eg, single ventricle or hypoplastic left heart) with palliation of single ventricle with aortic outflow obstruction and aortic arch hypoplasia, creation of cavopulmonary anastomosis, and removal of right and left pulmonary bands (eg, hybrid approach stage 2, Norwood, bidirectional Glenn, pulmonary artery debanding)

(Do not report 33622 in conjunction with 33619, 33767, 33822, 33840, 33845, 33851, 33853, 33917)

(For bilateral, bidirectional Glenn procedure, use 33622 in conjunction with 33768)

## Septal Defect

**33641**   Repair atrial septal defect, secundum, with cardiopulmonary bypass, with or without patch

**33645**   Direct or patch closure, sinus venosus, with or without anomalous pulmonary venous drainage

(Do not report 33645 in conjunction with 33724, 33726)

**33647**   Repair of atrial septal defect and ventricular septal defect, with direct or patch closure

(Do not report modifier 63 in conjunction with 33647)

(For repair of tricuspid atresia (eg, Fontan, Gago procedures), use 33615)

**33660**   Repair of incomplete or partial atrioventricular canal (ostium primum atrial septal defect), with or without atrioventricular valve repair

**33665**   Repair of intermediate or transitional atrioventricular canal, with or without atrioventricular valve repair

**33670**   Repair of complete atrioventricular canal, with or without prosthetic valve

(Do not report modifier 63 in conjunction with 33670)

**33675**   Closure of multiple ventricular septal defects;

**33676**       with pulmonary valvotomy or infundibular resection (acyanotic)

**33677**       with removal of pulmonary artery band, with or without gusset

(Do not report 33675-33677 in conjunction with 32100, 32422, 32551, 33210, 33681, 33684, 33688)

(For percutaneous closure, use 93581)

**33681**   Closure of single ventricular septal defect, with or without patch;

**33684**       with pulmonary valvotomy or infundibular resection (acyanotic)

**33688**       with removal of pulmonary artery band, with or without gusset

(For pulmonary vein repair requiring creation of atrial septal defect, use 33724)

**33690**   Banding of pulmonary artery

(For right and left pulmonary artery banding in a single ventricle [eg, hybrid approach stage 1], use 33620)

(Do not report modifier 63 in conjunction with 33690)

**33692**   Complete repair tetralogy of Fallot without pulmonary atresia;

**33694**       with transannular patch

(Do not report modifier 63 in conjunction with 33694)

(For ligation and takedown of a systemic-to-pulmonary artery shunt, performed in conjunction with a congenital heart procedure; see 33924)

**33697**   Complete repair tetralogy of Fallot with pulmonary atresia including construction of conduit from right ventricle to pulmonary artery and closure of ventricular septal defect

(For ligation and takedown of a systemic-to-pulmonary artery shunt, performed in conjunction with a congenital heart procedure; see 33924)

## Sinus of Valsalva

**33702**   Repair sinus of Valsalva fistula, with cardiopulmonary bypass;

**33710**       with repair of ventricular septal defect

**33720**   Repair sinus of Valsalva aneurysm, with cardiopulmonary bypass

**33722**   Closure of aortico-left ventricular tunnel

**Surgery: Cardiovascular System**

## Venous Anomalies

**33724** Repair of isolated partial anomalous pulmonary venous return (eg, Scimitar Syndrome)

(Do not report 33724 in conjunction with 32551, 33210, 33211)

**33726** Repair of pulmonary venous stenosis

(Do not report 33726 in conjunction with 32551, 33210, 33211)

**33730** Complete repair of anomalous pulmonary venous return (supracardiac, intracardiac, or infracardiac types)

(Do not report modifier 63 in conjunction with 33730)

(For partial anomalous pulmonary venous return, use 33724; for repair of pulmonary venous stenosis, use 33726)

**33732** Repair of cor triatriatum or supravalvular mitral ring by resection of left atrial membrane

(Do not report modifier 63 in conjunction with 33732)

## Shunting Procedures

**33735** Atrial septectomy or septostomy; closed heart (Blalock-Hanlon type operation)

**33736** open heart with cardiopulmonary bypass

(Do not report modifier 63 in conjunction with 33735, 33736)

**33737** open heart, with inflow occlusion

(For transvenous method cardiac catheterization balloon atrial septectomy or septostomy (Rashkind type), use 92992)

(For blade method cardiac catheterization atrial septectomy or septostomy (Sang-Park septostomy), use 92993)

**33750** Shunt; subclavian to pulmonary artery (Blalock-Taussig type operation)

**33755** ascending aorta to pulmonary artery (Waterston type operation)

**33762** descending aorta to pulmonary artery (Potts-Smith type operation)

(Do not report modifier 63 in conjunction with 33750, 33755, 33762)

**33764** central, with prosthetic graft

**33766** superior vena cava to pulmonary artery for flow to 1 lung (classical Glenn procedure)

**33767** superior vena cava to pulmonary artery for flow to both lungs (bidirectional Glenn procedure)

**+ 33768** Anastomosis, cavopulmonary, second superior vena cava (List separately in addition to primary procedure)

(Use 33768 in conjunction with 33478, 33617, 33622, 33767)

(Do not report 33768 in conjunction with 32551, 33210, 33211)

## Transposition of the Great Vessels

**33770** Repair of transposition of the great arteries with ventricular septal defect and subpulmonary stenosis; without surgical enlargement of ventricular septal defect

**33771** with surgical enlargement of ventricular septal defect

**33774** Repair of transposition of the great arteries, atrial baffle procedure (eg, Mustard or Senning type) with cardiopulmonary bypass;

**33775** with removal of pulmonary band

**33776** with closure of ventricular septal defect

**33777** with repair of subpulmonic obstruction

**33778** Repair of transposition of the great arteries, aortic pulmonary artery reconstruction (eg, Jatene type);

(Do not report modifier 63 in conjunction with 33778)

**33779** with removal of pulmonary band

**33780** with closure of ventricular septal defect

**33781** with repair of subpulmonic obstruction

**33782** Aortic root translocation with ventricular septal defect and pulmonary stenosis repair (ie, Nikaidoh procedure); without coronary ostium reimplantation

(Do not report 33782 in conjunction with 33412, 33413, 33608, 33681, 33770, 33771, 33778, 33780, 33920)

**33783** with reimplantation of 1 or both coronary ostia

## Truncus Arteriosus

**33786** Total repair, truncus arteriosus (Rastelli type operation)

(Do not report modifier 63 in conjunction with 33786)

**33788** Reimplantation of an anomalous pulmonary artery

(For pulmonary artery band, use 33690)

## Aortic Anomalies

**33800** Aortic suspension (aortopexy) for tracheal decompression (eg, for tracheomalacia) (separate procedure)

**33802** Division of aberrant vessel (vascular ring);

**33803** with reanastomosis

**33813** Obliteration of aortopulmonary septal defect; without cardiopulmonary bypass

**33814** with cardiopulmonary bypass

**33820** Repair of patent ductus arteriosus; by ligation

**33822** by division, younger than 18 years

**33824** by division, 18 years and older

**33840**   Excision of coarctation of aorta, with or without associated patent ductus arteriosus; with direct anastomosis

**33845**      with graft

**33851**      repair using either left subclavian artery or prosthetic material as gusset for enlargement

**33852**   Repair of hypoplastic or interrupted aortic arch using autogenous or prosthetic material; without cardiopulmonary bypass

**33853**      with cardiopulmonary bypass

(For repair of hypoplastic left heart syndrome (eg, Norwood type), via excision of coarctation of aorta, use 33619)

## Thoracic Aortic Aneurysm

**33860**   Ascending aorta graft, with cardiopulmonary bypass, includes valve suspension, when performed

(33861 has been deleted. To report, use 33864)

**33863**   Ascending aorta graft, with cardiopulmonary bypass, with aortic root replacement using valved conduit and coronary reconstruction (eg, Bentall)

(Do not report 33863 in conjunction with 33405, 33406, 33410, 33411, 33412, 33413, 33860)

**33864**   Ascending aorta graft, with cardiopulmonary bypass with valve suspension, with coronary reconstruction and valve-sparing aortic root remodeling (eg, David Procedure, Yacoub Procedure)

(Do not report 33864 in conjunction with 33400, 33860-33863)

**33870**   Transverse arch graft, with cardiopulmonary bypass

**33875**   Descending thoracic aorta graft, with or without bypass

**33877**   Repair of thoracoabdominal aortic aneurysm with graft, with or without cardiopulmonary bypass

## Endovascular Repair of Descending Thoracic Aorta

Codes 33880-33891 represent a family of procedures to report placement of an endovascular graft for repair of the descending thoracic aorta. These codes include all device introduction, manipulation, positioning, and deployment. All balloon angioplasty and/or stent deployment within the target treatment zone for the endoprosthesis, either before or after endograft deployment, are not separately reportable. Open arterial exposure and associated closure of the arteriotomy sites (eg, 34812, 34820, 34833, 34834), introduction of guidewires and catheters (eg, 36140, 36200-36218), and extensive repair or replacement of an artery (eg, 35226, 35286) should be additionally reported. Transposition of subclavian artery to carotid, and carotid-carotid bypass performed in conjunction with endovascular repair of the

descending thoracic aorta (eg, 33889, 33891) should be separately reported. The primary codes, 33880 and 33881, include placement of all distal extensions, if required, in the distal thoracic aorta, while proximal extensions, if needed, are reported separately.

For fluoroscopic guidance in conjunction with endovascular repair of the thoracic aorta, see codes 75956-75959 as appropriate. Codes 75956 and 75957 include all angiography of the thoracic aorta and its branches for diagnostic imaging prior to deployment of the primary endovascular devices (including all routine components of modular devices), fluoroscopic guidance in the delivery of the endovascular components, and intraprocedural arterial angiography (eg, confirm position, detect endoleak, evaluate runoff). Code 75958 includes the analogous services for placement of each proximal thoracic endovascular extension. Code 75959 includes the analogous services for placement of a distal thoracic endovascular extension(s) placed during a procedure after the primary repair.

Other interventional procedures performed at the time of endovascular repair of the descending thoracic aorta should be additionally reported (eg, innominate, carotid, subclavian, visceral, or iliac artery transluminal angioplasty or stenting, arterial embolization, intravascular ultrasound) when performed before or after deployment of the aortic prostheses.

(For transcatheter placement of wireless physiologic sensor in aneurysmal sac, use 34806)

(For analysis, interpretation, and report of implanted wireless pressure sensor in aneurysmal sac, use 93982)

**33880**   Endovascular repair of descending thoracic aorta (eg, aneurysm, pseudoaneurysm, dissection, penetrating ulcer, intramural hematoma, or traumatic disruption); involving coverage of left subclavian artery origin, initial endoprosthesis plus descending thoracic aortic extension(s), if required, to level of celiac artery origin

(For radiological supervision and interpretation, use 75956 in conjunction with 33880)

**33881**      not involving coverage of left subclavian artery origin, initial endoprosthesis plus descending thoracic aortic extension(s), if required, to level of celiac artery origin

(For radiological supervision and interpretation, use 75957 in conjunction with 33881)

**33883**   Placement of proximal extension prosthesis for endovascular repair of descending thoracic aorta (eg, aneurysm, pseudoaneurysm, dissection, penetrating ulcer, intramural hematoma, or traumatic disruption); initial extension

(For radiological supervision and interpretation, use 75958 in conjunction with 33883)

(Do not report 33881, 33883 when extension placement converts repair to cover left subclavian origin. Use only 33880)

**Surgery: Cardiovascular System**

**+ 33884** each additional proximal extension (List separately in addition to code for primary procedure)

(Use 33884 in conjunction with 33883)

(For radiological supervision and interpretation, use 75958 in conjunction with 33884)

**33886** Placement of distal extension prosthesis(s) delayed after endovascular repair of descending thoracic aorta

(Do not report 33886 in conjunction with 33880, 33881)

(Report 33886 once, regardless of number of modules deployed)

(For radiological supervision and interpretation, use 75959 in conjunction with 33886)

**33889** Open subclavian to carotid artery transposition performed in conjunction with endovascular repair of descending thoracic aorta, by neck incision, unilateral

(Do not report 33889 in conjunction with 35694)

**33891** Bypass graft, with other than vein, transcervical retropharyngeal carotid-carotid, performed in conjunction with endovascular repair of descending thoracic aorta, by neck incision

(Do not report 33891 in conjunction with 35509, 35601)

## Pulmonary Artery

**33910** Pulmonary artery embolectomy; with cardiopulmonary bypass

**33915** without cardiopulmonary bypass

**33916** Pulmonary endarterectomy, with or without embolectomy, with cardiopulmonary bypass

**33917** Repair of pulmonary artery stenosis by reconstruction with patch or graft

**33920** Repair of pulmonary atresia with ventricular septal defect, by construction or replacement of conduit from right or left ventricle to pulmonary artery

(For repair of other complex cardiac anomalies by construction or replacement of right or left ventricle to pulmonary artery conduit, use 33608)

**33922** Transection of pulmonary artery with cardiopulmonary bypass

(Do not report modifier 63 in conjunction with 33922)

**+ 33924** Ligation and takedown of a systemic-to-pulmonary artery shunt, performed in conjunction with a congenital heart procedure (List separately in addition to code for primary procedure)

(Use 33924 in conjunction with 33470-33475, 33600-33619, 33684-33688, 33692-33697, 33735-33767, 33770-33781, 33786, 33920-33922)

**33925** Repair of pulmonary artery arborization anomalies by unifocalization; without cardiopulmonary bypass

**33926** with cardiopulmonary bypass

## Heart/Lung Transplantation

Heart with or without lung allotransplantation involves three distinct components of physician work:

1. *Cadaver donor cardiectomy with or without pneumonectomy,* which includes harvesting the allograft and cold preservation of the allograft (perfusing with cold preservation solution and cold maintenance) (see 33930, 33940).

2. *Backbench work:*

Preparation of a cadaver donor heart and lung allograft prior to transplantation, including dissection of the allograft from surrounding soft tissues to prepare the aorta, superior vena cava, inferior vena cava, and trachea for implantation (use 33933).

Preparation of a cadaver donor heart allograft prior to transplantation, including dissection of the allograft from surrounding soft tissues to prepare aorta, superior vena cava, inferior vena cava, pulmonary artery, and left atrium for implantation (use 33944).

3. *Recipient heart with or without lung allotransplantation,* which includes transplantation of allograft and care of the recipient (see 33935, 33945).

(For implantation of a total replacement heart system (artificial heart) with recipient cardiectomy or heart replacement system components, see Category III codes 0051T-0053T)

**33930** Donor cardiectomy-pneumonectomy (including cold preservation)

**33933** Backbench standard preparation of cadaver donor heart/lung allograft prior to transplantation, including dissection of allograft from surrounding soft tissues to prepare aorta, superior vena cava, inferior vena cava, and trachea for implantation

**33935** Heart-lung transplant with recipient cardiectomy-pneumonectomy

**33940** Donor cardiectomy (including cold preservation)

**33944** Backbench standard preparation of cadaver donor heart allograft prior to transplantation, including dissection of allograft from surrounding soft tissues to prepare aorta, superior vena cava, inferior vena cava, pulmonary artery, and left atrium for implantation

(For repair or resection procedures on the donor heart, see 33300, 33310, 33320, 33400, 33463, 33464, 33510, 33641, 35216, 35276 or 35685)

**33945** Heart transplant, with or without recipient cardiectomy

## Cardiac Assist

The insertion of a ventricular assist device (VAD) can be performed via percutaneous (0048T) or transthoracic (33975, 33976, 33979) approach. The location of the ventricular assist device may be intracorporeal or extracorporeal.

Removal of a ventricular assist device (33977, 33978, 33980, 0050T) includes removal of the entire device, including the cannulas.

►Replacement of a ventricular assist device pump (ie, 33981-33983) includes the removal of the pump and insertion of a new pump, connection, de-airing, and initiation of the new pump.◄

►Replacement of the entire ventricular assist device system, ie, pump(s) and cannulas, is reported using the insertion codes (ie, 33975, 33976, 33979). Removal (ie, 33977, 33978, 33980) of the ventricular assist device system being replaced is not separately reported.◄

(For implantation or removal of ventricular assist device, extracorporeal, percutaneous transseptal access, see 0048T, 0050T. For replacement of a ventricular assist device, extracorporeal, percutaneous transseptal access, use 33999)

▲ **33960**   Prolonged extracorporeal circulation for cardiopulmonary insufficiency; initial day

▲ **33961**         each subsequent day

►[Do not use in conjunction with modifier 63, 33961]◄

**33961**   [Do not use in conjunction with modifier 63, 33961]

(Do not report modifier 63 in conjunction with 33960, 33961)

(For insertion of cannula for prolonged extracorporeal circulation, use 36822)

**33967**   Insertion of intra-aortic balloon assist device, percutaneous

**33968**   Removal of intra-aortic balloon assist device, percutaneous

**33970**   Insertion of intra-aortic balloon assist device through the femoral artery, open approach

**33971**   Removal of intra-aortic balloon assist device including repair of femoral artery, with or without graft

**33973**   Insertion of intra-aortic balloon assist device through the ascending aorta

**33974**   Removal of intra-aortic balloon assist device from the ascending aorta, including repair of the ascending aorta, with or without graft

**33975**   Insertion of ventricular assist device; extracorporeal, single ventricle

**33976**         extracorporeal, biventricular

**33977**   Removal of ventricular assist device; extracorporeal, single ventricle

**33978**         extracorporeal, biventricular

**33979**   Insertion of ventricular assist device, implantable intracorporeal, single ventricle

**33980**   Removal of ventricular assist device, implantable intracorporeal, single ventricle

**33981**   Replacement of extracorporeal ventricular assist device, single or biventricular, pump(s), single or each pump

**33982**   Replacement of ventricular assist device pump(s); implantable intracorporeal, single ventricle, without cardiopulmonary bypass

**33983**         implantable intracorporeal, single ventricle, with cardiopulmonary bypass

## Other Procedures

**33999**   Unlisted procedure, cardiac surgery

# Arteries and Veins

Primary vascular procedure listings include establishing both inflow and outflow by whatever procedures necessary. Also included is that portion of the operative arteriogram performed by the surgeon, as indicated. Sympathectomy, when done, is included in the listed aortic procedures. For unlisted vascular procedure, use 37799.

## Embolectomy/Thrombectomy

### Arterial, With or Without Catheter

**34001**   Embolectomy or thrombectomy, with or without catheter; carotid, subclavian or innominate artery, by neck incision

**34051**         innominate, subclavian artery, by thoracic incision

**34101**         axillary, brachial, innominate, subclavian artery, by arm incision

**34111**         radial or ulnar artery, by arm incision

**34151**         renal, celiac, mesentery, aortoiliac artery, by abdominal incision

**34201**         femoropopliteal, aortoiliac artery, by leg incision

**34203**         popliteal-tibio-peroneal artery, by leg incision

### Venous, Direct or With Catheter

**34401**   Thrombectomy, direct or with catheter; vena cava, iliac vein, by abdominal incision

**34421**         vena cava, iliac, femoropopliteal vein, by leg incision

**34451**         vena cava, iliac, femoropopliteal vein, by abdominal and leg incision

**34471**         subclavian vein, by neck incision

**34490**         axillary and subclavian vein, by arm incision

## Venous Reconstruction

**34501**   Valvuloplasty, femoral vein

**34502**   Reconstruction of vena cava, any method

**34510**   Venous valve transposition, any vein donor

**Surgery: Cardiovascular System**

34520    Cross-over vein graft to venous system

34530    Saphenopopliteal vein anastomosis

# Endovascular Repair of Abdominal Aortic Aneurysm

Codes 34800-34826 represent a family of component procedures to report placement of an endovascular graft for abdominal aortic aneurysm repair. These codes describe open femoral or iliac artery exposure, device manipulation and deployment, and closure of the arteriotomy sites. Balloon angioplasty and/or stent deployment within the target treatment zone for the endoprosthesis, either before or after endograft deployment, are not separately reportable. Introduction of guidewires and catheters should be reported separately (eg, 36200, 36245-36248, 36140). Extensive repair or replacement of an artery should be additionally reported (eg, 35226 or 35286).

For fluoroscopic guidance in conjunction with endovascular aneurysm repair, see code 75952 or 75953, as appropriate. Code 75952 includes angiography of the aorta and its branches for diagnostic imaging prior to deployment of the endovascular device (including all routine components of modular devices), fluoroscopic guidance in the delivery of the endovascular components, and intraprocedural arterial angiography (eg, confirm position, detect endoleak, evaluate runoff). Code 75953 includes the analogous services for placement of additional extension prostheses (not for routine components of modular devices).

Other interventional procedures performed at the time of endovascular abdominal aortic aneurysm repair should be additionally reported (eg, renal transluminal angioplasty, arterial embolization, intravascular ultrasound, balloon angioplasty or stenting of native artery[s] outside the endoprosthesis target zone, when done before or after deployment of graft).

(For transcatheter placement of wireless physiologic sensor in aneurysmal sac, use 34806)

(For analysis, interpretation and report of implanted wireless pressure sensor in aneurysmal sac, use 93982)

34800    Endovascular repair of infrarenal abdominal aortic aneurysm or dissection; using aorto-aortic tube prosthesis

34802        using modular bifurcated prosthesis (1 docking limb)

34803        using modular bifurcated prosthesis (2 docking limbs)

(For endovascular repair of abdominal aortic aneurysm or dissection involving visceral vessels using a fenestrated modular bifurcated prosthesis (2 docking limbs), use Category III codes 0078T, 0079T)

34804        using unibody bifurcated prosthesis

34805        using aorto-uniiliac or aorto-unifemoral prosthesis

►(For radiological supervision and interpretation, use 75952 in conjunction with 34800-34805)◄

+ 34806    Transcatheter placement of wireless physiologic sensor in aneurysmal sac during endovascular repair, including radiological supervision and interpretation, instrument calibration, and collection of pressure data (List separately in addition to code for primary procedure)

(Use 34806 in conjunction with 33880, 33881, 33886, 34800-34805, 34825, 34900)

(Do not report 34806 in conjunction with 93982)

+ 34808    Endovascular placement of iliac artery occlusion device (List separately in addition to code for primary procedure)

(Use 34808 in conjunction with 34800, 34805, 34813, 34825, 34826)

(For open arterial exposure, report 34812, 34820, 34833, 34834 as appropriate, in addition to 34800-34808)

34812    Open femoral artery exposure for delivery of endovascular prosthesis, by groin incision, unilateral

(For bilateral procedure, use modifier 50)

+ 34813    Placement of femoral-femoral prosthetic graft during endovascular aortic aneurysm repair (List separately in addition to code for primary procedure)

(Use 34813 in conjunction with 34812)

►(For femoral artery grafting, see 35521, 35533, 35539, 35540, 35556, 35558, 35566, 35621, 35646, 35654-35661, 35666, 35700)◄

34820    Open iliac artery exposure for delivery of endovascular prosthesis or iliac occlusion during endovascular therapy, by abdominal or retroperitoneal incision, unilateral

(For bilateral procedure, use modifier 50)

34825    Placement of proximal or distal extension prosthesis for endovascular repair of infrarenal abdominal aortic or iliac aneurysm, false aneurysm, or dissection; initial vessel

+ 34826        each additional vessel (List separately in addition to code for primary procedure)

(Use 34826 in conjunction with 34825)

►(Use 34825, 34826 in addition to 34800-34805, 34900 as appropriate)◄

(For radiological supervision and interpretation, use 75953)

34830    Open repair of infrarenal aortic aneurysm or dissection, plus repair of associated arterial trauma, following unsuccessful endovascular repair; tube prosthesis

34831        aorto-bi-iliac prosthesis

34832        aorto-bifemoral prosthesis

**34833**  Open iliac artery exposure with creation of conduit for delivery of aortic or iliac endovascular prosthesis, by abdominal or retroperitoneal incision, unilateral

(Do not report 34833 in addition to 34820)

(For bilateral procedure, use modifier 50)

**34834**  Open brachial artery exposure to assist in the deployment of aortic or iliac endovascular prosthesis by arm incision, unilateral

(For bilateral procedure, use modifier 50)

## Endovascular Repair of Iliac Aneurysm

►Code 34900 represents a procedure to report introduction, positioning, and deployment of an endovascular graft for treatment of aneurysm, pseudoaneurysm, or arteriovenous malformation or trauma of the iliac artery (common, hypogastric, external). All balloon angioplasty and/or stent deployments within the target treatment zone for the endoprosthesis, either before or after endograft deployment, are included in the work of 34900 and are not separately reportable. Open femoral or iliac artery exposure (eg, 34812, 34820), introduction of guidewires and catheters (eg, 36200, 36245-36248), and extensive repair or replacement of an artery (eg, 35206-35286) should be additionally reported.◄

For fluoroscopic guidance in conjunction with endovascular iliac aneurysm repair, see code 75954. Code 75954 includes angiography of the aorta and iliac arteries for diagnostic imaging prior to deployment of the endovascular device (including all routine components), fluoroscopic guidance in the delivery of the endovascular components, and intraprocedural arterial angiography to confirm appropriate position of the graft, detect endoleaks, and evaluate the status of the runoff vessels (eg, evaluation for dissection, stenosis, thrombosis, distal embolization, or iatrogenic injury).

Other interventional procedures performed at the time of endovascular iliac aneurysm repair should be additionally reported (eg, transluminal angioplasty outside the aneurysm target zone, arterial embolization, intravascular ultrasound).

**34900**  Endovascular repair of iliac artery (eg, aneurysm, pseudoaneurysm, arteriovenous malformation, trauma) using ilio-iliac tube endoprosthesis

(For endovascular repair of iliac artery bifurcation [eg, aneurysm, pseudoaneurysm, arteriovenous malformation, trauma] using bifurcated endoprosthesis, use 0254T)

(For radiological supervision and interpretation, use 75954)

(For placement of extension prosthesis during endovascular iliac artery repair, use 34825)

(For bilateral procedure, use modifier 50)

## Direct Repair of Aneurysm or Excision (Partial or Total) and Graft Insertion for Aneurysm, Pseudoaneurysm, Ruptured Aneurysm, and Associated Occlusive Disease

Procedures 35001-35152 include preparation of artery for anastomosis including endarterectomy.

(For direct repairs associated with occlusive disease only, see 35201-35286)

(For intracranial aneurysm, see 61700 et seq)

(For endovascular repair of abdominal aortic aneurysm, see 34800-34826)

(For endovascular repair of iliac artery aneurysm, see 34900)

(For thoracic aortic aneurysm, see 33860-33875)

(For endovascular repair of descending thoracic aorta, involving coverage of left subclavian artery origin, use 33880)

**35001**  Direct repair of aneurysm, pseudoaneurysm, or excision (partial or total) and graft insertion, with or without patch graft; for aneurysm and associated occlusive disease, carotid, subclavian artery, by neck incision

**35002**  for ruptured aneurysm, carotid, subclavian artery, by neck incision

**35005**  for aneurysm, pseudoaneurysm, and associated occlusive disease, vertebral artery

**35011**  for aneurysm and associated occlusive disease, axillary-brachial artery, by arm incision

**35013**  for ruptured aneurysm, axillary-brachial artery, by arm incision

**35021**  for aneurysm, pseudoaneurysm, and associated occlusive disease, innominate, subclavian artery, by thoracic incision

**35022**  for ruptured aneurysm, innominate, subclavian artery, by thoracic incision

**35045**  for aneurysm, pseudoaneurysm, and associated occlusive disease, radial or ulnar artery

**35081**  for aneurysm, pseudoaneurysm, and associated occlusive disease, abdominal aorta

**35082**  for ruptured aneurysm, abdominal aorta

**35091**  for aneurysm, pseudoaneurysm, and associated occlusive disease, abdominal aorta involving visceral vessels (mesenteric, celiac, renal)

**35092**  for ruptured aneurysm, abdominal aorta involving visceral vessels (mesenteric, celiac, renal)

**35102**  for aneurysm, pseudoaneurysm, and associated occlusive disease, abdominal aorta involving iliac vessels (common, hypogastric, external)

**35103** for ruptured aneurysm, abdominal aorta involving iliac vessels (common, hypogastric, external)

**35111** for aneurysm, pseudoaneurysm, and associated occlusive disease, splenic artery

**35112** for ruptured aneurysm, splenic artery

**35121** for aneurysm, pseudoaneurysm, and associated occlusive disease, hepatic, celiac, renal, or mesenteric artery

**35122** for ruptured aneurysm, hepatic, celiac, renal, or mesenteric artery

**35131** for aneurysm, pseudoaneurysm, and associated occlusive disease, iliac artery (common, hypogastric, external)

**35132** for ruptured aneurysm, iliac artery (common, hypogastric, external)

**35141** for aneurysm, pseudoaneurysm, and associated occlusive disease, common femoral artery (profunda femoris, superficial femoral)

**35142** for ruptured aneurysm, common femoral artery (profunda femoris, superficial femoral)

**35151** for aneurysm, pseudoaneurysm, and associated occlusive disease, popliteal artery

**35152** for ruptured aneurysm, popliteal artery

## Repair Arteriovenous Fistula

**35180** Repair, congenital arteriovenous fistula; head and neck

**35182** thorax and abdomen

**35184** extremities

**35188** Repair, acquired or traumatic arteriovenous fistula; head and neck

**35189** thorax and abdomen

**35190** extremities

## Repair Blood Vessel Other Than for Fistula, With or Without Patch Angioplasty

(For AV fistula repair, see 35180-35190)

**35201** Repair blood vessel, direct; neck

**35206** upper extremity

**35207** hand, finger

**35211** intrathoracic, with bypass

**35216** intrathoracic, without bypass

**35221** intra-abdominal

**35226** lower extremity

**35231** Repair blood vessel with vein graft; neck

**35236** upper extremity

**35241** intrathoracic, with bypass

**35246** intrathoracic, without bypass

**35251** intra-abdominal

**35256** lower extremity

**35261** Repair blood vessel with graft other than vein; neck

**35266** upper extremity

**35271** intrathoracic, with bypass

**35276** intrathoracic, without bypass

**35281** intra-abdominal

**35286** lower extremity

## Thromboendarterectomy

(For coronary artery, see 33510-33536 and 33572)

(35301-35372 include harvest of saphenous or upper extremity vein when performed)

**35301** Thromboendarterectomy, including patch graft, if performed; carotid, vertebral, subclavian, by neck incision

**35302** superficial femoral artery

**35303** popliteal artery

(Do not report 35302, 35303 in conjunction with 35500, 37225, 37227)

**35304** tibioperoneal trunk artery

**35305** tibial or peroneal artery, initial vessel

**+ 35306** each additional tibial or peroneal artery (List separately in addition to code for primary procedure)

(Use 35306 in conjunction with 35305)

(Do not report 35304, 35305, 35306 in conjunction with 35500, 37229, 37231, 37233, 37235)

**35311** subclavian, innominate, by thoracic incision

**35321** axillary-brachial

**35331** abdominal aorta

**35341** mesenteric, celiac, or renal

**35351** iliac

**35355** iliofemoral

**35361** combined aortoiliac

**35363** combined aortoiliofemoral

**35371** common femoral

**35372** deep (profunda) femoral

**+ 35390** Reoperation, carotid, thromboendarterectomy, more than 1 month after original operation (List separately in addition to code for primary procedure)

(Use 35390 in conjunction with 35301)

## Angioscopy

+ **35400**  Angioscopy (non-coronary vessels or grafts) during therapeutic intervention (List separately in addition to code for primary procedure)

## Transluminal Angioplasty

If done as part of another operation, use modifier 51 or use modifier 52.

(For radiological supervision and interpretation, see 75962-75968 and 75978)

### Open

**35450**  Transluminal balloon angioplasty, open; renal or other visceral artery

**35452**      aortic

(35454, 35456 have been deleted. To report, see 37220-37227)

**35458**      brachiocephalic trunk or branches, each vessel

(35459 has been deleted. To report, see 37228-37235)

**35460**      venous

### Percutaneous

Codes for catheter placement and the radiologic supervision and interpretation should also be reported, in addition to the code(s) for the therapeutic aspect of the procedure.

(35470 has been deleted. To report, see 37228-37235)

⊙ **35471**  Transluminal balloon angioplasty, percutaneous; renal or visceral artery

⊙ **35472**      aortic

(35473, 35474 have been deleted. To report, see 37220-37227)

⊙ **35475**      brachiocephalic trunk or branches, each vessel

⊙ **35476**      venous

(For radiological supervision and interpretation, use 75978)

## Transluminal Atherectomy

### Open

(35480 has been deleted. To report, see 0234T, 0235T)

(35481 has been deleted. To report, use 0236T)

(35482 has been deleted. To report, use 0238T)

(35483 has been deleted. To report, see 37225, 37227)

(35484 has been deleted. To report, use 0237T)

(35485 has been deleted. To report, see 37229, 37231, 37233, 37235)

### Percutaneous

(35490 has been deleted. To report, see 0234T, 0235T)

(35491 has been deleted. To report, use 0236T)

(35492 has been deleted. To report, use 0238T)

(35493 has been deleted. To report, see 37225, 37227)

(35494 has been deleted. To report, use 0237T)

(35495 has been deleted. To report, see 37229, 37231, 37233, 37235)

## Bypass Graft

### Vein

Procurement of the saphenous vein graft is included in the description of the work for 35501-35587 and should not be reported as a separate service or co-surgery. To report harvesting of an upper extremity vein, use 35500 in addition to the bypass procedure. To report harvesting of a femoropopliteal vein segment, use 35572 in addition to the bypass procedure. To report harvesting and construction of an autogenous composite graft of two segments from two distant locations, report 35682 in addition to the bypass procedure, for autogenous composite of three or more segments from distant sites, report 35683.

+ **35500**  Harvest of upper extremity vein, 1 segment, for lower extremity or coronary artery bypass procedure (List separately in addition to code for primary procedure)

►(Use 35500 in conjunction with 33510-33536, 35556, 35566, 35570, 35571, 35583-35587)◄

(For harvest of more than one vein segment, see 35682, 35683)

(For endoscopic procedure, use 33508)

**35501**  Bypass graft, with vein; common carotid-ipsilateral internal carotid

**35506**      carotid-subclavian or subclavian-carotid

**35508**      carotid-vertebral

**35509**      carotid-contralateral carotid

**35510**      carotid-brachial

**35511**      subclavian-subclavian

**35512**      subclavian-brachial

**35515**      subclavian-vertebral

**35516**      subclavian-axillary

**35518**      axillary-axillary

**Surgery: Cardiovascular System**

**35521**      axillary-femoral

(For bypass graft performed with synthetic graft, use 35621)

**35522**      axillary-brachial

**35523**      brachial-ulnar or -radial

(Do not report 35523 in conjunction with 35206, 35500, 35525, 36838)

(For bypass graft performed with synthetic conduit, use 37799)

**35525**      brachial-brachial

**35526**      aortosubclavian, aortoinnominate, or aortocarotid

(For bypass graft performed with synthetic graft, use 35626)

**35531**      aortoceliac or aortomesenteric

**35533**      axillary-femoral-femoral

(For bypass graft performed with synthetic graft, use 35654)

**35535**      hepatorenal

(Do not report 35535 in conjunction with 35221, 35251, 35281, 35500, 35536, 35560, 35631, 35636)

**35536**      splenorenal

**35537**      aortoiliac

(For bypass graft performed with synthetic graft, use 35637)

(Do not report 35537 in conjunction with 35538)

**35538**      aortobi-iliac

(For bypass graft performed with synthetic graft, use 35638)

(Do not report 35538 in conjunction with 35537)

**35539**      aortofemoral

(For bypass graft performed with synthetic graft, use 35647)

(Do not report 35539 in conjunction with 35540)

**35540**      aortobifemoral

(For bypass graft performed with synthetic graft, use 35646)

(Do not report 35540 in conjunction with 35539)

▶(35548 has been deleted. To report, see 35537, 35539, 35565)◀

▶(35549 has been deleted. To report, see 35537, 35538, 35539, 35540, 35565)◀

▶(35551 has been deleted. To report, see 35539, 35540, 35556, 35583)◀

**35556**      femoral-popliteal

**35558**      femoral-femoral

**35560**      aortorenal

**35563**      ilioiliac

**35565**      iliofemoral

**35566**      femoral-anterior tibial, posterior tibial, peroneal artery or other distal vessels

**35570**      tibial-tibial, peroneal-tibial, or tibial/peroneal trunk-tibial

(Do not report 35570 in conjunction with 35256, 35286)

**35571**      popliteal-tibial, -peroneal artery or other distal vessels

**+ 35572**   Harvest of femoropopliteal vein, 1 segment, for vascular reconstruction procedure (eg, aortic, vena caval, coronary, peripheral artery) (List separately in addition to code for primary procedure)

(Use 35572 in conjunction with 33510-33516, 33517-33523, 33533-33536, 34502, 34520, 35001, 35002, 35011-35022, 35102, 35103, 35121-35152, 35231-35256, 35501-35587, 35879-35907)

(For bilateral procedure, use modifier 50)

## In-Situ Vein

(To report aortobifemoral bypass using synthetic conduit, and femoral-popliteal bypass with vein conduit in-situ, use 35646 and 35583. To report aorto[uni]femoral bypass with synthetic conduit, and femoral-popliteal bypass with vein conduit in-situ, use 35647 and 35583. To report aortofemoral bypass using vein conduit, and femoral-popliteal bypass with vein conduit in-situ, use 35539 and 35583)

**35583**      In-situ vein bypass; femoral-popliteal

**35585**      femoral-anterior tibial, posterior tibial, or peroneal artery

**35587**      popliteal-tibial, peroneal

## Other Than Vein

(For arterial transposition and/or reimplantation, see 35691-35695)

**+ 35600**   Harvest of upper extremity artery, 1 segment, for coronary artery bypass procedure (List separately in addition to code for primary procedure)

(Use 35600 in conjunction with 33533–33536)

**35601**      Bypass graft, with other than vein; common carotid-ipsilateral internal carotid

**35606**      carotid-subclavian

(For open transcervical common carotid-common carotid bypass performed in conjunction with endovascular repair of descending thoracic aorta, use 33891)

(For open subclavian to carotid artery transposition performed in conjunction with endovascular thoracic aneurysm repair by neck incision, use 33889)

| | |
|---|---|
| **35612** | subclavian-subclavian |
| **35616** | subclavian-axillary |
| **35621** | axillary-femoral |
| **35623** | axillary-popliteal or -tibial |
| **35626** | aortosubclavian, aortoinnominate, or aortocarotid |
| **35631** | aortoceliac, aortomesenteric, aortorenal |
| **35632** | ilio-celiac |

(Do not report 35632 in conjunction with 35221, 35251, 35281, 35531, 35631)

| | |
|---|---|
| **35633** | ilio-mesenteric |

(Do not report 35633 in conjunction with 35221, 35251, 35281, 35531, 35631)

| | |
|---|---|
| **35634** | iliorenal |

(Do not report 35634 in conjunction with 35221, 35251, 35281, 35560, 35536, 35631)

| | |
|---|---|
| **35636** | splenorenal (splenic to renal arterial anastomosis) |
| **35637** | aortoiliac |

(Do not report 35637 in conjunction with 35638, 35646)

| | |
|---|---|
| **35638** | aortobi-iliac |

(Do not report 35638 in conjunction with 35637, 35646)

(For open placement of aortobi-iliac prosthesis following unsuccessful endovascular repair, use 34831)

| | |
|---|---|
| **35642** | carotid-vertebral |
| **35645** | subclavian-vertebral |
| **35646** | aortobifemoral |

(For bypass graft performed with vein graft, use 35540)

(For open placement of aortobifemoral prosthesis following unsuccessful endovascular repair, use 34832)

| | |
|---|---|
| **35647** | aortofemoral |

(For bypass graft performed with vein graft, use 35539)

| | |
|---|---|
| **35650** | axillary-axillary |

▶(35651 has been deleted. To report, see 35646, 35647, 35656)◀

| | |
|---|---|
| **35654** | axillary-femoral-femoral |
| **35656** | femoral-popliteal |
| **35661** | femoral-femoral |
| **35663** | ilioiliac |
| **35665** | iliofemoral |
| **35666** | femoral-anterior tibial, posterior tibial, or peroneal artery |
| **35671** | popliteal-tibial or -peroneal artery |

## Composite Grafts

Codes 35682-35683 are used to report harvest and anastomosis of multiple vein segments from distant sites for use as arterial bypass graft conduits. These codes are intended for use when the two or more vein segments are harvested from a limb other than that undergoing bypass.

**+ 35681**   Bypass graft; composite, prosthetic and vein (List separately in addition to code for primary procedure)

(Do not report 35681 in addition to 35682, 35683)

**+ 35682**        autogenous composite, 2 segments of veins from 2 locations (List separately in addition to code for primary procedure)

(Use 35682 in conjunction with 35556, 35566, 35570, 35571, 35583-35587)

(Do not report 35682 in addition to 35681, 35683)

**+ 35683**        autogenous composite, 3 or more segments of vein from 2 or more locations (List separately in addition to code for primary procedure)

(Use 35683 in conjunction with 35556, 35566, 35570, 35571, 35583-35587)

(Do not report 35683 in addition to 35681, 35682)

## Adjuvant Techniques

Adjuvant (additional) technique(s) may be required at the time a bypass graft is created to improve patency of the lower extremity autogenous or synthetic bypass graft (eg, femoral-popliteal, femoral-tibial, or popliteal-tibial arteries). Code 35685 should be reported in addition to the primary synthetic bypass graft procedure, when an interposition of venous tissue (vein patch or cuff) is placed at the anastomosis between the synthetic bypass conduit and the involved artery (includes harvest).

Code 35686 should be reported in addition to the primary bypass graft procedure, when autogenous vein is used to create a fistula between the tibial or peroneal artery and vein at or beyond the distal bypass anastomosis site of the involved artery.

(For composite graft(s), see 35681-35683)

**+ 35685**   Placement of vein patch or cuff at distal anastomosis of bypass graft, synthetic conduit (List separately in addition to code for primary procedure)

(Use 35685 in conjunction with 35656, 35666, or 35671)

**+ 35686**   Creation of distal arteriovenous fistula during lower extremity bypass surgery (non-hemodialysis) (List separately in addition to code for primary procedure)

▶(Use 35686 in conjunction with 35556, 35566, 35570, 35571, 35583-35587, 35623, 35656, 35666, 35671)◀

## Arterial Transposition

**35691**    Transposition and/or reimplantation; vertebral to carotid artery

**35693**        vertebral to subclavian artery

**35694**        subclavian to carotid artery

(For open subclavian to carotid artery transposition performed in conjunction with endovascular repair of descending thoracic aorta, use 33889)

**35695**        carotid to subclavian artery

**+ 35697**    Reimplantation, visceral artery to infrarenal aortic prosthesis, each artery (List separately in addition to code for primary procedure)

(Do not report 35697 in conjunction with 33877)

## Excision, Exploration, Repair, Revision

**+ 35700**    Reoperation, femoral-popliteal or femoral (popliteal)- anterior tibial, posterior tibial, peroneal artery, or other distal vessels, more than 1 month after original operation (List separately in addition to code for primary procedure)

▶(Use 35700 in conjunction with 35556, 35566, 35570, 35571, 35583, 35585, 35587, 35656, 35666, 35671)◀

**35701**    Exploration (not followed by surgical repair), with or without lysis of artery; carotid artery

**35721**        femoral artery

**35741**        popliteal artery

**35761**        other vessels

**35800**    Exploration for postoperative hemorrhage, thrombosis or infection; neck

**35820**        chest

**35840**        abdomen

**35860**        extremity

**35870**    Repair of graft-enteric fistula

**35875**    Thrombectomy of arterial or venous graft (other than hemodialysis graft or fistula);

**35876**        with revision of arterial or venous graft

(For thrombectomy of hemodialysis graft or fistula, see 36831, 36833)

Codes 35879 and 35881 describe open revision of graft-threatening stenoses of lower extremity arterial bypass graft(s) (previously constructed with autogenous vein conduit) using vein patch angioplasty or segmental vein interposition techniques. For thrombectomy with revision of any non-coronary arterial or venous graft, including those of the lower extremity, (other than hemodialysis graft or fistula), use 35876. For direct repair (other than for fistula) of a lower extremity blood vessel (with or without patch angioplasty), use 35226. For repair (other than for fistula) of a lower extremity blood vessel using a vein graft, use 35256.

**35879**    Revision, lower extremity arterial bypass, without thrombectomy, open; with vein patch angioplasty

**35881**        with segmental vein interposition

(For revision of femoral anastomosis of synthetic arterial bypass graft, see 35883, 35884)

(For excision of infected graft, see 35901-35907 and appropriate revascularization code)

**35883**    Revision, femoral anastomosis of synthetic arterial bypass graft in groin, open; with nonautogenous patch graft (eg, Dacron, ePTFE, bovine pericardium)

(For bilateral procedure, use modifier 50)

(Do not report 35883 in conjunction with 35700, 35875, 35876, 35884)

**35884**        with autogenous vein patch graft

(For bilateral procedure, use modifier 50)

(Do not report 35884 in conjunction with 35700, 35875, 35876, 35883)

**35901**    Excision of infected graft; neck

**35903**        extremity

**35905**        thorax

**35907**        abdomen

## Vascular Injection Procedures

Listed services for injection procedures include necessary local anesthesia, introduction of needles or catheter, injection of contrast media with or without automatic power injection, and/or necessary pre- and postinjection care specifically related to the injection procedure.

Selective vascular catheterization should be coded to include introduction and all lesser order selective catheterization used in the approach (eg, the description for a selective right middle cerebral artery catheterization includes the introduction and placement catheterization of the right common and internal carotid arteries).

Additional second and/or third order arterial catheterization within the same family of arteries or veins supplied by a single first order vessel should be expressed by 36012, 36218, or 36248.

Additional first order or higher catheterization in vascular families supplied by a first order vessel different from a previously selected and coded family should be separately coded using the conventions described above.

(For radiological supervision and interpretation, see **Radiology**)

(For injection procedures in conjunction with cardiac catheterization, see 93452-93461, 93563-93568)

(For chemotherapy of malignant disease, see 96401-96549)

## Intravenous

An intracatheter is a sheathed combination of needle and short catheter.

**36000**   Introduction of needle or intracatheter, vein

**36002**   Injection procedures (eg, thrombin) for percutaneous treatment of extremity pseudoaneurysm

(For imaging guidance, see 76942, 77002, 77012, 77021)

(For ultrasound guided compression repair of pseudoaneurysms, use 76936)

(Do not report 36002 for vascular sealant of an arteriotomy site)

**36005**   Injection procedure for extremity venography (including introduction of needle or intracatheter)

(For radiological supervision and interpretation, see 75820, 75822)

**36010**   Introduction of catheter, superior or inferior vena cava

**36011**   Selective catheter placement, venous system; first order branch (eg, renal vein, jugular vein)

**36012**       second order, or more selective, branch (eg, left adrenal vein, petrosal sinus)

**36013**   Introduction of catheter, right heart or main pulmonary artery

**36014**   Selective catheter placement, left or right pulmonary artery

**36015**   Selective catheter placement, segmental or subsegmental pulmonary artery

(For insertion of flow directed catheter (eg, Swan-Ganz), use 93503)

(For venous catheterization for selective organ blood sampling, use 36500)

## Intra-Arterial—Intra-Aortic

(For radiological supervision and interpretation, see **Radiology**)

**36100**   Introduction of needle or intracatheter, carotid or vertebral artery

(For bilateral procedure, report 36100 with modifier 50)

**36120**   Introduction of needle or intracatheter; retrograde brachial artery

**36140**       extremity artery

(For insertion of arteriovenous cannula, see 36810-36821)

(36145 has been deleted. To report see 36147, 36148)

▶*Diagnostic Studies of Arteriovenous (AV) Shunts for Dialysis:* For diagnostic studies, the arteriovenous (AV) dialysis shunt (AV shunt) is defined as beginning with the arterial anastomosis and extending to the right atrium. This definition includes all upper and lower extremity AV shunts (arteriovenous fistulae [AVF] and arteriovenous grafts [AVG]). Code 36147 includes the work of directly accessing and imaging the entire AV shunt. Antegrade and/or retrograde punctures of the AV shunt are typically used for imaging, and contrast may be injected directly through a needle or through a catheter placed into the AV shunt. Occasionally the catheter needs to be advanced further into the shunt to adequately visualize the arterial anastomosis or the central veins, and all manipulation of the catheter for diagnostic imaging of the AV shunt is included in 36147. Advancement of the catheter to the vena cava to adequately image that segment of the AV shunt is included in 36147 and is not separately reported. Advancement of the catheter tip through the arterial anastomosis to adequately visualize the anastomosis is also considered integral to the work of 36147 and is not separately reported.

Ultrasound guidance for puncture of the AV shunt is not included in 36147. Particularly in the case of new or failing AVF, ultrasound may be necessary to safely and effectively puncture the AV access for evaluation, and this may be reported separately with 76937 if all the appropriate elements for reporting 76937 are performed.

Evaluation of the peri-anastomotic portion of the inflow is considered an integral part of the dialysis fistulagram and is included in the work of 36147. The peri-anastomotic portion of the vessel at the arterial anastomosis includes the short segment of the artery immediately adjacent to the anastomosis, the anastomosis itself, and the portion of the vessel or graft immediately distal to the anastomosis.

The arterial inflow to the AV access is considered a separate vessel. If a more proximal inflow problem separate from the peri-anastomotic segment is suspected and additional catheter work and imaging must be done for adequate evaluation, this work is not included in 36147. If a catheter is selectively advanced from the AV shunt puncture into the inflow artery, an additional catheterization code may be reported. In the typical case of an upper extremity AV shunt, 36215 is used to report this work, and includes placement of the catheter retrograde into the inflow artery and into the aorta if necessary (ie, 36200 may not be also reported since that work is included in the work defined by 36215).◀

▶*Interventions for Arteriovenous (AV) Shunts Created for Dialysis (AV Grafts and AV Fistulae):* For the purposes of coding interventional procedures in arteriovenous (AV) shunts created for dialysis (both arteriovenous fistulae [AVF] and arteriovenous grafts [AVG]), the AV shunt is artificially divided into two vessel segments. The first segment is peripheral and extends from the peri-arterial anastomosis through the axillary vein (or entire cephalic vein in the case of cephalic venous outflow). The second segment includes the veins central to the axillary and cephalic veins, including the subclavian and innominate veins through the vena cava. Interventions performed in a single segment, regardless of

*Surgery: Cardiovascular System*

the number of lesions treated, are coded as a single intervention.

The AV shunt is considered to be venous and most interventions are coded with the venous intervention codes (ie, angioplasty is reported with venous angioplasty codes 35476, 75978). Codes 35476 and 75978 would be reported once to describe all angioplasty work performed in one segment of the AV dialysis shunt, regardless of the number of distinct lesions treated within that segment, the number of times the balloon is inflated, or the number of balloon catheters required to open all lesions.

There is an exception to the use of venous interventional codes. When there is a stenosis at the arterial anastomosis, it typically extends across the anastomosis and involves the artery just proximal to and at the anastomosis as well as the outflow vessel or graft. This segment is called the peri-anastomotic (or juxta-anastomotic) region, and even though the stenosis can involve multiple vessels, it is typically a single lesion with a single etiology crossing the anastomosis, and treatment to open this lesion crosses from the artery into the vein or venous graft. An intervention treated in this peri-anastomotic segment is coded as an arterial intervention (35475, 75962). Since the entire segment of the AV shunt from the peri-arterial anastomosis through the axillary vein is considered a single vessel for coding of interventions, the arterial angioplasty codes include the work of opening the peri-anastomotic stenosis, as well as all other stenoses treated within this segment of the vessel. Codes 35475 and 75962 are reported once to describe all work done to angioplasty any lesion from the peri-arterial anastomosis through the axillary vein in procedures that involve angioplasty of the peri-arterial anastomosis of the AV shunt. In these special instances, venous angioplasty codes would not be reported additionally for this first or most peripheral shunt segment, even if balloon angioplasty is performed on segments of the AV dialysis shunt that are purely venous anatomy within this specific vessel segment.

It is never appropriate to report removal of the arterial plug during a declot/thrombectomy procedure as an arterial or venous angioplasty (35475, 35476). Removal of the arterial plug is included in the work of a fistula thrombectomy (36870), even if a balloon catheter is used to mechanically dislodge the resistant thrombus.

The central veins (eg, subclavian, innominate, and cava) are considered an additional, separate venous vessel segment for purposes of interventional coding for AV dialysis shunt interventions. If one or more central venous stenoses are treated with angioplasty, this is reported as a single venous angioplasty (35476, 75978), regardless of the number of discrete lesions treated within this segment, and also independent of the number of balloon inflations or number of balloon catheters or sizes required. This additional work should be clearly documented in the patient record and in the recorded images.

The codes for stents placed in AV dialysis accesses are generic for intravascular work and not specific for arterial or venous anatomy. However, the same rules used for angioplasty apply to stent placements for AV dialysis shunts with respect to the number of interventions reported for each patient. Stent codes (37205, 75960) are reported once to describe all work of stenting lesions within the defined AV dialysis shunt segment from the peri-arterial anastomosis through the axillary and cephalic veins, regardless of the number of stents placed or the number of discrete lesions treated within that vessel segment. If additional stenting is required for central venous stenosis, this may be reported as an additional stent placement (37206, 75960), describing all the work of stent placement within the central venous segment.

The work of catheterizing all the veins in the dialysis AV shunt is included in 36147 (and, if appropriate, 36148). Selective catheterization of the inferior/superior vena cava and central veins cannot be separately reported when performed from a direct puncture of the AVF/AVG.

However, if additional venous side branches off of the conduit, known as accessory veins, are separately catheterized for intervention such as embolization of a large competing accessory vein, this additional work may be separately reported using the appropriate selective venous catheterization codes (36011 and 36012). The embolization may be reported using 37204, 75894.◀

⊙ **36147** Introduction of needle and/or catheter, arteriovenous shunt created for dialysis (graft/fistula); initial access with complete radiological evaluation of dialysis access, including fluoroscopy, image documentation and report (includes access of shunt, injection[s] of contrast, and all necessary imaging from the arterial anastomosis and adjacent artery through entire venous outflow including the inferior or superior vena cava)

(If 36147 indicates the need for a therapeutic intervention requiring a second catheterization of the shunt, use 36148)

(Do not report 36147 in conjunction with 75791)

⊙+ **36148** additional access for therapeutic intervention (List separately in addition to code for primary procedure)

(Use 36148 in conjunction with 36147)

**36160** Introduction of needle or intracatheter, aortic, translumbar

⊙▲ **36200** Introduction of catheter, aorta

**36215** Selective catheter placement, arterial system; each first order thoracic or brachiocephalic branch, within a vascular family

(For catheter placement for coronary angiography, see 93454-93461)

**36216** initial second order thoracic or brachiocephalic branch, within a vascular family

**36217** initial third order or more selective thoracic or brachiocephalic branch, within a vascular family

**+ 36218**      additional second order, third order, and beyond, thoracic or brachiocephalic branch, within a vascular family (List in addition to code for initial second or third order vessel as appropriate)

(Use 36218 in conjunction with 36216, 36217)

(For angiography, see 36147, 75600-75774, 75791)

(For angioplasty, see 37228-37235, 35471, 35472, 35475)

(For transcatheter therapies, see 37200-37208, 61624, 61626)

(When coronary artery, arterial conduit (eg, internal mammary, inferior epigastric or free radical artery) or venous bypass graft angiography is performed in conjunction with cardiac catheterization, see the appropriate cardiac catheterization, injection procedure, and imaging supervision code(s) (93451-93461, 93503-93533, 93563-93568) in the **Medicine** section of the CPT codebook. When coronary artery, arterial coronary conduit or venous bypass graft angiography is performed without concomitant left heart cardiac catheterization, see 93454-93457, 93563, 93564. When internal mammary artery angiography only is performed without a concomitant left heart cardiac catheterization, use 36216 or 36217 as appropriate.)

⊙▲ **36245**   Selective catheter placement, arterial system; each first order abdominal, pelvic, or lower extremity artery branch, within a vascular family

⊙▲ **36246**      initial second order abdominal, pelvic, or lower extremity artery branch, within a vascular family

⊙▲ **36247**      initial third order or more selective abdominal, pelvic, or lower extremity artery branch, within a vascular family

⊙+▲ **36248**      additional second order, third order, and beyond, abdominal, pelvic, or lower extremity artery branch, within a vascular family (List in addition to code for initial second or third order vessel as appropriate)

(Use 36248 in conjunction with 36246, 36247)

⊙● **36251**   Selective catheter placement (first-order), main renal artery and any accessory renal artery(s) for renal angiography, including arterial puncture and catheter placement(s), fluoroscopy, contrast injection(s), image postprocessing, permanent recording of images, and radiological supervision and interpretation, including pressure gradient measurements when performed, and flush aortogram when performed; unilateral

⊙● **36252**      bilateral

⊙● **36253**   Superselective catheter placement (one or more second order or higher renal artery branches) renal artery and any accessory renal artery(s) for renal angiography, including arterial puncture, catheterization, fluoroscopy, contrast injection(s), image postprocessing, permanent recording of images, and radiological supervision and interpretation, including pressure gradient measurements when performed, and flush aortogram when performed; unilateral

▶(Do not report 36253 in conjunction with 36251 when performed for the same kidney)◀

⊙● **36254**      bilateral

▶(Do not report 36254 in conjunction with 36252)◀

▶(Placement of closure device at the vascular access site is not separately reported with 36251-36254)◀

**36260**   Insertion of implantable intra-arterial infusion pump (eg, for chemotherapy of liver)

**36261**   Revision of implanted intra-arterial infusion pump

**36262**   Removal of implanted intra-arterial infusion pump

**36299**   Unlisted procedure, vascular injection

## Venous

Venipuncture, needle or catheter for diagnostic study or intravenous therapy, percutaneous. These codes are also used to report the therapy as specified. For collection of a specimen from an established catheter, use 36592. For collection of a specimen from a completely implantable venous access device, use 36591.

**36400**   Venipuncture, younger than age 3 years, necessitating physician's skill, not to be used for routine venipuncture; femoral or jugular vein

**36405**      scalp vein

**36406**      other vein

**36410**   Venipuncture, age 3 years or older, necessitating physician's skill (separate procedure), for diagnostic or therapeutic purposes (not to be used for routine venipuncture)

**36415**   Collection of venous blood by venipuncture

(Do not report modifier 63 in conjunction with 36415)

**36416**   Collection of capillary blood specimen (eg, finger, heel, ear stick)

**36420**   Venipuncture, cutdown; younger than age 1 year

(Do not report modifier 63 in conjunction with 36420)

**36425**      age 1 or over

**36430**   Transfusion, blood or blood components

**36440**   Push transfusion, blood, 2 years or younger

**36450**   Exchange transfusion, blood; newborn

(Do not report modifier 63 in conjunction with 36450)

**36455**      other than newborn

**36460**   Transfusion, intrauterine, fetal

(Do not report modifier 63 in conjunction with 36460)

(For radiological supervision and interpretation, use 76941)

**36468**   Single or multiple injections of sclerosing solutions, spider veins (telangiectasia); limb or trunk

## Surgery: Cardiovascular System

36469   face

36470   Injection of sclerosing solution; single vein

36471       multiple veins, same leg

36475   Endovenous ablation therapy of incompetent vein, extremity, inclusive of all imaging guidance and monitoring, percutaneous, radiofrequency; first vein treated

+ 36476       second and subsequent veins treated in a single extremity, each through separate access sites (List separately in addition to code for primary procedure)

(Use 36476 in conjunction with 36475)

▶(Do not report 29581, 29582, 36475, 36476 in conjunction with 36000-36005, 36410, 36425, 36478, 36479, 37204, 75894, 76000, 76001, 76937, 76942, 76998, 77022, 93970, 93971)◀

36478   Endovenous ablation therapy of incompetent vein, extremity, inclusive of all imaging guidance and monitoring, percutaneous, laser; first vein treated

+ 36479       second and subsequent veins treated in a single extremity, each through separate access sites (List separately in addition to code for primary procedure)

(Use 36479 in conjunction with 36478)

▶(Do not report 36478, 36479 in conjunction with 29581, 29582, 36000-36005, 36410, 36425, 36475, 36476, 37204, 75894, 76000, 76001, 76937, 76942, 76998, 77022, 93970, 93971)◀

⊙ 36481   Percutaneous portal vein catheterization by any method

(For radiological supervision and interpretation, see 75885, 75887)

36500   Venous catheterization for selective organ blood sampling

(For catheterization in superior or inferior vena cava, use 36010)

(For radiological supervision and interpretation, use 75893)

36510   Catheterization of umbilical vein for diagnosis or therapy, newborn

(Do not report modifier 63 in conjunction with 36510)

36511   Therapeutic apheresis; for white blood cells

36512       for red blood cells

36513       for platelets

36514       for plasma pheresis

36515       with extracorporeal immunoadsorption and plasma reinfusion

36516       with extracorporeal selective adsorption or selective filtration and plasma reinfusion

(For physician evaluation, use modifier 26)

36522   Photopheresis, extracorporeal

## Central Venous Access Procedures

To qualify as a central venous access catheter or device, the tip of the catheter/device must terminate in the subclavian, brachiocephalic (innominate) or iliac veins, the superior or inferior vena cava, or the right atrium. The venous access device may be either centrally inserted (jugular, subclavian, femoral vein or inferior vena cava catheter entry site) or peripherally inserted (eg, basilic or cephalic vein). The device may be accessed for use either via exposed catheter (external to the skin), via a subcutaneous port or via a subcutaneous pump.

The procedures involving these types of devices fall into five categories:

1. *Insertion* (placement of catheter through a newly established venous access)

2. *Repair* (fixing device without replacement of either catheter or port/pump, other than pharmacologic or mechanical correction of intracatheter or pericatheter occlusion [see 36595 or 36596])

3. *Partial replacement* of only the catheter component associated with a port/pump device, but not entire device

4. *Complete replacement* of entire device via same venous access site (complete exchange)

5. *Removal* of entire device.

There is no coding distinction between venous access achieved percutaneously versus by cutdown or based on catheter size.

For the repair, partial (catheter only) replacement, complete replacement, or removal of both catheters (placed from separate venous access sites) of a multi-catheter device, with or without subcutaneous ports/pumps, use the appropriate code describing the service with a frequency of two.

If an existing central venous access device is removed and a new one placed via a separate venous access site, appropriate codes for both procedures (removal of old, if code exists, and insertion of new device) should be reported.

When imaging is used for these procedures, either for gaining access to the venous entry site or for manipulating the catheter into final central position, use 76937, 77001.

(For refilling and maintenance of an implantable pump or reservoir for intravenous or intra-arterial drug delivery, use 96522)

### Insertion of Central Venous Access Device

⊙ 36555   Insertion of non-tunneled centrally inserted central venous catheter; younger than 5 years of age

(For peripherally inserted non-tunneled central venous catheter, younger than 5 years of age, use 36568)

# The Central Venous Access Procedures Table

| | Non-tunneled | Tunneled Without Port or Pump | Central Tunneled | Tunneled With Port | Tunneled With Pump | Peripheral | <5 years | ≥5 years | Any Age |
|---|---|---|---|---|---|---|---|---|---|
| **Insertion** | | | | | | | | | |
| Catheter | 36555 | | | | | | 36555 | | |
| | 36556 | | | | | | | 36556 | |
| | | 36557 | 36557 | | | | 36557 | | |
| | | 36558 | 36558 | | | | | 36558 | |
| | 36568 (w/o port or pump) | | | | | 36568 (w/o port or pump) | 36568 (w/o port or pump) | | |
| | 36569 (w/o port or pump) | | | | | 36569 (w/o port or pump) | | 36569 (w/o port or pump) | |
| Device | | | 36560 | 36560 | | | 36560 | | |
| | | | 36561 | 36561 | | | | 36561 | |
| | | | 36563 | | 36563 | | | | 36563 |
| | | 36565 | 36565 | | | | | | 36565 |
| | | | 36566 | 36566 | | | | | |
| | 36570 (w port) | | | 36570 (w port) | | 36570 (w port) | 36570 (w port) | | |
| | 36571 (w port) | | | 36571 (w port) | | 36571 (w port) | | 36571 (w port) | |
| **Repair** | | | | | | | | | |
| Catheter | 36575 (w/o port or pump) | 36575 (w/o port or pump) | 36575 (w/o port or pump) | | | 36575 (w/o port or pump) | | | 36575 |
| Device | 36576 (w port or pump) | | | | | 36576 (w port or pump) | | | 36576 |
| **Partial Replacement - Central Venous Access Device (Catheter only)** | | | | | | | | | |
| | | | 36578 | 36578 | 36578 | 36578 | | | 36578 |
| **Complete Replacement - Central Venous Access Device (Through Same Venous Access Site)** | | | | | | | | | |
| Catheter | 36580 (w/o port or pump) | | | | | | | | 36580 |
| | | 36581 | 36581 | | | | | | 36581 |
| | 36584 (w/o port or pump) | | | | | 36584 (w/o port or pump) | | | 36584 |
| Device | | | 36582 | 36582 | | | | | 36582 |
| | | | 36583 | | 36583 | | | | 36583 |
| | | | | 36585 (w port) | | 36585 (w port) | | | 36585 |
| **Removal** | | | | | | | | | |
| Catheter | | 36589 | | | | | | | 36589 |
| Device | | | 36590 | 36590 | 36590 | 36590 | | | 36590 |
| **Removal of Obstructive Material from Device** | | | | | | | | | |
| | 36595 (pericatheter) | 36595 (pericatheter) | 36595 (pericatheter) | 36595 (pericatheter) | 36595 (pericatheter) | 36595 (pericatheter) | | | 36595 (pericatheter) |
| | 36596 (intraluminal) | 36596 (intraluminal) | 36596 (intraluminal) | 36596 (intraluminal) | 36596 (intraluminal) | 36596 (intraluminal) | | | 36596 (intraluminal) |
| **Repositioning of Catheter** | | | | | | | | | |
| | 36597 | 36597 | 36597 | 36597 | 36597 | 36597 | 36597 | 36597 | 36597 |

**Surgery: Cardiovascular System**

**Surgery: Cardiovascular System**

36556    age 5 years or older

(For peripherally inserted non-tunneled central venous catheter, age 5 years or older, use 36569)

⊙ 36557    Insertion of tunneled centrally inserted central venous catheter, without subcutaneous port or pump; younger than 5 years of age

⊙ 36558    age 5 years or older

(For peripherally inserted central venous catheter with port, 5 years or older, use 36571)

⊙ 36560    Insertion of tunneled centrally inserted central venous access device, with subcutaneous port; younger than 5 years of age

(For peripherally inserted central venous access device with subcutaneous port, younger than 5 years of age, use 36570)

⊙ 36561    age 5 years or older

(For peripherally inserted central venous catheter with subcutaneous port, 5 years or older, use 36571)

⊙ 36563    Insertion of tunneled centrally inserted central venous access device with subcutaneous pump

⊙ 36565    Insertion of tunneled centrally inserted central venous access device, requiring 2 catheters via 2 separate venous access sites; without subcutaneous port or pump (eg, Tesio type catheter)

⊙ 36566    with subcutaneous port(s)

⊙ 36568    Insertion of peripherally inserted central venous catheter (PICC), without subcutaneous port or pump; younger than 5 years of age

(For placement of centrally inserted non-tunneled central venous catheter, without subcutaneous port or pump, younger than 5 years of age, use 36555)

36569    age 5 years or older

(For placement of centrally inserted non-tunneled central venous catheter, without subcutaneous port or pump, age 5 years or older, use 36556)

⊙ 36570    Insertion of peripherally inserted central venous access device, with subcutaneous port; younger than 5 years of age

(For insertion of tunneled centrally inserted central venous access device with subcutaneous port, younger than 5 years of age, use 36560)

⊙ 36571    age 5 years or older

(For insertion of tunneled centrally inserted central venous access device with subcutaneous port, age 5 years or older, use 36561)

## Repair of Central Venous Access Device

(For mechanical removal of pericatheter obstructive material, use 36595)

(For mechanical removal of intracatheter obstructive material, use 36596)

36575    Repair of tunneled or non-tunneled central venous access catheter, without subcutaneous port or pump, central or peripheral insertion site

⊙ 36576    Repair of central venous access device, with subcutaneous port or pump, central or peripheral insertion site

## Partial Replacement of Central Venous Access Device (Catheter Only)

⊙ 36578    Replacement, catheter only, of central venous access device, with subcutaneous port or pump, central or peripheral insertion site

(For complete replacement of entire device through same venous access, use 36582 or 36583)

## Complete Replacement of Central Venous Access Device Through Same Venous Access Site

36580    Replacement, complete, of a non-tunneled centrally inserted central venous catheter, without subcutaneous port or pump, through same venous access

⊙ 36581    Replacement, complete, of a tunneled centrally inserted central venous catheter, without subcutaneous port or pump, through same venous access

⊙ 36582    Replacement, complete, of a tunneled centrally inserted central venous access device, with subcutaneous port, through same venous access

⊙ 36583    Replacement, complete, of a tunneled centrally inserted central venous access device, with subcutaneous pump, through same venous access

36584    Replacement, complete, of a peripherally inserted central venous catheter (PICC), without subcutaneous port or pump, through same venous access

⊙ 36585    Replacement, complete, of a peripherally inserted central venous access device, with subcutaneous port, through same venous access

## Removal of Central Venous Access Device

36589    Removal of tunneled central venous catheter, without subcutaneous port or pump

⊙ 36590    Removal of tunneled central venous access device, with subcutaneous port or pump, central or peripheral insertion

(Do not report 36589 or 36590 for removal of non-tunneled central venous catheters)

### Other Central Venous Access Procedures

**36591**  Collection of blood specimen from a completely implantable venous access device

(Do not report 36591 in conjunction with other services except a laboratory service)

(For collection of venous blood specimen by venipuncture, use 36415)

(For collection of capillary blood specimen, use 36416)

**36592**  Collection of blood specimen using established central or peripheral catheter, venous, not otherwise specified

(For blood collection from an established arterial catheter, use 37799)

(Do not report 36592 in conjunction with other services except a laboratory service)

**36593**  Declotting by thrombolytic agent of implanted vascular access device or catheter

**36595**  Mechanical removal of pericatheter obstructive material (eg, fibrin sheath) from central venous device via separate venous access

(Do not report 36595 in conjunction with 36593)

(For venous catheterization, see 36010-36012)

(For radiological supervision and interpretation, use 75901)

**36596**  Mechanical removal of intraluminal (intracatheter) obstructive material from central venous device through device lumen

(Do not report 36596 in conjunction with 36593)

(For venous catheterization, see 36010-36012)

(For radiological supervision and interpretation, use 75902)

**36597**  Repositioning of previously placed central venous catheter under fluoroscopic guidance

(For fluoroscopic guidance, use 76000)

**36598**  Contrast injection(s) for radiologic evaluation of existing central venous access device, including fluoroscopy, image documentation and report

(Do not report 36598 in conjunction with 76000)

(Do not report 36598 in conjunction with 36595, 36596)

(For complete diagnostic studies, see 75820, 75825, 75827)

## Arterial

**36600**  Arterial puncture, withdrawal of blood for diagnosis

⊘ **36620**  Arterial catheterization or cannulation for sampling, monitoring or transfusion (separate procedure); percutaneous

**36625**  cutdown

**36640**  Arterial catheterization for prolonged infusion therapy (chemotherapy), cutdown

(See also 96420-96425)

(For arterial catheterization for occlusion therapy, see 75894)

**36660**  Catheterization, umbilical artery, newborn, for diagnosis or therapy

(Do not report modifier 63 in conjunction with 36660)

## Intraosseous

**36680**  Placement of needle for intraosseous infusion

## Hemodialysis Access, Intervascular Cannulation for Extracorporeal Circulation, or Shunt Insertion

**36800**  Insertion of cannula for hemodialysis, other purpose (separate procedure); vein to vein

**36810**      arteriovenous, external (Scribner type)

**36815**      arteriovenous, external revision, or closure

**36818**  Arteriovenous anastomosis, open; by upper arm cephalic vein transposition

(Do not report 36818 in conjunction with 36819, 36820, 36821, 36830 during a unilateral upper extremity procedure. For bilateral upper extremity open arteriovenous anastomoses performed at the same operative session, use modifier 50 or 59 as appropriate)

**36819**      by upper arm basilic vein transposition

(Do not report 36819 in conjunction with 36818, 36820, 36821, 36830 during a unilateral upper extremity procedure. For bilateral upper extremity open arteriovenous anastomoses performed at the same operative session, use modifier 50 or 59 as appropriate)

**36820**      by forearm vein transposition

**36821**      direct, any site (eg, Cimino type) (separate procedure)

**36822**  Insertion of cannula(s) for prolonged extracorporeal circulation for cardiopulmonary insufficiency (ECMO) (separate procedure)

(For maintenance of prolonged extracorporeal circulation, see 33960, 33961)

**36823**  Insertion of arterial and venous cannula(s) for isolated extracorporeal circulation including regional chemotherapy perfusion to an extremity, with or without hyperthermia, with removal of cannula(s) and repair of arteriotomy and venotomy sites

(36823 includes chemotherapy perfusion supported by a membrane oxygenator/perfusion pump. Do not report 96409-96425 in conjunction with 36823)

**36825** Creation of arteriovenous fistula by other than direct arteriovenous anastomosis (separate procedure); autogenous graft

(For direct arteriovenous anastomosis, use 36821)

**36830** nonautogenous graft (eg, biological collagen, thermoplastic graft)

(For direct arteriovenous anastomosis, use 36821)

**36831** Thrombectomy, open, arteriovenous fistula without revision, autogenous or nonautogenous dialysis graft (separate procedure)

**36832** Revision, open, arteriovenous fistula; without thrombectomy, autogenous or nonautogenous dialysis graft (separate procedure)

**36833** with thrombectomy, autogenous or nonautogenous dialysis graft (separate procedure)

(36834 has been deleted. To report an arteriovenous access fistula or graft revision, use 36832)

**36835** Insertion of Thomas shunt (separate procedure)

**36838** Distal revascularization and interval ligation (DRIL), upper extremity hemodialysis access (steal syndrome)

(Do not report 36838 in conjunction with 35512, 35522, 35523, 36832, 37607, 37618)

**36860** External cannula declotting (separate procedure); without balloon catheter

**36861** with balloon catheter

(If imaging guidance is performed, use 76000)

⊙ **36870** Thrombectomy, percutaneous, arteriovenous fistula, autogenous or nonautogenous graft (includes mechanical thrombus extraction and intra-graft thrombolysis)

(Do not report 36870 in conjunction with 36593)

(For catheterization, see 36147, 36148)

(For radiological supervision and interpretation, see 36147, 75791)

## Portal Decompression Procedures

**37140** Venous anastomosis, open; portocaval

(For peritoneal-venous shunt, use 49425)

**37145** renoportal

**37160** caval-mesenteric

**37180** splenorenal, proximal

**37181** splenorenal, distal (selective decompression of esophagogastric varices, any technique)

(For percutaneous procedure, use 37182)

**37182** Insertion of transvenous intrahepatic portosystemic shunt(s) (TIPS) (includes venous access, hepatic and portal vein catheterization, portography with hemodynamic evaluation, intrahepatic tract formation/dilatation, stent placement and all associated imaging guidance and documentation)

(Do not report 75885 or 75887 in conjunction with 37182)

(For open procedure, use 37140)

⊙ **37183** Revision of transvenous intrahepatic portosystemic shunt(s) (TIPS) (includes venous access, hepatic and portal vein catheterization, portography with hemodynamic evaluation, intrahepatic tract recanulization/dilatation, stent placement and all associated imaging guidance and documentation)

(Do not report 75885 or 75887 in conjunction with 37183)

(For repair of arteriovenous aneurysm, use 36832)

## Transcatheter Procedures

Codes for catheter placement and the radiologic supervision and interpretation should also be reported, in addition to the code(s) for the therapeutic aspect of the procedure.

### *Mechanical Thrombectomy*

Code(s) for catheter placement(s), diagnostic studies, and other percutaneous interventions (eg, transluminal balloon angioplasty, stent placement) provided are separately reportable.

Codes 37184-37188 specifically include intraprocedural fluoroscopic radiological supervision and interpretation services for guidance of the procedure.

Intraprocedural injection(s) of a thrombolytic agent is an included service and not separately reportable in conjunction with mechanical thrombectomy. However, subsequent or prior continuous infusion of a thrombolytic is not an included service and is separately reportable (see 37201, 75896, 75898).

For coronary mechanical thrombectomy, use 92973.

For mechanical thrombectomy for dialysis fistula, use 36870.

### *Arterial Mechanical Thrombectomy*

Arterial mechanical thrombectomy may be performed as a "primary" transcatheter procedure with pretreatment planning, performance of the procedure, and postprocedure evaluation focused on providing this service. Typically, the diagnosis of thrombus has been made prior to the procedure, and a mechanical thrombectomy is planned preoperatively. Primary mechanical thrombectomy is reported per vascular family using 37184 for the initial vessel treated and 37185 for second or all subsequent vessel(s) within the same vascular family. To report mechanical thrombectomy of an additional vascular family treated through a separate

Surgery: Cardiovascular System

access site, use modifier 51 in conjunction with 37184-37185.

Primary mechanical thrombectomy may precede or follow another percutaneous intervention. Most commonly primary mechanical thrombectomy will precede another percutaneous intervention with the decision regarding the need for other services not made until after mechanical thrombectomy has been performed. Occasionally, the performance of primary mechanical thrombectomy may follow another percutaneous intervention.

Do **NOT** report 37184-37185 for mechanical thrombectomy performed for the retrieval of short segments of thrombus or embolus evident during other percutaneous interventional procedures. See 37186 for these procedures.

Arterial mechanical thrombectomy is considered a "secondary" transcatheter procedure for removal or retrieval of short segments of thrombus or embolus when performed either before or after another percutaneous intervention (eg, percutaneous transluminal balloon angioplasty, stent placement). Secondary mechanical thrombectomy is reported using 37186. Do **NOT** report 37186 in conjunction with 37184-37185.

### *Venous Mechanical Thrombectomy*

Use 37187 to report the initial application of venous mechanical thrombectomy. To report bilateral venous mechanical thrombectomy performed through a separate access site(s), use modifier 50 in conjunction with 37187. For repeat treatment on a subsequent day during a course of thrombolytic therapy, use 37188.

## Arterial Mechanical Thrombectomy

⊙ **37184**    Primary percutaneous transluminal mechanical thrombectomy, noncoronary, arterial or arterial bypass graft, including fluoroscopic guidance and intraprocedural pharmacological thrombolytic injection(s); initial vessel

(Do not report 37184 in conjunction with 76000, 76001, 96374, 99143-99150)

⊙+ **37185**    second and all subsequent vessel(s) within the same vascular family (List separately in addition to code for primary mechanical thrombectomy procedure)

(Do not report 37185 in conjunction with 76000, 76001, 96375)

⊙+ **37186**    Secondary percutaneous transluminal thrombectomy (eg, nonprimary mechanical, snare basket, suction technique), noncoronary, arterial or arterial bypass graft, including fluoroscopic guidance and intraprocedural pharmacological thrombolytic injections, provided in conjunction with another percutaneous intervention other than primary mechanical thrombectomy (List separately in addition to code for primary procedure)

(Do not report 37186 in conjunction with 76000, 76001, 96375)

## Venous Mechanical Thrombectomy

⊙ **37187**    Percutaneous transluminal mechanical thrombectomy, vein(s), including intraprocedural pharmacological thrombolytic injections and fluoroscopic guidance

(Do not report 37187 in conjunction with 76000, 76001, 96375)

⊙ **37188**    Percutaneous transluminal mechanical thrombectomy, vein(s), including intraprocedural pharmacological thrombolytic injections and fluoroscopic guidance, repeat treatment on subsequent day during course of thrombolytic therapy

(Do not report 37188 in conjunction with 76000, 76001, 96375)

## Other Procedures

⊙● **37191**    Insertion of intravascular vena cava filter, endovascular approach including vascular access, vessel selection, and radiological supervision and interpretation, intraprocedural roadmapping, and imaging guidance (ultrasound and fluoroscopy), when performed

►(For open surgical interruption of the inferior vena cava through a laparotomy or retroperitoneal exposure, use 37619)◄

⊙● **37192**    Repositioning of intravascular vena cava filter, endovascular approach including vascular access, vessel selection, and radiological supervision and interpretation, intraprocedural roadmapping, and imaging guidance (ultrasound and fluoroscopy), when performed

►(Do not report 37192 in conjunction with 37191)◄

⊙● **37193**    Retrieval (removal) of intravascular vena cava filter, endovascular approach including vascular access, vessel selection, and radiological supervision and interpretation, intraprocedural roadmapping, and imaging guidance (ultrasound and fluoroscopy), when performed

►(Do not report 37193 in conjunction with 37203, 75961)◄

**37195**    Thrombolysis, cerebral, by intravenous infusion

**37200**    Transcatheter biopsy

(For radiological supervision and interpretation, use 75970)

**37201**    Transcatheter therapy, infusion for thrombolysis other than coronary

(For radiological supervision and interpretation, use 75896)

**37202**    Transcatheter therapy, infusion other than for thrombolysis, any type (eg, spasmolytic, vasoconstrictive)

(For thrombolysis of coronary vessels, see 92975, 92977)

(For radiological supervision and interpretation, use 75896)

⊙ **37203** Transcatheter retrieval, percutaneous, of intravascular foreign body (eg, fractured venous or arterial catheter)

(For radiological supervision and interpretation, use 75961)

▶(For removal of a vena cava filter, use 37193)◀

**37204** Transcatheter occlusion or embolization (eg, for tumor destruction, to achieve hemostasis, to occlude a vascular malformation), percutaneous, any method, non-central nervous system, non-head or neck

(See also 61624, 61626)

(For radiological supervision and interpretation, use 75894)

(For uterine fibroid embolization [uterine artery embolization performed to treat uterine fibroids], use 37210)

(For obstetrical and gynecologic embolization procedures other than uterine fibroid embolization [eg, embolization to treat obstetrical or postpartum hemorrhage], use 37204)

**37205** Transcatheter placement of an intravascular stent(s) (except coronary, carotid, vertebral, iliac, and lower extremity arteries), percutaneous; initial vessel

(For radiological supervision and interpretation, use 75960)

(For transcatheter placement of intravascular cervical carotid artery stent(s), see 37215, 37216)

(For transcatheter placement of intracranial stents, use 61635)

(For transcatherter coronary stent placement, see 92980, 92981)

(For transcatheter stent placement of extracranial vertebral or intrathoracic carotid artery stent(s), see Category III codes 0075T, 0076T)

(For stent placement in iliac, femoral, popliteal, and tibial/peroneal arteries, see 37221, 37223, 37226, 37227, 37230, 37231, 37234, 37235)

+ **37206** each additional vessel (List separately in addition to code for primary procedure)

(Use 37206 in conjunction with 37205)

(For radiological supervision and interpretation, use 75960)

**37207** Transcatheter placement of an intravascular stent(s) (except cornary, carotid, vertebral, iliac and lower extremity arteries), open; initial vessel

(For stent placement in iliac, femoral, popliteal, and tibial/peroneal arteries, see 37221, 37223, 37226, 37227, 37230, 37231, 37234, 37235)

+ **37208** each additional vessel (List separately in addition to code for primary procedure)

(Use 37208 in conjunction with 37207)

(For radiological supervision and interpretation, use 75960)

(For catheterizations, see 36215-36248)

(For transcatheter placement of intracoronary stent(s), see 92980, 92981)

**37209** Exchange of a previously placed intravascular catheter during thrombolytic therapy

(For radiological supervision and interpretation, use 75900)

⊙ **37210** Uterine fibroid embolization (UFE, embolization of the uterine arteries to treat uterine fibroids, leiomyomata), percutaneous approach inclusive of vascular access, vessel selection, embolization, and all radiological supervision and interpretation, intraprocedural roadmapping, and imaging guidance necessary to complete the procedure

(37210 includes all catheterizations and intraprocedural imaging required for a UFE procedure to confirm the presence of previously known fibroids and to roadmap vascular anatomy to enable appropriate therapy)

(Do not report 37210 in conjunction with 36200, 36245-36248, 37204, 75894, 75898)

(For all other non-central nervous system (CNS) embolization procedures, use 37204)

⊙ **37215** Transcatheter placement of intravascular stent(s), cervical carotid artery, percutaneous; with distal embolic protection

⊙ **37216** without distal embolic protection

(37215 and 37216 include all ipsilateral selective carotid catheterization, all diagnostic imaging for ipsilateral, cervical and cerebral carotid arteriography, and all related radiological supervision and interpretation. When ipsilateral carotid arteriogram (including imaging and selective catheterization) confirms the need for carotid stenting, 37215 and 37216 are inclusive of these services. If carotid stenting is not indicated, then the appropriate codes for carotid catheterization and imaging should be reported in lieu of 37215 and 37216)

(Do not report 37215, 37216 in conjunction with 75671, 75680)

(For transcatheter placement of extracranial vertebral or intrathoracic carotid artery stent(s), see Category III codes 0075T, 0076T)

(For percutaneous transcatheter placement of intravascular stents other than coronary, carotid, or vertebral, see 37205, 37206)

# Endovascular Revascularization (Open or Percutaneous, Transcatheter)

Codes 37220-37235 are to be used to describe lower extremity endovascular revascularization services performed for occlusive disease. These lower extremity codes are built on progressive hierarchies with more intensive services inclusive of lesser intensive services. The code inclusive of all of the services provided for that vessel should be reported (ie, use the code inclusive of the most intensive services provided). Only one code from this family (37220-37235) should be reported for each lower extremity vessel treated.

►These lower extremity endovascular revascularization codes all include the work of accessing and selectively catheterizing the vessel, traversing the lesion, radiological supervision and interpretation directly related to the intervention(s) performed, embolic protection if used, closure of the arteriotomy by pressure and application of an arterial closure device or standard closure of the puncture by suture, and imaging performed to document completion of the intervention in addition to the intervention(s) performed. Extensive repair or replacement of an artery may be additionally reported (eg, 35226 or 35286). These codes describe endovascular procedures performed percutaneously and/or through an open surgical exposure. These codes include balloon angioplasty (eg, low-profile, cutting balloon, cryoplasty), atherectomy (eg, directional, rotational, laser), and stenting (eg, balloon-expandable, self-expanding, bare metal, covered, drug-eluting). Each code in this family (37220-37235) includes balloon angioplasty, when performed.◄

These codes describe revascularization therapies (ie, transluminal angioplasty, atherectomy, and stent placement) provided in three arterial vascular territories: iliac, femoral/popliteal, and tibial/peroneal.

1. ***Iliac Vascular Territory***—The iliac territory is divided into 3 vessels: common iliac, internal iliac, and external iliac.

2. ***Femoral/Popliteal Vascular Territory***—The entire femoral/popliteal territory in 1 lower extremity is considered a single vessel for CPT reporting specifically for the endovascular lower extremity revascularization codes 37224-37227.

3. ***Tibial/Peroneal Territory***—The tibial/peroneal territory is divided into 3 vessels: anterior tibial, posterior tibial, and peroneal arteries.

There are specific coding guidelines for each of the 3 vascular territories.

1. ***Iliac Vascular Territory***—A single primary code is used for the initial iliac artery treated in each leg (37220 or 37221). If other iliac vessels are also treated in that leg, these interventions are reported with the appropriate add-on code(s) (37222, 37223). Up to 2 add-on codes can be used in a unilateral iliac vascular

territory since there are 3 vessels which could be treated. Add-on codes are used for different vessels, not distinct lesions within the same vessel.

2. ***Femoral/Popliteal Territory***—A single interventional code is used no matter what combination of angioplasty/stent/atherectomy is applied to all segments, including the common, deep and superficial femoral arteries as well as the popliteal artery (37224, 37225, 37226, or 37227). There are no add-on codes for additional vessels treated within the femoral/popliteal territory. Because only 1 service is reported when 2 lesions are treated in this territory, report the most complex service (eg, use 37227 if a stent is placed for 1 lesion and an atherectomy is performed on a second lesion)

3. ***Tibial/Peroneal Territory***—A single primary code is used for the initial tibial/peroneal artery treated in each leg (37228, 37229, 37230, or 37231). If other tibial/peroneal vessels are also treated in the same leg, these interventions are reported with the appropriate add-on code(s) (37232-37235). Up to 2 add-on codes could be used to describe services provided in a single leg since there are 3 tibial/peroneal vessels which could be treated. Add-on codes are used for different vessels, not distinct lesions within the same vessel. The common tibio-peroneal trunk is considered part of the tibial/peroneal territory, but is not considered a separate, fourth segment of vessel in the tibio-peroneal family for CPT reporting of endovascular lower extremity interventions. For instance, if lesions in the common tibio-peroneal trunk are treated in conjunction with lesions in the posterior tibial artery, a single code would be reported for treatment of this segment.

When treating multiple territories in the same leg, one primary lower extremity revascularization code is used for each territory treated. When second or third vessel(s) are treated in the iliac and/or tibial/peroneal territories, add-on code(s) are used to report the additional service(s). When more than one stent is placed in the same vessel, the code should be reported only once.

When multiple vessels in multiple territories in a single leg are treated at the same setting, the primary code for the treatment in the initial vessel in each vascular territory is reported. Add-on code(s) are reported when second and third iliac or tibial/peroneal arteries are treated in addition to the initial vessel in that vascular territory.

If a lesion extends across the margins of one vessel vascular territory into another, but can be opened with a single therapy, this intervention should be reported with a single code despite treating more than one vessel and/or vascular territory. For instance, if a stenosis extends from the common iliac artery into the proximal external iliac artery, and a single stent is placed to open the entire lesion, this therapy should be coded as a single stent placement in the iliac artery (37221). In this example, a code for an additional vessel treatment would not be used (do not report both 37221 and 37223).

For bifurcation lesions distal to the common iliac origins which require therapy of 2 distinct branches of the iliac or tibial/peroneal vascular territories, a primary code and an add-on code would be used to describe the intervention. In the femoral/popliteal territory, all branches are included in the primary code, so treatment of a bifurcation lesion would be reported as a single code.

When the same territor(ies) of both legs are treated in the same session, modifiers may be required to describe the interventions. Use modifier 59 to denote that different legs are being treated, even if the mode of therapy is different.

Mechanical thrombectomy and/or thrombolysis in the lower extremity vessels are sometimes necessary to aid in restoring flow to areas of occlusive disease, and are reported separately.

⊙ **37220**   Revascularization, endovascular, open or percutaneous, iliac artery, unilateral, initial vessel; with transluminal angioplasty

⊙ **37221**     with transluminal stent placement(s), includes angioplasty within the same vessel, when performed

⊙✚ **37222**   Revascularization, endovascular, open or percutaneous, iliac artery, each additional ipsilateral iliac vessel; with transluminal angioplasty (List separately in addition to code for primary procedure)

(Use 37222 in conjunction with 37220, 37221)

⊙✚ **37223**     with transluminal stent placement(s), includes angioplasty within the same vessel, when performed (List separately in addition to code for primary procedure)

►(Use 37223 in conjunction with 37221, 37229, 37231)◄

⊙ **37224**   Revascularization, endovascular, open or percutaneous, femoral, popliteal artery(s), unilateral; with transluminal angioplasty

⊙ **37225**     with atherectomy, includes angioplasty within the same vessel, when performed

⊙ **37226**     with transluminal stent placement(s), includes angioplasty within the same vessel, when performed

⊙ **37227**     with transluminal stent placement(s) and atherectomy, includes angioplasty within the same vessel, when performed

⊙ **37228**   Revascularization, endovascular, open or percutaneous, tibial, peroneal artery, unilateral, initial vessel; with transluminal angioplasty

⊙ **37229**     with atherectomy, includes angioplasty within the same vessel, when performed

⊙ **37230**     with transluminal stent placement(s), includes angioplasty within the same vessel, when performed

⊙ **37231**     with transluminal stent placement(s) and atherectomy, includes angioplasty within the same vessel, when performed

⊙✚ **37232**   Revascularization, endovascular, open or percutaneous, tibial/peroneal artery, unilateral, each additional vessel; with transluminal angioplasty (List separately in addition to code for primary procedure)

(Use 37232 in conjunction with 37228-37231)

⊙✚ **37233**     with atherectomy, includes angioplasty within the same vessel, when performed (List separately in addition to code for primary procedure)

►(Use 37233 in conjunction with 37229, 37231)◄

⊙✚ **37234**     with transluminal stent placement(s), includes angioplasty within the same vessel, when performed (List separately in addition to code for primary procedure)

►(Use 37234 in conjunction with 37229, 37230, 37231)◄

⊙✚ **37235**     with transluminal stent placement(s) and atherectomy, includes angioplasty within the same vessel, when performed (List separately in addition to code for primary procedure)

(Use 37235 in conjunction with 37231)

## Intravascular Ultrasound Services

Intravascular ultrasound services include all transducer manipulations and repositioning within the specific vessel being examined, both before and after therapeutic intervention (eg, stent placement).

Vascular access for intravascular ultrasound performed during a therapeutic intervention is not reported separately.

✚ **37250**   Intravascular ultrasound (non-coronary vessel) during diagnostic evaluation and/or therapeutic intervention; initial vessel (List separately in addition to code for primary procedure)

✚ **37251**     each additional vessel (List separately in addition to code for primary procedure)

(Use 37251 in conjunction with 37250)

(For catheterizations, see 36215-36248)

(For transcatheter therapies, see 37200-37208, 61624, 61626)

(For radiological supervision and interpretation see 75945, 75946)

## Endoscopy

Surgical vascular endoscopy always includes diagnostic endoscopy.

**37500**   Vascular endoscopy, surgical, with ligation of perforator veins, subfascial (SEPS)

(For open procedure, use 37760)

**37501**   Unlisted vascular endoscopy procedure

## Ligation

(For phleborraphy and arteriorraphy, see 35201-35286)

**37565**   Ligation, internal jugular vein

**37600**   Ligation; external carotid artery

**37605**      internal or common carotid artery

**37606**      internal or common carotid artery, with gradual occlusion, as with Selverstone or Crutchfield clamp

(For transcatheter permanent arterial occlusion or embolization, see 61624-61626)

(For endovascular temporary arterial balloon occlusion, use 61623)

(For ligation treatment of intracranial aneurysm, use 61703)

**37607**   Ligation or banding of angioaccess arteriovenous fistula

**37609**   Ligation or biopsy, temporal artery

**37615**   Ligation, major artery (eg, post-traumatic, rupture); neck

**37616**      chest

**37617**      abdomen

**37618**      extremity

● **37619**   Ligation of inferior vena cava

►(For endovascular delivery of an inferior vena cava filter, use 37191)◄

►(37620 has been deleted. To report, see 37191 for endovascular placement of intravascular filter or 37619 for open surgical ligation of the inferior vena cava)◄

**37650**   Ligation of femoral vein

(For bilateral procedure, report 37650 with modifier 50)

**37660**   Ligation of common iliac vein

**37700**   Ligation and division of long saphenous vein at saphenofemoral junction, or distal interruptions

(Do not report 37700 in conjunction with 37718, 37722)

(For bilateral procedure, report 37700 with modifier 50)

**37718**   Ligation, division, and stripping, short saphenous vein

(For bilateral procedure, use modifier 50)

(Do not report 37718 in conjunction with 37735, 37780)

**37722**   Ligation, division, and stripping, long (greater) saphenous veins from saphenofemoral junction to knee or below

(For ligation and stripping of the short saphenous vein, use 37718)

(For bilateral procedure, report 37722 with modifier 50)

(Do not report 37722 in conjunction with 37700, 37735)

(For ligation, division, and stripping of the greater saphenous vein, use 37722. For ligation, division, and stripping of the short saphenous vein, use 37718)

**37735**   Ligation and division and complete stripping of long or short saphenous veins with radical excision of ulcer and skin graft and/or interruption of communicating veins of lower leg, with excision of deep fascia

(Do not report 37735 in conjunction with 37700, 37718, 37722, 37780)

(For bilateral procedure, report 37735 with modifier 50)

**37760**   Ligation of perforator veins, subfascial, radical (Linton type), including skin graft, when performed, open,1 leg

(For endoscopic procedure, use 37500)

**37761**   Ligation of perforator vein(s), subfascial, open, including ultrasound guidance, when performed, 1 leg

(For bilateral procedure, report 37761 with modifier 50)

(Do not report 37760, 37761 in conjunction with 76937, 76942, 76998, 93971)

(For endoscopic ligation of subfascial perforator veins, use 37500)

**37765**   Stab phlebectomy of varicose veins, 1 extremity; 10-20 stab incisions

(For less than 10 incisions, use 37799)

(For more than 20 incisions, use 37766)

**37766**      more than 20 incisions

**37780**   Ligation and division of short saphenous vein at saphenopopliteal junction (separate procedure)

(For bilateral procedure, report 37780 with modifier 50)

**37785**   Ligation, division, and/or excision of varicose vein cluster(s), 1 leg

(For bilateral procedure, report 37785 with modifier 50)

## Other Procedures

**37788**   Penile revascularization, artery, with or without vein graft

**37790**   Penile venous occlusive procedure

**37799**   Unlisted procedure, vascular surgery

# Hemic and Lymphatic Systems

## Spleen

### Excision

**38100**   Splenectomy; total (separate procedure)

**38101**      partial (separate procedure)

+ **38102**      total, en bloc for extensive disease, in conjunction with other procedure (List in addition to code for primary procedure)

## Repair

**38115**    Repair of ruptured spleen (splenorrhaphy) with or without partial splenectomy

## Laparoscopy

Surgical laparoscopy always includes diagnostic laparoscopy. To report a diagnostic laparoscopy (peritoneoscopy) (separate procedure), use 49320.

**38120**    Laparoscopy, surgical, splenectomy

**38129**    Unlisted laparoscopy procedure, spleen

## Introduction

**38200**    Injection procedure for splenoportography

(For radiological supervision and interpretation, use 75810)

# General

## Bone Marrow or Stem Cell Services/ Procedures

Codes 38207-38215 describe various steps used to preserve, prepare and purify bone marrow/stem cells prior to transplantation or reinfusion. Each code may be reported only once per day regardless of the quantity of bone marrow/stem cells manipulated.

**38204**    Management of recipient hematopoietic progenitor cell donor search and cell acquisition

**38205**    Blood-derived hematopoietic progenitor cell harvesting for transplantation, per collection; allogeneic

**38206**      autologous

**38207**    Transplant preparation of hematopoietic progenitor cells; cryopreservation and storage

(For diagnostic cryopreservation and storage, use 88240)

▲ **38208**      thawing of previously frozen harvest, without washing, per donor

(For diagnostic thawing and expansion of frozen cells, use 88241)

▲ **38209**      thawing of previously frozen harvest, with washing, per donor

**38210**      specific cell depletion within harvest, T-cell depletion

**38211**      tumor cell depletion

**38212**      red blood cell removal

**38213**      platelet depletion

**38214**      plasma (volume) depletion

**38215**      cell concentration in plasma, mononuclear, or buffy coat layer

(Do not report 38207-38215 in conjunction with 88182, 88184-88189)

**38220**    Bone marrow; aspiration only

**38221**      biopsy, needle or trocar

(For bone marrow biopsy interpretation, use 88305)

▲ **38230**    Bone marrow harvesting for transplantation; allogeneic

● **38232**      autologous

(For autologous and allogeneic blood-derived peripheral stem cell harvesting for transplantation, see 38205-38206)

**38240**    Bone marrow or blood-derived peripheral stem cell transplantation; allogeneic

**38241**      autologous

**38242**      allogeneic donor lymphocyte infusions

(For bone marrow aspiration, use 38220)

(For modification, treatment, and processing of bone marrow or blood-derived stem cell specimens for transplantation, use 38210-38213)

(For cryopreservation, freezing, and storage of blood-derived stem cells for transplantation, use 38207)

(For thawing and expansion of blood-derived stem cells for transplantation, see 38208, 38209)

(For compatibility studies, see 86812-86822)

# Lymph Nodes and Lymphatic Channels

## Incision

**38300**    Drainage of lymph node abscess or lymphadenitis; simple

**38305**      extensive

**38308**    Lymphangiotomy or other operations on lymphatic channels

**38380**    Suture and/or ligation of thoracic duct; cervical approach

**38381**      thoracic approach

**38382**      abdominal approach

## Excision

(For injection for sentinel node identification, use 38792)

**38500**    Biopsy or excision of lymph node(s); open, superficial

(Do not report 38500 with 38700-38780)

**38505**      by needle, superficial (eg, cervical, inguinal, axillary)

(If imaging guidance is performed, see 76942, 77012, 77021)

(For fine needle aspiration, use 10021 or 10022)

(For evaluation of fine needle aspirate, see 88172, 88173)

| 38510 | open, deep cervical node(s) |
|---|---|

38520   open, deep cervical node(s) with excision scalene fat pad

38525   open, deep axillary node(s)

38530   open, internal mammary node(s)

(Do not report 38530 with 38720-38746)

(For percutaneous needle biopsy, retroperitoneal lymph node or mass, use 49180. For fine needle aspiration, use 10022)

38542   Dissection, deep jugular node(s)

(For radical cervical neck dissection, use 38720)

38550   Excision of cystic hygroma, axillary or cervical; without deep neurovascular dissection

38555   with deep neurovascular dissection

## Limited Lymphadenectomy for Staging

38562   Limited lymphadenectomy for staging (separate procedure); pelvic and para-aortic

(When combined with prostatectomy, use 55812 or 55842)

(When combined with insertion of radioactive substance into prostate, use 55862)

38564   retroperitoneal (aortic and/or splenic)

## Laparoscopy

Surgical laparoscopy always includes diagnostic laparoscopy. To report a diagnostic laparoscopy (peritoneoscopy) (separate procedure), use 49320.

38570   Laparoscopy, surgical; with retroperitoneal lymph node sampling (biopsy), single or multiple

38571   with bilateral total pelvic lymphadenectomy

38572   with bilateral total pelvic lymphadenectomy and peri-aortic lymph node sampling (biopsy), single or multiple

(For drainage of lymphocele to peritoneal cavity, use 49323)

38589   Unlisted laparoscopy procedure, lymphatic system

## Radical Lymphadenectomy (Radical Resection of Lymph Nodes)

(For limited pelvic and retroperitoneal lymphadenectomies, see 38562, 38564)

38700   Suprahyoid lymphadenectomy

(For bilateral procedure, report 38700 with modifier 50)

38720   Cervical lymphadenectomy (complete)

(For bilateral procedure, report 38720 with modifier 50)

38724   Cervical lymphadenectomy (modified radical neck dissection)

38740   Axillary lymphadenectomy; superficial

38745   complete

+▲ 38746   Thoracic lymphadenectomy by thoracotomy, mediastinal and regional lymphadenectomy (List separately in addition to code for primary procedure)

►(On the right, mediastinal lymph nodes include the paratracheal, subcarinal, paraesophageal, and inferior pulmonary ligament)◄

►(On the left, mediastinal lymph nodes include the aortopulmonary window, subcarinal, paraesophageal, and inferior pulmonary ligament)◄

►(Report 38746 in conjunction with 32440, 32442, 32445, 32480, 32482, 32484, 32486, 32488, 32503, 32504, 32505)◄

►(To report mediastinal and regional lymphadenectomy via thoracoscopy [VATS], see 32674)◄

+ 38747   Abdominal lymphadenectomy, regional, including celiac, gastric, portal, peripancreatic, with or without para-aortic and vena caval nodes (List separately in addition to code for primary procedure)

38760   Inguinofemoral lymphadenectomy, superficial, including Cloquets node (separate procedure)

(For bilateral procedure, report 38760 with modifier 50)

38765   Inguinofemoral lymphadenectomy, superficial, in continuity with pelvic lymphadenectomy, including external iliac, hypogastric, and obturator nodes (separate procedure)

(For bilateral procedure, report 38765 with modifier 50)

38770   Pelvic lymphadenectomy, including external iliac, hypogastric, and obturator nodes (separate procedure)

(For bilateral procedure, report 38770 with modifier 50)

38780   Retroperitoneal transabdominal lymphadenectomy, extensive, including pelvic, aortic, and renal nodes (separate procedure)

(For excision and repair of lymphedematous skin and subcutaneous tissue, see 15004-15005, 15570-15650)

## Introduction

38790   Injection procedure; lymphangiography

(For bilateral procedure, report 38790 with modifier 50)

(For radiological supervision and interpretation, see 75801-75807)

▲ 38792   radioactive tracer for identification of sentinel node

(For excision of sentinel node, see 38500-38542)

(For nuclear medicine lymphatics and lymph gland imaging, use 78195)

**Surgery: Cardiovascular System**

▶(For intraoperative identification (eg, mapping) of sentinel lymph node(s) including injection of non-radioactive dye, see 38900)◀

**38794**   Cannulation, thoracic duct

## Other Procedures

**+ 38900**   Intraoperative identification (eg, mapping) of sentinel lymph node(s) includes injection of non-radioactive dye, when performed (List separately in addition to code for primary procedure)

(Use 38900 in conjunction with 19302, 19307, 38500, 38510, 38520, 38525, 38530, 38542, 38740, 38745)

(For injection of radioactive tracer for identification of sentinel node, use 38792)

**38999**   Unlisted procedure, hemic or lymphatic system

# Mediastinum and Diaphragm

## Mediastinum

### Incision

**39000**   Mediastinotomy with exploration, drainage, removal of foreign body, or biopsy; cervical approach

**39010**       transthoracic approach, including either transthoracic or median sternotomy

▶(For VATS pericardial biopsy, use 32604)◀

### ▶Excision/Resection◀

▲ **39200**   Resection of mediastinal cyst

▲ **39220**   Resection of mediastinal tumor

(For substernal thyroidectomy, use 60270)

(For thymectomy, use 60520)

▶(For thoracoscopic [VATS] resection of mediastinal cyst, tumor, or mass, use 32662)◀

### Endoscopy

▲ **39400**   Mediastinoscopy, includes biopsy(ies), when performed

### Other Procedures

**39499**   Unlisted procedure, mediastinum

## Diaphragm

### Repair

(For transabdominal repair of diaphragmatic [esophageal hiatal] hernia, use 43325)

(For laparoscopic repair of diaphragmatic [esophageal hiatal] hernias and fundoplication, see 43280, 43281, 43282)

**39501**   Repair, laceration of diaphragm, any approach

(39502 has been deleted. To report transabdominal paraesophageal hiatal hernia repair with fundoplasty, vagotomy, and/or pyloroplasty when performed, see 43332, 43333, 43335, 43337)

(For laparoscopic paraesophageal hernia repair, see 43281, 43282)

**39503**   Repair, neonatal diaphragmatic hernia, with or without chest tube insertion and with or without creation of ventral hernia

(Do not report modifier 63 in conjunction with 39503)

(39520 has been deleted. To report transthoracic diaphragmatic [esophageal hiatal] hernia repair, see 43334, 43335)

(For laparoscopic paraesophageal hernia repair, see 43281, 43282)

(39530 has been deleted. To report thoracoabdominal diaphragmatic [esophageal hiatal] hernia repair, see 43336, 43337)?

(39531 has been deleted. To report thoracoabdominal diaphragmatic [esophageal hiatal] hernia repair, see 43336, 43337)

**39540**   Repair, diaphragmatic hernia (other than neonatal), traumatic; acute

**39541**       chronic

**39545**   Imbrication of diaphragm for eventration, transthoracic or transabdominal, paralytic or nonparalytic

**39560**   Resection, diaphragm; with simple repair (eg, primary suture)

**39561**       with complex repair (eg, prosthetic material, local muscle flap)

### Other Procedures

**39599**   Unlisted procedure, diaphragm

# Digestive System

## Lips

(For procedures on skin of lips, see 10040 et seq)

### Excision

**40490**  Biopsy of lip

**40500**  Vermilionectomy (lip shave), with mucosal advancement

**40510**  Excision of lip; transverse wedge excision with primary closure

**40520**  V-excision with primary direct linear closure

(For excision of mucous lesions, see 40810-40816)

**40525**  full thickness, reconstruction with local flap (eg, Estlander or fan)

**40527**  full thickness, reconstruction with cross lip flap (Abbe-Estlander)

**40530**  Resection of lip, more than one-fourth, without reconstruction

(For reconstruction, see 13131 et seq)

### Repair (Cheiloplasty)

**40650**  Repair lip, full thickness; vermilion only

**40652**  up to half vertical height

**40654**  over one-half vertical height, or complex

**40700**  Plastic repair of cleft lip/nasal deformity; primary, partial or complete, unilateral

**40701**  primary bilateral, 1-stage procedure

**40702**  primary bilateral, 1 of 2 stages

**40720**  secondary, by recreation of defect and reclosure

(For bilateral procedure, report 40720 with modifier 50)

(To report rhinoplasty only for nasal deformity secondary to congenital cleft lip, see 30460, 30462)

(For repair of cleft lip, with cross lip pedicle flap (Abbe-Estlander type), use 40527)

**40761**  with cross lip pedicle flap (Abbe-Estlander type), including sectioning and inserting of pedicle

(For repair cleft palate, see 42200 et seq)

(For other reconstructive procedures, see 14060, 14061, 15120-15261, 15574, 15576, 15630)

### Other Procedures

**40799**  Unlisted procedure, lips

## Vestibule of Mouth

The vestibule is the part of the oral cavity outside the dentoalveolar structures; it includes the mucosal and submucosal tissue of lips and cheeks.

### Incision

**40800**  Drainage of abscess, cyst, hematoma, vestibule of mouth; simple

**40801**  complicated

**40804**  Removal of embedded foreign body, vestibule of mouth; simple

**40805**  complicated

**40806**  Incision of labial frenum (frenotomy)

### Excision, Destruction

**40808**  Biopsy, vestibule of mouth

**40810**  Excision of lesion of mucosa and submucosa, vestibule of mouth; without repair

**40812**  with simple repair

**40814**  with complex repair

**40816**  complex, with excision of underlying muscle

**40818**  Excision of mucosa of vestibule of mouth as donor graft

**40819**  Excision of frenum, labial or buccal (frenumectomy, frenulectomy, frenectomy)

**40820**  Destruction of lesion or scar of vestibule of mouth by physical methods (eg, laser, thermal, cryo, chemical)

### Repair

**40830**  Closure of laceration, vestibule of mouth; 2.5 cm or less

**40831**  over 2.5 cm or complex

**40840**  Vestibuloplasty; anterior

**40842**  posterior, unilateral

**40843**  posterior, bilateral

**40844**  entire arch

**40845**  complex (including ridge extension, muscle repositioning)

(For skin grafts, see 15002 et seq)

### Other Procedures

**40899**  Unlisted procedure, vestibule of mouth

Surgery: Digestive System

# Tongue and Floor of Mouth

## Incision

**41000** Intraoral incision and drainage of abscess, cyst, or hematoma of tongue or floor of mouth; lingual

**41005**     sublingual, superficial

**41006**     sublingual, deep, supramylohyoid

**41007**     submental space

**41008**     submandibular space

**41009**     masticator space

**41010** Incision of lingual frenum (frenotomy)

**41015** Extraoral incision and drainage of abscess, cyst, or hematoma of floor of mouth; sublingual

**41016**     submental

**41017**     submandibular

**41018**     masticator space

(For frenoplasty, use 41520)

**41019** Placement of needles, catheters, or other device(s) into the head and/or neck region (percutaneous, transoral, or transnasal) for subsequent interstitial radioelement application

(For imaging guidance, see 76942, 77002, 77012, 77021)

(For stereotactic insertion of intracranial brachytherapy radiation sources, use 61770)

(For interstitial radioelement application, see 77776-77787)

## Excision

**41100** Biopsy of tongue; anterior two-thirds

**41105**     posterior one-third

**41108** Biopsy of floor of mouth

**41110** Excision of lesion of tongue without closure

**41112** Excision of lesion of tongue with closure; anterior two-thirds

**41113**     posterior one-third

**41114**     with local tongue flap

(Do not report 41114 in conjunction with 41112 or 41113)

**41115** Excision of lingual frenum (frenectomy)

**41116** Excision, lesion of floor of mouth

**41120** Glossectomy; less than one-half tongue

**41130**     hemiglossectomy

**41135**     partial, with unilateral radical neck dissection

**41140**     complete or total, with or without tracheostomy, without radical neck dissection

**41145**     complete or total, with or without tracheostomy, with unilateral radical neck dissection

**41150**     composite procedure with resection floor of mouth and mandibular resection, without radical neck dissection

**41153**     composite procedure with resection floor of mouth, with suprahyoid neck dissection

**41155**     composite procedure with resection floor of mouth, mandibular resection, and radical neck dissection (Commando type)

## Repair

**41250** Repair of laceration 2.5 cm or less; floor of mouth and/or anterior two-thirds of tongue

**41251**     posterior one-third of tongue

**41252** Repair of laceration of tongue, floor of mouth, over 2.6 cm or complex

## Other Procedures

**41500** Fixation of tongue, mechanical, other than suture (eg, K-wire)

**41510** Suture of tongue to lip for micrognathia (Douglas type procedure)

**41512** Tongue base suspension, permanent suture technique

(For fixation of tongue, mechanical, other than suture, use 41500)

(For suture of tongue to lip for micrognathia, use 41510)

**41520** Frenoplasty (surgical revision of frenum, eg, with Z-plasty)

(For frenotomy, see 40806, 41010)

**41530** Submucosal ablation of the tongue base, radiofrequency, 1 or more sites, per session

**41599** Unlisted procedure, tongue, floor of mouth

# Dentoalveolar Structures

## Incision

**41800** Drainage of abscess, cyst, hematoma from dentoalveolar structures

**41805** Removal of embedded foreign body from dentoalveolar structures; soft tissues

**41806**     bone

## Excision, Destruction

**41820** Gingivectomy, excision gingiva, each quadrant

**41821** Operculectomy, excision pericoronal tissues

**41822** Excision of fibrous tuberosities, dentoalveolar structures

Surgery: Digestive System

**41823**    Excision of osseous tuberosities, dentoalveolar structures

**41825**    Excision of lesion or tumor (except listed above), dentoalveolar structures; without repair

**41826**        with simple repair

**41827**        with complex repair

(For nonexcisional destruction, use 41850)

**41828**    Excision of hyperplastic alveolar mucosa, each quadrant (specify)

**41830**    Alveolectomy, including curettage of osteitis or sequestrectomy

**41850**    Destruction of lesion (except excision), dentoalveolar structures

## Other Procedures

**41870**    Periodontal mucosal grafting

**41872**    Gingivoplasty, each quadrant (specify)

**41874**    Alveoloplasty, each quadrant (specify)

(For closure of lacerations, see 40830, 40831)

(For segmental osteotomy, use 21206)

(For reduction of fractures, see 21421-21490)

**41899**    Unlisted procedure, dentoalveolar structures

# Palate and Uvula

## Incision

**42000**    Drainage of abscess of palate, uvula

## Excision, Destruction

**42100**    Biopsy of palate, uvula

**42104**    Excision, lesion of palate, uvula; without closure

**42106**        with simple primary closure

**42107**        with local flap closure

(For skin graft, see 14040-14302)

(For mucosal graft, use 40818)

**42120**    Resection of palate or extensive resection of lesion

(For reconstruction of palate with extraoral tissue, see 14040-14302, 15050, 15120, 15240, 15576)

**42140**    Uvulectomy, excision of uvula

**42145**    Palatopharyngoplasty (eg, uvulopalatopharyngoplasty, uvulopharyngoplasty)

(For removal of exostosis of the bony palate, see 21031, 21032)

**42160**    Destruction of lesion, palate or uvula (thermal, cryo or chemical)

## Repair

**42180**    Repair, laceration of palate; up to 2 cm

**42182**        over 2 cm or complex

**42200**    Palatoplasty for cleft palate, soft and/or hard palate only

**42205**    Palatoplasty for cleft palate, with closure of alveolar ridge; soft tissue only

**42210**        with bone graft to alveolar ridge (includes obtaining graft)

**42215**    Palatoplasty for cleft palate; major revision

**42220**        secondary lengthening procedure

**42225**        attachment pharyngeal flap

**42226**    Lengthening of palate, and pharyngeal flap

**42227**    Lengthening of palate, with island flap

**42235**    Repair of anterior palate, including vomer flap

(For repair of oronasal fistula, use 30600)

**42260**    Repair of nasolabial fistula

(For repair of cleft lip, see 40700 et seq)

**42280**    Maxillary impression for palatal prosthesis

**42281**    Insertion of pin-retained palatal prosthesis

## Other Procedures

**42299**    Unlisted procedure, palate, uvula

# Salivary Gland and Ducts

## Incision

**42300**    Drainage of abscess; parotid, simple

**42305**        parotid, complicated

**42310**    Drainage of abscess; submaxillary or sublingual, intraoral

**42320**        submaxillary, external

**42330**    Sialolithotomy; submandibular (submaxillary), sublingual or parotid, uncomplicated, intraoral

**42335**        submandibular (submaxillary), complicated, intraoral

**42340**        parotid, extraoral or complicated intraoral

## Excision

**42400**    Biopsy of salivary gland; needle

(For fine needle aspiration, see 10021, 10022)

(For evaluation of fine needle aspirate, see 88172, 88173)

(If imaging guidance is performed, see 76942, 77002, 77012, 77021)

**42405**        incisional

(If imaging guidance is performed, see 76942, 77002, 77012, 77021)

42408   Excision of sublingual salivary cyst (ranula)

42409   Marsupialization of sublingual salivary cyst (ranula)

42410   Excision of parotid tumor or parotid gland; lateral lobe, without nerve dissection

42415       lateral lobe, with dissection and preservation of facial nerve

42420       total, with dissection and preservation of facial nerve

42425       total, en bloc removal with sacrifice of facial nerve

42426       total, with unilateral radical neck dissection

        (For suture or grafting of facial nerve, see 64864, 64865, 69740, 69745)

42440   Excision of submandibular (submaxillary) gland

42450   Excision of sublingual gland

## Repair

42500   Plastic repair of salivary duct, sialodochoplasty; primary or simple

42505       secondary or complicated

42507   Parotid duct diversion, bilateral (Wilke type procedure);

42508       with excision of 1 submandibular gland

42509       with excision of both submandibular glands

42510       with ligation of both submandibular (Wharton's) ducts

## Other Procedures

42550   Injection procedure for sialography

        (For radiological supervision and interpretation, use 70390)

42600   Closure salivary fistula

42650   Dilation salivary duct

42660   Dilation and catheterization of salivary duct, with or without injection

42665   Ligation salivary duct, intraoral

42699   Unlisted procedure, salivary glands or ducts

# Pharynx, Adenoids, and Tonsils

## Incision

42700   Incision and drainage abscess; peritonsillar

42720       retropharyngeal or parapharyngeal, intraoral approach

42725       retropharyngeal or parapharyngeal, external approach

## Excision, Destruction

42800   Biopsy; oropharynx

42802       hypopharynx

42804       nasopharynx, visible lesion, simple

42806       nasopharynx, survey for unknown primary lesion

        (For laryngoscopic biopsy, see 31510, 31535, 31536)

42808   Excision or destruction of lesion of pharynx, any method

42809   Removal of foreign body from pharynx

42810   Excision branchial cleft cyst or vestige, confined to skin and subcutaneous tissues

42815   Excision branchial cleft cyst, vestige, or fistula, extending beneath subcutaneous tissues and/or into pharynx

42820   Tonsillectomy and adenoidectomy; younger than age 12

42821       age 12 or over

42825   Tonsillectomy, primary or secondary; younger than age 12

42826       age 12 or over

42830   Adenoidectomy, primary; younger than age 12

42831       age 12 or over

42835   Adenoidectomy, secondary; younger than age 12

42836       age 12 or over

42842   Radical resection of tonsil, tonsillar pillars, and/or retromolar trigone; without closure

42844       closure with local flap (eg, tongue, buccal)

42845       closure with other flap

        (For closure with other flap(s), use appropriate number for flap(s))

        (When combined with radical neck dissection, use also 38720)

42860   Excision of tonsil tags

42870   Excision or destruction lingual tonsil, any method (separate procedure)

        (For resection of the nasopharynx [eg, juvenile angiofibroma] by bicoronal and/or transzygomatic approach, see 61586 and 61600)

42890   Limited pharyngectomy

42892   Resection of lateral pharyngeal wall or pyriform sinus, direct closure by advancement of lateral and posterior pharyngeal walls

        (When combined with radical neck dissection, use also 38720)

42894   Resection of pharyngeal wall requiring closure with myocutaneous or fasciocutaneous flap or free muscle, skin, or fascial flap with microvascular anastamosis

        (When combined with radical neck dissection, use also 38720)

        (For limited pharyngectomy with radical neck dissection, use 38720 with 42890)

        (For flap used for reconstruction, see 15732, 15734, 15756, 15757, 15758)

## Repair

**42900**  Suture pharynx for wound or injury

**42950**  Pharyngoplasty (plastic or reconstructive operation on pharynx)

(For pharyngeal flap, use 42225)

**42953**  Pharyngoesophageal repair

(For closure with myocutaneous or other flap, use appropriate number in addition)

## Other Procedures

**42955**  Pharyngostomy (fistulization of pharynx, external for feeding)

**42960**  Control oropharyngeal hemorrhage, primary or secondary (eg, post-tonsillectomy); simple

**42961**      complicated, requiring hospitalization

**42962**      with secondary surgical intervention

**42970**  Control of nasopharyngeal hemorrhage, primary or secondary (eg, postadenoidectomy); simple, with posterior nasal packs, with or without anterior packs and/or cautery

**42971**      complicated, requiring hospitalization

**42972**      with secondary surgical intervention

**42999**  Unlisted procedure, pharynx, adenoids, or tonsils

# Esophagus

## Incision

(For esophageal intubation with laparotomy, use 43510)

**43020**  Esophagotomy, cervical approach, with removal of foreign body

**43030**  Cricopharyngeal myotomy

**43045**  Esophagotomy, thoracic approach, with removal of foreign body

## Excision

(For gastrointestinal reconstruction for previous esophagectomy, see 43360, 43361)

**43100**  Excision of lesion, esophagus, with primary repair; cervical approach

**43101**      thoracic or abdominal approach

(For wide excision of malignant lesion of cervical esophagus, with total laryngectomy without radical neck dissection, see 43107, 43116, 43124, and 31360)

(For wide excision of malignant lesion of cervical esophagus, with total laryngectomy with radical neck dissection, see 43107, 43116, 43124, and 31365)

**43107**  Total or near total esophagectomy, without thoracotomy; with pharyngogastrostomy or cervical esophagogastrostomy, with or without pyloroplasty (transhiatal)

**43108**      with colon interposition or small intestine reconstruction, including intestine mobilization, preparation and anastomosis(es)

**43112**  Total or near total esophagectomy, with thoracotomy; with pharyngogastrostomy or cervical esophagogastrostomy, with or without pyloroplasty

**43113**      with colon interposition or small intestine reconstruction, including intestine mobilization, preparation, and anastomosis(es)

**43116**  Partial esophagectomy, cervical, with free intestinal graft, including microvascular anastomosis, obtaining the graft and intestinal reconstruction

(Do not report 43116 in conjunction with 69990)

(Report 43116 with the modifier 52 appended if intestinal or free jejunal graft with microvascular anastomosis is performed by another physician)

(For free jejunal graft with microvascular anastomosis performed by another physician, use 43496)

**43117**  Partial esophagectomy, distal two-thirds, with thoracotomy and separate abdominal incision, with or without proximal gastrectomy; with thoracic esophagogastrostomy, with or without pyloroplasty (Ivor Lewis)

**43118**      with colon interposition or small intestine reconstruction, including intestine mobilization, preparation, and anastomosis(es)

(For total esophagectomy with gastropharyngostomy, see 43107, 43124)

(For esophagogastrectomy (lower third) and vagotomy, use 43122)

**43121**  Partial esophagectomy, distal two-thirds, with thoracotomy only, with or without proximal gastrectomy, with thoracic esophagogastrostomy, with or without pyloroplasty

**43122**  Partial esophagectomy, thoracoabdominal or abdominal approach, with or without proximal gastrectomy; with esophagogastrostomy, with or without pyloroplasty

**43123**      with colon interposition or small intestine reconstruction, including intestine mobilization, preparation, and anastomosis(es)

**43124**  Total or partial esophagectomy, without reconstruction (any approach), with cervical esophagostomy

**43130**  Diverticulectomy of hypopharynx or esophagus, with or without myotomy; cervical approach

**43135**      thoracic approach

Surgery: Digestive System

# Endoscopy

For endoscopic procedures, code appropriate endoscopy of each anatomic site examined.

Surgical endoscopy always includes diagnostic endoscopy.

⊙ **43200**  Esophagoscopy, rigid or flexible; diagnostic, with or without collection of specimen(s) by brushing or washing (separate procedure)

⊙ **43201**  with directed submucosal injection(s), any substance

(For injection sclerosis of esophageal varices, use 43204)

⊙ **43202**  with biopsy, single or multiple

⊙ **43204**  with injection sclerosis of esophageal varices

⊙ **43205**  with band ligation of esophageal varices

⊙ **43215**  with removal of foreign body

(For radiological supervision and interpretation, use 74235)

⊙ **43216**  with removal of tumor(s), polyp(s), or other lesion(s) by hot biopsy forceps or bipolar cautery

⊙ **43217**  with removal of tumor(s), polyp(s), or other lesion(s) by snare technique

⊙ **43219**  with insertion of plastic tube or stent

⊙ **43220**  with balloon dilation (less than 30 mm diameter)

(If imaging guidance is performed, use 74360)

(For endoscopic dilation with balloon 30 mm diameter or larger, use 43458)

(For dilation without visualization, use 43450-43453)

(For diagnostic fiberoptic esophagogastroscopy, use 43200, 43235)

(For fiberoptic esophagogastroscopy with biopsy or collection of specimen, use 43200, 43202, 43235, 43239)

(For fiberoptic esophagogastroscopy with removal of foreign body, use 43215, 43247)

(For fiberoptic esophagogastroscopy with removal of polyp(s), use 43217, 43251)

⊙ **43226**  with insertion of guide wire followed by dilation over guide wire

(For radiological supervision and interpretation, use 74360)

⊙ **43227**  with control of bleeding (eg, injection, bipolar cautery, unipolar cautery, laser, heater probe, stapler, plasma coagulator)

⊙ **43228**  with ablation of tumor(s), polyp(s), or other lesion(s), not amenable to removal by hot biopsy forceps, bipolar cautery or snare technique

(For esophagoscopic photodynamic therapy, report 43228 in addition to 96570, 96571 as appropriate)

⊙ **43231**  with endoscopic ultrasound examination

(Do not report 43231 in conjunction with 76975)

⊙ **43232**  with transendoscopic ultrasound-guided intramural or transmural fine needle aspiration/biopsy(s)

(Do not report 43232 in conjunction with 76942, 76975)

(For interpretation of specimen, see 88172-88173)

⊙ **43234**  Upper gastrointestinal endoscopy, simple primary examination (eg, with small diameter flexible endoscope) (separate procedure)

⊙ **43235**  Upper gastrointestinal endoscopy including esophagus, stomach, and either the duodenum and/or jejunum as appropriate; diagnostic, with or without collection of specimen(s) by brushing or washing (separate procedure)

⊙ **43236**  with directed submucosal injection(s), any substance

(For injection sclerosis of esophageal and/or gastric varices, use 43243)

⊙ **43237**  with endoscopic ultrasound examination limited to the esophagus

(Do not report 43237 in conjunction with 76942, 76975)

⊙ **43238**  with transendoscopic ultrasound-guided intramural or transmural fine needle aspiration/biopsy(s), esophagus (includes endoscopic ultrasound examination limited to the esophagus)

(Do not report 43238 in conjunction with 76942 or 76975)

⊙ **43239**  with biopsy, single or multiple

⊙ **43240**  with transmural drainage of pseudocyst

⊙ **43241**  with transendoscopic intraluminal tube or catheter placement

⊙ **43242**  with transendoscopic ultrasound-guided intramural or transmural fine needle aspiration/biopsy(s) (includes endoscopic ultrasound examination of the esophagus, stomach, and either the duodenum and/or jejunum as appropriate)

(Do not report 43242 in conjunction with 76942, 76975)

(For transendoscopic fine needle aspiration/biopsy limited to esophagus, use 43238)

(For interpretation of specimen, see 88172-88173)

⊙ **43243**  with injection sclerosis of esophageal and/or gastric varices

⊙ **43244**  with band ligation of esophageal and/or gastric varices

⊙ **43245**  with dilation of gastric outlet for obstruction (eg, balloon, guide wire, bougie)

(Do not report 43245 in conjunction with 43256)

⊙ **43246**  with directed placement of percutaneous gastrostomy tube

(For nonendoscopic percutaneous placement of gastrostomy tube, see 49440)

⊙ **43247**  with removal of foreign body

(For radiological supervision and interpretation, use 74235)

⊙ **43248**   with insertion of guide wire followed by dilation of esophagus over guide wire

⊙ **43249**   with balloon dilation of esophagus (less than 30 mm diameter)

⊙ **43250**   with removal of tumor(s), polyp(s), or other lesion(s) by hot biopsy forceps or bipolar cautery

⊙ **43251**   with removal of tumor(s), polyp(s), or other lesion(s) by snare technique

⊙ **43255**   with control of bleeding, any method

⊙ **43256**   with transendoscopic stent placement (includes predilation)

⊙ **43257**   with delivery of thermal energy to the muscle of lower esophageal sphincter and/or gastric cardia, for treatment of gastroesophageal reflux disease

⊙ **43258**   with ablation of tumor(s), polyp(s), or other lesion(s) not amenable to removal by hot biopsy forceps, bipolar cautery or snare technique

(For injection sclerosis of esophageal varices, use 43204, 43243)

⊙ **43259**   with endoscopic ultrasound examination, including the esophagus, stomach, and either the duodenum and/or jejunum as appropriate

(Do not report 43259 in conjunction with 76975)

⊙ **43260**   Endoscopic retrograde cholangiopancreatography (ERCP); diagnostic, with or without collection of specimen(s) by brushing or washing (separate procedure)

(For radiological supervision and interpretation, see 74328, 74329, 74330)

⊙ **43261**   with biopsy, single or multiple

(For radiological supervision and interpretation, see 74328, 74329, 74330)

⊙ **43262**   with sphincterotomy/papillotomy

(For radiological supervision and interpretation, see 74328, 74329, 74330)

⊙ **43263**   with pressure measurement of sphincter of Oddi (pancreatic duct or common bile duct)

(For radiological supervision and interpretation, see 74328, 74329, 74330)

⊙ **43264**   with endoscopic retrograde removal of calculus/calculi from biliary and/or pancreatic ducts

(When done with sphincterotomy, also use 43262)

(For radiological supervision and interpretation, see 74328, 74329, 74330)

⊙ **43265**   with endoscopic retrograde destruction, lithotripsy of calculus/calculi, any method

(When done with sphincterotomy, also use 43262)

(For radiological supervision and interpretation, see 74328, 74329, 74330)

⊙ **43267**   with endoscopic retrograde insertion of nasobiliary or nasopancreatic drainage tube

(When done with sphincterotomy, also use 43262)

(For radiological supervision and interpretation, see 74328, 74329, 74330)

⊙ **43268**   with endoscopic retrograde insertion of tube or stent into bile or pancreatic duct

(When done with sphincterotomy, also use 43262)

(For radiological supervision and interpretation, see 74328, 74329, 74330)

⊙ **43269**   with endoscopic retrograde removal of foreign body and/or change of tube or stent

(When done with sphincterotomy, also use 43262)

(For radiological supervision and interpretation, see 74328, 74329, 74330)

⊙ **43271**   with endoscopic retrograde balloon dilation of ampulla, biliary and/or pancreatic duct(s)

(When done with sphincterotomy, also use 43262)

(For radiological supervision and interpretation, see 74328, 74329, 74330)

⊙ **43272**   with ablation of tumor(s), polyp(s), or other lesion(s) not amenable to removal by hot biopsy forceps, bipolar cautery or snare technique

(For radiological supervision and interpretation, see 74328, 74329, 74330)

⊙+ **43273**   Endoscopic cannulation of papilla with direct visualization of common bile duct(s) and/or pancreatic duct(s) (List separately in addition to code(s) for primary procedure)

(Use 43273 in conjunction with 43260-43265, 43267-43272)

## Laparoscopy

Surgical laparoscopy always includes diagnostic laparoscopy. To report a diagnostic laparoscopy (peritoneoscopy) (separate procedure), use 49320.

**43279**   Laparoscopy, surgical, esophagomyotomy (Heller type), with fundoplasty, when performed

(For open approach, see 43330, 43331)

(Do not report 43279 in conjunction with 43280)

**43280**   Laparoscopy, surgical, esophagogastric fundoplasty (eg, Nissen, Toupet procedures)

(Do not report 43280 in conjunction with 43279)

(For open approach, see 43327, 43328)

**43281**   Laparoscopy, surgical, repair of paraesophageal hernia, includes fundoplasty, when performed; without implantation of mesh

**Surgery: Digestive System**

---

**43282**      with implantation of mesh

(To report transabdominal paraesophageal hiatal hernia repair, see 43332, 43333. To report transthoracic diaphragmatic hernia repair, see 43334, 43335)

(Do not report 43281, 43282 in conjunction with 43280, 43450, 43453, 43456, 43458, 49568)

**+ 43283**  Laparoscopy, surgical, esophageal lengthening procedure (eg, Collis gastroplasty or wedge gastroplasty) (List separately in addition to code for primary procedure)

(Use 43283 in conjunction with 43280, 43281, 43282)

**43289**  Unlisted laparoscopy procedure, esophagus

## Repair

**43300**  Esophagoplasty (plastic repair or reconstruction), cervical approach; without repair of tracheoesophageal fistula

**43305**      with repair of tracheoesophageal fistula

**43310**  Esophagoplasty (plastic repair or reconstruction), thoracic approach; without repair of tracheoesophageal fistula

**43312**      with repair of tracheoesophageal fistula

**43313**  Esophagoplasty for congenital defect (plastic repair or reconstruction), thoracic approach; without repair of congenital tracheoesophageal fistula

**43314**      with repair of congenital tracheoesophageal fistula

(Do not report modifier 63 in conjunction with 43313, 43314)

**43320**  Esophagogastrostomy (cardioplasty), with or without vagotomy and pyloroplasty, transabdominal or transthoracic approach

(43324 has been deleted. To report esophagogastric fundoplasty, see 43327, 43328)

(For laparoscopic procedure, use 43280)

**43325**  Esophagogastric fundoplasty; with fundic patch (Thal-Nissen procedure)

(For cricopharyngeal myotomy, use 43030)

(43326 has been deleted. To report esophagogastric fundoplasty with gastroplasty, see 43327, 43328, 43332-43338)

**43327**  Esophagogastric fundoplasty partial or complete; laparotomy

**43328**      thoracotomy

**43330**  Esophagomyotomy (Heller type); abdominal approach

(For laparoscopic esophagomyotomy procedure, use 43279)

**43331**      thoracic approach

(For thoracoscopic esophagomyotomy, use 32665)

**43332**  Repair, paraesophageal hiatal hernia (including fundoplication), via laparotomy, except neonatal; without implantation of mesh or other prosthesis

**43333**      with implantation of mesh or other prosthesis

(For neonatal diaphragmatic hernia repair, use 39503)

**43334**  Repair, paraesophageal hiatal hernia (including fundoplication), via thoracotomy, except neonatal; without implantation of mesh or other prosthesis

**43335**      with implantation of mesh or other prosthesis

(For neonatal diaphragmatic hernia repair, use 39503)

**43336**  Repair, paraesophageal hiatal hernia, (including fundoplication), via thoracoabdominal incision, except neonatal; without implantation of mesh or other prosthesis

**43337**      with implantation of mesh or other prosthesis

(For neonatal diaphragmatic hernia repair, use 39503)

**+ 43338**  Esophageal lengthening procedure (eg, Collis gastroplasty or wedge gastroplasty) (List separately in addition to code for primary procedure)

(Use 43338 in conjunction with 43280, 43327-43337)

**43340**  Esophagojejunostomy (without total gastrectomy); abdominal approach

**43341**      thoracic approach

**43350**  Esophagostomy, fistulization of esophagus, external; abdominal approach

**43351**      thoracic approach

**43352**      cervical approach

**43360**  Gastrointestinal reconstruction for previous esophagectomy, for obstructing esophageal lesion or fistula, or for previous esophageal exclusion; with stomach, with or without pyloroplasty

**43361**      with colon interposition or small intestine reconstruction, including intestine mobilization, preparation, and anastomosis(es)

**43400**  Ligation, direct, esophageal varices

**43401**  Transection of esophagus with repair, for esophageal varices

**43405**  Ligation or stapling at gastroesophageal junction for pre-existing esophageal perforation

**43410**  Suture of esophageal wound or injury; cervical approach

**43415**      transthoracic or transabdominal approach

**43420**  Closure of esophagostomy or fistula; cervical approach

**43425**      transthoracic or transabdominal approach

(To report transabdominal paraesophageal hiatal hernia repair, see 43332, 43333. To report transthoracic diaphragmatic hernia repair, see 43334, 43335)

## Manipulation

(For associated esophagogram, use 74220)

**43450**   Dilation of esophagus, by unguided sound or bougie, single or multiple passes

(For radiological supervision and interpretation, use 74360)

⊙ **43453**   Dilation of esophagus, over guide wire

(For dilation with direct visualization, use 43220)

(For dilation of esophagus, by balloon or dilator, see 43220, 43458, and 74360)

(For radiological supervision and interpretation, use 74360)

⊙ **43456**   Dilation of esophagus, by balloon or dilator, retrograde

(For radiological supervision and interpretation, use 74360)

⊙ **43458**   Dilation of esophagus with balloon (30 mm diameter or larger) for achalasia

(For dilation with balloon less than 30 mm diameter, use 43220)

(For radiological supervision and interpretation, use 74360)

**43460**   Esophagogastric tamponade, with balloon (Sengstaken type)

(For removal of esophageal foreign body by balloon catheter, see 43215, 43247, 74235)

## Other Procedures

**43496**   Free jejunum transfer with microvascular anastomosis

(Do not report code 69990 in addition to code 43496)

**43499**   Unlisted procedure, esophagus

## Stomach

### Incision

**43500**   Gastrotomy; with exploration or foreign body removal

**43501**        with suture repair of bleeding ulcer

**43502**        with suture repair of pre-existing esophagogastric laceration (eg, Mallory-Weiss)

**43510**        with esophageal dilation and insertion of permanent intraluminal tube (eg, Celestin or Mousseaux-Barbin)

**43520**   Pyloromyotomy, cutting of pyloric muscle (Fredet-Ramstedt type operation)

(Do not report modifier 63 in conjunction with 43520)

## Excision

(43600 has been deleted)

**43605**   Biopsy of stomach, by laparotomy

**43610**   Excision, local; ulcer or benign tumor of stomach

**43611**        malignant tumor of stomach

**43620**   Gastrectomy, total; with esophagoenterostomy

**43621**        with Roux-en-Y reconstruction

**43622**        with formation of intestinal pouch, any type

**43631**   Gastrectomy, partial, distal; with gastroduodenostomy

**43632**        with gastrojejunostomy

**43633**        with Roux-en-Y reconstruction

**43634**        with formation of intestinal pouch

✛ **43635**   Vagotomy when performed with partial distal gastrectomy (List separately in addition to code[s] for primary procedure)

(Use 43635 in conjunction with 43631, 43632, 43633, 43634)

**43640**   Vagotomy including pyloroplasty, with or without gastrostomy; truncal or selective

(For pyloroplasty, use 43800)

(For vagotomy, see 64752-64760)

**43641**        parietal cell (highly selective)

(For upper gastrointestinal endoscopy, see 43234-43259)

## Laparoscopy

Surgical laparoscopy always includes diagnostic laparoscopy. To report a diagnostic laparoscopy (peritoneoscopy) (separate procedure), use 49320.

(For upper gastrointestinal endoscopy including esophagus, stomach, and either the duodenum and/or jejunum, see 43235-43259)

**43644**   Laparoscopy, surgical, gastric restrictive procedure; with gastric bypass and Roux-en-Y gastroenterostomy (roux limb 150 cm or less)

(Do not report 43644 in conjunction with 43846, 49320)

(Esophagogastroduodenoscopy [EGD] performed for a separate condition should be reported with modifier 59)

(For greater than 150 cm, use 43645)

(For open procedure, use 43846)

**43645**        with gastric bypass and small intestine reconstruction to limit absorption

(Do not report 43645 in conjunction with 49320, 43847)

**43647**   Laparoscopy, surgical; implantation or replacement of gastric neurostimulator electrodes, antrum

**Surgery: Digestive System**

---

**43648**   revision or removal of gastric neurostimulator electrodes, antrum

(For open approach, see 43881, 43882)

(For insertion of gastric neurostimulator pulse generator, use 64590)

(For revision or removal of gastric neurostimulator pulse generator, use 64595)

(For electronic analysis and programming of gastric neurostimulator pulse generator, see 95980-95982)

►(For laparoscopic implantation, revision, or removal of gastric neurostimulator electrodes, lesser curvature [morbid obesity], use 43659)◄

**43651**   Laparoscopy, surgical; transection of vagus nerves, truncal

**43652**   transection of vagus nerves, selective or highly selective

**43653**   gastrostomy, without construction of gastric tube (eg, Stamm procedure) (separate procedure)

**43659**   Unlisted laparoscopy procedure, stomach

## Introduction

**43752**   Naso- or oro-gastric tube placement, requiring physician's skill and fluoroscopic guidance (includes fluoroscopy, image documentation and report)

(Do not report 43752 in conjunction with critical care codes 99291-99292, neonatal critical care codes 99468, 99469, pediatric critical care codes 99471, 99472 or low birth weight intensive care service codes 99478, 99479)

(For percutaneous placement of gastrostomy tube, use 49440)

(For enteric tube placement, see 44500, 74340)

**43753**   Gastric intubation and aspiration(s) therapeutic, necessitating physician's skill (eg, for gastrointestinal hemorrhage), including lavage if performed

**43754**   Gastric intubation and aspiration, diagnostic; single specimen (eg, acid analysis)

**43755**   collection of multiple fractional specimens with gastric stimulation, single or double lumen tube (gastric secretory study) (eg, histamine, insulin, pentagastrin, calcium, secretin), includes drug administration

(For gastric acid analysis, use 82930)

(For naso- or oro-gastric tube placement by physician with fluoroscopic guidance, use 43752)

(Report the drug[s] or substance[s] administered. The fluid used to administer the drug[s] is not separately reported)

**43756**   Duodenal intubation and aspiration, diagnostic, includes image guidance; single specimen (eg, bile study for crystals or afferent loop culture)

**43757**   collection of multiple fractional specimens with pancreatic or gallbladder stimulation, single or double lumen tube, includes drug administration

(For appropriate chemical analysis procedures, see 89049-89240)

(Report the substances[s] or drug[s] administered. The fluid used to administer the drug[s] is not separately reported)

**43760**   Change of gastrostomy tube, percutaneous, without imaging or endoscopic guidance

(To report fluoroscopically guided replacement of gastrostomy tube, use 49450)

(For endoscopic placement of gastrostomy tube, use 43246)

**43761**   Repositioning of a naso- or oro-gastric feeding tube, through the duodenum for enteric nutrition

(Do not report 43761 in conjunction with 44500, 49446)

(If imaging guidance is performed, use 76000)

(For endoscopic conversion of a gastrostomy tube to jejunostomy tube, use 44373)

(For placement of a long gastrointestinal tube into the duodenum, use 44500)

## Bariatric Surgery

Bariatric surgical procedures may involve the stomach, duodenum, jejunum, and/or the ileum.

### Laparoscopy

Surgical laparoscopy always includes diagnostic laparoscopy. To report a diagnostic laparoscopy (separate procedure), use 49320.

Typical postoperative follow-up care (see Surgery Guidelines, CPT Surgical Package Definition) after gastric restriction using the adjustable gastric restrictive device includes subsequent restrictive device adjustment(s) through the postoperative period for the typical patient. Adjustment consists of changing the gastric restrictive device component diameter by injection or aspiration of fluid through the subcutaneous port component.

**43770**   Laparoscopy, surgical, gastric restrictive procedure; placement of adjustable gastric restrictive device (eg, gastric band and subcutaneous port components)

(For individual component placement, report 43770 with modifier 52)

**43771**   revision of adjustable gastric restrictive device component only

**43772**   removal of adjustable gastric restrictive device component only

Surgery: Digestive System

**43773**    removal and replacement of adjustable gastric restrictive device component only

(Do not report 43773 in conjunction with 43772)

**43774**    removal of adjustable gastric restrictive device and subcutaneous port components

(For removal and replacement of both gastric band and subcutaneous port components, use 43659)

**43775**    longitudinal gastrectomy (ie, sleeve gastrectomy)

(For open gastric restrictive procedure, without gastric bypass, for morbid obesity, other than vertical-banded gastroplasty, use 43843)

## Other Procedures

**43800**    Pyloroplasty

(For pyloroplasty and vagotomy, use 43640)

**43810**    Gastroduodenostomy

**43820**    Gastrojejunostomy; without vagotomy

**43825**        with vagotomy, any type

**43830**    Gastrostomy, open; without construction of gastric tube (eg, Stamm procedure) (separate procedure)

**43831**        neonatal, for feeding

(For change of gastrostomy tube, use 43760)

(Do not report modifier 63 in conjunction with 43831)

**43832**        with construction of gastric tube (eg, Janeway procedure)

(For percutaneous endoscopic gastrostomy, use 43246)

**43840**    Gastrorrhaphy, suture of perforated duodenal or gastric ulcer, wound, or injury

**43842**    Gastric restrictive procedure, without gastric bypass, for morbid obesity; vertical-banded gastroplasty

**43843**        other than vertical-banded gastroplasty

(For laparoscopic longitudinal gastrectomy [ie, sleeve gastrectomy], use 43775)

**43845**    Gastric restrictive procedure with partial gastrectomy, pylorus-preserving duodenoileostomy and ileoileostomy (50 to 100 cm common channel) to limit absorption (biliopancreatic diversion with duodenal switch)

(Do not report 43845 in conjunction with 43633, 43847, 44130, 49000)

**43846**    Gastric restrictive procedure, with gastric bypass for morbid obesity; with short limb (150 cm or less) Roux-en-Y gastroenterostomy

(For greater than 150 cm, use 43847)

(For laparoscopic procedure, use 43644)

**43847**        with small intestine reconstruction to limit absorption

**43848**    Revision, open, of gastric restrictive procedure for morbid obesity, other than adjustable gastric restrictive device (separate procedure)

(For laparoscopic adjustable gastric restrictive procedures, see 43770-43774)

(For gastric restrictive port procedures, see 43886-43888)

**43850**    Revision of gastroduodenal anastomosis (gastroduodenostomy) with reconstruction; without vagotomy

**43855**        with vagotomy

**43860**    Revision of gastrojejunal anastomosis (gastrojejunostomy) with reconstruction, with or without partial gastrectomy or intestine resection; without vagotomy

**43865**        with vagotomy

**43870**    Closure of gastrostomy, surgical

**43880**    Closure of gastrocolic fistula

**43881**    Implantation or replacement of gastric neurostimulator electrodes, antrum, open

**43882**    Revision or removal of gastric neurostimulator electrodes, antrum, open

(For laparoscopic approach, see 43647, 43648)

(For insertion of gastric neurostimulator pulse generator, use 64590)

(For revision or removal of gastric neurostimulator pulse generator, use 64595)

(For electronic analysis and programming of gastric neurostimulator pulse generator, see 95980-95982)

►(For open implantation, revision, or removal of gastric neurostimulator electrodes, lesser curvature [morbid obesity], use 43999)◄

(For electronic analysis and programming of gastric neurostimulator, lesser curvature, use Category III code 0162T)

**43886**    Gastric restrictive procedure, open; revision of subcutaneous port component only

**43887**        removal of subcutaneous port component only

**43888**        removal and replacement of subcutaneous port component only

(Do not report 43888 in conjunction with 43774, 43887)

(For laparoscopic removal of both gastric restrictive device and subcutaneous port components, use 43774)

(For removal and replacement of both gastric restrictive device and subcutaneous port components, use 43659)

**43999**    Unlisted procedure, stomach

# Intestines (Except Rectum)

## Incision

**44005** Enterolysis (freeing of intestinal adhesion) (separate procedure)

(Do not report 44005 in addition to 45136)

(For laparoscopic approach, use 44180)

**44010** Duodenotomy, for exploration, biopsy(s), or foreign body removal

**+ 44015** Tube or needle catheter jejunostomy for enteral alimentation, intraoperative, any method (List separately in addition to primary procedure)

**44020** Enterotomy, small intestine, other than duodenum; for exploration, biopsy(s), or foreign body removal

**44021** for decompression (eg, Baker tube)

**44025** Colotomy, for exploration, biopsy(s), or foreign body removal

(For exteriorization of intestine (Mikulicz resection with crushing of spur), see 44602-44605)

**44050** Reduction of volvulus, intussusception, internal hernia, by laparotomy

**44055** Correction of malrotation by lysis of duodenal bands and/or reduction of midgut volvulus (eg, Ladd procedure)

(Do not report modifier 63 in conjunction with 44055)

## Excision

Intestinal allotransplantation involves three distinct components of physician work:

1. *Cadaver donor enterectomy,* which includes harvesting the intestine graft and cold preservation of the graft (perfusing with cold preservation solution and cold maintenance) (use 44132). *Living donor enterectomy,* which includes harvesting the intestine graft, cold preservation of the graft (perfusing with cold preservation solution and cold maintenance), and care of the donor (use 44133).

2. *Backbench work:*

   Standard preparation of an intestine allograft prior to transplantation includes mobilization and fashioning of the superior mesenteric artery and vein (see 44715).

   Additional reconstruction of an intestine allograft prior to transplantation may include venous and/or arterial anastomosis(es) (see 44720-44721).

3. *Recipient intestinal allotransplantation with or without recipient enterectomy,* which includes transplantation of allograft and care of the recipient (see 44135, 44136).

**44100** Biopsy of intestine by capsule, tube, peroral (1 or more specimens)

**44110** Excision of 1 or more lesions of small or large intestine not requiring anastomosis, exteriorization, or fistulization; single enterotomy

**44111** multiple enterotomies

**44120** Enterectomy, resection of small intestine; single resection and anastomosis

(Do not report 44120 in addition to 45136)

**+ 44121** each additional resection and anastomosis (List separately in addition to code for primary procedure)

(Use 44121 in conjunction with 44120)

**44125** with enterostomy

**44126** Enterectomy, resection of small intestine for congenital atresia, single resection and anastomosis of proximal segment of intestine; without tapering

**44127** with tapering

**+ 44128** each additional resection and anastomosis (List separately in addition to code for primary procedure)

(Use 44128 in conjunction with 44126, 44127)

(Do not report modifier 63 in conjunction with 44126, 44127, 44128)

**44130** Enteroenterostomy, anastomosis of intestine, with or without cutaneous enterostomy (separate procedure)

**44132** Donor enterectomy (including cold preservation), open; from cadaver donor

**44133** partial, from living donor

(For backbench intestinal graft preparation or reconstruction, see 44715, 44720, 44721)

**44135** Intestinal allotransplantation; from cadaver donor

**44136** from living donor

**44137** Removal of transplanted intestinal allograft, complete

(For partial removal of transplant allograft, see 44120, 44121, 44140)

**+ 44139** Mobilization (take-down) of splenic flexure performed in conjunction with partial colectomy (List separately in addition to primary procedure)

(Use 44139 in conjunction with 44140-44147)

**44140** Colectomy, partial; with anastomosis

(For laparoscopic procedure, use 44204)

**44141** with skin level cecostomy or colostomy

**44143** with end colostomy and closure of distal segment (Hartmann type procedure)

(For laparoscopic procedure, use 44206)

**44144** with resection, with colostomy or ileostomy and creation of mucofistula

**44145** with coloproctostomy (low pelvic anastomosis)

(For laparoscopic procedure, use 44207)

Surgery: Digestive System

**44146**     with coloproctostomy (low pelvic anastomosis), with colostomy

(For laparoscopic procedure, use 44208)

**44147**     abdominal and transanal approach

**44150**   Colectomy, total, abdominal, without proctectomy; with ileostomy or ileoproctostomy

(For laparoscopic procedure, use 44210)

**44151**     with continent ileostomy

**44155**   Colectomy, total, abdominal, with proctectomy; with ileostomy

(For laparoscopic procedure, use 44212)

**44156**     with continent ileostomy

**44157**     with ileoanal anastomosis, includes loop ileostomy, and rectal mucosectomy, when performed

**44158**     with ileoanal anastomosis, creation of ileal reservoir (S or J), includes loop ileostomy, and rectal mucosectomy, when performed

(For laparoscopic procedure, use 44211)

**44160**   Colectomy, partial, with removal of terminal ileum with ileocolostomy

(For laparoscopic procedure, use 44205)

## Laparoscopy

Surgical laparoscopy always includes diagnostic laparoscopy. To report a diagnostic laparoscopy (peritoneoscopy) (separate procedure), use 49320.

### Incision

**44180**   Laparoscopy, surgical, enterolysis (freeing of intestinal adhesion) (separate procedure)

(For laparoscopy with salpingolysis, ovariolysis, use 58660)

### Enterostomy—External Fistulization of Intestines

**44186**   Laparoscopy, surgical; jejunostomy (eg, for decompression or feeding)

**44187**     ileostomy or jejunostomy, non-tube

(For open procedure, use 44310)

**44188**   Laparoscopy, surgical, colostomy or skin level cecostomy

(For open procedure, use 44320)

(Do not report 44188 in conjunction with 44970)

### Excision

**44202**   Laparoscopy, surgical; enterectomy, resection of small intestine, single resection and anastomosis

**+ 44203**     each additional small intestine resection and anastomosis (List separately in addition to code for primary procedure)

(Use 44203 in conjunction with 44202)

(For open procedure, see 44120, 44121)

**44204**     colectomy, partial, with anastomosis

(For open procedure, use 44140)

**44205**     colectomy, partial, with removal of terminal ileum with ileocolostomy

(For open procedure, use 44160)

**44206**     colectomy, partial, with end colostomy and closure of distal segment (Hartmann type procedure)

(For open procedure, use 44143)

**44207**     colectomy, partial, with anastomosis, with coloproctostomy (low pelvic anastomosis)

(For open procedure, use 44145)

**44208**     colectomy, partial, with anastomosis, with coloproctostomy (low pelvic anastomosis) with colostomy

(For open procedure, use 44146)

**44210**     colectomy, total, abdominal, without proctectomy, with ileostomy or ileoproctostomy

(For open procedure, use 44150)

**44211**     colectomy, total, abdominal, with proctectomy, with ileoanal anastomosis, creation of ileal reservoir (S or J), with loop ileostomy, includes rectal mucosectomy, when performed

(For open procedure, see 44157, 44158)

**44212**     colectomy, total, abdominal, with proctectomy, with ileostomy

(For open procedure, use 44155)

**+ 44213**   Laparoscopy, surgical, mobilization (take-down) of splenic flexure performed in conjunction with partial colectomy (List separately in addition to primary procedure)

(Use 44213 in conjunction with 44204-44208)

(For open procedure, use 44139)

### Repair

**44227**   Laparoscopy, surgical, closure of enterostomy, large or small intestine, with resection and anastomosis

(For open procedure, see 44625, 44626)

### Other Procedures

**44238**   Unlisted laparoscopy procedure, intestine (except rectum)

## Enterostomy—External Fistulization of Intestines

**44300**    Placement, enterostomy or cecostomy, tube open (eg, for feeding or decompression) (separate procedure)

(For percutaneous placement of duodenostomy, jejunostomy, gastro-jejunostomy or cecostomy [or other colonic] tube including fluoroscopic imaging guidance, see 49441-49442)

**44310**    Ileostomy or jejunostomy, non-tube

(For laparoscopic procedure, use 44187)

(Do not report 44310 in conjunction with 44144, 44150-44151, 44155, 44156, 45113, 45119, 45136)

**44312**    Revision of ileostomy; simple (release of superficial scar) (separate procedure)

**44314**        complicated (reconstruction in-depth) (separate procedure)

**44316**    Continent ileostomy (Kock procedure) (separate procedure)

(For fiberoptic evaluation, use 44385)

**44320**    Colostomy or skin level cecostomy;

(For laparoscopic procedure, use 44188)

(Do not report 44320 in conjunction with 44141, 44144, 44146, 44605, 45110, 45119, 45126, 45563, 45805, 45825, 50810, 51597, 57307, or 58240)

**44322**        with multiple biopsies (eg, for congenital megacolon) (separate procedure)

**44340**    Revision of colostomy; simple (release of superficial scar) (separate procedure)

**44345**        complicated (reconstruction in-depth) (separate procedure)

**44346**        with repair of paracolostomy hernia (separate procedure)

## Endoscopy, Small Intestine and Stomal

Surgical endoscopy always includes diagnostic endoscopy.

(For upper gastrointestinal endoscopy, see 43234-43258)

⊙ **44360**    Small intestinal endoscopy, enteroscopy beyond second portion of duodenum, not including ileum; diagnostic, with or without collection of specimen(s) by brushing or washing (separate procedure)

⊙ **44361**        with biopsy, single or multiple

⊙ **44363**        with removal of foreign body

⊙ **44364**        with removal of tumor(s), polyp(s), or other lesion(s) by snare technique

⊙ **44365**        with removal of tumor(s), polyp(s), or other lesion(s) by hot biopsy forceps or bipolar cautery

⊙ **44366**        with control of bleeding (eg, injection, bipolar cautery, unipolar cautery, laser, heater probe, stapler, plasma coagulator)

⊙ **44369**        with ablation of tumor(s), polyp(s), or other lesion(s) not amenable to removal by hot biopsy forceps, bipolar cautery or snare technique

⊙ **44370**        with transendoscopic stent placement (includes predilation)

⊙ **44372**        with placement of percutaneous jejunostomy tube

⊙ **44373**        with conversion of percutaneous gastrostomy tube to percutaneous jejunostomy tube

(For fiberoptic jejunostomy through stoma, use 43235)

⊙ **44376**    Small intestinal endoscopy, enteroscopy beyond second portion of duodenum, including ileum; diagnostic, with or without collection of specimen(s) by brushing or washing (separate procedure)

⊙ **44377**        with biopsy, single or multiple

⊙ **44378**        with control of bleeding (eg, injection, bipolar cautery, unipolar cautery, laser, heater probe, stapler, plasma coagulator)

⊙ **44379**        with transendoscopic stent placement (includes predilation)

⊙ **44380**    Ileoscopy, through stoma; diagnostic, with or without collection of specimen(s) by brushing or washing (separate procedure)

⊙ **44382**        with biopsy, single or multiple

⊙ **44383**        with transendoscopic stent placement (includes predilation)

⊙ **44385**    Endoscopic evaluation of small intestinal (abdominal or pelvic) pouch; diagnostic, with or without collection of specimen(s) by brushing or washing (separate procedure)

⊙ **44386**        with biopsy, single or multiple

⊙ **44388**    Colonoscopy through stoma; diagnostic, with or without collection of specimen(s) by brushing or washing (separate procedure)

⊙ **44389**        with biopsy, single or multiple

⊙ **44390**        with removal of foreign body

⊙ **44391**        with control of bleeding (eg, injection, bipolar cautery, unipolar cautery, laser, heater probe, stapler, plasma coagulator)

⊙ **44392**        with removal of tumor(s), polyp(s), or other lesion(s) by hot biopsy forceps or bipolar cautery

⊙ **44393**        with ablation of tumor(s), polyp(s), or other lesion(s) not amenable to removal by hot biopsy forceps, bipolar cautery or snare technique

⊙ **44394**        with removal of tumor(s), polyp(s), or other lesion(s) by snare technique

(For colonoscopy per rectum, see 45330-45385)

⊙ **44397**        with transendoscopic stent placement (includes predilation)

# Introduction

⊙⊘ **44500**   Introduction of long gastrointestinal tube (eg, Miller-Abbott) (separate procedure)

(For radiological supervision and interpretation, use 74340)

(For naso- or oro-gastric tube placement, use 43752)

# Repair

**44602**   Suture of small intestine (enterorrhaphy) for perforated ulcer, diverticulum, wound, injury or rupture; single perforation

**44603**        multiple perforations

**44604**   Suture of large intestine (colorrhaphy) for perforated ulcer, diverticulum, wound, injury or rupture (single or multiple perforations); without colostomy

**44605**        with colostomy

**44615**   Intestinal stricturoplasty (enterotomy and enterorrhaphy) with or without dilation, for intestinal obstruction

**44620**   Closure of enterostomy, large or small intestine;

**44625**        with resection and anastomosis other than colorectal

**44626**        with resection and colorectal anastomosis (eg, closure of Hartmann type procedure)

(For laparoscopic procedure, use 44227)

**44640**   Closure of intestinal cutaneous fistula

**44650**   Closure of enteroenteric or enterocolic fistula

**44660**   Closure of enterovesical fistula; without intestinal or bladder resection

**44661**        with intestine and/or bladder resection

(For closure of renocolic fistula, see 50525, 50526)

(For closure of gastrocolic fistula, use 43880)

(For closure of rectovesical fistula, see 45800, 45805)

**44680**   Intestinal plication (separate procedure)

# Other Procedures

**44700**   Exclusion of small intestine from pelvis by mesh or other prosthesis, or native tissue (eg, bladder or omentum)

(For therapeutic radiation clinical treatment, see **Radiation Oncology** section)

+ **44701**   Intraoperative colonic lavage (List separately in addition to code for primary procedure)

(Use 44701 in conjunction with 44140, 44145, 44150, or 44604 as appropriate)

(Do not report 44701 in conjunction with 44300, 44950-44960)

**44715**   Backbench standard preparation of cadaver or living donor intestine allograft prior to transplantation, including mobilization and fashioning of the superior mesenteric artery and vein

**44720**   Backbench reconstruction of cadaver or living donor intestine allograft prior to transplantation; venous anastomosis, each

**44721**        arterial anastomosis, each

**44799**   Unlisted procedure, intestine

(For unlisted laparoscopic procedure, intestine except rectum, use 44238)

# Meckel's Diverticulum and the Mesentery

## Excision

**44800**   Excision of Meckel's diverticulum (diverticulectomy) or omphalomesenteric duct

**44820**   Excision of lesion of mesentery (separate procedure)

(With intestine resection, see 44120 or 44140 et seq)

## Suture

**44850**   Suture of mesentery (separate procedure)

(For reduction and repair of internal hernia, use 44050)

## Other Procedures

**44899**   Unlisted procedure, Meckel's diverticulum and the mesentery

# Appendix

## Incision

**44900**   Incision and drainage of appendiceal abscess; open

⊙ **44901**        percutaneous

(For radiological supervision and interpretation, use 75989)

## Excision

**44950**   Appendectomy;

(Incidental appendectomy during intra-abdominal surgery does not usually warrant a separate identification. If necessary to report, add modifier 52)

+ **44955**        when done for indicated purpose at time of other major procedure (not as separate procedure) (List separately in addition to code for primary procedure)

**44960**        for ruptured appendix with abscess or generalized peritonitis

---

## Laparoscopy

Surgical laparoscopy always includes diagnostic laparoscopy. To report a diagnostic laparoscopy (peritoneoscopy) (separate procedure), use 49320.

**44970**   Laparoscopy, surgical, appendectomy

**44979**   Unlisted laparoscopy procedure, appendix

# Rectum

## Incision

**45000**   Transrectal drainage of pelvic abscess

**45005**   Incision and drainage of submucosal abscess, rectum

**45020**   Incision and drainage of deep supralevator, pelvirectal, or retrorectal abscess

(See also 46050, 46060)

## Excision

**45100**   Biopsy of anorectal wall, anal approach (eg, congenital megacolon)

(For endoscopic biopsy, use 45305)

**45108**   Anorectal myomectomy

**45110**   Proctectomy; complete, combined abdominoperineal, with colostomy

(For laparoscopic procedure, use 45395)

**45111**       partial resection of rectum, transabdominal approach

**45112**   Proctectomy, combined abdominoperineal, pull-through procedure (eg, colo-anal anastomosis)

(For colo-anal anastomosis with colonic reservoir or pouch, use 45119)

**45113**   Proctectomy, partial, with rectal mucosectomy, ileoanal anastomosis, creation of ileal reservoir (S or J), with or without loop ileostomy

**45114**   Proctectomy, partial, with anastomosis; abdominal and transsacral approach

**45116**       transsacral approach only (Kraske type)

**45119**   Proctectomy, combined abdominoperineal pull-through procedure (eg, colo-anal anastomosis), with creation of colonic reservoir (eg, J-pouch), with diverting enterostomy when performed

(For laparoscopic procedure, use 45397)

**45120**   Proctectomy, complete (for congenital megacolon), abdominal and perineal approach; with pull-through procedure and anastomosis (eg, Swenson, Duhamel, or Soave type operation)

**45121**       with subtotal or total colectomy, with multiple biopsies

**45123**   Proctectomy, partial, without anastomosis, perineal approach

**45126**   Pelvic exenteration for colorectal malignancy, with proctectomy (with or without colostomy), with removal of bladder and ureteral transplantations, and/or hysterectomy, or cervicectomy, with or without removal of tube(s), with or without removal of ovary(s), or any combination thereof

**45130**   Excision of rectal procidentia, with anastomosis; perineal approach

**45135**       abdominal and perineal approach

**45136**   Excision of ileoanal reservoir with ileostomy

(Do not report 45136 in addition to 44005, 44120, 44310)

**45150**   Division of stricture of rectum

**45160**   Excision of rectal tumor by proctotomy, transsacral or transcoccygeal approach

(45170 has been deleted. To report excision of rectal tumor, transanal approach, see 45171, 45172)

**45171**   Excision of rectal tumor, transanal approach; not including muscularis propria (ie, partial thickness)

**45172**       including muscularis propria (ie, full thickness)

(For destruction of rectal tumor, transanal approach, use 45190)

(For transanal endoscopic microsurgical [ie, TEMS] excision of rectal tumor, including muscularis propria [ie, full thickness], use 0184T)

## Destruction

**45190**   Destruction of rectal tumor (eg, electrodesiccation, electrosurgery, laser ablation, laser resection, cryosurgery) transanal approach

(For excision of rectal tumor, transanal approach, see 45171, 45172)

(For transanal endoscopic microsurgical [ie, TEMS] excision of rectal tumor, including muscularis propria [ie, full thickness], use 0184T)

## Endoscopy

### Definitions

*Proctosigmoidoscopy* is the examination of the rectum and sigmoid colon.

*Sigmoidoscopy* is the examination of the entire rectum, sigmoid colon and may include examination of a portion of the descending colon.

*Colonoscopy* is the examination of the entire colon, from the rectum to the cecum, and may include the examination of the terminal ileum.

When performing an endoscopy on a patient who is scheduled and prepared for a total colonoscopy, if the physician is unable to advance the colonoscope beyond the splenic flexure, due to unforeseen circumstances, report the colonoscopy code with modifier 53 and appropriate documentation.

Surgical endoscopy always includes diagnostic endoscopy.

For computed tomographic colonography, see 74261-74263.

**45300**    Proctosigmoidoscopy, rigid; diagnostic, with or without collection of specimen(s) by brushing or washing (separate procedure)

⊙ **45303**    with dilation (eg, balloon, guide wire, bougie)

(For radiological supervision and interpretation, use 74360)

⊙ **45305**    with biopsy, single or multiple

⊙ **45307**    with removal of foreign body

⊙ **45308**    with removal of single tumor, polyp, or other lesion by hot biopsy forceps or bipolar cautery

⊙ **45309**    with removal of single tumor, polyp, or other lesion by snare technique

⊙ **45315**    with removal of multiple tumors, polyps, or other lesions by hot biopsy forceps, bipolar cautery or snare technique

⊙ **45317**    with control of bleeding (eg, injection, bipolar cautery, unipolar cautery, laser, heater probe, stapler, plasma coagulator)

⊙ **45320**    with ablation of tumor(s), polyp(s), or other lesion(s) not amenable to removal by hot biopsy forceps, bipolar cautery or snare technique (eg, laser)

⊙ **45321**    with decompression of volvulus

⊙ **45327**    with transendoscopic stent placement (includes predilation)

**45330**    Sigmoidoscopy, flexible; diagnostic, with or without collection of specimen(s) by brushing or washing (separate procedure)

**45331**    with biopsy, single or multiple

⊙ **45332**    with removal of foreign body

⊙ **45333**    with removal of tumor(s), polyp(s), or other lesion(s) by hot biopsy forceps or bipolar cautery

⊙ **45334**    with control of bleeding (eg, injection, bipolar cautery, unipolar cautery, laser, heater probe, stapler, plasma coagulator)

⊙ **45335**    with directed submucosal injection(s), any substance

⊙ **45337**    with decompression of volvulus, any method

⊙ **45338**    with removal of tumor(s), polyp(s), or other lesion(s) by snare technique

⊙ **45339**    with ablation of tumor(s), polyp(s), or other lesion(s) not amenable to removal by hot biopsy forceps, bipolar cautery or snare technique

⊙ **45340**    with dilation by balloon, 1 or more strictures

(Do not report 45340 in conjunction with 45345)

⊙ **45341**    with endoscopic ultrasound examination

⊙ **45342**    with transendoscopic ultrasound guided intramural or transmural fine needle aspiration/biopsy(s)

(Do not report 45341, 45342 in conjunction with 76942, 76975)

(For interpretation of specimen, see 88172-88173)

(For transrectal ultrasound utilizing rigid probe device, use 76872)

⊙ **45345**    with transendoscopic stent placement (includes predilation)

⊙ **45355**    Colonoscopy, rigid or flexible, transabdominal via colotomy, single or multiple

(For fiberoptic colonoscopy beyond 25cm to splenic flexure, see 45330-45345)

⊙ **45378**    Colonoscopy, flexible, proximal to splenic flexure; diagnostic, with or without collection of specimen(s) by brushing or washing, with or without colon decompression (separate procedure)

⊙ **45379**    with removal of foreign body

⊙ **45380**    with biopsy, single or multiple

⊙ **45381**    with directed submucosal injection(s), any substance

⊙ **45382**    with control of bleeding (eg, injection, bipolar cautery, unipolar cautery, laser, heater probe, stapler, plasma coagulator)

⊙ **45383**    with ablation of tumor(s), polyp(s), or other lesion(s) not amenable to removal by hot biopsy forceps, bipolar cautery or snare technique

⊙ **45384**    with removal of tumor(s), polyp(s), or other lesion(s) by hot biopsy forceps or bipolar cautery

⊙ **45385**    with removal of tumor(s), polyp(s), or other lesion(s) by snare technique

(For small intestine and stomal endoscopy, see 44360-44393)

⊙ **45386**    with dilation by balloon, 1 or more strictures

(Do not report 45386 in conjunction with 45387)

⊙ **45387**    with transendoscopic stent placement (includes predilation)

⊙ **45391**    with endoscopic ultrasound examination

(Do not report 45391 in conjunction with 45330, 45341, 45342, 45378, 76872)

⊙ **45392**    with transendoscopic ultrasound guided intramural or transmural fine needle aspiration/biopsy(s)

(Do not report 45392 in conjunction with 45330, 45341, 45342, 45378, 76872)

**Surgery: Digestive System**

# Laparoscopy

Surgical laparoscopy always includes diagnostic laparoscopy. To report a diagnostic laparoscopy (peritoneoscopy) (separate procedure), use 49320.

### Excision

**45395**  Laparoscopy, surgical; proctectomy, complete, combined abdominoperineal, with colostomy

(For open procedure, use 45110)

**45397**  proctectomy, combined abdominoperineal pull-through procedure (eg, colo-anal anastomosis), with creation of colonic reservoir (eg, J-pouch), with diverting enterostomy, when performed

(For open procedure, use 45119)

### Repair

**45400**  Laparoscopy, surgical; proctopexy (for prolapse)

(For open procedure, use 45540, 45541)

**45402**  proctopexy (for prolapse), with sigmoid resection

(For open procedure, use 45550)

**45499**  Unlisted laparoscopy procedure, rectum

# Repair

**45500**  Proctoplasty; for stenosis

**45505**  for prolapse of mucous membrane

**45520**  Perirectal injection of sclerosing solution for prolapse

**45540**  Proctopexy (eg, for prolapse); abdominal approach

(For laparoscopic procedure, use 45400)

**45541**  perineal approach

**45550**  with sigmoid resection, abdominal approach

(For laparoscopic procedure, use 45402)

**45560**  Repair of rectocele (separate procedure)

(For repair of rectocele with posterior colporrhaphy, use 57250)

**45562**  Exploration, repair, and presacral drainage for rectal injury;

**45563**  with colostomy

**45800**  Closure of rectovesical fistula;

**45805**  with colostomy

**45820**  Closure of rectourethral fistula;

**45825**  with colostomy

(For rectovaginal fistula closure, see 57300-57308)

# Manipulation

**45900**  Reduction of procidentia (separate procedure) under anesthesia

**45905**  Dilation of anal sphincter (separate procedure) under anesthesia other than local

**45910**  Dilation of rectal stricture (separate procedure) under anesthesia other than local

**45915**  Removal of fecal impaction or foreign body (separate procedure) under anesthesia

# Other Procedures

Surgical diagnostic anorectal exam (45990) includes the following elements: external perineal exam, digital rectal exam, pelvic exam (when performed), diagnostic anoscopy, and diagnostic rigid proctoscopy.

**45990**  Anorectal exam, surgical, requiring anesthesia (general, spinal, or epidural), diagnostic

(Do not report 45990 in conjunction with 45300-45327, 46600, 57410, 99170)

**45999**  Unlisted procedure, rectum

(For unlisted laparoscopic procedure, rectum, use 45499)

# Anus

For incision of thrombosed external hemorrhoid, use 46083. For ligation of internal hemorrhoid(s), see 46221, 46945, 46946. For excision of internal and/or external hemorrhoid(s), see 46250-46262, 46320. For injection of hemorrhoid(s), use 46500. For destruction of internal hemorrhoid(s) by thermal energy, use 46930. For destruction of hemorrhoid(s) by cryosurgery, use 46999. For hemorrhoidopexy, use 46947.

# Incision

(For subcutaneous fistulotomy, use 46270)

**46020**  Placement of seton

(Do not report 46020 in addition to 46060, 46280, 46600, 0249T)

**46030**  Removal of anal seton, other marker

**46040**  Incision and drainage of ischiorectal and/or perirectal abscess (separate procedure)

**46045**  Incision and drainage of intramural, intramuscular, or submucosal abscess, transanal, under anesthesia

**46050**  Incision and drainage, perianal abscess, superficial

(See also 45020, 46060)

**46060**  Incision and drainage of ischiorectal or intramural abscess, with fistulectomy or fistulotomy, submuscular, with or without placement of seton

(Do not report 46060 in addition to 46020)

(See also 45020)

**46070**   Incision, anal septum (infant)

(For anoplasty, see 46700-46705).

(Do not report modifier 63 in conjunction with 46070)

**46080**   Sphincterotomy, anal, division of sphincter (separate procedure)

**46083**   Incision of thrombosed hemorrhoid, external

## Excision

**46200**   Fissurectomy, including sphincterotomy, when performed

(46210, 46211 have been deleted. To report, use 46999)

**46220**   Code is out of numerical sequence. See 46200-46288

**46221**   Hemorrhoidectomy, internal, by rubber band ligation(s)

(For ligation, hemorrhoidal vascular bundle(s), including ultrasound guidance, use 0249T)

**# 46945**   Hemorrhoidectomy, internal, by ligation other than rubber band; single hemorrhoid column/group

**# 46946**      2 or more hemorrhoid columns/groups

(Do not report 46221, 46945, and 46946 in conjunction with 0249T)

**# 46220**   Excision of single external papilla or tag, anus

**46230**   Excision of multiple external papillae or tags, anus

**# 46320**   Excision of thrombosed hemorrhoid, external

**46250**   Hemorrhoidectomy, external, 2 or more columns/groups

(For hemorrhoidectomy, external, single column/group, use 46999)

**46255**   Hemorrhoidectomy, internal and external, single column/group;

**46257**      with fissurectomy

**46258**      with fistulectomy, including fissurectomy, when performed

**46260**   Hemorrhoidectomy, internal and external, 2 or more columns/groups;

**46261**      with fissurectomy

**46262**      with fistulectomy, including fissurectomy, when performed

(Do not report 46250-46262 in conjunction with 0249T)

**46270**   Surgical treatment of anal fistula (fistulectomy/fistulotomy); subcutaneous

**46275**      intersphincteric

**46280**      transsphincteric, suprasphincteric, extrasphincteric or multiple, including placement of seton, when performed

(Do not report 46280 in conjunction with 46020)

**46285**      second stage

**46288**   Closure of anal fistula with rectal advancement flap

**46320**   Code is out of numerical sequence. See 46200-46288

## Introduction

**46500**   Injection of sclerosing solution, hemorrhoids

**46505**   Chemodenervation of internal anal sphincter

(For chemodenervation of other muscles, see 64612-64614. For destruction of nerve by neurolytic agent, see 64630, 64640)

(Report the specific service in conjunction with the specific substance(s) or drug(s) provided)

## Endoscopy

Surgical endoscopy always includes diagnostic endoscopy.

**46600**   Anoscopy; diagnostic, with or without collection of specimen(s) by brushing or washing (separate procedure)

(Do not report 46600 in conjunction with 46020, 0249T)

(For diagnostic high resolution anoscopy [HRA], use 0226T)

**46604**      with dilation (eg, balloon, guide wire, bougie)

**46606**      with biopsy, single or multiple

(For high resolution anoscopy [HRA] with biopsy, use 0227T)

**46608**      with removal of foreign body

**46610**      with removal of single tumor, polyp, or other lesion by hot biopsy forceps or bipolar cautery

**46611**      with removal of single tumor, polyp, or other lesion by snare technique

**46612**      with removal of multiple tumors, polyps, or other lesions by hot biopsy forceps, bipolar cautery or snare technique

**46614**      with control of bleeding (eg, injection, bipolar cautery, unipolar cautery, laser, heater probe, stapler, plasma coagulator)

**46615**      with ablation of tumor(s), polyp(s), or other lesion(s) not amenable to removal by hot biopsy forceps, bipolar cautery or snare technique

▶(For delivery of thermal energy to the muscle of the anal canal, use 0288T)◀

## Repair

**46700**   Anoplasty, plastic operation for stricture; adult

**46705**      infant

(Do not report modifier 63 in conjunction with 46705)

(For simple incision of anal septum, use 46070)

**46706**   Repair of anal fistula with fibrin glue

**46707**   Repair of anorectal fistula with plug (eg, porcine small intestine submucosa [SIS])

**46710**   Repair of ileoanal pouch fistula/sinus (eg, perineal or vaginal), pouch advancement; transperineal approach

---

▲=Revised code   ●=New code   ▶ ◀=Contains new or revised text   ⦶=Modifier 51 exempt

| | |
|---|---|
| 46712 | combined transperineal and transabdominal approach |
| 46715 | Repair of low imperforate anus; with anoperineal fistula (cut-back procedure) |
| 46716 | with transposition of anoperineal or anovestibular fistula |

(Do not report modifier 63 in conjunction with 46715, 46716)

| | |
|---|---|
| 46730 | Repair of high imperforate anus without fistula; perineal or sacroperineal approach |
| 46735 | combined transabdominal and sacroperineal approaches |

(Do not report modifier 63 in conjunction with 46730, 46735)

| | |
|---|---|
| 46740 | Repair of high imperforate anus with rectourethral or rectovaginal fistula; perineal or sacroperineal approach |
| 46742 | combined transabdominal and sacroperineal approaches |

(Do not report modifier 63 in conjunction with 46740, 46742)

| | |
|---|---|
| 46744 | Repair of cloacal anomaly by anorectovaginoplasty and urethroplasty, sacroperineal approach |

(Do not report modifier 63 in conjunction with 46744)

| | |
|---|---|
| 46746 | Repair of cloacal anomaly by anorectovaginoplasty and urethroplasty, combined abdominal and sacroperineal approach; |
| 46748 | with vaginal lengthening by intestinal graft or pedicle flaps |
| 46750 | Sphincteroplasty, anal, for incontinence or prolapse; adult |
| 46751 | child |
| 46753 | Graft (Thiersch operation) for rectal incontinence and/or prolapse |
| 46754 | Removal of Thiersch wire or suture, anal canal |
| 46760 | Sphincteroplasty, anal, for incontinence, adult; muscle transplant |
| 46761 | levator muscle imbrication (Park posterior anal repair) |
| 46762 | implantation artificial sphincter |
| # 46947 | Hemorrhoidopexy (eg, for prolapsing internal hemorrhoids) by stapling |

## Destruction

| | |
|---|---|
| 46900 | Destruction of lesion(s), anus (eg, condyloma, papilloma, molluscum contagiosum, herpetic vesicle), simple; chemical |
| 46910 | electrodesiccation |
| 46916 | cryosurgery |
| 46917 | laser surgery |
| 46922 | surgical excision |

| | |
|---|---|
| 46924 | Destruction of lesion(s), anus (eg, condyloma, papilloma, molluscum contagiosum, herpetic vesicle), extensive (eg, laser surgery, electrosurgery, cryosurgery, chemosurgery) |
| 46930 | Destruction of internal hemorrhoid(s) by thermal energy (eg, infrared coagulation, cautery, radiofrequency) |

(46934-46936 have been deleted)

(46937, 46938 have been deleted. To report, use 45190)

| | |
|---|---|
| 46940 | Curettage or cautery of anal fissure, including dilation of anal sphincter (separate procedure); initial |
| 46942 | subsequent |
| 46945 | Code is out of numerical sequence. See 46200-46288 |
| 46946 | Code is out of numerical sequence. See 46200-46288 |
| 46947 | Code is out of numerical sequence. See 46700-46947 |

## Other Procedures

| | |
|---|---|
| 46999 | Unlisted procedure, anus |

# Liver

## Incision

| | |
|---|---|
| ⊙▲ 47000 | Biopsy of liver, needle; percutaneous |

(If imaging guidance is performed, see 76942, 77002, 77012, 77021)

| | |
|---|---|
| + 47001 | when done for indicated purpose at time of other major procedure (List separately in addition to code for primary procedure) |

(If imaging guidance is performed, see 76942, 77002)

(For fine needle aspiration in conjunction with 47000, 47001, see 10021, 10022)

(For evaluation of fine needle aspirate in conjunction with 47000, 47001, see 88172, 88173)

| | |
|---|---|
| 47010 | Hepatotomy; for open drainage of abscess or cyst, 1 or 2 stages |
| ⊙ 47011 | for percutaneous drainage of abscess or cyst, 1 or 2 stages |

(For radiological supervision and interpretation, use 75989)

| | |
|---|---|
| 47015 | Laparotomy, with aspiration and/or injection of hepatic parasitic (eg, amoebic or echinococcal) cyst(s) or abscess(es) |

## Excision

| | |
|---|---|
| 47100 | Biopsy of liver, wedge |
| 47120 | Hepatectomy, resection of liver; partial lobectomy |
| 47122 | trisegmentectomy |
| 47125 | total left lobectomy |
| 47130 | total right lobectomy |

Surgery: Digestive System

## Liver Transplantation

Liver allotransplantation involves three distinct components of physician work:

1. ***Cadaver donor hepatectomy,*** which includes harvesting the graft and cold preservation of the graft (perfusing with cold preservation solution and cold maintenance) (use 47133). ***Living donor hepatectomy,*** which includes harvesting the graft, cold preservation of the graft (perfusing with cold preservation solution and cold maintenance), and care of the donor (see 47140-47142).

2. ***Backbench work:***

   Standard preparation of the whole liver graft will include one of the following:

   Preparation of whole liver graft (including cholecystectomy, if necessary, and dissection and removal of surrounding soft tissues to prepare vena cava, portal vein, hepatic artery, and common bile duct for implantation) (use 47143).

   Preparation as described for whole liver graft, plus trisegment split into two partial grafts (use 47144).

   Preparation as described for whole liver graft, plus lobe split into two partial grafts (use 47145).

   Additional reconstruction of the liver graft may include venous and/or arterial anastomosis(es) (see 47146, 47147).

3. ***Recipient liver allotransplantation,*** which includes recipient hepatectomy (partial or whole), transplantation of the allograft (partial or whole), and care of the recipient (see 47135, 47136).

**47133**   Donor hepatectomy (including cold preservation), from cadaver donor

**47135**   Liver allotransplantation; orthotopic, partial or whole, from cadaver or living donor, any age

**47136**      heterotopic, partial or whole, from cadaver or living donor, any age

**47140**   Donor hepatectomy (including cold preservation), from living donor; left lateral segment only (segments II and III)

**47141**      total left lobectomy (segments II, III and IV)

**47142**      total right lobectomy (segments V, VI, VII and VIII)

**47143**   Backbench standard preparation of cadaver donor whole liver graft prior to allotransplantation, including cholecystectomy, if necessary, and dissection and removal of surrounding soft tissues to prepare the vena cava, portal vein, hepatic artery, and common bile duct for implantation; without trisegment or lobe split

**47144**      with trisegment split of whole liver graft into 2 partial liver grafts (ie, left lateral segment [segments II and III] and right trisegment [segments I and IV through VIII])

**47145**      with lobe split of whole liver graft into 2 partial liver grafts (ie, left lobe [segments II, III, and IV] and right lobe [segments I and V through VIII])

**47146**   Backbench reconstruction of cadaver or living donor liver graft prior to allotransplantation; venous anastomosis, each

**47147**      arterial anastomosis, each

(Do not report 47143-47147 in conjunction with 47120-47125, 47600, 47610)

## Repair

**47300**   Marsupialization of cyst or abscess of liver

**47350**   Management of liver hemorrhage; simple suture of liver wound or injury

**47360**      complex suture of liver wound or injury, with or without hepatic artery ligation

**47361**      exploration of hepatic wound, extensive debridement, coagulation and/or suture, with or without packing of liver

**47362**      re-exploration of hepatic wound for removal of packing

## Laparoscopy

Surgical laparoscopy always includes diagnostic laparoscopy. To report a diagnostic laparoscopy (peritoneoscopy) (separate procedure), use 49320.

**47370**   Laparoscopy, surgical, ablation of 1 or more liver tumor(s); radiofrequency

(For imaging guidance, use 76940)

**47371**      cryosurgical

(For imaging guidance, use 76940)

**47379**   Unlisted laparoscopic procedure, liver

## Other Procedures

**47380**   Ablation, open, of 1 or more liver tumor(s); radiofrequency

(For imaging guidance, use 76940)

**47381**      cryosurgical

(For imaging guidance, use 76940)

⊙ **47382**   Ablation, 1 or more liver tumor(s), percutaneous, radiofrequency

(For imaging guidance and monitoring, see 76940, 77013, 77022)

**47399**   Unlisted procedure, liver

Surgery: Digestive System

# Biliary Tract

## Incision

**47400**   Hepaticotomy or hepaticostomy with exploration, drainage, or removal of calculus

**47420**   Choledochotomy or choledochostomy with exploration, drainage, or removal of calculus, with or without cholecystotomy; without transduodenal sphincterotomy or sphincteroplasty

**47425**   with transduodenal sphincterotomy or sphincteroplasty

**47460**   Transduodenal sphincterotomy or sphincteroplasty, with or without transduodenal extraction of calculus (separate procedure)

**47480**   Cholecystotomy or cholecystostomy, open, with exploration, drainage, or removal of calculus (separate procedure)

(For percutaneous cholecystostomy, use 47490)

## Introduction

**47490**   Cholecystostomy, percutaneous, complete procedure, including imaging guidance, catheter placement, cholecystogram when performed, and radiological supervision and interpretation

(Do not report 47490 in conjunction with 47505, 74305, 75989, 76942, 77002, 77012, 77021)

**47500**   Injection procedure for percutaneous transhepatic cholangiography

(For radiological supervision and interpretation, use 74320)

**47505**   Injection procedure for cholangiography through an existing catheter (eg, percutaneous transhepatic or T-tube)

(For radiological supervision and interpretation, use 74305)

**47510**   Introduction of percutaneous transhepatic catheter for biliary drainage

(For radiological supervision and interpretation, use 75980)

**47511**   Introduction of percutaneous transhepatic stent for internal and external biliary drainage

(For radiological supervision and interpretation, use 75982)

⊙ **47525**   Change of percutaneous biliary drainage catheter

(For radiological supervision and interpretation, use 75984)

**47530**   Revision and/or reinsertion of transhepatic tube

(For radiological supervision and interpretation, use 75984)

## Endoscopy

Surgical endoscopy always includes diagnostic endoscopy.

+ **47550**   Biliary endoscopy, intraoperative (choledochoscopy) (List separately in addition to code for primary procedure)

**47552**   Biliary endoscopy, percutaneous via T-tube or other tract; diagnostic, with or without collection of specimen(s) by brushing and/or washing (separate procedure)

**47553**   with biopsy, single or multiple

**47554**   with removal of calculus/calculi

**47555**   with dilation of biliary duct stricture(s) without stent

**47556**   with dilation of biliary duct stricture(s) with stent

(For ERCP, see 43260-43272, 74363)

(If imaging guidance is performed, see 74363, 75982)

## Laparoscopy

Surgical laparoscopy always includes diagnostic laparoscopy. To report a diagnostic laparoscopy (peritoneoscopy) (separate procedure), use 49320.

**47560**   Laparoscopy, surgical; with guided transhepatic cholangiography, without biopsy

**47561**   with guided transhepatic cholangiography with biopsy

**47562**   cholecystectomy

**47563**   cholecystectomy with cholangiography

**47564**   cholecystectomy with exploration of common duct

**47570**   cholecystoenterostomy

**47579**   Unlisted laparoscopy procedure, biliary tract

## Excision

**47600**   Cholecystectomy;

**47605**   with cholangiography

(For laparoscopic approach, see 47562-47564)

**47610**   Cholecystectomy with exploration of common duct;

(For cholecystectomy with exploration of common duct with biliary endoscopy, use 47610 with 47550)

**47612**   with choledochoenterostomy

**47620**   with transduodenal sphincterotomy or sphincteroplasty, with or without cholangiography

**47630**   Biliary duct stone extraction, percutaneous via T-tube tract, basket, or snare (eg, Burhenne technique)

(For radiological supervision and interpretation, use 74327)

**47700**   Exploration for congenital atresia of bile ducts, without repair, with or without liver biopsy, with or without cholangiography

(Do not report modifier 63 in conjunction with 47700)

**47701**    Portoenterostomy (eg, Kasai procedure)

       (Do not report modifier 63 in conjunction with 47701)

**47711**    Excision of bile duct tumor, with or without primary repair of bile duct; extrahepatic

**47712**       intrahepatic

       (For anastomosis, see 47760-47800)

**47715**    Excision of choledochal cyst

## Repair

**47720**    Cholecystoenterostomy; direct

       (For laparoscopic approach, use 47570)

**47721**       with gastroenterostomy

**47740**       Roux-en-Y

**47741**       Roux-en-Y with gastroenterostomy

**47760**    Anastomosis, of extrahepatic biliary ducts and gastrointestinal tract

**47765**    Anastomosis, of intrahepatic ducts and gastrointestinal tract

**47780**    Anastomosis, Roux-en-Y, of extrahepatic biliary ducts and gastrointestinal tract

**47785**    Anastomosis, Roux-en-Y, of intrahepatic biliary ducts and gastrointestinal tract

**47800**    Reconstruction, plastic, of extrahepatic biliary ducts with end-to-end anastomosis

**47801**    Placement of choledochal stent

**47802**    U-tube hepaticoenterostomy

**47900**    Suture of extrahepatic biliary duct for pre-existing injury (separate procedure)

## Other Procedures

**47999**    Unlisted procedure, biliary tract

# Pancreas

       (For peroral pancreatic endoscopic procedures, see 43260-43272)

## Incision

**48000**    Placement of drains, peripancreatic, for acute pancreatitis;

**48001**       with cholecystostomy, gastrostomy, and jejunostomy

**48020**    Removal of pancreatic calculus

## Excision

**48100**    Biopsy of pancreas, open (eg, fine needle aspiration, needle core biopsy, wedge biopsy)

**48102**    Biopsy of pancreas, percutaneous needle

       (For radiological supervision and interpretation, see 76942, 77002, 77012, 77021)

       (For fine needle aspiration, use 10022)

       (For evaluation of fine needle aspirate, see 88172, 88173)

**48105**    Resection or debridement of pancreas and peripancreatic tissue for acute necrotizing pancreatitis

**48120**    Excision of lesion of pancreas (eg, cyst, adenoma)

**48140**    Pancreatectomy, distal subtotal, with or without splenectomy; without pancreaticojejunostomy

**48145**       with pancreaticojejunostomy

**48146**    Pancreatectomy, distal, near-total with preservation of duodenum (Child-type procedure)

**48148**    Excision of ampulla of Vater

**48150**    Pancreatectomy, proximal subtotal with total duodenectomy, partial gastrectomy, choledochoenterostomy and gastrojejunostomy (Whipple-type procedure); with pancreatojejunostomy

**48152**       without pancreatojejunostomy

**48153**    Pancreatectomy, proximal subtotal with near-total duodenectomy, choledochoenterostomy and duodenojejunostomy (pylorus-sparing, Whipple-type procedure); with pancreatojejunostomy

**48154**       without pancreatojejunostomy

**48155**    Pancreatectomy, total

**48160**    Pancreatectomy, total or subtotal, with autologous transplantation of pancreas or pancreatic islet cells

## Introduction

+ **48400**    Injection procedure for intraoperative pancreatography (List separately in addition to code for primary procedure)

       (For radiological supervision and interpretation, see 74300-74305)

## Repair

**48500**    Marsupialization of pancreatic cyst

**48510**    External drainage, pseudocyst of pancreas; open

⊙ **48511**       percutaneous

       (For radiological supervision and interpretation, use 75989)

**48520**    Internal anastomosis of pancreatic cyst to gastrointestinal tract; direct

**48540**       Roux-en-Y

**48545**    Pancreatorrhaphy for injury

**48547**    Duodenal exclusion with gastrojejunostomy for pancreatic injury

**48548**    Pancreaticojejunostomy, side-to-side anastomosis (Puestow-type operation)

**Surgery: Digestive System**

## Pancreas Transplantation

Pancreas allotransplantation involves three distinct components of physician work:

1. *Cadaver donor pancreatectomy,* which includes harvesting the pancreas graft, with or without duodenal segment, and cold preservation of the graft (perfusing with cold preservation solution and cold maintenance) (use 48550).

2. *Backbench work:*

Standard preparation of a cadaver donor pancreas allograft prior to transplantation includes dissection of the allograft from surrounding soft tissues, splenectomy, duodenotomy, ligation of bile duct, ligation of mesenteric vessels, and Y-graft arterial anastomoses from the iliac artery to the superior mesenteric artery and to the splenic artery (use 48551).

Additional reconstruction of a cadaver donor pancreas allograft prior to transplantation may include venous anastomosis(es) (use 48552).

3. *Recipient pancreas allotransplantation,* which includes transplantation of allograft, and care of the recipient (use 48554).

48550    Donor pancreatectomy (including cold preservation), with or without duodenal segment for transplantation

48551    Backbench standard preparation of cadaver donor pancreas allograft prior to transplantation, including dissection of allograft from surrounding soft tissues, splenectomy, duodenotomy, ligation of bile duct, ligation of mesenteric vessels, and Y-graft arterial anastomoses from iliac artery to superior mesenteric artery and to splenic artery

48552    Backbench reconstruction of cadaver donor pancreas allograft prior to transplantation, venous anastomosis, each

(Do not report 48551 and 48552 in conjunction with 35531, 35563, 35685, 38100-38102, 44010, 44820, 44850, 47460, 47505-47525, 47550-47556, 48100-48120, 48545)

48554    Transplantation of pancreatic allograft

48556    Removal of transplanted pancreatic allograft

## Other Procedures

48999    Unlisted procedure, pancreas

# Abdomen, Peritoneum, and Omentum

## Incision

49000    Exploratory laparotomy, exploratory celiotomy with or without biopsy(s) (separate procedure)

(To report wound exploration due to penetrating trauma without laparotomy, use 20102)

49002    Reopening of recent laparotomy

(To report re-exploration of hepatic wound for removal of packing, use 47362)

49010    Exploration, retroperitoneal area with or without biopsy(s) (separate procedure)

(To report wound exploration due to penetrating trauma without laparotomy, use 20102)

49020    Drainage of peritoneal abscess or localized peritonitis, exclusive of appendiceal abscess; open

(For appendiceal abscess, use 44900)

⊙ 49021        percutaneous

(For radiological supervision and interpretation, use 75989)

49040    Drainage of subdiaphragmatic or subphrenic abscess; open

⊙ 49041        percutaneous

(For radiological supervision and interpretation, use 75989)

49060    Drainage of retroperitoneal abscess; open

⊙ 49061        percutaneous

(For laparoscopic drainage, use 49323)

(For radiological supervision and interpretation, use 75989)

49062    Drainage of extraperitoneal lymphocele to peritoneal cavity, open

▶(49080, 49081 have been deleted. To report, see 49082-49084)◀

● 49082    Abdominal paracentesis (diagnostic or therapeutic); without imaging guidance

● 49083        with imaging guidance

▶(Do not report 49083 in conjunction with 76942, 77002, 77012, 77021)◀

● 49084    Peritoneal lavage, including imaging guidance, when performed

▶(Do not report 49084 in conjunction with 76942, 77002, 77012, 77021)◀

## Excision, Destruction

(For lysis of intestinal adhesions, use 44005)

49180    Biopsy, abdominal or retroperitoneal mass, percutaneous needle

(If imaging guidance is performed, see 76942, 77002, 77012, 77021)

(For fine needle aspiration, use 10021 or 10022)

(For evaluation of fine needle aspirate, see 88172, 88173)

**49203**   Excision or destruction, open, intra-abdominal tumors, cysts or endometriomas, 1 or more peritoneal, mesenteric, or retroperitoneal primary or secondary tumors; largest tumor 5 cm diameter or less

**49204**   largest tumor 5.1-10.0 cm diameter

**49205**   largest tumor greater than 10.0 cm diameter

(Do not report 49203-49205 in conjunction with 38770, 38780, 49000, 49010, 49215, 50010, 50205, 50225, 50236, 50250, 50290, 58900-58960)

(For partial or total nephrectomy, use 50220 or 50240 in conjunction with 49203-49205)

(For colectomy, use 44140 in conjunction with 49203-49205)

(For small bowel resection, use 44120 in conjunction with 49203-49205)

(For vena caval resection with reconstruction, use 49203-49205 in conjunction with 37799)

(For resection of recurrent ovarian, tubal, primary peritoneal, or uterine malignancy, see 58957, 58958)

(For cryoablation of renal tumors, see 50250, 50593)

**49215**   Excision of presacral or sacrococcygeal tumor

(Do not report modifier 63 in conjunction with 49215)

**49220**   Staging laparotomy for Hodgkins disease or lymphoma (includes splenectomy, needle or open biopsies of both liver lobes, possibly also removal of abdominal nodes, abdominal node and/or bone marrow biopsies, ovarian repositioning)

**49250**   Umbilectomy, omphalectomy, excision of umbilicus (separate procedure)

**49255**   Omentectomy, epiploectomy, resection of omentum (separate procedure)

## Laparoscopy

Surgical laparoscopy always includes diagnostic laparoscopy. To report a diagnostic laparoscopy (peritoneoscopy), (separate procedure), use 49320.

For laparoscopic fulguration or excision of lesions of the ovary, pelvic viscera, or peritoneal surface use 58662.

**49320**   Laparoscopy, abdomen, peritoneum, and omentum, diagnostic, with or without collection of specimen(s) by brushing or washing (separate procedure)

**49321**   Laparoscopy, surgical; with biopsy (single or multiple)

**49322**   with aspiration of cavity or cyst (eg, ovarian cyst) (single or multiple)

**49323**   with drainage of lymphocele to peritoneal cavity

(For percutaneous or open drainage, see 49060, 49061)

**49324**   with insertion of tunneled intraperitoneal catheter

(For subcutaneous extension of intraperitoneal catheter with remote chest exit site, use 49435 in conjunction with 49324)

(For open insertion of tunneled intraperitoneal catheter, use 49421)

**49325**   with revision of previously placed intraperitoneal cannula or catheter, with removal of intraluminal obstructive material if performed

**+ 49326**   with omentopexy (omental tacking procedure) (List separately in addition to code for primary procedure)

(Use 49326 in conjunction with 49324, 49325)

**+ 49327**   with placement of interstitial device(s) for radiation therapy guidance (eg, fiducial markers, dosimeter), intra-abdominal, intrapelvic, and/or retroperitoneum, including imaging guidance, if performed, single or multiple (List separately in addition to code for primary procedure)

(Use 49327 in conjunction with laparoscopic abdominal, pelvic, or retroperitoneal procedure[s] performed concurrently)

(For placement of interstitial device[s] for intra-abdominal, intrapelvic, and/or retroperitoneal radiation therapy guidance concurrent with open procedure, use 49412)

(For percutaneous placement of interstitial device[s] for intra-abdominal, intrapelvic, and/or retroperitoneal radiation therapy guidance, use 49411)

**49329**   Unlisted laparoscopy procedure, abdomen, peritoneum and omentum

## Introduction, Revision, Removal

**49400**   Injection of air or contrast into peritoneal cavity (separate procedure)

(For radiological supervision and interpretation, use 74190)

**49402**   Removal of peritoneal foreign body from peritoneal cavity

(For lysis of intestinal adhesions, use 44005)

⊙ **49411**   Placement of interstitial device(s) for radiation therapy guidance (eg, fiducial markers, dosimeter), percutaneous, intra-abdominal, intra-pelvic (except prostate), and/or retroperitoneum, single or multiple

(Report supply of device separately)

(For imaging guidance, see 76942, 77002, 77012, 77021)

(For percutaneous placement of interstitial device[s] for intra-thoracic radiation therapy guidance, use 32553)

**+ 49412**   Placement of interstitial device(s) for radiation therapy guidance (eg, fiducial markers, dosimeter), open, intra-abdominal, intrapelvic, and/or retroperitoneum, including image guidance, if performed, single or multiple (List separately in addition to code for primary procedure)

(Use 49412 in conjunction with open abdominal, pelvic, or retroperitoneal procedure[s] performed concurrently)

*Surgery: Digestive System*

(For placement of interstitial device[s] for intra-abdominal, intrapelvic, and/or retroperitoneal radiation therapy guidance concurrent with laparoscopic procedure, use 49327)

(For percutaneous placement of interstitial device[s] for intra-abdominal, intrapelvic, and/or retroperitoneal radiation therapy guidance, use 49411)

⊙ **49418** Insertion of tunneled intraperitoneal catheter (eg, dialysis, intraperitoneal chemotherapy instillation, management of ascites), complete procedure, including imaging guidance, catheter placement, contrast injection when performed, and radiological supervision and interpretation, percutaneous

**49419** Insertion of tunneled intraperitoneal catheter, with subcutaneous port (ie, totally implantable)

(For removal, use 49422)

▶(49420 has been deleted. To report open placement of a tunneled intraperitoneal catheter for dialysis, use 49421. To report open or percutaneous peritoneal drainage or lavage, see 49020, 49021, 49040, 49041, 49082-49084, as appropriate. To report percutaneous insertion of a tunneled intraperitoneal catheter without subcutaneous port, use 49418)◀

**49421** Insertion of tunneled intraperitoneal catheter for dialysis, open

(For laparoscopic insertion of tunneled intraperitoneal catheter, use 49324)

(For subcutaneous extension of intraperitoneal catheter with remote chest exit site, use 49435 in conjunction with 49421)

**49422** Removal of tunneled intraperitoneal catheter

(For removal of a non-tunneled catheter, use appropriate E/M code)

**49423** Exchange of previously placed abscess or cyst drainage catheter under radiological guidance (separate procedure)

(For radiological supervision and interpretation, use 75984)

**49424** Contrast injection for assessment of abscess or cyst via previously placed drainage catheter or tube (separate procedure)

(For radiological supervision and interpretation, use 76080)

**49425** Insertion of peritoneal-venous shunt

**49426** Revision of peritoneal-venous shunt

(For shunt patency test, use 78291)

**49427** Injection procedure (eg, contrast media) for evaluation of previously placed peritoneal-venous shunt

(For radiological supervision and interpretation, see 75809, 78291)

**49428** Ligation of peritoneal-venous shunt

**49429** Removal of peritoneal-venous shunt

+ **49435** Insertion of subcutaneous extension to intraperitoneal cannula or catheter with remote chest exit site (List separately in addition to code for primary procedure)

(Use 49435 in conjunction with 49324, 49421)

**49436** Delayed creation of exit site from embedded subcutaneous segment of intraperitoneal cannula or catheter

## Initial Placement

Do not additionally report 43752 for placement of a nasogastric (NG) or orogastric (OG) tube to insufflate the stomach prior to percutaneous gastrointestinal tube placement. NG or OG tube placement is considered part of the procedure in this family of codes.

⊙ **49440** Insertion of gastrostomy tube, percutaneous, under fluoroscopic guidance including contrast injection(s), image documentation and report

(For conversion to a gastro-jejunostomy tube at the time of initial gastrostomy tube placement, use 49440 in conjunction with 49446)

⊙ **49441** Insertion of duodenostomy or jejunostomy tube, percutaneous, under fluoroscopic guidance including contrast injection(s), image documentation and report

(For conversion of gastrostomy tube to gastro-jejunostomy tube, use 49446)

⊙ **49442** Insertion of cecostomy or other colonic tube, percutaneous, under fluoroscopic guidance including contrast injection(s), image documentation and report

## Conversion

⊙ **49446** Conversion of gastrostomy tube to gastro-jejunostomy tube, percutaneous, under fluoroscopic guidance including contrast injection(s), image documentation and report

(For conversion to a gastro-jejunostomy tube at the time of initial gastrostomy tube placement, use 49446 in conjunction with 49440)

## Replacement

If an existing gastrostomy, duodenostomy, jejunostomy, gastro-jejunostomy, or cecostomy (or other colonic) tube is removed and a new tube is placed via a separate percutaneous access site, the placement of the new tube is not considered a replacement and would be reported using the appropriate initial placement codes 49440-49442.

**49450** Replacement of gastrostomy or cecostomy (or other colonic) tube, percutaneous, under fluoroscopic guidance including contrast injection(s), image documentation and report

⊙=Moderate sedation   ✚=Add-on code   ✗=FDA approval pending   #=Resequenced code   ○=Recycled/reinstated code

(To report a percutaneous change of a gastrostomy tube without imaging or endoscopic guidance, use 43760)

**49451**   Replacement of duodenostomy or jejunostomy tube, percutaneous, under fluoroscopic guidance including contrast injection(s), image documentation and report

**49452**   Replacement of gastro-jejunostomy tube, percutaneous, under fluoroscopic guidance including contrast injection(s), image documentation and report

## Mechanical Removal of Obstructive Material

**49460**   Mechanical removal of obstructive material from gastrostomy, duodenostomy, jejunostomy, gastro-jejunostomy, or cecostomy (or other colonic) tube, any method, under fluoroscopic guidance including contrast injection(s), if performed, image documentation and report

(Do not report 49460 in conjunction with 49450-49452, 49465)

## Other

**49465**   Contrast injection(s) for radiological evaluation of existing gastrostomy, duodenostomy, jejunostomy, gastro-jejunostomy, or cecostomy (or other colonic) tube, from a percutaneous approach including image documentation and report

(Do not report 49465 in conjunction with 49450-49460)

# Repair

### Hernioplasty, Herniorrhaphy, Herniotomy

The hernia repair codes in this section are categorized primarily by the type of hernia (inguinal, femoral, incisional, etc).

Some types of hernias are further categorized as "initial" or "recurrent" based on whether or not the hernia has required previous repair(s).

Additional variables accounted for by some of the codes include patient age and clinical presentation (reducible vs. incarcerated or strangulated).

With the exception of the incisional hernia repairs (see 49560-49566) the use of mesh or other prostheses is not separately reported.

The excision/repair of strangulated organs or structures such as testicle(s), intestine, ovaries are reported by using the appropriate code for the excision/repair (eg, 44120, 54520, and 58940) in addition to the appropriate code for the repair of the strangulated hernia.

(For reduction and repair of intra-abdominal hernia, use 44050)

(For debridement of abdominal wall, see 11042, 11043)

(Codes 49491-49651 are unilateral procedures. To report bilateral procedure, report modifier 50 with the appropriate procedure code)

**49491**   Repair, initial inguinal hernia, preterm infant (younger than 37 weeks gestation at birth), performed from birth up to 50 weeks postconception age, with or without hydrocelectomy; reducible

**49492**        incarcerated or strangulated

(Do not report modifier 63 in conjunction with 49491, 49492)

(Postconception age equals gestational age at birth plus age of infant in weeks at the time of the hernia repair. Initial inguinal hernia repairs that are performed on preterm infants who are older than 50 weeks postconception age and younger than age 6 months at the time of surgery, should be reported using codes 49495, 49496)

**49495**   Repair, initial inguinal hernia, full term infant younger than age 6 months, or preterm infant older than 50 weeks postconception age and younger than age 6 months at the time of surgery, with or without hydrocelectomy; reducible

**49496**        incarcerated or strangulated

(Do not report modifier 63 in conjunction with 49495, 49496)

(Postconception age equals gestational age at birth plus age in weeks at the time of the hernia repair. Initial inguinal hernia repairs that are performed on preterm infants who are younger than or up to 50 weeks postconception age but younger than 6 months of age since birth, should be reported using codes 49491, 49492. Inguinal hernia repairs on infants age 6 months to younger than 5 years should be reported using codes 49500-49501)

**49500**   Repair initial inguinal hernia, age 6 months to younger than 5 years, with or without hydrocelectomy; reducible

**49501**        incarcerated or strangulated

**49505**   Repair initial inguinal hernia, age 5 years or older; reducible

**49507**        incarcerated or strangulated

(For inguinal hernia repair, with simple orchiectomy, see 49505 or 49507 and 54520)

(For inguinal hernia repair, with excision of hydrocele or spermatocele, see 49505 or 49507 and 54840 or 55040)

**49520**   Repair recurrent inguinal hernia, any age; reducible

**49521**        incarcerated or strangulated

**49525**   Repair inguinal hernia, sliding, any age

(For incarcerated or strangulated inguinal hernia repair, see 49496, 49501, 49507, 49521)

**49540**   Repair lumbar hernia

**49550**   Repair initial femoral hernia, any age; reducible

---

**Surgery: Digestive System**

| | |
|---|---|
| 49553 | incarcerated or strangulated |
| 49555 | Repair recurrent femoral hernia; reducible |
| 49557 | incarcerated or strangulated |
| 49560 | Repair initial incisional or ventral hernia; reducible |
| 49561 | incarcerated or strangulated |
| 49565 | Repair recurrent incisional or ventral hernia; reducible |
| 49566 | incarcerated or strangulated |

+ 49568   Implantation of mesh or other prosthesis for open incisional or ventral hernia repair or mesh for closure of debridement for necrotizing soft tissue infection (List separately in addition to code for the incisional or ventral hernia repair)

(Use 49568 in conjunction with 11004-11006, 49560-49566)

| | |
|---|---|
| 49570 | Repair epigastric hernia (eg, preperitoneal fat); reducible (separate procedure) |
| 49572 | incarcerated or strangulated |
| 49580 | Repair umbilical hernia, younger than age 5 years; reducible |
| 49582 | incarcerated or strangulated |
| 49585 | Repair umbilical hernia, age 5 years or older; reducible |
| 49587 | incarcerated or strangulated |
| 49590 | Repair spigelian hernia |
| 49600 | Repair of small omphalocele, with primary closure |

(Do not report modifier 63 in conjunction with 49600)

49605   Repair of large omphalocele or gastroschisis; with or without prosthesis

49606   with removal of prosthesis, final reduction and closure, in operating room

(Do not report modifier 63 in conjunction with 49605, 49606)

| | |
|---|---|
| 49610 | Repair of omphalocele (Gross type operation); first stage |
| 49611 | second stage |

(Do not report modifier 63 in conjunction with 49610, 49611)

(For diaphragmatic or hiatal hernia repair, see 39503, 43332)

(For surgical repair of omentum, use 49999)

### Laparoscopy

Surgical laparoscopy always includes diagnostic laparoscopy. To report a diagnostic laparoscopy (peritoneoscopy) (separate procedure), use 49320.

| | |
|---|---|
| 49650 | Laparoscopy, surgical; repair initial inguinal hernia |
| 49651 | repair recurrent inguinal hernia |

49652   Laparoscopy, surgical, repair, ventral, umbilical, spigelian or epigastric hernia (includes mesh insertion, when performed); reducible

(Do not report 49652 in conjunction with 44180, 49568)

49653   incarcerated or strangulated

(Do not report 49653 in conjunction with 44180, 49568)

49654   Laparoscopy, surgical, repair, incisional hernia (includes mesh insertion, when performed); reducible

(Do not report 49654 in conjunction with 44180, 49568)

49655   incarcerated or strangulated

(Do not report 49655 in conjunction with 44180, 49568)

49656   Laparoscopy, surgical, repair, recurrent incisional hernia (includes mesh insertion, when performed); reducible

(Do not report 49656 in conjunction with 44180, 49568)

49657   incarcerated or strangulated

(Do not report 49657 in conjunction with 44180, 49568)

49659   Unlisted laparoscopy procedure, hernioplasty, herniorrhaphy, herniotomy

## Suture

49900   Suture, secondary, of abdominal wall for evisceration or dehiscence

(For suture of ruptured diaphragm, see 39540, 39541)

(For debridement of abdominal wall, see 11042, 11043)

## Other Procedures

49904   Omental flap, extra-abdominal (eg, for reconstruction of sternal and chest wall defects)

(Code 49904 includes harvest and transfer. If a second surgeon harvests the omental flap, then the 2 surgeons should code 49904 as co-surgeons, using modifier 62)

+ 49905   Omental flap, intra-abdominal (List separately in addition to code for primary procedure)

(Do not report 49905 in conjunction with 44700)

49906   Free omental flap with microvascular anastomosis

(Do not report code 69990 in addition to 49906)

49999   Unlisted procedure, abdomen, peritoneum and omentum

# Urinary System

(For provision of chemotherapeutic agents, report both the specific service in addition to code(s) for the specific substance(s) or drug(s) provided)

## Kidney

### Incision

(For retroperitoneal exploration, abscess, tumor, or cyst, see 49010, 49060, 49203-49205)

**50010**    Renal exploration, not necessitating other specific procedures

(For laparoscopic ablation of renal mass lesion(s), use 50542)

**50020**    Drainage of perirenal or renal abscess; open

⊙ **50021**        percutaneous

(For radiological supervision and interpretation, use 75989)

**50040**    Nephrostomy, nephrotomy with drainage

**50045**    Nephrotomy, with exploration

(For renal endoscopy performed in conjunction with this procedure, see 50570-50580)

**50060**    Nephrolithotomy; removal of calculus

**50065**        secondary surgical operation for calculus

**50070**        complicated by congenital kidney abnormality

**50075**        removal of large staghorn calculus filling renal pelvis and calyces (including anatrophic pyelolithotomy)

**50080**    Percutaneous nephrostolithotomy or pyelostolithotomy, with or without dilation, endoscopy, lithotripsy, stenting, or basket extraction; up to 2 cm

**50081**        over 2 cm

(For establishment of nephrostomy without nephrostolithotomy, see 50040, 50395, 52334)

(For fluoroscopic guidance, see 76000, 76001)

**50100**    Transection or repositioning of aberrant renal vessels (separate procedure)

**50120**    Pyelotomy; with exploration

(For renal endoscopy performed in conjunction with this procedure, see 50570-50580)

**50125**        with drainage, pyelostomy

**50130**        with removal of calculus (pyelolithotomy, pelviolithotomy, including coagulum pyelolithotomy)

**50135**        complicated (eg, secondary operation, congenital kidney abnormality)

(For supply of anticarcinogenic agents, use 99070 in addition to code for primary procedure)

## Excision

(For excision of retroperitoneal tumor or cyst, see 49203-49205)

(For laparoscopic ablation of renal mass lesion(s), use 50542)

⊙ **50200**    Renal biopsy; percutaneous, by trocar or needle

(For radiological supervision and interpretation, see 76942, 77002, 77012, 77021)

(For fine needle aspiration, use 10022)

(For evaluation of fine needle aspirate, see 88172, 88173)

**50205**        by surgical exposure of kidney

**50220**    Nephrectomy, including partial ureterectomy, any open approach including rib resection;

**50225**        complicated because of previous surgery on same kidney

**50230**        radical, with regional lymphadenectomy and/or vena caval thrombectomy

(When vena caval resection with reconstruction is necessary, use 37799)

**50234**    Nephrectomy with total ureterectomy and bladder cuff; through same incision

**50236**        through separate incision

**50240**    Nephrectomy, partial

(For laparoscopic partial nephrectomy, use 50543)

**50250**    Ablation, open, 1 or more renal mass lesion(s), cryosurgical, including intraoperative ultrasound guidance and monitoring, if performed

(For laparoscopic ablation of renal mass lesions, use 50542)

(For percutaneous ablation of renal tumors, see 50592, 50593)

**50280**    Excision or unroofing of cyst(s) of kidney

(For laparoscopic ablation of renal cysts, use 50541)

**50290**    Excision of perinephric cyst

## Renal Transplantation

Renal *auto*transplantation includes reimplantation of the autograft as the primary procedure, along with secondary extra-corporeal procedure(s) (eg, partial nephrectomy, nephrolithotomy) reported with modifier 51 (see 50380 and applicable secondary procedure(s)).

Renal *allo*transplantation involves three distinct components of physician work:

1. ***Cadaver donor nephrectomy, unilateral or bilateral,*** which includes harvesting the graft(s) and cold preservation of the graft(s) (perfusing with cold preservation solution and cold maintenance) (use

50300). ***Living donor nephrectomy,*** which includes harvesting the graft, cold preservation of the graft (perfusing with cold preservation solution and cold maintenance), and care of the donor (see 50320, 50547).

2. ***Backbench work:***

Standard preparation of a cadaver donor renal allograft prior to transplantation including dissection and removal of perinephric fat, diaphragmatic and retroperitoneal attachments; excision of adrenal gland; and preparation of ureter(s), renal vein(s), and renal artery(s), ligating branches, as necessary (use 50323).

Standard preparation of a living donor renal allograft (open or laparoscopic) prior to transplantation including dissection and removal of perinephric fat and preparation of ureter(s), renal vein(s), and renal artery(s), ligating branches, as necessary (use 50325).

Additional reconstruction of a cadaver or living donor renal allograft prior to transplantation may include venous, arterial, and/or ureteral anastomosis(es) necessary for implantation (see 50327-50329).

3. ***Recipient renal allotransplantation,*** which includes transplantation of the allograft (with or without recipient nephrectomy) and care of the recipient (see 50360, 50365).

(For dialysis, see 90935-90999)

(For laparoscopic donor nephrectomy, use 50547)

(For laparoscopic drainage of lymphocele to peritoneal cavity, use 49323)

**50300**   Donor nephrectomy (including cold preservation); from cadaver donor, unilateral or bilateral

**50320**      open, from living donor

**50323**   Backbench standard preparation of cadaver donor renal allograft prior to transplantation, including dissection and removal of perinephric fat, diaphragmatic and retroperitoneal attachments, excision of adrenal gland, and preparation of ureter(s), renal vein(s), and renal artery(s), ligating branches, as necessary

(Do not report 50323 in conjunction with 60540, 60545)

**50325**   Backbench standard preparation of living donor renal allograft (open or laparoscopic) prior to transplantation, including dissection and removal of perinephric fat and preparation of ureter(s), renal vein(s), and renal artery(s), ligating branches, as necessary

**50327**   Backbench reconstruction of cadaver or living donor renal allograft prior to transplantation; venous anastomosis, each

**50328**      arterial anastomosis, each

**50329**      ureteral anastomosis, each

**50340**   Recipient nephrectomy (separate procedure)

(For bilateral procedure, report 50340 with modifier 50)

**50360**   Renal allotransplantation, implantation of graft; without recipient nephrectomy

**50365**      with recipient nephrectomy

(For bilateral procedure, report 50365 with modifier 50)

**50370**   Removal of transplanted renal allograft

**50380**   Renal autotransplantation, reimplantation of kidney

(For renal autotransplantation extra-corporeal [bench] surgery, use autotransplantation as the primary procedure and report secondary procedure[s] [eg, partial nephrectomy, nephrolithotomy] with modifier 51)

## Introduction

### Renal Pelvis Catheter Procedures

*Internally Dwelling*

⊙ **50382**   Removal (via snare/capture) and replacement of internally dwelling ureteral stent via percutaneous approach, including radiological supervision and interpretation

(For bilateral procedure, use modifier 50)

(For removal and replacement of an internally dwelling ureteral stent via a transurethral approach, use 50385)

⊙ **50384**   Removal (via snare/capture) of internally dwelling ureteral stent via percutaneous approach, including radiological supervision and interpretation

(For bilateral procedure, use modifier 50)

(Do not report 50382, 50384 in conjunction with 50395)

(For removal of an internally dwelling ureteral stent via a transurethral approach, use 50386)

⊙ **50385**   Removal (via snare/capture) and replacement of internally dwelling ureteral stent via transurethral approach, without use of cystoscopy, including radiological supervision and interpretation

⊙ **50386**   Removal (via snare/capture) of internally dwelling ureteral stent via transurethral approach, without use of cystoscopy, including radiological supervision and interpretation

*Externally Accessible*

⊙ **50387**   Removal and replacement of externally accessible transnephric ureteral stent (eg, external/internal stent) requiring fluoroscopic guidance, including radiological supervision and interpretation

(For bilateral procedure, use modifier 50)

(For removal and replacement of externally accessible ureteral stent via ureterostomy or ilieal conduit, use 50688)

(For removal without replacement of an externally accessible ureteral stent not requiring fluoroscopic guidance, see **Evaluation and Management** services codes)

**50389**   Removal of nephrostomy tube, requiring fluoroscopic guidance (eg, with concurrent indwelling ureteral stent)

(Removal of nephrostomy tube not requiring fluoroscopic guidance is considered inherent to E/M services. Report the appropriate level of E/M service provided)

## Other Introduction Procedures

**50390**   Aspiration and/or injection of renal cyst or pelvis by needle, percutaneous

(For radiological supervision and interpretation, see 74425, 74470, 76942, 77002, 77012, 77021)

(For evaluation of fine needle aspirate, see 88172, 88173)

**50391**   Instillation(s) of therapeutic agent into renal pelvis and/or ureter through established nephrostomy, pyelostomy or ureterostomy tube (eg, anticarcinogenic or antifungal agent)

**50392**   Introduction of intracatheter or catheter into renal pelvis for drainage and/or injection, percutaneous

(For radiological supervision and interpretation, see 74475, 76942, 77012)

**50393**   Introduction of ureteral catheter or stent into ureter through renal pelvis for drainage and/or injection, percutaneous

(For radiological supervision and interpretation, see 74480, 76942, 77002, 77012)

**50394**   Injection procedure for pyelography (as nephrostogram, pyelostogram, antegrade pyeloureterograms) through nephrostomy or pyelostomy tube, or indwelling ureteral catheter

(For radiological supervision and interpretation, use 74425)

**50395**   Introduction of guide into renal pelvis and/or ureter with dilation to establish nephrostomy tract, percutaneous

(For radiological supervision and interpretation, see 74475, 74480, 74485)

(For nephrostolithotomy, see 50080, 50081)

(For retrograde percutaneous nephrostomy, use 52334)

(For endoscopic surgery, see 50551-50561)

**50396**   Manometric studies through nephrostomy or pyelostomy tube, or indwelling ureteral catheter

(For radiological supervision and interpretation, see 74425, 74475, 74480)

**50398**   Change of nephrostomy or pyelostomy tube

(For radiological supervision and interpretation, use 75984)

## Repair

**50400**   Pyeloplasty (Foley Y-pyeloplasty), plastic operation on renal pelvis, with or without plastic operation on ureter, nephropexy, nephrostomy, pyelostomy, or ureteral splinting; simple

**50405**       complicated (congenital kidney abnormality, secondary pyeloplasty, solitary kidney, calycoplasty)

(For laparoscopic approach, use 50544)

**50500**   Nephrorrhaphy, suture of kidney wound or injury

**50520**   Closure of nephrocutaneous or pyelocutaneous fistula

**50525**   Closure of nephrovisceral fistula (eg, renocolic), including visceral repair; abdominal approach

**50526**       thoracic approach

**50540**   Symphysiotomy for horseshoe kidney with or without pyeloplasty and/or other plastic procedure, unilateral or bilateral (1 operation)

## Laparoscopy

Surgical laparoscopy always includes diagnostic laparoscopy. To report a diagnostic laparoscopy (peritoneoscopy) (separate procedure), use 49320.

**50541**   Laparoscopy, surgical; ablation of renal cysts

**50542**       ablation of renal mass lesion(s), including intraoperative ultrasound guidance and monitoring, when performed

(For open procedure, use 50250)

(For percutaneous ablation of renal tumors, see 50592, 50593)

**50543**       partial nephrectomy

(For open procedure, use 50240)

**50544**       pyeloplasty

**50545**       radical nephrectomy (includes removal of Gerota's fascia and surrounding fatty tissue, removal of regional lymph nodes, and adrenalectomy)

(For open procedure, use 50230)

**50546**       nephrectomy, including partial ureterectomy

**50547**       donor nephrectomy (including cold preservation), from living donor

(For open procedure, use 50320)

(For backbench renal allograft standard preparation prior to transplantation, use 50325)

(For backbench renal allograft reconstruction prior to transplantation, see 50327-50329)

**50548**       nephrectomy with total ureterectomy

(For open procedure, see 50234, 50236)

**50549**   Unlisted laparoscopy procedure, renal

Surgery: Urinary System

(For laparoscopic drainage of lymphocele to peritoneal cavity, use 49323)

## Endoscopy

(For supplies and materials, use 99070)

**50551**  Renal endoscopy through established nephrostomy or pyelostomy, with or without irrigation, instillation, or ureteropyelography, exclusive of radiologic service;

**50553**  with ureteral catheterization, with or without dilation of ureter

**50555**  with biopsy

**50557**  with fulguration and/or incision, with or without biopsy

**50561**  with removal of foreign body or calculus

**50562**  with resection of tumor

(When procedures 50570-50580 provide a significant identifiable service, they may be added to 50045 and 50120)

**50570**  Renal endoscopy through nephrotomy or pyelotomy, with or without irrigation, instillation, or ureteropyelography, exclusive of radiologic service;

(For nephrotomy, use 50045)

(For pyelotomy, use 50120)

**50572**  with ureteral catheterization, with or without dilation of ureter

**50574**  with biopsy

**50575**  with endopyelotomy (includes cystoscopy, ureteroscopy, dilation of ureter and ureteral pelvic junction, incision of ureteral pelvic junction and insertion of endopyelotomy stent)

**50576**  with fulguration and/or incision, with or without biopsy

**50580**  with removal of foreign body or calculus

## Other Procedures

**50590**  Lithotripsy, extracorporeal shock wave

⊙ **50592**  Ablation, 1 or more renal tumor(s), percutaneous, unilateral, radiofrequency

(50592 is a unilateral procedure. For bilateral procedure, report 50592 with modifier 50)

(For imaging guidance and monitoring, see 76940, 77013, 77022)

⊙ **50593**  Ablation, renal tumor(s), unilateral, percutaneous, cryotherapy

(50593 is a unilateral procedure. For bilateral procedure, report 50593 with modifier 50)

(For imaging guidance and monitoring, see codes 76940, 77013, 77022)

# Ureter

## Incision

**50600**  Ureterotomy with exploration or drainage (separate procedure)

(For ureteral endoscopy performed in conjunction with this procedure, see 50970-50980)

**50605**  Ureterotomy for insertion of indwelling stent, all types

**50610**  Ureterolithotomy; upper one-third of ureter

**50620**  middle one-third of ureter

**50630**  lower one-third of ureter

(For laparoscopic approach, use 50945)

(For transvesical ureterolithotomy, use 51060)

(For cystotomy with stone basket extraction of ureteral calculus, use 51065)

(For endoscopic extraction or manipulation of ureteral calculus, see 50080, 50081, 50561, 50961, 50980, 52320-52330, 52352, 52353)

## Excision

(For ureterocele, see 51535, 52300)

**50650**  Ureterectomy, with bladder cuff (separate procedure)

**50660**  Ureterectomy, total, ectopic ureter, combination abdominal, vaginal and/or perineal approach

## Introduction

**50684**  Injection procedure for ureterography or ureteropyelography through ureterostomy or indwelling ureteral catheter

(For radiological supervision and interpretation, use 74425)

**50686**  Manometric studies through ureterostomy or indwelling ureteral catheter

**50688**  Change of ureterostomy tube or externally accessible ureteral stent via ileal conduit

(If imaging guidance is performed, use 75984)

**50690**  Injection procedure for visualization of ileal conduit and/or ureteropyelography, exclusive of radiologic service

(For radiological supervision and interpretation, use 74425)

## Repair

**50700**  Ureteroplasty, plastic operation on ureter (eg, stricture)

**50715**  Ureterolysis, with or without repositioning of ureter for retroperitoneal fibrosis

(For bilateral procedure, report 50715 with modifier 50)

Surgery: Urinary System

**50722**   Ureterolysis for ovarian vein syndrome

**50725**   Ureterolysis for retrocaval ureter, with reanastomosis of upper urinary tract or vena cava

**50727**   Revision of urinary-cutaneous anastomosis (any type urostomy);

**50728**       with repair of fascial defect and hernia

**50740**   Ureteropyelostomy, anastomosis of ureter and renal pelvis

**50750**   Ureterocalycostomy, anastomosis of ureter to renal calyx

**50760**   Ureteroureterostomy

**50770**   Transureteroureterostomy, anastomosis of ureter to contralateral ureter

(Codes 50780-50785 include minor procedures to prevent vesicoureteral reflux)

**50780**   Ureteroneocystostomy; anastomosis of single ureter to bladder

(For bilateral procedure, report 50780 with modifier 50)

(When combined with cystourethroplasty or vesical neck revision, use 51820)

**50782**       anastomosis of duplicated ureter to bladder

**50783**       with extensive ureteral tailoring

**50785**       with vesico-psoas hitch or bladder flap

(For bilateral procedure, report 50785 with modifier 50)

**50800**   Ureteroenterostomy, direct anastomosis of ureter to intestine

(For bilateral procedure, report 50800 with modifier 50)

**50810**   Ureterosigmoidostomy, with creation of sigmoid bladder and establishment of abdominal or perineal colostomy, including intestine anastomosis

**50815**   Ureterocolon conduit, including intestine anastomosis

(For bilateral procedure, report 50815 with modifier 50)

**50820**   Ureteroileal conduit (ileal bladder), including intestine anastomosis (Bricker operation)

(For bilateral procedure, report 50820 with modifier 50)

(For combination of 50800-50820 with cystectomy, see 51580-51595)

**50825**   Continent diversion, including intestine anastomosis using any segment of small and/or large intestine (Kock pouch or Camey enterocystoplasty)

**50830**   Urinary undiversion (eg, taking down of ureteroileal conduit, ureterosigmoidostomy or ureteroenterostomy with ureteroureterostomy or ureteroneocystostomy)

**50840**   Replacement of all or part of ureter by intestine segment, including intestine anastomosis

(For bilateral procedure, report 50840 with modifier 50)

**50845**   Cutaneous appendico-vesicostomy

**50860**   Ureterostomy, transplantation of ureter to skin

(For bilateral procedure, report 50860 with modifier 50)

**50900**   Ureterorrhaphy, suture of ureter (separate procedure)

**50920**   Closure of ureterocutaneous fistula

**50930**   Closure of ureterovisceral fistula (including visceral repair)

**50940**   Deligation of ureter

(For ureteroplasty, ureterolysis, see 50700-50860)

## Laparoscopy

Surgical laparoscopy always includes diagnostic laparoscopy. To report a diagnostic laparoscopy (peritoneoscopy) (separate procedure), use 49320.

**50945**   Laparoscopy, surgical; ureterolithotomy

**50947**       ureteroneocystostomy with cystoscopy and ureteral stent placement

**50948**       ureteroneocystostomy without cystoscopy and ureteral stent placement

(For open ureteroneocystostomy, see 50780-50785)

**50949**   Unlisted laparoscopy procedure, ureter

## Endoscopy

**50951**   Ureteral endoscopy through established ureterostomy, with or without irrigation, instillation, or ureteropyelography, exclusive of radiologic service;

**50953**       with ureteral catheterization, with or without dilation of ureter

**50955**       with biopsy

**50957**       with fulguration and/or incision, with or without biopsy

**50961**       with removal of foreign body or calculus

(When procedures 50970-50980 provide a significant identifiable service, they may be added to 50600)

**50970**   Ureteral endoscopy through ureterotomy, with or without irrigation, instillation, or ureteropyelography, exclusive of radiologic service;

(For ureterotomy, use 50600)

**50972**       with ureteral catheterization, with or without dilation of ureter

**50974**       with biopsy

**50976**       with fulguration and/or incision, with or without biopsy

**50980**       with removal of foreign body or calculus

Surgery: Urinary System

# Bladder

## Incision

**51020**   Cystotomy or cystostomy; with fulguration and/or insertion of radioactive material

**51030**       with cryosurgical destruction of intravesical lesion

**51040**   Cystostomy, cystotomy with drainage

**51045**   Cystotomy, with insertion of ureteral catheter or stent (separate procedure)

**51050**   Cystolithotomy, cystotomy with removal of calculus, without vesical neck resection

**51060**   Transvesical ureterolithotomy

**51065**   Cystotomy, with calculus basket extraction and/or ultrasonic or electrohydraulic fragmentation of ureteral calculus

**51080**   Drainage of perivesical or prevesical space abscess

## Removal

**51100**   Aspiration of bladder; by needle

**51101**       by trocar or intracatheter

**51102**       with insertion of suprapubic catheter

(For imaging guidance, see 76942, 77002, 77012)

## Excision

**51500**   Excision of urachal cyst or sinus, with or without umbilical hernia repair

**51520**   Cystotomy; for simple excision of vesical neck (separate procedure)

**51525**       for excision of bladder diverticulum, single or multiple (separate procedure)

**51530**       for excision of bladder tumor

(For transurethral resection, see 52234-52240, 52305)

**51535**   Cystotomy for excision, incision, or repair of ureterocele

(For bilateral procedure, report 51535 with modifier 50)

(For transurethral excision, use 52300)

**51550**   Cystectomy, partial; simple

**51555**       complicated (eg, postradiation, previous surgery, difficult location)

**51565**   Cystectomy, partial, with reimplantation of ureter(s) into bladder (ureteroneocystostomy)

**51570**   Cystectomy, complete; (separate procedure)

**51575**       with bilateral pelvic lymphadenectomy, including external iliac, hypogastric, and obturator nodes

**51580**   Cystectomy, complete, with ureterosigmoidostomy or ureterocutaneous transplantations;

**51585**       with bilateral pelvic lymphadenectomy, including external iliac, hypogastric, and obturator nodes

**51590**   Cystectomy, complete, with ureteroileal conduit or sigmoid bladder, including intestine anastomosis;

**51595**       with bilateral pelvic lymphadenectomy, including external iliac, hypogastric, and obturator nodes

**51596**   Cystectomy, complete, with continent diversion, any open technique, using any segment of small and/or large intestine to construct neobladder

**51597**   Pelvic exenteration, complete, for vesical, prostatic or urethral malignancy, with removal of bladder and ureteral transplantations, with or without hysterectomy and/or abdominoperineal resection of rectum and colon and colostomy, or any combination thereof

(For pelvic exenteration for gynecologic malignancy, use 58240)

## Introduction

**51600**   Injection procedure for cystography or voiding urethrocystography

(For radiological supervision and interpretation, see 74430, 74455)

**51605**   Injection procedure and placement of chain for contrast and/or chain urethrocystography

(For radiological supervision and interpretation, use 74430)

**51610**   Injection procedure for retrograde urethrocystography

(For radiological supervision and interpretation, use 74450)

**51700**   Bladder irrigation, simple, lavage and/or instillation

(Codes 51701-51702 are reported only when performed independently. Do not report 51701-51702 when catheter insertion is an inclusive component of another procedure.)

**51701**   Insertion of non-indwelling bladder catheter (eg, straight catheterization for residual urine)

**51702**   Insertion of temporary indwelling bladder catheter; simple (eg, Foley)

**51703**       complicated (eg, altered anatomy, fractured catheter/balloon)

**51705**   Change of cystostomy tube; simple

**51710**       complicated

(If imaging guidance is performed, use 75984)

**51715**   Endoscopic injection of implant material into the submucosal tissues of the urethra and/or bladder neck

**51720**   Bladder instillation of anticarcinogenic agent (including retention time)

Surgery: Urinary System

## Urodynamics

The following section (51725-51792) lists procedures that may be used separately or in many and varied combinations.

When multiple procedures are performed in the same investigative session, modifier 51 should be employed.

All procedures in this section imply that these services are performed by, or are under the direct supervision of, a physician and that all instruments, equipment, fluids, gases, probes, catheters, technician's fees, medications, gloves, trays, tubing and other sterile supplies be provided by the physician. When the physician only interprets the results and/or operates the equipment, a professional component, modifier 26, should be used to identify physicians' services.

**51725**   Simple cystometrogram (CMG) (eg, spinal manometer)

**51726**   Complex cystometrogram (ie, calibrated electronic equipment);

**51727**       with urethral pressure profile studies (ie, urethral closure pressure profile), any technique

**51728**       with voiding pressure studies (ie, bladder voiding pressure), any technique

**51729**       with voiding pressure studies (ie, bladder voiding pressure) and urethral pressure profile studies (ie, urethral closure pressure profile), any technique

#+ **51797**   Voiding pressure studies, intra-abdominal (ie, rectal, gastric, intraperitoneal) (List separately in addition to code for primary procedure)

           (Use 51797 in conjunction with 51728, 51729)

**51736**   Simple uroflowmetry (UFR) (eg, stop-watch flow rate, mechanical uroflowmeter)

**51741**   Complex uroflowmetry (eg, calibrated electronic equipment)

           (51772 has been deleted. To report urethral pressure profile studies, see 51727, 51729)

**51784**   Electromyography studies (EMG) of anal or urethral sphincter, other than needle, any technique

**51785**   Needle electromyography studies (EMG) of anal or urethral sphincter, any technique

**51792**   Stimulus evoked response (eg, measurement of bulbocavernosus reflex latency time)

           (51795 has been deleted. To report bladder voiding pressure studies, see 51728, 51729)

**51797**   Code is out of numerical sequence. See 51725-51798

**51798**   Measurement of post-voiding residual urine and/or bladder capacity by ultrasound, non-imaging

## Repair

**51800**   Cystoplasty or cystourethroplasty, plastic operation on bladder and/or vesical neck (anterior Y-plasty, vesical fundus resection), any procedure, with or without wedge resection of posterior vesical neck

**51820**   Cystourethroplasty with unilateral or bilateral ureteroneocystostomy

**51840**   Anterior vesicourethropexy, or urethropexy (eg, Marshall-Marchetti-Krantz, Burch); simple

**51841**       complicated (eg, secondary repair)

           (For urethropexy (Pereyra type), use 57289)

**51845**   Abdomino-vaginal vesical neck suspension, with or without endoscopic control (eg, Stamey, Raz, modified Pereyra)

**51860**   Cystorrhaphy, suture of bladder wound, injury or rupture; simple

**51865**       complicated

**51880**   Closure of cystostomy (separate procedure)

**51900**   Closure of vesicovaginal fistula, abdominal approach

           (For vaginal approach, see 57320-57330)

**51920**   Closure of vesicouterine fistula;

**51925**       with hysterectomy

           (For closure of vesicoenteric fistula, see 44660, 44661)

           (For closure of rectovesical fistula, see 45800-45805)

**51940**   Closure, exstrophy of bladder

           (See also 54390)

**51960**   Enterocystoplasty, including intestinal anastomosis

**51980**   Cutaneous vesicostomy

## Laparoscopy

Surgical laparoscopy always includes diagnostic laparoscopy. To report a diagnostic laparoscopy (peritoneoscopy) (separate procedure), use 49320.

**51990**   Laparoscopy, surgical; urethral suspension for stress incontinence

**51992**       sling operation for stress incontinence (eg, fascia or synthetic)

           (For open sling operation for stress incontinence, use 57288)

           (For reversal or removal of sling operation for stress incontinence, use 57287)

**51999**   Unlisted laparoscopy procedure, bladder

# Endoscopy—Cystoscopy, Urethroscopy, Cystourethroscopy

Endoscopic descriptions are listed so that the main procedure can be identified without having to list all the minor related functions performed at the same time. For example: meatotomy, urethral calibration and/or dilation, urethroscopy, and cystoscopy prior to a transurethral resection of prostate; ureteral catheterization following extraction of ureteral calculus; internal urethrotomy and bladder neck fulguration when performing a cystourethroscopy for the female urethral syndrome. When the secondary procedure requires significant additional time and effort, it may be identified by the addition of modifier 22.

For example: urethrotomy performed for a documented pre-existing stricture or bladder neck contracture.

**52000**   Cystourethroscopy (separate procedure)

**52001**   Cystourethroscopy with irrigation and evacuation of multiple obstructing clots

   (Do not report 52001 in conjunction with 52000)

**52005**   Cystourethroscopy, with ureteral catheterization, with or without irrigation, instillation, or ureteropyelography, exclusive of radiologic service;

**52007**      with brush biopsy of ureter and/or renal pelvis

**52010**   Cystourethroscopy, with ejaculatory duct catheterization, with or without irrigation, instillation, or duct radiography, exclusive of radiologic service

   (For radiological supervision and interpretation, use 74440)

## Transurethral Surgery

### Urethra and Bladder

**52204**   Cystourethroscopy, with biopsy(s)

**52214**   Cystourethroscopy, with fulguration (including cryosurgery or laser surgery) of trigone, bladder neck, prostatic fossa, urethra, or periurethral glands

   (For transurethral fulguration of prostate tissue performed within the postoperative period of 52601 or 52630 performed by the same physician, append modifier 78)

   (For transurethral fulguration of prostate tissue performed within the postoperative period of a related procedure performed by the same physician, append modifier 78)

   (For transurethral fulguration of prostate for postoperative bleeding performed by the same physician, append modifier 78)

**52224**   Cystourethroscopy, with fulguration (including cryosurgery or laser surgery) or treatment of MINOR (less than 0.5 cm) lesion(s) with or without biopsy

**52234**   Cystourethroscopy, with fulguration (including cryosurgery or laser surgery) and/or resection of; SMALL bladder tumor(s) (0.5 up to 2.0 cm)

**52235**      MEDIUM bladder tumor(s) (2.0 to 5.0 cm)

**52240**      LARGE bladder tumor(s)

**52250**   Cystourethroscopy with insertion of radioactive substance, with or without biopsy or fulguration

**52260**   Cystourethroscopy, with dilation of bladder for interstitial cystitis; general or conduction (spinal) anesthesia

**52265**      local anesthesia

**52270**   Cystourethroscopy, with internal urethrotomy; female

**52275**      male

**52276**   Cystourethroscopy with direct vision internal urethrotomy

**52277**   Cystourethroscopy, with resection of external sphincter (sphincterotomy)

**52281**   Cystourethroscopy, with calibration and/or dilation of urethral stricture or stenosis, with or without meatotomy, with or without injection procedure for cystography, male or female

**52282**   Cystourethroscopy, with insertion of permanent urethral stent

   (For placement of temporary prostatic urethral stent, use 53855)

**52283**   Cystourethroscopy, with steroid injection into stricture

**52285**   Cystourethroscopy for treatment of the female urethral syndrome with any or all of the following: urethral meatotomy, urethral dilation, internal urethrotomy, lysis of urethrovaginal septal fibrosis, lateral incisions of the bladder neck, and fulguration of polyp(s) of urethra, bladder neck, and/or trigone

**52290**   Cystourethroscopy; with ureteral meatotomy, unilateral or bilateral

**52300**      with resection or fulguration of orthotopic ureterocele(s), unilateral or bilateral

**52301**      with resection or fulguration of ectopic ureterocele(s), unilateral or bilateral

**52305**      with incision or resection of orifice of bladder diverticulum, single or multiple

**52310**   Cystourethroscopy, with removal of foreign body, calculus, or ureteral stent from urethra or bladder (separate procedure); simple

**52315**      complicated

**52317**   Litholapaxy: crushing or fragmentation of calculus by any means in bladder and removal of fragments; simple or small (less than 2.5 cm)

**52318**      complicated or large (over 2.5 cm)

## Ureter and Pelvis

Therapeutic cystourethroscopy always includes diagnostic cystourethroscopy. To report a diagnostic cystourethroscopy, use 52000. Therapeutic cystourethroscopy with ureteroscopy and/or pyeloscopy always includes diagnostic cystourethroscopy with ureteroscopy and/or pyeloscopy. To report a diagnostic cystourethroscopy with ureteroscopy and/or pyeloscopy, use 52351.

Do not report 52000 in conjunction with 52320-52343.

Do not report 52351 in conjunction with 52344-52346, 52352-52355.

The insertion and removal of a temporary ureteral catheter (52005) during diagnostic or therapeutic cystourethroscopic with ureteroscopy and/or pyeloscopy is included in 52320-52355 and should not be reported separately.

To report insertion of a self-retaining, indwelling stent performed during diagnostic or therapeutic cystourethroscopy with ureteroscopy and/or pyeloscopy, report 52332, in addition to primary procedure(s) performed (52320-52355), and append modifier 51. 52332 is used to report a unilateral procedure unless otherwise specified.

For bilateral insertion of self-retaining, indwelling ureteral stents, use code 52332, and append modifier 50.

To report cystourethroscopic removal of a self-retaining, indwelling ureteral stent, see 52310, 52315, and append modifier 58, if appropriate.

**52320**   Cystourethroscopy (including ureteral catheterization); with removal of ureteral calculus

**52325**   with fragmentation of ureteral calculus (eg, ultrasonic or electro-hydraulic technique)

**52327**   with subureteric injection of implant material

**52330**   with manipulation, without removal of ureteral calculus

**52332**   Cystourethroscopy, with insertion of indwelling ureteral stent (eg, Gibbons or double-J type)

**52334**   Cystourethroscopy with insertion of ureteral guide wire through kidney to establish a percutaneous nephrostomy, retrograde

(For percutaneous nephrostolithotomy, see 50080, 50081; for establishment of nephrostomy tract only, use 50395)

(For cystourethroscopy, with ureteroscopy and/or pyeloscopy, see 52351-52355)

(For cystourethroscopy with incision, fulguration, or resection of congenital posterior urethral valves or obstructive hypertrophic mucosal folds, use 52400)

**52341**   Cystourethroscopy; with treatment of ureteral stricture (eg, balloon dilation, laser, electrocautery, and incision)

**52342**   with treatment of ureteropelvic junction stricture (eg, balloon dilation, laser, electrocautery, and incision)

**52343**   with treatment of intra-renal stricture (eg, balloon dilation, laser, electrocautery, and incision)

**52344**   Cystourethroscopy with ureteroscopy; with treatment of ureteral stricture (eg, balloon dilation, laser, electrocautery, and incision)

**52345**   with treatment of ureteropelvic junction stricture (eg, balloon dilation, laser, electrocautery, and incision)

**52346**   with treatment of intra-renal stricture (eg, balloon dilation, laser, electrocautery, and incision)

(For transurethral resection or incision of ejaculatory ducts, use 52402)

**52351**   Cystourethroscopy, with ureteroscopy and/or pyeloscopy; diagnostic

(For radiological supervision and interpretation, use 74485)

(Do not report 52351 in conjunction with 52341-52346, 52352-52355)

**52352**   with removal or manipulation of calculus (ureteral catheterization is included)

**52353**   with lithotripsy (ureteral catheterization is included)

**52354**   with biopsy and/or fulguration of ureteral or renal pelvic lesion

**52355**   with resection of ureteral or renal pelvic tumor

## Vesical Neck and Prostate

**52400**   Cystourethroscopy with incision, fulguration, or resection of congenital posterior urethral valves, or congenital obstructive hypertrophic mucosal folds

**52402**   Cystourethroscopy with transurethral resection or incision of ejaculatory ducts

**52450**   Transurethral incision of prostate

**52500**   Transurethral resection of bladder neck (separate procedure)

**52601**   Transurethral electrosurgical resection of prostate, including control of postoperative bleeding, complete (vasectomy, meatotomy, cystourethroscopy, urethral calibration and/or dilation, and internal urethrotomy are included)

(For other approaches, see 55801-55845)

(52606 has been deleted. For transurethral fulguration of prostate, use 52214)

(52612, 52614, 52620 have been deleted. For first stage transurethral partial resection of prostate, use 52601. For second stage partial resection of prostate, use 52601 with modifier 58. For transurethral resection of residual or regrowth of obstructive prostate tissue, use 52630)

Surgery: Urinary System

**52630** Transurethral resection; residual or regrowth of obstructive prostate tissue including control of postoperative bleeding, complete (vasectomy, meatotomy, cystourethroscopy, urethral calibration and/or dilation, and internal urethrotomy are included)

(For resection of residual prostate tissue performed within the postoperative period of a related procedure performed by the same physician, append modifier 78)

**52640** of postoperative bladder neck contracture

**52647** Laser coagulation of prostate, including control of postoperative bleeding, complete (vasectomy, meatotomy, cystourethroscopy, urethral calibration and/or dilation, and internal urethrotomy are included if performed)

**52648** Laser vaporization of prostate, including control of postoperative bleeding, complete (vasectomy, meatotomy, cystourethroscopy, urethral calibration and/or dilation, internal urethrotomy and transurethral resection of prostate are included if performed)

**52649** Laser enucleation of the prostate with morcellation, including control of postoperative bleeding, complete (vasectomy, meatotomy, cystourethroscopy, urethral calibration and/or dilation, internal urethrotomy and transurethral resection of prostate are included if performed)

(Do not report 52649 in conjunction with 52000, 52276, 52281, 52601, 52647, 52648, 53020, 55250)

**52700** Transurethral drainage of prostatic abscess

(For litholapaxy, use 52317, 52318)

# Urethra

(For endoscopy, see cystoscopy, urethroscopy, cystourethroscopy, 52000-52700)

(For injection procedure for urethrocystography, see 51600-51610)

## Incision

**53000** Urethrotomy or urethrostomy, external (separate procedure); pendulous urethra

**53010** perineal urethra, external

**53020** Meatotomy, cutting of meatus (separate procedure); except infant

**53025** infant

(Do not report modifier 63 in conjunction with 53025)

**53040** Drainage of deep periurethral abscess

(For subcutaneous abscess, see 10060, 10061)

**53060** Drainage of Skene's gland abscess or cyst

**53080** Drainage of perineal urinary extravasation; uncomplicated (separate procedure)

**53085** complicated

# Excision

**53200** Biopsy of urethra

**53210** Urethrectomy, total, including cystostomy; female

**53215** male

**53220** Excision or fulguration of carcinoma of urethra

**53230** Excision of urethral diverticulum (separate procedure); female

**53235** male

**53240** Marsupialization of urethral diverticulum, male or female

**53250** Excision of bulbourethral gland (Cowper's gland)

**53260** Excision or fulguration; urethral polyp(s), distal urethra

(For endoscopic approach, see 52214, 52224)

**53265** urethral caruncle

**53270** Skene's glands

**53275** urethral prolapse

# Repair

(For hypospadias, see 54300-54352)

**53400** Urethroplasty; first stage, for fistula, diverticulum, or stricture (eg, Johannsen type)

**53405** second stage (formation of urethra), including urinary diversion

**53410** Urethroplasty, 1-stage reconstruction of male anterior urethra

**53415** Urethroplasty, transpubic or perineal, 1-stage, for reconstruction or repair of prostatic or membranous urethra

**53420** Urethroplasty, 2-stage reconstruction or repair of prostatic or membranous urethra; first stage

**53425** second stage

**53430** Urethroplasty, reconstruction of female urethra

**53431** Urethroplasty with tubularization of posterior urethra and/or lower bladder for incontinence (eg, Tenago, Leadbetter procedure)

**53440** Sling operation for correction of male urinary incontinence (eg, fascia or synthetic)

**53442** Removal or revision of sling for male urinary incontinence (eg, fascia or synthetic)

**53444** Insertion of tandem cuff (dual cuff)

**53445** Insertion of inflatable urethral/bladder neck sphincter, including placement of pump, reservoir, and cuff

**53446** Removal of inflatable urethral/bladder neck sphincter, including pump, reservoir, and cuff

**53447** Removal and replacement of inflatable urethral/bladder neck sphincter including pump, reservoir, and cuff at the same operative session

Surgery: Urinary System

**53448**   Removal and replacement of inflatable urethral/bladder neck sphincter including pump, reservoir, and cuff through an infected field at the same operative session including irrigation and debridement of infected tissue

(Do not report 11042, 11043 in addition to 53448)

**53449**   Repair of inflatable urethral/bladder neck sphincter, including pump, reservoir, and cuff

**53450**   Urethromeatoplasty, with mucosal advancement

(For meatotomy, see 53020, 53025)

**53460**   Urethromeatoplasty, with partial excision of distal urethral segment (Richardson type procedure)

**53500**   Urethrolysis, transvaginal, secondary, open, including cystourethroscopy (eg, postsurgical obstruction, scarring)

(For urethrolysis by retropubic approach, use 53899)

(Do not report 53500 in conjunction with 52000)

**53502**   Urethrorrhaphy, suture of urethral wound or injury, female

**53505**   Urethrorrhaphy, suture of urethral wound or injury; penile

**53510**        perineal

**53515**        prostatomembranous

**53520**   Closure of urethrostomy or urethrocutaneous fistula, male (separate procedure)

(For closure of urethrovaginal fistula, use 57310)

(For closure of urethrorectal fistula, see 45820, 45825)

## Manipulation

(For radiological supervision and interpretation, use 74485)

**53600**   Dilation of urethral stricture by passage of sound or urethral dilator, male; initial

**53601**        subsequent

**53605**   Dilation of urethral stricture or vesical neck by passage of sound or urethral dilator, male, general or conduction (spinal) anesthesia

(For dilation of urethral stricture, male, performed under local anesthesia, see 53600, 53601, 53620, 53621)

**53620**   Dilation of urethral stricture by passage of filiform and follower, male; initial

**53621**        subsequent

**53660**   Dilation of female urethra including suppository and/or instillation; initial

**53661**        subsequent

**53665**   Dilation of female urethra, general or conduction (spinal) anesthesia

(For urethral catheterization, see 51701-51703)

(For dilation of urethra performed under local anesthesia, female, see 53660, 53661)

## Other Procedures

(For 2 or 3 glass urinalysis, use 81020)

**53850**   Transurethral destruction of prostate tissue; by microwave thermotherapy

**53852**        by radiofrequency thermotherapy

(53853 has been deleted. To report, use 55899)

**53855**   Insertion of a temporary prostatic urethral stent, including urethral measurement

(For insertion of permanent urethral stent, use 52282)

**53860**   Transurethral radiofrequency micro-remodeling of the female bladder neck and proximal urethra for stress urinary incontinence

**53899**   Unlisted procedure, urinary system

**Surgery: Urinary System**

# Male Genital System

## Penis

### Incision

(For abdominal perineal gangrene debridement, see 11004-11006)

**54000**  Slitting of prepuce, dorsal or lateral (separate procedure); newborn

(Do not report modifier 63 in conjunction with 54000)

**54001**      except newborn

**54015**  Incision and drainage of penis, deep

(For skin and subcutaneous abscess, see 10060-10160)

### Destruction

**54050**  Destruction of lesion(s), penis (eg, condyloma, papilloma, molluscum contagiosum, herpetic vesicle), simple; chemical

**54055**      electrodesiccation

**54056**      cryosurgery

**54057**      laser surgery

**54060**      surgical excision

**54065**  Destruction of lesion(s), penis (eg, condyloma, papilloma, molluscum contagiosum, herpetic vesicle), extensive (eg, laser surgery, electrosurgery, cryosurgery, chemosurgery)

(For destruction or excision of other lesions, see **Integumentary System**)

### Excision

**54100**  Biopsy of penis; (separate procedure)

**54105**      deep structures

**54110**  Excision of penile plaque (Peyronie disease);

**54111**      with graft to 5 cm in length

**54112**      with graft greater than 5 cm in length

**54115**  Removal foreign body from deep penile tissue (eg, plastic implant)

**54120**  Amputation of penis; partial

**54125**      complete

**54130**  Amputation of penis, radical; with bilateral inguinofemoral lymphadenectomy

**54135**      in continuity with bilateral pelvic lymphadenectomy, including external iliac, hypogastric and obturator nodes

(For lymphadenectomy (separate procedure), see 38760-38770)

**54150**  Circumcision, using clamp or other device with regional dorsal penile or ring block

(Do not report modifier 63 in conjunction with 54150)

(Report 54150 with modifier 52 when performed without dorsal penile or ring block)

**54160**  Circumcision, surgical excision other than clamp, device, or dorsal slit; neonate (28 days of age or less)

(Do not report modifier 63 in conjunction with 54160)

**54161**      older than 28 days of age

**54162**  Lysis or excision of penile post-circumcision adhesions

**54163**  Repair incomplete circumcision

**54164**  Frenulotomy of penis

(Do not report 54164 with circumcision codes 54150-54161, 54162, 54163)

### Introduction

**54200**  Injection procedure for Peyronie disease;

**54205**      with surgical exposure of plaque

**54220**  Irrigation of corpora cavernosa for priapism

**54230**  Injection procedure for corpora cavernosography

(For radiological supervision and interpretation, use 74445)

**54231**  Dynamic cavernosometry, including intracavernosal injection of vasoactive drugs (eg, papaverine, phentolamine)

**54235**  Injection of corpora cavernosa with pharmacologic agent(s) (eg, papaverine, phentolamine)

**54240**  Penile plethysmography

**54250**  Nocturnal penile tumescence and/or rigidity test

### Repair

(For other urethroplasties, see 53400-53430)

(For penile revascularization, use 37788)

**54300**  Plastic operation of penis for straightening of chordee (eg, hypospadias), with or without mobilization of urethra

**54304**  Plastic operation on penis for correction of chordee or for first stage hypospadias repair with or without transplantation of prepuce and/or skin flaps

**54308**  Urethroplasty for second stage hypospadias repair (including urinary diversion); less than 3 cm

**54312**      greater than 3 cm

**54316**  Urethroplasty for second stage hypospadias repair (including urinary diversion) with free skin graft obtained from site other than genitalia

**54318**  Urethroplasty for third stage hypospadias repair to release penis from scrotum (eg, third stage Cecil repair)

Surgery: Male Genital System

**54322** 1-stage distal hypospadias repair (with or without chordee or circumcision); with simple meatal advancement (eg, Magpi, V-flap)

**54324** with urethroplasty by local skin flaps (eg, flip-flap, prepucial flap)

**54326** with urethroplasty by local skin flaps and mobilization of urethra

**54328** with extensive dissection to correct chordee and urethroplasty with local skin flaps, skin graft patch, and/or island flap

(For urethroplasty and straightening of chordee, use 54308)

**54332** 1-stage proximal penile or penoscrotal hypospadias repair requiring extensive dissection to correct chordee and urethroplasty by use of skin graft tube and/or island flap

**54336** 1-stage perineal hypospadias repair requiring extensive dissection to correct chordee and urethroplasty by use of skin graft tube and/or island flap

**54340** Repair of hypospadias complications (ie, fistula, stricture, diverticula); by closure, incision, or excision, simple

**54344** requiring mobilization of skin flaps and urethroplasty with flap or patch graft

**54348** requiring extensive dissection and urethroplasty with flap, patch or tubed graft (includes urinary diversion)

**54352** Repair of hypospadias cripple requiring extensive dissection and excision of previously constructed structures including re-release of chordee and reconstruction of urethra and penis by use of local skin as grafts and island flaps and skin brought in as flaps or grafts

**54360** Plastic operation on penis to correct angulation

**54380** Plastic operation on penis for epispadias distal to external sphincter;

**54385** with incontinence

**54390** with exstrophy of bladder

**54400** Insertion of penile prosthesis; non-inflatable (semi-rigid)

**54401** inflatable (self-contained)

(For removal or replacement of penile prosthesis, see 54415, 54416)

**54405** Insertion of multi-component, inflatable penile prosthesis, including placement of pump, cylinders, and reservoir

(For reduced services, report 54405 with modifier 52)

**54406** Removal of all components of a multi-component, inflatable penile prosthesis without replacement of prosthesis

(For reduced services, report 54406 with modifier 52)

**54408** Repair of component(s) of a multi-component, inflatable penile prosthesis

**54410** Removal and replacement of all component(s) of a multi-component, inflatable penile prosthesis at the same operative session

**54411** Removal and replacement of all components of a multi-component inflatable penile prosthesis through an infected field at the same operative session, including irrigation and debridement of infected tissue

(For reduced services, report 54411 with modifier 52)

(Do not report 11042, 11043 in addition to 54411)

**54415** Removal of non-inflatable (semi-rigid) or inflatable (self-contained) penile prosthesis, without replacement of prosthesis

**54416** Removal and replacement of non-inflatable (semi-rigid) or inflatable (self-contained) penile prosthesis at the same operative session

**54417** Removal and replacement of non-inflatable (semi-rigid) or inflatable (self-contained) penile prosthesis through an infected field at the same operative session, including irrigation and debridement of infected tissue

(Do not report 11042, 11043 in addition to 54417)

**54420** Corpora cavernosa-saphenous vein shunt (priapism operation), unilateral or bilateral

**54430** Corpora cavernosa-corpus spongiosum shunt (priapism operation), unilateral or bilateral

**54435** Corpora cavernosa-glans penis fistulization (eg, biopsy needle, Winter procedure, rongeur, or punch) for priapism

**54440** Plastic operation of penis for injury

## Manipulation

**54450** Foreskin manipulation including lysis of preputial adhesions and stretching

# Testis

## Excision

(For abdominal perineal gangrene debridement, see 11004-11006)

**54500** Biopsy of testis, needle (separate procedure)

(For fine needle aspiration, see 10021, 10022)

(For evaluation of fine needle aspirate, see 88172, 88173)

**54505** Biopsy of testis, incisional (separate procedure)

(For bilateral procedure, report 54505 with modifier 50)

(When combined with vasogram, seminal vesiculogram, or epididymogram, use 55300)

**54512** Excision of extraparenchymal lesion of testis

**54520** Orchiectomy, simple (including subcapsular), with or without testicular prosthesis, scrotal or inguinal approach

(For bilateral procedure, report 54520 with modifier 50)

*Surgery: Male Genital System*

**Surgery: Male Genital System**

54522    Orchiectomy, partial

54530    Orchiectomy, radical, for tumor; inguinal approach

54535        with abdominal exploration

(For orchiectomy with repair of hernia, see 49505 or 49507 and 54520)

(For radical retroperitoneal lymphadenectomy, use 38780)

## Exploration

54550    Exploration for undescended testis (inguinal or scrotal area)

(For bilateral procedure, report 54550 with modifier 50)

54560    Exploration for undescended testis with abdominal exploration

(For bilateral procedure, report 54560 with modifier 50)

## Repair

54600    Reduction of torsion of testis, surgical, with or without fixation of contralateral testis

54620    Fixation of contralateral testis (separate procedure)

54640    Orchiopexy, inguinal approach, with or without hernia repair

(For bilateral procedure, report 54640 with modifier 50)

(For inguinal hernia repair performed in conjunction with inguinal orchiopexy, see 49495-49525)

54650    Orchiopexy, abdominal approach, for intra-abdominal testis (eg, Fowler-Stephens)

(For laparoscopic approach, use 54692)

54660    Insertion of testicular prosthesis (separate procedure)

(For bilateral procedure, report 54660 with modifier 50)

54670    Suture or repair of testicular injury

54680    Transplantation of testis(es) to thigh (because of scrotal destruction)

## Laparoscopy

Surgical laparoscopy always includes diagnostic laparoscopy. To report a diagnostic laparoscopy (peritoneoscopy) (separate procedure), use 49320.

54690    Laparoscopy, surgical; orchiectomy

54692        orchiopexy for intra-abdominal testis

54699    Unlisted laparoscopy procedure, testis

# Epididymis

## Incision

54700    Incision and drainage of epididymis, testis and/or scrotal space (eg, abscess or hematoma)

(For debridement of necrotizing soft tissue infection of external genitalia, see 11004-11006)

## Excision

54800    Biopsy of epididymis, needle

(For fine needle aspiration, see 10021, 10022)

(For evaluation of fine needle aspirate, see 88172, 88173)

54830    Excision of local lesion of epididymis

54840    Excision of spermatocele, with or without epididymectomy

54860    Epididymectomy; unilateral

54861        bilateral

## Exploration

54865    Exploration of epididymis, with or without biopsy

## Repair

54900    Epididymovasostomy, anastomosis of epididymis to vas deferens; unilateral

54901        bilateral

(For operating microscope, use 69990)

# Tunica Vaginalis

## Incision

55000    Puncture aspiration of hydrocele, tunica vaginalis, with or without injection of medication

## Excision

55040    Excision of hydrocele; unilateral

55041        bilateral

(With hernia repair, see 49495-49501)

## Repair

55060    Repair of tunica vaginalis hydrocele (Bottle type)

# Scrotum

## Incision

**55100**    Drainage of scrotal wall abscess

(See also 54700)

(For debridement of necrotizing soft tissue infection of external genitalia, see 11004-11006)

**55110**    Scrotal exploration

**55120**    Removal of foreign body in scrotum

## Excision

(For excision of local lesion of skin of scrotum, see **Integumentary System**)

**55150**    Resection of scrotum

## Repair

**55175**    Scrotoplasty; simple

**55180**        complicated

# Vas Deferens

## Incision

**55200**    Vasotomy, cannulization with or without incision of vas, unilateral or bilateral (separate procedure)

## Excision

**55250**    Vasectomy, unilateral or bilateral (separate procedure), including postoperative semen examination(s)

## Introduction

**55300**    Vasotomy for vasograms, seminal vesiculograms, or epididymograms, unilateral or bilateral

(For radiological supervision and interpretation, use 74440)

(When combined with biopsy of testis, see 54505 and use modifier 51)

## Repair

**55400**    Vasovasostomy, vasovasorrhaphy

(For bilateral procedure, report 55400 with modifier 50)

(For operating microscope, use 69990)

## Suture

**55450**    Ligation (percutaneous) of vas deferens, unilateral or bilateral (separate procedure)

# Spermatic Cord

## Excision

**55500**    Excision of hydrocele of spermatic cord, unilateral (separate procedure)

**55520**    Excision of lesion of spermatic cord (separate procedure)

**55530**    Excision of varicocele or ligation of spermatic veins for varicocele; (separate procedure)

**55535**        abdominal approach

**55540**        with hernia repair

## Laparoscopy

Surgical laparoscopy always includes diagnostic laparoscopy. To report a diagnostic laparoscopy (peritoneoscopy) (separate procedure), use 49320.

**55550**    Laparoscopy, surgical, with ligation of spermatic veins for varicocele

**55559**    Unlisted laparoscopy procedure, spermatic cord

# Seminal Vesicles

## Incision

**55600**    Vesiculotomy;

(For bilateral procedure, report 55600 with modifier 50)

**55605**        complicated

## Excision

**55650**    Vesiculectomy, any approach

(For bilateral procedure, report 55650 with modifier 50)

**55680**    Excision of Mullerian duct cyst

(For injection procedure, see 52010, 55300)

# Prostate

## Incision

**55700**    Biopsy, prostate; needle or punch, single or multiple, any approach

(If imaging guidance is performed, use 76942)

(For fine needle aspiration, see 10021, 10022)

(For evaluation of fine needle aspirate, see 88172, 88173)

(For transperineal stereotactic template guided saturation prostate biopsies, use 55706)

**55705**        incisional, any approach

**Surgery: Male Genital System**

**55706** Biopsies, prostate, needle, transperineal, stereotactic template guided saturation sampling, including imaging guidance

(Do not report 55706 in conjunction with 55700)

**55720** Prostatotomy, external drainage of prostatic abscess, any approach; simple

**55725** complicated

(For transurethral drainage, use 52700)

## Excision

(For transurethral removal of prostate, see 52601-52640)

(For transurethral destruction of prostate, see 53850-53852)

(For limited pelvic lymphadenectomy for staging (separate procedure), use 38562)

(For independent node dissection, see 38770-38780)

**55801** Prostatectomy, perineal, subtotal (including control of postoperative bleeding, vasectomy, meatotomy, urethral calibration and/or dilation, and internal urethrotomy)

**55810** Prostatectomy, perineal radical;

**55812** with lymph node biopsy(s) (limited pelvic lymphadenectomy)

**55815** with bilateral pelvic lymphadenectomy, including external iliac, hypogastric and obturator nodes

(If 55815 is carried out on separate days, use 38770 with modifier 50 and 55810)

**55821** Prostatectomy (including control of postoperative bleeding, vasectomy, meatotomy, urethral calibration and/or dilation, and internal urethrotomy); suprapubic, subtotal, 1 or 2 stages

**55831** retropubic, subtotal

**55840** Prostatectomy, retropubic radical, with or without nerve sparing;

**55842** with lymph node biopsy(s) (limited pelvic lymphadenectomy)

**55845** with bilateral pelvic lymphadenectomy, including external iliac, hypogastric, and obturator nodes

(If 55845 is carried out on separate days, use 38770 with modifier 50 and 55840)

(For laparoscopic retropubic radical prostatectomy, use 55866)

**55860** Exposure of prostate, any approach, for insertion of radioactive substance;

(For application of interstitial radioelement, see 77776-77778)

**55862** with lymph node biopsy(s) (limited pelvic lymphadenectomy)

**55865** with bilateral pelvic lymphadenectomy, including external iliac, hypogastric and obturator nodes

## Laparoscopy

Surgical laparoscopy always includes diagnostic laparoscopy. To report a diagnostic laparoscopy (peritoneoscopy) (separate procedure), use 49320.

**55866** Laparoscopy, surgical prostatectomy, retropubic radical, including nerve sparing, includes robotic assistance, when performed

(For open procedure, use 55840)

## Other Procedures

(For artificial insemination, see 58321, 58322)

**55870** Electroejaculation

**55873** Cryosurgical ablation of the prostate (includes ultrasonic guidance and monitoring)

**55875** Transperineal placement of needles or catheters into prostate for interstitial radioelement application, with or without cystoscopy

(For placement of needles or catheters into pelvic organs and/or genitalia [except prostate] for interstitial radioelement application, use 55920)

(For interstitial radioelement application, see 77776-77787)

(For ultrasonic guidance for interstitial radioelement application, use 76965)

**55876** Placement of interstitial device(s) for radiation therapy guidance (eg, fiducial markers, dosimeter), prostate (via needle, any approach), single or multiple

(Report supply of device separately)

(For imaging guidance, see 76942, 77002, 77012, 77021)

**55899** Unlisted procedure, male genital system

# Reproductive System Procedures

**55920** Placement of needles or catheters into pelvic organs and/or genitalia (except prostate) for subsequent interstitial radioelement application

(For placement of needles or catheters into prostate, use 55875)

(For insertion of uterine tandems and/or vaginal ovoids for clinical brachytherapy, use 57155)

(For insertion of Heyman capsules for clinical brachytherapy, use 58346)

# Intersex Surgery

**55970** Intersex surgery; male to female

**55980** female to male

# Female Genital System

(For pelvic laparotomy, use 49000)

(For excision or destruction of endometriomas, open method, see 49203-49205, 58957, 58958)

►(For paracentesis, see 49082, 49083, 49084)◄

(For secondary closure of abdominal wall evisceration or disruption, use 49900)

(For fulguration or excision of lesions, laparoscopic approach, use 58662)

(For chemotherapy, see 96401-96549)

## Vulva, Perineum, and Introitus

### Definitions

The following definitions apply to the vulvectomy codes (56620-56640):

A *simple* procedure is the removal of skin and superficial subcutaneous tissues.

A *radical* procedure is the removal of skin and deep subcutaneous tissue.

A *partial* procedure is the removal of less than 80% of the vulvar area.

A *complete* procedure is the removal of greater than 80% of the vulvar area.

## Incision

(For incision and drainage of sebaceous cyst, furuncle, or abscess, see 10040, 10060, 10061)

56405    Incision and drainage of vulva or perineal abscess

56420    Incision and drainage of Bartholin's gland abscess

(For incision and drainage of Skene's gland abscess or cyst, use 53060)

56440    Marsupialization of Bartholin's gland cyst

56441    Lysis of labial adhesions

56442    Hymenotomy, simple incision

## Destruction

56501    Destruction of lesion(s), vulva; simple (eg, laser surgery, electrosurgery, cryosurgery, chemosurgery)

56515        extensive (eg, laser surgery, electrosurgery, cryosurgery, chemosurgery)

(For destruction of Skene's gland cyst or abscess, use 53270)

(For cautery destruction of urethral caruncle, use 53265)

## Excision

56605    Biopsy of vulva or perineum (separate procedure); 1 lesion

+ 56606        each separate additional lesion (List separately in addition to code for primary procedure)

(Use 56606 in conjunction with 56605)

(For excision of local lesion, see 11420-11426, 11620-11626)

56620    Vulvectomy simple; partial

56625        complete

(For skin graft, see 15002 et seq)

56630    Vulvectomy, radical, partial;

(For skin graft, if used, see 15004-15005, 15120, 15121, 15240, 15241)

56631        with unilateral inguinofemoral lymphadenectomy

56632        with bilateral inguinofemoral lymphadenectomy

56633    Vulvectomy, radical, complete;

56634        with unilateral inguinofemoral lymphadenectomy

56637        with bilateral inguinofemoral lymphadenectomy

56640    Vulvectomy, radical, complete, with inguinofemoral, iliac, and pelvic lymphadenectomy

(For bilateral procedure, report 56640 with modifier 50)

(For lymphadenectomy, see 38760-38780)

56700    Partial hymenectomy or revision of hymenal ring

56740    Excision of Bartholin's gland or cyst

(For excision of Skene's gland, use 53270)

(For excision of urethral caruncle, use 53265)

(For excision or fulguration of urethral carcinoma, use 53220)

(For excision or marsupialization of urethral diverticulum, see 53230, 53240)

## Repair

(For repair of urethra for mucosal prolapse, use 53275)

56800    Plastic repair of introitus

56805    Clitoroplasty for intersex state

56810    Perineoplasty, repair of perineum, nonobstetrical (separate procedure)

(See also 56800)

(For repair of wounds to genitalia, see 12001-12007, 12041-12047, 13131-13133)

(For repair of recent injury of vagina and perineum, nonobstetrical, use 57210)

**Surgery: Female Genital System**

(For anal sphincteroplasty, see 46750, 46751)

(For episiorrhaphy, episioperineorrhaphy for recent injury of vulva and/or perineum, nonobstetrical, use 57210)

## Endoscopy

**56820**   Colposcopy of the vulva;

**56821**       with biopsy(s)

(For colposcopic examinations/procedures involving the vagina, see 57420, 57421; cervix, see 57452-57461)

# Vagina

## Incision

**57000**   Colpotomy; with exploration

**57010**       with drainage of pelvic abscess

**57020**   Colpocentesis (separate procedure)

**57022**   Incision and drainage of vaginal hematoma; obstetrical/postpartum

**57023**       non-obstetrical (eg, post-trauma, spontaneous bleeding)

## Destruction

**57061**   Destruction of vaginal lesion(s); simple (eg, laser surgery, electrosurgery, cryosurgery, chemosurgery)

**57065**       extensive (eg, laser surgery, electrosurgery, cryosurgery, chemosurgery)

## Excision

**57100**   Biopsy of vaginal mucosa; simple (separate procedure)

**57105**       extensive, requiring suture (including cysts)

**57106**   Vaginectomy, partial removal of vaginal wall;

**57107**       with removal of paravaginal tissue (radical vaginectomy)

**57109**       with removal of paravaginal tissue (radical vaginectomy) with bilateral total pelvic lymphadenectomy and para-aortic lymph node sampling (biopsy)

**57110**   Vaginectomy, complete removal of vaginal wall;

**57111**       with removal of paravaginal tissue (radical vaginectomy)

**57112**       with removal of paravaginal tissue (radical vaginectomy) with bilateral total pelvic lymphadenectomy and para-aortic lymph node sampling (biopsy)

**57120**   Colpocleisis (Le Fort type)

**57130**   Excision of vaginal septum

**57135**   Excision of vaginal cyst or tumor

## Introduction

**57150**   Irrigation of vagina and/or application of medicament for treatment of bacterial, parasitic, or fungoid disease

⊙ **57155**   Insertion of uterine tandems and/or vaginal ovoids for clinical brachytherapy

(For placement of needles or catheters into pelvic organs and/or genitalia [except prostate] for interstitial radioelement application, use 55920)

(For insertion of radioelement sources or ribbons, see 77761-77763, 77785-77787)

**57156**   Insertion of a vaginal radiation afterloading apparatus for clinical brachytherapy

**57160**   Fitting and insertion of pessary or other intravaginal support device

**57170**   Diaphragm or cervical cap fitting with instructions

**57180**   Introduction of any hemostatic agent or pack for spontaneous or traumatic nonobstetrical vaginal hemorrhage (separate procedure)

## Repair

(For urethral suspension, Marshall-Marchetti-Krantz type, abdominal approach, see 51840, 51841)

(For laparoscopic suspension, use 51990)

**57200**   Colporrhaphy, suture of injury of vagina (nonobstetrical)

**57210**   Colpoperineorrhaphy, suture of injury of vagina and/or perineum (nonobstetrical)

**57220**   Plastic operation on urethral sphincter, vaginal approach (eg, Kelly urethral plication)

**57230**   Plastic repair of urethrocele

**57240**   Anterior colporrhaphy, repair of cystocele with or without repair of urethrocele

**57250**   Posterior colporrhaphy, repair of rectocele with or without perineorrhaphy

(For repair of rectocele (separate procedure) without posterior colporrhaphy, use 45560)

**57260**   Combined anteroposterior colporrhaphy;

**57265**       with enterocele repair

+ **57267**   Insertion of mesh or other prosthesis for repair of pelvic floor defect, each site (anterior, posterior compartment), vaginal approach (List separately in addition to code for primary procedure)

(Use 57267 in conjunction with 45560, 57240-57265, 57285)

**57268**   Repair of enterocele, vaginal approach (separate procedure)

**57270**   Repair of enterocele, abdominal approach (separate procedure)

**57280**   Colpopexy, abdominal approach

Surgery: Female Genital System

**57282**    Colpopexy, vaginal; extra-peritoneal approach (sacrospinous, iliococcygeus)

**57283**        intra-peritoneal approach (uterosacral, levator myorrhaphy)

▶(Do not report 57283 in conjunction with 57556, 58263, 58270, 58280, 58292, 58294)◀

**57284**    Paravaginal defect repair (including repair of cystocele, if performed); open abdominal approach

(Do not report 57284 in conjunction with 51840, 51841, 51990, 57240, 57260, 57265, 58152, 58267)

**57285**        vaginal approach

(Do not report 57285 in conjunction with 51990, 57240, 57260, 57265, 58267)

**57287**    Removal or revision of sling for stress incontinence (eg, fascia or synthetic)

**57288**    Sling operation for stress incontinence (eg, fascia or synthetic)

(For laparoscopic approach, use 51992)

**57289**    Pereyra procedure, including anterior colporrhaphy

**57291**    Construction of artificial vagina; without graft

**57292**        with graft

**57295**    Revision (including removal) of prosthetic vaginal graft; vaginal approach

**57296**        open abdominal approach

(For laparoscopic approach, use 57426)

**57300**    Closure of rectovaginal fistula; vaginal or transanal approach

**57305**        abdominal approach

**57307**        abdominal approach, with concomitant colostomy

**57308**        transperineal approach, with perineal body reconstruction, with or without levator plication

**57310**    Closure of urethrovaginal fistula;

**57311**        with bulbocavernosus transplant

**57320**    Closure of vesicovaginal fistula; vaginal approach

(For concomitant cystostomy, see 51020-51040, 51101, 51102)

**57330**        transvesical and vaginal approach

(For abdominal approach, use 51900)

**57335**    Vaginoplasty for intersex state

## Manipulation

**57400**    Dilation of vagina under anesthesia (other than local)

**57410**    Pelvic examination under anesthesia (other than local)

**57415**    Removal of impacted vaginal foreign body (separate procedure) under anesthesia (other than local)

(For removal without anesthesia of an impacted vaginal foreign body, use the appropriate E/M code)

## Endoscopy/Laparoscopy

**57420**    Colposcopy of the entire vagina, with cervix if present;

**57421**        with biopsy(s) of vagina/cervix

(For colposcopic visualization of cervix and adjacent upper vagina, use 57452)

(When reporting colposcopies of multiple sites, use modifier 51 as appropriate. For colposcopic examinations/procedures involving the vulva, see 56820, 56821; cervix, see 57452-57461)

(For endometrial sampling (biopsy) performed in conjunction with colposcopy, use 58110)

**57423**    Paravaginal defect repair (including repair of cystocele, if performed), laparoscopic approach

(Do not report 57423 in conjunction with 49320, 51840, 51841, 51990, 57240, 57260, 58152, 58267)

**57425**    Laparoscopy, surgical, colpopexy (suspension of vaginal apex)

**57426**    Revision (including removal) of prosthetic vaginal graft, laparoscopic approach

(For vaginal approach, see 57295. For open abdominal approach, see 57296)

# Cervix Uteri

(For cervicography, use Category III code 0003T)

## Endoscopy

(For colposcopic examinations/procedures involving the vulva, see 56820, 56821; vagina, see 57420, 57421)

**57452**    Colposcopy of the cervix including upper/adjacent vagina;

(Do not report 57452 in addition to 57454-57461)

**57454**        with biopsy(s) of the cervix and endocervical curettage

**57455**        with biopsy(s) of the cervix

**57456**        with endocervical curettage

**57460**        with loop electrode biopsy(s) of the cervix

**57461**        with loop electrode conization of the cervix

(Do not report 57461 in addition to 57456)

(For endometrial sampling [biopsy] performed in conjunction with colposcopy, use 58110)

*Surgery: Female Genital System*

# Excision

(For radical surgical procedures, see 58200-58240)

**57500** Biopsy of cervix, single or multiple, or local excision of lesion, with or without fulguration (separate procedure)

**57505** Endocervical curettage (not done as part of a dilation and curettage)

**57510** Cautery of cervix; electro or thermal

**57511** cryocautery, initial or repeat

**57513** laser ablation

**57520** Conization of cervix, with or without fulguration, with or without dilation and curettage, with or without repair; cold knife or laser

(See also 58120)

**57522** loop electrode excision

**57530** Trachelectomy (cervicectomy), amputation of cervix (separate procedure)

**57531** Radical trachelectomy, with bilateral total pelvic lymphadenectomy and para-aortic lymph node sampling biopsy, with or without removal of tube(s), with or without removal of ovary(s)

(For radical abdominal hysterectomy, use 58210)

**57540** Excision of cervical stump, abdominal approach;

**57545** with pelvic floor repair

**57550** Excision of cervical stump, vaginal approach;

**57555** with anterior and/or posterior repair

**57556** with repair of enterocele

(For insertion of intrauterine device, use 58300)

(For insertion of any hemostatic agent or pack for control of spontaneous non-obstetrical hemorrhage, see 57180)

**57558** Dilation and curettage of cervical stump

# Repair

**57700** Cerclage of uterine cervix; nonobstetrical

**57720** Trachelorrhaphy, plastic repair of uterine cervix, vaginal approach

# Manipulation

**57800** Dilation of cervical canal, instrumental (separate procedure)

# Corpus Uteri

## Excision

**58100** Endometrial sampling (biopsy) with or without endocervical sampling (biopsy), without cervical dilation, any method (separate procedure)

(For endocervical curettage only, use 57505)

(For endometrial sampling (biopsy) performed in conjunction with colposcopy (57420, 57421, 57452-57461), use 58110)

**+ 58110** Endometrial sampling (biopsy) performed in conjunction with colposcopy (List separately in addition to code for primary procedure)

(Use 58110 in conjunction with 57420, 57421, 57452-57461)

**58120** Dilation and curettage, diagnostic and/or therapeutic (nonobstetrical)

(For postpartum hemorrhage, use 59160)

**58140** Myomectomy, excision of fibroid tumor(s) of uterus, 1 to 4 intramural myoma(s) with total weight of 250 g or less and/or removal of surface myomas; abdominal approach

**58145** vaginal approach

**58146** Myomectomy, excision of fibroid tumor(s) of uterus, 5 or more intramural myomas and/or intramural myomas with total weight greater than 250 g, abdominal approach

(Do not report 58146 in addition to 58140-58145, 58150-58240)

## Hysterectomy Procedures

**58150** Total abdominal hysterectomy (corpus and cervix), with or without removal of tube(s), with or without removal of ovary(s);

**58152** with colpo-urethrocystopexy (eg, Marshall-Marchetti-Krantz, Burch)

(For urethrocystopexy without hysterectomy, see 51840, 51841)

**58180** Supracervical abdominal hysterectomy (subtotal hysterectomy), with or without removal of tube(s), with or without removal of ovary(s)

**58200** Total abdominal hysterectomy, including partial vaginectomy, with para-aortic and pelvic lymph node sampling, with or without removal of tube(s), with or without removal of ovary(s)

**58210** Radical abdominal hysterectomy, with bilateral total pelvic lymphadenectomy and para-aortic lymph node sampling (biopsy), with or without removal of tube(s), with or without removal of ovary(s)

(For radical hysterectomy with ovarian transposition, use also 58825)

**58240**    Pelvic exenteration for gynecologic malignancy, with total abdominal hysterectomy or cervicectomy, with or without removal of tube(s), with or without removal of ovary(s), with removal of bladder and ureteral transplantations, and/or abdominoperineal resection of rectum and colon and colostomy, or any combination thereof

(For pelvic exenteration for lower urinary tract or male genital malignancy, use 51597)

**58260**    Vaginal hysterectomy, for uterus 250 g or less;

**58262**        with removal of tube(s), and/or ovary(s)

**58263**        with removal of tube(s), and/or ovary(s), with repair of enterocele

**58267**        with colpo-urethrocystopexy (Marshall-Marchetti-Krantz type, Pereyra type) with or without endoscopic control

**58270**        with repair of enterocele

(For repair of enterocele with removal of tubes and/or ovaries, use 58263)

**58275**    Vaginal hysterectomy, with total or partial vaginectomy;

**58280**        with repair of enterocele

**58285**    Vaginal hysterectomy, radical (Schauta type operation)

**58290**    Vaginal hysterectomy, for uterus greater than 250 g;

**58291**        with removal of tube(s) and/or ovary(s)

**58292**        with removal of tube(s) and/or ovary(s), with repair of enterocele

**58293**        with colpo-urethrocystopexy (Marshall-Marchetti-Krantz type, Pereyra type) with or without endoscopic control

**58294**        with repair of enterocele

## Introduction

▶(To report insertion of non-biodegradable drug delivery implant for contraception, use 11981. To report removal of implantable contraceptive capsules with subsequent insertion of non-biodegradable drug delivery implant, use 11976 and 11981)◀

**58300**    Insertion of intrauterine device (IUD)

**58301**    Removal of intrauterine device (IUD)

**58321**    Artificial insemination; intra-cervical

**58322**        intra-uterine

**58323**    Sperm washing for artificial insemination

**58340**    Catheterization and introduction of saline or contrast material for saline infusion sonohysterography (SIS) or hysterosalpingography

(For radiological supervision and interpretation of saline infusion sonohysterography, use 76831)

(For radiological supervision and interpretation of hysterosalpingography, use 74740)

**58345**    Transcervical introduction of fallopian tube catheter for diagnosis and/or re-establishing patency (any method), with or without hysterosalpingography

(For radiological supervision and interpretation, use 74742)

**58346**    Insertion of Heyman capsules for clinical brachytherapy

(For placement of needles or catheters into pelvic organs and/or genitalia [except prostate] for interstitial radioelement application, use 55920)

(For insertion of radioelement sources or ribbons, see 77761-77763, 77785-77787)

**58350**    Chromotubation of oviduct, including materials

(For materials supplied by physician, use 99070)

**58353**    Endometrial ablation, thermal, without hysteroscopic guidance

(For hysteroscopic procedure, use 58563)

**58356**    Endometrial cryoablation with ultrasonic guidance, including endometrial curettage, when performed

(Do not report 58356 in conjunction with 58100, 58120, 58340, 76700, 76856)

## Repair

**58400**    Uterine suspension, with or without shortening of round ligaments, with or without shortening of sacrouterine ligaments; (separate procedure)

**58410**        with presacral sympathectomy

(For anastomosis of tubes to uterus, use 58752)

**58520**    Hysterorrhaphy, repair of ruptured uterus (nonobstetrical)

**58540**    Hysteroplasty, repair of uterine anomaly (Strassman type)

(For closure of vesicouterine fistula, use 51920)

## Laparoscopy/Hysteroscopy

Surgical laparoscopy always includes diagnostic laparoscopy. To report a diagnostic laparoscopy (peritoneoscopy) (separate procedure), use 49320. To report a diagnostic hysteroscopy (separate procedure), use 58555.

**58541**    Laparoscopy, surgical, supracervical hysterectomy, for uterus 250 g or less;

**58542**        with removal of tube(s) and/or ovary(s)

(Do not report 58541, 58542 in conjunction with 49320, 57000, 57180, 57410, 58140-58146, 58545, 58546, 58561, 58661, 58670, 58671)

**58543**    Laparoscopy, surgical, supracervical hysterectomy, for uterus greater than 250 g;

Surgery: Female Genital System

**58544**    with removal of tube(s) and/or ovary(s)

(Do not report 58543-58544 in conjunction with 49320, 57000, 57180, 57410, 58140-58146, 58545, 58546, 58561, 58661, 58670, 58671)

**58545**    Laparoscopy, surgical, myomectomy, excision; 1 to 4 intramural myomas with total weight of 250 g or less and/or removal of surface myomas

**58546**    5 or more intramural myomas and/or intramural myomas with total weight greater than 250 g

**58548**    Laparoscopy, surgical, with radical hysterectomy, with bilateral total pelvic lymphadenectomy and para-aortic lymph node sampling (biopsy), with removal of tube(s) and ovary(s), if performed

(Do not report 58548 in conjunction with 38570-38572, 58210, 58285, 58550-58554)

**58550**    Laparoscopy, surgical, with vaginal hysterectomy, for uterus 250 g or less;

**58552**    with removal of tube(s) and/or ovary(s)

(Do not report 58550-58552 in conjunction with 49320, 57000, 57180, 57410, 58140-58146, 58545, 58546, 58561, 58661, 58670, 58671)

**58553**    Laparoscopy, surgical, with vaginal hysterectomy, for uterus greater than 250 g;

**58554**    with removal of tube(s) and/or ovary(s)

(Do not report 58553-58554 in conjunction with 49320, 57000, 57180, 57410, 58140-58146, 58545, 58546, 58561, 58661, 58670, 58671)

**58555**    Hysteroscopy, diagnostic (separate procedure)

**58558**    Hysteroscopy, surgical; with sampling (biopsy) of endometrium and/or polypectomy, with or without D & C

**58559**    with lysis of intrauterine adhesions (any method)

**58560**    with division or resection of intrauterine septum (any method)

**58561**    with removal of leiomyomata

**58562**    with removal of impacted foreign body

**58563**    with endometrial ablation (eg, endometrial resection, electrosurgical ablation, thermoablation)

**58565**    with bilateral fallopian tube cannulation to induce occlusion by placement of permanent implants

(Do not report 58565 in conjunction with 58555 or 57800)

(For unilateral procedure, use modifier 52)

**58570**    Laparoscopy, surgical, with total hysterectomy, for uterus 250 g or less;

**58571**    with removal of tube(s) and/or ovary(s)

**58572**    Laparoscopy, surgical, with total hysterectomy, for uterus greater than 250 g;

**58573**    with removal of tube(s) and/or ovary(s)

(Do not report 58570-58573 in conjunction with 49320, 57000, 57180, 57410, 58140-58146, 58150, 58545, 58546, 58561, 58661, 58670, 58671)

**58578**    Unlisted laparoscopy procedure, uterus

**58579**    Unlisted hysteroscopy procedure, uterus

# Oviduct/Ovary

## Incision

**58600**    Ligation or transection of fallopian tube(s), abdominal or vaginal approach, unilateral or bilateral

**58605**    Ligation or transection of fallopian tube(s), abdominal or vaginal approach, postpartum, unilateral or bilateral, during same hospitalization (separate procedure)

(For laparoscopic procedures, use 58670, 58671)

+ **58611**    Ligation or transection of fallopian tube(s) when done at the time of cesarean delivery or intra-abdominal surgery (not a separate procedure) (List separately in addition to code for primary procedure)

**58615**    Occlusion of fallopian tube(s) by device (eg, band, clip, Falope ring) vaginal or suprapubic approach

(For laparoscopic approach, use 58671)

(For lysis of adnexal adhesions, use 58740)

## Laparoscopy

Surgical laparoscopy always includes diagnostic laparoscopy. To report a diagnostic laparoscopy (peritoneoscopy) (separate procedure), use 49320.

**58660**    Laparoscopy, surgical; with lysis of adhesions (salpingolysis, ovariolysis) (separate procedure)

**58661**    with removal of adnexal structures (partial or total oophorectomy and/or salpingectomy)

**58662**    with fulguration or excision of lesions of the ovary, pelvic viscera, or peritoneal surface by any method

**58670**    with fulguration of oviducts (with or without transection)

**58671**    with occlusion of oviducts by device (eg, band, clip, or Falope ring)

**58672**    with fimbrioplasty

**58673**    with salpingostomy (salpingoneostomy)

(Codes 58672 and 58673 are used to report unilateral procedures. For bilateral procedure, use modifier 50)

**58679**    Unlisted laparoscopy procedure, oviduct, ovary

(For laparoscopic aspiration of ovarian cyst, use 49322)

(For laparoscopic biopsy of the ovary or fallopian tube, use 49321)

Surgery: Female Genital System

# Excision

**58700**   Salpingectomy, complete or partial, unilateral or bilateral (separate procedure)

**58720**   Salpingo-oophorectomy, complete or partial, unilateral or bilateral (separate procedure)

# Repair

**58740**   Lysis of adhesions (salpingolysis, ovariolysis)

(For laparoscopic approach, use 58660)

(For excision or destruction of endometriomas, open method, see 49203-49205, 58957, 58958)

(For fulguration or excision of lesions, laparoscopic approach, use 58662)

**58750**   Tubotubal anastomosis

**58752**   Tubouterine implantation

**58760**   Fimbrioplasty

(For laparoscopic approach, use 58672)

**58770**   Salpingostomy (salpingoneostomy)

(For laparoscopic approach, use 58673)

# Ovary

## Incision

**58800**   Drainage of ovarian cyst(s), unilateral or bilateral (separate procedure); vaginal approach

**58805**          abdominal approach

**58820**   Drainage of ovarian abscess; vaginal approach, open

**58822**          abdominal approach

⊙ **58823**   Drainage of pelvic abscess, transvaginal or transrectal approach, percutaneous (eg, ovarian, pericolic)

(For radiological supervision and interpretation, use 75989)

**58825**   Transposition, ovary(s)

## Excision

**58900**   Biopsy of ovary, unilateral or bilateral (separate procedure)

(For laparoscopic biopsy of the ovary or fallopian tube, use 49321)

**58920**   Wedge resection or bisection of ovary, unilateral or bilateral

**58925**   Ovarian cystectomy, unilateral or bilateral

**58940**   Oophorectomy, partial or total, unilateral or bilateral;

(For oophorectomy with concomitant debulking for ovarian malignancy, use 58952)

**58943**   for ovarian, tubal or primary peritoneal malignancy, with para-aortic and pelvic lymph node biopsies, peritoneal washings, peritoneal biopsies, diaphragmatic assessments, with or without salpingectomy(s), with or without omentectomy

**58950**   Resection (initial) of ovarian, tubal or primary peritoneal malignancy with bilateral salpingo-oophorectomy and omentectomy;

**58951**          with total abdominal hysterectomy, pelvic and limited para-aortic lymphadenectomy

**58952**          with radical dissection for debulking (ie, radical excision or destruction, intra-abdominal or retroperitoneal tumors)

(For resection of recurrent ovarian, tubal, primary peritoneal, or uterine malignancy, see 58957, 58958)

**58953**   Bilateral salpingo-oophorectomy with omentectomy, total abdominal hysterectomy and radical dissection for debulking;

**58954**          with pelvic lymphadenectomy and limited para-aortic lymphadenectomy

**58956**   Bilateral salpingo-oophorectomy with total omentectomy, total abdominal hysterectomy for malignancy

(Do not report 58956 in conjunction with 49255, 58150, 58180, 58262, 58263, 58550, 58661, 58700, 58720, 58900, 58925, 58940, 58957, 58958)

**58957**   Resection (tumor debulking) of recurrent ovarian, tubal, primary peritoneal, uterine malignancy (intra-abdominal, retroperitoneal tumors), with omentectomy, if performed;

**58958**          with pelvic lymphadenectomy and limited para-aortic lymphadenectomy

(Do not report 58957, 58958 in conjunction with 38770, 38780, 44005, 49000, 49203-49215, 49255, 58900-58960)

**58960**   Laparotomy, for staging or restaging of ovarian, tubal, or primary peritoneal malignancy (second look), with or without omentectomy, peritoneal washing, biopsy of abdominal and pelvic peritoneum, diaphragmatic assessment with pelvic and limited para-aortic lymphadenectomy

(Do not report 58960 in conjunction with 58957, 58958)

# In Vitro Fertilization

**58970**   Follicle puncture for oocyte retrieval, any method

(For radiological supervision and interpretation, use 76948)

**58974**   Embryo transfer, intrauterine

**58976**   Gamete, zygote, or embryo intrafallopian transfer, any method

(For laparoscopic adnexal procedures, see 58660-58673)

Surgery: Female Genital System

## Other Procedures

**58999**   Unlisted procedure, female genital system
(nonobstetrical)

# Maternity Care and Delivery

The services normally provided in uncomplicated maternity cases include antepartum care, delivery, and postpartum care.

Antepartum care includes the initial and subsequent history, physical examinations, recording of weight, blood pressures, fetal heart tones, routine chemical urinalysis, and monthly visits up to 28 weeks gestation, biweekly visits to 36 weeks gestation, and weekly visits until delivery. Any other visits or services within this time period should be coded separately.

Postpartum care only services (59430) include office or other outpatient visits following vaginal or cesarean section delivery.

Delivery services include admission to the hospital, the admission history and physical examination, management of uncomplicated labor, vaginal delivery (with or without episiotomy, with or without forceps), or cesarean delivery. When reporting delivery only services (59409, 59514, 59612, 59620), report inpatient post delivery management and discharge services using Evaluation and Management Services codes. Delivery and postpartum services (59410, 59515, 59614, 59622) include delivery services and all inpatient and outpatient postpartum services. Medical problems complicating labor and delivery management may require additional resources and should be identified by utilizing the codes in the **Medicine** and **Evaluation and Management Services** section in addition to codes for maternity care.

For medical complications of pregnancy (eg, cardiac problems, neurological problems, diabetes, hypertension, toxemia, hyperemesis, pre-term labor, premature rupture of membranes), see services in the **Medicine** and **Evaluation and Management Services** section.

For surgical complications of pregnancy (eg, appendectomy, hernia, ovarian cyst, Bartholin cyst), see services in the **Surgery** section.

If a physician provides all or part of the antepartum and/or postpartum patient care but does not perform delivery due to termination of pregnancy by abortion or referral to another physician for delivery, see the antepartum and postpartum care codes 59425-59426 and 59430.

(For circumcision of newborn, see 54150, 54160)

## Antepartum and Fetal Invasive Services

(For fetal intrauterine transfusion, use 36460)

(For unlisted fetal invasive procedure, use 59897)

**59000**   Amniocentesis; diagnostic

(For radiological supervision and interpretation, use 76946)

**59001**      therapeutic amniotic fluid reduction (includes ultrasound guidance)

**59012**   Cordocentesis (intrauterine), any method

(For radiological supervision and interpretation, use 76941)

**59015**   Chorionic villus sampling, any method

(For radiological supervision and interpretation, use 76945)

**59020**   Fetal contraction stress test

**59025**   Fetal non-stress test

**59030**   Fetal scalp blood sampling

(For repeat fetal scalp blood sampling, use 59030 and see modifiers 76 and 77)

**59050**   Fetal monitoring during labor by consulting physician (ie, non-attending physician) with written report; supervision and interpretation

**59051**      interpretation only

**59070**   Transabdominal amnioinfusion, including ultrasound guidance

**59072**   Fetal umbilical cord occlusion, including ultrasound guidance

**59074**   Fetal fluid drainage (eg, vesicocentesis, thoracocentesis, paracentesis), including ultrasound guidance

**59076**   Fetal shunt placement, including ultrasound guidance

## Excision

**59100**   Hysterotomy, abdominal (eg, for hydatidiform mole, abortion)

(When tubal ligation is performed at the same time as hysterotomy, use 58611 in addition to 59100)

**59120**   Surgical treatment of ectopic pregnancy; tubal or ovarian, requiring salpingectomy and/or oophorectomy, abdominal or vaginal approach

**59121**      tubal or ovarian, without salpingectomy and/or oophorectomy

**59130**      abdominal pregnancy

**59135**      interstitial, uterine pregnancy requiring total hysterectomy

**59136**      interstitial, uterine pregnancy with partial resection of uterus

**59140**      cervical, with evacuation

**59150** Laparoscopic treatment of ectopic pregnancy; without salpingectomy and/or oophorectomy

**59151** with salpingectomy and/or oophorectomy

**59160** Curettage, postpartum

## Introduction

(For intrauterine fetal transfusion, use 36460)

(For introduction of hypertonic solution and/or prostaglandins to initiate labor, see 59850-59857)

**59200** Insertion of cervical dilator (eg, laminaria, prostaglandin) (separate procedure)

## Repair

(For tracheloplasty, use 57700)

**59300** Episiotomy or vaginal repair, by other than attending physician

**59320** Cerclage of cervix, during pregnancy; vaginal

**59325** abdominal

**59350** Hysterorrhaphy of ruptured uterus

## Vaginal Delivery, Antepartum and Postpartum Care

**59400** Routine obstetric care including antepartum care, vaginal delivery (with or without episiotomy, and/or forceps) and postpartum care

**59409** Vaginal delivery only (with or without episiotomy and/or forceps);

**59410** including postpartum care

**59412** External cephalic version, with or without tocolysis

(Use 59412 in addition to code[s] for delivery)

**59414** Delivery of placenta (separate procedure);

(For antepartum care only, see 59425, 59426 or appropriate E/M code(s))

(For 1-3 antepartum care visits, see appropriate E/M code(s))

**59425** Antepartum care only; 4-6 visits

**59426** 7 or more visits

**59430** Postpartum care only (separate procedure)

## Cesarean Delivery

(For standby attendance for infant, use 99360)

(For low cervical cesarean section, see 59510, 59515, 59525)

**59510** Routine obstetric care including antepartum care, cesarean delivery, and postpartum care

**59514** Cesarean delivery only;

**59515** including postpartum care

(For classic cesarean section, see 59510, 59515, 59525)

**+ 59525** Subtotal or total hysterectomy after cesarean delivery (List separately in addition to code for primary procedure)

(Use 59525 in conjunction with 59510, 59514, 59515, 59618, 59620, 59622)

(For extraperitoneal cesarean section, or cesarean section with subtotal or total hysterectomy, see 59510, 59515, 59525)

## Delivery After Previous Cesarean Delivery

Patients who have had a previous cesarean delivery and now present with the expectation of a vaginal delivery are coded using codes 59610-59622. If the patient has a successful vaginal delivery after a previous cesarean delivery (VBAC), use codes 59610-59614. If the attempt is unsuccessful and another cesarean delivery is carried out, use codes 59618-59622. To report elective cesarean deliveries use code 59510, 59514 or 59515.

**59610** Routine obstetric care including antepartum care, vaginal delivery (with or without episiotomy, and/or forceps) and postpartum care, after previous cesarean delivery

**59612** Vaginal delivery only, after previous cesarean delivery (with or without episiotomy and/or forceps);

**59614** including postpartum care

**59618** Routine obstetric care including antepartum care, cesarean delivery, and postpartum care, following attempted vaginal delivery after previous cesarean delivery

**59620** Cesarean delivery only, following attempted vaginal delivery after previous cesarean delivery;

**59622** including postpartum care

## Abortion

(For medical treatment of spontaneous complete abortion, any trimester, use E/M codes 99201-99233)

(For surgical treatment of spontaneous abortion, use 59812)

**59812** Treatment of incomplete abortion, any trimester, completed surgically

**59820** Treatment of missed abortion, completed surgically; first trimester

**59821** second trimester

**59830** Treatment of septic abortion, completed surgically

**59840** Induced abortion, by dilation and curettage

**59841** Induced abortion, by dilation and evacuation

**59850** Induced abortion, by 1 or more intra-amniotic injections (amniocentesis-injections), including hospital admission and visits, delivery of fetus and secundines;

**Surgery: Female Genital System**

| 59851 | with dilation and curettage and/or evacuation |
|---|---|
| 59852 | with hysterotomy (failed intra-amniotic injection) |

(For insertion of cervical dilator, use 59200)

| 59855 | Induced abortion, by 1 or more vaginal suppositories (eg, prostaglandin) with or without cervical dilation (eg, laminaria), including hospital admission and visits, delivery of fetus and secundines; |
|---|---|
| 59856 | with dilation and curettage and/or evacuation |
| 59857 | with hysterotomy (failed medical evacuation) |

## Other Procedures

| 59866 | Multifetal pregnancy reduction(s) (MPR) |
|---|---|
| 59870 | Uterine evacuation and curettage for hydatidiform mole |
| 59871 | Removal of cerclage suture under anesthesia (other than local) |
| 59897 | Unlisted fetal invasive procedure, including ultrasound guidance, when performed |
| 59898 | Unlisted laparoscopy procedure, maternity care and delivery |
| 59899 | Unlisted procedure, maternity care and delivery |

# Endocrine System

(For pituitary and pineal surgery, see **Nervous System**)

## Thyroid Gland

### Incision

| 60000 | Incision and drainage of thyroglossal duct cyst, infected |
|---|---|

### Excision

| 60100 | Biopsy thyroid, percutaneous core needle |
|---|---|

(If imaging guidance is performed, see 76942, 77002, 77012, 77021)

(For fine needle aspiration, use 10021 or 10022)

(For evaluation of fine needle aspirate, see 88172, 88173)

| 60200 | Excision of cyst or adenoma of thyroid, or transection of isthmus |
|---|---|
| 60210 | Partial thyroid lobectomy, unilateral; with or without isthmusectomy |
| 60212 | with contralateral subtotal lobectomy, including isthmusectomy |
| 60220 | Total thyroid lobectomy, unilateral; with or without isthmusectomy |
| 60225 | with contralateral subtotal lobectomy, including isthmusectomy |

| 60240 | Thyroidectomy, total or complete |
|---|---|

(For thyroidectomy, subtotal or partial, use 60271)

| 60252 | Thyroidectomy, total or subtotal for malignancy; with limited neck dissection |
|---|---|
| 60254 | with radical neck dissection |
| 60260 | Thyroidectomy, removal of all remaining thyroid tissue following previous removal of a portion of thyroid |

(For bilateral procedure, report 60260 with modifier 50)

| 60270 | Thyroidectomy, including substernal thyroid; sternal split or transthoracic approach |
|---|---|
| 60271 | cervical approach |
| 60280 | Excision of thyroglossal duct cyst or sinus; |
| 60281 | recurrent |

(For thyroid ultrasonography, use 76536)

## Removal

| 60300 | Aspiration and/or injection, thyroid cyst |
|---|---|

(For fine needle aspiration, see 10021, 10022)

(If imaging guidance is performed, see 76942, 77012)

# Parathyroid, Thymus, Adrenal Glands, Pancreas, and Carotid Body

## Excision

(For pituitary and pineal surgery, see **Nervous System**)

| 60500 | Parathyroidectomy or exploration of parathyroid(s); |
|---|---|
| 60502 | re-exploration |
| 60505 | with mediastinal exploration, sternal split or transthoracic approach |
| + 60512 | Parathyroid autotransplantation (List separately in addition to code for primary procedure) |

(Use 60512 in conjunction with 60500, 60502, 60505, 60212, 60225, 60240, 60252, 60254, 60260, 60270, 60271)

| 60520 | Thymectomy, partial or total; transcervical approach (separate procedure) |
|---|---|
| 60521 | sternal split or transthoracic approach, without radical mediastinal dissection (separate procedure) |
| 60522 | sternal split or transthoracic approach, with radical mediastinal dissection (separate procedure) |

►(For thoracoscopic [VATS] thymectomy, see 32673)◄

| 60540 | Adrenalectomy, partial or complete, or exploration of adrenal gland with or without biopsy, transabdominal, lumbar or dorsal (separate procedure); |
|---|---|

**60545**          with excision of adjacent retroperitoneal tumor

                   (Do not report 60540, 60545 in conjunction with 50323)

                   (For bilateral procedure, report 60540 with modifier 50)

                   (For excision of remote or disseminated
                   pheochromocytoma, see 49203-49205)

                   (For laparoscopic approach, use 60650)

**60600**      Excision of carotid body tumor; without excision of
               carotid artery

**60605**          with excision of carotid artery

## Laparoscopy

Surgical laparoscopy always includes diagnostic
laparoscopy. To report a diagnostic laparoscopy
(peritoneoscopy) (separate procedure), use 49320.

**60650**      Laparoscopy, surgical, with adrenalectomy, partial or
               complete, or exploration of adrenal gland with or without
               biopsy, transabdominal, lumbar or dorsal

**60659**      Unlisted laparoscopy procedure, endocrine system

## Other Procedures

**60699**      Unlisted procedure, endocrine system

Surgery: Endocrine System

# Nervous System

## Skull, Meninges, and Brain

(For injection procedure for cerebral angiography, see 36100-36218)

(For injection procedure for ventriculography, see 61026, 61120)

(For injection procedure for pneumoencephalography, use 61055)

### Injection, Drainage, or Aspiration

**61000**  Subdural tap through fontanelle, or suture, infant, unilateral or bilateral; initial

**61001**      subsequent taps

**61020**  Ventricular puncture through previous burr hole, fontanelle, suture, or implanted ventricular catheter/reservoir; without injection

**61026**      with injection of medication or other substance for diagnosis or treatment

**61050**  Cisternal or lateral cervical (C1-C2) puncture; without injection (separate procedure)

**61055**      with injection of medication or other substance for diagnosis or treatment (eg, C1-C2)

(For radiological supervision and interpretation, see **Radiology**)

**61070**  Puncture of shunt tubing or reservoir for aspiration or injection procedure

(For radiological supervision and interpretation, use 75809)

### Twist Drill, Burr Hole(s), or Trephine

**61105**  Twist drill hole for subdural or ventricular puncture

⊘ **61107**  Twist drill hole(s) for subdural, intracerebral, or ventricular puncture; for implanting ventricular catheter, pressure recording device, or other intracerebral monitoring device

(For intracranial neuroendoscopic ventricular catheter placement, use 62160)

**61108**      for evacuation and/or drainage of subdural hematoma

**61120**  Burr hole(s) for ventricular puncture (including injection of gas, contrast media, dye, or radioactive material)

**61140**  Burr hole(s) or trephine; with biopsy of brain or intracranial lesion

**61150**      with drainage of brain abscess or cyst

**61151**      with subsequent tapping (aspiration) of intracranial abscess or cyst

**61154**  Burr hole(s) with evacuation and/or drainage of hematoma, extradural or subdural

(For bilateral procedure, report 61154 with modifier 50)

**61156**  Burr hole(s); with aspiration of hematoma or cyst, intracerebral

**61210**      for implanting ventricular catheter, reservoir, EEG electrode(s), pressure recording device, or other cerebral monitoring device (separate procedure)

(For intracranial neuroendoscopic ventricular catheter placement, use 62160)

**61215**  Insertion of subcutaneous reservoir, pump or continuous infusion system for connection to ventricular catheter

(For refilling and maintenance of an implantable infusion pump for spinal or brain drug therapy, use 95990)

(For chemotherapy, use 96450)

**61250**  Burr hole(s) or trephine, supratentorial, exploratory, not followed by other surgery

(For bilateral procedure, report 61250 with modifier 50)

**61253**  Burr hole(s) or trephine, infratentorial, unilateral or bilateral

(If burr hole[s] or trephine are followed by craniotomy at same operative session, use 61304-61321; do not use 61250 or 61253)

## Craniectomy or Craniotomy

**61304**  Craniectomy or craniotomy, exploratory; supratentorial

**61305**      infratentorial (posterior fossa)

**61312**  Craniectomy or craniotomy for evacuation of hematoma, supratentorial; extradural or subdural

**61313**      intracerebral

**61314**  Craniectomy or craniotomy for evacuation of hematoma, infratentorial; extradural or subdural

**61315**      intracerebellar

**+ 61316**  Incision and subcutaneous placement of cranial bone graft (List separately in addition to code for primary procedure)

(Use 61316 in conjunction with 61304, 61312, 61313, 61322, 61323, 61340, 61570, 61571, 61680-61705)

**61320**  Craniectomy or craniotomy, drainage of intracranial abscess; supratentorial

**61321**      infratentorial

**61322**  Craniectomy or craniotomy, decompressive, with or without duraplasty, for treatment of intracranial hypertension, without evacuation of associated intraparenchymal hematoma; without lobectomy

(Do not report 61313 in addition to 61322)

(For subtemporal decompression, use 61340)

**61323**    with lobectomy

(Do not report 61313 in addition to 61323)

(For subtemporal decompression, use 61340)

**61330**    Decompression of orbit only, transcranial approach

(For bilateral procedure, report 61330 with modifier 50)

**61332**    Exploration of orbit (transcranial approach); with biopsy

**61333**    with removal of lesion

**61334**    with removal of foreign body

**61340**    Subtemporal cranial decompression (pseudotumor cerebri, slit ventricle syndrome)

(For bilateral procedure, report 61340 with modifier 50)

(For decompressive craniotomy or craniectomy for intracranial hypertension, without hematoma evacuation, see 61322, 61323)

**61343**    Craniectomy, suboccipital with cervical laminectomy for decompression of medulla and spinal cord, with or without dural graft (eg, Arnold-Chiari malformation)

**61345**    Other cranial decompression, posterior fossa

(For orbital decompression by lateral wall approach, Kroenlein type, use 67445)

**61440**    Craniotomy for section of tentorium cerebelli (separate procedure)

**61450**    Craniectomy, subtemporal, for section, compression, or decompression of sensory root of gasserian ganglion

**61458**    Craniectomy, suboccipital; for exploration or decompression of cranial nerves

**61460**    for section of 1 or more cranial nerves

**61470**    for medullary tractotomy

**61480**    for mesencephalic tractotomy or pedunculotomy

**61490**    Craniotomy for lobotomy, including cingulotomy

(For bilateral procedure, report 61490 with modifier 50)

**61500**    Craniectomy; with excision of tumor or other bone lesion of skull

**61501**    for osteomyelitis

**61510**    Craniectomy, trephination, bone flap craniotomy; for excision of brain tumor, supratentorial, except meningioma

**61512**    for excision of meningioma, supratentorial

**61514**    for excision of brain abscess, supratentorial

**61516**    for excision or fenestration of cyst, supratentorial

(For excision of pituitary tumor or craniopharyngioma, see 61545, 61546, 61548)

**+ 61517**    Implantation of brain intracavitary chemotherapy agent (List separately in addition to code for primary procedure)

(Use 61517 only in conjunction with 61510 or 61518)

(Do not report 61517 for brachytherapy insertion. For intracavitary insertion of radioelement sources or ribbons, see 77785-77787)

**61518**    Craniectomy for excision of brain tumor, infratentorial or posterior fossa; except meningioma, cerebellopontine angle tumor, or midline tumor at base of skull

**61519**    meningioma

**61520**    cerebellopontine angle tumor

**61521**    midline tumor at base of skull

**61522**    Craniectomy, infratentorial or posterior fossa; for excision of brain abscess

**61524**    for excision or fenestration of cyst

**61526**    Craniectomy, bone flap craniotomy, transtemporal (mastoid) for excision of cerebellopontine angle tumor;

**61530**    combined with middle/posterior fossa craniotomy/craniectomy

**61531**    Subdural implantation of strip electrodes through 1 or more burr or trephine hole(s) for long-term seizure monitoring

(For stereotactic implantation of electrodes, use 61760)

(For craniotomy for excision of intracranial arteriovenous malformation, see 61680-61692)

**61533**    Craniotomy with elevation of bone flap; for subdural implantation of an electrode array, for long-term seizure monitoring

(For continuous EEG monitoring, see 95950-95954)

**61534**    for excision of epileptogenic focus without electrocorticography during surgery

**61535**    for removal of epidural or subdural electrode array, without excision of cerebral tissue (separate procedure)

**61536**    for excision of cerebral epileptogenic focus, with electrocorticography during surgery (includes removal of electrode array)

**61537**    for lobectomy, temporal lobe, without electrocorticography during surgery

**61538**    for lobectomy, temporal lobe, with electrocorticography during surgery

**61539**    for lobectomy, other than temporal lobe, partial or total, with electrocorticography during surgery

**61540**    for lobectomy, other than temporal lobe, partial or total, without electrocorticography during surgery

**61541**    for transection of corpus callosum

**61542**    for total hemispherectomy

**61543**    for partial or subtotal (functional) hemispherectomy

**61544**    for excision or coagulation of choroid plexus

**Surgery: Nervous System**

**Surgery: Nervous System**

**61545**    for excision of craniopharyngioma

(For craniotomy for selective amygdalohippocampectomy, use 61566)

(For craniotomy for multiple subpial transections during surgery, use 61567)

**61546**    Craniotomy for hypophysectomy or excision of pituitary tumor, intracranial approach

**61548**    Hypophysectomy or excision of pituitary tumor, transnasal or transseptal approach, nonstereotactic

(Do not report code 69990 in addition to code 61548)

**61550**    Craniectomy for craniosynostosis; single cranial suture

**61552**       multiple cranial sutures

(For cranial reconstruction for orbital hypertelorism, see 21260-21263)

(For reconstruction, see 21172-21180)

**61556**    Craniotomy for craniosynostosis; frontal or parietal bone flap

**61557**       bifrontal bone flap

**61558**    Extensive craniectomy for multiple cranial suture craniosynostosis (eg, cloverleaf skull); not requiring bone grafts

**61559**       recontouring with multiple osteotomies and bone autografts (eg, barrel-stave procedure) (includes obtaining grafts)

(For reconstruction, see 21172-21180)

**61563**    Excision, intra and extracranial, benign tumor of cranial bone (eg, fibrous dysplasia); without optic nerve decompression

**61564**       with optic nerve decompression

(For reconstruction, see 21181-21183)

**61566**    Craniotomy with elevation of bone flap; for selective amygdalohippocampectomy

**61567**       for multiple subpial transections, with electrocorticography during surgery

**61570**    Craniectomy or craniotomy; with excision of foreign body from brain

**61571**       with treatment of penetrating wound of brain

(For sequestrectomy for osteomyelitis, use 61501)

**61575**    Transoral approach to skull base, brain stem or upper spinal cord for biopsy, decompression or excision of lesion;

**61576**       requiring splitting of tongue and/or mandible (including tracheostomy)

(For arthrodesis, use 22548)

## Surgery of Skull Base

The surgical management of lesions involving the skull base (base of anterior, middle, and posterior cranial fossae) often requires the skills of several surgeons of different surgical specialties working together or in tandem during the operative session. These operations are usually not staged because of the need for definitive closure of dura, subcutaneous tissues, and skin to avoid serious infections such as osteomyelitis and/or meningitis.

The procedures are categorized according to

(1) *approach procedure* necessary to obtain adequate exposure to the lesion (pathologic entity), (2) *definitive procedure(s)* necessary to biopsy, excise or otherwise treat the lesion, and (3) *repair/reconstruction* of the defect present following the definitive procedure(s).

The *approach procedure* is described according to anatomical area involved, ie, anterior cranial fossa, middle cranial fossa, posterior cranial fossa, and brain stem or upper spinal cord.

The *definitive procedure(s)* describes the repair, biopsy, resection, or excision of various lesions of the skull base and, when appropriate, primary closure of the dura, mucous membranes, and skin.

The *repair/reconstruction procedure(s)* is reported separately if extensive dural grafting, cranioplasty, local or regional myocutaneous pedicle flaps, or extensive skin grafts are required.

For primary closure, see the appropriate codes (ie, 15732, 15756-15758).

When one surgeon performs the approach procedure, another surgeon performs the definitive procedure, and another surgeon performs the repair/reconstruction procedure, each surgeon reports only the code for the specific procedure performed.

If one surgeon performs more than one procedure (ie, approach procedure and definitive procedure), then both codes are reported, adding modifier 51 to the secondary, additional procedure(s).

### Approach Procedures

#### Anterior Cranial Fossa

**61580**    Craniofacial approach to anterior cranial fossa; extradural, including lateral rhinotomy, ethmoidectomy, sphenoidectomy, without maxillectomy or orbital exenteration

**61581**       extradural, including lateral rhinotomy, orbital exenteration, ethmoidectomy, sphenoidectomy and/or maxillectomy

**61582**     extradural, including unilateral or bifrontal craniotomy, elevation of frontal lobe(s), osteotomy of base of anterior cranial fossa

**61583**     intradural, including unilateral or bifrontal craniotomy, elevation or resection of frontal lobe, osteotomy of base of anterior cranial fossa

**61584**     Orbitocranial approach to anterior cranial fossa, extradural, including supraorbital ridge osteotomy and elevation of frontal and/or temporal lobe(s); without orbital exenteration

**61585**        with orbital exenteration

**61586**     Bicoronal, transzygomatic and/or LeFort I osteotomy approach to anterior cranial fossa with or without internal fixation, without bone graft

## Middle Cranial Fossa

**61590**     Infratemporal pre-auricular approach to middle cranial fossa (parapharyngeal space, infratemporal and midline skull base, nasopharynx), with or without disarticulation of the mandible, including parotidectomy, craniotomy, decompression and/or mobilization of the facial nerve and/or petrous carotid artery

**61591**     Infratemporal post-auricular approach to middle cranial fossa (internal auditory meatus, petrous apex, tentorium, cavernous sinus, parasellar area, infratemporal fossa) including mastoidectomy, resection of sigmoid sinus, with or without decompression and/or mobilization of contents of auditory canal or petrous carotid artery

**61592**     Orbitocranial zygomatic approach to middle cranial fossa (cavernous sinus and carotid artery, clivus, basilar artery or petrous apex) including osteotomy of zygoma, craniotomy, extra- or intradural elevation of temporal lobe

## Posterior Cranial Fossa

**61595**     Transtemporal approach to posterior cranial fossa, jugular foramen or midline skull base, including mastoidectomy, decompression of sigmoid sinus and/or facial nerve, with or without mobilization

**61596**     Transcochlear approach to posterior cranial fossa, jugular foramen or midline skull base, including labyrinthectomy, decompression, with or without mobilization of facial nerve and/or petrous carotid artery

**61597**     Transcondylar (far lateral) approach to posterior cranial fossa, jugular foramen or midline skull base, including occipital condylectomy, mastoidectomy, resection of C1-C3 vertebral body(s), decompression of vertebral artery, with or without mobilization

**61598**     Transpetrosal approach to posterior cranial fossa, clivus or foramen magnum, including ligation of superior petrosal sinus and/or sigmoid sinus

## Definitive Procedures

### Base of Anterior Cranial Fossa

**61600**     Resection or excision of neoplastic, vascular or infectious lesion of base of anterior cranial fossa; extradural

**61601**        intradural, including dural repair, with or without graft

### Base of Middle Cranial Fossa

**61605**     Resection or excision of neoplastic, vascular or infectious lesion of infratemporal fossa, parapharyngeal space, petrous apex; extradural

**61606**        intradural, including dural repair, with or without graft

**61607**     Resection or excision of neoplastic, vascular or infectious lesion of parasellar area, cavernous sinus, clivus or midline skull base; extradural

**61608**        intradural, including dural repair, with or without graft

Codes 61609-61612 are reported in addition to code(s) for primary procedure(s) 61605-61608. Report only one transection or ligation of carotid artery code per operative session.

**+ 61609**     Transection or ligation, carotid artery in cavernous sinus; without repair (List separately in addition to code for primary procedure)

**+ 61610**        with repair by anastomosis or graft (List separately in addition to code for primary procedure)

**+ 61611**     Transection or ligation, carotid artery in petrous canal; without repair (List separately in addition to code for primary procedure)

**+ 61612**        with repair by anastomosis or graft (List separately in addition to code for primary procedure)

**61613**     Obliteration of carotid aneurysm, arteriovenous malformation, or carotid-cavernous fistula by dissection within cavernous sinus

### Base of Posterior Cranial Fossa

**61615**     Resection or excision of neoplastic, vascular or infectious lesion of base of posterior cranial fossa, jugular foramen, foramen magnum, or C1-C3 vertebral bodies; extradural

**61616**        intradural, including dural repair, with or without graft

## Repair and/or Reconstruction of Surgical Defects of Skull Base

**61618**     Secondary repair of dura for cerebrospinal fluid leak, anterior, middle or posterior cranial fossa following surgery of the skull base; by free tissue graft (eg, pericranium, fascia, tensor fascia lata, adipose tissue, homologous or synthetic grafts)

**Surgery: Nervous System**

**61619**    by local or regionalized vascularized pedicle flap or myocutaneous flap (including galea, temporalis, frontalis or occipitalis muscle)

## Endovascular Therapy

**61623**    Endovascular temporary balloon arterial occlusion, head or neck (extracranial/intracranial) including selective catheterization of vessel to be occluded, positioning and inflation of occlusion balloon, concomitant neurological monitoring, and radiologic supervision and interpretation of all angiography required for balloon occlusion and to exclude vascular injury post occlusion

(If selective catheterization and angiography of arteries other than artery to be occluded is performed, use appropriate catheterization and radiologic supervision and interpretation codes)

(If complete diagnostic angiography of the artery to be occluded is performed immediately prior to temporary occlusion, use appropriate radiologic supervision and interpretation codes only)

**61624**    Transcatheter permanent occlusion or embolization (eg, for tumor destruction, to achieve hemostasis, to occlude a vascular malformation), percutaneous, any method; central nervous system (intracranial, spinal cord)

(See also 37204)

(For radiological supervision and interpretation, use 75894)

**61626**        non-central nervous system, head or neck (extracranial, brachiocephalic branch)

(See also 37204)

(For radiological supervision and interpretation, use 75894)

**61630**    Balloon angioplasty, intracranial (eg, atherosclerotic stenosis), percutaneous

**61635**    Transcatheter placement of intravascular stent(s), intracranial (eg, atherosclerotic stenosis), including balloon angioplasty, if performed

(61630 and 61635 include all selective vascular catheterization of the target vascular family, all diagnostic imaging for arteriography of the target vascular family, and all related radiological supervision and interpretation. When diagnostic arteriogram (including imaging and selective catheterization) confirms the need for angioplasty or stent placement, 61630 and 61635 are inclusive of these services. If angioplasty or stenting are not indicated, then the appropriate codes for selective catheterization and imaging should be reported in lieu of 61630 and 61635)

**61640**    Balloon dilatation of intracranial vasospasm, percutaneous; initial vessel

**+ 61641**        each additional vessel in same vascular family (List separately in addition to code for primary procedure)

**+ 61642**        each additional vessel in different vascular family (List separately in addition to code for primary procedure)

(Use 61641 and 61642 in conjunction with 61640)

(61640, 61641, 61642 include all selective vascular catheterization of the target vessel, contrast injection(s), vessel measurement, roadmapping, postdilatation angiography, and fluoroscopic guidance for the balloon dilatation)

## Surgery for Aneurysm, Arteriovenous Malformation, or Vascular Disease

Includes craniotomy when appropriate for procedure.

**61680**    Surgery of intracranial arteriovenous malformation; supratentorial, simple

**61682**        supratentorial, complex

**61684**        infratentorial, simple

**61686**        infratentorial, complex

**61690**        dural, simple

**61692**        dural, complex

**61697**    Surgery of complex intracranial aneurysm, intracranial approach; carotid circulation

**61698**        vertebrobasilar circulation

(61697, 61698 involve aneurysms that are larger than 15 mm or with calcification of the aneurysm neck, or with incorporation of normal vessels into the aneurysm neck, or a procedure requiring temporary vessel occlusion, trapping or cardiopulmonary bypass to successfully treat the aneurysm)

**61700**    Surgery of simple intracranial aneurysm, intracranial approach; carotid circulation

**61702**        vertebrobasilar circulation

**61703**    Surgery of intracranial aneurysm, cervical approach by application of occluding clamp to cervical carotid artery (Selverstone-Crutchfield type)

(For cervical approach for direct ligation of carotid artery, see 37600-37606)

**61705**    Surgery of aneurysm, vascular malformation or carotid-cavernous fistula; by intracranial and cervical occlusion of carotid artery

**61708**        by intracranial electrothrombosis

(For ligation or gradual occlusion of internal/common carotid artery, see 37605, 37606)

**61710**        by intra-arterial embolization, injection procedure, or balloon catheter

**61711**   Anastomosis, arterial, extracranial-intracranial (eg, middle cerebral/cortical) arteries

(For carotid or vertebral thromboendarterectomy, use 35301)

(Use 69990 when the surgical microscope is employed for the microsurgical procedure. Do not use 69990 for visualization with magnifying loupes or corrected vision)

## Stereotaxis

**61720**   Creation of lesion by stereotactic method, including burr hole(s) and localizing and recording techniques, single or multiple stages; globus pallidus or thalamus

**61735**       subcortical structure(s) other than globus pallidus or thalamus

**61750**   Stereotactic biopsy, aspiration, or excision, including burr hole(s), for intracranial lesion;

**61751**       with computed tomography and/or magnetic resonance guidance

(For radiological supervision and interpretation of computerized tomography, see 70450, 70460, or 70470 as appropriate)

(For radiological supervision and interpretation of magnetic resonance imaging, see 70551, 70552, or 70553 as appropriate)

**61760**   Stereotactic implantation of depth electrodes into the cerebrum for long-term seizure monitoring

**61770**   Stereotactic localization, including burr hole(s), with insertion of catheter(s) or probe(s) for placement of radiation source

**+ 61781**   Stereotactic computer-assisted (navigational) procedure; cranial, intradural (List separately in addition to code for primary procedure)

(Do not report 61781 in conjunction with 61720-61791, 61796-61799, 61863-61868, 62201, 77371-77373, 77432)

**+ 61782**       cranial, extradural (List separately in addition to code for primary procedure)

(Do not report 61781, 61782 by the same provider during the same surgical session)

**+ 61783**       spinal (List separately in addition to code for primary procedure)

(Do not report 61783 in conjunction with 63620, 63621)

**61790**   Creation of lesion by stereotactic method, percutaneous, by neurolytic agent (eg, alcohol, thermal, electrical, radiofrequency); gasserian ganglion

**61791**       trigeminal medullary tract

(61793 has been deleted. To report, see 61796-61800, 63620-63621)

## Stereotactic Radiosurgery (Cranial)

Cranial stereotactic radiosurgery is a distinct procedure that utilizes externally generated ionizing radiation to inactivate or eradicate defined target(s) in the head without the need to make an incision. The target is defined by and the treatment is delivered using high-resolution stereotactic imaging. Stereotactic radiosurgery codes and headframe application procedures are reported by the neurosurgeon. The radiation oncologist reports the appropriate code(s) for clinical treatment planning, physics and dosimetry, treatment delivery, and management from the **Radiation Oncology** section (77261-77790). Any necessary planning, dosimetry, targeting, positioning, or blocking by the neurosurgeon is included in the stereotactic radiation surgery services. The same physician should not report stereotactic radiosurgery services with radiation treatment management codes (77427-77435).

Cranial stereotactic radiosurgery is typically performed in a single planning and treatment session, using a rigidly attached stereotactic guiding device, other immobilization technology and/or a stereotactic image-guidance system, but can be performed with more than one planning session and in a limited number of treatment sessions, up to a maximum of five sessions. Do not report stereotactic radiosurgery more than once per lesion per course of treatment when the treatment requires more than one session.

Codes 61796 and 61797 involve stereotactic radiosurgery for simple cranial lesions. Simple cranial lesions are lesions less than 3.5 cm in maximum dimension that do not meet the definition of a complex lesion provided below. Report code 61796 when all lesions are simple.

Codes 61798 and 61799 involve stereotactic radiosurgery for complex cranial lesions and procedures that create therapeutic lesions (eg, thalamotomy or pallidotomy). All lesions 3.5 cm in maximum dimension or greater are complex. When performing therapeutic lesion creation procedures, report code 61798 only once regardless of the number of lesions created. Schwannomas, arterio-venous malformations, pituitary tumors, glomus tumors, pineal region tumors and cavernous sinus/parasellar/petroclival tumors are complex. Any lesion that is adjacent (5mm or less) to the optic nerve/optic chasm/optic tract or within the brainstem is complex. If treating multiple lesions, and any single lesion treated is complex, use 61798.

Do not report codes 61796-61800 in conjunction with code 20660.

Codes 61796-61799 include computer-assisted planning. Do not report codes 61796-61799 in conjunction with 61781-61783.

(For intensity modulated beam delivery plan and treatment, see 77301, 77418. For stereotactic body radiation therapy, see 77373, 77435)

Surgery: Nervous System

---

(61795 has been deleted. To report, see 61781, 61782, 61783)

**61796** Stereotactic radiosurgery (particle beam, gamma ray, or linear accelerator); 1 simple cranial lesion

(Do not report 61796 more than once per course of treatment)

(Do not report 61796 in conjunction with 61798)

**+ 61797** each additional cranial lesion, simple (List separately in addition to code for primary procedure)

(Use 61797 in conjunction with 61796, 61798)

(For each course of treatment, 61797 and 61799 may be reported no more than once per lesion. Do not report any combination of 61797 and 61799 more than 4 times for entire course of treatment regardless of number of lesions treated)

**61798** 1 complex cranial lesion

(Do not report 61798 more than once per course of treatment)

(Do not report 61798 in conjunction with 61796)

**+ 61799** each additional cranial lesion, complex (List separately in addition to code for primary procedure)

(Use 61799 in conjunction with 61798)

(For each course of treatment, 61797 and 61799 may be reported no more than once per lesion. Do not report any combination of 61797 and 61799 more than 4 times for entire course of treatment regardless of number of lesions treated)

**+ 61800** Application of stereotactic headframe for stereotactic radiosurgery (List separately in addition to code for primary procedure)

(Use 61800 in conjunction with 61796, 61798)

## Neurostimulators (Intracranial)

Codes 61850-61888 apply to both simple and complex neurostimulators. For initial or subsequent electronic analysis and programming of neurostimulator pulse generators, see codes 95970-95975.

Microelectrode recording, when performed by the operating surgeon in association with implantation of neurostimulator electrode arrays, is an inclusive service and should not be reported separately. If another physician participates in neurophysiological mapping during a deep brain stimulator implantation procedure, this service may be reported by the other physician with codes 95961-95962.

**61850** Twist drill or burr hole(s) for implantation of neurostimulator electrodes, cortical

**61860** Craniectomy or craniotomy for implantation of neurostimulator electrodes, cerebral, cortical

**61863** Twist drill, burr hole, craniotomy, or craniectomy with stereotactic implantation of neurostimulator electrode array in subcortical site (eg, thalamus, globus pallidus, subthalamic nucleus, periventricular, periaqueductal gray), without use of intraoperative microelectrode recording; first array

**+ 61864** each additional array (List separately in addition to primary procedure)

(Use 61864 in conjunction with 61863)

**61867** Twist drill, burr hole, craniotomy, or craniectomy with stereotactic implantation of neurostimulator electrode array in subcortical site (eg, thalamus, globus pallidus, subthalamic nucleus, periventricular, periaqueductal gray), with use of intraoperative microelectrode recording; first array

**+ 61868** each additional array (List separately in addition to primary procedure)

(Use 61868 in conjunction with 61867)

**61870** Craniectomy for implantation of neurostimulator electrodes, cerebellar; cortical

**61875** subcortical

**61880** Revision or removal of intracranial neurostimulator electrodes

**61885** Insertion or replacement of cranial neurostimulator pulse generator or receiver, direct or inductive coupling; with connection to a single electrode array

**61886** with connection to 2 or more electrode arrays

(For percutaneous placement of cranial nerve (eg, vagal, trigeminal) neurostimulator electrode(s), use 64553)

▶(For revision or removal of cranial nerve (eg, vagal, trigeminal) neurostimulator electrode array, use 64569)◀

**61888** Revision or removal of cranial neurostimulator pulse generator or receiver

(Do not report 61888 in conjunction with 61885 or 61886 for the same pulse generator)

## Repair

**62000** Elevation of depressed skull fracture; simple, extradural

**62005** compound or comminuted, extradural

**62010** with repair of dura and/or debridement of brain

**62100** Craniotomy for repair of dural/cerebrospinal fluid leak, including surgery for rhinorrhea/otorrhea

(For repair of spinal dural/CSF leak, see 63707, 63709)

**62115** Reduction of craniomegalic skull (eg, treated hydrocephalus); not requiring bone grafts or cranioplasty

**62116** with simple cranioplasty

**62117** requiring craniotomy and reconstruction with or without bone graft (includes obtaining grafts)

**62120** Repair of encephalocele, skull vault, including cranioplasty

**62121** Craniotomy for repair of encephalocele, skull base

**62140** Cranioplasty for skull defect; up to 5 cm diameter

**62141** larger than 5 cm diameter

**62142** Removal of bone flap or prosthetic plate of skull

**62143** Replacement of bone flap or prosthetic plate of skull

**62145** Cranioplasty for skull defect with reparative brain surgery

**62146** Cranioplasty with autograft (includes obtaining bone grafts); up to 5 cm diameter

**62147** larger than 5 cm diameter

**+ 62148** Incision and retrieval of subcutaneous cranial bone graft for cranioplasty (List separately in addition to code for primary procedure)

(Use 62148 in conjunction with 62140-62147)

## Neuroendoscopy

Surgical endoscopy always includes diagnostic endoscopy.

**+ 62160** Neuroendoscopy, intracranial, for placement or replacement of ventricular catheter and attachment to shunt system or external drainage (List separately in addition to code for primary procedure)

(Use 62160 only in conjunction with 61107, 61210, 62220-62230, 62258)

**62161** Neuroendoscopy, intracranial; with dissection of adhesions, fenestration of septum pellucidum or intraventricular cysts (including placement, replacement, or removal of ventricular catheter)

**62162** with fenestration or excision of colloid cyst, including placement of external ventricular catheter for drainage

**62163** with retrieval of foreign body

**62164** with excision of brain tumor, including placement of external ventricular catheter for drainage

**62165** with excision of pituitary tumor, transnasal or trans-sphenoidal approach

## Cerebrospinal Fluid (CSF) Shunt

**62180** Ventriculocisternostomy (Torkildsen type operation)

**62190** Creation of shunt; subarachnoid/subdural-atrial, -jugular, -auricular

**62192** subarachnoid/subdural-peritoneal, -pleural, other terminus

**62194** Replacement or irrigation, subarachnoid/subdural catheter

**62200** Ventriculocisternostomy, third ventricle;

**62201** stereotactic, neuroendoscopic method

(For intracranial neuroendoscopic procedures, see 62161-62165)

**62220** Creation of shunt; ventriculo-atrial, -jugular, -auricular

(For intracranial neuroendoscopic ventricular catheter placement, use 62160)

**62223** ventriculo-peritoneal, -pleural, other terminus

(For intracranial neuroendoscopic ventricular catheter placement, use 62160)

**62225** Replacement or irrigation, ventricular catheter

(For intracranial neuroendoscopic ventricular catheter placement, use 62160)

**62230** Replacement or revision of cerebrospinal fluid shunt, obstructed valve, or distal catheter in shunt system

(For intracranial neuroendoscopic ventricular catheter placement, use 62160)

**62252** Reprogramming of programmable cerebrospinal shunt

**62256** Removal of complete cerebrospinal fluid shunt system; without replacement

**62258** with replacement by similar or other shunt at same operation

(For percutaneous irrigation or aspiration of shunt reservoir, use 61070)

(For reprogramming of programmable CSF shunt, use 62252)

(For intracranial neuroendoscopic ventricular catheter placement, use 62160)

## Spine and Spinal Cord

(For application of caliper or tongs, use 20660)

(For treatment of fracture or dislocation of spine, see 22305-22327)

## Injection, Drainage, or Aspiration

Injection of contrast during fluoroscopic guidance and localization is an inclusive component of 62263, 62264, 62267, 62270-62273, 62280-62282, 62310-62319. Fluoroscopic guidance and localization is reported with 77003, unless a formal contrast study (myelography, epidurography, or arthrography) is performed, in which case the use of fluoroscopy is included in the supervision and interpretation codes.

For radiologic supervision and interpretation of epidurography, use 72275. Code 72275 is only to be used when an epidurogram is performed, images documented, and a formal radiologic report is issued.

Code 62263 describes a catheter-based treatment involving targeted injection of various substances (eg, hypertonic saline, steroid, anesthetic) via an indwelling epidural catheter. Code 62263 includes percutaneous insertion and removal of an epidural catheter (remaining

Surgery: Nervous System

in place over a several-day period), for the administration of multiple injections of a neurolytic agent(s) performed during serial treatment sessions (ie, spanning two or more treatment days). If required, adhesions or scarring may also be lysed by mechanical means. Code 62263 is **not** reported for each adhesiolysis treatment, but should be reported **once** to describe the entire series of injections/infusions spanning two or more treatment days.

Code 62264 describes multiple adhesiolysis treatment sessions performed on the same day. Adhesions or scarring may be lysed by injections of neurolytic agent(s). If required, adhesions or scarring may also be lysed mechanically using a percutaneously-deployed catheter.

Codes 62263 and 62264 include the procedure of injections of contrast for epidurography (72275) and fluoroscopic guidance and localization (77003) during initial or subsequent sessions.

▶Fluoroscopy (for localization) may be used in the placement of injections reported with 62310-62319, but is not required. If used, fluoroscopy should be reported with 77003. For epidurography, use 72275.

The placement and use of a catheter to administer one or more epidural or subarachnoid injections on a single calendar day should be reported in the same manner as if a needle had been used, ie, as a single injection using either 62310 or 62311. Such injections should not be reported with 62318 or 62319.

Threading a catheter into the epidural space, injecting substances at one or more levels and then removing the catheter should be treated as a single injection (62310, 62311). If the catheter is left in place to deliver substance(s) over a prolonged period (ie, more than a single calendar day) either continuously or via intermittent bolus, use 62318, 62319 as appropriate.

When reporting 62310-62319, code choice is based on the region at which the needle or catheter entered the body (eg, lumbar). Codes 62310-62319 should be reported only once, when the substance injected spreads or catheter tip insertion moves into another spinal region (eg, 62311 is reported only once for injection or catheter insertion at L3-4 with spread of the substance or placement of the catheter tip to the thoracic region).

Percutaneous spinal procedures are done with indirect visualization (eg, image guidance or endoscopic approaches) and without direct visualization (including through a microscope). Endoscopic assistance during an open procedure with direct visualization is reported using excision codes (eg, 63020-63035).◀

(Report 01996 for daily hospital management of continuous epidural or subarachnoid drug administration performed in conjunction with 62318-62319)

**62263**  Percutaneous lysis of epidural adhesions using solution injection (eg, hypertonic saline, enzyme) or mechanical means (eg, catheter) including radiologic localization (includes contrast when administered), multiple adhesiolysis sessions; 2 or more days

(62263 includes codes 72275 and 77003)

**62264**      1 day

(Do not report 62264 with 62263)

(62264 includes codes 72275 and 77003)

**62267**  Percutaneous aspiration within the nucleus pulposus, intervertebral disc, or paravertebral tissue for diagnostic purposes

(For imaging, use 77003)

(Do not report 62267 in conjunction with 10022, 20225, 62287, 62290, 62291)

**62268**  Percutaneous aspiration, spinal cord cyst or syrinx

(For radiological supervision and interpretation, see 76942, 77002, 77012)

**62269**  Biopsy of spinal cord, percutaneous needle

(For radiological supervision and interpretation, see 76942, 77002, 77012)

(For fine needle aspiration, see 10021, 10022)

(For evaluation of fine needle aspirate, see 88172, 88173)

**62270**  Spinal puncture, lumbar, diagnostic

**62272**  Spinal puncture, therapeutic, for drainage of cerebrospinal fluid (by needle or catheter)

**62273**  Injection, epidural, of blood or clot patch

(For injection of diagnostic or therapeutic substance(s), see 62310, 62311, 62318, 62319)

**62280**  Injection/infusion of neurolytic substance (eg, alcohol, phenol, iced saline solutions), with or without other therapeutic substance; subarachnoid

**62281**      epidural, cervical or thoracic

**62282**      epidural, lumbar, sacral (caudal)

**62284**  Injection procedure for myelography and/or computed tomography, spinal (other than C1-C2 and posterior fossa)

(For injection procedure at C1-C2, use 61055)

(For radiological supervision and interpretation, see **Radiology**)

▲ **62287**  Decompression procedure, percutaneous, of nucleus pulposus of intervertebral disc, any method utilizing needle based technique to remove disc material under fluoroscopic imaging or other form of indirect visualization, with the use of an endoscope, with discography and/or epidural injection(s) at the treated level(s), when performed, single or multiple levels, lumbar

►(This includes endoscopic approach)◄

►(Do not report 62287 in conjunction with 62267, 62290, 62311, 77003, 77012, 72295, when performed at same level)◄

►(For non-needle based technique for percutaneous decompression of nucleus pulposus of intervertebral disc, see codes 0276T, 0277T)◄

**62290**    Injection procedure for discography, each level; lumbar

**62291**        cervical or thoracic

(For radiological supervision and interpretation, see 72285, 72295)

**62292**    Injection procedure for chemonucleolysis, including discography, intervertebral disc, single or multiple levels, lumbar

**62294**    Injection procedure, arterial, for occlusion of arteriovenous malformation, spinal

▲ **62310**    Injection(s), of diagnostic or therapeutic substance(s) (including anesthetic, antispasmodic, opioid, steroid, other solution), not including neurolytic substances, including needle or catheter placement, includes contrast for localization when performed, epidural or subarachnoid; cervical or thoracic

▲ **62311**        lumbar or sacral (caudal)

▲ **62318**    Injection(s), including indwelling catheter placement, continuous infusion or intermittent bolus, of diagnostic or therapeutic substance(s) (including anesthetic, antispasmodic, opioid, steroid, other solution), not including neurolytic substances, includes contrast for localization when performed, epidural or subarachnoid; cervical or thoracic

▲ **62319**        lumbar or sacral (caudal)

(For transforaminal epidural injection, see 64479-64484)

(Report 01996 for daily hospital management of continuous epidural or subarachnoid drug administration performed in conjunction with 62318-62319)

## Catheter Implantation

(For percutaneous placement of intrathecal or epidural catheter, see codes 62270-62273, 62280-62284, 62310-62319)

**62350**    Implantation, revision or repositioning of tunneled intrathecal or epidural catheter, for long-term medication administration via an external pump or implantable reservoir/infusion pump; without laminectomy

**62351**        with laminectomy

(For refilling and maintenance of an implantable infusion pump for spinal or brain drug therapy, see 95990, 95991)

**62355**    Removal of previously implanted intrathecal or epidural catheter

## Reservoir/Pump Implantation

**62360**    Implantation or replacement of device for intrathecal or epidural drug infusion; subcutaneous reservoir

**62361**        nonprogrammable pump

**62362**        programmable pump, including preparation of pump, with or without programming

**62365**    Removal of subcutaneous reservoir or pump, previously implanted for intrathecal or epidural infusion

▲ **62367**    Electronic analysis of programmable, implanted pump for intrathecal or epidural drug infusion (includes evaluation of reservoir status, alarm status, drug prescription status); without reprogramming or refill

**62368**        with reprogramming

(For refilling and maintenance of an implantable infusion pump for spinal or brain drug therapy, see 95990-95991)

● **62369**        with reprogramming and refill

● **62370**        with reprogramming and refill (requiring physician's skill)

►(Do not report 62367-62370 in conjunction with 95990, 95991. For refilling and maintenance of a reservoir or an implantable infusion pump for spinal or brain drug delivery without reprogramming, see 95990, 95991)◄

## Posterior Extradural Laminotomy or Laminectomy for Exploration/ Decompression of Neural Elements or Excision of Herniated Intervertebral Discs

►Endoscopically assisted laminotomy (hemilaminectomy) requires open and direct visualization. When visualization is only endoscopic and/or image guidance, the procedure is percutaneous and reported using 0274T, 0275T.◄

(When 63001-63048 are followed by arthrodesis, see 22590-22614)

**63001**    Laminectomy with exploration and/or decompression of spinal cord and/or cauda equina, without facetectomy, foraminotomy or discectomy (eg, spinal stenosis), 1 or 2 vertebral segments; cervical

**63003**        thoracic

**63005**        lumbar, except for spondylolisthesis

**63011**        sacral

**63012**    Laminectomy with removal of abnormal facets and/or pars inter-articularis with decompression of cauda equina and nerve roots for spondylolisthesis, lumbar (Gill type procedure)

**63015**    Laminectomy with exploration and/or decompression of spinal cord and/or cauda equina, without facetectomy, foraminotomy or discectomy (eg, spinal stenosis), more than 2 vertebral segments; cervical

**63016**        thoracic

**Surgery: Nervous System**

**63017**        lumbar

▲ **63020**    Laminotomy (hemilaminectomy), with decompression of nerve root(s), including partial facetectomy, foraminotomy and/or excision of herniated intervertebral disc; 1 interspace, cervical

(For bilateral procedure, report 63020 with modifier 50)

▲ **63030**        1 interspace, lumbar

(For bilateral procedure, report 63030 with modifier 50)

+▲ **63035**        each additional interspace, cervical or lumbar (List separately in addition to code for primary procedure)

(Use 63035 in conjunction with 63020-63030)

(For bilateral procedure, report 63035 with modifier 50)

►(For percutaneous endoscopic approach, see 0274T, 0275T)◄

**63040**    Laminotomy (hemilaminectomy), with decompression of nerve root(s), including partial facetectomy, foraminotomy and/or excision of herniated intervertebral disc, reexploration, single interspace; cervical

(For bilateral procedure, report 63040 with modifier 50)

**63042**        lumbar

(For bilateral procedure, report 63042 with modifier 50)

+ **63043**        each additional cervical interspace (List separately in addition to code for primary procedure)

(Use 63043 in conjunction with 63040)

(For bilateral procedure, report 63043 with modifier 50)

+ **63044**        each additional lumbar interspace (List separately in addition to code for primary procedure)

(Use 63044 in conjunction with 63042)

(For bilateral procedure, report 63044 with modifier 50)

**63045**    Laminectomy, facetectomy and foraminotomy (unilateral or bilateral with decompression of spinal cord, cauda equina and/or nerve root[s], [eg, spinal or lateral recess stenosis]), single vertebral segment; cervical

**63046**        thoracic

**63047**        lumbar

+ **63048**        each additional segment, cervical, thoracic, or lumbar (List separately in addition to code for primary procedure)

(Use 63048 in conjunction with 63045-63047)

**63050**    Laminoplasty, cervical, with decompression of the spinal cord, 2 or more vertebral segments;

**63051**        with reconstruction of the posterior bony elements (including the application of bridging bone graft and non-segmental fixation devices (eg, wire, suture, mini-plates), when performed)

(Do not report 63050 or 63051 in conjunction with 22600, 22614, 22840-22842, 63001, 63015, 63045, 63048, 63295 for the same vertebral segment(s))

## Transpedicular or Costovertebral Approach for Posterolateral Extradural Exploration/Decompression

**63055**    Transpedicular approach with decompression of spinal cord, equina and/or nerve root(s) (eg, herniated intervertebral disc), single segment; thoracic

**63056**        lumbar (including transfacet, or lateral extraforaminal approach) (eg, far lateral herniated intervertebral disc)

+ **63057**        each additional segment, thoracic or lumbar (List separately in addition to code for primary procedure)

(Use 63057 in conjunction with 63055, 63056)

**63064**    Costovertebral approach with decompression of spinal cord or nerve root(s) (eg, herniated intervertebral disc), thoracic; single segment

+ **63066**        each additional segment (List separately in addition to code for primary procedure)

(Use 63066 in conjunction with 63064)

(For excision of thoracic intraspinal lesions by laminectomy, see 63266, 63271, 63276, 63281, 63286)

## Anterior or Anterolateral Approach for Extradural Exploration/Decompression

For the following codes, when two surgeons work together as primary surgeons performing distinct part(s) of spinal cord exploration/decompression operation, each surgeon should report his/her distinct operative work by appending modifier 62 to the procedure code (and any associated add-on codes for that procedure code as long as both surgeons continue to work together as primary surgeons). In this situation, modifier 62 may be appended to the definitive procedure code(s) 63075, 63077, 63081, 63085, 63087, 63090 and, as appropriate, to associated additional interspace add-on code(s) 63076, 63078 or additional segment add-on code(s) 63082, 63086, 63088, 63091 as long as both surgeons continue to work together as primary surgeons.

**63075**    Discectomy, anterior, with decompression of spinal cord and/or nerve root(s), including osteophytectomy; cervical, single interspace

(Do not report 63075 in conjunction with 22554, even if performed by separate providers. To report anterior cervical discectomy and interbody fusion at the same level during the same session, use 22551)

+ **63076**        cervical, each additional interspace (List separately in addition to code for primary procedure)

(Do not report 63076 in conjunction with 22554, even if performed by separate providers. To report anterior cervical discectomy and interbody fusion at the same level during the same session, use 22552)

(Use 63076 in conjunction with 63075)

**Surgery: Nervous System**

**63077**  thoracic, single interspace

**+ 63078**  thoracic, each additional interspace (List separately in addition to code for primary procedure)

(Use 63078 in conjunction with 63077)

(Do not report code 69990 in addition to codes 63075-63078)

**63081**  Vertebral corpectomy (vertebral body resection), partial or complete, anterior approach with decompression of spinal cord and/or nerve root(s); cervical, single segment

**+ 63082**  cervical, each additional segment (List separately in addition to code for primary procedure)

(Use 63082 in conjunction with 63081)

(For transoral approach, see 61575, 61576)

**63085**  Vertebral corpectomy (vertebral body resection), partial or complete, transthoracic approach with decompression of spinal cord and/or nerve root(s); thoracic, single segment

**+ 63086**  thoracic, each additional segment (List separately in addition to code for primary procedure)

(Use 63086 in conjunction with 63085)

**63087**  Vertebral corpectomy (vertebral body resection), partial or complete, combined thoracolumbar approach with decompression of spinal cord, cauda equina or nerve root(s), lower thoracic or lumbar; single segment

**+ 63088**  each additional segment (List separately in addition to code for primary procedure)

(Use 63088 in conjunction with 63087)

**63090**  Vertebral corpectomy (vertebral body resection), partial or complete, transperitoneal or retroperitoneal approach with decompression of spinal cord, cauda equina or nerve root(s), lower thoracic, lumbar, or sacral; single segment

**+ 63091**  each additional segment (List separately in addition to code for primary procedure)

(Use 63091 in conjunction with 63090)

(Procedures 63081-63091 include discectomy above and/or below vertebral segment)

(If followed by arthrodesis, see 22548-22812)

(For reconstruction of spine, use appropriate vertebral corpectomy codes 63081-63091, bone graft codes 20930-20938, arthrodesis codes 22548-22812, and spinal instrumentation codes 22840-22855)

## Lateral Extracavitary Approach for Extradural Exploration/Decompression

**63101**  Vertebral corpectomy (vertebral body resection), partial or complete, lateral extracavitary approach with decompression of spinal cord and/or nerve root(s) (eg, for tumor or retropulsed bone fragments); thoracic, single segment

**63102**  lumbar, single segment

**+ 63103**  thoracic or lumbar, each additional segment (List separately in addition to code for primary procedure)

(Use 63103 in conjunction with 63101 and 63102)

## Incision

**63170**  Laminectomy with myelotomy (eg, Bischof or DREZ type), cervical, thoracic, or thoracolumbar

**63172**  Laminectomy with drainage of intramedullary cyst/syrinx; to subarachnoid space

**63173**  to peritoneal or pleural space

**63180**  Laminectomy and section of dentate ligaments, with or without dural graft, cervical; 1 or 2 segments

**63182**  more than 2 segments

**63185**  Laminectomy with rhizotomy; 1 or 2 segments

**63190**  more than 2 segments

**63191**  Laminectomy with section of spinal accessory nerve

(For bilateral procedure, report 63191 with modifier 50)

(For resection of sternocleidomastoid muscle, use 21720)

**63194**  Laminectomy with cordotomy, with section of 1 spinothalamic tract, 1 stage; cervical

**63195**  thoracic

**63196**  Laminectomy with cordotomy, with section of both spinothalamic tracts, 1 stage; cervical

**63197**  thoracic

**63198**  Laminectomy with cordotomy with section of both spinothalamic tracts, 2 stages within 14 days; cervical

**63199**  thoracic

**63200**  Laminectomy, with release of tethered spinal cord, lumbar

## Excision by Laminectomy of Lesion Other Than Herniated Disc

**63250**  Laminectomy for excision or occlusion of arteriovenous malformation of spinal cord; cervical

**63251**  thoracic

**63252**  thoracolumbar

**63265**  Laminectomy for excision or evacuation of intraspinal lesion other than neoplasm, extradural; cervical

**63266**  thoracic

**63267**  lumbar

**63268**  sacral

**63270**  Laminectomy for excision of intraspinal lesion other than neoplasm, intradural; cervical

**63271**  thoracic

**63272**  lumbar

Surgery: Nervous System

| | |
|---|---|
| 63273 | sacral |
| 63275 | Laminectomy for biopsy/excision of intraspinal neoplasm; extradural, cervical |
| 63276 | extradural, thoracic |
| 63277 | extradural, lumbar |
| 63278 | extradural, sacral |
| 63280 | intradural, extramedullary, cervical |
| 63281 | intradural, extramedullary, thoracic |
| 63282 | intradural, extramedullary, lumbar |
| 63283 | intradural, sacral |
| 63285 | intradural, intramedullary, cervical |
| 63286 | intradural, intramedullary, thoracic |
| 63287 | intradural, intramedullary, thoracolumbar |
| 63290 | combined extradural-intradural lesion, any level |

(For drainage of intramedullary cyst/syrinx, use 63172, 63173)

+ 63295    Osteoplastic reconstruction of dorsal spinal elements, following primary intraspinal procedure (List separately in addition to code for primary procedure)

(Use 63295 in conjunction with 63172, 63173, 63185, 63190, 63200-63290)

(Do not report 63295 in conjunction with 22590-22614, 22840-22844, 63050, 63051 for the same vertebral segment(s))

## Excision, Anterior or Anterolateral Approach, Intraspinal Lesion

For the following codes, when two surgeons work together as primary surgeons performing distinct part(s) of an anterior approach for an intraspinal excision, each surgeon should report his/her distinct operative work by appending modifier 62 to the single definitive procedure code. In this situation, modifier 62 may be appended to the definitive procedure code(s) 63300-63307 and, as appropriate, to the associated additional segment add-on code 63308 as long as both surgeons continue to work together as primary surgeons.

(For arthrodesis, see 22548-22585)

(For reconstruction of spine, see 20930-20938)

| | |
|---|---|
| 63300 | Vertebral corpectomy (vertebral body resection), partial or complete, for excision of intraspinal lesion, single segment; extradural, cervical |
| 63301 | extradural, thoracic by transthoracic approach |
| 63302 | extradural, thoracic by thoracolumbar approach |
| 63303 | extradural, lumbar or sacral by transperitoneal or retroperitoneal approach |
| 63304 | intradural, cervical |
| 63305 | intradural, thoracic by transthoracic approach |
| 63306 | intradural, thoracic by thoracolumbar approach |
| 63307 | intradural, lumbar or sacral by transperitoneal or retroperitoneal approach |
| + 63308 | each additional segment (List separately in addition to codes for single segment) |

(Use 63308 in conjunction with 63300-63307)

## Stereotaxis

| | |
|---|---|
| 63600 | Creation of lesion of spinal cord by stereotactic method, percutaneous, any modality (including stimulation and/or recording) |
| 63610 | Stereotactic stimulation of spinal cord, percutaneous, separate procedure not followed by other surgery |
| 63615 | Stereotactic biopsy, aspiration, or excision of lesion, spinal cord |

## Stereotactic Radiosurgery (Spinal)

Spinal stereotactic radiosurgery is a distinct procedure that utilizes externally generated ionizing radiation to inactivate or eradicate defined target(s) in the spine without the need to make an incision. The target is defined by and the treatment is delivered using high-resolution stereotactic imaging. These codes are reported by the surgeon. The radiation oncologist reports the appropriate code(s) for clinical treatment planning, physics and dosimetry, treatment delivery and management from the **Radiation Oncology** section (77261-77790). Any necessary planning, dosimetry, targeting, positioning, or blocking by the neurosurgeon is included in the stereotactic radiation surgery services. The same physician should not report stereotactic radiosurgery services with radiation treatment management codes (77427-77432).

Spinal stereotactic radiosurgery is typically performed in a single planning and treatment session using a stereotactic image-guidance system, but can be performed with a planning session and in a limited number of treatment sessions, up to a maximum of five sessions. Do not report stereotactic radiosurgery more than once per lesion per course of treatment when the treatment requires greater than one session.

Stereotactic spinal surgery is only used when the tumor being treated affects spinal neural tissue or abuts the dura mater. Arteriovenous malformations must be subdural. For other radiation services of the spine, see **Radiation Oncology** services.

Codes 63620, 63621 include computer-assisted planning. Do not report 63620, 63621 in conjunction with 61781-61783.

(For intensity modulated beam delivery plan and treatment, see 77301, 77418. For stereotactic body radiation therapy, see 77373, 77435)

**63620**  Stereotactic radiosurgery (particle beam, gamma ray, or linear accelerator); 1 spinal lesion

(Do not report 63620 more than once per course of treatment)

**+ 63621**  each additional spinal lesion (List separately in addition to code for primary procedure)

(Report 63621 in conjunction with 63620)

(For each course of treatment, 63621 may be reported no more than once per lesion. Do not report 63621 more than 2 times for entire course of treatment regardless of number of lesions treated)

## Neurostimulators (Spinal)

Codes 63650-63688 apply to both simple and complex neurostimulators. For initial or subsequent electronic analysis and programming of neurostimulator pulse generators, see codes 95970-95975.

Codes 63650, 63655, and 63661-63664 describe the operative placement, revision, replacement, or removal of the spinal neurostimulator system components to provide spinal electrical stimulation. A neurostimulator system includes an implanted neurostimulator, external controller, extension, and collection of contacts. Multiple contacts or electrodes (4 or more) provide the actual electrical stimulation in the epidural space.

For percutaneously placed neurostimulator systems (63650, 63661, 63663), the contacts are on a catheter-like lead. An array defines the collection of contacts that are on one catheter.

For systems placed via an open surgical exposure (63655, 63662, 63664), the contacts are on a plate or paddle-shaped surface.

Do not report 63661 or 63663 when removing or replacing a temporary percutaneously placed array for an external generator.

**63650**  Percutaneous implantation of neurostimulator electrode array, epidural

**63655**  Laminectomy for implantation of neurostimulator electrodes, plate/paddle, epidural

(63660 has been deleted. To report, see 63661-63664)

**63661**  Removal of spinal neurostimulator electrode percutaneous array(s), including fluoroscopy, when performed

**63662**  Removal of spinal neurostimulator electrode plate/paddle(s) placed via laminotomy or laminectomy, including fluoroscopy, when performed

**63663**  Revision including replacement, when performed, of spinal neurostimulator electrode percutaneous array(s), including fluoroscopy, when performed

(Do not report 63663 in conjunction with 63661, 63662 for the same spinal level)

**63664**  Revision including replacement, when performed, of spinal neurostimulator electrode plate/paddle(s) placed via laminotomy or laminectomy, including fluoroscopy, when performed

(Do not report 63664 in conjunction with 63661, 63662 for the same spinal level)

**63685**  Insertion or replacement of spinal neurostimulator pulse generator or receiver, direct or inductive coupling

(Do not report 63685 in conjunction with 63688 for the same pulse generator or receiver)

**63688**  Revision or removal of implanted spinal neurostimulator pulse generator or receiver

(For electronic analysis of implanted neurostimulator pulse generator system, see 95970-95975)

## Repair

**63700**  Repair of meningocele; less than 5 cm diameter

**63702**  larger than 5 cm diameter

(Do not use modifier 63 in conjunction with 63700, 63702)

**63704**  Repair of myelomeningocele; less than 5 cm diameter

**63706**  larger than 5 cm diameter

(Do not use modifier 63 in conjunction with 63704, 63706)

(For complex skin closure, see **Integumentary System**)

**63707**  Repair of dural/cerebrospinal fluid leak, not requiring laminectomy

**63709**  Repair of dural/cerebrospinal fluid leak or pseudomeningocele, with laminectomy

**63710**  Dural graft, spinal

(For laminectomy and section of dentate ligaments, with or without dural graft, cervical, see 63180, 63182)

## Shunt, Spinal CSF

**63740**  Creation of shunt, lumbar, subarachnoid-peritoneal, -pleural, or other; including laminectomy

**63741**  percutaneous, not requiring laminectomy

**63744**  Replacement, irrigation or revision of lumbosubarachnoid shunt

**63746**  Removal of entire lumbosubarachnoid shunt system without replacement

(For insertion of subarachnoid catheter with reservoir and/or pump for intermittent or continuous infusion of drug including laminectomy, see 62351 and 62360, 62361 or 62362)

(For insertion or replacement of subarachnoid or epidural catheter, with reservoir and/or pump for drug infusion without laminectomy, see 62350 and 62360, 62361 or 62362)

# Extracranial Nerves, Peripheral Nerves, and Autonomic Nervous System

(For intracranial surgery on cranial nerves, see 61450, 61460, 61790)

## Introduction/Injection of Anesthetic Agent (Nerve Block), Diagnostic or Therapeutic

(For destruction by neurolytic agent or chemodenervation, see 62280-62282, 64600-64681)

(For epidural or subarachnoid injection, see 62310-62319)

(64479-64495 are unilateral procedures. For bilateral procedures, use modifier 50)

### Somatic Nerves

**64400**  Injection, anesthetic agent; trigeminal nerve, any division or branch

**64402**  facial nerve

**64405**  greater occipital nerve

**64408**  vagus nerve

**64410**  phrenic nerve

**64412**  spinal accessory nerve

**64413**  cervical plexus

**64415**  brachial plexus, single

**64416**  brachial plexus, continuous infusion by catheter (including catheter placement)

(Do not report 64416 in conjunction with 01996)

**64417**  axillary nerve

**64418**  suprascapular nerve

**64420**  intercostal nerve, single

**64421**  intercostal nerves, multiple, regional block

**64425**  ilioinguinal, iliohypogastric nerves

**64430**  pudendal nerve

**64435**  paracervical (uterine) nerve

**64445**  sciatic nerve, single

**64446**  sciatic nerve, continuous infusion by catheter (including catheter placement)

(Do not report 64446 in conjunction with 01996)

**64447**  femoral nerve, single

(Do not report 64447 in conjunction with 01996)

**64448**  femoral nerve, continuous infusion by catheter (including catheter placement)

(Do not report 64448 in conjunction with 01996)

**64449**  lumbar plexus, posterior approach, continuous infusion by catheter (including catheter placement)

(Do not report 64449 in conjunction with 01996)

**64450**  other peripheral nerve or branch

**64455**  Injection(s), anesthetic agent and/or steroid, plantar common digital nerve(s) (eg, Morton's neuroma)

(Do not report 64455 in conjunction with 64632)

(Imaging guidance [fluoroscopy or CT] and any injection of contrast are inclusive components of 64479-64484. Imaging guidance and localization are required for the performance of 64479-64484)

(64470-64476 have been deleted. To report, see 64490-64495)

**64479**  Injection, anesthetic agent and/or steroid, transforaminal epidural, with imaging guidance (fluoroscopy or CT); cervical or thoracic, single level

(For transforaminal epidural injection under ultrasound guidance, use 0228T)

**+ 64480**  cervical or thoracic, each additional level (List separately in addition to code for primary procedure)

(Use 64480 in conjunction with 64479)

(For transforaminal epidural injection under ultrasound guidance, use 0229T)

(For transforaminal epidural injection at the T12-L1 level, use 64479)

**64483**  lumbar or sacral, single level

(For transforaminal epidural injection under ultrasound guidance, use 0230T)

**+ 64484**  lumbar or sacral, each additional level (List separately in addition to code for primary procedure)

(Use 64484 in conjunction with 64483)

(For transforaminal epidural injection under ultrasound guidance, use 0231T)

(64479-64484 are unilateral procedures. For bilateral procedures, use modifier 50)

### Paravertebral Spinal Nerves and Branches

►(Image guidance [fluoroscopy or CT] and any injection of contrast are inclusive components of 64490-64495. Imaging guidance and localization are required for the performance of paravertebral facet joint injections described by codes 64490-64495. If imaging is not used, report 20552-20553. If ultrasound guidance is used, report 0213T-0218T)◄

(For bilateral paravertebral facet injection procedures, use modifier 50)

(For paravertebral facet injection of the T12-L1 joint, or nerves innervating that joint, use 64490)

Surgery: Nervous System

**64490**    Injection(s), diagnostic or therapeutic agent, paravertebral facet (zygapophyseal) joint (or nerves innervating that joint) with image guidance (fluoroscopy or CT), cervical or thoracic; single level

**+ 64491**    second level (List separately in addition to code for primary procedure)

**+ 64492**    third and any additional level(s) (List separately in addition to code for primary procedure)

(Do not report 64492 more than once per day)

(Use 64491, 64492 in conjunction with 64490)

**64493**    Injection(s), diagnostic or therapeutic agent, paravertebral facet (zygapophyseal) joint (or nerves innervating that joint) with image guidance (fluoroscopy or CT), lumbar or sacral; single level

**+ 64494**    second level (List separately in addition to code for primary procedure)

**+ 64495**    third and any additional level(s) (List separately in addition to code for primary procedure)

(Do not report 64495 more than once per day)

(Use 64494, 64495 in conjunction with 64493)

### Autonomic Nerves

**64505**    Injection, anesthetic agent; sphenopalatine ganglion

**64508**    carotid sinus (separate procedure)

**64510**    stellate ganglion (cervical sympathetic)

**64517**    superior hypogastric plexus

**64520**    lumbar or thoracic (paravertebral sympathetic)

**64530**    celiac plexus, with or without radiologic monitoring

## Neurostimulators (Peripheral Nerve)

►Codes 64553-64595 apply to both simple and complex neurostimulators. For initial or subsequent electronic analysis and programming of neurostimulator pulse generators, see codes 95970-95975. An electrode array is a catheter or other device with more than one contact. The function of each contact may be capable of being adjusted during programming services.◄

►(For implantation of trial or permanent electrode arrays or pulse generators for peripheral subcutaneous field stimulation, see 0282T-0284T)◄

**64550**    Application of surface (transcutaneous) neurostimulator

▲ **64553**    Percutaneous implantation of neurostimulator electrode array; cranial nerve

(For open placement of cranial nerve (eg, vagal, trigeminal) neurostimulator pulse generator or receiver, see 61885, 61886, as appropriate)

▲ **64555**    peripheral nerve (excludes sacral nerve)

(Do not report 64555 in conjunction with 64566)

►(64560 has been deleted)◄

▲ **64561**    sacral nerve (transforaminal placement)

▲ **64565**    neuromuscular

**64566**    Posterior tibial neurostimulation, percutaneous needle electrode, single treatment, includes programming

(Do not report 64566 in conjunction with 64555, 95970-95972)

**64568**    Incision for implantation of cranial nerve (eg, vagus nerve) neurostimulator electrode array and pulse generator

(Do not report 64568 in conjunction with 61885, 61886, 64570)

**64569**    Revision or replacement of cranial nerve (eg, vagus nerve) neurostimulator electrode array, including connection to existing pulse generator

(Do not report 64569 in conjunction with 64570 or 61888)

(For replacement of pulse generator, use 61885)

**64570**    Removal of cranial nerve (eg, vagus nerve) neurostimulator electrode array and pulse generator

(Do not report 64570 in conjunction with 61888)

(64573 has been deleted)

▲ **64575**    Incision for implantation of neurostimulator electrode array; peripheral nerve (excludes sacral nerve)

►(64577 has been deleted)◄

▲ **64580**    neuromuscular

▲ **64581**    sacral nerve (transforaminal placement)

▲ **64585**    Revision or removal of peripheral neurostimulator electrode array

**64590**    Insertion or replacement of peripheral or gastric neurostimulator pulse generator or receiver, direct or inductive coupling

(Do not report 64590 in conjunction with 64595)

**64595**    Revision or removal of peripheral or gastric neurostimulator pulse generator or receiver

## Destruction by Neurolytic Agent (eg, Chemical, Thermal, Electrical or Radiofrequency)

►Codes 64600-64681 include the injection of other therapeutic agents (eg, corticosteroids). Do not report diagnostic/therapeutic injections separately. (For therapies that are not destructive of the target nerve [eg, pulsed radiofrequency], use 64999)◄

### Somatic Nerves

**64600**    Destruction by neurolytic agent, trigeminal nerve; supraorbital, infraorbital, mental, or inferior alveolar branch

---

**64605**       second and third division branches at foramen ovale

**64610**       second and third division branches at foramen ovale under radiologic monitoring

**64611**  Chemodenervation of parotid and submandibular salivary glands, bilateral

(Report 64611 with modifier 52 if fewer than four salivary glands are injected)

**64612**  Chemodenervation of muscle(s); muscle(s) innervated by facial nerve (eg, for blepharospasm, hemifacial spasm)

**64613**       neck muscle(s) (eg, for spasmodic torticollis, spasmodic dysphonia)

**64614**       extremity(s) and/or trunk muscle(s) (eg, for dystonia, cerebral palsy, multiple sclerosis)

(For chemodenervation guided by needle electromyography or muscle electrical stimulation, see 95873, 95874)

(For chemodenervation for strabismus involving the extraocular muscles, use 67345)

(For chemodenervation of internal anal sphincter, use 46505)

**64620**  Destruction by neurolytic agent, intercostal nerve

▶(64622-64627 have been deleted. For image guided neurolysis of facet joint nerve(s), see 64633-64636)◀

▶(Imaging guidance [fluoroscopy, CT] are inclusive components of 64633-64636)◀

▶(Image guidance [fluoroscopy or CT] and any injection of contrast are inclusive components of 64633-64636. Image guidance and localization are required for the performance of paravertebral facet joint nerve destruction by neurolytic agent described by 64633-64636. If CT or fluoroscopic imaging is not used, report 64999)◀

▶(For paravertebral facet destruction by neurolysis of the T12-L1 joint, or nerves innervating that joint, use 64633)◀

#● **64633**  Destruction by neurolytic agent, paravertebral facet joint nerve(s), with imaging guidance (fluoroscopy or CT); cervical or thoracic, single facet joint

▶(For bilateral procedure, report 64633 with modifier 50)◀

#+● **64634**       cervical or thoracic, each additional facet joint (List separately in addition to code for primary procedure)

▶(Use 64634 in conjunction with 64633)◀

▶(For bilateral procedure, report 64634 with modifier 50)◀

#● **64635**       lumbar or sacral, single facet joint

▶(For bilateral procedure, report 64635 with modifier 50)◀

#+● **64636**       lumbar or sacral, each additional facet joint (List separately in addition to code for primary procedure)

▶(Use 64636 in conjunction with 64635)◀

▶(For bilateral procedure, report 64636 with modifier 50)◀

▶(Do not report 64633-64636 in conjunction with 77003, 77012)◀

**64630**  Destruction by neurolytic agent; pudendal nerve

**64632**       plantar common digital nerve

(Do not report 64632 in conjunction with 64455)

**64633**  ▶Code is out of numerical sequence. See 64600-64640◀

**64634**  ▶Code is out of numerical sequence. See 64600-64640◀

**64635**  ▶Code is out of numerical sequence. See 64600-64640◀

**64636**  ▶Code is out of numerical sequence. See 64600-64640◀

**64640**       other peripheral nerve or branch

## Sympathetic Nerves

**64650**  Chemodenervation of eccrine glands; both axillae

**64653**       other area(s) (eg, scalp, face, neck), per day

(Report the specific service in conjunction with code(s) for the specific substance(s) or drug(s) provided)

(For chemodenervation of extremities (eg, hands or feet), use 64999)

**64680**  Destruction by neurolytic agent, with or without radiologic monitoring; celiac plexus

**64681**       superior hypogastric plexus

## Neuroplasty (Exploration, Neurolysis or Nerve Decompression)

Neuroplasty is the surgical decompression or freeing of intact nerve from scar tissue, including external neurolysis and/or transposition to repair or restore the nerve.

(For percutaneous neurolysis, see 62263, 62264, 62280-62282)

(For internal neurolysis requiring use of operating microscope, use 64727)

(For facial nerve decompression, use 69720)

(For neuroplasty with nerve wrapping, see 64702-64727, 64999)

**64702**  Neuroplasty; digital, 1 or both, same digit

**64704**       nerve of hand or foot

**64708**  Neuroplasty, major peripheral nerve, arm or leg, open; other than specified

**64712**       sciatic nerve

**64713**       brachial plexus

**64714**       lumbar plexus

**64716**  Neuroplasty and/or transposition; cranial nerve (specify)

| | |
|---|---|
| **64718** | ulnar nerve at elbow |
| **64719** | ulnar nerve at wrist |
| **64721** | · median nerve at carpal tunnel |

(For arthroscopic procedure, use 29848)

| | |
|---|---|
| **64722** | Decompression; unspecified nerve(s) (specify) |
| **64726** | plantar digital nerve |
| **+ 64727** | Internal neurolysis, requiring use of operating microscope (List separately in addition to code for neuroplasty) (Neuroplasty includes external neurolysis) |

(Do not report code 69990 in addition to code 64727)

## Transection or Avulsion

(For stereotactic lesion of gasserian ganglion, use 61790)

| | |
|---|---|
| **64732** | Transection or avulsion of; supraorbital nerve |
| **64734** | infraorbital nerve |
| **64736** | mental nerve |
| **64738** | inferior alveolar nerve by osteotomy |
| **64740** | lingual nerve |
| **64742** | facial nerve, differential or complete |
| **64744** | greater occipital nerve |
| **64746** | phrenic nerve |

(For section of recurrent laryngeal nerve, use 31595)

| | |
|---|---|
| **64752** | vagus nerve (vagotomy), transthoracic |
| **64755** | vagus nerves limited to proximal stomach (selective proximal vagotomy, proximal gastric vagotomy, parietal cell vagotomy, supra- or highly selective vagotomy) |

(For laparoscopic approach, use 43652)

| | |
|---|---|
| **64760** | vagus nerve (vagotomy), abdominal |

(For laparoscopic approach, use 43651)

| | |
|---|---|
| **64761** | pudendal nerve |

(For bilateral procedure, report 64761 with modifier 50)

| | |
|---|---|
| **64763** | Transection or avulsion of obturator nerve, extrapelvic, with or without adductor tenotomy |

(For bilateral procedure, report 64763 with modifier 50)

| | |
|---|---|
| **64766** | Transection or avulsion of obturator nerve, intrapelvic, with or without adductor tenotomy |

(For bilateral procedure, report 64766 with modifier 50)

| | |
|---|---|
| **64771** | Transection or avulsion of other cranial nerve, extradural |
| **64772** | Transection or avulsion of other spinal nerve, extradural |

(For excision of tender scar, skin and subcutaneous tissue, with or without tiny neuroma, see 11400-11446, 13100-13153)

## Excision

### Somatic Nerves

(For Morton neurectomy, use 28080)

| | |
|---|---|
| **64774** | Excision of neuroma; cutaneous nerve, surgically identifiable |
| **64776** | digital nerve, 1 or both, same digit |
| **+ 64778** | digital nerve, each additional digit (List separately in addition to code for primary procedure) |

(Use 64778 in conjunction with 64776)

| | |
|---|---|
| **64782** | hand or foot, except digital nerve |
| **+ 64783** | hand or foot, each additional nerve, except same digit (List separately in addition to code for primary procedure) |

(Use 64783 in conjunction with 64782)

| | |
|---|---|
| **64784** | major peripheral nerve, except sciatic |
| **64786** | sciatic nerve |
| **+ 64787** | Implantation of nerve end into bone or muscle (List separately in addition to neuroma excision) |

(Use 64787 in conjunction with 64774-64786)

| | |
|---|---|
| **64788** | Excision of neurofibroma or neurolemmoma; cutaneous nerve |
| **64790** | major peripheral nerve |
| **64792** | extensive (including malignant type) |
| **64795** | Biopsy of nerve |

### Sympathetic Nerves

| | |
|---|---|
| **64802** | Sympathectomy, cervical |

(For bilateral procedure, report 64802 with modifier 50)

| | |
|---|---|
| **64804** | Sympathectomy, cervicothoracic |

(For bilateral procedure, report 64804 with modifier 50)

| | |
|---|---|
| **64809** | Sympathectomy, thoracolumbar |

(For bilateral procedure, report 64809 with modifier 50)

| | |
|---|---|
| **64818** | Sympathectomy, lumbar |

(For bilateral procedure, report 64818 with modifier 50)

| | |
|---|---|
| **64820** | Sympathectomy; digital arteries, each digit |

(Do not report 69990 in addition to code 64820)

| | |
|---|---|
| **64821** | radial artery |

(Do not report 69990 in addition to code 64821)

| | |
|---|---|
| **64822** | ulnar artery |

(Do not report 69990 in addition to code 64822)

| | |
|---|---|
| **64823** | superficial palmar arch |

(Do not report 69990 in addition to code 64823)

---

▲=Revised code   ●=New code   ▶◀=Contains new or revised text   ⊘=Modifier 51 exempt

## Neurorrhaphy

**64831**  Suture of digital nerve, hand or foot; 1 nerve

**+ 64832**  each additional digital nerve (List separately in addition to code for primary procedure)

(Use 64832 in conjunction with 64831)

**64834**  Suture of 1 nerve; hand or foot, common sensory nerve

**64835**  median motor thenar

**64836**  ulnar motor

**+ 64837**  Suture of each additional nerve, hand or foot (List separately in addition to code for primary procedure)

(Use 64837 in conjunction with 64834-64836)

**64840**  Suture of posterior tibial nerve

**64856**  Suture of major peripheral nerve, arm or leg, except sciatic; including transposition

**64857**  without transposition

**64858**  Suture of sciatic nerve

**+ 64859**  Suture of each additional major peripheral nerve (List separately in addition to code for primary procedure)

(Use 64859 in conjunction with 64856, 64857)

**64861**  Suture of; brachial plexus

**64862**  lumbar plexus

**64864**  Suture of facial nerve; extracranial

**64865**  infratemporal, with or without grafting

**64866**  Anastomosis; facial-spinal accessory

**64868**  facial-hypoglossal

**64870**  facial-phrenic

**+ 64872**  Suture of nerve; requiring secondary or delayed suture (List separately in addition to code for primary neurorrhaphy)

(Use 64872 in conjunction with 64831-64865)

**+ 64874**  requiring extensive mobilization, or transposition of nerve (List separately in addition to code for nerve suture)

(Use 64874 in conjunction with 64831-64865)

**+ 64876**  requiring shortening of bone of extremity (List separately in addition to code for nerve suture)

(Use 64876 in conjunction with 64831-64865)

## Neurorrhaphy With Nerve Graft, Vein Graft, or Conduit

**64885**  Nerve graft (includes obtaining graft), head or neck; up to 4 cm in length

**64886**  more than 4 cm length

**64890**  Nerve graft (includes obtaining graft), single strand, hand or foot; up to 4 cm length

**64891**  more than 4 cm length

**64892**  Nerve graft (includes obtaining graft), single strand, arm or leg; up to 4 cm length

**64893**  more than 4 cm length

**64895**  Nerve graft (includes obtaining graft), multiple strands (cable), hand or foot; up to 4 cm length

**64896**  more than 4 cm length

**64897**  Nerve graft (includes obtaining graft), multiple strands (cable), arm or leg; up to 4 cm length

**64898**  more than 4 cm length

**+ 64901**  Nerve graft, each additional nerve; single strand (List separately in addition to code for primary procedure)

(Use 64901 in conjunction with 64885-64893)

**+ 64902**  multiple strands (cable) (List separately in addition to code for primary procedure)

(Use 64902 in conjunction with 64885, 64886, 64895-64898)

**64905**  Nerve pedicle transfer; first stage

**64907**  second stage

**64910**  Nerve repair; with synthetic conduit or vein allograft (eg, nerve tube), each nerve

**64911**  with autogenous vein graft (includes harvest of vein graft), each nerve

(Do not report 69990 in addition to 64910, 64911)

## Other Procedures

**64999**  Unlisted procedure, nervous system

# Eye and Ocular Adnexa

(For diagnostic and treatment ophthalmological services, see **Medicine, Ophthalmology,** and 92002 et seq)

(Do not report code 69990 in addition to codes 65091-68850)

## Eyeball

### Removal of Eye

**65091** Evisceration of ocular contents; without implant

**65093** with implant

**65101** Enucleation of eye; without implant

**65103** with implant, muscles not attached to implant

**65105** with implant, muscles attached to implant

(For conjunctivoplasty after enucleation, see 68320 et seq)

**65110** Exenteration of orbit (does not include skin graft), removal of orbital contents; only

**65112** with therapeutic removal of bone

**65114** with muscle or myocutaneous flap

(For skin graft to orbit (split skin), see 15120, 15121; free, full thickness, see 15260, 15261)

(For eyelid repair involving more than skin, see 67930 et seq)

### Secondary Implant(s) Procedures

An ocular implant is an implant inside muscular cone; an orbital implant is an implant outside muscular cone.

**65125** Modification of ocular implant with placement or replacement of pegs (eg, drilling receptacle for prosthesis appendage) (separate procedure)

**65130** Insertion of ocular implant secondary; after evisceration, in scleral shell

**65135** after enucleation, muscles not attached to implant

**65140** after enucleation, muscles attached to implant

**65150** Reinsertion of ocular implant; with or without conjunctival graft

**65155** with use of foreign material for reinforcement and/or attachment of muscles to implant

**65175** Removal of ocular implant

(For orbital implant (implant outside muscle cone) insertion, use 67550; removal, use 67560)

### Removal of Foreign Body

(For removal of implanted material: ocular implant, use 65175; anterior segment implant, use 65920; posterior segment implant, use 67120; orbital implant, use 67560)

(For diagnostic x-ray for foreign body, use 70030)

(For diagnostic echography for foreign body, use 76529)

(For removal of foreign body from orbit: frontal approach, use 67413; lateral approach, use 67430; transcranial approach, use 61334)

(For removal of foreign body from eyelid, embedded, use 67938)

(For removal of foreign body from lacrimal system, use 68530)

**65205** Removal of foreign body, external eye; conjunctival superficial

**65210** conjunctival embedded (includes concretions), subconjunctival, or scleral nonperforating

**65220** corneal, without slit lamp

**65222** corneal, with slit lamp

(For repair of corneal laceration with foreign body, use 65275)

**65235** Removal of foreign body, intraocular; from anterior chamber of eye or lens

(For removal of implanted material from anterior segment, use 65920)

**65260** from posterior segment, magnetic extraction, anterior or posterior route

**65265** from posterior segment, nonmagnetic extraction

(For removal of implanted material from posterior segment, use 67120)

### Repair of Laceration

(For fracture of orbit, see 21385 et seq)

(For repair of wound of eyelid, skin, linear, simple, see 12011-12018; intermediate, layered closure, see 12051-12057; linear, complex, see 13150-13160; other, see 67930, 67935)

(For repair of wound of lacrimal system, use 68700)

(For repair of operative wound, use 66250)

**65270** Repair of laceration; conjunctiva, with or without nonperforating laceration sclera, direct closure

**65272** conjunctiva, by mobilization and rearrangement, without hospitalization

**65273** conjunctiva, by mobilization and rearrangement, with hospitalization

**65275** cornea, nonperforating, with or without removal foreign body

**Surgery: Ocular System**

| | |
|---|---|
| 65280 | cornea and/or sclera, perforating, not involving uveal tissue |
| 65285 | cornea and/or sclera, perforating, with reposition or resection of uveal tissue |

►(65280 and 65285 are not used for repair of a surgical wound)◄

| | |
|---|---|
| 65286 | application of tissue glue, wounds of cornea and/or sclera |

(Repair of laceration includes use of conjunctival flap and restoration of anterior chamber, by air or saline injection when indicated)

(For repair of iris or ciliary body, use 66680)

| | |
|---|---|
| 65290 | Repair of wound, extraocular muscle, tendon and/or Tenon's capsule |

# Anterior Segment

## Cornea

### Excision

| | |
|---|---|
| 65400 | Excision of lesion, cornea (keratectomy, lamellar, partial), except pterygium |
| 65410 | Biopsy of cornea |
| 65420 | Excision or transposition of pterygium; without graft |
| 65426 | with graft |

### Removal or Destruction

| | |
|---|---|
| 65430 | Scraping of cornea, diagnostic, for smear and/or culture |
| 65435 | Removal of corneal epithelium; with or without chemocauterization (abrasion, curettage) |
| 65436 | with application of chelating agent (eg, EDTA) |
| 65450 | Destruction of lesion of cornea by cryotherapy, photocoagulation or thermocauterization |
| 65600 | Multiple punctures of anterior cornea (eg, for corneal erosion, tattoo) |

### Keratoplasty

Corneal transplant includes use of fresh or preserved grafts. The preparation of donor material is included for penetrating or anterior lamellar keratoplasty, but reported separately for endothelial keratoplasty. Do not report 65710-65757 in conjunction with 92025.

(Keratoplasty excludes refractive keratoplasty procedures, 65760, 65765, and 65767)

| | |
|---|---|
| 65710 | Keratoplasty (corneal transplant); anterior lamellar |
| 65730 | penetrating (except in aphakia or pseudophakia) |
| 65750 | penetrating (in aphakia) |
| 65755 | penetrating (in pseudophakia) |
| 65756 | endothelial |
| + 65757 | Backbench preparation of corneal endothelial allograft prior to transplantation (List separately in addition to code for primary procedure) |

(Use 65757 in conjunction with 65756)

### Other Procedures

Do not report 65760-65771 in conjunction with 92025.

| | |
|---|---|
| 65760 | Keratomileusis |
| 65765 | Keratophakia |
| 65767 | Epikeratoplasty |
| 65770 | Keratoprosthesis |
| 65771 | Radial keratotomy |
| 65772 | Corneal relaxing incision for correction of surgically induced astigmatism |
| 65775 | Corneal wedge resection for correction of surgically induced astigmatism |

►(For fitting of contact lens for treatment of disease, see 92071, 92072)◄

(For unlisted procedures on cornea, use 66999)

| | |
|---|---|
| 65778 | Placement of amniotic membrane on the ocular surface for wound healing; self-retaining |
| 65779 | single layer, sutured |

(Do not report 65778, 65779 in conjunction with 65430, 65435, 65780)

(For placement of amniotic membrane using tissue glue, use 66999)

| | |
|---|---|
| 65780 | Ocular surface reconstruction; amniotic membrane transplantation, multiple layers |

(For placement of amniotic membrane without reconstruction using self-retaining or single layer suture technique, see 65778, 65779)

| | |
|---|---|
| 65781 | limbal stem cell allograft (eg, cadaveric or living donor) |
| 65782 | limbal conjunctival autograft (includes obtaining graft) |

(For harvesting conjunctival allograft, living donor, use 68371)

## Anterior Chamber

### Incision

| | |
|---|---|
| 65800 | Paracentesis of anterior chamber of eye (separate procedure); with diagnostic aspiration of aqueous |
| 65805 | with therapeutic release of aqueous |

**65810**    with removal of vitreous and/or discission of anterior hyaloid membrane, with or without air injection

**65815**    with removal of blood, with or without irrigation and/or air injection

(For injection, see 66020-66030)

(For removal of blood clot, use 65930)

**65820**    Goniotomy

(Do not report modifier 63 in conjunction with 65820)

(For use of ophthalmic endoscope with 65820, use 66990)

**65850**    Trabeculotomy ab externo

**65855**    Trabeculoplasty by laser surgery, 1 or more sessions (defined treatment series)

(If re-treatment is necessary after several months because of disease progression, a new treatment or treatment series should be reported with a modifier, if necessary, to indicate lesser or greater complexity)

(For trabeculectomy, use 66170)

**65860**    Severing adhesions of anterior segment, laser technique (separate procedure)

**65865**    Severing adhesions of anterior segment of eye, incisional technique (with or without injection of air or liquid) (separate procedure); goniosynechiae

(For trabeculoplasty by laser surgery, use 65855)

**65870**    anterior synechiae, except goniosynechiae

**65875**    posterior synechiae

(For use of ophthalmic endoscope with 65875, use 66990)

**65880**    corneovitreal adhesions

(For laser surgery, use 66821)

### Removal

**65900**    Removal of epithelial downgrowth, anterior chamber of eye

**65920**    Removal of implanted material, anterior segment of eye

(For use of ophthalmic endoscope with 65920, use 66990)

**65930**    Removal of blood clot, anterior segment of eye

### Introduction

**66020**    Injection, anterior chamber of eye (separate procedure); air or liquid

**66030**    medication

(For unlisted procedures on anterior segment, use 66999)

## Anterior Sclera

### Excision

(For removal of intraocular foreign body, use 65235)

(For operations on posterior sclera, use 67250, 67255)

**66130**    Excision of lesion, sclera

**66150**    Fistulization of sclera for glaucoma; trephination with iridectomy

**66155**    thermocauterization with iridectomy

**66160**    sclerectomy with punch or scissors, with iridectomy

**66165**    iridencleisis or iridotasis

**66170**    trabeculectomy ab externo in absence of previous surgery

(For trabeculotomy ab externo, use 65850)

(For repair of operative wound, use 66250)

**66172**    trabeculectomy ab externo with scarring from previous ocular surgery or trauma (includes injection of antifibrotic agents)

**66174**    Transluminal dilation of aqueous outflow canal; without retention of device or stent

**66175**    with retention of device or stent

### Aqueous Shunt

**66180**    Aqueous shunt to extraocular reservoir (eg, Molteno, Schocket, Denver-Krupin)

**66185**    Revision of aqueous shunt to extraocular reservoir

(For removal of implanted shunt, use 67120)

### Repair or Revision

(For scleral procedures in retinal surgery, see 67101 et seq)

**66220**    Repair of scleral staphyloma; without graft

**66225**    with graft

(For scleral reinforcement, see 67250, 67255)

**66250**    Revision or repair of operative wound of anterior segment, any type, early or late, major or minor procedure

(For unlisted procedures on anterior sclera, use 66999)

## Iris, Ciliary Body

### Incision

**66500**    Iridotomy by stab incision (separate procedure); except transfixion

**Surgery: Ocular System**

**66505**    with transfixion as for iris bombe

(For iridotomy by photocoagulation, use 66761)

## Excision

**66600**    Iridectomy, with corneoscleral or corneal section; for removal of lesion

**66605**    with cyclectomy

**66625**    peripheral for glaucoma (separate procedure)

**66630**    sector for glaucoma (separate procedure)

**66635**    optical (separate procedure)

(For coreoplasty by photocoagulation, use 66762)

## Repair

**66680**    Repair of iris, ciliary body (as for iridodialysis)

(For reposition or resection of uveal tissue with perforating wound of cornea or sclera, use 65285)

**66682**    Suture of iris, ciliary body (separate procedure) with retrieval of suture through small incision (eg, McCannel suture)

## Destruction

**66700**    Ciliary body destruction; diathermy

**66710**    cyclophotocoagulation, transscleral

**66711**    cyclophotocoagulation, endoscopic

(Do not report 66711 in conjunction with 66990)

⊙ **66720**    cryotherapy

**66740**    cyclodialysis

**66761**    Iridotomy/iridectomy by laser surgery (eg, for glaucoma) (per session)

**66762**    Iridoplasty by photocoagulation (1 or more sessions) (eg, for improvement of vision, for widening of anterior chamber angle)

**66770**    Destruction of cyst or lesion iris or ciliary body (nonexcisional procedure)

(For excision lesion iris, ciliary body, see 66600, 66605; for removal of epithelial downgrowth, use 65900)

(For unlisted procedures on iris, ciliary body, use 66999)

## Lens

### Incision

**66820**    Discission of secondary membranous cataract (opacified posterior lens capsule and/or anterior hyaloid); stab incision technique (Ziegler or Wheeler knife)

**66821**    laser surgery (eg, YAG laser) (1 or more stages)

**66825**    Repositioning of intraocular lens prosthesis, requiring an incision (separate procedure)

## Removal

Lateral canthotomy, iridectomy, iridotomy, anterior capsulotomy, posterior capsulotomy, the use of viscoelastic agents, enzymatic zonulysis, use of other pharmacologic agents, and subconjunctival or sub-tenon injections are included as part of the code for the extraction of lens.

**66830**    Removal of secondary membranous cataract (opacified posterior lens capsule and/or anterior hyaloid) with corneo-scleral section, with or without iridectomy (iridocapsulotomy, iridocapsulectomy)

**66840**    Removal of lens material; aspiration technique, 1 or more stages

**66850**    phacofragmentation technique (mechanical or ultrasonic) (eg, phacoemulsification), with aspiration

**66852**    pars plana approach, with or without vitrectomy

**66920**    intracapsular

**66930**    intracapsular, for dislocated lens

**66940**    extracapsular (other than 66840, 66850, 66852)

(For removal of intralenticular foreign body without lens extraction, use 65235)

(For repair of operative wound, use 66250)

## Intraocular Lens Procedures

**66982**    Extracapsular cataract removal with insertion of intraocular lens prosthesis (1-stage procedure), manual or mechanical technique (eg, irrigation and aspiration or phacoemulsification), complex, requiring devices or techniques not generally used in routine cataract surgery (eg, iris expansion device, suture support for intraocular lens, or primary posterior capsulorrhexis) or performed on patients in the amblyogenic developmental stage

**66983**    Intracapsular cataract extraction with insertion of intraocular lens prosthesis (1 stage procedure)

**66984**    Extracapsular cataract removal with insertion of intraocular lens prosthesis (1 stage procedure), manual or mechanical technique (eg, irrigation and aspiration or phacoemulsification)

(For complex extracapsular cataract removal, use 66982)

**66985**    Insertion of intraocular lens prosthesis (secondary implant), not associated with concurrent cataract removal

(To code implant at time of concurrent cataract surgery, see 66982, 66983, 66984)

(For intraocular lens prosthesis supplied by physician, use 99070)

(For ultrasonic determination of intraocular lens power, use 76519)

Surgery: Ocular System

(For removal of implanted material from anterior segment, use 65920)

(For secondary fixation (separate procedure), use 66682)

(For use of ophthalmic endoscope with 66985, use 66990)

**66986**    Exchange of intraocular lens

(For use of ophthalmic endoscope with 66986, use 66990)

## Other Procedures

**+ 66990**    Use of ophthalmic endoscope (List separately in addition to code for primary procedure)

(66990 may be used only with codes 65820, 65875, 65920, 66985, 66986, 67036, 67039, 67040, 67041, 67042, 67043, 67112, 67113)

**66999**    Unlisted procedure, anterior segment of eye

## Posterior Segment

### Vitreous

**67005**    Removal of vitreous, anterior approach (open sky technique or limbal incision); partial removal

**67010**          subtotal removal with mechanical vitrectomy

(For removal of vitreous by paracentesis of anterior chamber, use 65810)

(For removal of corneovitreal adhesions, use 65880)

**67015**    Aspiration or release of vitreous, subretinal or choroidal fluid, pars plana approach (posterior sclerotomy)

**67025**    Injection of vitreous substitute, pars plana or limbal approach (fluid-gas exchange), with or without aspiration (separate procedure)

**67027**    Implantation of intravitreal drug delivery system (eg, ganciclovir implant), includes concomitant removal of vitreous

(For removal, use 67121)

**67028**    Intravitreal injection of a pharmacologic agent (separate procedure)

**67030**    Discission of vitreous strands (without removal), pars plana approach

**67031**    Severing of vitreous strands, vitreous face adhesions, sheets, membranes or opacities, laser surgery (1 or more stages)

**67036**    Vitrectomy, mechanical, pars plana approach;

(For application of intraocular epiretinal radiation with 67036, use 0190T)

**67039**          with focal endolaser photocoagulation

**67040**          with endolaser panretinal photocoagulation

**67041**          with removal of preretinal cellular membrane (eg, macular pucker)

**67042**          with removal of internal limiting membrane of retina (eg, for repair of macular hole, diabetic macular edema), includes, if performed, intraocular tamponade (ie, air, gas or silicone oil)

**67043**          with removal of subretinal membrane (eg, choroidal neovascularization), includes, if performed, intraocular tamponade (ie, air, gas or silicone oil) and laser photocoagulation

(For use of ophthalmic endoscope with 67036, 67039, 67040-67043, use 66990)

(For associated lensectomy, use 66850)

(For use of vitrectomy in retinal detachment surgery, see 67108, 67113)

(For associated removal of foreign body, see 65260, 65265)

(For unlisted procedures on vitreous, use 67299)

### Retina or Choroid

#### Repair

(If diathermy, cryotherapy and/or photocoagulation are combined, report under principal modality used)

**67101**    Repair of retinal detachment, 1 or more sessions; cryotherapy or diathermy, with or without drainage of subretinal fluid

**67105**          photocoagulation, with or without drainage of subretinal fluid

**67107**    Repair of retinal detachment; scleral buckling (such as lamellar scleral dissection, imbrication or encircling procedure), with or without implant, with or without cryotherapy, photocoagulation, and drainage of subretinal fluid

**67108**          with vitrectomy, any method, with or without air or gas tamponade, focal endolaser photocoagulation, cryotherapy, drainage of subretinal fluid, scleral buckling, and/or removal of lens by same technique

**67110**          by injection of air or other gas (eg, pneumatic retinopexy)

**67112**          by scleral buckling or vitrectomy, on patient having previous ipsilateral retinal detachment repair(s) using scleral buckling or vitrectomy techniques

(For aspiration or drainage of subretinal or subchoroidal fluid, use 67015)

(For use of ophthalmic endoscope with 67112, use 66990)

**67113**    Repair of complex retinal detachment (eg, proliferative vitreoretinopathy, stage C-1 or greater, diabetic traction retinal detachment, retinopathy of prematurity, retinal tear of greater than 90 degrees), with vitrectomy and membrane peeling, may include air, gas, or silicone oil tamponade, cryotherapy, endolaser photocoagulation, drainage of subretinal fluid, scleral buckling, and/or removal of lens

**Surgery: Ocular System**

(To report vitrectomy, pars plana approach, other than in retinal detachment surgery, see 67036-67043)

(For use of ophthalmic endoscope with 67113, use 66990)

**67115** Release of encircling material (posterior segment)

**67120** Removal of implanted material, posterior segment; extraocular

**67121** intraocular

(For removal from anterior segment, use 65920)

(For removal of foreign body, see 65260, 65265)

### Prophylaxis

Codes 67141, 67145 include treatment at one or more sessions that may occur at different encounters. These codes should be reported once during a defined treatment period.

Repetitive services. The services listed below are often performed in multiple sessions or groups of sessions. The methods of reporting vary.

The following descriptors are intended to include all sessions in a defined treatment period.

**67141** Prophylaxis of retinal detachment (eg, retinal break, lattice degeneration) without drainage, 1 or more sessions; cryotherapy, diathermy

**67145** photocoagulation (laser or xenon arc)

### Destruction

Codes 67208, 67210, 67218, 67220, 67227, 67228, 67229 include treatment at one or more sessions that may occur at different encounters. These codes should be reported once during a defined treatment period.

**67208** Destruction of localized lesion of retina (eg, macular edema, tumors), 1 or more sessions; cryotherapy, diathermy

**67210** photocoagulation

**67218** radiation by implantation of source (includes removal of source)

**67220** Destruction of localized lesion of choroid (eg, choroidal neovascularization); photocoagulation (eg, laser), 1 or more sessions

**67221** photodynamic therapy (includes intravenous infusion)

**+ 67225** photodynamic therapy, second eye, at single session (List separately in addition to code for primary eye treatment)

(Use 67225 in conjunction with 67221)

**67227** Destruction of extensive or progressive retinopathy (eg, diabetic retinopathy), 1 or more sessions; cryotherapy, diathermy

**67228** Treatment of extensive or progressive retinopathy, 1 or more sessions; (eg, diabetic retinopathy), photocoagulation

**67229** preterm infant (less than 37 weeks gestation at birth), performed from birth up to 1 year of age (eg, retinopathy of prematurity), photocoagulation or cryotherapy

(For bilateral procedure, use modifier 50)

(For unlisted procedures on retina, use 67299)

## Posterior Sclera

### Repair

(For excision lesion sclera, use 66130)

**67250** Scleral reinforcement (separate procedure); without graft

**67255** with graft

(For repair scleral staphyloma, see 66220, 66225)

## Other Procedures

**67299** Unlisted procedure, posterior segment

# Ocular Adnexa

## Extraocular Muscles

**67311** Strabismus surgery, recession or resection procedure; 1 horizontal muscle

**67312** 2 horizontal muscles

**67314** 1 vertical muscle (excluding superior oblique)

**67316** 2 or more vertical muscles (excluding superior oblique)

(For adjustable sutures, use 67335 in addition to codes 67311-67334 for primary procedure reflecting number of muscles operated on)

**67318** Strabismus surgery, any procedure, superior oblique muscle

**+ 67320** Transposition procedure (eg, for paretic extraocular muscle), any extraocular muscle (specify) (List separately in addition to code for primary procedure)

(Use 67320 in conjunction with 67311-67318)

**+ 67331** Strabismus surgery on patient with previous eye surgery or injury that did not involve the extraocular muscles (List separately in addition to code for primary procedure)

(Use 67331 in conjunction with 67311-67318)

**Surgery: Ocular System**

+ 67332  Strabismus surgery on patient with scarring of extraocular muscles (eg, prior ocular injury, strabismus or retinal detachment surgery) or restrictive myopathy (eg, dysthyroid ophthalmopathy) (List separately in addition to code for primary procedure)

(Use 67332 in conjunction with 67311-67318)

+ 67334  Strabismus surgery by posterior fixation suture technique, with or without muscle recession (List separately in addition to code for primary procedure)

(Use 67334 in conjunction with 67311-67318)

+ 67335  Placement of adjustable suture(s) during strabismus surgery, including postoperative adjustment(s) of suture(s) (List separately in addition to code for specific strabismus surgery)

(Use 67335 in conjunction with 67311-67334)

+ 67340  Strabismus surgery involving exploration and/or repair of detached extraocular muscle(s) (List separately in addition to code for primary procedure)

(Use 67340 in conjunction with 67311-67334)

67343  Release of extensive scar tissue without detaching extraocular muscle (separate procedure)

(Use 67343 in conjunction with 67311-67340, when such procedures are performed other than on the affected muscle)

67345  Chemodenervation of extraocular muscle

(For chemodenervation for blepharospasm and other neurological disorders, see 64612 and 64613)

67346  Biopsy of extraocular muscle

(For repair of wound, extraocular muscle, tendon or Tenon's capsule, use 65290)

## Other Procedures

67399  Unlisted procedure, ocular muscle

# Orbit

## Exploration, Excision, Decompression

67400  Orbitotomy without bone flap (frontal or transconjunctival approach); for exploration, with or without biopsy

67405      with drainage only

67412      with removal of lesion

67413      with removal of foreign body

67414      with removal of bone for decompression

67415  Fine needle aspiration of orbital contents

(For exenteration, enucleation, and repair, see 65101 et seq; for optic nerve decompression, use 67570)

67420  Orbitotomy with bone flap or window, lateral approach (eg, Kroenlein); with removal of lesion

67430      with removal of foreign body

67440      with drainage

67445      with removal of bone for decompression

(For optic nerve sheath decompression, use 67570)

67450      for exploration, with or without biopsy

(For orbitotomy, transcranial approach, see 61330-61334)

(For orbital implant, see 67550, 67560)

(For removal of eyeball or for repair after removal, see 65091-65175)

## Other Procedures

67500  Retrobulbar injection; medication (separate procedure, does not include supply of medication)

67505      alcohol

67515  Injection of medication or other substance into Tenon's capsule

(For subconjunctival injection, use 68200)

67550  Orbital implant (implant outside muscle cone); insertion

67560      removal or revision

(For ocular implant (implant inside muscle cone), see 65093-65105, 65130-65175)

(For treatment of fractures of malar area, orbit, see 21355 et seq)

67570  Optic nerve decompression (eg, incision or fenestration of optic nerve sheath)

67599  Unlisted procedure, orbit

# Eyelids

## Incision

67700  Blepharotomy, drainage of abscess, eyelid

67710  Severing of tarsorrhaphy

67715  Canthotomy (separate procedure)

(For canthoplasty, use 67950)

(For division of symblepharon, use 68340)

## Excision, Destruction

Codes for removal of lesion include more than skin (ie, involving lid margin, tarsus, and/or palpebral conjunctiva).

(For removal of lesion, involving mainly skin of eyelid, see 11310-11313; 11440-11446, 11640-11646; 17000-17004)

(For repair of wounds, blepharoplasty, grafts, reconstructive surgery, see 67930-67975)

67800  Excision of chalazion; single

**Surgery: Ocular System**

67801    multiple, same lid

67805    multiple, different lids

67808    under general anesthesia and/or requiring hospitalization, single or multiple

67810    Biopsy of eyelid

67820    Correction of trichiasis; epilation, by forceps only

67825    epilation by other than forceps (eg, by electrosurgery, cryotherapy, laser surgery)

67830    incision of lid margin

67835    incision of lid margin, with free mucous membrane graft

67840    Excision of lesion of eyelid (except chalazion) without closure or with simple direct closure

(For excision and repair of eyelid by reconstructive surgery, see 67961, 67966)

67850    Destruction of lesion of lid margin (up to 1 cm)

(For Mohs micrographic surgery, see 17311-17315)

(For initiation or follow-up care of topical chemotherapy (eg, 5-FU or similar agents), see appropriate office visits)

## Tarsorrhaphy

67875    Temporary closure of eyelids by suture (eg, Frost suture)

67880    Construction of intermarginal adhesions, median tarsorrhaphy, or canthorrhaphy;

67882    with transposition of tarsal plate

(For severing of tarsorrhaphy, use 67710)

(For canthoplasty, reconstruction canthus, use 67950)

(For canthotomy, use 67715)

## Repair (Brow Ptosis, Blepharoptosis, Lid Retraction, Ectropion, Entropion)

67900    Repair of brow ptosis (supraciliary, mid-forehead or coronal approach)

(For forehead rhytidectomy, use 15824)

67901    Repair of blepharoptosis; frontalis muscle technique with suture or other material (eg, banked fascia)

67902    frontalis muscle technique with autologous fascial sling (includes obtaining fascia)

67903    (tarso) levator resection or advancement, internal approach

67904    (tarso) levator resection or advancement, external approach

67906    superior rectus technique with fascial sling (includes obtaining fascia)

67908    conjunctivo-tarso-Muller's muscle-levator resection (eg, Fasanella-Servat type)

67909    Reduction of overcorrection of ptosis

67911    Correction of lid retraction

(For obtaining autogenous graft materials, see 20920, 20922 or 20926)

(For correction of trichiasis by mucous membrane graft, use 67835)

67912    Correction of lagophthalmos, with implantation of upper eyelid lid load (eg, gold weight)

67914    Repair of ectropion; suture

67915    thermocauterization

67916    excision tarsal wedge

67917    extensive (eg, tarsal strip operations)

(For correction of everted punctum, use 68705)

67921    Repair of entropion; suture

67922    thermocauterization

67923    excision tarsal wedge

67924    extensive (eg, tarsal strip or capsulopalpebral fascia repairs operation)

(For repair of cicatricial ectropion or entropion requiring scar excision or skin graft, see also 67961 et seq)

## Reconstruction

Codes for blepharoplasty involve more than skin (ie, involving lid margin, tarsus, and/or palpebral conjunctiva).

67930    Suture of recent wound, eyelid, involving lid margin, tarsus, and/or palpebral conjunctiva direct closure; partial thickness

67935    full thickness

67938    Removal of embedded foreign body, eyelid

(For repair of skin of eyelid, see 12011-12018; 12051-12057; 13150-13153)

(For tarsorrhaphy, canthorrhaphy, see 67880, 67882)

(For repair of blepharoptosis and lid retraction, see 67901-67911)

(For blepharoplasty for entropion, ectropion, see 67916, 67917, 67923, 67924)

(For correction of blepharochalasis (blepharorhytidectomy), see 15820-15823)

(For repair of skin of eyelid, adjacent tissue transfer, see 14060, 14061; preparation for graft, use 15004; free graft, see 15120, 15121, 15260, 15261)

(For excision of lesion of eyelid, use 67800 et seq)

(For repair of lacrimal canaliculi, use 68700)

67950    Canthoplasty (reconstruction of canthus)

**67961** Excision and repair of eyelid, involving lid margin, tarsus, conjunctiva, canthus, or full thickness, may include preparation for skin graft or pedicle flap with adjacent tissue transfer or rearrangement; up to one-fourth of lid margin

**67966** over one-fourth of lid margin

(For canthoplasty, use 67950)

(For free skin grafts, see 15120, 15121, 15260, 15261)

(For tubed pedicle flap preparation, use 15576; for delay, use 15630; for attachment, use 15650)

**67971** Reconstruction of eyelid, full thickness by transfer of tarsoconjunctival flap from opposing eyelid; up to two-thirds of eyelid, 1 stage or first stage

**67973** total eyelid, lower, 1 stage or first stage

**67974** total eyelid, upper, 1 stage or first stage

**67975** second stage

### Other Procedures

**67999** Unlisted procedure, eyelids

# Conjunctiva

(For removal of foreign body, see 65205 et seq)

## Incision and Drainage

**68020** Incision of conjunctiva, drainage of cyst

**68040** Expression of conjunctival follicles (eg, for trachoma)

## Excision and/or Destruction

**68100** Biopsy of conjunctiva

**68110** Excision of lesion, conjunctiva; up to 1 cm

**68115** over 1 cm

**68130** with adjacent sclera

**68135** Destruction of lesion, conjunctiva

## Injection

(For injection into Tenon's capsule or retrobulbar injection, see 67500-67515)

**68200** Subconjunctival injection

## Conjunctivoplasty

(For wound repair, see 65270-65273)

**68320** Conjunctivoplasty; with conjunctival graft or extensive rearrangement

**68325** with buccal mucous membrane graft (includes obtaining graft)

**68326** Conjunctivoplasty, reconstruction cul-de-sac; with conjunctival graft or extensive rearrangement

**68328** with buccal mucous membrane graft (includes obtaining graft)

**68330** Repair of symblepharon; conjunctivoplasty, without graft

**68335** with free graft conjunctiva or buccal mucous membrane (includes obtaining graft)

**68340** division of symblepharon, with or without insertion of conformer or contact lens

## Other Procedures

**68360** Conjunctival flap; bridge or partial (separate procedure)

**68362** total (such as Gunderson thin flap or purse string flap)

(For conjunctival flap for perforating injury, see 65280, 65285)

(For repair of operative wound, use 66250)

(For removal of conjunctival foreign body, see 65205, 65210)

**68371** Harvesting conjunctival allograft, living donor

**68399** Unlisted procedure, conjunctiva

# Lacrimal System

## Incision

**68400** Incision, drainage of lacrimal gland

**68420** Incision, drainage of lacrimal sac (dacryocystotomy or dacryocystostomy)

**68440** Snip incision of lacrimal punctum

## Excision

**68500** Excision of lacrimal gland (dacryoadenectomy), except for tumor; total

**68505** partial

**68510** Biopsy of lacrimal gland

**68520** Excision of lacrimal sac (dacryocystectomy)

**68525** Biopsy of lacrimal sac

**68530** Removal of foreign body or dacryolith, lacrimal passages

**68540** Excision of lacrimal gland tumor; frontal approach

**68550** involving osteotomy

## Repair

**68700** Plastic repair of canaliculi

**68705** Correction of everted punctum, cautery

**68720** Dacryocystorhinostomy (fistulization of lacrimal sac to nasal cavity)

**Surgery: Ocular System**

**68745** Conjunctivorhinostomy (fistulization of conjunctiva to nasal cavity); without tube

**68750**     with insertion of tube or stent

**68760** Closure of the lacrimal punctum; by thermocauterization, ligation, or laser surgery

**68761**     by plug, each

**68770** Closure of lacrimal fistula (separate procedure)

## Probing and/or Related Procedures

**68801** Dilation of lacrimal punctum, with or without irrigation

(To report a bilateral procedure, use 68801 with modifier 50)

**68810** Probing of nasolacrimal duct, with or without irrigation;

(For bilateral procedure, report 68810 with modifier 50)

**68811**     requiring general anesthesia

(For bilateral procedure, report 68811 with modifier 50)

**68815**     with insertion of tube or stent

(See also 92018)

(For bilateral procedure, report 68815 with modifier 50)

**68816**     with transluminal balloon catheter dilation

(Do not report 68816 in conjunction with 68810, 68811, 68815)

(For bilateral procedure, report 68816 with modifier 50)

**68840** Probing of lacrimal canaliculi, with or without irrigation

**68850** Injection of contrast medium for dacryocystography

(For radiological supervision and interpretation, see 70170, 78660)

## Other Procedures

**68899** Unlisted procedure, lacrimal system

# Auditory System

(For diagnostic services (eg, audiometry, vestibular tests), see 92502 et seq)

## External Ear

### Incision

**69000**   Drainage external ear, abscess or hematoma; simple

**69005**        complicated

**69020**   Drainage external auditory canal, abscess

**69090**   Ear piercing

### Excision

**69100**   Biopsy external ear

**69105**   Biopsy external auditory canal

**69110**   Excision external ear; partial, simple repair

**69120**        complete amputation

(For reconstruction of ear, see 15120 et seq)

**69140**   Excision exostosis(es), external auditory canal

**69145**   Excision soft tissue lesion, external auditory canal

**69150**   Radical excision external auditory canal lesion; without neck dissection

**69155**        with neck dissection

(For resection of temporal bone, use 69535)

(For skin grafting, see 15004-15261)

### Removal

**69200**   Removal foreign body from external auditory canal; without general anesthesia

**69205**        with general anesthesia

**69210**   Removal impacted cerumen (separate procedure), 1 or both ears

**69220**   Debridement, mastoidectomy cavity, simple (eg, routine cleaning)

(For bilateral procedure, report 69220 with modifier 50)

**69222**   Debridement, mastoidectomy cavity, complex (eg, with anesthesia or more than routine cleaning)

(For bilateral procedure, report 69222 with modifier 50)

### Repair

(For suture of wound or injury of external ear, see 12011-14302)

⊙ **69300**   Otoplasty, protruding ear, with or without size reduction

(For bilateral procedure, report 69300 with modifier 50)

**69310**   Reconstruction of external auditory canal (meatoplasty) (eg, for stenosis due to injury, infection) (separate procedure)

**69320**   Reconstruction external auditory canal for congenital atresia, single stage

(For combination with middle ear reconstruction, see 69631, 69641)

(For other reconstructive procedures with grafts (eg, skin, cartilage, bone), see 13150-15760, 21230-21235)

## Other Procedures

(For otoscopy under general anesthesia, use 92502)

**69399**   Unlisted procedure, external ear

## Middle Ear

### Introduction

**69400**   Eustachian tube inflation, transnasal; with catheterization

**69401**        without catheterization

**69405**   Eustachian tube catheterization, transtympanic

### Incision

**69420**   Myringotomy including aspiration and/or eustachian tube inflation

**69421**   Myringotomy including aspiration and/or eustachian tube inflation requiring general anesthesia

**69424**   Ventilating tube removal requiring general anesthesia

(For bilateral procedure, report 69424 with modifier 50)

(Do not report code 69424 in conjunction with 69205, 69210, 69420, 69421, 69433-69676, 69710-69745, 69801-69930)

**69433**   Tympanostomy (requiring insertion of ventilating tube), local or topical anesthesia

(For bilateral procedure, report 69433 with modifier 50)

**69436**   Tympanostomy (requiring insertion of ventilating tube), general anesthesia

(For bilateral procedure, report 69436 with modifier 50)

**69440**   Middle ear exploration through postauricular or ear canal incision

(For atticotomy, see 69601 et seq)

**69450**   Tympanolysis, transcanal

### Excision

**69501**   Transmastoid antrotomy (simple mastoidectomy)

**69502**   Mastoidectomy; complete

**69505**        modified radical

Surgery: Auditory System

**69511**  radical

(For skin graft, see 15004 et seq)

(For mastoidectomy cavity debridement, see 69220, 69222)

**69530**  Petrous apicectomy including radical mastoidectomy

**69535**  Resection temporal bone, external approach

(For middle fossa approach, see 69950-69970)

**69540**  Excision aural polyp

**69550**  Excision aural glomus tumor; transcanal

**69552**  transmastoid

**69554**  extended (extratemporal)

## Repair

**69601**  Revision mastoidectomy; resulting in complete mastoidectomy

**69602**  resulting in modified radical mastoidectomy

**69603**  resulting in radical mastoidectomy

**69604**  resulting in tympanoplasty

(For planned secondary tympanoplasty after mastoidectomy, see 69631, 69632)

**69605**  with apicectomy

(For skin graft, see 15120, 15121, 15260, 15261)

**69610**  Tympanic membrane repair, with or without site preparation of perforation for closure, with or without patch

**69620**  Myringoplasty (surgery confined to drumhead and donor area)

**69631**  Tympanoplasty without mastoidectomy (including canalplasty, atticotomy and/or middle ear surgery), initial or revision; without ossicular chain reconstruction

**69632**  with ossicular chain reconstruction (eg, postfenestration)

**69633**  with ossicular chain reconstruction and synthetic prosthesis (eg, partial ossicular replacement prosthesis [PORP], total ossicular replacement prosthesis [TORP])

**69635**  Tympanoplasty with antrotomy or mastoidotomy (including canalplasty, atticotomy, middle ear surgery, and/or tympanic membrane repair); without ossicular chain reconstruction

**69636**  with ossicular chain reconstruction

**69637**  with ossicular chain reconstruction and synthetic prosthesis (eg, partial ossicular replacement prosthesis [PORP], total ossicular replacement prosthesis [TORP])

**69641**  Tympanoplasty with mastoidectomy (including canalplasty, middle ear surgery, tympanic membrane repair); without ossicular chain reconstruction

**69642**  with ossicular chain reconstruction

**69643**  with intact or reconstructed wall, without ossicular chain reconstruction

**69644**  with intact or reconstructed canal wall, with ossicular chain reconstruction

**69645**  radical or complete, without ossicular chain reconstruction

**69646**  radical or complete, with ossicular chain reconstruction

**69650**  Stapes mobilization

**69660**  Stapedectomy or stapedotomy with reestablishment of ossicular continuity, with or without use of foreign material;

**69661**  with footplate drill out

**69662**  Revision of stapedectomy or stapedotomy

**69666**  Repair oval window fistula

**69667**  Repair round window fistula

**69670**  Mastoid obliteration (separate procedure)

**69676**  Tympanic neurectomy

(For bilateral procedure, report 69676 with modifier 50)

## Other Procedures

**69700**  Closure postauricular fistula, mastoid (separate procedure)

**69710**  Implantation or replacement of electromagnetic bone conduction hearing device in temporal bone

(Replacement procedure includes removal of old device)

**69711**  Removal or repair of electromagnetic bone conduction hearing device in temporal bone

**69714**  Implantation, osseointegrated implant, temporal bone, with percutaneous attachment to external speech processor/cochlear stimulator; without mastoidectomy

**69715**  with mastoidectomy

**69717**  Replacement (including removal of existing device), osseointegrated implant, temporal bone, with percutaneous attachment to external speech processor/cochlear stimulator; without mastoidectomy

**69718**  with mastoidectomy

**69720**  Decompression facial nerve, intratemporal; lateral to geniculate ganglion

**69725**  including medial to geniculate ganglion

**69740**  Suture facial nerve, intratemporal, with or without graft or decompression; lateral to geniculate ganglion

**69745**  including medial to geniculate ganglion

(For extracranial suture of facial nerve, use 64864)

**69799**  Unlisted procedure, middle ear

**Surgery: Auditory System**

# Inner Ear

## Incision and/or Destruction

**69801**   Labyrinthotomy, with perfusion of vestibuloactive drug(s); transcanal

(Do not report 69801 more than once per day)

(Do not report 69801 in conjunction with 69420, 69421, 69433, 69436 when performed on the same ear)

▶(69802 has been deleted)◀

**69805**   Endolymphatic sac operation; without shunt

**69806**       with shunt

**69820**   Fenestration semicircular canal

**69840**   Revision fenestration operation

## Excision

**69905**   Labyrinthectomy; transcanal

**69910**       with mastoidectomy

**69915**   Vestibular nerve section, translabyrinthine approach

(For transcranial approach, use 69950)

## Introduction

**69930**   Cochlear device implantation, with or without mastoidectomy

## Other Procedures

**69949**   Unlisted procedure, inner ear

# Temporal Bone, Middle Fossa Approach

(For external approach, use 69535)

**69950**   Vestibular nerve section, transcranial approach

**69955**   Total facial nerve decompression and/or repair (may include graft)

**69960**   Decompression internal auditory canal

**69970**   Removal of tumor, temporal bone

## Other Procedures

**69979**   Unlisted procedure, temporal bone, middle fossa approach

# Operating Microscope

The surgical microscope is employed when the surgical services are performed using the techniques of microsurgery. Code 69990 should be reported (without modifier 51 appended) in addition to the code for the primary procedure performed. Do not use 69990 for visualization with magnifying loupes or corrected vision. Do not report 69990 in addition to procedures where use of the operating microscope is an inclusive component (15756-15758, 15842, 19364, 19368, 20955-20962, 20969-20973, 22551, 22552, 22856-22861, 26551-26554, 26556, 31526, 31531, 31536, 31541, 31545, 31546, 31561, 31571, 43116, 43496, 49906, 61548, 63075-63078, 64727, 64820-64823, 65091-68850, 0184T, 0226T, 0227T).

**+ 69990**   Microsurgical techniques, requiring use of operating microscope (List separately in addition to code for primary procedure)

**Surgery: Auditory System**

# Notes

⊙=Moderate sedation    ✚=Add-on code    ✗=FDA approval pending    #=Resequenced code    ○=Recycled/reinstated code

# Radiology Guidelines (Including Nuclear Medicine and Diagnostic Ultrasound)

Items used by all physicians in reporting their services are presented in the **Introduction.** Some of the commonalities are repeated here for the convenience of those physicians referring to this section on **Radiology (Including Nuclear Medicine and Diagnostic Ultrasound).** Other definitions and items unique to Radiology are also listed.

## Subject Listings

Subject listings apply when radiological services are performed by or under the responsible supervision of a physician.

## Separate Procedures

Some of the procedures or services listed in the CPT codebook that are commonly carried out as an integral component of a total service or procedure have been identified by the inclusion of the term "separate procedure." The codes designated as "separate procedure" should not be reported in addition to the code for the total procedure or service of which it is considered an integral component.

However, when a procedure or service that is designated as a "separate procedure" is carried out independently or considered to be unrelated or distinct from other procedures/services provided at that time, it may be reported by itself, or in addition to other procedures/services by appending modifier 59 to the specific "separate procedure" code to indicate that the procedure is not considered to be a component of another procedure, but is a distinct, independent procedure. This may represent a different session or patient encounter, different procedure or surgery, different site or organ system, separate incision/excision, separate lesion, separate injury, or area of injury in extensive injuries.

## Unlisted Service or Procedure

A service or procedure may be provided that is not listed in this edition of the CPT codebook. When reporting such a service, the appropriate "Unlisted Procedure" code may be used to indicate the service, identifying it by "Special Report" as discussed below. The "Unlisted Procedures" and accompanying codes for **Radiology (Including Nuclear Medicine and Diagnostic Ultrasound)** are as follows:

| | |
|---|---|
| 76496 | Unlisted fluoroscopic procedure (eg, diagnostic, interventional) |
| 76497 | Unlisted computed tomography procedure (eg, diagnostic, interventional) |
| 76498 | Unlisted magnetic resonance procedure (eg, diagnostic, interventional) |
| 76499 | Unlisted diagnostic radiographic procedure |
| 76999 | Unlisted ultrasound procedure (eg, diagnostic, interventional) |
| 77299 | Unlisted procedure, therapeutic radiology clinical treatment planning |
| 77399 | Unlisted procedure, medical radiation physics, dosimetry and treatment devices, and special services |
| 77499 | Unlisted procedure, therapeutic radiology treatment management |
| 77799 | Unlisted procedure, clinical brachytherapy |
| 78099 | Unlisted endocrine procedure, diagnostic nuclear medicine |
| 78199 | Unlisted hematopoietic, reticuloendothelial and lymphatic procedure, diagnostic nuclear medicine |
| 78299 | Unlisted gastrointestinal procedure, diagnostic nuclear medicine |
| 78399 | Unlisted musculoskeletal procedure, diagnostic nuclear medicine |
| 78499 | Unlisted cardiovascular procedure, diagnostic nuclear medicine |
| 78599 | Unlisted respiratory procedure, diagnostic nuclear medicine |

**78699**  Unlisted nervous system procedure, diagnostic nuclear medicine

**78799**  Unlisted genitourinary procedure, diagnostic nuclear medicine

**78999**  Unlisted miscellaneous procedure, diagnostic nuclear medicine

**79999**  Radiopharmaceutical therapy, unlisted procedure

# Special Report

A service that is rarely provided, unusual, variable, or new may require a special report. Pertinent information should include an adequate definition or description of the nature, extent, and need for the procedure; and the time, effort, and equipment necessary to provide the service.

# Supervision and Interpretation

When a procedure is performed by two physicians, the radiologic portion of the procedure is designated as "radiological supervision and interpretation." When a physician performs both the procedure and provides imaging supervision and interpretation, a combination of procedure codes outside the 70000 series and imaging supervision and interpretation codes are to be used.

(The Radiological Supervision and Interpretation codes are not applicable to the Radiation Oncology subsection.)

# Administration of Contrast Material(s)

The phrase "with contrast" used in the codes for procedures performed using contrast for imaging enhancement represents contrast material administered intravascularly, intra-articularly or intrathecally.

For intra-articular injection, use the appropriate joint injection code. If radiographic arthrography is performed, also use the arthrography supervision and interpretation code for the appropriate joint (which includes fluoroscopy). If computed tomography (CT) or magnetic resonance (MR) arthrography are performed without radiographic arthrography, use the appropriate joint injection code, the appropriate CT or MR code ("with contrast" or "without followed by contrast"), and the appropriate imaging guidance code for needle placement for contrast injection.

For spine examinations using computed tomography, magnetic resonance imaging, magnetic resonance angiography, "with contrast" includes intrathecal or intravascular injection. For intrathecal injection, use also 61055 or 62284.

Injection of intravascular contrast material is part of the "with contrast" CT, computed tomographic angiography (CTA), magnetic resonance imaging (MRI), and magnetic resonance angiography (MRA) procedures.

Oral and/or rectal contrast administration alone does not qualify as a study "with contrast."

# Written Report(s)

A written report signed by the interpreting physician should be considered an integral part of a radiologic procedure or interpretation.

# Radiology

## Diagnostic Radiology (Diagnostic Imaging)

### Head and Neck

**70010** Myelography, posterior fossa, radiological supervision and interpretation

**70015** Cisternography, positive contrast, radiological supervision and interpretation

**70030** Radiologic examination, eye, for detection of foreign body

**70100** Radiologic examination, mandible; partial, less than 4 views

**70110** complete, minimum of 4 views

**70120** Radiologic examination, mastoids; less than 3 views per side

**70130** complete, minimum of 3 views per side

**70134** Radiologic examination, internal auditory meati, complete

**70140** Radiologic examination, facial bones; less than 3 views

**70150** complete, minimum of 3 views

**70160** Radiologic examination, nasal bones, complete, minimum of 3 views

**70170** Dacryocystography, nasolacrimal duct, radiological supervision and interpretation

**70190** Radiologic examination; optic foramina

**70200** orbits, complete, minimum of 4 views

**70210** Radiologic examination, sinuses, paranasal, less than 3 views

**70220** Radiologic examination, sinuses, paranasal, complete, minimum of 3 views

**70240** Radiologic examination, sella turcica

**70250** Radiologic examination, skull; less than 4 views

**70260** complete, minimum of 4 views

**70300** Radiologic examination, teeth; single view

**70310** partial examination, less than full mouth

**70320** complete, full mouth

**70328** Radiologic examination, temporomandibular joint, open and closed mouth; unilateral

**70330** bilateral

**70332** Temporomandibular joint arthrography, radiological supervision and interpretation

(Do not report 70332 in conjunction with 77002)

**70336** Magnetic resonance (eg, proton) imaging, temporomandibular joint(s)

**70350** Cephalogram, orthodontic

▲ **70355** Orthopantogram (eg, panoramic x-ray)

**70360** Radiologic examination; neck, soft tissue

**70370** pharynx or larynx, including fluoroscopy and/or magnification technique

**70371** Complex dynamic pharyngeal and speech evaluation by cine or video recording

**70373** Laryngography, contrast, radiological supervision and interpretation

**70380** Radiologic examination, salivary gland for calculus

**70390** Sialography, radiological supervision and interpretation

**70450** Computed tomography, head or brain; without contrast material

**70460** with contrast material(s)

**70470** without contrast material, followed by contrast material(s) and further sections

(To report 3D rendering, see 76376, 76377)

**70480** Computed tomography, orbit, sella, or posterior fossa or outer, middle, or inner ear; without contrast material

**70481** with contrast material(s)

**70482** without contrast material, followed by contrast material(s) and further sections

(To report 3D rendering, see 76376, 76377)

**70486** Computed tomography, maxillofacial area; without contrast material

**70487** with contrast material(s)

**70488** without contrast material, followed by contrast material(s) and further sections

(To report 3D rendering, see 76376, 76377)

**70490** Computed tomography, soft tissue neck; without contrast material

**70491** with contrast material(s)

**70492** without contrast material followed by contrast material(s) and further sections

(To report 3D rendering, see 76376, 76377)

(For cervical spine, see 72125, 72126)

**70496** Computed tomographic angiography, head, with contrast material(s), including noncontrast images, if performed, and image postprocessing

**70498** Computed tomographic angiography, neck, with contrast material(s), including noncontrast images, if performed, and image postprocessing

**70540**  Magnetic resonance (eg, proton) imaging, orbit, face, and/or neck; without contrast material(s)

(For head or neck magnetic resonance angiography studies, see 70544-70546, 70547-70549)

**70542**  with contrast material(s)

**70543**  without contrast material(s), followed by contrast material(s) and further sequences

(Report 70540-70543 once per imaging session)

**70544**  Magnetic resonance angiography, head; without contrast material(s)

**70545**  with contrast material(s)

**70546**  without contrast material(s), followed by contrast material(s) and further sequences

**70547**  Magnetic resonance angiography, neck; without contrast material(s)

**70548**  with contrast material(s)

**70549**  without contrast material(s), followed by contrast material(s) and further sequences

**70551**  Magnetic resonance (eg, proton) imaging, brain (including brain stem); without contrast material

**70552**  with contrast material(s)

**70553**  without contrast material, followed by contrast material(s) and further sequences

(For magnetic spectroscopy, use 76390)

Functional MRI involves identification and mapping of stimulation of brain function. When neurofunctional tests are administered by a technologist or other non-physician or non-psychologist, use 70554. When neurofunctional tests are entirely administered by a physician or psychologist, use 70555.

**70554**  Magnetic resonance imaging, brain, functional MRI; including test selection and administration of repetitive body part movement and/or visual stimulation, not requiring physician or psychologist administration

(Do not report 70554 in conjunction with 96020)

**70555**  requiring physician or psychologist administration of entire neurofunctional testing

(Do not report 70555 unless 96020 is performed)

(Do not report 70554, 70555 in conjunction with 70551-70553 unless a separate diagnostic MRI is performed)

**70557**  Magnetic resonance (eg, proton) imaging, brain (including brain stem and skull base), during open intracranial procedure (eg, to assess for residual tumor or residual vascular malformation); without contrast material

**70558**  with contrast material(s)

**70559**  without contrast material(s), followed by contrast material(s) and further sequences

(For stereotactic biopsy of intracranial lesion with magnetic resonance guidance, use 61751. 70557, 70558 or 70559 may be reported only if a separate report is generated. Report only 1 of the above codes once per operative session. Do not use these codes in conjunction with 61751, 77021, 77022)

## Chest

(For fluoroscopic or ultrasonic guidance for needle placement procedures (eg, biopsy, aspiration, injection, localization device) of the thorax, see 76942, 77002)

**71010**  Radiologic examination, chest; single view, frontal

**71015**  stereo, frontal

**71020**  Radiologic examination, chest, 2 views, frontal and lateral;

**71021**  with apical lordotic procedure

**71022**  with oblique projections

**71023**  with fluoroscopy

**71030**  Radiologic examination, chest, complete, minimum of 4 views;

(For concurrent computer-aided detection [CAD] performed in addition to codes 71010, 71020, 71021, 71022, and 71030, use 0174T. Do not report 71010, 71020, 71021, 71022, and 71030 in conjunction with 0175T for CAD performed remotely from the primary interpretation)

**71034**  with fluoroscopy

(For separate chest fluoroscopy, use 76000)

**71035**  Radiologic examination, chest, special views (eg, lateral decubitus, Bucky studies)

**71040**  Bronchography, unilateral, radiological supervision and interpretation

**71060**  Bronchography, bilateral, radiological supervision and interpretation

▶(71090 has been deleted. To report pacemaker or pacing cardioverter-defibrillator lead insertion, replacement, or revision procedures with fluoroscopic guidance, see 33206-33249. To report fluoroscopic guidance for diagnostic lead evaluation without lead insertion, replacement, or revision procedures, use 76000)◀

**71100**  Radiologic examination, ribs, unilateral; 2 views

**71101**  including posteroanterior chest, minimum of 3 views

**71110**  Radiologic examination, ribs, bilateral; 3 views

**71111**  including posteroanterior chest, minimum of 4 views

**71120**  Radiologic examination; sternum, minimum of 2 views

**71130**  sternoclavicular joint or joints, minimum of 3 views

**71250**  Computed tomography, thorax; without contrast material

**71260**  with contrast material(s)

**Radiology**

**71270**      without contrast material, followed by contrast material(s) and further sections

(For cardiac computed tomography of the heart, see 75571-75574)

(To report 3D rendering, see 76376, 76377)

**71275**    Computed tomographic angiography, chest (noncoronary), with contrast material(s), including noncontrast images, if performed, and image postprocessing

(For coronary artery computed tomographic angiography including calcification score and/or cardiac morphology, use 75574)

**71550**    Magnetic resonance (eg, proton) imaging, chest (eg, for evaluation of hilar and mediastinal lymphadenopathy); without contrast material(s)

**71551**      with contrast material(s)

**71552**      without contrast material(s), followed by contrast material(s) and further sequences

(For breast MRI, see 77058, 77059)

**71555**    Magnetic resonance angiography, chest (excluding myocardium), with or without contrast material(s)

# Spine and Pelvis

**72010**    Radiologic examination, spine, entire, survey study, anteroposterior and lateral

**72020**    Radiologic examination, spine, single view, specify level

**72040**    Radiologic examination, spine, cervical; 2 or 3 views

**72050**      minimum of 4 views

**72052**      complete, including oblique and flexion and/or extension studies

**72069**    Radiologic examination, spine, thoracolumbar, standing (scoliosis)

**72070**    Radiologic examination, spine; thoracic, 2 views

**72072**      thoracic, 3 views

**72074**      thoracic, minimum of 4 views

**72080**      thoracolumbar, 2 views

**72090**      scoliosis study, including supine and erect studies

**72100**    Radiologic examination, spine, lumbosacral; 2 or 3 views

**72110**      minimum of 4 views

▲ **72114**      complete, including bending views, minimum of 6 views

▲ **72120**      bending views only, 2 or 3 views

(Contrast material in CT of spine is either by intrathecal or intravenous injection. For intrathecal injection, use also 61055 or 62284. IV injection of contrast material is part of the CT procedure)

**72125**    Computed tomography, cervical spine; without contrast material

**72126**      with contrast material

**72127**      without contrast material, followed by contrast material(s) and further sections

(For intrathecal injection procedure, see 61055, 62284)

**72128**    Computed tomography, thoracic spine; without contrast material

**72129**      with contrast material

(For intrathecal injection procedure, see 61055, 62284)

**72130**      without contrast material, followed by contrast material(s) and further sections

(For intrathecal injection procedure, see 61055, 62284)

**72131**    Computed tomography, lumbar spine; without contrast material

**72132**      with contrast material

**72133**      without contrast material, followed by contrast material(s) and further sections

(For intrathecal injection procedure, see 61055, 62284)

(To report 3D rendering, see 76376, 76377)

**72141**    Magnetic resonance (eg, proton) imaging, spinal canal and contents, cervical; without contrast material

**72142**      with contrast material(s)

(For cervical spinal canal imaging without contrast material followed by contrast material, use 72156)

**72146**    Magnetic resonance (eg, proton) imaging, spinal canal and contents, thoracic; without contrast material

**72147**      with contrast material(s)

(For thoracic spinal canal imaging without contrast material followed by contrast material, use 72157)

**72148**    Magnetic resonance (eg, proton) imaging, spinal canal and contents, lumbar; without contrast material

**72149**      with contrast material(s)

(For lumbar spinal canal imaging without contrast material followed by contrast material, use 72158)

**72156**    Magnetic resonance (eg, proton) imaging, spinal canal and contents, without contrast material, followed by contrast material(s) and further sequences; cervical

**72157**      thoracic

**72158**      lumbar

**72159**    Magnetic resonance angiography, spinal canal and contents, with or without contrast material(s)

**72170**    Radiologic examination, pelvis; 1 or 2 views

**72190**      complete, minimum of 3 views

(For pelvimetry, use 74710)

►(For a combined computed tomography (CT) or computed tomographic angiography abdomen and pelvis study, see 74174, 74176-74178)◄

**Radiology**

**72191** Computed tomographic angiography, pelvis, with contrast material(s), including noncontrast images, if performed, and image postprocessing

▶(Do not report 72191 in conjunction with 73706 or 75635. For CTA aorto-iliofemoral runoff, use 75635)◄

▶(Do not report 72191 in conjunction with 74175. For a combined computed tomographic angiography abdomen and pelvis study, use 74174)◄

**72192** Computed tomography, pelvis; without contrast material

**72193**      with contrast material(s)

**72194**      without contrast material, followed by contrast material(s) and further sections

(For a combined CT abdomen and pelvis study, see 74176-74178)

(To report 3D rendering, see 76376, 76377)

(For computed tomographic colonography, diagnostic, see 74261-74262. For computed tomographic colonography, screening, use 74263)

(Do not report 72192-72194 in conjunction with 74261-74263)

**72195** Magnetic resonance (eg, proton) imaging, pelvis; without contrast material(s)

**72196**      with contrast material(s)

**72197**      without contrast material(s), followed by contrast material(s) and further sequences

**72198** Magnetic resonance angiography, pelvis, with or without contrast material(s)

**72200** Radiologic examination, sacroiliac joints; less than 3 views

**72202**      3 or more views

**72220** Radiologic examination, sacrum and coccyx, minimum of 2 views

**72240** Myelography, cervical, radiological supervision and interpretation

(For complete cervical myelography, see 61055, 62284, 72240)

**72255** Myelography, thoracic, radiological supervision and interpretation

(For complete thoracic myelography, see 61055, 62284, 72255)

**72265** Myelography, lumbosacral, radiological supervision and interpretation

(For complete lumbosacral myelography, see 61055, 62284, 72265)

**72270** Myelography, 2 or more regions (eg, lumbar/thoracic, cervical/thoracic, lumbar/cervical, lumbar/thoracic/cervical), radiological supervision and interpretation

(For complete myelography of entire spinal canal, see 61055, 62284, 72270)

**72275** Epidurography, radiological supervision and interpretation

(72275 includes 77003)

(For injection procedure, see 62280-62282, 62310-62319, 64479-64484)

(Use 72275 only when an epidurogram is performed, images documented, and a formal radiologic report is issued)

**72285** Discography, cervical or thoracic, radiological supervision and interpretation

**72291** Radiological supervision and interpretation, percutaneous vertebroplasty, vertebral augmentation, or sacral augmentation (sacroplasty), including cavity creation, per vertebral body or sacrum; under fluoroscopic guidance

**72292**      under CT guidance

(For procedure, see 22520-22525, 0200T, 0201T)

**72295** Discography, lumbar, radiological supervision and interpretation

## Upper Extremities

(For stress views, any joint, use 77071)

**73000** Radiologic examination; clavicle, complete

**73010**      scapula, complete

**73020** Radiologic examination, shoulder; 1 view

**73030**      complete, minimum of 2 views

**73040** Radiologic examination, shoulder, arthrography, radiological supervision and interpretation

(Do not report 77002 in conjunction with 73040)

**73050** Radiologic examination; acromioclavicular joints, bilateral, with or without weighted distraction

**73060**      humerus, minimum of 2 views

**73070** Radiologic examination, elbow; 2 views

**73080**      complete, minimum of 3 views

**73085** Radiologic examination, elbow, arthrography, radiological supervision and interpretation

(Do not report 77002 in conjunction with 73085)

**73090** Radiologic examination; forearm, 2 views

**73092**      upper extremity, infant, minimum of 2 views

**73100** Radiologic examination, wrist; 2 views

**73110**      complete, minimum of 3 views

**73115** Radiologic examination, wrist, arthrography, radiological supervision and interpretation

(Do not report 77002 in conjunction with 73115)

**73120** Radiologic examination, hand; 2 views

**73130**      minimum of 3 views

**73140** Radiologic examination, finger(s), minimum of 2 views

Radiology

**73200**　Computed tomography, upper extremity; without contrast material

**73201**　　with contrast material(s)

**73202**　　without contrast material, followed by contrast material(s) and further sections

　　(To report 3D rendering, see 76376, 76377)

**73206**　Computed tomographic angiography, upper extremity, with contrast material(s), including noncontrast images, if performed, and image postprocessing

**73218**　Magnetic resonance (eg, proton) imaging, upper extremity, other than joint; without contrast material(s)

**73219**　　with contrast material(s)

**73220**　　without contrast material(s), followed by contrast material(s) and further sequences

**73221**　Magnetic resonance (eg, proton) imaging, any joint of upper extremity; without contrast material(s)

**73222**　　with contrast material(s)

**73223**　　without contrast material(s), followed by contrast material(s) and further sequences

**73225**　Magnetic resonance angiography, upper extremity, with or without contrast material(s)

## Lower Extremities

　　(For stress views, any joint, use 77071)

**73500**　Radiologic examination, hip, unilateral; 1 view

**73510**　　complete, minimum of 2 views

**73520**　Radiologic examination, hips, bilateral, minimum of 2 views of each hip, including anteroposterior view of pelvis

**73525**　Radiologic examination, hip, arthrography, radiological supervision and interpretation

　　(Do not report 73525 in conjunction with 77002)

**73530**　Radiologic examination, hip, during operative procedure

**73540**　Radiologic examination, pelvis and hips, infant or child, minimum of 2 views

　　▶(73542 has been deleted, for arthrography use 27096)◀

**73550**　Radiologic examination, femur, 2 views

**73560**　Radiologic examination, knee; 1 or 2 views

**73562**　　3 views

**73564**　　complete, 4 or more views

**73565**　　both knees, standing, anteroposterior

**73580**　Radiologic examination, knee, arthrography, radiological supervision and interpretation

　　(Do not report 73580 in conjunction with 77002)

**73590**　Radiologic examination; tibia and fibula, 2 views

**73592**　　lower extremity, infant, minimum of 2 views

**73600**　Radiologic examination, ankle; 2 views

**73610**　　complete, minimum of 3 views

**73615**　Radiologic examination, ankle, arthrography, radiological supervision and interpretation

　　(Do not report 73615 in conjunction with 77002)

**73620**　Radiologic examination, foot; 2 views

**73630**　　complete, minimum of 3 views

**73650**　Radiologic examination; calcaneus, minimum of 2 views

**73660**　　toe(s), minimum of 2 views

**73700**　Computed tomography, lower extremity; without contrast material

**73701**　　with contrast material(s)

**73702**　　without contrast material, followed by contrast material(s) and further sections

　　(To report 3D rendering, see 76376, 76377)

**73706**　Computed tomographic angiography, lower extremity, with contrast material(s), including noncontrast images, if performed, and image postprocessing

　　(For CTA aorto-iliofemoral runoff, use 75635)

**73718**　Magnetic resonance (eg, proton) imaging, lower extremity other than joint; without contrast material(s)

**73719**　　with contrast material(s)

**73720**　　without contrast material(s), followed by contrast material(s) and further sequences

**73721**　Magnetic resonance (eg, proton) imaging, any joint of lower extremity; without contrast material

**73722**　　with contrast material(s)

**73723**　　without contrast material(s), followed by contrast material(s) and further sequences

**73725**　Magnetic resonance angiography, lower extremity, with or without contrast material(s)

## Abdomen

**74000**　Radiologic examination, abdomen; single anteroposterior view

**74010**　　anteroposterior and additional oblique and cone views

**74020**　　complete, including decubitus and/or erect views

**74022**　　complete acute abdomen series, including supine, erect, and/or decubitus views, single view chest

**74150**　Computed tomography, abdomen; without contrast material

**74160**　　with contrast material(s)

**74170**　　without contrast material, followed by contrast material(s) and further sections

　　(For a combined CT abdomen and pelvis study, see 74176-74178)

**Radiology**

(To report 3D rendering, see 76376, 76377)

(For computed tomographic colonography, diagnostic, see 74261-74262. For computed tomographic colonography, screening, use 74263)

(Do not report 74150-74170 in conjunction with 74261-74263)

● **74174** Computed tomographic angiography, abdomen and pelvis, with contrast material(s), including noncontrast images, if performed, and image postprocessing

▶(Do not report 74174 in conjunction with 72191, 73706, 74175, 75635, 76376, 76377)◄

▶(For CTA aorto-iliofemoral runoff, use 75635)◄

**74175** Computed tomographic angiography, abdomen, with contrast material(s), including noncontrast images, if performed, and image postprocessing

▶(Do not report 74175 in conjunction with 73706 or 75635. For CTA aorto-iliofemoral runoff, use 75635)◄

▶(Do not report 74175 in conjunction with 72191. For a combined computed tomographic angiography abdomen and pelvis study, use 74174)◄

For combinations of CT of the abdomen with CT of the pelvis performed at the same session, use the following table. Do not report more than one CT of the abdomen or CT of the pelvis for any session.

| Stand Alone Code | 74150 CT Abdomen WO Contrast | 74160 CT Abdomen W Contrast | 74170 CT Abdomen WO/W Contrast |
|---|---|---|---|
| 72192 CT Pelvis WO Contrst | 74176 | 74178 | 74178 |
| 72193 CT Pelvis W Contrast | 74178 | 74177 | 74178 |
| 72194 CT Pelvis WO/W Contrast | 74178 | 74178 | 74178 |

**74176** Computed tomography, abdomen and pelvis; without contrast material

**74177** with contrast material(s)

**74178** without contrast material in one or both body regions, followed by contrast material(s) and further sections in one or both body regions

(Do not report 74176-74178 in conjunction with 72192-72194, 74150-74170)

(Report 74176, 74177, or 74178 only once per CT abdomen and pelvis examination)

**74181** Magnetic resonance (eg, proton) imaging, abdomen; without contrast material(s)

**74182** with contrast material(s)

**74183** without contrast material(s), followed by with contrast material(s) and further sequences

**74185** Magnetic resonance angiography, abdomen, with or without contrast material(s)

**74190** Peritoneogram (eg, after injection of air or contrast), radiological supervision and interpretation

(For procedure, use 49400)

(For computed tomography, see 72192 or 74150)

## Gastrointestinal Tract

(For percutaneous placement of gastrostomy tube, use 43246)

**74210** Radiologic examination; pharynx and/or cervical esophagus

**74220** esophagus

**74230** Swallowing function, with cineradiography/videoradiography

**74235** Removal of foreign body(s), esophageal, with use of balloon catheter, radiological supervision and interpretation

(For procedure, see 43215, 43247)

**74240** Radiologic examination, gastrointestinal tract, upper; with or without delayed films, without KUB

**74241** with or without delayed films, with KUB

**74245** with small intestine, includes multiple serial films

**74246** Radiological examination, gastrointestinal tract, upper, air contrast, with specific high density barium, effervescent agent, with or without glucagon; with or without delayed films, without KUB

**74247** with or without delayed films, with KUB

**74249** with small intestine follow-through

**74250** Radiologic examination, small intestine, includes multiple serial films;

**74251** via enteroclysis tube

**74260** Duodenography, hypotonic

**74261** Computed tomographic (CT) colonography, diagnostic, including image postprocessing; without contrast material

**74262** with contrast material(s) including non-contrast images, if performed

(Do not report 74261, 74262 in conjunction with 72192-72194, 74150-74170, 74263, 76376, 76377)

**74263** Computed tomographic (CT) colonography, screening, including image postprocessing

(Do not report 74263 in conjunction with 72192-72194, 74150-74170, 74261, 74262, 76376, 76377)

**74270** Radiologic examination, colon; contrast (eg, barium) enema, with or without KUB

⊙=Moderate sedation  ✚=Add-on code  ✒=FDA approval pending  #=Resequenced code  ○=Recycled/reinstated code

Radiology

**74280**     air contrast with specific high density barium, with or without glucagon

**74283**     Therapeutic enema, contrast or air, for reduction of intussusception or other intraluminal obstruction (eg, meconium ileus)

**74290**     Cholecystography, oral contrast;

**74291**     additional or repeat examination or multiple day examination

**74300**     Cholangiography and/or pancreatography; intraoperative, radiological supervision and interpretation

**+ 74301**     additional set intraoperative, radiological supervision and interpretation (List separately in addition to code for primary procedure)

      (Use 74301 in conjunction with 74300)

**74305**     through existing catheter, radiological supervision and interpretation

      (For procedure, see 47505, 48400, 47560-47561, 47563)

      (For biliary duct stone extraction, percutaneous, see 47630, 74327)

**74320**     Cholangiography, percutaneous, transhepatic, radiological supervision and interpretation

**74327**     Postoperative biliary duct calculus removal, percutaneous via T-tube tract, basket, or snare (eg, Burhenne technique), radiological supervision and interpretation

      (For procedure, use 47630)

**74328**     Endoscopic catheterization of the biliary ductal system, radiological supervision and interpretation

      (For procedure, see 43260-43272 as appropriate)

**74329**     Endoscopic catheterization of the pancreatic ductal system, radiological supervision and interpretation

      (For procedure, see 43260-43272 as appropriate)

**74330**     Combined endoscopic catheterization of the biliary and pancreatic ductal systems, radiological supervision and interpretation

      (For procedure, see 43260-43272 as appropriate)

**74340**     Introduction of long gastrointestinal tube (eg, Miller-Abbott), including multiple fluoroscopies and films, radiological supervision and interpretation

      (For tube placement, use 44500)

**74355**     Percutaneous placement of enteroclysis tube, radiological supervision and interpretation

**74360**     Intraluminal dilation of strictures and/or obstructions (eg, esophagus), radiological supervision and interpretation

**74363**     Percutaneous transhepatic dilation of biliary duct stricture with or without placement of stent, radiological supervision and interpretation

      (For procedure, see 47510, 47511, 47555, 47556)

## Urinary Tract

**74400**     Urography (pyelography), intravenous, with or without KUB, with or without tomography

**74410**     Urography, infusion, drip technique and/or bolus technique;

**74415**     with nephrotomography

**74420**     Urography, retrograde, with or without KUB

**74425**     Urography, antegrade (pyelostogram, nephrostogram, loopogram), radiological supervision and interpretation

**74430**     Cystography, minimum of 3 views, radiological supervision and interpretation

**74440**     Vasography, vesiculography, or epididymography, radiological supervision and interpretation

**74445**     Corpora cavernosography, radiological supervision and interpretation

**74450**     Urethrocystography, retrograde, radiological supervision and interpretation

**74455**     Urethrocystography, voiding, radiological supervision and interpretation

**74470**     Radiologic examination, renal cyst study, translumbar, contrast visualization, radiological supervision and interpretation

**74475**     Introduction of intracatheter or catheter into renal pelvis for drainage and/or injection, percutaneous, radiological supervision and interpretation

**74480**     Introduction of ureteral catheter or stent into ureter through renal pelvis for drainage and/or injection, percutaneous, radiological supervision and interpretation

      (For transurethral surgery [ureter and pelvis], see 52320-52355)

**74485**     Dilation of nephrostomy, ureters, or urethra, radiological supervision and interpretation

      (For dilation of ureter without radiologic guidance, use 52341, 52344)

      (For change of nephrostomy or pyelostomy tube, use 50398)

## Gynecological and Obstetrical

      (For abdomen and pelvis, see 72170-72190, 74000-74170)

**74710**     Pelvimetry, with or without placental localization

**74740**     Hysterosalpingography, radiological supervision and interpretation

      (For introduction of saline or contrast for hysterosalpingography, see 58340)

**74742**     Transcervical catheterization of fallopian tube, radiological supervision and interpretation

      (For procedure, use 58345)

**74775**     Perineogram (eg, vaginogram, for sex determination or extent of anomalies)

**Radiology**

---

△=Revised code    ●=New code    ▶ ◀=Contains new or revised text    ⃠=Modifier 51 exempt      

# Heart

Cardiac magnetic imaging differs from traditional magnetic resonance imaging (MRI) in its ability to provide a physiologic evaluation of cardiac function. Traditional MRI relies on static images to obtain clinical diagnoses based upon anatomic information. Improvement in spatial and temporal resolution has expanded the application from an anatomic test and includes physiologic evaluation of cardiac function. Flow and velocity assessment for valves and intracardiac shunts is performed in addition to a function and morphologic evaluation. Use 75559 with 75565 to report flow with pharmacologic wall motion stress evaluation without contrast. Use 75563 with 75565 to report flow with pharmacologic perfusion stress with contrast.

Cardiac MRI for velocity flow mapping can be reported in conjunction with 75557, 75559, 75561, or 75563.

Listed procedures may be performed independently or in the course of overall medical care. If the physician providing these services is also responsible for diagnostic workup and/or follow-up care of the patient, see appropriate sections also. Only one procedure in the series 75557-75563 is appropriately reported per session. Only one add-on code for flow velocity can be reported per session.

Cardiac MRI studies may be performed at rest and/or during pharmacologic stress. Therefore, the appropriate stress testing code from the 93015-93018 series should be reported in addition to 75559 or 75563.

Cardiac computed tomography (CT) and coronary computed tomographic angiography (CTA) include the axial source images of the pre-contrast, arterial phase sequence, and venous phase sequence (if performed), as well as the two-dimensional and three-dimensional reformatted images resulting from the study, including cine review. Contrast enhanced cardiac CT and coronary CTA codes 75571-75574 include any quantitative assessment when performed as part of the same encounter. Report only one computed tomography heart service per encounter.

> (For separate injection procedures for vascular radiology, see **Surgery** section, 36000-36299)
>
> (For cardiac catheterization procedures, see 93451-93572)
>
> (75552-75556 have been deleted. To report, see 75557, 75559, 75561, 75563, 75565)

**75557**  Cardiac magnetic resonance imaging for morphology and function without contrast material;

**75559**      with stress imaging

**75561**  Cardiac magnetic resonance imaging for morphology and function without contrast material(s), followed by contrast material(s) and further sequences;

**75563**      with stress imaging

> (75558, 75560, 75562, 75564 have been deleted. To report flow velocity, use 75565)

**+ 75565**  Cardiac magnetic resonance imaging for velocity flow mapping (List separately in addition to code for primary procedure)

> (Use 75565 in conjunction with 75557, 75559, 75561, 75563)
>
> (Do not report 75557, 75559, 75561, 75563, 75565 in conjunction with 76376, 76377)

**75571**  Computed tomography, heart, without contrast material, with quantitative evaluation of coronary calcium

**75572**  Computed tomography, heart, with contrast material, for evaluation of cardiac structure and morphology (including 3D image postprocessing, assessment of cardiac function, and evaluation of venous structures, if performed)

**75573**  Computed tomography, heart, with contrast material, for evaluation of cardiac structure and morphology in the setting of congenital heart disease (including 3D image postprocessing, assessment of LV cardiac function, RV structure and function and evaluation of venous structures, if performed)

**75574**  Computed tomographic angiography, heart, coronary arteries and bypass grafts (when present), with contrast material, including 3D image postprocessing (including evaluation of cardiac structure and morphology, assessment of cardiac function, and evaluation of venous structures, if performed)

# Vascular Procedures

## Aorta and Arteries

Selective vascular catheterizations should be coded to include introduction and all lesser order selective catheterizations used in the approach (eg, the description for a selective right middle cerebral artery catheterization includes the introduction and placement catheterization of the right common and internal carotid arteries).

Additional second and/or third order arterial catheterizations within the same family of arteries supplied by a single first order artery should be expressed by 36218 or 36248. Additional first order or higher catheterizations in vascular families supplied by a first order vessel different from a previously selected and coded family should be separately coded using the conventions described above.

The lower extremity endovascular revascularization codes describing services performed for occlusive disease (37220-37235) include catheterization (36200, 36140, 36245-36248) in the work described by the codes. Catheterization codes are not additionally reported for diagnostic lower extremity angiography when performed through the same access site as the therapy (37220-37235) performed in the same session. However,

Radiology

catheterization for the diagnostic lower extremity angiogram may be reported separately if a different arterial puncture site is necessary.

For angiography performed in conjunction with therapeutic transcatheter radiological supervision and interpretation services, see the **Radiology Transcatheter Procedures** guidelines.

Diagnostic angiography (radiological supervision and interpretation) codes should NOT be used with interventional procedures for:

1. Contrast injections, angiography, roadmapping, and/or fluoroscopic guidance for the intervention,

2. Vessel measurement, and

3. Post-angioplasty/stent/atherectomy angiography, as this work is captured in the radiological supervision and interpretation code(s). In those therapeutic codes that include radiological supervision and interpretation, this work is captured in the therapeutic code.

Diagnostic angiography performed at the time of an interventional procedure is separately reportable if:

1. No prior catheter-based angiographic study is available and a full diagnostic study is performed, and the decision to intervene is based on the diagnostic study, OR

2. A prior study is available, but as documented in the medical record:

   a. The patient's condition with respect to the clinical indication has changed since the prior study, OR

   b. There is inadequate visualization of the anatomy and/or pathology, OR

   c. There is a clinical change during the procedure that requires new evaluation outside the target area of intervention.

Diagnostic angiography performed at a separate sessions from an interventional procedure is separately reported.

If diagnostic angiography is necessary, is performed at the same session as the interventional procedure and meets the above criteria, modifier 59 must be appended to the diagnostic radiological supervision and interpretation code(s) to denote that diagnostic work has been done following these guidelines.

Diagnostic angiography performed at the time of an interventional procedure is NOT separately reportable if it is specifically included in the interventional code descriptor.

(For intravenous procedure, see 36000, 36005-36015, and for intra-arterial procedure, see 36100-36248)

(For radiological supervision and interpretation, see 75600-75893)

**75600** Aortography, thoracic, without serialography, radiological supervision and interpretation

(For injection procedure, use 93567, which includes imaging supervision, interpretation, and report)

**75605** Aortography, thoracic, by serialography, radiological supervision and interpretation

(For injection procedure, use 93567, which includes imaging supervision, interpretation, and report)

**75625** Aortography, abdominal, by serialography, radiological supervision and interpretation

(For injection procedure, use 93567, which includes imaging supervision, interpretation, and report)

**75630** Aortography, abdominal plus bilateral iliofemoral lower extremity, catheter, by serialography, radiological supervision and interpretation

**75635** Computed tomographic angiography, abdominal aorta and bilateral iliofemoral lower extremity runoff, with contrast material(s), including noncontrast images, if performed, and image postprocessing

►(Do not report 75635 in conjunction with 72191, 73706, 74175 or 74174)◄

**75650** Angiography, cervicocerebral, catheter, including vessel origin, radiological supervision and interpretation

**75658** Angiography, brachial, retrograde, radiological supervision and interpretation

**75660** Angiography, external carotid, unilateral, selective, radiological supervision and interpretation

**75662** Angiography, external carotid, bilateral, selective, radiological supervision and interpretation

**75665** Angiography, carotid, cerebral, unilateral, radiological supervision and interpretation

**75671** Angiography, carotid, cerebral, bilateral, radiological supervision and interpretation

**75676** Angiography, carotid, cervical, unilateral, radiological supervision and interpretation

**75680** Angiography, carotid, cervical, bilateral, radiological supervision and interpretation

**75685** Angiography, vertebral, cervical, and/or intracranial, radiological supervision and interpretation

**75705** Angiography, spinal, selective, radiological supervision and interpretation

**75710** Angiography, extremity, unilateral, radiological supervision and interpretation

**75716** Angiography, extremity, bilateral, radiological supervision and interpretation

►(75722 has been deleted. To report, see 36251, 36253)◄

►(75724 has been deleted. To report, see 36252, 36254)◄

**75726** Angiography, visceral, selective or supraselective (with or without flush aortogram), radiological supervision and interpretation

(For selective angiography, each additional visceral vessel studied after basic examination, use 75774)

**75731**   Angiography, adrenal, unilateral, selective, radiological supervision and interpretation

**75733**   Angiography, adrenal, bilateral, selective, radiological supervision and interpretation

**75736**   Angiography, pelvic, selective or supraselective, radiological supervision and interpretation

**75741**   Angiography, pulmonary, unilateral, selective, radiological supervision and interpretation

(For injection procedure, use 93568, which includes imaging supervision, interpretation, and report)

**75743**   Angiography, pulmonary, bilateral, selective, radiological supervision and interpretation

(For injection procedure, use 93568, which includes imaging supervision, interpretation, and report)

**75746**   Angiography, pulmonary, by nonselective catheter or venous injection, radiological supervision and interpretation

(For injection procedure, use 93568, which includes imaging supervision, interpretation, and report)

(For introduction of catheter, injection procedure, see 93451, 93453-93461, 93530-93533, 93563, 93564, 93568)

**75756**   Angiography, internal mammary, radiological supervision and interpretation

(For introduction of catheter, injection procedure, see 93451-93462, 93530-93533, 93563, 93564, 93567, 93568, which includes imaging supervision, interpretation, and report)

**+ 75774**   Angiography, selective, each additional vessel studied after basic examination, radiological supervision and interpretation (List separately in addition to code for primary procedure)

(Use 75774 in addition to code for specific initial vessel studied)

(For angiography, see 36147, 75600-75756, 75791)

(For catheterizations, see codes 36215-36248)

(For introduction of catheter, injection procedure, see 93451-93462, 93530-93533, 93563-93568)

(75790 has been deleted. To report, see 36147, 75791)

**75791**   Angiography, arteriovenous shunt (eg, dialysis patient fistula/graft), complete evaluation of dialysis access, including fluoroscopy, image documentation and report (includes injections of contrast and all necessary imaging from the arterial anastomosis and adjacent artery through entire venous outflow including the inferior or superior vena cava), radiological supervision and interpretation

(Do not report 75791 in conjunction with 36147, 36148)

(For introduction of catheter, if necessary, see 36140, 36215-36217, 36245-36247)

(Use 75791 only if radiological evaluation is performed through an already existing access into the shunt or from an access that is not a direct puncture of the shunt)

(For radiological evaluation with needle/catheter introduction, AV dialysis shunt, complete procedure, use 36147)

## Veins and Lymphatics

For venography performed in conjunction with therapeutic transcatheter radiological supervision and interpretation services, see the **Radiology Transcatheter Procedures** guidelines.

Diagnostic venography (radiological supervision and interpretation) codes should NOT be used with interventional procedures for:

1. Contrast injections, venography, roadmapping, and/ or fluoroscopic guidance for the intervention,

2. Vessel measurement, and

3. Post-angioplasty/stent venography, as this work is captured in the radiological supervision and intrepretation code(s).

Diagnostic venography performed at the time of an interventional procedure is separately reportable if:

1. No prior catheter-based venographic study is available and a full diagnostic study is performed, and decision to intervene is based on the diagnostic study, OR

2. A prior study is available, but as documented in the medical record:

   a. The patient's condition with respect to the clinical indication has changed since the prior study, OR

   b. There is inadequate visualization of the anatomy and/or pathology, OR

   c. There is a clinical change during the procedure that requires new evaluation outside the target area of intervention.

Diagnostic venography performed at a separate setting from an interventional procedure is separately reported.

Diagnostic venography performed at the time of an interventional procedure is NOT separately reportable if it is specifically included in the interventional code descriptor.

(For injection procedure for venous system, see 36000-36015, 36400-36510)

(For injection procedure for lymphatic system, use 38790)

**75801**   Lymphangiography, extremity only, unilateral, radiological supervision and interpretation

**75803**   Lymphangiography, extremity only, bilateral, radiological supervision and interpretation

**75805**   Lymphangiography, pelvic/abdominal, unilateral, radiological supervision and interpretation

| | |
|---|---|
| 75807 | Lymphangiography, pelvic/abdominal, bilateral, radiological supervision and interpretation |
| 75809 | Shuntogram for investigation of previously placed indwelling nonvascular shunt (eg, LeVeen shunt, ventriculoperitoneal shunt, indwelling infusion pump), radiological supervision and interpretation |

(For procedure, see 49427 or 61070)

| | |
|---|---|
| 75810 | Splenoportography, radiological supervision and interpretation |
| 75820 | Venography, extremity, unilateral, radiological supervision and interpretation |
| 75822 | Venography, extremity, bilateral, radiological supervision and interpretation |
| 75825 | Venography, caval, inferior, with serialography, radiological supervision and interpretation |
| 75827 | Venography, caval, superior, with serialography, radiological supervision and interpretation |
| 75831 | Venography, renal, unilateral, selective, radiological supervision and interpretation |
| 75833 | Venography, renal, bilateral, selective, radiological supervision and interpretation |
| 75840 | Venography, adrenal, unilateral, selective, radiological supervision and interpretation |
| 75842 | Venography, adrenal, bilateral, selective, radiological supervision and interpretation |
| 75860 | Venography, venous sinus (eg, petrosal and inferior sagittal) or jugular, catheter, radiological supervision and interpretation |
| 75870 | Venography, superior sagittal sinus, radiological supervision and interpretation |
| 75872 | Venography, epidural, radiological supervision and interpretation |
| 75880 | Venography, orbital, radiological supervision and interpretation |
| 75885 | Percutaneous transhepatic portography with hemodynamic evaluation, radiological supervision and interpretation |
| 75887 | Percutaneous transhepatic portography without hemodynamic evaluation, radiological supervision and interpretation |
| 75889 | Hepatic venography, wedged or free, with hemodynamic evaluation, radiological supervision and interpretation |
| 75891 | Hepatic venography, wedged or free, without hemodynamic evaluation, radiological supervision and interpretation |
| 75893 | Venous sampling through catheter, with or without angiography (eg, for parathyroid hormone, renin), radiological supervision and interpretation |

(For procedure, use 36500)

## Transcatheter Procedures

Therapeutic transcatheter radiological supervision and interpretation code(s) include the following services associated with that intervention:

1. Contrast injections, angiography/venography, roadmapping, and fluoroscopic guidance for the intervention,

2. Vessel measurement, and

3. Completion angiography/venography (except for those uses permitted by 75898).

Unless specifically included in the code descriptor, diagnostic angiography/venography performed at the time of transcatheter therapeutic radiological and interpretation service(s) is separately reportable (eg, no prior catheter-based diagnostic angiography/venography study of the target vessel is available, prior diagnostic study is inadequate, patient's condition with respect to the clinical indication has changed since the prior study or during the intervention). See 75600-75893.

Codes 75956 and 75957 include all angiography of the thoracic aorta and its branches for diagnostic imaging prior to deployment of the primary endovascular devices (including all routine components of modular devices), fluoroscopic guidance in the delivery of the endovascular components, and intraprocedural arterial angiography (eg, confirm position, detect endoleak, evaluate runoff).

Code 75958 includes the analogous services for placement of each proximal thoracic endovascular extension. Code 75959 includes the analogous services for placement of a distal thoracic endovascular extension(s) placed during a procedure after the primary repair.

| | |
|---|---|
| 75894 | Transcatheter therapy, embolization, any method, radiological supervision and interpretation |

(For uterine fibroid embolization [uterine artery embolization performed to treat uterine fibroids], use 37210)

(For obstetrical and gynecologic embolization procedures other than uterine fibroid embolization [eg, embolization to treat obstetrical or postpartum hemorrhage], use 37204)

| | |
|---|---|
| 75896 | Transcatheter therapy, infusion, any method (eg, thrombolysis other than coronary), radiological supervision and interpretation |

(For infusion for coronary disease, see 92975, 92977)

| | |
|---|---|
| 75898 | Angiography through existing catheter for follow-up study for transcatheter therapy, embolization or infusion |
| 75900 | Exchange of a previously placed intravascular catheter during thrombolytic therapy with contrast monitoring, radiological supervision and interpretation |

(For procedure, use 37209)

Radiology

**75901**    Mechanical removal of pericatheter obstructive material (eg, fibrin sheath) from central venous device via separate venous access, radiologic supervision and interpretation

(For procedure, use 36595)

(For venous catheterization, see 36010-36012)

**75902**    Mechanical removal of intraluminal (intracatheter) obstructive material from central venous device through device lumen, radiologic supervision and interpretation

(For procedure, use 36596)

(For venous catheterization, see 36010-36012)

▶(75940 has been deleted. To report, use 37191)◀

**75945**    Intravascular ultrasound (non-coronary vessel), radiological supervision and interpretation; initial vessel

**+ 75946**       each additional non-coronary vessel (List separately in addition to code for primary procedure)

(Use 75946 in conjunction with 75945)

(For catheterizations, see codes 36215-36248)

(For transcatheter therapies, see codes 37200-37208, 61624, 61626)

(For procedure, see 37250, 37251)

**75952**    Endovascular repair of infrarenal abdominal aortic aneurysm or dissection, radiological supervision and interpretation

▶(For implantation of endovascular grafts, see 34800-34805)◀

▶(For radiologic supervision and interpretation of endovascular repair of abdominal aortic aneurysm involving visceral vessels, see Category III codes 0080T, 0081T)◀

**75953**    Placement of proximal or distal extension prosthesis for endovascular repair of infrarenal aortic or iliac artery aneurysm, pseudoaneurysm, or dissection, radiological supervision and interpretation

(For implantation of endovascular extension prostheses, see 34825, 34826)

**75954**    Endovascular repair of iliac artery aneurysm, pseudoaneurysm, arteriovenous malformation, or trauma, using ilio-iliac tube endoprosthesis, radiological supervision and interpretation

(For implantation of endovascular graft, see 34900)

(For endovascular repair of iliac artery bifurcation [eg, aneurysm, pseudoaneurysm, arteriovenous malformation, trauma] using bifurcated endoprosthesis, radiological supervision and interpretation, use 0255T)

**75956**    Endovascular repair of descending thoracic aorta (eg, aneurysm, pseudoaneurysm, dissection, penetrating ulcer, intramural hematoma, or traumatic disruption); involving coverage of left subclavian artery origin, initial endoprosthesis plus descending thoracic aortic extension(s), if required, to level of celiac artery origin, radiological supervision and interpretation

(For implantation of endovascular graft, use 33880)

**75957**       not involving coverage of left subclavian artery origin, initial endoprosthesis plus descending thoracic aortic extension(s), if required, to level of celiac artery origin, radiological supervision and interpretation

(For implantation of endovascular graft, use 33881)

**75958**    Placement of proximal extension prosthesis for endovascular repair of descending thoracic aorta (eg, aneurysm, pseudoaneurysm, dissection, penetrating ulcer, intramural hematoma, or traumatic disruption), radiological supervision and interpretation

(Report 75958 for each proximal extension)

(For implantation of proximal endovascular extension, see 33883, 33884)

**75959**    Placement of distal extension prosthesis(s) (delayed) after endovascular repair of descending thoracic aorta, as needed, to level of celiac origin, radiological supervision and interpretation

(Do not report 75959 in conjunction with 75956, 75957)

(Report 75959 once, regardless of number of modules deployed)

(For implantation of distal endovascular extension, use 33886)

**75960**    Transcatheter introduction of intravascular stent(s) (except coronary, carotid, vertebral, iliac, and lower extremity artery), percutaneous and/or open, radiological supervision and interpretation, each vessel

(For stent placement, including radiological supervision and interpretation, in iliac, femoral, popliteal, and tibial/peroneal arteries, see 37221, 37223, 37226, 37227, 37230, 37231, 37234, 37235)

(For procedure, see 37205-37208)

(For radiologic supervision and interpretation for transcatheter placement of extracranial vertebral or intrathoracic carotid artery stent(s), see Category III codes 0075T, 0076T)

**75961**    Transcatheter retrieval, percutaneous, of intravascular foreign body (eg, fractured venous or arterial catheter), radiological supervision and interpretation

(For procedure, use 37203)

▶(For removal of a vena cava filter, use 37193)◀

▲ **75962**    Transluminal balloon angioplasty, peripheral artery other than renal, or other visceral artery, iliac or lower extremity, radiological supervision and interpretation

(For radiological supervision and interpretation for transluminal balloon angioplasty in iliac, femoral, popliteal, and tibial/peroneal arteries, see 37220-37235)

►(For procedure, see 35458, 35475)◄

**+▲ 75964** Transluminal balloon angioplasty, each additional peripheral artery other than renal, or other visceral artery, iliac or lower extremity, radiological supervision and interpretation (List separately in addition to code for primary procedure)

(Use 75964 in conjunction with 75962)

**75966** Transluminal balloon angioplasty, renal or other visceral artery, radiological supervision and interpretation

**+ 75968** Transluminal balloon angioplasty, each additional visceral artery, radiological supervision and interpretation (List separately in addition to code for primary procedure)

(Use 75968 in conjunction with 75966)

(For percutaneous transluminal coronary angioplasty, see 92982-92984)

**75970** Transcatheter biopsy, radiological supervision and interpretation

(For injection procedure only for transcatheter therapy or biopsy, see 36100-36299)

(For transcatheter renal and ureteral biopsy, use 52007)

(For percutaneous needle biopsy of pancreas, use 48102; of retroperitoneal lymph node or mass, use 49180)

**75978** Transluminal balloon angioplasty, venous (eg, subclavian stenosis), radiological supervision and interpretation

**75980** Percutaneous transhepatic biliary drainage with contrast monitoring, radiological supervision and interpretation

**75982** Percutaneous placement of drainage catheter for combined internal and external biliary drainage or of a drainage stent for internal biliary drainage in patients with an inoperable mechanical biliary obstruction, radiological supervision and interpretation

**75984** Change of percutaneous tube or drainage catheter with contrast monitoring (eg, genitourinary system, abscess), radiological supervision and interpretation

(For percutaneous replacement of gastrostomy, duodenostomy, jejunostomy, gastro-jejunostomy, or cecostomy [or other colonic] tube including fluoroscopic imaging guidance, see 49450-49452)

(For change of nephrostomy or pyelostomy tube only, use 50398)

(For introduction procedure only for percutaneous biliary drainage, see 47510, 47511)

(For percutaneous cholecystostomy, use 47490)

(For change of percutaneous biliary drainage catheter only, use 47525)

(For percutaneous nephrostolithotomy or pyelostolithotomy, see 50080, 50081)

(For removal and/or replacement of an internally dwelling ureteral stent via a transurethral approach, see 50385-50386)

**75989** Radiological guidance (ie, fluoroscopy, ultrasound, or computed tomography), for percutaneous drainage (eg, abscess, specimen collection), with placement of catheter, radiological supervision and interpretation

(Do not report 75989 in conjunction with 47490)

## Transluminal Atherectomy

(75992 has been deleted. To report, see 37225, 37227, 37229, 37231, 0238T)

(75993 has been deleted. To report, see 37233, 37235, 0238T)

(75994 has been deleted. To report, use 0234T)

(75995 has been deleted. To report, use 0235T)

(75996 has been deleted. To report, use 0235T)

## Other Procedures

(For computed tomography cerebral perfusion analysis, see Category III code 0042T)

(For arthrography of shoulder, use 73040; elbow, use 73085; wrist, use 73115; hip, use 73525; knee, use 73580; ankle, use 73615)

**76000** Fluoroscopy (separate procedure), up to 1 hour physician time, other than 71023 or 71034 (eg, cardiac fluoroscopy)

**76001** Fluoroscopy, physician time more than 1 hour, assisting a nonradiologic physician (eg, nephrostolithotomy, ERCP, bronchoscopy, transbronchial biopsy)

**76010** Radiologic examination from nose to rectum for foreign body, single view, child

**76080** Radiologic examination, abscess, fistula or sinus tract study, radiological supervision and interpretation

(For contrast injection[s] and radiological assessment of gastrostomy, duodenostomy, jejunostomy, gastro-jejunostomy, or cecostomy [or other colonic] tube including fluoroscopic imaging guidance, use 49465)

**76098** Radiological examination, surgical specimen

**76100** Radiologic examination, single plane body section (eg, tomography), other than with urography

**76101** Radiologic examination, complex motion (ie, hypercycloidal) body section (eg, mastoid polytomography), other than with urography; unilateral

**76102** bilateral

►(Do not report 76101, 76102 more than once per day)◄

►(For panoramic X-ray, use 70355)◄

(For nephrotomography, use 74415)

**76120** Cineradiography/videoradiography, except where specifically included

**Radiology**

**+ 76125**   Cineradiography/videoradiography to complement routine examination (List separately in addition to code for primary procedure)

**76140**   Consultation on X-ray examination made elsewhere, written report

(76150 has been deleted)

(76350 has been deleted)

(2D reformatting is no longer separately reported. To report 3D rendering, see 76376, 76377)

(76376, 76377 require concurrent physician supervision of image postprocessing 3D manipulation of volumetric data set and image rendering)

**76376**   3D rendering with interpretation and reporting of computed tomography, magnetic resonance imaging, ultrasound, or other tomographic modality; not requiring image postprocessing on an independent workstation

(Use 76376 in conjunction with code[s] for base imaging procedure[s])

▶(Do not report 76376 in conjunction with 31627, 70496, 70498, 70544-70549, 71275, 71555, 72159, 72191, 72198, 73206, 73225, 73706, 73725, 74174, 74175, 74185, 74261-74263, 75557, 75559, 75561, 75563, 75565, 75571-75574, 75635, 76377, 78000-78999, 0159T)◀

**76377**   requiring image postprocessing on an independent workstation

(Use 76377 in conjunction with code[s] for base imaging procedure[s])

▶(Do not report 76377 in conjunction with 70496, 70498, 70544-70549, 71275, 71555, 72159, 72191, 72198, 73206, 73225, 73706, 73725, 74174, 74175, 74185, 74261-74263, 75557, 75559, 75561, 75563, 75565, 75571-75574, 75635, 76376, 78000-78999, 0159T)◀

(To report computer-aided detection, including computer algorithm analysis of MRI data for lesion detection/characterization, pharmacokinetic analysis, breast MRI, use Category III code 0159T)

**76380**   Computed tomography, limited or localized follow-up study

**76390**   Magnetic resonance spectroscopy

(For magnetic resonance imaging, use appropriate MRI body site code)

**76496**   Unlisted fluoroscopic procedure (eg, diagnostic, interventional)

**76497**   Unlisted computed tomography procedure (eg, diagnostic, interventional)

**76498**   Unlisted magnetic resonance procedure (eg, diagnostic, interventional)

**76499**   Unlisted diagnostic radiographic procedure

# Diagnostic Ultrasound

All diagnostic ultrasound examinations require permanently recorded images with measurements, when such measurements are clinically indicated. For those codes whose sole diagnostic goal is a biometric measure (ie, 76514, 76516, and 76519), permanently recorded images are not required. A final, written report should be issued for inclusion in the patient's medical record. The prescription form for the intraocular lens satisfies the written report requirement for 76519. For those anatomic regions that have "complete" and "limited" ultrasound codes, note the elements that comprise a "complete" exam. The report should contain a description of these elements or the reason that an element could not be visualized (eg, obscured by bowel gas, surgically absent).

If less than the required elements for a "complete" exam are reported (eg, limited number of organs or limited portion of region evaluated), the "limited" code for that anatomic region should be used once per patient exam session. A "limited" exam of an anatomic region should not be reported for the same exam session as a "complete" exam of that same region.

▶Evaluation of vascular structures using both color and spectral Doppler is separately reportable. To report, see **Noninvasive Vascular Diagnostic Studies** (93880-93990). However, color Doppler alone, when performed for anatomic structure identification in conjunction with a real-time ultrasound examination, is not reported separately.◀

Ultrasound guidance procedures also require permanently recorded images of the site to be localized, as well as a documented description of the localization process, either separately or within the report of the procedure for which the guidance is utilized.

Use of ultrasound, without thorough evaluation of organ(s) or anatomic region, image documentation, and final, written report, is not separately reportable.

**Definitions**

*A-mode* implies a one-dimensional ultrasonic measurement procedure.

*M-mode* implies a one-dimensional ultrasonic measurement procedure with movement of the trace to record amplitude and velocity of moving echo-producing structures.

*B-scan* implies a two-dimensional ultrasonic scanning procedure with a two-dimensional display.

*Real-time scan* implies a two-dimensional ultrasonic scanning procedure with display of both two-dimensional structure and motion with time.

▶(To report diagnostic vascular ultrasound studies, see 93880-93990)◀

(For focused ultrasound ablation treatment of uterine leiomyomata, see Category III codes 0071T, 0072T)

⊙=Moderate sedation   +=Add-on code   ⁄=FDA approval pending   #=Resequenced code   ○=Recycled/reinstated code

# Head and Neck

**76506**　Echoencephalography, real time with image documentation (gray scale) (for determination of ventricular size, delineation of cerebral contents, and detection of fluid masses or other intracranial abnormalities), including A-mode encephalography as secondary component where indicated

**76510**　Ophthalmic ultrasound, diagnostic; B-scan and quantitative A-scan performed during the same patient encounter

**76511**　　　quantitative A-scan only

**76512**　　　B-scan (with or without superimposed non-quantitative A-scan)

**76513**　　　anterior segment ultrasound, immersion (water bath) B-scan or high resolution biomicroscopy

(For scanning computerized ophthalmic diagnostic imaging of the anterior and posterior segments using technology other than ultrasound, see 92132, 92133, 92134)

**76514**　　　corneal pachymetry, unilateral or bilateral (determination of corneal thickness)

**76516**　Ophthalmic biometry by ultrasound echography, A-scan;

**76519**　　　with intraocular lens power calculation

(For partial coherence interferometry, use 92136)

**76529**　Ophthalmic ultrasonic foreign body localization

**76536**　Ultrasound, soft tissues of head and neck (eg, thyroid, parathyroid, parotid), real time with image documentation

# Chest

**76604**　Ultrasound, chest (includes mediastinum), real time with image documentation

**76645**　Ultrasound, breast(s) (unilateral or bilateral), real time with image documentation

# Abdomen and Retroperitoneum

A complete ultrasound examination of the abdomen (76700) consists of real time scans of the liver, gall bladder, common bile duct, pancreas, spleen, kidneys, and the upper abdominal aorta and inferior vena cava including any demonstrated abdominal abnormality.

A complete ultrasound examination of the retroperitoneum (76770) consists of real time scans of the kidneys, abdominal aorta, common iliac artery origins, and inferior vena cava, including any demonstrated retroperitoneal abnormality. Alternatively, if clinical history suggests urinary tract pathology, complete evaluation of the kidneys and urinary bladder also comprises a complete retroperitoneal ultrasound.

Use of ultrasound, without thorough evaluation of organ(s) or anatomic region, image documentation and final, written report, is not separately reportable.

**76700**　Ultrasound, abdominal, real time with image documentation; complete

**76705**　　　limited (eg, single organ, quadrant, follow-up)

**76770**　Ultrasound, retroperitoneal (eg, renal, aorta, nodes), real time with image documentation; complete

**76775**　　　limited

**76776**　Ultrasound, transplanted kidney, real time and duplex Doppler with image documentation

(For ultrasound of transplanted kidney without duplex Doppler, use 76775)

►(For ultrasound and duplex Doppler of a transplanted kidney, do not report 76776 in conjunction with 93975, 93976)◄

# Spinal Canal

**76800**　Ultrasound, spinal canal and contents

# Pelvis

## Obstetrical

Codes 76801 and 76802 include determination of the number of gestational sacs and fetuses, gestational sac/fetal measurements appropriate for gestation (younger than 14 weeks 0 days), survey of visible fetal and placental anatomic structure, qualitative assessment of amniotic fluid volume/gestational sac shape and examination of the maternal uterus and adnexa.

Codes 76805 and 76810 include determination of number of fetuses and amniotic/chorionic sacs, measurements appropriate for gestational age (older than or equal to 14 weeks 0 days), survey of intracranial/spinal/abdominal anatomy, 4 chambered heart, umbilical cord insertion site, placenta location and amniotic fluid assessment and, when visible, examination of maternal adnexa.

Codes 76811 and 76812 include all elements of codes 76805 and 76810 plus detailed anatomic evaluation of the fetal brain/ventricles, face, heart/outflow tracts and chest anatomy, abdominal organ specific anatomy, number/length/architecture of limbs and detailed evaluation of the umbilical cord and placenta and other fetal anatomy as clinically indicated.

Report should document the results of the evaluation of each element described above or the reason for non-visualization.

Code 76815 represents a focused "quick look" exam limited to the assessment of one or more of the elements listed in code 76815.

Code 76816 describes an examination designed to reassess fetal size and interval growth or reevaluate one or more anatomic abnormalities of a fetus previously demonstrated on ultrasound, and should be coded once

**Radiology**

for each fetus requiring reevaluation using modifier 59 for each fetus after the first.

Code 76817 describes a transvaginal obstetric ultrasound performed separately or in addition to one of the transabdominal examinations described above. For transvaginal examinations performed for non-obstetrical purposes, use code 76830.

**76801**   Ultrasound, pregnant uterus, real time with image documentation, fetal and maternal evaluation, first trimester (< 14 weeks 0 days), transabdominal approach; single or first gestation

(To report first trimester fetal nuchal translucency measurement, use 76813)

**+ 76802**   each additional gestation (List separately in addition to code for primary procedure)

(Use 76802 in conjunction with 76801)

(To report first trimester fetal nuchal translucency measurement, use 76814)

**76805**   Ultrasound, pregnant uterus, real time with image documentation, fetal and maternal evaluation, after first trimester (> or = 14 weeks 0 days), transabdominal approach; single or first gestation

**+ 76810**   each additional gestation (List separately in addition to code for primary procedure)

(Use 76810 in conjunction with 76805)

**76811**   Ultrasound, pregnant uterus, real time with image documentation, fetal and maternal evaluation plus detailed fetal anatomic examination, transabdominal approach; single or first gestation

**+ 76812**   each additional gestation (List separately in addition to code for primary procedure)

(Use 76812 in conjunction with 76811)

**76813**   Ultrasound, pregnant uterus, real time with image documentation, first trimester fetal nuchal translucency measurement, transabdominal or transvaginal approach; single or first gestation

**+ 76814**   each additional gestation (List separately in addition to code for primary procedure)

(Use 76814 in conjunction with 76813)

**76815**   Ultrasound, pregnant uterus, real time with image documentation, limited (eg, fetal heart beat, placental location, fetal position and/or qualitative amniotic fluid volume), 1 or more fetuses

(Use 76815 only once per exam and not per element)

(To report first trimester fetal nuchal translucency measurement, see 76813, 76814)

**76816**   Ultrasound, pregnant uterus, real time with image documentation, follow-up (eg, re-evaluation of fetal size by measuring standard growth parameters and amniotic fluid volume, re-evaluation of organ system(s) suspected or confirmed to be abnormal on a previous scan), transabdominal approach, per fetus

(Report 76816 with modifier 59 for each additional fetus examined in a multiple pregnancy)

**76817**   Ultrasound, pregnant uterus, real time with image documentation, transvaginal

(For non-obstetrical transvaginal ultrasound, use 76830)

(If transvaginal examination is done in addition to transabdominal obstetrical ultrasound exam, use 76817 in addition to appropriate transabdominal exam code)

**76818**   Fetal biophysical profile; with non-stress testing

**76819**      without non-stress testing

(Fetal biophysical profile assessments for the second and any additional fetuses, should be reported separately by code 76818 or 76819 with the modifier 59 appended)

(For amniotic fluid index without non-stress test, use 76815)

**76820**   Doppler velocimetry, fetal; umbilical artery

**76821**      middle cerebral artery

**76825**   Echocardiography, fetal, cardiovascular system, real time with image documentation (2D), with or without M-mode recording;

**76826**      follow-up or repeat study

**76827**   Doppler echocardiography, fetal, pulsed wave and/or continuous wave with spectral display; complete

**76828**      follow-up or repeat study

(To report the use of color mapping, use 93325)

## Nonobstetrical

Code 76856 includes the complete evaluation of the female pelvic anatomy. Elements of this examination include a description and measurements of the uterus and adnexal structures, measurement of the endometrium, measurement of the bladder (when applicable), and a description of any pelvic pathology (eg, ovarian cysts, uterine leiomyomata, free pelvic fluid).

Code 76856 is also applicable to a complete evaluation of the male pelvis. Elements of the examination include evaluation and measurement (when applicable) of the urinary bladder, evaluation of the prostate and seminal vesicles to the extent that they are visualized transabdominally, and any pelvic pathology (eg, bladder tumor, enlarged prostate, free pelvic fluid, pelvic abscess).

Code 76857 represents a focused examination limited to the assessment of one or more elements listed in code 76856 and/or the reevaluation of one or more pelvic abnormalities previously demonstrated on ultrasound. Code 76857, rather than 76770, should be utilized if the urinary bladder alone (ie, not including the kidneys) is imaged, whereas code 51798 should be utilized if a bladder volume or post-void residual measurement is obtained without imaging the bladder.

**Radiology**

Use of ultrasound, without thorough evaluation of organ(s) or anatomic region, image documentation, and final, written report, is not separately reportable.

**76830**    Ultrasound, transvaginal

(For obstetrical transvaginal ultrasound, use 76817)

(If transvaginal examination is done in addition to transabdominal non-obstetrical ultrasound exam, use 76830 in addition to appropriate transabdominal exam code)

**76831**    Saline infusion sonohysterography (SIS), including color flow Doppler, when performed

(For introduction of saline for saline infusion sonohysterography, use 58340)

**76856**    Ultrasound, pelvic (nonobstetric), real time with image documentation; complete

**76857**        limited or follow-up (eg, for follicles)

## Genitalia

**76870**    Ultrasound, scrotum and contents

**76872**    Ultrasound, transrectal;

(Do not report 76872 in conjunction with 0249T)

**76873**        prostate volume study for brachytherapy treatment planning (separate procedure)

## Extremities

A complete ultrasound examination of an extremity (76881) consists of real time scans of a specific joint that includes examination of the muscles, tendons, joint, other soft tissue structures, and any identifiable abnormality.

Code 76882 refers to an examination of an extremity that would be performed primarily for evaluation of muscles, tendons, joints, and/or soft tissues. This is a limited examination of the extremity where a specific anatomic structure such as a tendon or muscle is assessed. In addition, the code would be used to evaluate a soft-tissue mass that may be present in an extremity where knowledge of its cystic or solid characteristics is needed.

For spectral and color Doppler evaluation of the extremities, use 93925, 93926, 93930, 93931, 93970, or 93971 as appropriate.

(76880 has been deleted. To report ultrasound examination of an extremity, see 76881, 76882)

**76881**    Ultrasound, extremity, nonvascular, real-time with image documentation; complete

**76882**        limited, anatomic specific

**76885**    Ultrasound, infant hips, real time with imaging documentation; dynamic (requiring physician manipulation)

**76886**        limited, static (not requiring physician manipulation)

## Ultrasonic Guidance Procedures

**76930**    Ultrasonic guidance for pericardiocentesis, imaging supervision and interpretation

**76932**    Ultrasonic guidance for endomyocardial biopsy, imaging supervision and interpretation

**76936**    Ultrasound guided compression repair of arterial pseudoaneurysm or arteriovenous fistulae (includes diagnostic ultrasound evaluation, compression of lesion and imaging)

**+ 76937**    Ultrasound guidance for vascular access requiring ultrasound evaluation of potential access sites, documentation of selected vessel patency, concurrent realtime ultrasound visualization of vascular needle entry, with permanent recording and reporting (List separately in addition to code for primary procedure)

►(Do not report 76937 in conjunction with 37191, 37192, 37193, 37760, 37761, 76942)◄

(If extremity venous non-invasive vascular diagnostic study is performed separate from venous access guidance, use 93965, 93970 or 93971)

**76940**    Ultrasound guidance for, and monitoring of, parenchymal tissue ablation

(Do not report 76940 in conjunction with 50250, 50542, 76942, 76998)

(For ablation, see 32998, 47370-47382, 50592, 50593)

**76941**    Ultrasonic guidance for intrauterine fetal transfusion or cordocentesis, imaging supervision and interpretation

(For procedure, see 36460, 59012)

**76942**    Ultrasonic guidance for needle placement (eg, biopsy, aspiration, injection, localization device), imaging supervision and interpretation

►(Do not report 76942 in conjunction with 27096, 37760, 37761, 43232, 43237, 43242, 45341, 45342, 64479-64484, 64490-64495, 76975, 0228T-0231T, 0232T, 0249T)◄

(For injection(s) of platelet rich plasma, use 0232T)

**76945**    Ultrasonic guidance for chorionic villus sampling, imaging supervision and interpretation

(For procedure, use 59015)

**76946**    Ultrasonic guidance for amniocentesis, imaging supervision and interpretation

**76948**    Ultrasonic guidance for aspiration of ova, imaging supervision and interpretation

**76950**    Ultrasonic guidance for placement of radiation therapy fields

(For placement of interstitial device[s] for radiation therapy guidance, see 31627, 32553, 49411, 55876)

**76965**    Ultrasonic guidance for interstitial radioelement application

**Radiology**

## Other Procedures

**76970** Ultrasound study follow-up (specify)

**76975** Gastrointestinal endoscopic ultrasound, supervision and interpretation

(Do not report 76975 in conjunction with 43231, 43232, 43237, 43238, 43242, 43259, 45341, 45342, or 76942)

**76977** Ultrasound bone density measurement and interpretation, peripheral site(s), any method

**76998** Ultrasonic guidance, intraoperative

(Do not report 76998 in conjunction with 36475-36479, 37760, 37761, 47370-47382, 0249T)

(For ultrasound guidance for open and laparoscopic radiofrequency tissue ablation, use 76940)

**76999** Unlisted ultrasound procedure (eg, diagnostic, interventional)

# Radiologic Guidance

## Fluoroscopic Guidance

(Do not report guidance codes 77001, 77002, 77003 for services in which fluoroscopic guidance is included in the descriptor)

**+ 77001** Fluoroscopic guidance for central venous access device placement, replacement (catheter only or complete), or removal (includes fluoroscopic guidance for vascular access and catheter manipulation, any necessary contrast injections through access site or catheter with related venography radiologic supervision and interpretation, and radiographic documentation of final catheter position) (List separately in addition to code for primary procedure)

(Do not use 77001 in conjunction with 77002)

(If formal extremity venography is performed from separate venous access and separately interpreted, use 36005 and 75820, 75822, 75825, or 75827)

**77002** Fluoroscopic guidance for needle placement (eg, biopsy, aspiration, injection, localization device)

(See appropriate surgical code for procedure and anatomic location)

(77002 includes all radiographic arthrography with the exception of supervision and interpretation for CT and MR arthrography)

(Do not report 77002 in addition to 70332, 73040, 73085, 73115, 73525, 73580, 73615, 0232T)

(For injection(s) of platelet rich plasma, use 0232T)

(77002 is included in the organ/anatomic specific radiological supervision and interpretation procedures 49440, 74320, 74355, 74445, 74470, 74475, 75809, 75810, 75885, 75887, 75980, 75982, 75989)

▲ **77003** Fluoroscopic guidance and localization of needle or catheter tip for spine or paraspinous diagnostic or therapeutic injection procedures (epidural or subarachnoid)

►(Injection of contrast during fluoroscopic guidance and localization [77003] is included in 22526, 22527, 27096, 62263, 62264, 62267, 62270-62282, 62310-62319)◄

(Fluoroscopic guidance for subarachnoid puncture for diagnostic radiographic myelography is included in supervision and interpretation codes 72240-72270)

(For epidural or subarachnoid needle or catheter placement and injection, see 62270-62282, 62310-62319)

►(For sacroiliac joint arthrography, see 27096)◄

►(For paravertebral facet joint injection, see 64490-64495. For paravertebral facet joint nerve destruction by neurolysis, see 64633-64636. For transforaminal epidural needle placement and injection, see 64479-64484)◄

►(Do not report 77003 in conjunction with 27096, 64479–64484, 64490-64495, 64633-64636)◄

(For percutaneous or endoscopic lysis of epidural adhesions, 62263, 62264 include fluoroscopic guidance and localization)

## Computed Tomography Guidance

**77011** Computed tomography guidance for stereotactic localization

**77012** Computed tomography guidance for needle placement (eg, biopsy, aspiration, injection, localization device), radiological supervision and interpretation

►(Do not report 77012 in conjunction with 27096, 64479-64484, 64490-64495, 64633-64636, 0232T)◄

(For injection(s) of platelet rich plasma, use 0232T)

**77013** Computed tomography guidance for, and monitoring of, parenchymal tissue ablation

(Do not report 77013 in conjunction with 20982)

(For percutaneous radiofrequency ablation, see 32998, 47382, 50592, 50593)

**77014** Computed tomography guidance for placement of radiation therapy fields

(For placement of interstitial device[s] for radiation therapy guidance, see 31627, 32553, 49411, 55876)

## Magnetic Resonance Guidance

**77021** Magnetic resonance guidance for needle placement (eg, for biopsy, needle aspiration, injection, or placement of localization device) radiological supervision and interpretation

(For procedure, see appropriate organ or site)

(Do not report 77021 in conjunction with 0232T)

(For injection(s) of platelet rich plasma, use 0232T)

Radiology

77022   Magnetic resonance guidance for, and monitoring of, parenchymal tissue ablation

(For percutaneous radiofrequency ablation, see 32998, 47382, 50592, 50593)

(For focused ultrasound ablation treatment of uterine leiomyomata, see Category III codes 0071T, 0072T)

## Other Radiologic Guidance

77031   Stereotactic localization guidance for breast biopsy or needle placement (eg, for wire localization or for injection), each lesion, radiological supervision and interpretation

(For procedure, see 10022, 19000-19103, 19290, 19291)

(For injection for sentinel node localization without lymphoscintigraphy, use 38792)

77032   Mammographic guidance for needle placement, breast (eg, for wire localization or for injection), each lesion, radiological supervision and interpretation

(For procedure, see 10022, 19000, 19102, 19103, 19290, 19291)

(For injection for sentinel node localization without lymphoscintigraphy, use 38792)

## Breast, Mammography

(For mammographic guidance for needle placement of breast lesion, use 77032)

+ 77051   Computer-aided detection (computer algorithm analysis of digital image data for lesion detection) with further physician review for interpretation, with or without digitization of film radiographic images; diagnostic mammography (List separately in addition to code for primary procedure)

(Use 77051 in conjunction with 77055, 77056)

+ 77052       screening mammography (List separately in addition to code for primary procedure)

(Use 77052 in conjunction with 77057)

77053   Mammary ductogram or galactogram, single duct, radiological supervision and interpretation

(For mammary ductogram or galactogram injection, use 19030)

77054   Mammary ductogram or galactogram, multiple ducts, radiological supervision and interpretation

77055   Mammography; unilateral

77056       bilateral

(Use 77055, 77056 in conjunction with 77051 for computer-aided detection applied to a diagnostic mammogram)

77057   Screening mammography, bilateral (2-view film study of each breast)

(Use 77057 in conjunction with 77052 for computer-aided detection applied to a screening mammogram)

(For electrical impedance breast scan, use 76499)

77058   Magnetic resonance imaging, breast, without and/or with contrast material(s); unilateral

77059       bilateral

## Bone/Joint Studies

77071   Manual application of stress performed by physician for joint radiography, including contralateral joint if indicated

(For radiographic interpretation of stressed images, see appropriate anatomic site and number of views)

77072   Bone age studies

77073   Bone length studies (orthoroentgenogram, scanogram)

77074   Radiologic examination, osseous survey; limited (eg, for metastases)

77075       complete (axial and appendicular skeleton)

77076   Radiologic examination, osseous survey, infant

77077   Joint survey, single view, 2 or more joints (specify)

77078   Computed tomography, bone mineral density study, 1 or more sites; axial skeleton (eg, hips, pelvis, spine)

►(77079  has been deleted)◄

77080   Dual-energy X-ray absorptiometry (DXA), bone density study, 1 or more sites; axial skeleton (eg, hips, pelvis, spine)

77081       appendicular skeleton (peripheral) (eg, radius, wrist, heel)

77082       vertebral fracture assessment

(For dual energy x-ray absorptiometry [DXA] body composition study, use 76499)

►(77083  has been deleted)◄

77084   Magnetic resonance (eg, proton) imaging, bone marrow blood supply

## Radiation Oncology

Listings for Radiation Oncology provide for teletherapy and brachytherapy to include initial consultation, clinical treatment planning, simulation, medical radiation physics, dosimetry, treatment devices, special services, and clinical treatment management procedures. They include normal follow-up care during course of treatment and for three months following its completion.

When a service or procedure is provided that is not listed in this edition of the CPT codebook it should be identified by a Special Report (see page 244) and one of the following unlisted procedure codes:

Radiology

77299 Unlisted procedure, therapeutic radiology clinical treatment planning

77399 Unlisted procedure, medical radiation physics, dosimetry and treatment devices, and special services

77499 Unlisted procedure, therapeutic radiology treatment management

77799 Unlisted procedure, clinical brachytherapy

**For treatment by injectable or ingestible isotopes, see subsection Nuclear Medicine.**

## Consultation: Clinical Management

Preliminary consultation, evaluation of patient prior to decision to treat, or full medical care (in addition to treatment management) when provided by the therapeutic radiologist may be identified by the appropriate procedure codes from **Evaluation and Management, Medicine,** or **Surgery** sections.

## Clinical Treatment Planning (External and Internal Sources)

The clinical treatment planning process is a complex service including interpretation of special testing, tumor localization, treatment volume determination, treatment time/dosage determination, choice of treatment modality, determination of number and size of treatment ports, selection of appropriate treatment devices, and other procedures.

**Definitions**

*Simple* planning requires a single treatment area of interest encompassed in a single port or simple parallel opposed ports with simple or no blocking.

*Intermediate* planning requires 3 or more converging ports, 2 separate treatment areas, multiple blocks, or special time dose constraints.

*Complex* planning requires highly complex blocking, custom shielding blocks, tangential ports, special wedges or compensators, three or more separate treatment areas, rotational or special beam considerations, combination of therapeutic modalities.

| 77261 | Therapeutic radiology treatment planning; simple |
|---|---|
| 77262 | intermediate |
| 77263 | complex |

**Definitions**

*Simple* simulation of a single treatment area with either a single port or parallel opposed ports. Simple or no blocking.

*Intermediate* simulation of three or more converging ports, two separate treatment areas, multiple blocks.

*Complex* simulation of tangential portals, three or more treatment areas, rotation or arc therapy, complex blocking, custom shielding blocks, brachytherapy source

verification, hyperthermia probe verification, any use of contrast materials.

***Three-dimensional (3D)*** computer-generated 3D reconstruction of tumor volume and surrounding critical normal tissue structures from direct CT scans and/or MRI data in preparation for non-coplanar or coplanar therapy. The simulation uses documented 3D beam's eye view volume-dose displays of multiple or moving beams. Documentation with 3D volume reconstruction and dose distribution is required.

Simulation may be carried out on a dedicated simulator, a radiation therapy treatment unit, or diagnostic X-ray machine.

| 77280 | Therapeutic radiology simulation-aided field setting; simple |
|---|---|
| 77285 | intermediate |
| 77290 | complex |
| 77295 | 3-dimensional |
| 77299 | Unlisted procedure, therapeutic radiology clinical treatment planning |

## Medical Radiation Physics, Dosimetry, Treatment Devices, and Special Services

| 77300 | Basic radiation dosimetry calculation, central axis depth dose calculation, TDF, NSD, gap calculation, off axis factor, tissue inhomogeneity factors, calculation of non-ionizing radiation surface and depth dose, as required during course of treatment, only when prescribed by the treating physician |
|---|---|
| 77301 | Intensity modulated radiotherapy plan, including dose-volume histograms for target and critical structure partial tolerance specifications |
|  | (Dose plan is optimized using inverse or forward planning technique for modulated beam delivery [eg, binary, dynamic MLC] to create highly conformal dose distribution. Computer plan distribution must be verified for positional accuracy based on dosimetric verification of the intensity map with verification of treatment set-up and interpretation of verification methodology) |
| 77305 | Teletherapy, isodose plan (whether hand or computer calculated); simple (1 or 2 parallel opposed unmodified ports directed to a single area of interest) |
| 77310 | intermediate (3 or more treatment ports directed to a single area of interest) |
| 77315 | complex (mantle or inverted Y, tangential ports, the use of wedges, compensators, complex blocking, rotational beam, or special beam considerations) |
|  | (Only 1 teletherapy isodose plan may be reported for a given course of therapy to a specific treatment area) |
| 77321 | Special teletherapy port plan, particles, hemibody, total body |

Radiology

**77326**    Brachytherapy isodose plan; simple (calculation made from single plane, 1 to 4 sources/ribbon application, remote afterloading brachytherapy, 1 to 8 sources)

(For definition of source/ribbon, see page 329)

**77327**       intermediate (multiplane dosage calculations, application involving 5 to 10 sources/ribbons, remote afterloading brachytherapy, 9 to 12 sources)

**77328**       complex (multiplane isodose plan, volume implant calculations, over 10 sources/ribbons used, special spatial reconstruction, remote afterloading brachytherapy, over 12 sources)

**77331**    Special dosimetry (eg, TLD, microdosimetry) (specify), only when prescribed by the treating physician

**77332**    Treatment devices, design and construction; simple (simple block, simple bolus)

**77333**       intermediate (multiple blocks, stents, bite blocks, special bolus)

**77334**       complex (irregular blocks, special shields, compensators, wedges, molds or casts)

**77336**    Continuing medical physics consultation, including assessment of treatment parameters, quality assurance of dose delivery, and review of patient treatment documentation in support of the radiation oncologist, reported per week of therapy

**77338**    Multi-leaf collimator (MLC) device(s) for intensity modulated radiation therapy (IMRT), design and construction per IMRT plan

(Do not report 77338 more than once per IMRT plan)

(For immobilization in IMRT treatment, see 77332-77334)

(Do not report 77338 in conjunction with 0073T, compensator based IMRT)

**77370**    Special medical radiation physics consultation

## Stereotactic Radiation Treatment Delivery

⊙ **77371**    Radiation treatment delivery, stereotactic radiosurgery (SRS), complete course of treatment of cranial lesion(s) consisting of 1 session; multi-source Cobalt 60 based

**77372**       linear accelerator based

(For radiation treatment management, use 77432)

**77373**    Stereotactic body radiation therapy, treatment delivery, per fraction to 1 or more lesions, including image guidance, entire course not to exceed 5 fractions

(Do not report 77373 in conjunction with 77401-77416, 77418)

(For single fraction cranial lesion[s], see 77371, 77372)

## Other Procedures

**77399**    Unlisted procedure, medical radiation physics, dosimetry and treatment devices, and special services

## Radiation Treatment Delivery

(Radiation treatment delivery [77401-77416] recognizes the technical component and the various energy levels)

(For intra-fraction localization and tracking of target, use 0197T)

**77401**    Radiation treatment delivery, superficial and/or ortho voltage

**77402**    Radiation treatment delivery, single treatment area, single port or parallel opposed ports, simple blocks or no blocks; up to 5 MeV

**77403**       6-10 MeV

**77404**       11-19 MeV

**77406**       20 MeV or greater

**77407**    Radiation treatment delivery, 2 separate treatment areas, 3 or more ports on a single treatment area, use of multiple blocks; up to 5 MeV

**77408**       6-10 MeV

**77409**       11-19 MeV

**77411**       20 MeV or greater

**77412**    Radiation treatment delivery, 3 or more separate treatment areas, custom blocking, tangential ports, wedges, rotational beam, compensators, electron beam; up to 5 MeV

**77413**       6-10 MeV

**77414**       11-19 MeV

**77416**       20 MeV or greater

**77417**    Therapeutic radiology port film(s)

**77418**    Intensity modulated treatment delivery, single or multiple fields/arcs, via narrow spatially and temporally modulated beams, binary, dynamic MLC, per treatment session

(For intensity modulated treatment planning, use 77301)

(For compensator-based beam modulation treatment delivery, use Category III code 0073T)

**77421**    Stereoscopic X-ray guidance for localization of target volume for the delivery of radiation therapy

(Do not report 77421 in conjunction with 77432, 77435)

►(Do not report 77421 more than once per treatment delivery session)◄

(For placement of interstitial device[s] for radiation therapy guidance, see 31627, 32553, 49411, 55876)

#● **77424**    Intraoperative radiation treatment delivery, x-ray, single treatment session

#● **77425**    Intraoperative radiation treatment delivery, electrons, single treatment session

# Neutron Beam Treatment Delivery

**77422**    High energy neutron radiation treatment delivery; single treatment area using a single port or parallel-opposed ports with no blocks or simple blocking

**77423**         1 or more isocenter(s) with coplanar or non-coplanar geometry with blocking and/or wedge, and/or compensator(s)

**77424**    ▶Code is out of numerical sequence. See 77401-77425◀

**77425**    ▶Code is out of numerical sequence. See 77401-77425◀

# Radiation Treatment Management

▶Radiation treatment management is reported in units of five fractions or treatment sessions, regardless of the actual time period in which the services are furnished. The services need not be furnished on consecutive days. Multiple fractions representing two or more treatment sessions furnished on the same day may be counted separately as long as there has been a distinct break in therapy sessions, and the fractions are of the character usually furnished on different days. Code 77427 is also reported if there are three or four fractions beyond a multiple of five at the end of a course of treatment; one or two fractions beyond a multiple of five at the end of a course of treatment are not reported separately.

Radiation treatment management requires **and includes** a minimum of one examination of the patient by the physician for medical evaluation and management (eg, assessment of the patient's response to treatment, coordination of care and treatment, review of imaging and/or lab test results with documentation) for each reporting of the radiation treatment management service. Code 77469 represents only the intraoperative session management and does not include medical evaluation and management outside of that session.

The professional services furnished during treatment management typically include:

■ Review of port films;

■ Review of dosimetry, dose delivery, and treatment parameters;

■ Review of patient treatment set-up.◀

**77427**    Radiation treatment management, 5 treatments

**77431**    Radiation therapy management with complete course of therapy consisting of 1 or 2 fractions only

(77431 is not to be used to fill in the last week of a long course of therapy)

**77432**    Stereotactic radiation treatment management of cranial lesion(s) (complete course of treatment consisting of 1 session)

(The same physician should not report both stereotactic radiosurgery services [61796-61800] and radiation treatment management [77432 or 77435] for cranial lesions)

(For stereotactic body radiation therapy treatment, use 77435)

**77435**    Stereotactic body radiation therapy, treatment management, per treatment course, to 1 or more lesions, including image guidance, entire course not to exceed 5 fractions

(Do not report 77435 in conjunction with 77427-77432)

(The same physician should not report both stereotactic radiosurgery services [63620, 63621] and radiation treatment management [77435] for extracranial lesions)

● **77469**    Intraoperative radiation treatment management

▲ **77470**    Special treatment procedure (eg, total body irradiation, hemibody radiation, per oral or endocavitary irradiation)

(77470 assumes that the procedure is performed 1 or more times during the course of therapy, in addition to daily or weekly patient management)

▶(For intraoperative radiation treatment delivery and management, see 77424, 77425, 77469)◀

**77499**    Unlisted procedure, therapeutic radiology treatment management

# Proton Beam Treatment Delivery

### Definitions

*Simple* proton treatment delivery to a single treatment area utilizing a single non-tangential/oblique port, custom block with compensation (77522) and without compensation (77520).

*Intermediate* proton treatment delivery to one or more treatment areas utilizing two or more ports or one or more tangential/oblique ports, with custom blocks and compensators.

*Complex* proton treatment delivery to one or more treatment areas utilizing two or more ports per treatment area with matching or patching fields and/or multiple isocenters, with custom blocks and compensators.

**77520**    Proton treatment delivery; simple, without compensation

**77522**         simple, with compensation

**77523**         intermediate

**77525**         complex

# Hyperthermia

Hyperthermia treatments as listed in this section include external (superficial and deep), interstitial, and intracavitary.

Radiation therapy when given concurrently is listed separately.

Hyperthermia is used only as an adjunct to radiation therapy or chemotherapy. It may be induced by a variety of sources (eg, microwave, ultrasound, low energy radio-frequency conduction, or by probes).

Radiology

The listed treatments include management during the course of therapy and follow-up care for three months after completion.

Preliminary consultation is not included (see **Evaluation and Management** 99241-99255).

Physics planning and interstitial insertion of temperature sensors, and use of external or interstitial heat generating sources are included.

The following descriptors are included in the treatment schedule:

⊙ **77600**    Hyperthermia, externally generated; superficial (ie, heating to a depth of 4 cm or less)

⊙ **77605**        deep (ie, heating to depths greater than 4 cm)

⊙ **77610**    Hyperthermia generated by interstitial probe(s); 5 or fewer interstitial applicators

⊙ **77615**        more than 5 interstitial applicators

## Clinical Intracavitary Hyperthermia

**77620**    Hyperthermia generated by intracavitary probe(s)

## Clinical Brachytherapy

Clinical brachytherapy requires the use of either natural or man-made radioelements applied into or around a treatment field of interest. The supervision of radioelements and dose interpretation are performed solely by the therapeutic radiologist.

Services 77750-77799 include admission to the hospital and daily visits.

For insertion of ovoids and tandems, use 57155.

For insertion of Heyman capsules, use 58346.

### Definitions

(Sources refer to intracavitary placement or permanent interstitial placement; ribbons refer to temporary interstitial placement)

*A simple* application has one to four sources/ribbons.

*An intermediate* application has five to 10 sources/ribbons.

*A complex* application has greater than 10 sources/ribbons.

        (For high dose rate electronic brachytherapy, per fraction, use Category III code 0182T)

**77750**    Infusion or instillation of radioelement solution (includes 3-month follow-up care)

        (For administration of radiolabeled monoclonal antibodies, use 79403)

        (For non-antibody radiopharmaceutical therapy by intravenous administration only, not including 3-month follow-up care, use 79101)

**77761**    Intracavitary radiation source application; simple

**77762**        intermediate

**77763**        complex

        (Do not report 77761-77763 in conjunction with Category III code 0182T)

**77776**    Interstitial radiation source application; simple

**77777**        intermediate

**77778**        complex

        (Do not report 77776-77778 in conjunction with Category III code 0182T)

        (77781 has been deleted. To report, see 77785, 77786)

        (77782-77784 have been deleted. To report, see 77785-77787)

**77785**    Remote afterloading high dose rate radionuclide brachytherapy; 1 channel

**77786**        2-12 channels

**77787**        over 12 channels

        (Do not report 77785-77787 in conjunction with Category III code 0182T)

**77789**    Surface application of radiation source

        (Do not report 77789 in conjunction with Category III code 0182T)

**77790**    Supervision, handling, loading of radiation source

**77799**    Unlisted procedure, clinical brachytherapy

# Nuclear Medicine

Listed procedures may be performed independently or in the course of overall medical care. If the physician providing these services is also responsible for diagnostic work-up and/or follow-up care of patient, see appropriate sections also.

Radioimmunoassay tests are found in the **Clinical Pathology** section (codes 82000-84999). These codes can be appropriately used by any specialist performing such tests in a laboratory licensed and/or certified for radioimmunoassays. The reporting of these tests is not confined to clinical pathology laboratories alone.

The services listed do not include the radiopharmaceutical or drug. Diagnostic and therapeutic radiopharmaceuticals and drugs supplied by the physician should be reported separately using the appropriate supply code(s), in addition to the procedure code.

## Diagnostic

### Endocrine System

**78000**    Thyroid uptake; single determination

**78001**        multiple determinations

Radiology

78003        stimulation, suppression or discharge (not including initial uptake studies)

78006    Thyroid imaging, with uptake; single determination

78007        multiple determinations

78010    Thyroid imaging; only

78011        with vascular flow

78015    Thyroid carcinoma metastases imaging; limited area (eg, neck and chest only)

78016        with additional studies (eg, urinary recovery)

78018        whole body

+ 78020    Thyroid carcinoma metastases uptake (List separately in addition to code for primary procedure)

     (Use 78020 in conjunction with 78018 only)

78070    Parathyroid imaging

78075    Adrenal imaging, cortex and/or medulla

78099    Unlisted endocrine procedure, diagnostic nuclear medicine

     (For chemical analysis, see **Chemistry** section)

## Hematopoietic, Reticuloendothelial and Lymphatic System

78102    Bone marrow imaging; limited area

78103        multiple areas

78104        whole body

78110    Plasma volume, radiopharmaceutical volume-dilution technique (separate procedure); single sampling

78111        multiple samplings

78120    Red cell volume determination (separate procedure); single sampling

78121        multiple samplings

78122    Whole blood volume determination, including separate measurement of plasma volume and red cell volume (radiopharmaceutical volume-dilution technique)

78130    Red cell survival study;

78135        differential organ/tissue kinetics (eg, splenic and/or hepatic sequestration)

78140    Labeled red cell sequestration, differential organ/tissue (eg, splenic and/or hepatic)

78185    Spleen imaging only, with or without vascular flow

     (If combined with liver study, use procedures 78215 and 78216)

78190    Kinetics, study of platelet survival, with or without differential organ/tissue localization

78191    Platelet survival study

78195    Lymphatics and lymph nodes imaging

     (For sentinel node identification without scintigraphy imaging, use 38792)

     (For sentinel node excision, see 38500-38542)

78199    Unlisted hematopoietic, reticuloendothelial and lymphatic procedure, diagnostic nuclear medicine

     (For chemical analysis, see **Chemistry** section)

## Gastrointestinal System

78201    Liver imaging; static only

78202        with vascular flow

     (For spleen imaging only, use 78185)

78205    Liver imaging (SPECT);

78206        with vascular flow

78215    Liver and spleen imaging; static only

78216        with vascular flow

     ►(78220 has been deleted)◄

     ►(78223 has been deleted. To report hepatobiliary system imaging, see 78226, 78227)◄

● 78226    Hepatobiliary system imaging, including gallbladder when present;

● 78227        with pharmacologic intervention, including quantitative measurement(s) when performed

78230    Salivary gland imaging;

78231        with serial images

78232    Salivary gland function study

78258    Esophageal motility

78261    Gastric mucosa imaging

78262    Gastroesophageal reflux study

78264    Gastric emptying study

78267    Urea breath test, C-14 (isotopic); acquisition for analysis

78268        analysis

78270    Vitamin B-12 absorption study (eg, Schilling test); without intrinsic factor

78271        with intrinsic factor

78272    Vitamin B-12 absorption studies combined, with and without intrinsic factor

78278    Acute gastrointestinal blood loss imaging

78282    Gastrointestinal protein loss

78290    Intestine imaging (eg, ectopic gastric mucosa, Meckel's localization, volvulus)

78291    Peritoneal-venous shunt patency test (eg, for LeVeen, Denver shunt)

     (For injection procedure, use 49427)

78299    Unlisted gastrointestinal procedure, diagnostic nuclear medicine

**Radiology**

  ⊙=Moderate sedation    ✚=Add-on code    ✗=FDA approval pending    #=Resequenced code    ○=Recycled/reinstated code

## Musculoskeletal System

Bone and joint imaging can be used in the diagnosis of a variety of inflammatory processes (eg, osteomyelitis), as well as for localization of primary and/or metastatic neoplasms.

**78300** Bone and/or joint imaging; limited area

**78305** multiple areas

**78306** whole body

**78315** 3 phase study

**78320** tomographic (SPECT)

**78350** Bone density (bone mineral content) study, 1 or more sites; single photon absorptiometry

**78351** dual photon absorptiometry, 1 or more sites

**78399** Unlisted musculoskeletal procedure, diagnostic nuclear medicine

## Cardiovascular System

Myocardial perfusion and cardiac blood pool imaging studies may be performed at rest and/or during stress. When performed during exercise and/or pharmacologic stress, the appropriate stress testing code from the 93015-93018 series should be reported in addition to 78451-78454, 78472-78492.

**78414** Determination of central c-v hemodynamics (non-imaging) (eg, ejection fraction with probe technique) with or without pharmacologic intervention or exercise, single or multiple determinations

**78428** Cardiac shunt detection

**78445** Non-cardiac vascular flow imaging (ie, angiography, venography)

**78451** Myocardial perfusion imaging, tomographic (SPECT) (including attenuation correction, qualitative or quantitative wall motion, ejection fraction by first pass or gated technique, additional quantification, when performed); single study, at rest or stress (exercise or pharmacologic)

**78452** multiple studies, at rest and/or stress (exercise or pharmacologic) and/or redistribution and/or rest reinjection

**78453** Myocardial perfusion imaging, planar (including qualitative or quantitative wall motion, ejection fraction by first pass or gated technique, additional quantification, when performed); single study, at rest or stress (exercise or pharmacologic)

**78454** multiple studies, at rest and/or stress (exercise or pharmacologic) and/or redistribution and/or rest reinjection

**78456** Acute venous thrombosis imaging, peptide

**78457** Venous thrombosis imaging, venogram; unilateral

**78458** bilateral

**78459** Myocardial imaging, positron emission tomography (PET), metabolic evaluation

(For myocardial perfusion study, see 78491-78492)

(78460-78465 have been deleted. To report, see 78451-78454)

**78466** Myocardial imaging, infarct avid, planar; qualitative or quantitative

**78468** with ejection fraction by first pass technique

**78469** tomographic SPECT with or without quantification

**78472** Cardiac blood pool imaging, gated equilibrium; planar, single study at rest or stress (exercise and/or pharmacologic), wall motion study plus ejection fraction, with or without additional quantitative processing

(For assessment of right ventricular ejection fraction by first pass technique, use 78496)

**78473** multiple studies, wall motion study plus ejection fraction, at rest and stress (exercise and/or pharmacologic), with or without additional quantification

(Do not report 78472, 78473 in conjunction with 78451-78454, 78481, 78483, 78494)

(78478, 78480 have been deleted. To report, see 78451-78454)

**78481** Cardiac blood pool imaging (planar), first pass technique; single study, at rest or with stress (exercise and/or pharmacologic), wall motion study plus ejection fraction, with or without quantification

**78483** multiple studies, at rest and with stress (exercise and/or pharmacologic), wall motion study plus ejection fraction, with or without quantification

(For cerebral blood flow study, use 78610)

(Do not report 78481-78483 in conjunction with 78451-78454)

**78491** Myocardial imaging, positron emission tomography (PET), perfusion; single study at rest or stress

**78492** multiple studies at rest and/or stress

**78494** Cardiac blood pool imaging, gated equilibrium, SPECT, at rest, wall motion study plus ejection fraction, with or without quantitative processing

**+ 78496** Cardiac blood pool imaging, gated equilibrium, single study, at rest, with right ventricular ejection fraction by first pass technique (List separately in addition to code for primary procedure)

(Use 78496 in conjunction with 78472)

**78499** Unlisted cardiovascular procedure, diagnostic nuclear medicine

**Radiology**

## Respiratory System

● **78579**  Pulmonary ventilation imaging (eg, aerosol or gas)

▲ **78580**  Pulmonary perfusion imaging (eg, particulate)

● **78582**  Pulmonary ventilation (eg, aerosol or gas) and perfusion imaging

● **78597**  Quantitative differential pulmonary perfusion, including imaging when performed

● **78598**  Quantitative differential pulmonary perfusion and ventilation (eg, aerosol or gas), including imaging when performed

▶(Report 78579, 78580, 78582-78598 only once per imaging session)◀

▶(Do not report 78580, 78582-78598 in conjunction with 78451-78454)◀

▶(78584-78596 have been deleted. To report, see 78579, 78582-78598)◀

**78599**  Unlisted respiratory procedure, diagnostic nuclear medicine

## Nervous System

**78600**  Brain imaging, less than 4 static views;

**78601**  with vascular flow

**78605**  Brain imaging, minimum 4 static views;

**78606**  with vascular flow

**78607**  Brain imaging, tomographic (SPECT)

**78608**  Brain imaging, positron emission tomography (PET); metabolic evaluation

**78609**  perfusion evaluation

**78610**  Brain imaging, vascular flow only

**78630**  Cerebrospinal fluid flow, imaging (not including introduction of material); cisternography

(For injection procedure, see 61000-61070, 62270-62319)

**78635**  ventriculography

(For injection procedure, see 61000-61070, 62270-62294)

**78645**  shunt evaluation

(For injection procedure, see 61000-61070, 62270-62294)

**78647**  tomographic (SPECT)

**78650**  Cerebrospinal fluid leakage detection and localization

(For injection procedure, see 61000-61070, 62270-62294)

**78660**  Radiopharmaceutical dacryocystography

**78699**  Unlisted nervous system procedure, diagnostic nuclear medicine

## Genitourinary System

**78700**  Kidney imaging morphology;

**78701**  with vascular flow

**78707**  with vascular flow and function, single study without pharmacological intervention

**78708**  with vascular flow and function, single study, with pharmacological intervention (eg, angiotensin converting enzyme inhibitor and/or diuretic)

**78709**  with vascular flow and function, multiple studies, with and without pharmacological intervention (eg, angiotensin converting enzyme inhibitor and/or diuretic)

(For introduction of radioactive substance in association with renal endoscopy, see 77776-77778)

**78710**  tomographic (SPECT)

**78725**  Kidney function study, non-imaging radioisotopic study

+ **78730**  Urinary bladder residual study (List separately in addition to code for primary procedure)

(Use 78730 in conjunction with 78740)

(For measurement of postvoid residual urine and/or bladder capacity by ultrasound, nonimaging, use 51798)

(For ultrasound imaging of the bladder only, with measurement of postvoid residual urine when performed, use 76857)

**78740**  Ureteral reflux study (radiopharmaceutical voiding cystogram)

(Use 78740 in conjunction with 78730 for urinary bladder residual study)

(For catheterization, see 51701, 51702, 51703)

**78761**  Testicular imaging with vascular flow

**78799**  Unlisted genitourinary procedure, diagnostic nuclear medicine

(For chemical analysis, see **Chemistry** section)

## Other Procedures

(For specific organ, see appropriate heading)

(For radiophosphorus tumor identification, ocular, see 78800)

**78800**  Radiopharmaceutical localization of tumor or distribution of radiopharmaceutical agent(s); limited area

(For specific organ, see appropriate heading)

**78801**  multiple areas

**78802**  whole body, single day imaging

**78803**  tomographic (SPECT)

**78804**  whole body, requiring 2 or more days imaging

**Radiology**

⊙=Moderate sedation  ✚=Add-on code  ✔=FDA approval pending  #=Resequenced code  ○=Recycled/reinstated code

**78805**  Radiopharmaceutical localization of inflammatory process; limited area

**78806**    whole body

**78807**    tomographic (SPECT)

(For imaging bone infectious or inflammatory disease with a bone imaging radiopharmaceutical, see 78300, 78305, 78306)

**78808**  Injection procedure for radiopharmaceutical localization by non-imaging probe study, intravenous (eg, parathyroid adenoma)

(For sentinel lymph node identification, use 38792)

(For PET of brain, see 78608, 78609)

(For PET myocardial imaging, see 78459, 78491, 78492)

**78811**  Positron emission tomography (PET) imaging; limited area (eg, chest, head/neck)

**78812**    skull base to mid-thigh

**78813**    whole body

**78814**  Positron emission tomography (PET) with concurrently acquired computed tomography (CT) for attenuation correction and anatomical localization imaging; limited area (eg, chest, head/neck)

**78815**    skull base to mid-thigh

**78816**    whole body

(Report 78811-78816 only once per imaging session)

(Computed tomography [CT] performed for other than attenuation correction and anatomical localization is reported using the appropriate site specific CT code with modifier 59)

(78890, 78891 have been deleted)

**78999**  Unlisted miscellaneous procedure, diagnostic nuclear medicine

# Therapeutic

The oral and intravenous administration codes in this section are inclusive of the mode of administration. For intra-arterial, intra-cavitary, and intra-articular administration, also use the appropriate injection and/or procedure codes, as well as imaging guidance and radiological supervision and interpretation codes, when appropriate.

**79005**  Radiopharmaceutical therapy, by oral administration

(For monoclonal antibody therapy, use 79403)

**79101**  Radiopharmaceutical therapy, by intravenous administration

(Do not report 79101 in conjunction with 36400, 36410, 79403, 96360, 96374 or 96375, 96409)

(For radiolabeled monoclonal antibody by intravenous infusion, use 79403)

(For infusion or instillation of non-antibody radioelement solution that includes 3 months follow-up care, use 77750)

**79200**  Radiopharmaceutical therapy, by intracavitary administration

**79300**  Radiopharmaceutical therapy, by interstitial radioactive colloid administration

**79403**  Radiopharmaceutical therapy, radiolabeled monoclonal antibody by intravenous infusion

(For pre-treatment imaging, see 78802, 78804)

(Do not report 79403 in conjunction with 79101)

**79440**  Radiopharmaceutical therapy, by intra-articular administration

**79445**  Radiopharmaceutical therapy, by intra-arterial particulate administration

(Do not report 79445 in conjunction with 96373, 96420)

(Use appropriate procedural and radiological supervision and interpretation codes for the angiographic and interventional procedures provided prerequisite to intra-arterial radiopharmaceutical therapy)

**79999**  Radiopharmaceutical therapy, unlisted procedure

**Radiology**

# Notes

# Pathology and Laboratory Guidelines

Items used by all physicians in reporting their services are presented in the **Introduction.** Some of the commonalities are repeated here for the convenience of those physicians referring to this section on **Pathology and Laboratory.** Other definitions and items unique to Pathology and Laboratory are also listed.

## Services in Pathology and Laboratory

Services in Pathology and Laboratory are provided by a physician or by technologists under responsible supervision of a physician.

## Separate or Multiple Procedures

It is appropriate to designate multiple procedures that are rendered on the same date by separate entries.

## Unlisted Service or Procedure

A service or procedure may be provided that is not listed in this edition of the CPT codebook. When reporting such a service, the appropriate "Unlisted Procedure" code may be used to indicate the service, identifying it by "Special Report" as discussed below. The "Unlisted Procedures" and accompanying codes for **Pathology and Laboratory** are as follows:

| | |
|---|---|
| **81099** | Unlisted urinalysis procedure |
| **84999** | Unlisted chemistry procedure |
| **85999** | Unlisted hematology and coagulation procedure |
| **86486** | unlisted antigen, each |
| **86849** | Unlisted immunology procedure |
| **86999** | Unlisted transfusion medicine procedure |
| **87999** | Unlisted microbiology procedure |
| **88099** | Unlisted necropsy (autopsy) procedure |
| **88199** | Unlisted cytopathology procedure |
| **88299** | Unlisted cytogenetic study |
| **88399** | Unlisted surgical pathology procedure |
| **88749** | Unlisted in vivo (eg, transcutaneous) laboratory service |
| **89240** | Unlisted miscellaneous pathology test |
| **89398** | Unlisted reproductive medicine laboratory procedure |

## Special Report

A service that is rarely provided, unusual, variable, or new may require a special report. Pertinent information should include an adequate definition or description of the nature, extent, and need for the procedure; and the time, effort, and equipment necessary to provide the service.

# Pathology and Laboratory

## Organ or Disease-Oriented Panels

These panels were developed for coding purposes only and should not be interpreted as clinical parameters. The tests listed with each panel identify the defined components of that panel.

These panel components are not intended to limit the performance of other tests. If one performs tests in addition to those specifically indicated for a particular panel, those tests should be reported separately in addition to the panel code.

Do not report two or more panel codes that include any of the same constituent tests performed from the same patient collection. If a group of tests overlaps two or more panels, report the panel that incorporates the greater number of tests to fulfill the code definition and report the remaining tests using individual test codes (eg, do not report 80047 in conjunction with 80053)

**80047**   Basic metabolic panel (Calcium, ionized)

This panel must include the following:

Calcium, ionized (82330)

Carbon dioxide (82374)

Chloride (82435)

Creatinine (82565)

Glucose (82947)

Potassium (84132)

Sodium (84295)

Urea Nitrogen (BUN) (84520)

**80048**   Basic metabolic panel (Calcium, total)

This panel must include the following:

Calcium, total (82310)

Carbon dioxide (82374)

Chloride (82435)

Creatinine (82565)

Glucose (82947)

Potassium (84132)

Sodium (84295)

Urea nitrogen (BUN) (84520)

**80050**   General health panel

This panel must include the following:

Comprehensive metabolic panel (80053)

Blood count, complete (CBC), automated and automated differential WBC count (85025 or 85027 and 85004)

OR

Blood count, complete (CBC), automated (85027) and appropriate manual differential WBC count (85007 or 85009)

Thyroid stimulating hormone (TSH) (84443)

**80051**   Electrolyte panel

This panel must include the following:

Carbon dioxide (82374)

Chloride (82435)

Potassium (84132)

Sodium (84295)

**80053**   Comprehensive metabolic panel

This panel must include the following:

Albumin (82040)

Bilirubin, total (82247)

Calcium, total (82310)

Carbon dioxide (bicarbonate) (82374)

Chloride (82435)

Creatinine (82565)

Glucose (82947)

Phosphatase, alkaline (84075)

Potassium (84132)

Protein, total (84155)

Sodium (84295)

Transferase, alanine amino (ALT) (SGPT) (84460)

Transferase, aspartate amino (AST) (SGOT) (84450)

Urea nitrogen (BUN) (84520)

**80055**   Obstetric panel

This panel must include the following:

Blood count, complete (CBC), automated and automated differential WBC count (85025 or 85027 and 85004)

OR

Blood count, complete (CBC), automated (85027) and appropriate manual differential WBC count (85007 or 85009)

Hepatitis B surface antigen (HBsAg) (87340)

Antibody, rubella (86762)

Pathology and Laboratory

Syphilis test, non-treponemal antibody; qualitative (eg, VDRL, RPR, ART) (86592)

Antibody screen, RBC, each serum technique (86850)

Blood typing, ABO (86900) AND

Blood typing, Rh (D) (86901)

(When syphilis screening is performed using a treponemal antibody approach [86780], do not use 80055. Use the individual codes for the tests performed in the obstetric panel)

**80061**    Lipid panel

This panel must include the following:

Cholesterol, serum, total (82465)

Lipoprotein, direct measurement, high density cholesterol (HDL cholesterol) (83718)

Triglycerides (84478)

**80069**    Renal function panel

This panel must include the following:

Albumin (82040)

Calcium, total (82310)

Carbon dioxide (bicarbonate) (82374)

Chloride (82435)

Creatinine (82565)

Glucose (82947)

Phosphorus inorganic (phosphate) (84100)

Potassium (84132)

Sodium (84295)

Urea nitrogen (BUN) (84520)

**80074**    Acute hepatitis panel

This panel must include the following:

Hepatitis A antibody (HAAb), IgM antibody (86709)

Hepatitis B core antibody (HBcAb), IgM antibody (86705)

Hepatitis B surface antigen (HBsAg) (87340)

Hepatitis C antibody (86803)

**80076**    Hepatic function panel

This panel must include the following:

Albumin (82040)

Bilirubin, total (82247)

Bilirubin, direct (82248)

Phosphatase, alkaline (84075)

Protein, total (84155)

Transferase, alanine amino (ALT) (SGPT) (84460)

Transferase, aspartate amino (AST) (SGOT) (84450)

# Drug Testing

The following list contains examples of drugs or classes of drugs that are commonly assayed by qualitative screen, followed by confirmation with a second method:

- Alcohols
- Amphetamines
- Barbiturates
- Benzodiazepines
- Cocaine and metabolites
- Methadones
- Methaqualones
- Opiates
- Phencyclidines
- Phenothiazines
- Propoxyphenes
- Tetrahydrocannabinoids
- Tricyclic antidepressants

Confirmed drugs may also be quantitated.

Use 80100 for each multiple drug class chromatographic procedure. Use 80102 for each procedure necessary for confirmation. For chromatography, each combination of stationary and mobile phase is to be counted as one procedure. For example, if detection of three drugs by chromatography requires one stationary phase with three mobile phases, use 80100 three times. However, if multiple drugs can be detected using a single analysis (eg, one stationary phase with one mobile phase), use 80100 only once.

For quantitation of drugs screened, use appropriate code in **Chemistry** section (82000-84999) or **Therapeutic Drug Assay** section (80150-80299).

**80100**    Drug screen, qualitative; multiple drug classes chromatographic method, each procedure

**80101**      single drug class method (eg, immunoassay, enzyme assay), each drug class

(For qualitative analysis by multiplexed screening kit for multiple drugs or drug classes, use 80104)

**# 80104**      multiple drug classes other than chromatographic method, each procedure

**80102**    Drug confirmation, each procedure

**80103**    Tissue preparation for drug analysis

**80104**    Code is out of numerical sequence. See 80100-80103

**Pathology and Laboratory**

# Therapeutic Drug Assays

The material for examination may be from any source. Examination is quantitative. For nonquantitative testing, see Drug Testing (80100-80103).

| | |
|---|---|
| 80150 | Amikacin |
| 80152 | Amitriptyline |
| 80154 | Benzodiazepines |
| 80156 | Carbamazepine; total |
| 80157 | free |
| 80158 | Cyclosporine |
| 80160 | Desipramine |
| 80162 | Digoxin |
| 80164 | Dipropylacetic acid (valproic acid) |
| 80166 | Doxepin |
| 80168 | Ethosuximide |
| 80170 | Gentamicin |
| 80172 | Gold |
| 80173 | Haloperidol |
| 80174 | Imipramine |
| 80176 | Lidocaine |
| 80178 | Lithium |
| 80182 | Nortriptyline |
| 80184 | Phenobarbital |
| 80185 | Phenytoin; total |
| 80186 | free |
| 80188 | Primidone |
| 80190 | Procainamide; |
| 80192 | with metabolites (eg, n-acetyl procainamide) |
| 80194 | Quinidine |
| 80195 | Sirolimus |
| 80196 | Salicylate |
| 80197 | Tacrolimus |
| 80198 | Theophylline |
| 80200 | Tobramycin |
| 80201 | Topiramate |
| 80202 | Vancomycin |
| 80299 | Quantitation of drug, not elsewhere specified |

# Evocative/Suppression Testing

The following test panels involve the administration of evocative or suppressive agents, and the baseline and subsequent measurement of their effects on chemical constituents. These codes are to be used for the reporting of the laboratory component of the overall testing protocol. For the physician's administration of the evocative or suppressive agents, see 96360, 96361, 96372-96374, 96375; for the supplies and drugs, see 99070. To report physician attendance and monitoring during the testing, use the appropriate evaluation and management code, including the prolonged physician care codes if required. Prolonged physician care codes are not separately reported when evocative/suppression testing involves prolonged infusions reported with 96360, 96361. In the code descriptors where reference is made to a particular analyte (eg, Cortisol: 82533 x 2) the "x 2" refers to the number of times the test for that particular analyte is performed.

80400 ACTH stimulation panel; for adrenal insufficiency

This panel must include the following:

Cortisol (82533 x 2)

80402 for 21 hydroxylase deficiency

This panel must include the following:

Cortisol (82533 x 2)

17 hydroxyprogesterone (83498 x 2)

80406 for 3 beta-hydroxydehydrogenase deficiency

This panel must include the following:

Cortisol (82533 x 2)

17 hydroxypregnenolone (84143 x 2)

80408 Aldosterone suppression evaluation panel (eg, saline infusion)

This panel must include the following:

Aldosterone (82088 x 2)

Renin (84244 x 2)

80410 Calcitonin stimulation panel (eg, calcium, pentagastrin)

This panel must include the following:

Calcitonin (82308 x 3)

80412 Corticotropic releasing hormone (CRH) stimulation panel

This panel must include the following:

Cortisol (82533 x 6)

Adrenocorticotropic hormone (ACTH) (82024 x 6)

80414 Chorionic gonadotropin stimulation panel; testosterone response

This panel must include the following:

Testosterone (84403 x 2 on 3 pooled blood samples)

Pathology and Laboratory

**80415**     estradiol response

This panel must include the following:

Estradiol (82670 x 2 on 3 pooled blood samples)

**80416**     Renal vein renin stimulation panel (eg, captopril)

This panel must include the following:

Renin (84244 x 6)

**80417**     Peripheral vein renin stimulation panel (eg, captopril)

This panel must include the following:

Renin (84244 x 2)

**80418**     Combined rapid anterior pituitary evaluation panel

This panel must include the following:

Adrenocorticotropic hormone (ACTH) (82024 x 4)

Luteinizing hormone (LH) (83002 x 4)

Follicle stimulating hormone (FSH) (83001 x 4)

Prolactin (84146 x 4)

Human growth hormone (HGH) (83003 x 4)

Cortisol (82533 x 4)

Thyroid stimulating hormone (TSH) (84443 x 4)

**80420**     Dexamethasone suppression panel, 48 hour

This panel must include the following:

Free cortisol, urine (82530 x 2)

Cortisol (82533 x 2)

Volume measurement for timed collection (81050 x 2)

(For single dose dexamethasone, use 82533)

**80422**     Glucagon tolerance panel; for insulinoma

This panel must include the following:

Glucose (82947 x 3)

Insulin (83525 x 3)

**80424**     for pheochromocytoma

This panel must include the following:

Catecholamines, fractionated (82384 x 2)

**80426**     Gonadotropin releasing hormone stimulation panel

This panel must include the following:

Follicle stimulating hormone (FSH) (83001 x 4)

Luteinizing hormone (LH) (83002 x 4)

**80428**     Growth hormone stimulation panel (eg, arginine infusion, l-dopa administration)

This panel must include the following:

Human growth hormone (HGH) (83003 x 4)

**80430**     Growth hormone suppression panel (glucose administration)

This panel must include the following:

Glucose (82947 x 3)

Human growth hormone (HGH) (83003 x 4)

**80432**     Insulin-induced C-peptide suppression panel

This panel must include the following:

Insulin (83525)

C-peptide (84681 x 5)

Glucose (82947 x 5)

**80434**     Insulin tolerance panel; for ACTH insufficiency

This panel must include the following:

Cortisol (82533 x 5)

Glucose (82947 x 5)

**80435**     for growth hormone deficiency

This panel must include the following:

Glucose (82947 x 5)

Human growth hormone (HGH) (83003 x 5)

**80436**     Metyrapone panel

This panel must include the following:

Cortisol (82533 x 2)

11 deoxycortisol (82634 x 2)

**80438**     Thyrotropin releasing hormone (TRH) stimulation panel; 1 hour

This panel must include the following:

Thyroid stimulating hormone (TSH) (84443 x 3)

**80439**     2 hour

This panel must include the following:

Thyroid stimulating hormone (TSH) (84443 x 4)

**80440**     for hyperprolactinemia

This panel must include the following:

Prolactin (84146 x 3)

# Consultations (Clinical Pathology)

A clinical pathology consultation is a service, including a written report, rendered by the pathologist in response to a request from an attending physician in relation to a test result(s) requiring additional medical interpretive judgment.

Reporting of a test result(s) without medical interpretive judgment is not considered a clinical pathology consultation.

**80500**     Clinical pathology consultation; limited, without review of patient's history and medical records

Pathology and Laboratory

**Pathology and Laboratory**

80502     comprehensive, for a complex diagnostic problem, with review of patient's history and medical records

(These codes may also be used for pharmacokinetic consultations)

(For consultations involving the examination and evaluation of the patient, see 99241-99255)

# Urinalysis

For specific analyses, see appropriate section.

81000     Urinalysis, by dip stick or tablet reagent for bilirubin, glucose, hemoglobin, ketones, leukocytes, nitrite, pH, protein, specific gravity, urobilinogen, any number of these constituents; non-automated, with microscopy

81001     automated, with microscopy

81002     non-automated, without microscopy

81003     automated, without microscopy

81005     Urinalysis; qualitative or semiquantitative, except immunoassays

(For non-immunoassay reagent strip urinalysis, see 81000, 81002)

(For immunoassay, qualitative or semiquantitative, use 83518)

(For microalbumin, see 82043, 82044)

81007     bacteriuria screen, except by culture or dipstick

(For culture, see 87086-87088)

(For dipstick, use 81000 or 81002)

81015     microscopic only

(For sperm evaluation for retrograde ejaculation, use 89331)

81020     2 or 3 glass test

81025     Urine pregnancy test, by visual color comparison methods

81050     Volume measurement for timed collection, each

81099     Unlisted urinalysis procedure

# ►Molecular Pathology◄

►Molecular pathology procedures are medical laboratory procedures involving the analyses of nucleic acid to detect variants in genes that may be indicative of germline (eg, constitutional disorders) or somatic (eg, neoplasia) conditions, or to test for histocompatibility antigens (eg, HLA). Code selection is typically based on the specific gene(s) that is being analyzed. Genes are described using Human Genome Organization (HUGO) approved gene names and are italicized in the code descriptors. Gene names were taken from tables of the HUGO Gene Nomenclature Commmittee (HGNC) at the time the

CPT codes were developed. For the most part, Human Genome Variation Society (HGVS) recommendations were followed for the names of specific molecular variants. The familiar name is used for some variants because defined criteria were not in place when the variant was first described or because HGVS recommendations were changed over time (eg, intronic variants, processed proteins). When the gene name is represented by an abbreviation, the abbreviation is listed first, followed by the full gene name italicized in parentheses (eg, "F5 [coagulation Factor V]"), except for the HLA series of codes. Proteins or diseases commonly associated with the genes are listed as examples in the code descriptors. The examples do not represent all conditions in which testing of the gene may be indicated.

Codes that describe tests to assess for the presence of gene variants (see definitions) use common gene variant names. Typically, all of the listed variants would be tested. However, these lists are not exclusive. If other variants are also tested in the analysis, they would be included in the procedure and not reported separately. Full gene sequencing should not be reported using codes that assess for the presence of gene variants unless specifically stated in the code descriptor.

The molecular pathology codes include all analytical services performed in the test (eg, cell lysis, nucleic acid stabilization, extraction, digestion, amplification, and detection). Any procedures required prior to cell lysis (eg, microdissection, codes 88380 and 88381) should be reported separately.

The results of the procedure may require interpretation by a physician or other qualified health care professional. When only the interpretation and report are performed, modifier 26 may be appended to the specific molecular pathology code.

All analyses are qualitative unless otherwise noted.

For microbial identification, see 87149-87153 and 87470-87801, and 87900-87904. For in situ hybridization analyses, see 88271-88275 and 88365-88368.

Molecular pathology procedures that are not specified in 81200-81350 should be reported using either the appropriate Tier 2 code (81400-81408) or the appropriate methodology codes in the 83890-83914 and 88384-88386 series.

**Definitions**

For purposes of CPT reporting, the following definitions apply:

*Abnormal allele:* an alternative form of a gene that contains a disease-related variation from the normal sequence.

*Breakpoint:* the region at which a chromosome breaks during a translocation (defined elsewhere). These regions are often consistent for a given translocation.

**Codon:** a discrete unit of three nucleotides of a DNA or mRNA sequence that encodes a specific amino acid within, or signals the termination of, a polypeptide.

**Common variants:** variants (as defined elsewhere) that are associated with compromised gene function and are interrogated in a single round of laboratory testing (in a single, typically multiplex, assay format or using more than one assay to encompass all variants to be tested). These variants typically fit the definition of a "mutation," and are usually the predominant ones causing disease. Testing for additional uncommon variants may provide additional limited value in assessment of a patient. Often there are professional society recommendations or guidelines for which variants are most appropriate to test (eg, American College of Medical Genetics/American College of Obstetrics and Gynecology guidelines for variants used in population screening for cystic fibrosis).

**Constitutional:** synonymous with germline, often used in reference to the genetic code that is present at birth.

**Cytogenomic:** chromosome analysis using molecular techniques.

**Duplication/Deletion(Dup/Del):** terms that are usually used together with the '/' to refer to molecular testing, which assesses the dosage of a particular genomic region. The region tested is typically of modest to substantial size - from several dozen to several million or more nucleotides. Normal gene dosage is two copies per cell, except for the sex chromosomes (X and Y). Thus, zero or one copy represents a deletion, and three (or more) copies represent a duplication.

**Dynamic mutation:** polynucleotide (eg, trinucleotide) repeats that are in or associated with genes that can undergo disease-producing increases or decreases in the numbers of repeats within tissues and across generations.

**Exon:** typically, one of multiple nucleic acid sequences used to encode information for a gene product (polypeptide or protein). Exons are separated from each other by non-protein-coding sequences known as introns. Exons at the respective ends of a gene also contain nucleic acid sequence that does not code for the gene's protein product.

**Gene:** a nucleic acid sequence that typically contains information for coding a protein as well as for the regulated expression of that protein. Human genes usually contain multiple protein coding regions (exons) separated by non-protein coding regions (introns). See also *exon*, *intron*, and *polypeptide*.

**Intron:** a nucleic acid sequence found between exons in human genes. An intron contains essential sequences for its proper removal (by a process known as *splicing*) to join exons together and thus facilitate production of a functional protein from a gene. An intron is sometimes referred to as an intervening sequence (IVS).

**Microarray:** surface(s) on which multiple specific nucleic acid sequences are attached in a known arrangement. Sometimes referred to as a 'gene chip'. Examples of uses of microarrays include evaluation of a patient specimen for gains or losses of DNA sequences (copy number variants, CNVs), identification of the presence of specific nucleotide sequence variants (also known as single nucleotide polymorphisms, SNPs), mRNA expression levels, or DNA sequence analysis.

**Mutations:** typically are variants associated with altered gene function that lead to functional deficits or disease (pathogenic).

**Mutation scanning:** a technique (eg, single strand conformation polymorphism, temperature gradient gel electrophoresis, etc.) typically employed on multiple PCR amplicons to indicate the presence of DNA sequence variants by differences in physical properties compared to normal. Variants are then further characterized by DNA sequence analysis only in amplicons which demonstrate differences.

**Polymorphisms:** typically are variants that do not compromise gene function or produce disease (benign).

**Polypeptide:** a sequence of amino acids covalently linked in a specified order. Polypeptides alone or in combination with other polypeptide subunits are the building blocks of proteins.

**Short Tandem Repeat (STR):** a region of DNA where a pattern of two or more nucleotides are repeated. The number of repeating segments can be used as genetic markers for human identity testing.

**Single-nucleotide polymorphism (SNP):** a DNA sequence variation existing at a significant frequency in the population, in which a single nucleotide (A, T, C, or G) differs between individuals and/or within an individual's paired chromosomes,

**Somatic:** synonymous with acquired, referring to genetic code alterations that develop after birth (eg, occurring in neoplastic cells)

**Translocation:** an abnormality resulting from the breakage of a chromosome and the relocation of a portion of that chromosome's DNA sequence to the same or another chromosome. Most common translocations involve a reciprocal exchange of DNA sequences between two differently numbered (ie, non-homologous) chromosomes, with or without a clinically significant loss of DNA.

**Variant:** a nucleotide sequence difference from the "normal" (predominant) sequence for a given region. Variants are typically of two types: substitutions of one nucleotide for another, and deletions or insertions of nucleotides. Occasionally, variants reflect several nucleotide sequence changes in reasonably close proximity on the same chromosomal strand of DNA (a haplotype). These nucleotide sequence variants often result in amino acid changes in the protein made by the gene. The term *variant* does not itself carry a functional implication for those protein changes.

Variants in introns are typically described in one of two ways. The altered nucleotide(s) within a defined intervening sequence (eg, IVS3-2A>G) of a gene is listed with a "+" or "-" sign, which indicates the position relative to the first or last nucleotide of the intron. Or, the variant position is indicated relative to the last nucleotide of the preceding exon or first nucleotide of the following exon (eg, c.171+1G>A c.172-1G>T are single nucleotide changes at the first and last nucleotide of a given intron for a specific gene).

The majority of the variants described here are listed by the amino acid change using the single letter amino acid code for the original amino acid followed by the numerical position in the protein product and the amino acid substitution, eg, for *ASPA* E285A, Glutamic acid (E) at position 285 is replaced with an alanine (A). A few of the variants are described by the DNA change using the numerical position followed by the original nucleotide, a greater than sign (>) and the new nucleotide, eg, *MTHFR*. 677C>T.

A known familial variant is a specific mutation that has previously been identified within a patient's family.◄

## ►Tier 1 Molecular Pathology Procedures◄

►The following codes represent gene-specific and genomic procedures:◄

● **81200**  *ASPA (aspartoacylase)* (eg, Canavan disease) gene analysis, common variants (eg, E285A, Y231X)

● **81205**  *BCKDHB (branched-chain keto acid dehydrogenase E1, beta polypeptide)* (eg, Maple syrup urine disease) gene analysis, common variants (eg, R183P, G278S, E422X)

● **81206**  *BCR/ABL1 (t(9;22))* (eg, chronic myelogenous leukemia) translocation analysis; major breakpoint, qualitative or quantitative

● **81207**     minor breakpoint, qualitative or quantitative

● **81208**     other breakpoint, qualitative or quantitative

● **81209**  *BLM (Bloom syndrome, RecQ helicase-like)* (eg, Bloom syndrome) gene analysis, 2281del6ins7 variant

● **81210**  *BRAF (v-raf murine sarcoma viral oncogene homolog B1)* (eg, colon cancer), gene analysis, V600E variant

● **81211**  *BRCA1, BRCA2 (breast cancer 1 and 2)* (eg, hereditary breast and ovarian cancer) gene analysis; full sequence analysis and common duplication/deletion variants in BRCA1 (ie, exon 13 del 3.835kb, exon 13 dup 6kb, exon 14-20 del 26kb, exon 22 del 510bp, exon 8-9 del 7.1kb)

● **81212**     185delAG, 5385insC, 6174delT variants

● **81213**     uncommon duplication/deletion variants

● **81214**  *BRCA1 (breast cancer 1)* (eg, hereditary breast and ovarian cancer) gene analysis; full sequence analysis and common duplication/deletion variants (ie, exon 13 del 3.835kb, exon 13 dup 6kb, exon 14-20 del 26kb, exon 22 del 510bp, exon 8-9 del 7.1kb)

►(When performing *BRCA1* full sequence analysis with *BRCA2* full sequence analysis, use 81211)◄

● **81215**     known familial variant

● **81216**  *BRCA2 (breast cancer 2)* (eg, hereditary breast and ovarian cancer) gene analysis; full sequence analysis

►(When performing *BRCA2* full sequence analysis with *BRCA1* full sequence analysis, use 81211)◄

● **81217**     known familial variant

● **81220**  *CFTR (cystic fibrosis transmembrane conductance regulator)* (eg, cystic fibrosis) gene analysis; common variants (eg, ACMG/ACOG guidelines)

►(When Intron 8 poly-T analysis is performed in conjunction with 81220 in a R117H positive patient, do not report 81224)◄

● **81221**     known familial variants

● **81222**     duplication/deletion variants

● **81223**     full gene sequence

● **81224**     intron 8 poly-T analysis (eg, male infertility)

● **81225**  *CYP2C19 (cytochrome P450, family 2, subfamily C, polypeptide 19)* (eg, drug metabolism), gene analysis, common variants (eg, *2, *3, *4, *8, *17)

● **81226**  *CYP2D6 (cytochrome P450, family 2, subfamily D, polypeptide 6)* (eg, drug metabolism), gene analysis, common variants (eg, *2, *3, *4, *5, *6, *9, *10, *17, *19, *29, *35, *41, *1XN, *2XN, *4XN)

● **81227**  *CYP2C9 (cytochrome P450, family 2, subfamily C, polypeptide 9)* (eg, drug metabolism), gene analysis, common variants (eg, *2, *3, *5, *6)

● **81228**  Cytogenomic constitutional (genome-wide) microarray analysis; interrogation of genomic regions for copy number variants (eg, Bacterial Artificial Chromosome [BAC] or oligo-based comparative genomic hybridization [CGH] microarray analysis)

● **81229**     interrogation of genomic regions for copy number and single nucleotide polymorphism (SNP) variants for chromosomal abnormalities

►(Do not report 81228 in conjunction with 81229)◄

● **81240**  *F2 (prothrombin, coagulation factor II)* (eg, hereditary hypercoagulability) gene analysis, 20210G>A variant

● **81241**  *F5 (coagulation Factor V)* (eg, hereditary hypercoagulability) gene analysis, Leiden variant

● **81242**  *FANCC (Fanconi anemia, complementation group C)* (eg, Fanconi anemia, type C) gene analysis, common variant (eg, IVS4+4A>T)

● **81243**    *FMR1 (Fragile X mental retardation 1)* (eg, fragile X mental retardation) gene analysis; evaluation to detect abnormal (eg, expanded) alleles

▶(For evaluation to detect and characterize abnormal alleles, see 81243, 81244)◀

▶(For evaluation to detect and characterize abnormal alleles using a single assay [eg, PCR], use 81243)◀

● **81244**    characterization of alleles (eg, expanded size and methylation status)

● **81245**    *FLT3 (fms-related tyrosine kinase 3)* (eg, acute myeloid leukemia), gene analysis, internal tandem duplication (ITD) variants (ie, exons 14, 15)

● **81250**    *G6PC (glucose-6-phosphatase, catalytic subunit)* (eg, Glycogen storage disease, Type 1a, von Gierke disease) gene analysis, common variants (eg, R83C, Q347X)

● **81251**    *GBA (glucosidase, beta, acid)* (eg, Gaucher disease) gene analysis, common variants (eg, N370S, 84GG, L444P, IVS2+1G>A)

● **81255**    *HEXA (hexosaminidase A [alpha polypeptide])* (eg, Tay-Sachs disease) gene analysis, common variants (eg, 1278insTATC, 1421+1G>C, G269S)

● **81256**    *HFE (hemochromatosis)* (eg, hereditary hemochromatosis) gene analysis, common variants (eg, C282Y, H63D)

● **81257**    *HBA1/HBA2 (alpha globin 1 and alpha globin 2)* (eg, alpha thalassemia, Hb Bart hydrops fetalis syndrome, HbH disease), gene analysis, for common deletions or variant (eg, Southeast Asian, Thai, Filipino, Mediterranean, alpha3.7, alpha4.2, alpha20.5, and Constant Spring)

● **81260**    *IKBKAP (inhibitor of kappa light polypeptide gene enhancer in B-cells, kinase complex-associated protein)* (eg, familial dysautonomia) gene analysis, common variants (eg, 2507+6T>C, R696P)

● **81261**    *IGH@ (Immunoglobulin heavy chain locus)* (eg, leukemias and lymphomas, B-cell), gene rearrangement analysis to detect abnormal clonal population(s); amplified methodology (eg, polymerase chain reaction)

● **81262**    direct probe methodology (eg, Southern blot)

● **81263**    *IGH@ (Immunoglobulin heavy chain locus)* (eg, leukemia and lymphoma, B-cell), variable region somatic mutation analysis

● **81264**    *IGK@ (Immunoglobulin kappa light chain locus)* (eg, leukemia and lymphoma, B-cell), gene rearrangement analysis, evaluation to detect abnormal clonal population(s)

▶(For immunoglobulin lambda gene *[IGL@]* rearrangement or immunoglobulin kappa deleting element, *[IGKDEL]* analysis, report the appropriate methodology code[s] in the 83890-83914 series)◀

● **81265**    Comparative analysis using Short Tandem Repeat (STR) markers; patient and comparative specimen (eg, pre-transplant recipient and donor germline testing, post-transplant non-hematopoietic recipient germline [eg, buccal swab or other germline tissue sample] and donor testing, twin zygosity testing, or maternal cell contamination of fetal cells)

+● **81266**    each additional specimen (eg, additional cord blood donor, additional fetal samples from different cultures, or additional zygosity in multiple birth pregnancies) (List separately in addition to code for primary procedure)

▶(Use 81266 in conjunction with 81265)◀

● **81267**    Chimerism (engraftment) analysis, post transplantation specimen (eg, hematopoietic stem cell), includes comparison to previously performed baseline analyses; without cell selection

● **81268**    with cell selection (eg, CD3, CD33), each cell type

▶(If comparative STR analysis of recipient [using buccal swab or other germline tissue sample] and donor are performed after hematopoietic stem cell transplantation, report 81265, 81266 in conjunction with 81267, 81268 for chimerism testing)◀

● **81270**    *JAK2 (Janus kinase 2)* (eg, myeloproliferative disorder) gene analysis, p.Val617Phe (V617F) variant

● **81275**    *KRAS (v-Ki-ras2 Kirsten rat sarcoma viral oncogene)* (eg, carcinoma) gene analysis, variants in codons 12 and 13

● **81280**    Long QT syndrome gene analyses (eg, *KCNQ1, KCNH2, SCN5A, KCNE1, KCNE2, KCNJ2, CACNA1C, CAV3, SCN4B, AKAP, SNTA1, and ANK2*); full sequence analysis

● **81281**    known familial sequence variant

● **81282**    duplication/deletion variants

● **81290**    *MCOLN1 (mucolipin 1)* (eg, Mucolipidosis, type IV) gene analysis, common variants (eg, IVS3-2A>G, del6.4kb)

● **81291**    *MTHFR (5,10-methylenetetrahydrofolate reductase)* (eg, hereditary hypercoagulability) gene analysis, common variants (eg, 677T, 1298C)

● **81292**    *MLH1 (mutL homolog 1, colon cancer, nonpolyposis type 2)* (eg, hereditary non-polyposis colorectal cancer, Lynch syndrome) gene analysis; full sequence analysis

● **81293**    known familial variants

● **81294**    duplication/deletion variants

● **81295**    *MSH2 (mutS homolog 2, colon cancer, nonpolyposis type 1)* (eg, hereditary non-polyposis colorectal cancer, Lynch syndrome) gene analysis; full sequence analysis

● **81296**    known familial variants

● **81297**    duplication/deletion variants

● **81298**    *MSH6 (mutS homolog 6 [E. coli])* (eg, hereditary non-polyposis colorectal cancer, Lynch syndrome) gene analysis; full sequence analysis

**Pathology and Laboratory**

---

▲=Revised code   ●=New code   ▶ ◀=Contains new or revised text   ⊘=Modifier 51 exempt

● **81299**          known familial variants

● **81300**          duplication/deletion variants

● **81301**   Microsatellite instability analysis (eg, hereditary non-polyposis colorectal cancer, Lynch syndrome) of markers for mismatch repair deficiency (eg, BAT25, BAT26), includes comparison of neoplastic and normal tissue, if performed

● **81302**   *MECP2 (methyl CpG binding protein 2)* (eg, Rett syndrome) gene analysis; full sequence analysis

● **81303**          known familial variant

● **81304**          duplication/deletion variants

● **81310**   *NPM1 (nucleophosmin)* (eg, acute myeloid leukemia) gene analysis, exon 12 variants

● **81315**   *PML/RARalpha, (t(15;17)), (promyelocytic leukemia/retinoic acid receptor alpha)* (eg, promyelocytic leukemia) translocation analysis; common breakpoints (eg, intron 3 and intron 6), qualitative or quantitative

● **81316**          single breakpoint (eg, intron 3, intron 6 or exon 6), qualitative or quantitative

   ►(For intron 3 and intron 6 [including exon 6 if performed] analysis, use 81315)◄

   ►(If both intron 6 and exon 6 are analyzed, without intron 3, use one unit of 81316)◄

● **81317**   *PMS2 (postmeiotic segregation increased 2 [S. cerevisiae])* (eg, hereditary non-polyposis colorectal cancer, Lynch syndrome) gene analysis; full sequence analysis

● **81318**          known familial variants

● **81319**          duplication/deletion variants

● **81330**   *SMPD1(sphingomyelin phosphodiesterase 1, acid lysosomal)* (eg, Niemann-Pick disease, Type A) gene analysis, common variants (eg, R496L, L302P, fsP330)

● **81331**   *SNRPN/UBE3A (small nuclear ribonucleoprotein polypeptide N and ubiquitin protein ligase E3A)* (eg, Prader-Willi syndrome and/or Angelman syndrome), methylation analysis

● **81332**   *SERPINA1 (serpin peptidase inhibitor, clade A, alpha-1 antiproteinase, antitrypsin, member 1)* (eg, alpha-1-antitrypsin deficiency), gene analysis, common variants (eg, *S and *Z)

● **81340**   *TRB@ (T cell antigen receptor, beta)* (eg, leukemia and lymphoma), gene rearrangement analysis to detect abnormal clonal population(s); using amplification methodology (eg, polymerase chain reaction)

● **81341**          using direct probe methodology (eg, Southern blot)

● **81342**   *TRG@ (T cell antigen receptor, gamma)* (eg, leukemia and lymphoma), gene rearrangement analysis, evaluation to detect abnormal clonal population(s)

   ►(For T cell antigen alpha [*TRA@*] gene rearrangement analysis, report the appropriate methodology code(s) in the 83890-83914 series)◄

   ►(For T cell antigen delta [*TCD@*] gene rearrangement analysis, report 81401)◄

● **81350**   *UGT1A1 (UDP glucuronosyltransferase 1 family, polypeptide A1)* (eg, irinotecan metabolism), gene analysis, common variants (eg, *28, *36, *37)

● **81355**   *VKORC1 (vitamin K epoxide reductase complex, subunit 1)* (eg, warfarin metabolism), gene analysis, common variants (eg, -1639/3673)

►Human Leukocyte Antigen (HLA) typing is performed to assess compatibility of recipients and potential donors as a part of solid organ and hematopoietic stem cell pretransplant testing. HLA testing is also performed to identify HLA alleles and allele groups (antigen equivalents) associated with specific diseases and individualized responses to drug therapy (eg, HLA-B*27 and ankylosing spondylitis and HLA-B*57:01 and abacavir hypersensitivity), as well as other clinical uses. One or more HLA genes may be tested in specific clinical situations (eg, HLA-DQB1 for narcolepsy and HLA-A, -B, -C, -DRB1 and -DQB1 for kidney transplantation). Each HLA gene typically has multiple variant alleles or allele groups that can be identified by typing. For HLA result reporting, a low resolution HLA type is denoted by a two digit HLA name (eg, A*02) and intermediate resolution typing by a string of alleles or an NMDP (National Marrow Donor Program) code (eg, B*14:01/07N/08/12/14, B*39CKGN). Both low and intermediate resolution are considered low resolution for code assignment. High resolution typing resolves the common well defined (CWD) alleles and is usually denoted by at least 4 digits (eg, A*02:02, *03:01:01:01, A*26:01:01G, and C*03:04P), however, high resolution typing may include some ambiguities for rare alleles, which may be reported as a string of alleles or an NMDP code.

If additional testing is required to resolve ambiguous allele combinations for high resolution typing, this is included in the base HLA typing codes below. The gene names have been italicized similar to the other molecular pathology codes.◄

   ►(For HLA antigen typing by non-molecular pathology techniques, see 86812-86822)◄

● **81370**   HLA Class I and II typing, low resolution (eg, antigen equivalents); *HLA-A, -B, -C, -DRB1/3/4/5, and -DQB1*

● **81371**          *HLA-A, -B, and -DRB1/3/4/5* (eg, verification typing)

● **81372**   HLA Class I typing, low resolution (eg, antigen equivalents); complete *(ie, HLA-A, -B, and -C)*

   ►(When performing both Class I and II low resolution *HLA typing for HLA-A,-B,-C, -DRB1/3/4/5,* and *-DQB1,* use 81370)◄

● **81373**          one locus *(eg, HLA-A, -B, or -C),* each

   ►(When performing a complete Class I *[HLA-A,-B,* and *-C]* low resolution HLA typing, use 81372)◄

●81374          one antigen equivalent (eg, *B\*27*), each

►(When the presence or absence of a single antigen equivalent is reported using low resolution testing, use 81374)◄

►(When testing for presence or absence of more than 2 antigen equivalents at a locus, use 81373 for each locus tested)◄

●81375    HLA Class II typing, low resolution (eg, antigen equivalents); *HLA-DRB1/3/4/5* and *-DQB1*

►(When performing both Class I and II low resolution HLA typing *for HLA-A,-B,-C, -DRB1/3/4/5,* and *—DQB1,* use 81370)◄

●81376          one locus (eg, *HLA-DRB1/3/4/5, -DQB1, -DQA1, -DPB1,* or *-DPA1*), each

►(When low resolution typing is performed for *HLA-DRB1/3/4/5* and *-DQB1,* use 81375)◄

►(For low resolution typing, *HLA-DRB1/3/4/5* should be treated as a single locus)◄

●81377          one antigen equivalent, each

►(When testing for presence or absence of more than 2 antigen equivalents at a locus, use 81376 for each locus)◄

●81378    HLA Class I and II typing, high resolution (ie, alleles or allele groups), *HLA-A, -B, -C,* and *-DRB1*

●81379    HLA Class I typing, high resolution (ie, alleles or allele groups); complete (ie, *HLA-A, -B,* and *-C*)

●81380          one locus (eg, *HLA-A, -B,* or *-C*), each

►(When a complete Class I high resolution typing for *HLA-A,-B,* and *-C* is performed, use 81379)◄

►(When the presence or absence of a single allele or allele group is reported using high resolution testing, use 81381)◄

●81381          one allele or allele group (eg, *B\*57:01P*), each

►(When testing for the presence or absence of more than 2 alleles or allele groups at a locus, use 81380 for each locus)◄

●81382    HLA Class II typing, high resolution (ie, alleles or allele groups); one locus (eg, *HLA-DRB1, -DRB3, -DRB4, -DRB5, -DQB1, -DQA1, -DPB1,* or *-DPA1*), each

►(When only the presence or absence of a single allele or allele group is reported using high resolution testing, use 81383)◄

●81383          one allele or allele group (eg, *HLA-DQB1\*06:02P*), each

►(When testing for the presence or absence of more than 2 alleles or allele groups at a locus, use 81382 for each locus)◄

## ►Tier 2 Molecular Pathology Procedures◄

►The following molecular pathology procedure (Tier 2) codes are used to report procedures not listed in the Tier 1 molecular pathology codes (81200-81350). They represent medically useful procedures that are generally performed in lower volumes than Tier 1 procedures (eg, the incidence of the disease being tested is rare). They are arranged by level of technical resources and interpretive work by the physician or other qualified health care professional. The individual analyses listed under each code (ie, level of procedure) utilize the definitions and coding principles as described in the introduction preceding the Tier 1 molecular pathology codes. The parenthetical examples of methodologies presented near the beginning of each code provide general guidelines used to group procedures for a given level and are not all-inclusive.

Use the appropriate molecular pathology procedure level code that includes the specific analyte listed after the code descriptor. If the analyte tested is not listed under one of the Tier 2 codes or is not represented by a Tier 1 code, use the appropriate methodology codes in the 83890-83914 and 88384-88386 series.◄

●81400    Molecular pathology procedure, Level 1 (eg, identification of single germline variant [eg, SNP] by techniques such as restriction enzyme digestion or melt curve analysis)

*ACADM (acyl-CoA dehydrogenase, C-4 to C-12 straight chain, MCAD)* (eg, medium chain acyl dehydrogenase deficiency), K304E variant

*ACE (angiotensin converting enzyme)* (eg, hereditary blood pressure regulation), insertion/deletion variant

*AGTR1 (angiotensin II receptor, type 1)* (eg, essential hypertension), 1166A>C variant

*CCR5 (chemokine C-C motif receptor 5)* (eg, HIV resistance), 32-bp deletion mutation/794 825del32 deletion

*DPYD (dihydropyrimidine dehydrogenase)* (eg, 5-fluorouracil/5-FU and capecitabine drug metabolism), IVS14+1G>A variant

*F2 (coagulation factor 2)* (eg, hereditary hypercoagulability), 1199G>A variant

*F5 (coagulation factor V)* (eg, hereditary hypercoagulability), HR2 variant

*F7 (coagulation factor VII [serum prothrombin conversion accelerator])* (eg, hereditary hypercoagulability), R353Q variant

*F13B (coagulation factor XIII, B polypeptide)* (eg, hereditary hypercoagulability), V34L variant

*FGB (fibrinogen beta chain)* (eg, hereditary ischemic heart disease), -455G>A variant

**Pathology and Laboratory**

**Pathology and Laboratory**

Human Platelet Antigen 1 genotyping (HPA-1), *ITGB3 (integrin, beta 3 [platelet glycoprotein IIIa], antigen CD61 [GPIIIa])* (eg, neonatal alloimmune thrombocytopenia [NAIT], post-transfusion purpura), HPA-1a/b (L33P)

Human Platelet Antigen 2 genotyping (HPA-2), *GP1BA (glycoprotein Ib [platelet], alpha polypeptide [GPIbα])* (eg, neonatal alloimmune thrombocytopenia [NAIT], post-transfusion purpura), HPA-2a/b (T145M)

Human Platelet Antigen 3 genotyping (HPA-3), *ITGA2B (integrin, alpha 2b [platelet glycoprotein IIb of IIb/IIIa complex], antigen CD41 [GPIIb])* (eg, neonatal alloimmune thrombocytopenia [NAIT], post-transfusion purpura), HPA-3a/b (I843S)

Human Platelet Antigen 4 genotyping (HPA-4), *ITGB3 (integrin, beta 3 [platelet glycoprotein IIIa], antigen CD61 [GPIIIa])* (eg, neonatal alloimmune thrombocytopenia [NAIT], post-transfusion purpura), HPA-4a/b (R143Q)

Human Platelet Antigen 5 genotyping (HPA-5), *ITGA2 (integrin, alpha 2 [CD49B, alpha 2 subunit of VLA-2 receptor] [GPIa])* (eg, neonatal alloimmune thrombocytopenia [NAIT], post-transfusion purpura), HPA-5a/b (K505E)

Human Platelet Antigen 6 genotyping (HPA-6w), *ITGB3 (integrin, beta 3 [platelet glycoprotein IIIa, antigen CD61] [GPIIIa])* (eg, neonatal alloimmune thrombocytopenia [NAIT], post-transfusion purpura), HPA-6a/b (R489Q)

Human Platelet Antigen 9 genotyping (HPA-9w), *ITGA2B (integrin, alpha 2b [platelet glycoprotein IIb of IIb/IIIa complex, antigen CD41] [GPIIb])* (eg, neonatal alloimmune thrombocytopenia [NAIT], post-transfusion purpura), HPA-9a/b (V837M)

Human Platelet Antigen 15 genotyping (HPA-15), *CD109 (CD109 molecule)* (eg, neonatal alloimmune thrombocytopenia [NAIT], post-transfusion purpura), HPA-15a/b(S682Y)

*SERPINE1 (serpine peptidase inhibitor clade E, member 1, plasminogen activator inhibitor -1, PAI-1)* (eg, thrombophilia), 4G variant

● **81401**  Molecular pathology procedure, Level 2 (eg, 2-10 SNPs, 1 methylated variant, or 1 somatic variant [typically using nonsequencing target variant analysis], or detection of a dynamic mutation disorder/triplet repeat)

*ABL (c-abl oncogene 1, receptor tyrosine kinase)* (eg, acquired imatinib resistance), T315I variant

*ACADM (acyl-CoA dehydrogenase, C-4 to C-12 straight chain, MCAD)* (eg, medium chain acyl dehydrogenase deficiency), commons variants (eg, K304E, Y42H)

*ADRB2 (adrenergic beta-2 receptor surface)* (eg, drug metabolism), common variants (eg, G16R, Q27E)

*APOE (apolipoprotein E)* (eg, hyperlipoproteinemia type III, cardiovascular disease, Alzheimer disease), common variants (eg, *2, *3, *4)

*CBFB/MYH11 (inv(16))* (eg, acute myeloid leukemia), qualitative, and quantitative, if performed

*CCND1/IGH (BCL1/IgH, t(11;14))* (eg, mantle cell lymphoma) translocation analysis, major breakpoint, qualitative, and quantitative, if performed

*CFH/ARMS2 (complement factor H/age-related maculopathy susceptibility 2)* (eg, macular degeneration), common variants (eg, Y402H [CFH], A69S [ARMS2])

*CYP3A4 (cytochrome P450, family 3, subfamily A, polypeptide 4)* (eg, drug metabolism), common variants (eg, *2, *3, *4, *5, *6)

*CYP3A5 (cytochrome P450, family 3, subfamily A, polypeptide 5)* (eg, drug metabolism), common variants (eg, *2, *3, *4, *5, *6)

*DMPK (dystrophia myotonica-protein kinase)* (eg, myotonic dystrophy, type 1), evaluation to detect abnormal (eg, expanded) alleles

*F11 (coagulation factor XI)* (eg, coagulation disorder), common variants (eg, E117X [Type II], F283L [Type III], IVS14del14, and IVS14+1G>A [Type I])

*FGFR3 (fibroblast growth factor receptor 3)* (eg, achondroplasia), common variants (eg, 1138G>A, 1138G>C)

*FIP1L1/PDGFRA (del[4q12])* (eg, imatinib-sensitive chronic eosinophilic leukemia), qualitative, and quantitative, if performed

*GALT (galactose-1-phosphate uridylyltransferase)* (eg, galactosemia), common variants (eg, Q188R, S135L, K285N, T138M, L195P, Y209C, IVS2-2A>G, P171S, del5kb, N314D, L218L/N314D)

*HBB (hemoglobin, beta)* (eg, sickle cell anemia, hemoglobin C, hemoglobin E), common variants (eg, HbS, HbC, HbE)

*HTT (huntingtin)* (eg, Huntington disease), evaluation to detect abnormal (eg, expanded) alleles

*RUNX1/RUNX1T1 (t(8;21))* (eg, acute myeloid leukemia) translocation analysis, qualitative, and quantitative, if performed

*SEPT9 (Septin 9)* (eg, colon cancer), methylation analysis

*TPMT (thiopurine S-methyltransferase)* (eg, drug metabolism), common variants (eg, *2, *3)

*VWF (von Willebrand factor)* (eg, von Willebrand disease type 2N), common variants (eg, T791M, R816W, R854Q)

● **81402**  Molecular pathology procedure, Level 3 (eg, >10 SNPs, 2-10 methylated variants, or 2-10 somatic variants [typically using non-sequencing target variant analysis], immunoglobulin and T-cell receptor gene rearrangements, duplication/deletion variants 1 exon)

*CYP21A2 (cytochrome P450, family 21, subfamily A, polypeptide 2)* (eg, congenital adrenal hyperplasia, 21-hydroxylase deficiency), common variants (eg, IVS2-13G, P30L, I172N, exon 6 mutation cluster [I235N, V236E, M238K], V281L, L307FfsX6, Q318X, R356W, P453S, G110VfsX21, 30-kb deletion variant)

*ESR1/PGR (receptor 1/progesterone receptor)* ratio (eg, breast cancer)

*KIT (v-kit Hardy-Zuckerman 4 feline sarcoma viral oncogene homolog)* (eg, mastocytosis), common variants (eg, D816V, D816Y, D816F)

*MEFV (Mediterranean fever) (eg, familial Mediterranean fever)*, common variants (eg, E148Q, P369S, F479L, M680I, I692del, M694V, M694I, K695R, V726A, A744S, R761H)

*MPL (myeloproliferative leukemia virus oncogene, thrombopoietin receptor, TPOR)* (eg, myeloproliferative disorder), common variants (eg, W515A, W515K, W515L, W515R)

*TCD@ (T cell antigen receptor, delta)* (eg, leukemia and lymphoma), gene rearrangement analysis, evaluation to detect abnormal clonal population

● **81403**   Molecular pathology procedure, Level 4 (eg, analysis of single exon by DNA sequence analysis, analysis of >10 amplicons using multiplex PCR in 2 or more independent reactions, mutation scanning or duplication/deletion variants of 2-5 exons)

*ABL1 (c-abl oncogene 1, receptor tyrosine kinase)* (eg, acquired imatinib tyrosine kinase inhibitor resistance), variants in the kinase domain

*DAZ/SRY (deleted in azoospermia and sex determining region Y)* (eg, male infertility), common deletions (eg, AZFa, AZFb, AZFc, AZFd)

*GJB1 (gap junction protein, beta 1)* (eg, Charcot-Marie-Tooth X-linked), full gene sequence

*JAK2 (Janus kinase 2)* (eg, myeloproliferative disorder), exon 12 sequence and exon 13 sequence, if performed

*KRAS (v-Ki-ras2 Kirsten rat sarcoma viral oncogene)* (eg, carcinoma), gene analysis, variant(s) in exon 2

*MPL (myeloproliferative leukemia virus oncogene, thrombopoietin receptor, TPOR)* (eg, myeloproliferative disorder), exon 10 sequence

*VHL (von Hippel-Lindau tumor suppressor)* (eg, von Hippel-Lindau familial cancer syndrome), deletion/duplication analysis

*VWF (von Willebrand factor)* (eg, von Willebrand disease types 2A, 2B, 2M), targeted sequence analysis (eg, exon 28)

● **81404**   Molecular pathology procedure, Level 5 (eg, analysis of 2-5 exons by DNA sequence analysis, mutation scanning or duplication/deletion variants of 6-10 exons, or characterization of a dynamic mutation disorder/triplet repeat by Southern blot analysis)

*BTD (biotinidase)* (eg, biotinidase deficiency), full gene sequence

*CYP1B1 (cytochrome P450, family 1, subfamily B, polypeptide 1)* (eg, primary congenital glaucoma), full gene sequence

*DMPK (dystrophia myotonica-protein kinase)* (eg, myotonic dystrophy type 1), characterization of abnormal (eg, expanded) alleles

*EGR2 (early growth response 2)* (eg, Charcot-Marie-Tooth), full gene sequence

*FKRP (Fukutin related protein)* (eg, congenital muscular dystrophy type 1C [MDC1C], limb-girdle muscular dystrophy [LGMD] type 2I), full gene sequence

*FOXG1 (forkhead box G1)* (eg, Rett syndrome), full gene sequence

*FSHMD1A (facioscapulohumeral muscular dystrophy 1A)* (eg, facioscapulohumeral muscular dystrophy), evaluation to detect abnormal (eg, deleted) alleles

*FSHMD1A (facioscapulohumeral muscular dystrophy 1A)* (eg, facioscapulohumeral muscular dystrophy), characterization of haplotype(s) (ie, chromosome 4A and 4B haplotypes)

*HBB (hemoglobin, beta, Beta-Globin)* (eg, thalassemia), full gene sequence

*KIT (C-kit) (v-kit Hardy-Zuckerman 4 feline sarcoma viral oncogene homolog)* (eg, GIST, acute myeloid leukemia, melanoma), targeted gene analysis (eg, exons 8, 11, 13, 17, 18)

*LITAF (lipopolysaccharide-induced TNF factor)* (eg, Charcot-Marie-Tooth), full gene sequence

*MEFV (Mediterranean fever)* (eg, familial Mediterranean fever), full gene sequence

*NRAS (neuroblastoma RAS viral oncogene homolog)* (eg, colorectal carcinoma), exon 1 and exon 2 sequences

*PDGFRA (platelet-derived growth factor receptor alpha polypeptide)* (eg, gastrointestinal stromal tumor), targeted sequence analysis (eg, exons 12, 18)

*RET (ret proto-oncogene)* (eg, multiple endocrine neoplasia, type 2B and familial medullary thyroid carcinoma), common variants (eg, M918T, 2647_2648delinsTT, A883F)

*SDHD (succinate dehydrogenase complex, subunit D, integral membrane protein)* (eg, hereditary paraganglioma), full gene sequence

*VHL (von Hippel-Lindau tumor suppressor)* (eg, von Hippel-Lindau familial cancer syndrome), full gene sequence

*VWF (von Willebrand factor)* (eg, von Willebrand disease type 1C), targeted sequence analysis (eg, exons 26, 27, 37)

● **81405**   Molecular pathology procedure, Level 6 (eg, analysis of 6-10 exons by DNA sequence analysis, mutation scanning or duplication/deletion variants of 11-25 exons)

*CYP21A2 (cytochrome P450, family 21, subfamily A, polypeptide2)* (eg, steroid 21-hydroxylase isoform, congenital adrenal hyperplasia), full gene sequence

**Pathology and Laboratory**

*FKTN (fukutin)* (eg, limb-girdle muscular dystrophy [LGMD] type 2M or 2L), full gene sequence

*MPZ (myelin protein zero)* (eg, Charcot-Marie-Tooth), full gene sequence

*NEFL (neurofilament, light polypeptide)* (eg, Charcot-Marie-Tooth), full gene sequence

*RET (ret proto-oncogene)* (eg, multiple endocrine neoplasia, type 2A and familial medullary thyroid carcinoma), targeted sequence analysis (eg, exons 10, 11, 13-16)

*SDHB (succinate dehydrogenase complex, subunit B, iron sulfur)* (eg, hereditary paraganglioma), full gene sequence

*TGFBR1 (transforming growth factor, beta receptor 1)* (eg, Marfan syndrome), full gene sequence

*TGFBR2 (transforming growth factor, beta receptor 2)* (eg, Marfan syndrome), full gene sequence

*THRB (thyroid hormone receptor, beta)* (eg, thyroid hormone resistance, thyroid hormone beta receptor deficiency), full gene sequence or targeted sequence analysis of >5 exons

*TP53 (tumor protein 53)* (eg, Li-Fraumeni syndrome, tumor samples), full gene sequence or targeted sequence analysis of >5 exons

*VWF (von Willebrand factor)* (eg, von Willebrand disease type 2N), targeted sequence analysis (eg, exons 18-20, 23-25)

● **81406**  Molecular pathology procedure, Level 7 (eg, analysis of 11-25 exons by DNA sequence analysis, mutation scanning or duplication/deletion variants of 26-50 exons, cytogenomic array analysis for neoplasia)

*CAPN3 (Calpain 3)* (eg, limb-girdle muscular dystrophy [LGMD] type 2A, calpainopathy), full gene sequence

Cytogenomic microarray analysis, neoplasia (eg, interrogation of copy number, and loss-of-heterozygosity via single nucleotide polymorphism [SNP]-based comparative genomic hybridization [CGH] microarray analysis)

*GALT (galactose-1-phosphate uridylyltransferase)* (eg, galactosemia), full gene sequence

*HEXA (hexosaminidase A, alpha polypeptide)* (eg, Tay-Sachs disease), full gene sequence

*LMNA (lamin A/C)* (eg, Emery-Dreifuss muscular dystrophy [EDMD1, 2 and 3] limb-girdle muscular dystrophy [LGMD] type 1B, dilated cardiomyopathy [CMD1A], familial partial lipodystrophy [FPLD2]), full gene sequence

*PAH (phenylalanine hydroxylase)* (eg, phenylketonuria), full gene sequence

*POLG (polymerase [DNA directed], gamma)* (eg, Alpers-Huttenlocher syndrome, autosomal dominant progressive external ophthalmoplegia), full gene sequence

*POMGNT1 (protein O-linked mannose beta1,2-N acetylglucosaminyltransferase)* (eg, muscle-eye-brain disease, Walker-Warburg syndrome), full gene sequence

*POMT1 (protein-O-mannosyltransferase 1)* (eg, limb-girdle muscular dystrophy [LGMD] type 2K, Walker-Warburg syndrome), full gene sequence

*POMT2 (protein-O-mannosyltransferase 2)* (eg, limb-girdle muscular dystrophy [LGMD] type 2N, Walker-Warburg syndrome), full gene sequence

*RYR1 (ryanodine receptor 1, skeletal)* (eg, malignant hyperthermia), targeted sequence analysis of exons with functionally-confirmed mutations

*VWF (von Willebrand factor)* (von Willebrand disease type 2A), extended targeted sequence analysis (eg, exons 11-16, 24-26, 51, 52)

● **81407**  Molecular pathology procedure, Level 8 (eg, analysis of 26-50 exons by DNA sequence analysis, mutation scanning or duplication/deletion variants of >50 exons, sequence analysis of multiple genes on one platform)

*SCN1A (sodium channel, voltage-gated, type 1, alpha subunit)* (eg, generalized epilepsy with febrile seizures), full gene sequence

● **81408**  Molecular pathology procedure, Level 9 (eg, analysis of >50 exons in a single gene by DNA sequence analysis)

*FBN1 (fibrillin 1)* (eg, Marfan syndrome), full gene sequence

*NF1 (neurofibromin 1)* (eg, neurofibromatosis, type 1), full gene sequence

*RYR1 (ryanodine receptor 1, skeletal)* (eg, malignant hyperthermia), full gene sequence

*VWF (von Willebrand factor)* (eg, von Willebrand disease types 1 and 3), full gene sequence

# Chemistry

The material for examination may be from any source unless otherwise specified in the code descriptor. When an analyte is measured in multiple specimens from different sources, or in specimens that are obtained at different times, the analyte is reported separately for each source and for each specimen. The examination is quantitative unless specified. To report an organ or disease oriented panel, see codes 80048-80076.

When a code describes a method where measurement of multiple analytes may require one or several procedures, each procedure is coded separately (eg, 82491-82492, 82541-82544). For example, if two analytes are measured using column chromatography using a single stationary or mobile phase, use 82492. If the same two analytes are measured using different stationary or mobile phase conditions, 82491 would be used twice. If a total of four analytes are measured where two analytes are measured with a single stationary and mobile phase, and the other two analytes are measured using a different stationary and mobile phase, use 82492 twice. If a total of three analytes are measured where two analytes are measured using a single stationary or mobile phase condition, and the third analyte is measured separately using a different stationary or mobile phase procedure, use 82492 once for the two analytes measured under the same condition, and use 82491 once for the third analyte measured separately.

Clinical information derived from the results of laboratory data that is mathematically calculated (eg, free thyroxine index [T7]) is considered part of the test procedure and therefore is not a separately reportable service.

| 82000 | Acetaldehyde, blood |
|---|---|
| 82003 | Acetaminophen |
| 82009 | Acetone or other ketone bodies, serum; qualitative |
| 82010 | quantitative |
| 82013 | Acetylcholinesterase |

(For gastric acid analysis, use 82930)

(Acid phosphatase, see 84060-84066)

| 82016 | Acylcarnitines; qualitative, each specimen |
|---|---|
| 82017 | quantitative, each specimen |

(For carnitine, use 82379)

| 82024 | Adrenocorticotropic hormone (ACTH) |
|---|---|
| 82030 | Adenosine, 5-monophosphate, cyclic (cyclic AMP) |
| 82040 | Albumin; serum, plasma or whole blood |
| 82042 | urine or other source, quantitative, each specimen |
| 82043 | urine, microalbumin, quantitative |
| 82044 | urine, microalbumin, semiquantitative (eg, reagent strip assay) |

(For prealbumin, use 84134)

| 82045 | ischemia modified |
|---|---|
| 82055 | Alcohol (ethanol); any specimen except breath |

(For other volatiles, alcohol, use 84600)

| 82075 | breath |
|---|---|
| 82085 | Aldolase |
| 82088 | Aldosterone |

(Alkaline phosphatase, see 84075, 84080)

| 82101 | Alkaloids, urine, quantitative |
|---|---|

(Alphaketoglutarate, see 82009, 82010)

(Alpha tocopherol [Vitamin E], use 84446)

| 82103 | Alpha-1-antitrypsin; total |
|---|---|
| 82104 | phenotype |
| 82105 | Alpha-fetoprotein (AFP); serum |
| 82106 | amniotic fluid |

| 82107 | AFP-L3 fraction isoform and total AFP (including ratio) |
|---|---|
| 82108 | Aluminum |
| 82120 | Amines, vaginal fluid, qualitative |

(For combined pH and amines test for vaginitis, use 82120 and 83986)

| 82127 | Amino acids; single, qualitative, each specimen |
|---|---|
| 82128 | multiple, qualitative, each specimen |
| 82131 | single, quantitative, each specimen |
| 82135 | Aminolevulinic acid, delta (ALA) |
| 82136 | Amino acids, 2 to 5 amino acids, quantitative, each specimen |
| 82139 | Amino acids, 6 or more amino acids, quantitative, each specimen |
| 82140 | Ammonia |
| 82143 | Amniotic fluid scan (spectrophotometric) |

(For L/S ratio, use 83661)

(Amobarbital, see 80100-80103 for qualitative analysis, 82205 for quantitative analysis)

| 82145 | Amphetamine or methamphetamine |
|---|---|

(For qualitative analysis, see 80100-80103)

| 82150 | Amylase |
|---|---|
| 82154 | Androstanediol glucuronide |
| 82157 | Androstenedione |
| 82160 | Androsterone |
| 82163 | Angiotensin II |
| 82164 | Angiotensin I - converting enzyme (ACE) |

(Antidiuretic hormone (ADH), use 84588)

(Antimony, use 83015)

(Antitrypsin, alpha-1-, see 82103, 82104)

| 82172 | Apolipoprotein, each |
|---|---|
| 82175 | Arsenic |

(For heavy metal screening, use 83015)

| 82180 | Ascorbic acid (Vitamin C), blood |
|---|---|

(Aspirin, see acetylsalicylic acid, 80196)

(Atherogenic index, blood, ultracentrifugation, quantitative, use 83701)

| 82190 | Atomic absorption spectroscopy, each analyte |
|---|---|
| 82205 | Barbiturates, not elsewhere specified |

(For qualitative analysis, see 80100-80103)

(For B-Natriuretic peptide, use 83880)

| 82232 | Beta-2 microglobulin |
|---|---|

(Bicarbonate, use 82374)

| 82239 | Bile acids; total |
|---|---|

**Pathology and Laboratory**

82240      cholylglycine

(For bile pigments, urine, see 81000-81005)

82247      Bilirubin; total

82248         direct

82252         feces, qualitative

82261      Biotinidase, each specimen

82270      Blood, occult, by peroxidase activity (eg, guaiac), qualitative; feces, consecutive collected specimens with single determination, for colorectal neoplasm screening (ie, patient was provided 3 cards or single triple card for consecutive collection)

82271         other sources

82272      Blood, occult, by peroxidase activity (eg, guaiac), qualitative, feces, 1-3 simultaneous determinations, performed for other than colorectal neoplasm screening

(Blood urea nitrogen [BUN], see 84520, 84525)

82274      Blood, occult, by fecal hemoglobin determination by immunoassay, qualitative, feces, 1-3 simultaneous determinations

82286      Bradykinin

82300      Cadmium

82306      Vitamin D; 25 hydroxy, includes fraction(s), if performed

# 82652         1, 25 dihydroxy, includes fraction(s), if performed

(82307 has been deleted. For 25 hydroxy vitamin D, use 82306)

82308      Calcitonin

82310      Calcium; total

82330         ionized

82331         after calcium infusion test

82340         urine quantitative, timed specimen

82355      Calculus; qualitative analysis

82360         quantitative analysis, chemical

82365         infrared spectroscopy

82370         X-ray diffraction

(Carbamates, see individual listings)

82373      Carbohydrate deficient transferrin

82374      Carbon dioxide (bicarbonate)

(See also 82803)

82375      Carboxyhemoglobin; quantitative

82376         qualitative

(For transcutaneous measurement of carboxyhemoglobin, use 88740)

82378      Carcinoembryonic antigen (CEA)

82379      Carnitine (total and free), quantitative, each specimen

(For acylcarnitine, see 82016, 82017)

82380      Carotene

82382      Catecholamines; total urine

82383         blood

82384         fractionated

(For urine metabolites, see 83835, 84585)

82387      Cathepsin-D

82390      Ceruloplasmin

82397      Chemiluminescent assay

82415      Chloramphenicol

82435      Chloride; blood

82436         urine

82438         other source

(For sweat collection by iontophoresis, use 89230)

82441      Chlorinated hydrocarbons, screen

(Chlorpromazine, use 84022)

(Cholecalciferol [Vitamin D], use 82306)

82465      Cholesterol, serum or whole blood, total

(For high density lipoprotein [HDL], use 83718)

82480      Cholinesterase; serum

82482         RBC

82485      Chondroitin B sulfate, quantitative

(Chorionic gonadotropin, see gonadotropin, 84702, 84703)

82486      Chromatography, qualitative; column (eg, gas liquid or HPLC), analyte not elsewhere specified

82487         paper, 1-dimensional, analyte not elsewhere specified

82488         paper, 2-dimensional, analyte not elsewhere specified

82489         thin layer, analyte not elsewhere specified

82491      Chromatography, quantitative, column (eg, gas liquid or HPLC); single analyte not elsewhere specified, single stationary and mobile phase

82492         multiple analytes, single stationary and mobile phase

82495      Chromium

82507      Citrate

82520      Cocaine or metabolite

(Cocaine, qualitative analysis, see 80100-80103)

(Codeine, qualitative analysis, see 80100-80103)

(Codeine, quantitative analysis, see 82101)

(Complement, see 86160-86162)

82523      Collagen cross links, any method

| 82525 | Copper |
|---|---|

(Coproporphyrin, see 84119, 84120)

(Corticosteroids, use 83491)

| 82528 | Corticosterone |
|---|---|
| 82530 | Cortisol; free |
| 82533 | total |

(C-peptide, use 84681)

| 82540 | Creatine |
|---|---|
| 82541 | Column chromatography/mass spectrometry (eg, GC/MS, or HPLC/MS), analyte not elsewhere specified; qualitative, single stationary and mobile phase |
| 82542 | quantitative, single stationary and mobile phase |
| 82543 | stable isotope dilution, single analyte, quantitative, single stationary and mobile phase |
| 82544 | stable isotope dilution, multiple analytes, quantitative, single stationary and mobile phase |
| 82550 | Creatine kinase (CK), (CPK); total |
| 82552 | isoenzymes |
| 82553 | MB fraction only |
| 82554 | isoforms |
| 82565 | Creatinine; blood |
| 82570 | other source |
| 82575 | clearance |
| 82585 | Cryofibrinogen |
| 82595 | Cryoglobulin, qualitative or semi-quantitative (eg, cryocrit) |

(For quantitative, cryoglobulin, see 82784, 82785)

(Crystals, pyrophosphate vs urate, use 89060)

| 82600 | Cyanide |
|---|---|
| 82607 | Cyanocobalamin (Vitamin B-12); |
| 82608 | unsaturated binding capacity |

(Cyclic AMP, use 82030)

(Cyclic GMP, use 83008)

(Cyclosporine, use 80158)

| 82610 | Cystatin C |
|---|---|
| 82615 | Cystine and homocystine, urine, qualitative |
| 82626 | Dehydroepiandrosterone (DHEA) |
| 82627 | Dehydroepiandrosterone-sulfate (DHEA-S) |

(Delta-aminolevulinic acid (ALA), use 82135)

| 82633 | Desoxycorticosterone, 11- |
|---|---|
| 82634 | Deoxycortisol, 11- |

(Dexamethasone suppression test, use 80420)

(Diastase, urine, use 82150)

| 82638 | Dibucaine number |
|---|---|

(Dichloroethane, use 84600)

(Dichloromethane, use 84600)

(Diethylether, use 84600)

| 82646 | Dihydrocodeinone |
|---|---|

(For qualitative analysis, see 80100-80103)

| 82649 | Dihydromorphinone |
|---|---|

(For qualitative analysis, see 80100-80103)

| 82651 | Dihydrotestosterone (DHT) |
|---|---|
| 82652 | Code is out of numerical sequence. See 82000-84999 |
| 82654 | Dimethadione |

(For qualitative analysis, see 80100-80103)

(Diphenylhydantoin, use 80185)

(Dipropylacetic acid, use 80164)

(Dopamine, see 82382-82384)

(Duodenal contents, see individual enzymes; for intubation and collection, see 43756, 43757)

| 82656 | Elastase, pancreatic (EL-1), fecal, qualitative or semi-quantitative |
|---|---|
| 82657 | Enzyme activity in blood cells, cultured cells, or tissue, not elsewhere specified; nonradioactive substrate, each specimen |
| 82658 | radioactive substrate, each specimen |
| 82664 | Electrophoretic technique, not elsewhere specified |

(Endocrine receptor assays, see 84233-84235)

| 82666 | Epiandrosterone |
|---|---|

(Epinephrine, see 82382-82384)

| 82668 | Erythropoietin |
|---|---|
| 82670 | Estradiol |
| 82671 | Estrogens; fractionated |
| 82672 | total |

(Estrogen receptor assay, use 84233)

| 82677 | Estriol |
|---|---|
| 82679 | Estrone |

(Ethanol, see 82055 and 82075)

| 82690 | Ethchlorvynol |
|---|---|

(Ethyl alcohol, see 82055 and 82075)

| 82693 | Ethylene glycol |
|---|---|
| 82696 | Etiocholanolone |

(For fractionation of ketosteroids, use 83593)

| 82705 | Fat or lipids, feces; qualitative |
|---|---|
| 82710 | quantitative |

| | |
|---|---|
| 82715 | Fat differential, feces, quantitative |
| 82725 | Fatty acids, nonesterified |
| 82726 | Very long chain fatty acids |

(For long-chain [C20-22] omega-3 fatty acids in red blood cell [RBC] membranes, use Category III code 0111T)

| | |
|---|---|
| 82728 | Ferritin |

(Fetal hemoglobin, see hemoglobin 83030, 83033, and 85460)

(Fetoprotein, alpha-1, see 82105, 82106)

| | |
|---|---|
| 82731 | Fetal fibronectin, cervicovaginal secretions, semi-quantitative |
| 82735 | Fluoride |
| 82742 | Flurazepam |

(For qualitative analysis, see 80100-80103)

(Foam stability test, use 83662)

| | |
|---|---|
| 82746 | Folic acid; serum |
| 82747 | RBC |

(Follicle stimulating hormone [FSH], use 83001)

| | |
|---|---|
| 82757 | Fructose, semen |

(Fructosamine, use 82985)

(Fructose, TLC screen, use 84375)

| | |
|---|---|
| 82759 | Galactokinase, RBC |
| 82760 | Galactose |
| 82775 | Galactose-1-phosphate uridyl transferase; quantitative |
| 82776 | screen |
| 82784 | Gammaglobulin (immunoglobulin); IgA, IgD, IgG, IgM, each |
| 82785 | IgE |

(For allergen specific IgE, see 86003, 86005)

| | |
|---|---|
| 82787 | immunoglobulin subclasses (eg, IgG1, 2, 3, or 4), each |

(Gamma-glutamyltransferase [GGT], use 82977)

| | |
|---|---|
| 82800 | Gases, blood, pH only |
| 82803 | Gases, blood, any combination of pH, $pCO_2$, $pO_2$, $CO_2$, $HCO_3$ (including calculated $O_2$ saturation); |

(Use 82803 for 2 or more of the above listed analytes)

| | |
|---|---|
| 82805 | with $O_2$ saturation, by direct measurement, except pulse oximetry |
| 82810 | Gases, blood, $O_2$ saturation only, by direct measurement, except pulse oximetry |

(For pulse oximetry, use 94760)

| | |
|---|---|
| 82820 | Hemoglobin-oxygen affinity ($pO_2$ for 50% hemoglobin saturation with oxygen) |

(82926, 82928 have been deleted)

(For gastric acid analysis, use 82930)

| | |
|---|---|
| 82930 | Gastric acid analysis, includes pH if performed, each specimen |
| 82938 | Gastrin after secretin stimulation |
| 82941 | Gastrin |

(Gentamicin, use 80170)

(GGT, use 82977)

(GLC, gas liquid chromatography, use 82486)

| | |
|---|---|
| 82943 | Glucagon |
| 82945 | Glucose, body fluid, other than blood |
| 82946 | Glucagon tolerance test |
| 82947 | Glucose; quantitative, blood (except reagent strip) |
| 82948 | blood, reagent strip |
| 82950 | post glucose dose (includes glucose) |
| 82951 | tolerance test (GTT), 3 specimens (includes glucose) |
| + 82952 | tolerance test, each additional beyond 3 specimens (List separately in addition to code for primary procedure) |

(Use 82952 in conjunction with 82951)

| | |
|---|---|
| 82953 | tolbutamide tolerance test |

(For insulin tolerance test, see 80434, 80435)

(For leucine tolerance test, use 80428)

(For semiquantitative urine glucose, see 81000, 81002, 81005, 81099)

| | |
|---|---|
| 82955 | Glucose-6-phosphate dehydrogenase (G6PD); quantitative |
| 82960 | screen |

(For glucose tolerance test with medication, use 96374 in addition)

| | |
|---|---|
| 82962 | Glucose, blood by glucose monitoring device(s) cleared by the FDA specifically for home use |
| 82963 | Glucosidase, beta |
| 82965 | Glutamate dehydrogenase |
| 82975 | Glutamine (glutamic acid amide) |
| 82977 | Glutamyltransferase, gamma (GGT) |
| 82978 | Glutathione |
| 82979 | Glutathione reductase, RBC |
| 82980 | Glutethimide |

(Glycohemoglobin, use 83036)

| | |
|---|---|
| 82985 | Glycated protein |

(Gonadotropin, chorionic, see 84702, 84703)

| | |
|---|---|
| 83001 | Gonadotropin; follicle stimulating hormone (FSH) |
| 83002 | luteinizing hormone (LH) |

(For luteinizing releasing factor [LRH], use 83727)

Pathology and Laboratory

**83003**     Growth hormone, human (HGH) (somatotropin)

          (For antibody to human growth hormone, use 86277)

**83008**     Guanosine monophosphate (GMP), cyclic

**83009**     Helicobacter pylori, blood test analysis for urease
          activity, non-radioactive isotope (eg, C-13)

          (For H. pylori, breath test analysis for urease activity, see
          83013, 83014)

**83010**     Haptoglobin; quantitative

**83012**          phenotypes

**83013**     Helicobacter pylori; breath test analysis for urease
          activity, non-radioactive isotope (eg, C-13)

**83014**          drug administration

          (For H. pylori, stool, use 87338. For H. pylori, liquid
          scintillation counter, see 78267, 78268. For H. pylori,
          enzyme immunoassay, use 87339)

          (For H. pylori, blood test analysis for urease activity, use
          83009)

**83015**     Heavy metal (eg, arsenic, barium, beryllium, bismuth,
          antimony, mercury); screen

**83018**          quantitative, each

**83020**     Hemoglobin fractionation and quantitation;
          electrophoresis (eg, A2, S, C, and/or F)

**83021**          chromatography (eg, A2, S, C, and/or F)

          (For glycosylated [A1c] hemoglobin analysis, by
          chromatography, in the absence of an identified
          hemoglobin variant, use 83036)

**83026**     Hemoglobin; by copper sulfate method, non-automated

**83030**          F (fetal), chemical

**83033**          F (fetal), qualitative

**83036**          glycosylated (A1C)

          (For glycosylated [A1c] hemoglobin analysis, by
          chromatography, in the setting of an identified
          hemoglobin variant, use 83021)

          (For fecal hemoglobin detection by immunoassay, use
          82274)

**83037**          glycosylated (A1C) by device cleared by FDA for home
          use

**83045**          methemoglobin, qualitative

**83050**          methemoglobin, quantitative

          (For transcutaneous quantitative methemoglobin
          determination, use 88741)

**83051**          plasma

**83055**          sulfhemoglobin, qualitative

**83060**          sulfhemoglobin, quantitative

**83065**          thermolabile

**83068**          unstable, screen

**83069**          urine

**83070**     Hemosiderin; qualitative

**83071**          quantitative

          (Heroin, see 80100-80103)

          (HIAA, use 83497)

          (High performance liquid chromatography [HPLC], use
          82486)

**83080**     b-Hexosaminidase, each assay

**83088**     Histamine

          (Hollander test, see 43754, 43755)

**83090**     Homocysteine

**83150**     Homovanillic acid (HVA)

          (Hormones, see individual alphabetic listings in
          **Chemistry** section)

          (Hydrogen breath test, use 91065)

**83491**     Hydroxycorticosteroids, 17- (17-OHCS)

          (For cortisol, see 82530, 82533. For deoxycortisol, use
          82634)

**83497**     Hydroxyindolacetic acid, 5-(HIAA)

          (For urine qualitative test, use 81005)

          (5-Hydroxytryptamine, use 84260)

**83498**     Hydroxyprogesterone, 17-d

**83499**     Hydroxyprogesterone, 20-

**83500**     Hydroxyproline; free

**83505**          total

**83516**     Immunoassay for analyte other than infectious agent
          antibody or infectious agent antigen; qualitative or
          semiquantitative, multiple step method

**83518**          qualitative or semiquantitative, single step method
          (eg, reagent strip)

**83519**          quantitative, by radioimmunoassay (eg, RIA)

**83520**          quantitative, not otherwise specified

          (For immunoassays for antibodies to infectious agent
          antigens, see analyte and method specific codes in the
          **Immunology** section)

          (For immunoassay of tumor antigen not elsewhere
          specified, use 86316)

          (Immunoglobulins, see 82784, 82785)

**83525**     Insulin; total

          (For proinsulin, use 84206)

**83527**          free

**83528**     Intrinsic factor

          (For intrinsic factor antibodies, use 86340)

**83540**     Iron

Pathology and Laboratory

**Pathology and Laboratory**

| | |
|---|---|
| 83550 | Iron binding capacity |
| 83570 | Isocitric dehydrogenase (IDH) |

(Isonicotinic acid hydrazide, INH, see code for specific method)

(Isopropyl alcohol, use 84600)

**83582** Ketogenic steroids, fractionation

(Ketone bodies, for serum, see 82009, 82010; for urine, see 81000-81003)

**83586** Ketosteroids, 17- (17-KS); total

**83593**     fractionation

**83605** Lactate (lactic acid)

**83615** Lactate dehydrogenase (LD), (LDH);

**83625**     isoenzymes, separation and quantitation

**83630** Lactoferrin, fecal; qualitative

**83631**     quantitative

**83632** Lactogen, human placental (HPL) human chorionic somatomammotropin

**83633** Lactose, urine; qualitative

**83634**     quantitative

(For tolerance, see 82951, 82952)

(For breath hydrogen test for lactase deficiency, use 91065)

**83655** Lead

**83661** Fetal lung maturity assessment; lecithin sphingomyelin (L/S) ratio

**83662**     foam stability test

**83663**     fluorescence polarization

**83664**     lamellar body density

(For phosphatidylglycerol, use 84081)

**83670** Leucine aminopeptidase (LAP)

**83690** Lipase

**83695** Lipoprotein (a)

**83698** Lipoprotein-associated phospholipase $A_2$ (Lp-$PLA_2$)

**83700** Lipoprotein, blood; electrophoretic separation and quantitation

**83701**     high resolution fractionation and quantitation of lipoproteins including lipoprotein subclasses when performed (eg, electrophoresis, ultracentrifugation)

**83704**     quantitation of lipoprotein particle numbers and lipoprotein particle subclasses (eg, by nuclear magnetic resonance spectroscopy)

**83718** Lipoprotein, direct measurement; high density cholesterol (HDL cholesterol)

**83719**     VLDL cholesterol

**83721**     LDL cholesterol

(For fractionation by high resolution electrophoresis or ultracentrifugation, use 83701)

(For lipoprotein particle numbers and subclasses analysis by nuclear magnetic resonance spectroscopy, use 83704)

**83727** Luteinizing releasing factor (LRH)

(Luteinizing hormone [LH], use 83002)

(For qualitative analysis, see 80100-80103)

(Macroglobulins, alpha-2, use 86329)

**83735** Magnesium

**83775** Malate dehydrogenase

(Maltose tolerance, see 82951, 82952)

(Mammotropin, use 84146)

**83785** Manganese

(Marijuana, see 80100-80103)

**83788** Mass spectrometry and tandem mass spectrometry (MS, MS/MS), analyte not elsewhere specified; qualitative, each specimen

**83789**     quantitative, each specimen

**83805** Meprobamate

(For qualitative analysis, see 80100-80103)

**83825** Mercury, quantitative

(Mercury screen, use 83015)

**83835** Metanephrines

(For catecholamines, see 82382-82384)

**83840** Methadone

(For methadone qualitative analysis, see 80100-80103)

(Methamphetamine, see 80100-80103, 82145)

(Methanol, use 84600)

**83857** Methemalbumin

(Methemoglobin, see hemoglobin 83045, 83050)

**83858** Methsuximide

(Methyl alcohol, use 84600)

(Microalbumin, see 82043 for quantitative, see 82044 for semiquantitative)

**83861** Microfluidic analysis utilizing an integrated collection and analysis device, tear osmolarity

(Microglobulin, beta-2, use 82232)

(For microfluidic tear osmolarity of both eyes, report 83861 twice)

**83864** Mucopolysaccharides, acid; quantitative

**83866**     screen

**83872** Mucin, synovial fluid (Ropes test)

| | |
|---|---|
| **83873** | Myelin basic protein, cerebrospinal fluid |
| | (For oligoclonal bands, use 83916) |
| **83874** | Myoglobin |
| | (Nalorphine, use 83925) |
| **83876** | Myeloperoxidase (MPO) |
| **83880** | Natriuretic peptide |
| **83883** | Nephelometry, each analyte not elsewhere specified |
| **83885** | Nickel |
| **83887** | Nicotine |

Codes 83890-83914 are intended for use with molecular diagnostic techniques for analysis of nucleic acids.

Codes 83890-83914 are coded by procedure rather than analyte.

Code separately for each procedure used in an analysis. For example, a procedure requiring isolation of DNA, restriction endonuclease digestion, electrophoresis, and nucleic acid probe amplification would be coded 83890, 83892, 83894, and 83898.

When molecular diagnostic procedures are performed to test for oncology, hematology, neurology or inherited disorder, use the appropriate modifier to specify probe type or condition tested. (See **Appendix I** for a listing of appropriate modifiers to report with molecular diagnostic and cytogenetic procedures.)

Each nucleic acid preparation may include a digestate, undigested nucleic acid, or other uniquely modified nucleic acid sample (eg, newly synthesized oligonucleotide).

(For microbial identification, see 87149, 87150, 87152, 87153, 87470-87801)

(For array technology using more than 10 probes, see 88384-88386)

| | |
|---|---|
| **83890** | Molecular diagnostics; molecular isolation or extraction, each nucleic acid type (ie, DNA or RNA) |
| **83891** | isolation or extraction of highly purified nucleic acid, each nucleic acid type (ie, DNA or RNA) |
| **83892** | enzymatic digestion, each enzyme treatment |
| **83893** | dot/slot blot production, each nucleic acid preparation |
| **83894** | separation by gel electrophoresis (eg, agarose, polyacrylamide), each nucleic acid preparation |
| **83896** | nucleic acid probe, each |
| **83897** | nucleic acid transfer (eg, Southern, Northern), each nucleic acid preparation |
| **83898** | amplification, target, each nucleic acid sequence |
| | (For multiplex target amplification, see 83900, 83901) |
| | (For signal amplification, use 83908) |
| **83900** | amplification, target, multiplex, first 2 nucleic acid sequences |

| | |
|---|---|
| **+ 83901** | amplification, target, multiplex, each additional nucleic acid sequence beyond 2 (List separately in addition to code for primary procedure) |
| | (Use 83901 in conjunction with 83900) |
| **83902** | reverse transcription |
| **83903** | mutation scanning, by physical properties (eg, single strand conformational polymorphisms [SSCP], heteroduplex, denaturing gradient gel electrophoresis [DGGE], RNA'ase A), single segment, each |
| **83904** | mutation identification by sequencing, single segment, each segment |
| **83905** | mutation identification by allele specific transcription, single segment, each segment |
| **83906** | mutation identification by allele specific translation, single segment, each segment |
| **83907** | lysis of cells prior to nucleic acid extraction (eg, stool specimens, paraffin embedded tissue), each specimen |
| **83908** | amplification, signal, each nucleic acid sequence |
| | (For target amplification, see 83898, 83900, 83901) |
| **83909** | separation and identification by high resolution technique (eg, capillary electrophoresis), each nucleic acid preparation |
| **83912** | interpretation and report |
| **83913** | RNA stabilization |
| **83914** | Mutation identification by enzymatic ligation or primer extension, single segment, each segment (eg, oligonucleotide ligation assay [OLA], single base chain extension [SBCE], or allele-specific primer extension [ASPE]) |
| **83915** | Nucleotidase 5'- |
| **83916** | Oligoclonal immune (oligoclonal bands) |
| **83918** | Organic acids; total, quantitative, each specimen |
| **83919** | qualitative, each specimen |
| **83921** | Organic acid, single, quantitative |
| **83925** | Opiate(s), drug and metabolites, each procedure |
| **83930** | Osmolality; blood |
| **83935** | urine |
| | (For tear osmolarity using microfluidic analysis, use 83861) |
| **83937** | Osteocalcin (bone g1a protein) |
| **83945** | Oxalate |
| **83950** | Oncoprotein; HER-2/neu |
| | (For tissue, see 88342, 88365) |
| **83951** | des-gamma-carboxy-prothrombin (DCP) |

**Pathology and Laboratory**

| | |
|---|---|
| **83970** | Parathormone (parathyroid hormone) |
| | (Pesticide, quantitative, see code for specific method. For screen for chlorinated hydrocarbons, use 82441) |
| **83986** | pH; body fluid, not otherwise specified |
| **83987** | exhaled breath condensate |
| | (For blood pH, see 82800, 82803) |
| **83992** | Phencyclidine (PCP) |
| | (For qualitative analysis, see 80100-80103) |
| | (Phenobarbital, use 80184) |
| **83993** | Calprotectin, fecal |
| **84022** | Phenothiazine |
| | (For qualitative analysis, see 80100, 80101) |
| **84030** | Phenylalanine (PKU), blood |
| | (Phenylalanine-tyrosine ratio, see 84030, 84510) |
| **84035** | Phenylketones, qualitative |
| **84060** | Phosphatase, acid; total |
| **84061** | forensic examination |
| **84066** | prostatic |
| **84075** | Phosphatase, alkaline; |
| **84078** | heat stable (total not included) |
| **84080** | isoenzymes |
| **84081** | Phosphatidylglycerol |
| | (Phosphates inorganic, use 84100) |
| | (Phosphates, organic, see code for specific method. For cholinesterase, see 82480, 82482) |
| **84085** | Phosphogluconate, 6-, dehydrogenase, RBC |
| **84087** | Phosphohexose isomerase |
| **84100** | Phosphorus inorganic (phosphate); |
| **84105** | urine |
| | (Pituitary gonadotropins, see 83001-83002) |
| | (PKU, see 84030, 84035) |
| **84106** | Porphobilinogen, urine; qualitative |
| **84110** | quantitative |
| **84112** | Placental alpha microglobulin-1 (PAMG-1), cervicovaginal secretion, qualitative |
| **84119** | Porphyrins, urine; qualitative |
| **84120** | quantitation and fractionation |
| **84126** | Porphyrins, feces; quantitative |
| **84127** | qualitative |
| | (Porphyrin precursors, see 82135, 84106, 84110) |
| | (For protoporphyrin, RBC, see 84202, 84203) |
| **84132** | Potassium; serum, plasma or whole blood |

| | |
|---|---|
| **84133** | urine |
| **84134** | Prealbumin |
| | (For microalbumin, see 82043, 82044) |
| **84135** | Pregnanediol |
| **84138** | Pregnanetriol |
| **84140** | Pregnenolone |
| **84143** | 17-hydroxypregnenolone |
| **84144** | Progesterone |
| | (Progesterone receptor assay, use 84234) |
| | (For proinsulin, use 84206) |
| **84145** | Procalcitonin (PCT) |
| **84146** | Prolactin |
| **84150** | Prostaglandin, each |
| **84152** | Prostate specific antigen (PSA); complexed (direct measurement) |
| **84153** | total |
| **84154** | free |
| **84155** | Protein, total, except by refractometry; serum, plasma or whole blood |
| **84156** | urine |
| **84157** | other source (eg, synovial fluid, cerebrospinal fluid) |
| **84160** | Protein, total, by refractometry, any source |
| | (For urine total protein by dipstick method, use 81000-81003) |
| **84163** | Pregnancy-associated plasma protein-A (PAPP-A) |
| **84165** | Protein; electrophoretic fractionation and quantitation, serum |
| **84166** | electrophoretic fractionation and quantitation, other fluids with concentration (eg, urine, CSF) |
| **84181** | Western Blot, with interpretation and report, blood or other body fluid |
| **84182** | Western Blot, with interpretation and report, blood or other body fluid, immunological probe for band identification, each |
| | (For Western Blot tissue analysis, use 88371) |
| **84202** | Protoporphyrin, RBC; quantitative |
| **84203** | screen |
| **84206** | Proinsulin |
| | (Pseudocholinesterase, use 82480) |
| **84207** | Pyridoxal phosphate (Vitamin B-6) |
| **84210** | Pyruvate |
| **84220** | Pyruvate kinase |
| **84228** | Quinine |
| **84233** | Receptor assay; estrogen |

| | |
|---|---|
| 84234 | progesterone |
| 84235 | endocrine, other than estrogen or progesterone (specify hormone) |
| 84238 | non-endocrine (specify receptor) |
| 84244 | Renin |
| 84252 | Riboflavin (Vitamin B-2) |

(Salicylates, use 80196)

(Secretin test, see 99070, 43756, 43757 and appropriate analyses)

| | |
|---|---|
| 84255 | Selenium |
| 84260 | Serotonin |

(For urine metabolites (HIAA), use 83497)

| | |
|---|---|
| 84270 | Sex hormone binding globulin (SHBG) |
| 84275 | Sialic acid |

(Sickle hemoglobin, use 85660)

| | |
|---|---|
| 84285 | Silica |
| 84295 | Sodium; serum, plasma or whole blood |
| 84300 | urine |
| 84302 | other source |

(Somatomammotropin, use 83632)

(Somatotropin, use 83003)

| | |
|---|---|
| 84305 | Somatomedin |
| 84307 | Somatostatin |
| 84311 | Spectrophotometry, analyte not elsewhere specified |
| 84315 | Specific gravity (except urine) |

(For specific gravity, urine, see 81000-81003)

(Stone analysis, see 82355-82370)

| | |
|---|---|
| 84375 | Sugars, chromatographic, TLC or paper chromatography |
| 84376 | Sugars (mono-, di-, and oligosaccharides); single qualitative, each specimen |
| 84377 | multiple qualitative, each specimen |
| 84378 | single quantitative, each specimen |
| 84379 | multiple quantitative, each specimen |
| 84392 | Sulfate, urine |

(Sulfhemoglobin, see hemoglobin, 83055, 83060)

(T-3, see 84479-84481)

(T-4, see 84436-84439)

| | |
|---|---|
| 84402 | Testosterone; free |
| 84403 | total |
| 84425 | Thiamine (Vitamin B-1) |
| 84430 | Thiocyanate |

| | |
|---|---|
| 84431 | Thromboxane metabolite(s), including thromboxane if performed, urine |

(For concurrent urine creatinine determination, use 84431 in conjunction with 82570)

| | |
|---|---|
| 84432 | Thyroglobulin |

(Thyroglobulin, antibody, use 86800)

(Thyrotropin releasing hormone [TRH] test, see 80438, 80439)

| | |
|---|---|
| 84436 | Thyroxine; total |
| 84437 | requiring elution (eg, neonatal) |
| 84439 | free |
| 84442 | Thyroxine binding globulin (TBG) |
| 84443 | Thyroid stimulating hormone (TSH) |
| 84445 | Thyroid stimulating immune globulins (TSI) |

(Tobramycin, use 80200)

| | |
|---|---|
| 84446 | Tocopherol alpha (Vitamin E) |

(Tolbutamide tolerance, use 82953)

| | |
|---|---|
| 84449 | Transcortin (cortisol binding globulin) |
| 84450 | Transferase; aspartate amino (AST) (SGOT) |
| 84460 | alanine amino (ALT) (SGPT) |
| 84466 | Transferrin |

(Iron binding capacity, use 83550)

| | |
|---|---|
| 84478 | Triglycerides |
| 84479 | Thyroid hormone (T3 or T4) uptake or thyroid hormone binding ratio (THBR) |
| 84480 | Triiodothyronine T3; total (TT-3) |
| 84481 | free |
| 84482 | reverse |
| 84484 | Troponin, quantitative |

(For troponin, qualitative assay, use 84512)

| | |
|---|---|
| 84485 | Trypsin; duodenal fluid |
| 84488 | feces, qualitative |
| 84490 | feces, quantitative, 24-hour collection |
| 84510 | Tyrosine |

(Urate crystal identification, use 89060)

| | |
|---|---|
| 84512 | Troponin, qualitative |

(For troponin, quantitative assay, use 84484)

| | |
|---|---|
| 84520 | Urea nitrogen; quantitative |
| 84525 | semiquantitative (eg, reagent strip test) |
| 84540 | Urea nitrogen, urine |
| 84545 | Urea nitrogen, clearance |
| 84550 | Uric acid; blood |

---

▲=Revised code   ●=New code   ► ◄=Contains new or revised text   ⊘=Modifier 51 exempt

**84560**     other source

**84577** Urobilinogen, feces, quantitative

**84578** Urobilinogen, urine; qualitative

**84580**     quantitative, timed specimen

**84583**     semiquantitative

(Uroporphyrins, use 84120)

(Valproic acid [dipropylacetic acid], use 80164)

**84585** Vanillylmandelic acid (VMA), urine

**84586** Vasoactive intestinal peptide (VIP)

**84588** Vasopressin (antidiuretic hormone, ADH)

**84590** Vitamin A

(Vitamin B-1, use 84425)

(Vitamin B-2, use 84252)

(Vitamin B-6, use 84207)

(Vitamin B-12, use 82607)

(Vitamin B-12, absorption (Schilling), see 78270, 78271)

(Vitamin C, use 82180)

(Vitamin D, see 82306, 82652)

(Vitamin E, use 84446)

**84591** Vitamin, not otherwise specified

**84597** Vitamin K

(VMA, use 84585)

**84600** Volatiles (eg, acetic anhydride, carbon tetrachloride, dichloroethane, dichloromethane, diethylether, isopropyl alcohol, methanol)

(For acetaldehyde, use 82000)

(Volume, blood, RISA or Cr-51, see 78110, 78111)

**84620** Xylose absorption test, blood and/or urine

(For administration, use 99070)

**84630** Zinc

**84681** C-peptide

**84702** Gonadotropin, chorionic (hCG); quantitative

**84703**     qualitative

(For urine pregnancy test by visual color comparison, use 81025)

**84704**     free beta chain

**84830** Ovulation tests, by visual color comparison methods for human luteinizing hormone

**84999** Unlisted chemistry procedure

# Hematology and Coagulation

(For blood banking procedures, see **Transfusion Medicine**)

(Agglutinins, see **Immunology**)

(Antiplasmin, use 85410)

(Antithrombin III, see 85300, 85301)

**85002** Bleeding time

**85004** Blood count; automated differential WBC count

**85007**     blood smear, microscopic examination with manual differential WBC count

**85008**     blood smear, microscopic examination without manual differential WBC count

(For other fluids [eg, CSF], see 89050, 89051)

**85009**     manual differential WBC count, buffy coat

(Eosinophils, nasal smear, use 89190)

**85013**     spun microhematocrit

**85014**     hematocrit (Hct)

**85018**     hemoglobin (Hgb)

(For other hemoglobin determination, see 83020-83069)

(For immunoassay, hemoglobin, fecal, use 82274)

(For transcutaneous hemoglobin measurement, use 88738)

**85025**     complete (CBC), automated (Hgb, Hct, RBC, WBC and platelet count) and automated differential WBC count

**85027**     complete (CBC), automated (Hgb, Hct, RBC, WBC and platelet count)

**85032**     manual cell count (erythrocyte, leukocyte, or platelet) each

**85041**     red blood cell (RBC), automated

(Do not report code 85041 in conjunction with 85025 or 85027)

**85044**     reticulocyte, manual

**85045**     reticulocyte, automated

**85046**     reticulocytes, automated, including 1 or more cellular parameters (eg, reticulocyte hemoglobin content [CHr], immature reticulocyte fraction [IRF], reticulocyte volume [MRV], RNA content), direct measurement

**85048**     leukocyte (WBC), automated

**85049**     platelet, automated

**85055** Reticulated platelet assay

**85060** Blood smear, peripheral, interpretation by physician with written report

Pathology and Laboratory

**85097**    Bone marrow, smear interpretation

     (For special stains, see 88312, 88313)

     (For bone biopsy, see 20220, 20225, 20240, 20245, 20250, 20251)

**85130**    Chromogenic substrate assay

     (Circulating anti-coagulant screen [mixing studies], see 85611, 85732)

**85170**    Clot retraction

**85175**    Clot lysis time, whole blood dilution

     (Clotting factor I [fibrinogen], see 85384, 85385)

**85210**    Clotting; factor II, prothrombin, specific

     (See also 85610-85613)

**85220**      factor V (AcG or proaccelerin), labile factor

**85230**      factor VII (proconvertin, stable factor)

**85240**      factor VIII (AHG), 1-stage

**85244**      factor VIII related antigen

**85245**      factor VIII, VW factor, ristocetin cofactor

**85246**      factor VIII, VW factor antigen

**85247**      factor VIII, von Willebrand factor, multimetric analysis

**85250**      factor IX (PTC or Christmas)

**85260**      factor X (Stuart-Prower)

**85270**      factor XI (PTA)

**85280**      factor XII (Hageman)

**85290**      factor XIII (fibrin stabilizing)

**85291**      factor XIII (fibrin stabilizing), screen solubility

**85292**      prekallikrein assay (Fletcher factor assay)

**85293**      high molecular weight kininogen assay (Fitzgerald factor assay)

**85300**    Clotting inhibitors or anticoagulants; antithrombin III, activity

**85301**      antithrombin III, antigen assay

**85302**      protein C, antigen

**85303**      protein C, activity

**85305**      protein S, total

**85306**      protein S, free

**85307**    Activated Protein C (APC) resistance assay

**85335**    Factor inhibitor test

**85337**    Thrombomodulin

     (For mixing studies for inhibitors, use 85732)

**85345**    Coagulation time; Lee and White

**85347**      activated

**85348**      other methods

     (Differential count, see 85007 et seq)

     (Duke bleeding time, use 85002)

     (Eosinophils, nasal smear, use 89190)

**85360**    Euglobulin lysis

     (Fetal hemoglobin, see 83030, 83033, 85460)

**85362**    Fibrin(ogen) degradation (split) products (FDP) (FSP); agglutination slide, semiquantitative

     (Immunoelectrophoresis, use 86320)

**85366**      paracoagulation

**85370**      quantitative

**85378**    Fibrin degradation products, D-dimer; qualitative or semiquantitative

**85379**      quantitative

     (For ultrasensitive and standard sensitivity quantitative D-dimer, use 85379)

**85380**      ultrasensitive (eg, for evaluation for venous thromboembolism), qualitative or semiquantitative

**85384**    Fibrinogen; activity

**85385**      antigen

**85390**    Fibrinolysins or coagulopathy screen, interpretation and report

**85396**    Coagulation/fibrinolysis assay, whole blood (eg, viscoelastic clot assessment), including use of any pharmacologic additive(s), as indicated, including interpretation and written report, per day

**85397**    Coagulation and fibrinolysis, functional activity, not otherwise specified (eg, ADAMTS-13), each analyte

**85400**    Fibrinolytic factors and inhibitors; plasmin

**85410**      alpha-2 antiplasmin

**85415**      plasminogen activator

**85420**      plasminogen, except antigenic assay

**85421**      plasminogen, antigenic assay

     (Fragility, red blood cell, see 85547, 85555-85557)

**85441**    Heinz bodies; direct

**85445**      induced, acetyl phenylhydrazine

     (Hematocrit [PCV], see 85014, 85025, 85027)

     (Hemoglobin, see 83020-83068, 85018, 85025, 85027)

**85460**    Hemoglobin or RBCs, fetal, for fetomaternal hemorrhage; differential lysis (Kleihauer-Betke)

     (See also 83030, 83033)

     (Hemolysins, see 86940, 86941)

**85461**      rosette

**Pathology and Laboratory**

**85475** Hemolysin, acid

(See also 86940, 86941)

**85520** Heparin assay

**85525** Heparin neutralization

**85530** Heparin-protamine tolerance test

**85536** Iron stain, peripheral blood

(For iron stains on bone marrow or other tissues with physician evaluation, use 88313)

**85540** Leukocyte alkaline phosphatase with count

**85547** Mechanical fragility, RBC

**85549** Muramidase

(Nitroblue tetrazolium dye test, use 86384)

**85555** Osmotic fragility, RBC; unincubated

**85557** incubated

(Packed cell volume, use 85013)

(Partial thromboplastin time, see 85730, 85732)

(Parasites, blood [eg, malaria smears], use 87207)

(Plasmin, use 85400)

(Plasminogen, use 85420)

(Plasminogen activator, use 85415)

**85576** Platelet, aggregation (in vitro), each agent

(For thromboxane metabolite[s], including thromboxane, if performed, measurement[s] in urine, use 84431)

**85597** Phospholipid neutralization; platelet

**85598** hexagonal phospholipid

**85610** Prothrombin time;

**85611** substitution, plasma fractions, each

**85612** Russell viper venom time (includes venom); undiluted

**85613** diluted

(Red blood cell count, see 85025, 85027, 85041)

**85635** Reptilase test

(Reticulocyte count, see 85044, 85045)

**85651** Sedimentation rate, erythrocyte; non-automated

**85652** automated

**85660** Sickling of RBC, reduction

(Hemoglobin electrophoresis, use 83020)

(Smears [eg, for parasites, malaria], use 87207)

**85670** Thrombin time; plasma

**85675** titer

**85705** Thromboplastin inhibition, tissue

(For individual clotting factors, see 85245-85247)

**85730** Thromboplastin time, partial (PTT); plasma or whole blood

**85732** substitution, plasma fractions, each

**85810** Viscosity

(von Willebrand factor assay, see 85245-85247)

(WBC count, see 85025, 85027, 85048, 89050)

**85999** Unlisted hematology and coagulation procedure

# Immunology

(Acetylcholine receptor antibody, see 83519, 86255, 86256)

(Actinomyces, antibodies to, use 86602)

(Adrenal cortex antibodies, see 86255, 86256)

**86000** Agglutinins, febrile (eg, Brucella, Francisella, Murine typhus, Q fever, Rocky Mountain spotted fever, scrub typhus), each antigen

(For antibodies to infectious agents, see 86602-86804)

**86001** Allergen specific IgG quantitative or semiquantitative, each allergen

(Agglutinins and autohemolysins, see 86940, 86941)

**86003** Allergen specific IgE; quantitative or semiquantitative, each allergen

(For total quantitative IgE, use 82785)

**86005** qualitative, multiallergen screen (dipstick, paddle, or disk)

(For total qualitative IgE, use 83518)

(Alpha-1 antitrypsin, see 82103, 82104)

(Alpha-1 feto-protein, see 82105, 82106)

(Anti-AChR [acetylcholine receptor] antibody titer, see 86255, 86256)

(Anticardiolipin antibody, use 86147)

(Anti-DNA, use 86225)

(Anti-deoxyribonuclease titer, use 86215)

**86021** Antibody identification; leukocyte antibodies

**86022** platelet antibodies

**86023** platelet associated immunoglobulin assay

**86038** Antinuclear antibodies (ANA);

**86039** titer

(Antistreptococcal antibody, ie, anti-DNAse, use 86215)

(Antistreptokinase titer, use 86590)

**86060** Antistreptolysin O; titer

(For antibodies to infectious agents, see 86602-86804)

Pathology and Laboratory

86063        screen

(For antibodies to infectious agents, see 86602-86804)

(Blastomyces, antibodies to, use 86612)

86077    Blood bank physician services; difficult cross match and/ or evaluation of irregular antibody(s), interpretation and written report

86078        investigation of transfusion reaction including suspicion of transmissible disease, interpretation and written report

86079        authorization for deviation from standard blood banking procedures (eg, use of outdated blood, transfusion of Rh incompatible units), with written report

(Brucella, antibodies to, use 86622)

(Candida, antibodies to, use 86628. For skin testing, use 86485)

86140    C-reactive protein

(Candidiasis, use 86628)

86141        high sensitivity (hsCRP)

86146    Beta 2 Glycoprotein I antibody, each

86147    Cardiolipin (phospholipid) antibody, each Ig class

86148    Anti-phosphatidylserine (phospholipid) antibody

(To report antiprothrombin [phospholipid cofactor] antibody, use Category III code 0030T)

►(For cell enumeration using immunologic selection and identification in fluid specimen [eg, circulating tumor cells in blood], see 0279T, 0280T)◄

86155    Chemotaxis assay, specify method

(Clostridium difficile toxin, use 87230)

(Coccidioides, antibodies to, see 86635. For skin testing, use 86490)

86156    Cold agglutinin; screen

86157        titer

86160    Complement; antigen, each component

86161        functional activity, each component

86162        total hemolytic (CH50)

86171    Complement fixation tests, each antigen

(Coombs test, see 86880-86886)

86185    Counterimmunoelectrophoresis, each antigen

(Cryptococcus, antibodies to, use 86641)

86200    Cyclic citrullinated peptide (CCP), antibody

86215    Deoxyribonuclease, antibody

86225    Deoxyribonucleic acid (DNA) antibody; native or double stranded

(Echinococcus, antibodies to, see code for specific method)

(For HIV antibody tests, see 86701-86703)

86226        single stranded

(Anti D.S., DNA, IFA, eg, using C.Lucilae, see 86255 and 86256)

86235    Extractable nuclear antigen, antibody to, any method (eg, nRNP, SS-A, SS-B, Sm, RNP, Sc170, J01), each antibody

86243    Fc receptor

(Filaria, antibodies to, see code for specific method)

86255    Fluorescent noninfectious agent antibody; screen, each antibody

86256        titer, each antibody

(Fluorescent technique for antigen identification in tissue, use 88346; for indirect fluorescence, use 88347)

(FTA, use 86780)

(Gel [agar] diffusion tests, use 86331)

86277    Growth hormone, human (HGH), antibody

86280    Hemagglutination inhibition test (HAI)

(For rubella, use 86762)

(For antibodies to infectious agents, see 86602-86804)

86294    Immunoassay for tumor antigen, qualitative or semiquantitative (eg, bladder tumor antigen)

►(For qualitative NMP22 protein, use 86386)◄

86300    Immunoassay for tumor antigen, quantitative; CA 15-3 (27.29)

86301        CA 19-9

86304        CA 125

(For measurement of serum HER-2/neu oncoprotein, see 83950)

(For hepatitis delta agent, antibody, use 86692)

86305    Human epididymis protein 4 (HE4)

86308    Heterophile antibodies; screening

(For antibodies to infectious agents, see 86602-86804)

86309        titer

(For antibodies to infectious agents, see 86602-86804)

86310        titers after absorption with beef cells and guinea pig kidney

(Histoplasma, antibodies to, use 86698. For skin testing, use 86510)

(For antibodies to infectious agents, see 86602-86804)

(Human growth hormone antibody, use 86277)

86316    Immunoassay for tumor antigen, other antigen, quantitative (eg, CA 50, 72-4, 549), each

**Pathology and Laboratory**

86317 Immunoassay for infectious agent antibody, quantitative, not otherwise specified

(For immunoassay techniques for antigens, see 83516, 83518, 83519, 83520, 87301-87450, 87810-87899)

(For particle agglutination procedures, use 86403)

86318 Immunoassay for infectious agent antibody, qualitative or semiquantitative, single step method (eg, reagent strip)

86320 Immunoelectrophoresis; serum

86325 other fluids (eg, urine, cerebrospinal fluid) with concentration

86327 crossed (2-dimensional assay)

86329 Immunodiffusion; not elsewhere specified

86331 gel diffusion, qualitative (Ouchterlony), each antigen or antibody

86332 Immune complex assay

86334 Immunofixation electrophoresis; serum

86335 other fluids with concentration (eg, urine, CSF)

86336 Inhibin A

86337 Insulin antibodies

86340 Intrinsic factor antibodies

(Leptospira, antibodies to, use 86720)

(Leukoagglutinins, use 86021)

86341 Islet cell antibody

86343 Leukocyte histamine release test (LHR)

86344 Leukocyte phagocytosis

86352 Cellular function assay involving stimulation (eg, mitogen or antigen) and detection of biomarker (eg, ATP)

86353 Lymphocyte transformation, mitogen (phytomitogen) or antigen induced blastogenesis

(Malaria antibodies, use 86750)

(For cellular function assay involving stimulation and detection of biomarker, use 86352)

86355 B cells, total count

86356 Mononuclear cell antigen, quantitative (eg, flow cytometry), not otherwise specified, each antigen

(Do not report 88187-88189 for interpretation of 86355, 86356, 86357, 86359, 86360, 86361, 86367)

86357 Natural killer (NK) cells, total count

86359 T cells; total count

86360 absolute CD4 and CD8 count, including ratio

86361 absolute CD4 count

86367 Stem cells (ie, CD34), total count

(For flow cytometric immunophenotyping for the assessment of potential hematolymphoid neoplasia, see 88184-88189)

86376 Microsomal antibodies (eg, thyroid or liver-kidney), each

86378 Migration inhibitory factor test (MIF)

(Mitochondrial antibody, liver, see 86255, 86256)

(Mononucleosis, see 86308-86310)

86382 Neutralization test, viral

86384 Nitroblue tetrazolium dye test (NTD)

● 86386 Nuclear Matrix Protein 22 (NMP22), qualitative

(Ouchterlony diffusion, use 86331)

(Platelet antibodies, see 86022, 86023)

86403 Particle agglutination; screen, each antibody

86406 titer, each antibody

(Pregnancy test, see 84702, 84703)

(Rapid plasma reagin test (RPR), see 86592, 86593)

86430 Rheumatoid factor; qualitative

86431 quantitative

(Serologic test for syphilis, see 86592, 86593)

86480 Tuberculosis test, cell mediated immunity antigen response measurement; gamma interferon

86481 enumeration of gamma interferon-producing T-cells in cell suspension

86485 Skin test; candida

(For antibody, candida, use 86628)

86486 unlisted antigen, each

86490 coccidioidomycosis

86510 histoplasmosis

(For histoplasma, antibody, use 86698)

86580 tuberculosis, intradermal

(For tuberculosis test, cell mediated immunity measurement of gamma interferon antigen response, use 86480)

(For skin tests for allergy, see 95010-95199)

(Smooth muscle antibody, see 86255, 86256)

(Sporothrix, antibodies to, see code for specific method)

(For skin testing, unlisted antigen, use 86486. For flow cytometry, quantitative, not otherwise specified, use 86356)

86590 Streptokinase, antibody

(For antibodies to infectious agents, see 86602-86804)

(Streptolysin O antibody, see antistreptolysin O, 86060, 86063)

86592 Syphilis test, non-treponemal antibody; qualitative (eg, VDRL, RPR, ART)

(For antibodies to infectious agents, see 86602-86804)

⊙=Moderate sedation  +=Add-on code  ✗=FDA approval pending  #=Resequenced code  ○=Recycled/reinstated code

| 86593 | quantitative |
|---|---|

(For antibodies to infectious agents, see 86602-86804)

(Tetanus antibody, use 86774)

(Thyroglobulin antibody, use 86800)

(Thyroglobulin, use 84432)

(Thyroid microsomal antibody, use 86376)

(For toxoplasma antibody, see 86777-86778)

The following codes (86602-86804) are qualitative or semiquantitative immunoassays performed by multiple-step methods for the detection of antibodies to infectious agents. For immunoassays by single-step method (eg, reagent strips), use code 86318. Procedures for the identification of antibodies should be coded as precisely as possible. For example, an antibody to a virus could be coded with increasing specificity for virus, family, genus, species, or type. In some cases, further precision may be added to codes by specifying the class of immunoglobulin being detected. When multiple tests are done to detect antibodies to organisms classified more precisely than the specificity allowed by available codes, it is appropriate to code each as a separate service. For example, a test for antibody to an enterovirus is coded as 86658. Coxsackie viruses are enteroviruses, but there are no codes for the individual species of enterovirus. If assays are performed for antibodies to coxsackie A and B species, each assay should be separately coded. Similarly, if multiple assays are performed for antibodies of different immunoglobulin classes, each assay should be coded separately. When a coding option exists for reporting IgM specific antibodies (eg, 86632), the corresponding nonspecific code (eg, 86631) may be reported for performance of either an antibody analysis not specific for a particular immunoglobulin class or for an IgG analysis.

(For the detection of antibodies other than those to infectious agents, see specific antibody [eg, 86021-86023, 86376, 86800, 86850-86870] or specific method [eg, 83516, 86255, 86256]).

(For infectious agent/antigen detection, see 87260-87899)

| 86602 | Antibody; actinomyces |
|---|---|
| 86603 | adenovirus |
| 86606 | Aspergillus |
| 86609 | bacterium, not elsewhere specified |
| 86611 | Bartonella |
| 86612 | Blastomyces |
| 86615 | Bordetella |
| 86617 | Borrelia burgdorferi (Lyme disease) confirmatory test (eg, Western Blot or immunoblot) |
| 86618 | Borrelia burgdorferi (Lyme disease) |
| 86619 | Borrelia (relapsing fever) |

| 86622 | Brucella |
|---|---|
| 86625 | Campylobacter |
| 86628 | Candida |

(For skin test, candida, use 86485)

| 86631 | Chlamydia |
|---|---|
| 86632 | Chlamydia, IgM |

(For chlamydia antigen, see 87270, 87320. For fluorescent antibody technique, see 86255, 86256)

| 86635 | Coccidioides |
|---|---|
| 86638 | Coxiella burnetii (Q fever) |
| 86641 | Cryptococcus |
| 86644 | cytomegalovirus (CMV) |
| 86645 | cytomegalovirus (CMV), IgM |
| 86648 | Diphtheria |
| 86651 | encephalitis, California (La Crosse) |
| 86652 | encephalitis, Eastern equine |
| 86653 | encephalitis, St. Louis |
| 86654 | encephalitis, Western equine |
| 86658 | enterovirus (eg, coxsackie, echo, polio) |

(Trichinella, antibodies to, use 86784)

(Trypanosoma, antibodies to, see code for specific method)

(Tuberculosis, use 86580 for skin testing)

(Viral antibodies, see code for specific method)

| 86663 | Epstein-Barr (EB) virus, early antigen (EA) |
|---|---|
| 86664 | Epstein-Barr (EB) virus, nuclear antigen (EBNA) |
| 86665 | Epstein-Barr (EB) virus, viral capsid (VCA) |
| 86666 | Ehrlichia |
| 86668 | Francisella tularensis |
| 86671 | fungus, not elsewhere specified |
| 86674 | Giardia lamblia |
| 86677 | Helicobacter pylori |
| 86682 | helminth, not elsewhere specified |
| 86684 | Haemophilus influenza |
| 86687 | HTLV-I |
| 86688 | HTLV-II |
| 86689 | HTLV or HIV antibody, confirmatory test (eg, Western Blot) |
| 86692 | hepatitis, delta agent |

(For hepatitis delta agent, antigen, use 87380)

| 86694 | herpes simplex, non-specific type test |
|---|---|
| 86695 | herpes simplex, type 1 |

▲=Revised code   ●=New code   ▶ ◀=Contains new or revised text   ⊘=Modifier 51 exempt

| 86696 | herpes simplex, type 2 |
|-------|------------------------|
| 86698 | histoplasma |
| 86701 | HIV-1 |
| 86702 | HIV-2 |
| ▲ 86703 | HIV-1 and HIV-2, single result |

►(For HIV-1 antigen(s) with HIV-1 and HIV-2 antibodies, single result, use 87389)◄

►(When HIV immunoassay [HIV testing 86701-86703 or 87389] is performed using a kit or transportable instrument that wholly or in part consists of a single use, disposable analytical chamber, the service may be identified by adding modifier 92 to the usual code)◄

(For HIV-1 antigen, use 87390)

(For HIV-2 antigen, use 87391)

(For confirmatory test for HIV antibody (eg, Western Blot), use 86689)

| 86704 | Hepatitis B core antibody (HBcAb); total |
|-------|------------------------------------------|
| 86705 | IgM antibody |
| 86706 | Hepatitis B surface antibody (HBsAb) |
| 86707 | Hepatitis Be antibody (HBeAb) |
| 86708 | Hepatitis A antibody (HAAb); total |
| 86709 | IgM antibody |
| 86710 | Antibody; influenza virus |
| 86713 | Legionella |
| 86717 | Leishmania |
| 86720 | Leptospira |
| 86723 | Listeria monocytogenes |
| 86727 | lymphocytic choriomeningitis |
| 86729 | lymphogranuloma venereum |
| 86732 | mucormycosis |
| 86735 | mumps |
| 86738 | mycoplasma |
| 86741 | Neisseria meningitidis |
| 86744 | Nocardia |
| 86747 | parvovirus |
| 86750 | Plasmodium (malaria) |
| 86753 | protozoa, not elsewhere specified |
| 86756 | respiratory syncytial virus |
| 86757 | Rickettsia |
| 86759 | rotavirus |
| 86762 | rubella |
| 86765 | rubeola |

| 86768 | Salmonella |
|-------|------------|
| 86771 | Shigella |
| 86774 | tetanus |
| 86777 | Toxoplasma |
| 86778 | Toxoplasma, IgM |
| 86780 | Treponema pallidum |

(86781 has been deleted)

(For syphilis testing by non-treponemal antibody analysis, see 86592-86593)

| 86784 | Trichinella |
|-------|-------------|
| 86787 | varicella-zoster |
| 86788 | West Nile virus, IgM |
| 86789 | West Nile virus |
| 86790 | virus, not elsewhere specified |
| 86793 | Yersinia |
| 86800 | Thyroglobulin antibody |

(For thyroglobulin, use 84432)

| 86803 | Hepatitis C antibody; |
|-------|----------------------|
| 86804 | confirmatory test (eg, immunoblot) |

## Tissue Typing

| 86805 | Lymphocytotoxicity assay, visual crossmatch; with titration |
|-------|-------------------------------------------------------------|
| 86806 | without titration |
| 86807 | Serum screening for cytotoxic percent reactive antibody (PRA); standard method |
| 86808 | quick method |
| 86812 | HLA typing; A, B, or C (eg, A10, B7, B27), single antigen |
| 86813 | A, B, or C, multiple antigens |
| 86816 | DR/DQ, single antigen |
| 86817 | DR/DQ, multiple antigens |
| 86821 | lymphocyte culture, mixed (MLC) |
| 86822 | lymphocyte culture, primed (PLC) |

►(For HLA typing by molecular pathology techniques, see 81370-81383)◄

| 86825 | Human leukocyte antigen (HLA) crossmatch, non-cytotoxic (eg, using flow cytometry); first serum sample or dilution |
|-------|-------------------------------------------------------------------------------------------------------------------|
| + 86826 | each additional serum sample or sample dilution (List separately in addition to primary procedure) |

(Use 86826 in conjunction with 86825)

(Do not report 86825, 86826 in conjunction with 86355, 86359, 88184-88189 for antibody surface markers integral to crossmatch testing)

Pathology and Laboratory

(For autologous HLA crossmatch, see 86825, 86826)

(For lymphocytotoxicity visual crossmatch, see 86805, 86806)

**86849**    Unlisted immunology procedure

# Transfusion Medicine

(For apheresis, use 36511, 36512)

(For therapeutic phlebotomy, use 99195)

**86850**    Antibody screen, RBC, each serum technique

**86860**    Antibody elution (RBC), each elution

**86870**    Antibody identification, RBC antibodies, each panel for each serum technique

**86880**    Antihuman globulin test (Coombs test); direct, each antiserum

**86885**      indirect, qualitative, each reagent red cell

**86886**      indirect, each antibody titer

(For indirect antihuman globulin [Coombs] test for RBC antibody screening, use 86850)

(For indirect antihuman globulin [Coombs] test for RBC antibody identification using reagent red cell panels, use 86870)

**86890**    Autologous blood or component, collection processing and storage; predeposited

**86891**      intra- or postoperative salvage

(For physician services to autologous donors, see 99201-99204)

**86900**    Blood typing; ABO

**86901**      Rh (D)

**86902**      antigen testing of donor blood using reagent serum, each antigen test

(If multiple blood units are tested for the same antigen, 86902 should be reported once for each antigen for each unit tested)

(86903 has been deleted. To report, use 86902)

**86904**      antigen screening for compatible unit using patient serum, per unit screened

**86905**      RBC antigens, other than ABO or Rh (D), each

**86906**      Rh phenotyping, complete

**86910**    Blood typing, for paternity testing, per individual; ABO, Rh and MN

**86911**      each additional antigen system

**86920**    Compatibility test each unit; immediate spin technique

**86921**      incubation technique

**86922**      antiglobulin technique

**86923**      electronic

(Do not use 86923 in conjunction with 86920-86922 for same unit crossmatch)

**86927**    Fresh frozen plasma, thawing, each unit

**86930**    Frozen blood, each unit; freezing (includes preparation)

**86931**      thawing

**86932**      freezing (includes preparation) and thawing

**86940**    Hemolysins and agglutinins; auto, screen, each

**86941**      incubated

**86945**    Irradiation of blood product, each unit

**86950**    Leukocyte transfusion

(For leukapheresis, use 36511)

**86960**    Volume reduction of blood or blood product (eg, red blood cells or platelets), each unit

**86965**    Pooling of platelets or other blood products

(For injection(s) of platelet rich plasma, use 0232T)

**86970**    Pretreatment of RBCs for use in RBC antibody detection, identification, and/or compatibility testing; incubation with chemical agents or drugs, each

**86971**      incubation with enzymes, each

**86972**      by density gradient separation

**86975**    Pretreatment of serum for use in RBC antibody identification; incubation with drugs, each

**86976**      by dilution

**86977**      incubation with inhibitors, each

**86978**      by differential red cell absorption using patient RBCs or RBCs of known phenotype, each absorption

**86985**    Splitting of blood or blood products, each unit

**86999**    Unlisted transfusion medicine procedure

# Microbiology

Includes bacteriology, mycology, parasitology, and virology.

Presumptive identification of microorganisms is defined as identification by colony morphology, growth on selective media, Gram stains, or up to three tests (eg, catalase, oxidase, indole, urease). Definitive identification of microorganisms is defined as an identification to the genus or species level that requires additional tests (eg, biochemical panels, slide cultures). If additional studies involve molecular probes, nucleic acid sequencing, chromatography, or immunologic techniques, these should be separately coded using 87140-87158, in addition to definitive identification codes. The molecular diagnostic codes (eg, 83890-83914) are not to be used in combination with or instead of the procedures

**Pathology and Laboratory**

represented by 87140-87158. For multiple specimens/sites use modifier 59. For repeat laboratory tests performed on the same day, use modifier 91.

**87001** Animal inoculation, small animal; with observation

**87003**     with observation and dissection

**87015** Concentration (any type), for infectious agents

(Do not report 87015 in conjunction with 87177)

**87040** Culture, bacterial; blood, aerobic, with isolation and presumptive identification of isolates (includes anaerobic culture, if appropriate)

**87045**     stool, aerobic, with isolation and preliminary examination (eg, KIA, LIA), Salmonella and Shigella species

**87046**     stool, aerobic, additional pathogens, isolation and presumptive identification of isolates, each plate

**87070**     any other source except urine, blood or stool, aerobic, with isolation and presumptive identification of isolates

(For urine, use 87088)

**87071**     quantitative, aerobic with isolation and presumptive identification of isolates, any source except urine, blood or stool

(For urine, use 87088)

**87073**     quantitative, anaerobic with isolation and presumptive identification of isolates, any source except urine, blood or stool

(For definitive identification of isolates, use 87076 or 87077. For typing of isolates see 87140-87158)

**87075**     any source, except blood, anaerobic with isolation and presumptive identification of isolates

**87076**     anaerobic isolate, additional methods required for definitive identification, each isolate

**87077**     aerobic isolate, additional methods required for definitive identification, each isolate

**87081** Culture, presumptive, pathogenic organisms, screening only;

**87084**     with colony estimation from density chart

**87086** Culture, bacterial; quantitative colony count, urine

**87088**     with isolation and presumptive identification of each isolate, urine

**87101** Culture, fungi (mold or yeast) isolation, with presumptive identification of isolates; skin, hair, or nail

**87102**     other source (except blood)

**87103**     blood

**87106** Culture, fungi, definitive identification, each organism; yeast

**87107**     mold

**87109** Culture, mycoplasma, any source

**87110** Culture, chlamydia, any source

(For immunofluorescence staining of shell vials, use 87140)

**87116** Culture, tubercle or other acid-fast bacilli (eg, TB, AFB, mycobacteria) any source, with isolation and presumptive identification of isolates

(For concentration, use 87015)

**87118** Culture, mycobacterial, definitive identification, each isolate

**87140** Culture, typing; immunofluorescent method, each antiserum

**87143**     gas liquid chromatography (GLC) or high pressure liquid chromatography (HPLC) method

**87147**     immunologic method, other than immunofluoresence (eg, agglutination grouping), per antiserum

**87149**     identification by nucleic acid (DNA or RNA) probe, direct probe technique, per culture or isolate, each organism probed

(Do not report 87149 in conjunction with 83890-83914)

**87150**     identification by nucleic acid (DNA or RNA) probe, amplified probe technique, per culture or isolate, each organism probed

(Do not report 87150 in conjunction with 83890-83914)

**87152**     identification by pulse field gel typing

(Do not report 87152 in conjunction with 83890-83914)

**87153**     identification by nucleic acid sequencing method, each isolate (eg, sequencing of the 16S rRNA gene)

**87158**     other methods

**87164** Dark field examination, any source (eg, penile, vaginal, oral, skin); includes specimen collection

**87166**     without collection

**87168** Macroscopic examination; arthropod

**87169**     parasite

**87172** Pinworm exam (eg, cellophane tape prep)

**87176** Homogenization, tissue, for culture

**87177** Ova and parasites, direct smears, concentration and identification

(Do not report 87177 in conjunction with 87015)

(For direct smears from a primary source, use 87207)

(For coccidia or microsporidia exam, use 87207)

(For complex special stain (trichrome, iron hematoxylin), use 87209)

(For nucleic acid probes in cytologic material, use 88365)

**87181** Susceptibility studies, antimicrobial agent; agar dilution method, per agent (eg, antibiotic gradient strip)

**87184**     disk method, per plate (12 or fewer agents)

87185    enzyme detection (eg, beta lactamase), per enzyme

87186    microdilution or agar dilution (minimum inhibitory concentration [MIC] or breakpoint), each multi-antimicrobial, per plate

+ 87187    microdilution or agar dilution, minimum lethal concentration (MLC), each plate (List separately in addition to code for primary procedure)

(Use 87187 in conjunction with 87186 or 87188)

87188    macrobroth dilution method, each agent

87190    mycobacteria, proportion method, each agent

(For other mycobacterial susceptibility studies, see 87181, 87184, 87186, or 87188)

87197    Serum bactericidal titer (Schlicter test)

87205    Smear, primary source with interpretation; Gram or Giemsa stain for bacteria, fungi, or cell types

87206    fluorescent and/or acid fast stain for bacteria, fungi, parasites, viruses or cell types

87207    special stain for inclusion bodies or parasites (eg, malaria, coccidia, microsporidia, trypanosomes, herpes viruses)

(For direct smears with concentration and identification, use 87177)

(For thick smear preparation, use 87015)

(For fat, meat, fibers, nasal eosinophils, and starch, see miscellaneous section)

87209    complex special stain (eg, trichrome, iron hemotoxylin) for ova and parasites

87210    wet mount for infectious agents (eg, saline, India ink, KOH preps)

(For KOH examination of skin, hair or nails, see 87220)

87220    Tissue examination by KOH slide of samples from skin, hair, or nails for fungi or ectoparasite ova or mites (eg, scabies)

87230    Toxin or antitoxin assay, tissue culture (eg, Clostridium difficile toxin)

87250    Virus isolation; inoculation of embryonated eggs, or small animal, includes observation and dissection

87252    tissue culture inoculation, observation, and presumptive identification by cytopathic effect

87253    tissue culture, additional studies or definitive identification (eg, hemabsorption, neutralization, immunofluoresence stain), each isolate

(Electron microscopy, use 88348)

(Inclusion bodies in tissue sections, see 88304-88309; in smears, see 87207-87210; in fluids, use 88106)

87254    centrifuge enhanced (shell vial) technique, includes identification with immunofluorescence stain, each virus

(Report 87254 in addition to 87252 as appropriate)

87255    including identification by non-immunologic method, other than by cytopathic effect (eg, virus specific enzymatic activity)

These codes are intended for primary source only. For similar studies on culture material, refer to codes 87140-87158. Infectious agents by antigen detection, immunofluorescence microscopy, or nucleic acid probe techniques should be reported as precisely as possible. The molecular diagnostic codes (eg, 83890-83914) are not to be used in combination with or instead of the procedures represented by 87470-87801. The most specific code possible should be reported. If there is no specific agent code, the general methodology code (eg, 87299, 87449, 87450, 87797, 87798, 87799, 87899) should be used. For identification of antibodies to many of the listed infectious agents, see 86602-86804. When separate results are reported for different species or strain of organisms, each result should be coded separately. Use modifier 59 when separate results are reported for different species or strains that are described by the same code.

87260    Infectious agent antigen detection by immunofluorescent technique; adenovirus

87265    Bordetella pertussis/parapertussis

87267    Enterovirus, direct fluorescent antibody (DFA)

87269    giardia

87270    Chlamydia trachomatis

87271    Cytomegalovirus, direct fluorescent antibody (DFA)

87272    cryptosporidium

87273    Herpes simplex virus type 2

87274    Herpes simplex virus type 1

87275    influenza B virus

87276    influenza A virus

87277    Legionella micdadei

87278    Legionella pneumophila

87279    Parainfluenza virus, each type

87280    respiratory syncytial virus

87281    Pneumocystis carinii

87283    Rubeola

87285    Treponema pallidum

87290    Varicella zoster virus

87299    not otherwise specified, each organism

87300    Infectious agent antigen detection by immunofluorescent technique, polyvalent for multiple organisms, each polyvalent antiserum

(For physician evaluation of infectious disease agents by immunofluorescence, use 88346)

**Pathology and Laboratory**

87301   Infectious agent antigen detection by enzyme immunoassay technique, qualitative or semiquantitative, multiple-step method; adenovirus enteric types 40/41

87305       Aspergillus

87320       Chlamydia trachomatis

87324       Clostridium difficile toxin(s)

87327       Cryptococcus neoformans

(For Cryptococcus latex agglutination, use 86403)

87328       cryptosporidium

87329       giardia

87332       cytomegalovirus

87335       Escherichia coli O157

(For giardia antigen, use 87329)

87336       Entamoeba histolytica dispar group

87337       Entamoeba histolytica group

87338       Helicobacter pylori, stool

87339       Helicobacter pylori

(For H. pylori, stool, use 87338. For H. pylori, breath and blood by mass spectrometry, see 83013, 83014. For H. pylori, liquid scintillation counter, see 78267, 78268)

87340       hepatitis B surface antigen (HBsAg)

87341       hepatitis B surface antigen (HBsAg) neutralization

87350       hepatitis Be antigen (HBeAg)

87380       hepatitis, delta agent

87385       Histoplasma capsulatum

● 87389     HIV-1 antigen(s), with HIV-1 and HIV-2 antibodies, single result

87390       HIV-1

87391       HIV-2

87400       Influenza, A or B, each

87420       respiratory syncytial virus

87425       rotavirus

87427       Shiga-like toxin

87430       Streptococcus, group A

87449   Infectious agent antigen detection by enzyme immunoassay technique qualitative or semiquantitative; multiple step method, not otherwise specified, each organism

87450       single step method, not otherwise specified, each organism

87451       multiple step method, polyvalent for multiple organisms, each polyvalent antiserum

87470   Infectious agent detection by nucleic acid (DNA or RNA); Bartonella henselae and Bartonella quintana, direct probe technique

87471   Bartonella henselae and Bartonella quintana, amplified probe technique

87472   Bartonella henselae and Bartonella quintana, quantification

87475   Borrelia burgdorferi, direct probe technique

87476   Borrelia burgdorferi, amplified probe technique

87477   Borrelia burgdorferi, quantification

87480   Candida species, direct probe technique

87481   Candida species, amplified probe technique

87482   Candida species, quantification

87485   Chlamydia pneumoniae, direct probe technique

87486   Chlamydia pneumoniae, amplified probe technique

87487   Chlamydia pneumoniae, quantification

87490   Chlamydia trachomatis, direct probe technique

87491   Chlamydia trachomatis, amplified probe technique

87492   Chlamydia trachomatis, quantification

87493   Clostridium difficile, toxin gene(s), amplified probe technique

87495   cytomegalovirus, direct probe technique

87496   cytomegalovirus, amplified probe technique

87497   cytomegalovirus, quantification

87498   enterovirus, amplified probe technique

87500   vancomycin resistance (eg, enterococcus species van A, van B), amplified probe technique

87501   influenza virus, reverse transcription and amplified probe technique, each type or subtype

87502   influenza virus, for multiple types or sub-types, multiplex reverse transcription and amplified probe technique, first 2 types or sub-types

+ 87503   influenza virus, for multiple types or sub-types, multiplex reverse transcription and amplified probe technique, each additional influenza virus type or sub-type beyond 2 (List separately in addition to code for primary procedure)

(Use 87503 in conjunction with 87502)

87510   Gardnerella vaginalis, direct probe technique

87511   Gardnerella vaginalis, amplified probe technique

87512   Gardnerella vaginalis, quantification

87515   hepatitis B virus, direct probe technique

87516   hepatitis B virus, amplified probe technique

87517   hepatitis B virus, quantification

87520   hepatitis C, direct probe technique

87521   hepatitis C, amplified probe technique

87522   hepatitis C, quantification

87525   hepatitis G, direct probe technique

| | |
|---|---|
| 87526 | hepatitis G, amplified probe technique |
| 87527 | hepatitis G, quantification |
| 87528 | Herpes simplex virus, direct probe technique |
| 87529 | Herpes simplex virus, amplified probe technique |
| 87530 | Herpes simplex virus, quantification |
| 87531 | Herpes virus-6, direct probe technique |
| 87532 | Herpes virus-6, amplified probe technique |
| 87533 | Herpes virus-6, quantification |
| 87534 | HIV-1, direct probe technique |
| 87535 | HIV-1, amplified probe technique |
| 87536 | HIV-1, quantification |
| 87537 | HIV-2, direct probe technique |
| 87538 | HIV-2, amplified probe technique |
| 87539 | HIV-2, quantification |
| 87540 | Legionella pneumophila, direct probe technique |
| 87541 | Legionella pneumophila, amplified probe technique |
| 87542 | Legionella pneumophila, quantification |
| 87550 | Mycobacteria species, direct probe technique |
| 87551 | Mycobacteria species, amplified probe technique |
| 87552 | Mycobacteria species, quantification |
| 87555 | Mycobacteria tuberculosis, direct probe technique |
| 87556 | Mycobacteria tuberculosis, amplified probe technique |
| 87557 | Mycobacteria tuberculosis, quantification |
| 87560 | Mycobacteria avium-intracellulare, direct probe technique |
| 87561 | Mycobacteria avium-intracellulare, amplified probe technique |
| 87562 | Mycobacteria avium-intracellulare, quantification |
| 87580 | Mycoplasma pneumoniae, direct probe technique |
| 87581 | Mycoplasma pneumoniae, amplified probe technique |
| 87582 | Mycoplasma pneumoniae, quantification |
| 87590 | Neisseria gonorrhoeae, direct probe technique |
| 87591 | Neisseria gonorrhoeae, amplified probe technique |
| 87592 | Neisseria gonorrhoeae, quantification |
| 87620 | papillomavirus, human, direct probe technique |
| 87621 | papillomavirus, human, amplified probe technique |
| 87622 | papillomavirus, human, quantification |
| 87640 | Staphylococcus aureus, amplified probe technique |
| 87641 | Staphylococcus aureus, methicillin resistant, amplified probe technique |

(For assays that detect methicillin resistance and identify Staphylococcus aureus using a single nucleic acid sequence, use 87641)

| | |
|---|---|
| 87650 | Streptococcus, group A, direct probe technique |
| 87651 | Streptococcus, group A, amplified probe technique |
| 87652 | Streptococcus, group A, quantification |
| 87653 | Streptococcus, group B, amplified probe technique |
| 87660 | Trichomonas vaginalis, direct probe technique |
| 87797 | Infectious agent detection by nucleic acid (DNA or RNA), not otherwise specified; direct probe technique, each organism |
| 87798 | amplified probe technique, each organism |
| 87799 | quantification, each organism |
| 87800 | Infectious agent detection by nucleic acid (DNA or RNA), multiple organisms; direct probe(s) technique |
| 87801 | amplified probe(s) technique |

(For each specific organism nucleic acid detection from a primary source, see 87470-87660. For detection of specific infectious agents not otherwise specified, see 87797, 87798, or 87799 1 time for each agent)

| | |
|---|---|
| 87802 | Infectious agent antigen detection by immunoassay with direct optical observation; Streptococcus, group B |
| 87803 | Clostridium difficile toxin A |
| 87804 | Influenza |
| 87807 | respiratory syncytial virus |
| 87808 | Trichomonas vaginalis |
| 87809 | adenovirus |
| 87810 | Chlamydia trachomatis |
| 87850 | Neisseria gonorrhoeae |
| 87880 | Streptococcus, group A |
| 87899 | not otherwise specified |
| 87900 | Infectious agent drug susceptibility phenotype prediction using regularly updated genotypic bioinformatics |
| 87901 | Infectious agent genotype analysis by nucleic acid (DNA or RNA); HIV-1, reverse transcriptase and protease regions |
| # 87906 | HIV-1, other region (eg, integrase, fusion) |

(For infectious agent drug susceptibility phenotype prediction for HIV-1, use 87900)

| | |
|---|---|
| 87902 | Hepatitis C virus |
| 87903 | Infectious agent phenotype analysis by nucleic acid (DNA or RNA) with drug resistance tissue culture analysis, HIV 1; first through 10 drugs tested |
| + 87904 | each additional drug tested (List separately in addition to code for primary procedure) |

(Use 87904 in conjunction with 87903)

| | |
|---|---|
| 87905 | Infectious agent enzymatic activity other than virus (eg, sialidase activity in vaginal fluid) |

(For virus isolation including identification by non-immunologic method, other than by cytopathic effect, use 87255)

**87906**   Code is out of numerical sequence. See 87001-87999

**87999**   Unlisted microbiology procedure

# Anatomic Pathology

## Postmortem Examination

Procedures 88000 through 88099 represent physician services only. Use modifier 90 for outside laboratory services.

**88000**   Necropsy (autopsy), gross examination only; without CNS

**88005**   with brain

**88007**   with brain and spinal cord

**88012**   infant with brain

**88014**   stillborn or newborn with brain

**88016**   macerated stillborn

**88020**   Necropsy (autopsy), gross and microscopic; without CNS

**88025**   with brain

**88027**   with brain and spinal cord

**88028**   infant with brain

**88029**   stillborn or newborn with brain

**88036**   Necropsy (autopsy), limited, gross and/or microscopic; regional

**88037**   single organ

**88040**   Necropsy (autopsy); forensic examination

**88045**   coroner's call

**88099**   Unlisted necropsy (autopsy) procedure

## Cytopathology

**88104**   Cytopathology, fluids, washings or brushings, except cervical or vaginal; smears with interpretation

**88106**   simple filter method with interpretation

▶(Do not report 88106 in conjunction with 88104)◀

▶(88107 has been deleted. To report smears and simple filter preparation, see 88104, 88106)◀

(For nongynecological selective cellular enhancement including filter transfer techniques, use 88112)

**88108**   Cytopathology, concentration technique, smears and interpretation (eg, Saccomanno technique)

(For cervical or vaginal smears, see 88150-88155)

(For gastric intubation with lavage, see 43754, 43755)

(For x-ray localization, use 74340)

**88112**   Cytopathology, selective cellular enhancement technique with interpretation (eg, liquid based slide preparation method), except cervical or vaginal

(Do not report 88112 with 88108)

**88120**   Cytopathology, in situ hybridization (eg, FISH), urinary tract specimen with morphometric analysis, 3-5 molecular probes, each specimen; manual

**88121**   using computer-assisted technology

(For morphometric in situ hybridization on cytologic specimens other than urinary tract, see 88367, 88368)

(For more than 5 probes, use 88399)

**88125**   Cytopathology, forensic (eg, sperm)

**88130**   Sex chromatin identification; Barr bodies

**88140**   peripheral blood smear, polymorphonuclear drumsticks

(For Guard stain, use 88313)

Codes 88141-88155, 88164-88167, 88174-88175 are used to report cervical or vaginal screening by various methods and to report physician interpretation services. Use codes 88150-88154 to report conventional Pap smears that are examined using non-Bethesda reporting. Use codes 88164-88167 to report conventional Pap smears that are examined using the Bethesda System of reporting. Use codes 88142-88143 to report liquid-based specimens processed as thin-layer preparations that are examined using any system of reporting (Bethesda or non-Bethesda). Use codes 88174-88175 to report automated screening of liquid-based specimens that are examined using any system of reporting (Bethesda or non-Bethesda). Within each of these three code families choose the one code that describes the screening method(s) used. Codes 88141 and 88155 should be reported in addition to the screening code chosen when the additional services are provided. Manual rescreening requires a complete visual reassessment of the entire slide initially screened by either an automated or manual process. Manual review represents an assessment of selected cells or regions of a slide identified by initial automated review.

**88141**   Cytopathology, cervical or vaginal (any reporting system), requiring interpretation by physician

(Use 88141 in conjunction with 88142-88154, 88164-88167, 88174-88175)

**88142**   Cytopathology, cervical or vaginal (any reporting system), collected in preservative fluid, automated thin layer preparation; manual screening under physician supervision

**88143**   with manual screening and rescreening under physician supervision

(For automated screening of automated thin layer preparation, see 88174, 88175)

**88147**   Cytopathology smears, cervical or vaginal; screening by automated system under physician supervision

**88148**      screening by automated system with manual rescreening under physician supervision

**88150**   Cytopathology, slides, cervical or vaginal; manual screening under physician supervision

**88152**      with manual screening and computer-assisted rescreening under physician supervision

**88153**      with manual screening and rescreening under physician supervision

**88154**      with manual screening and computer-assisted rescreening using cell selection and review under physician supervision

**+ 88155**   Cytopathology, slides, cervical or vaginal, definitive hormonal evaluation (eg, maturation index, karyopyknotic index, estrogenic index) (List separately in addition to code[s] for other technical and interpretation services)

(Use 88155 in conjunction with 88142-88154, 88164-88167, 88174-88175)

**88160**   Cytopathology, smears, any other source; screening and interpretation

**88161**      preparation, screening and interpretation

**88162**      extended study involving over 5 slides and/or multiple stains

(For aerosol collection of sputum, use 89220)

(For special stains, see 88312-88314)

**88164**   Cytopathology, slides, cervical or vaginal (the Bethesda System); manual screening under physician supervision

**88165**      with manual screening and rescreening under physician supervision

**88166**      with manual screening and computer-assisted rescreening under physician supervision

**88167**      with manual screening and computer-assisted rescreening using cell selection and review under physician supervision

(To report collection of specimen via fine needle aspiration, see 10021, 10022)

**88172**   Cytopathology, evaluation of fine needle aspirate; immediate cytohistologic study to determine adequacy for diagnosis, first evaluation episode, each site

(The evaluation episode represents a complete set of cytologic material submitted for evaluation and is independent of the number of needle passes or slides prepared. A separate evaluation episode occurs if the proceduralist provider obtains additional material from the same site, based on the prior immediate adequacy assessment, or a separate lesion is aspirated)

**88173**      interpretation and report

(Report one unit of 88173 for the interpretation and report from each anatomic site, regardless of the number of passes or evaluation episodes performed during the aspiration procedure)

(For fine needle aspirate, see 10021, 10022)

(Do not report 88172, 88173 in conjunction with 88333 and 88334 for the same specimen)

**#+ 88177**      immediate cytohistologic study to determine adequacy for diagnosis, each separate additional evaluation episode, same site (List separately in addition to code for primary procedure)

(When repeat immediate evaluation episode(s) is required on subsequent cytologic material from the same site, eg, following determination the prior sampling that was not adequate for diagnosis, use 1 unit of 88177 for each additional evaluation episode)

(Use 88177 in conjunction with 88172)

**88174**   Cytopathology, cervical or vaginal (any reporting system), collected in preservative fluid, automated thin layer preparation; screening by automated system, under physician supervision

**88175**      with screening by automated system and manual rescreening or review, under physician supervision

(For manual screening, see 88142, 88143)

**88177**   Code is out of numerical sequence. See 88104-88199

**88182**   Flow cytometry, cell cycle or DNA analysis

(For DNA ploidy analysis by morphometric technique, use 88358)

**88184**   Flow cytometry, cell surface, cytoplasmic, or nuclear marker, technical component only; first marker

**+ 88185**      each additional marker (List separately in addition to code for first marker)

(Report 88185 in conjunction with 88184)

**88187**   Flow cytometry, interpretation; 2 to 8 markers

**88188**      9 to 15 markers

**88189**      16 or more markers

(Do not report 88187-88189 for interpretation of 86355, 86356, 86357, 86359, 86360, 86361, 86367)

►(For cell enumeration using immunologic selection and identification in fluid specimen [eg, circulating tumor cells in blood], see 0279T, 0280T)◄

**88199**   Unlisted cytopathology procedure

(For electron microscopy, see 88348, 88349)

# Cytogenetic Studies

When molecular diagnostic procedures are performed to test for oncologic or inherited disorder, use the appropriate modifier to specify probe type or condition tested. (See **Appendix I** for a listing of appropriate modifiers to report with molecular diagnostic and cytogenetic procedures.)

(For acetylcholinesterase, use 82013)

**Pathology and Laboratory**

(For alpha-fetoprotein, serum or amniotic fluid, see 82105, 82106)

(For laser microdissection of cells from tissue sample, see 88380)

**88230** Tissue culture for non-neoplastic disorders; lymphocyte

**88233** skin or other solid tissue biopsy

**88235** amniotic fluid or chorionic villus cells

**88237** Tissue culture for neoplastic disorders; bone marrow, blood cells

**88239** solid tumor

**88240** Cryopreservation, freezing and storage of cells, each cell line

(For therapeutic cryopreservation and storage, use 38207)

**88241** Thawing and expansion of frozen cells, each aliquot

(For therapeutic thawing of previous harvest, use 38208)

**88245** Chromosome analysis for breakage syndromes; baseline Sister Chromatid Exchange (SCE), 20-25 cells

**88248** baseline breakage, score 50-100 cells, count 20 cells, 2 karyotypes (eg, for ataxia telangiectasia, Fanconi anemia, fragile X)

**88249** score 100 cells, clastogen stress (eg, diepoxybutane, mitomycin C, ionizing radiation, UV radiation)

**88261** Chromosome analysis; count 5 cells, 1 karyotype, with banding

**88262** count 15-20 cells, 2 karyotypes, with banding

**88263** count 45 cells for mosaicism, 2 karyotypes, with banding

**88264** analyze 20-25 cells

**88267** Chromosome analysis, amniotic fluid or chorionic villus, count 15 cells, 1 karyotype, with banding

**88269** Chromosome analysis, in situ for amniotic fluid cells, count cells from 6-12 colonies, 1 karyotype, with banding

**88271** Molecular cytogenetics; DNA probe, each (eg, FISH)

**88272** chromosomal in situ hybridization, analyze 3-5 cells (eg, for derivatives and markers)

**88273** chromosomal in situ hybridization, analyze 10-30 cells (eg, for microdeletions)

**88274** interphase in situ hybridization, analyze 25-99 cells

**88275** interphase in situ hybridization, analyze 100-300 cells

**88280** Chromosome analysis; additional karyotypes, each study

**88283** additional specialized banding technique (eg, NOR, C-banding)

**88285** additional cells counted, each study

**88289** additional high resolution study

**88291** Cytogenetics and molecular cytogenetics, interpretation and report

**88299** Unlisted cytogenetic study

# Surgical Pathology

Services 88300 through 88309 include accession, examination, and reporting. They do not include the services designated in codes 88311 through 88365 and 88399, which are coded in addition when provided.

The unit of service for codes 88300 through 88309 is the specimen.

A specimen is defined as tissue or tissues that is (are) submitted for individual and separate attention, requiring individual examination and pathologic diagnosis. Two or more such specimens from the same patient (eg, separately identified endoscopic biopsies, skin lesions) are each appropriately assigned an individual code reflective of its proper level of service.

Service code 88300 is used for any specimen that in the opinion of the examining pathologist can be accurately diagnosed without microscopic examination. Service code 88302 is used when gross and microscopic examination is performed on a specimen to confirm identification and the absence of disease. Service codes 88304 through 88309 describe all other specimens requiring gross and microscopic examination, and represent additional ascending levels of physician work. Levels 88302 through 88309 are specifically defined by the assigned specimens.

Any unlisted specimen should be assigned to the code which most closely reflects the physician work involved when compared to other specimens assigned to that code.

(Do not report 88302-88309 on the same specimen as part of Mohs surgery)

**88300** **Level I** - Surgical pathology, gross examination only

**88302** **Level II** - Surgical pathology, gross and microscopic examination

Appendix, incidental

Fallopian tube, sterilization

Fingers/toes, amputation, traumatic

Foreskin, newborn

Hernia sac, any location

Hydrocele sac

Nerve

Skin, plastic repair

Sympathetic ganglion

Testis, castration

Vaginal mucosa, incidental

Vas deferens, sterilization

**88304** **Level III** - Surgical pathology, gross and microscopic examination

Abortion, induced

Abscess

⊙=Moderate sedation  ✚=Add-on code  ✂=FDA approval pending  #=Resequenced code  ⭕=Recycled/reinstated code

Aneurysm - arterial/ventricular

Anus, tag

Appendix, other than incidental

Artery, atheromatous plaque

Bartholin's gland cyst

Bone fragment(s), other than pathologic fracture

Bursa/synovial cyst

Carpal tunnel tissue

Cartilage, shavings

Cholesteatoma

Colon, colostomy stoma

Conjunctiva - biopsy/pterygium

Cornea

Diverticulum - esophagus/small intestine

Dupuytren's contracture tissue

Femoral head, other than fracture

Fissure/fistula

Foreskin, other than newborn

Gallbladder

Ganglion cyst

Hematoma

Hemorrhoids

Hydatid of Morgagni

Intervertebral disc

Joint, loose body

Meniscus

Mucocele, salivary

Neuroma - Morton's/traumatic

Pilonidal cyst/sinus

Polyps, inflammatory - nasal/sinusoidal

Skin - cyst/tag/debridement

Soft tissue, debridement

Soft tissue, lipoma

Spermatocele

Tendon/tendon sheath

Testicular appendage

Thrombus or embolus

Tonsil and/or adenoids

Varicocele

Vas deferens, other than sterilization

Vein, varicosity

**88305**   **Level IV** - Surgical pathology, gross and microscopic examination

Abortion - spontaneous/missed

Artery, biopsy

Bone marrow, biopsy

Bone exostosis

Brain/meninges, other than for tumor resection

Breast, biopsy, not requiring microscopic evaluation of surgical margins

Breast, reduction mammoplasty

Bronchus, biopsy

Cell block, any source

Cervix, biopsy

Colon, biopsy

Duodenum, biopsy

Endocervix, curettings/biopsy

Endometrium, curettings/biopsy

Esophagus, biopsy

Extremity, amputation, traumatic

Fallopian tube, biopsy

Fallopian tube, ectopic pregnancy

Femoral head, fracture

Fingers/toes, amputation, non-traumatic

Gingiva/oral mucosa, biopsy

Heart valve

Joint, resection

Kidney, biopsy

Larynx, biopsy

Leiomyoma(s), uterine myomectomy - without uterus

Lip, biopsy/wedge resection

Lung, transbronchial biopsy

Lymph node, biopsy

Muscle, biopsy

Nasal mucosa, biopsy

Nasopharynx/oropharynx, biopsy

Nerve, biopsy

Odontogenic/dental cyst

Omentum, biopsy

Ovary with or without tube, non-neoplastic

Ovary, biopsy/wedge resection

Parathyroid gland

Peritoneum, biopsy

Pituitary tumor

Placenta, other than third trimester

Pleura/pericardium - biopsy/tissue

Polyp, cervical/endometrial

Polyp, colorectal

Polyp, stomach/small intestine

Prostate, needle biopsy

Prostate, TUR

Salivary gland, biopsy

Sinus, paranasal biopsy

Skin, other than cyst/tag/debridement/plastic repair

Small intestine, biopsy

Soft tissue, other than tumor/mass/lipoma/debridement

Spleen

Stomach, biopsy

Synovium

Testis, other than tumor/biopsy/castration

Thyroglossal duct/brachial cleft cyst

Tongue, biopsy

Tonsil, biopsy

Trachea, biopsy

Ureter, biopsy

Urethra, biopsy

Urinary bladder, biopsy

Uterus, with or without tubes and ovaries, for prolapse

Vagina, biopsy

Vulva/labia, biopsy

**88307**  **Level V** - Surgical pathology, gross and microscopic examination

Adrenal, resection

Bone - biopsy/curettings

Bone fragment(s), pathologic fracture

Brain, biopsy

Brain/meninges, tumor resection

Breast, excision of lesion, requiring microscopic evaluation of surgical margins

Breast, mastectomy - partial/simple

Cervix, conization

Colon, segmental resection, other than for tumor

Extremity, amputation, non-traumatic

Eye, enucleation

Kidney, partial/total nephrectomy

Larynx, partial/total resection

Liver, biopsy - needle/wedge

Liver, partial resection

Lung, wedge biopsy

Lymph nodes, regional resection

Mediastinum, mass

Myocardium, biopsy

Odontogenic tumor

Ovary with or without tube, neoplastic

Pancreas, biopsy

Placenta, third trimester

Prostate, except radical resection

Salivary gland

Sentinel lymph node

Small intestine, resection, other than for tumor

Soft tissue mass (except lipoma) - biopsy/simple excision

Stomach - subtotal/total resection, other than for tumor

Testis, biopsy

Thymus, tumor

Thyroid, total/lobe

Ureter, resection

Urinary bladder, TUR

Uterus, with or without tubes and ovaries, other than neoplastic/prolapse

**88309**  **Level VI** - Surgical pathology, gross and microscopic examination

Bone resection

Breast, mastectomy - with regional lymph nodes

Colon, segmental resection for tumor

Colon, total resection

Esophagus, partial/total resection

Extremity, disarticulation

Fetus, with dissection

Larynx, partial/total resection - with regional lymph nodes

Lung - total/lobe/segment resection

Pancreas, total/subtotal resection

Prostate, radical resection

Small intestine, resection for tumor

Soft tissue tumor, extensive resection

Stomach - subtotal/total resection for tumor

Testis, tumor

Tongue/tonsil -resection for tumor

Urinary bladder, partial/total resection

Uterus, with or without tubes and ovaries, neoplastic

Vulva, total/subtotal resection

(For fine needle aspiration, see 10021, 10022)

(For evaluation of fine needle aspirate, see 88172-88173)

(Do not report 88302-88309 on the same specimen as part of Mohs surgery)

**+ 88311**  Decalcification procedure (List separately in addition to code for surgical pathology examination)

**▲ 88312**  Special stain including interpretation and report; Group I for microorganisms (eg, acid fast, methenamine silver)

►(Report one unit of 88312 for each special stain, on each surgical pathology block, cytologic specimen, or hematologic smear)◄

**▲ 88313**  Group II, all other (eg, iron, trichrome), except stain for microorganisms, stains for enzyme constituents, or immunocytochemistry and immunohistochemistry

►(Report one unit of 88313 for each special stain, on each surgical pathology block, cytologic specimen, or hematologic smear)◄

►(For immunocytochemistry and immunohistochemistry, use 88342)◄

**+▲ 88314**  histochemical stain on frozen tissue block (List separately in addition to code for primary procedure)

►(Use 88314 in conjunction with 17311-17315, 88302-88309, 88331, 88332)◄

►(Do not report 88314 with 17311-17315 for routine frozen section stain [eg, hematoxylin and eosin, toluidine blue], performed during Mohs surgery. When a nonroutine histochemical stain on frozen tissue during Mohs surgery is utilized, report 88314 with modifier 59)◄

►(Report one unit of 88314 for each special stain on each frozen surgical pathology block)◄

►(For a special stain performed on frozen tissue section material to identify enzyme constituents, use 88319)◄

►(88318 has been deleted)◄

►(For determinative histochemistry to identify chemical components, use 88313)◄

**▲ 88319**  Group III, for enzyme constituents

►(For each stain on each surgical pathology block, cytologic specimen, or hematologic smear, use one unit of 88319)◄

►(For detection of enzyme constituents by immunohistochemical or immunocytochemical technique, use 88342)◄

**88321**  Consultation and report on referred slides prepared elsewhere

**88323**  Consultation and report on referred material requiring preparation of slides

**88325**  Consultation, comprehensive, with review of records and specimens, with report on referred material

**88329**  Pathology consultation during surgery;

**88331**      first tissue block, with frozen section(s), single specimen

**+ 88332**      each additional tissue block with frozen section(s) (List separately in addition to code for primary procedure)

(Use 88332 in conjunction with 88331)

**88333**      cytologic examination (eg, touch prep, squash prep), initial site

**+ 88334**      cytologic examination (eg, touch prep, squash prep), each additional site (List separately in addition to code for primary procedure)

(Use 88334 in conjunction with 88331, 88333)

(For intraoperative consultation on a specimen requiring both frozen section and cytologic evaluation, use 88331 and 88334)

(For percutaneous needle biopsy requiring intraprocedural cytologic examination, use 88333)

(Do not report 88333 and 88334 for non-intraoperative cytologic examination, see 88160-88162)

(Do not report 88333 and 88334 for intraprocedural cytologic evaluation of fine needle aspirate, see 88172)

**88342**  Immunohistochemistry (including tissue immunoperoxidase), each antibody

(Do not report 88342 in conjunction with 88360 or 88361 for the same antibody)

(For quantitative or semiquantitative immunohistochemistry, see 88360, 88361)

**88346**  Immunofluorescent study, each antibody; direct method

**88347**      indirect method

**88348**  Electron microscopy; diagnostic

**88349**      scanning

**88355**  Morphometric analysis; skeletal muscle

**88356**      nerve

**88358**      tumor (eg, DNA ploidy)

(Do not report 88358 with 88313 unless each procedure is for a different special stain)

**88360**  Morphometric analysis, tumor immunohistochemistry (eg, Her-2/neu, estrogen receptor/progesterone receptor), quantitative or semiquantitative, each antibody; manual

**88361**      using computer-assisted technology

(Do not report 88360, 88361 with 88342 unless each procedure is for a different antibody)

**Pathology and Laboratory**

(For morphometric analysis using in situ hybridization techniques, see 88367, 88368)

(When semi-thin plastic-embedded sections are performed in conjunction with morphometric analysis, only the morphometric analysis should be reported; if performed as an independent procedure, see codes 88300-88309 for surgical pathology.)

**88362**   Nerve teasing preparations

**88363**   Examination and selection of retrieved archival (ie, previously diagnosed) tissue(s) for molecular analysis (eg, KRAS mutational analysis)

**88365**   In situ hybridization (eg, FISH), each probe

(Do not report 88365 in conjunction with 88367, 88368 for the same probe)

**88367**   Morphometric analysis, in situ hybridization (quantitative or semi-quantitative) each probe; using computer-assisted technology

**88368**      manual

(For morphometric in situ hybridization evaluation of urinary tract cytologic specimens, see 88120, 88121)

**88371**   Protein analysis of tissue by Western Blot, with interpretation and report;

**88372**      immunological probe for band identification, each

**88380**   Microdissection (ie, sample preparation of microscopically identified target); laser capture

**88381**      manual

(Do not report 88380 in conjunction with 88381)

**88384**   Array-based evaluation of multiple molecular probes; 11 through 50 probes

**88385**      51 through 250 probes

**88386**      251 through 500 probes

(For preparation of array-based evaluation, see 83890-83892, 83898-83901)

(For preparation and analyses of less than 11 probes, see 83890-83914)

**88387**   Macroscopic examination, dissection, and preparation of tissue for non-microscopic analytical studies (eg, nucleic acid-based molecular studies); each tissue preparation (eg, a single lymph node)

(Do not report 88387 for tissue preparation for microbiologic cultures or flow cytometric studies)

(Do not report 88387 in conjunction with 88388, 88329-88334)

**+ 88388**      in conjunction with a touch imprint, intraoperative consultation, or frozen section, each tissue preparation (eg, a single lymph node) (List separately in addition to code for primary procedure)

(Use 88388 in conjunction with 88329-88334)

(Do not report 88387 or 88388 for tissue preparation for microbiologic cultures or flow cytometric studies)

**88399**   Unlisted surgical pathology procedure

(88400 has been deleted. To report, use 88720)

# In Vivo (eg, Transcutaneous) Laboratory Procedures

(For all in vivo measurements not specifically listed, use 88749)

(For wavelength fluorescent spectroscopy of advanced glycation end products (skin), use 0233T)

►(For transcutaneous oxyhemoglobin measurement in a lower extremity wound by near infrared spectroscopy, use 0286T)◄

**88720**   Bilirubin, total, transcutaneous

(For transdermal oxygen saturation, see 94760-94762)

**88738**   Hemoglobin (Hgb), quantitative, transcutaneous

(For in vitro hemoglobin measurement, use 85018)

**88740**   Hemoglobin, quantitative, transcutaneous, per day; carboxyhemoglobin

(For in vitro carboxyhemoglobin measurement, use 82375)

**88741**      methemoglobin

(For in vitro quantitative methemoglobin determination, use 83050)

**88749**   Unlisted in vivo (eg, transcutaneous) laboratory service

# Other Procedures

**89049**   Caffeine halothane contracture test (CHCT) for malignant hyperthermia susceptibility, including interpretation and report

**89050**   Cell count, miscellaneous body fluids (eg, cerebrospinal fluid, joint fluid), except blood;

**89051**      with differential count

**89055**   Leukocyte assessment, fecal, qualitative or semiquantitative

**89060**   Crystal identification by light microscopy with or without polarizing lens analysis, tissue or any body fluid (except urine)

(Do not report 89060 for crystal identification on paraffin-embedded tissue)

(89100, 89105 have been deleted. To report, see 43756, 43757)

**89125**   Fat stain, feces, urine, or respiratory secretions

(89130-89141 have been deleted. To report, see 43754, 43755)

**89160**    Meat fibers, feces

**89190**    Nasal smear for eosinophils

     (Occult blood, feces, use 82270)

     (Paternity tests, use 86910)

**89220**    Sputum, obtaining specimen, aerosol induced technique (separate procedure)

     (89225 has been deleted)

**89230**    Sweat collection by iontophoresis

     (89235 has been deleted)

**89240**    Unlisted miscellaneous pathology test

# Reproductive Medicine Procedures

**89250**    Culture of oocyte(s)/embryo(s), less than 4 days;

**89251**      with co-culture of oocyte(s)/embryos

     (For extended culture of oocyte[s]/embryo[s], see 89272)

**89253**    Assisted embryo hatching, microtechniques (any method)

**89254**    Oocyte identification from follicular fluid

**89255**    Preparation of embryo for transfer (any method)

**89257**    Sperm identification from aspiration (other than seminal fluid)

     (For semen analysis, see 89300-89320)

     (For sperm identification from testis tissue, use 89264)

**89258**    Cryopreservation; embryo(s)

**89259**      sperm

     (For cryopreservation of reproductive tissue, testicular, use 89335).

**89260**    Sperm isolation; simple prep (eg, sperm wash and swim-up) for insemination or diagnosis with semen analysis

**89261**      complex prep (eg, Percoll gradient, albumin gradient) for insemination or diagnosis with semen analysis

     (For semen analysis without sperm wash or swim-up, use 89320)

**89264**    Sperm identification from testis tissue, fresh or cryopreserved

     (For biopsy of testis, see 54500, 54505)

     (For sperm identification from aspiration, use 89257)

     (For semen analysis, see 89300-89320)

**89268**    Insemination of oocytes

**89272**    Extended culture of oocyte(s)/embryo(s), 4-7 days

**89280**    Assisted oocyte fertilization, microtechnique; less than or equal to 10 oocytes

**89281**      greater than 10 oocytes

**89290**    Biopsy, oocyte polar body or embryo blastomere, microtechnique (for pre-implantation genetic diagnosis); less than or equal to 5 embryos

**89291**      greater than 5 embryos

**89300**    Semen analysis; presence and/or motility of sperm including Huhner test (post coital)

**89310**      motility and count (not including Huhner test)

**89320**      volume, count, motility, and differential

     (Skin tests, see 86485-86580 and 95010-95199)

**89321**      sperm presence and motility of sperm, if performed

     (To report Hyaluronan binding assay [HBA], use 89398)

**89322**      volume, count, motility, and differential using strict morphologic criteria (eg, Kruger)

**89325**    Sperm antibodies

     (For medicolegal identification of sperm, use 88125)

**89329**    Sperm evaluation; hamster penetration test

**89330**      cervical mucus penetration test, with or without spinnbarkeit test

**89331**    Sperm evaluation, for retrograde ejaculation, urine (sperm concentration, motility, and morphology, as indicated)

     (For semen analysis on concurrent semen specimen, see 89300-89322 in conjunction with 89331)

     (For detection of sperm in urine, use 81015)

**89335**    Cryopreservation, reproductive tissue, testicular

     (For cryopreservation of embryo[s], use 89258. For cryopreservation of sperm, use 89259)

     (For cryopreservation, ovarian reproductive tissue, oocytes, use 89240)

**89342**    Storage (per year); embryo(s)

**89343**      sperm/semen

**89344**      reproductive tissue, testicular/ovarian

**89346**      oocyte(s)

**89352**    Thawing of cryopreserved; embryo(s)

**89353**      sperm/semen, each aliquot

**89354**      reproductive tissue, testicular/ovarian

**89356**      oocytes, each aliquot

**89398**    Unlisted reproductive medicine laboratory procedure

**Pathology and Laboratory**

# Notes

# Medicine Guidelines

In addition to the definitions and commonly used terms presented in the **Introduction**, several other items unique to this section on **Medicine** are defined or identified here.

## Multiple Procedures

It is appropriate to designate multiple procedures that are rendered on the same date by separate entries. For example: If individual medical psychotherapy (90829) is rendered in addition to subsequent hospital care (eg, 99231), the psychotherapy would be reported separately from the hospital visit. In this instance, both 99231 and 90829 would be reported.

## Add-on Codes

Some of the listed procedures are commonly carried out in addition to the primary procedure performed. All add-on codes found in the CPT codebook are exempt from the multiple procedure concept. They are exempt from the use of modifier 51, as these procedures are not reported as stand-alone codes. These additional or supplemental procedures are designated as "add-on" codes. Add-on codes in the CPT codebook can be readily identified by specific descriptor nomenclature which includes phrases such as "each additional" or "(List separately in addition to primary procedure)."

## Separate Procedures

Some of the procedures or services listed in the CPT codebook that are commonly carried out as an integral component of a total service or procedure have been identified by the inclusion of the term "separate procedure." The codes designated as "separate procedure" should not be reported in addition to the code for the total procedure or service of which it is considered an integral component.

However, when a procedure or service that is designated as a "separate procedure" is carried out independently or considered to be unrelated or distinct from other procedures/services provided at that time, it may be reported by itself, or in addition to other procedures/services by appending modifier 59 to the specific "separate procedure" code to indicate that the procedure is not considered to be a component of another procedure, but is a distinct, independent procedure. This may represent a different session or patient encounter, different procedure or surgery, different site or organ system, separate incision/excision, separate lesion, or separate injury (or area of injury in extensive injuries).

## Unlisted Service or Procedure

A service or procedure may be provided that is not listed in this edition of the CPT codebook. When reporting such a service, the appropriate "Unlisted Procedure" code may be used to indicate the service, identifying it by "Special Report" as discussed on this page. The "Unlisted Procedures" and accompanying codes for **Medicine** are as follows:

| Code | Description |
|---|---|
| 90399 | Unlisted immune globulin |
| 90749 | Unlisted vaccine/toxoid |
| 90899 | Unlisted psychiatric service or procedure |
| 90999 | Unlisted dialysis procedure, inpatient or outpatient |
| 91299 | Unlisted diagnostic gastroenterology procedure |
| 92499 | Unlisted ophthalmological service or procedure |
| 92700 | Unlisted otorhinolaryngological service or procedure |
| 93799 | Unlisted cardiovascular service or procedure |
| ● 93998 | Unlisted noninvasive vascular diagnostic study |
| 94799 | Unlisted pulmonary service or procedure |
| 95199 | Unlisted allergy/clinical immunologic service or procedure |
| 95999 | Unlisted neurological or neuromuscular diagnostic procedure |
| 96379 | Unlisted therapeutic, prophylactic, or diagnostic intravenous or intra-arterial injection or infusion |
| 96549 | Unlisted chemotherapy procedure |
| 96999 | Unlisted special dermatological service or procedure |
| 97039 | Unlisted modality (specify type and time if constant attendance) |
| 97139 | Unlisted therapeutic procedure (specify) |
| 97799 | Unlisted physical medicine/rehabilitation service or procedure |
| 99199 | Unlisted special service, procedure or report |
| 99600 | Unlisted home visit service or procedure |

# Special Report

A service that is rarely provided, unusual, variable, or new may require a special report. Pertinent information should include an adequate definition or description of the nature, extent, and need for the procedure; and the time, effort, and equipment necessary to provide the service.

# Materials Supplied by Physician

Supplies and materials provided by the physician (eg, sterile trays/drugs), over and above those usually included with the procedure(s) rendered are reported separately. List drugs, trays, supplies, and materials provided. Identify as 99070 or specific supply code.

# Medicine

## Immune Globulins, Serum or Recombinant Products

Codes 90281-90399 identify the serum globulins, extracted from human blood; or recombinant immune globulin products created in a laboratory through genetic modification of human and/or animal proteins. Both are reported in addition to the administration codes 96365-96368, 96372, 96374, 96375 as appropriate. Modifier 51 should not be reported with this section of products codes when performed with another procedure. The serum or recombinant globulin products listed here include broad-spectrum anti-infective immune globulins, antitoxins, various isoantibodies, and monoclonal antibodies.

| | |
|---|---|
| **90281** | Immune globulin (Ig), human, for intramuscular use |
| **90283** | Immune globulin (IgIV), human, for intravenous use |
| **90284** | Immune globulin (SCIg), human, for use in subcutaneous infusions, 100 mg, each |
| **90287** | Botulinum antitoxin, equine, any route |
| **90288** | Botulism immune globulin, human, for intravenous use |
| **90291** | Cytomegalovirus immune globulin (CMV-IgIV), human, for intravenous use |
| **90296** | Diphtheria antitoxin, equine, any route |
| **90371** | Hepatitis B immune globulin (HBIg), human, for intramuscular use |
| **90375** | Rabies immune globulin (RIg), human, for intramuscular and/or subcutaneous use |
| **90376** | Rabies immune globulin, heat-treated (RIg-HT), human, for intramuscular and/or subcutaneous use |
| **90378** | Respiratory syncytial virus, monoclonal antibody, recombinant, for intramuscular use, 50 mg, each |
| | (90379 has been deleted) |
| **90384** | Rho(D) immune globulin (RhIg), human, full-dose, for intramuscular use |
| **90385** | Rho(D) immune globulin (RhIg), human, mini-dose, for intramuscular use |
| **90386** | Rho(D) immune globulin (RhIgIV), human, for intravenous use |
| **90389** | Tetanus immune globulin (TIg), human, for intramuscular use |
| **90393** | Vaccinia immune globulin, human, for intramuscular use |
| **90396** | Varicella-zoster immune globulin, human, for intramuscular use |
| **90399** | Unlisted immune globulin |

## Immunization Administration for Vaccines/Toxoids

►Report vaccine immunization administration codes 90460, 90461, 90471-90474 in addition to the vaccine and toxoid code(s) 90476-90749.◄

►Report codes 90460 and 90461 only when the physician or qualified health care professional provides face-to-face counseling of the patient/family during the administration of a vaccine. For immunization administration of any vaccine that is not accompanied by face-to-face physician or qualified health care professional counseling to the patient/family or for administration of vaccines to patients over 18 years of age, report codes 90471-90474.◄

If a significant separately identifiable Evaluation and Management service (eg, office or other outpatient services, preventive medicine services) is performed, the appropriate E/M service code should be reported in addition to the vaccine and toxoid administration codes.

►A component refers to all antigens in a vaccine that prevent disease(s) caused by one organism (90460 and 90461). Multi-valent antigens or multiple serotypes of antigens against a single organism are considered a single component of vaccines. Combination vaccines are those vaccines that contain multiple vaccine components. Conjugates or adjuvants contained in vaccines are not considered to be component parts of the vaccine as defined above.◄

(For allergy testing, see 95004 et seq)

(For skin testing of bacterial, viral, fungal extracts, see 86485-86580)

(For therapeutic or diagnostic injections, see 96372-96379)

| | |
|---|---|
| ▲ **90460** | Immunization administration through 18 years of age via any route of administration, with counseling by physician or other qualified health care professional; first or only component of each vaccine or toxoid administered |
| + ▲ **90461** | each additional vaccine or toxoid component administered (List separately in addition to code for primary procedure) |

(Use 90460 for each vaccine administered. For vaccines with multiple components [combination vaccines], report 90460 in conjunction with 90461 for each additional component in a given vaccine)

(90465-90468 have been deleted. To report, see 90460, 90461, 90471-90474)

►(90470 has been deleted)◄

Medicine

**90471**    Immunization administration (includes percutaneous, intradermal, subcutaneous, or intramuscular injections); 1 vaccine (single or combination vaccine/toxoid)

      (Do not report 90471 in conjunction with 90473)

**+ 90472**    each additional vaccine (single or combination vaccine/toxoid) (List separately in addition to code for primary procedure)

      (Use 90472 in conjunction with 90471 or 90473)

      (For administration of immune globulins, see 90281-90399, 96360, 96361, 96365-96368, 96374)

      (For intravesical administration of BCG vaccine, see 51720, 90586)

**90473**    Immunization administration by intranasal or oral route; 1 vaccine (single or combination vaccine/toxoid)

      (Do not report 90473 in conjunction with 90471)

**+ 90474**    each additional vaccine (single or combination vaccine/toxoid) (List separately in addition to code for primary procedure)

      (Use 90474 in conjunction with 90471 or 90473)

# Vaccines, Toxoids

To assist users to report the most recent new or revised vaccine product codes, the American Medical Association (AMA) currently uses the CPT Website, which features updates of CPT Editorial Panel actions regarding these products. Once approved by the CPT Editorial Panel, these codes will be made available for release on a semi-annual (twice a year: July 1 and January 1) basis. As part of the electronic distribution, there is a six-month implementation period from the initial release date (ie, codes released on January 1 are eligible for use on July 1 and codes released on July 1 are eligible for use January 1).

The CPT Editorial Panel, in recognition of the public health interest in vaccine products, has chosen to publish new vaccine product codes prior to approval by the U. S. Food and Drug Administration (FDA). These codes are indicated with the ✗ symbol and will be tracked by the AMA to monitor FDA approval status. Once the FDA status changes to approval, the ✗ symbol will be removed. CPT users should refer to the AMA Internet site (www.ama-assn.org/ama/pub/category/10902.html) for the most up-to-date information on codes with the ✗ symbol.

Codes 90476-90748 identify the vaccine product **only.** To report the administration of a vaccine/toxoid, the vaccine/toxoid product codes 90476-90749 must be used in addition to an immunization administration code(s) 90460-90474. Modifier 51 should not be reported for the vaccines, toxoids when performed with these administration procedures.

If a significantly separately identifiable Evaluation and Management (E/M) service (eg, office or other outpatient services, preventive medicine services) is performed, the appropriate E/M service code should be reported in addition to the vaccine and toxoid administration codes.

To meet the reporting requirements of immunization registries, vaccine distribution programs, and reporting systems (eg, Vaccine Adverse Event Reporting System) the exact vaccine product administered needs to be reported. Multiple codes for a particular vaccine are provided in the CPT codebook when the schedule (number of doses or timing) differs for two or more products of the same vaccine type (eg, hepatitis A, Hib) or the vaccine product is available in more than one chemical formulation, dosage, or route of administration.

The "when administered to" age descriptions included in CPT vaccine codes are not intended to identify a product's licensed age indication. The term "preservative free" includes use for vaccines that contain no preservative and vaccines that contain trace amounts of preservative agents that are not present in a sufficient concentration for the purpose of preserving the final vaccine formulation. The absence of a designation regarding a preservative does not necessarily indicate the presence or absence of preservative in the vaccine. Refer to the product's prescribing information (PI) for the licensed age indication before administering vaccine to a patient.

Separate codes are available for combination vaccines (eg, DTP-Hib, DtaP-Hib, HepB-Hib). It is inappropriate to code each component of a combination vaccine separately. If a specific vaccine code is not available, the unlisted procedure code should be reported, until a new code becomes available.

      (For immune globulins, see codes 90281-90399, 96365-96368, 96372-96375 for administration of immune globulins)

**90476**    Adenovirus vaccine, type 4, live, for oral use

**90477**    Adenovirus vaccine, type 7, live, for oral use

▲ **90581**    Anthrax vaccine, for subcutaneous or intramuscular use

**90585**    Bacillus Calmette-Guerin vaccine (BCG) for tuberculosis, live, for percutaneous use

**90586**    Bacillus Calmette-Guerin vaccine (BCG) for bladder cancer, live, for intravesical use

**90632**    Hepatitis A vaccine, adult dosage, for intramuscular use

**90633**    Hepatitis A vaccine, pediatric/adolescent dosage-2 dose schedule, for intramuscular use

**90634**    Hepatitis A vaccine, pediatric/adolescent dosage-3 dose schedule, for intramuscular use

**90636**    Hepatitis A and hepatitis B vaccine (HepA-HepB), adult dosage, for intramuscular use

Medicine

↗ ▲ **90644**　Meningococcal conjugate vaccine, serogroups C & Y and Hemophilus influenza B vaccine (Hib-MenCY), 4 dose schedule, when administered to children 2-15 months of age, for intramuscular use

**90645**　Hemophilus influenza b vaccine (Hib), HbOC conjugate (4 dose schedule), for intramuscular use

**90646**　Hemophilus influenza b vaccine (Hib), PRP-D conjugate, for booster use only, intramuscular use

**90647**　Hemophilus influenza b vaccine (Hib), PRP-OMP conjugate (3 dose schedule), for intramuscular use

**90648**　Hemophilus influenza b vaccine (Hib), PRP-T conjugate (4 dose schedule), for intramuscular use

**90649**　Human Papilloma virus (HPV) vaccine, types 6, 11, 16, 18 (quadrivalent), 3 dose schedule, for intramuscular use

**90650**　Human Papilloma virus (HPV) vaccine, types 16, 18, bivalent, 3 dose schedule, for intramuscular use

● **90654**　Influenza virus vaccine, split virus, preservative-free, for intradermal use

**90655**　Influenza virus vaccine, split virus, preservative free, when administered to children 6-35 months of age, for intramuscular use

**90656**　Influenza virus vaccine, split virus, preservative free, when administered to individuals 3 years and older, for intramuscular use

**90657**　Influenza virus vaccine, split virus, when administered to children 6-35 months of age, for intramuscular use

**90658**　Influenza virus vaccine, split virus, when administered to individuals 3 years of age and older, for intramuscular use

**90660**　Influenza virus vaccine, live, for intranasal use

↗ **90661**　Influenza virus vaccine, derived from cell cultures, subunit, preservative and antibiotic free, for intramuscular use

**90662**　Influenza virus vaccine, split virus, preservative free, enhanced immunogenicity via increased antigen content, for intramuscular use

►(90663 has been deleted)◄

↗ **90664**　Influenza virus vaccine, pandemic formulation, live, for intranasal use

**90665**　Code is out of numerical sequence. See 90476-90749

↗ **90666**　Influenza virus vaccine, pandemic formulation, split virus, preservative free, for intramuscular use

↗ **90667**　Influenza virus vaccine, pandemic formulation, split virus, adjuvanted, for intramuscular use

↗ **90668**　Influenza virus vaccine, pandemic formulation, split virus, for intramuscular use

\# **90665**　Lyme disease vaccine, adult dosage, for intramuscular use

**90669**　Pneumococcal conjugate vaccine, 7 valent, for intramuscular use

**90670**　Pneumococcal conjugate vaccine, 13 valent, for intramuscular use

**90675**　Rabies vaccine, for intramuscular use

**90676**　Rabies vaccine, for intradermal use

**90680**　Rotavirus vaccine, pentavalent, 3 dose schedule, live, for oral use

**90681**　Rotavirus vaccine, human, attenuated, 2 dose schedule, live, for oral use

**90690**　Typhoid vaccine, live, oral

**90691**　Typhoid vaccine, Vi capsular polysaccharide (ViCPs), for intramuscular use

**90692**　Typhoid vaccine, heat- and phenol-inactivated (H-P), for subcutaneous or intradermal use

**90693**　Typhoid vaccine, acetone-killed, dried (AKD), for subcutaneous use (U.S. military)

**90696**　Diphtheria, tetanus toxoids, acellular pertussis vaccine and poliovirus vaccine, inactivated (DTaP-IPV), when administered to children 4 through 6 years of age, for intramuscular use

**90698**　Diphtheria, tetanus toxoids, acellular pertussis vaccine, haemophilus influenza Type B, and poliovirus vaccine, inactivated (DTaP - Hib - IPV), for intramuscular use

**90700**　Diphtheria, tetanus toxoids, and acellular pertussis vaccine (DTaP), when administered to individuals younger than 7 years, for intramuscular use

**90701**　Diphtheria, tetanus toxoids, and whole cell pertussis vaccine (DTP), for intramuscular use

**90702**　Diphtheria and tetanus toxoids (DT) adsorbed when administered to individuals younger than 7 years, for intramuscular use

**90703**　Tetanus toxoid adsorbed, for intramuscular use

**90704**　Mumps virus vaccine, live, for subcutaneous use

**90705**　Measles virus vaccine, live, for subcutaneous use

**90706**　Rubella virus vaccine, live, for subcutaneous use

**90707**　Measles, mumps and rubella virus vaccine (MMR), live, for subcutaneous use

**90708**　Measles and rubella virus vaccine, live, for subcutaneous use

**90710**　Measles, mumps, rubella, and varicella vaccine (MMRV), live, for subcutaneous use

**90712**　Poliovirus vaccine, (any type[s]) (OPV), live, for oral use

**90713**　Poliovirus vaccine, inactivated (IPV), for subcutaneous or intramuscular use

**90714**　Tetanus and diphtheria toxoids (Td) adsorbed, preservative free, when administered to individuals

7 years or older, for intramuscular use

**90715**　Tetanus, diphtheria toxoids and acellular pertussis vaccine (Tdap), when administered to individuals 7 years or older, for intramuscular use

**Medicine**

---

▲=Revised code　　●=New code　　►◄=Contains new or revised text　　⊘=Modifier 51 exempt

**Medicine**

**90716**  Varicella virus vaccine, live, for subcutaneous use

**90717**  Yellow fever vaccine, live, for subcutaneous use

**90718**  Tetanus and diphtheria toxoids (Td) adsorbed when administered to individuals 7 years or older, for intramuscular use

**90719**  Diphtheria toxoid, for intramuscular use

**90720**  Diphtheria, tetanus toxoids, and whole cell pertussis vaccine and Hemophilus influenza B vaccine (DTP-Hib), for intramuscular use

**90721**  Diphtheria, tetanus toxoids, and acellular pertussis vaccine and Hemophilus influenza B vaccine (DtaP-Hib), for intramuscular use

**90723**  Diphtheria, tetanus toxoids, acellular pertussis vaccine, Hepatitis B, and poliovirus vaccine, inactivated (DtaP-HepB-IPV), for intramuscular use

**90725**  Cholera vaccine for injectable use

**90727**  Plague vaccine, for intramuscular use

**90732**  Pneumococcal polysaccharide vaccine, 23-valent, adult or immunosuppressed patient dosage, when administered to individuals 2 years or older, for subcutaneous or intramuscular use

**90733**  Meningococcal polysaccharide vaccine (any group(s)), for subcutaneous use

**90734**  Meningococcal conjugate vaccine, serogroups A, C, Y and W-135 (tetravalent), for intramuscular use

**90735**  Japanese encephalitis virus vaccine, for subcutaneous use

**90736**  Zoster (shingles) vaccine, live, for subcutaneous injection

**90738**  Japanese encephalitis virus vaccine, inactivated, for intramuscular use

**90740**  Hepatitis B vaccine, dialysis or immunosuppressed patient dosage (3 dose schedule), for intramuscular use

**90743**  Hepatitis B vaccine, adolescent (2 dose schedule), for intramuscular use

**90744**  Hepatitis B vaccine, pediatric/adolescent dosage (3 dose schedule), for intramuscular use

**90746**  Hepatitis B vaccine, adult dosage, for intramuscular use

**90747**  Hepatitis B vaccine, dialysis or immunosuppressed patient dosage (4 dose schedule), for intramuscular use

**90748**  Hepatitis B and Hemophilus influenza b vaccine (HepB-Hib), for intramuscular use

**90749**  Unlisted vaccine/toxoid

(90760 has been deleted. To report, use 96360)

(90761 has been deleted. To report, use 96361)

(90765 has been deleted. To report, use 96365)

(90766 has been deleted. To report, use 96366)

(90767 has been deleted. To report, use 96367)

(90768 has been deleted. To report, use 96368)

(90769 has been deleted. To report, use 96369)

(90770 has been deleted. To report, use 96370)

(90771 has been deleted. To report, use 96371)

(90772 has been deleted. To report, use 96372)

(90773 has been deleted. To report, use 96373)

(90774 has been deleted. To report, use 96374)

(90775 has been deleted. To report, use 96375)

(90776 has been deleted. To report, use 96376)

(90779 has been deleted. To report, use 96379)

# Psychiatry

Hospital care by the attending physician in treating a psychiatric inpatient or partial hospitalization may be initial or subsequent in nature (see 99221-99233) and may include exchanges with nursing and ancillary personnel. Hospital care services involve a variety of responsibilities unique to the medical management of inpatients, such as physician hospital orders, interpretation of laboratory or other medical diagnostic studies and observations.

Some patients receive hospital evaluation and management services only and others receive evaluation and management services and other procedures. If other procedures such as electroconvulsive therapy or psychotherapy are rendered in addition to hospital evaluation and management services, these should be listed separately (ie, hospital care service plus electroconvulsive therapy or when psychotherapy is done, an appropriate code defining psychotherapy with medical evaluation and management services). Modifier 22 may be used to indicate a more extensive service. Modifier 52 may be used to signify a service that is reduced or less extensive than the usual procedure.

Other evaluation and management services, such as office medical service or other patient encounters, may be described as listed in the section on **Evaluation and Management,** if appropriate.

The evaluation and management services should not be reported separately, when reporting codes 90805, 90807, 90809, 90811, 90813, 90815, 90817, 90819, 90822, 90824, 90827, 90829.

Consultation for psychiatric evaluation of a patient includes examination of a patient and exchange of information with the primary physician and other informants such as nurses or family members, and preparation of a report. These consultation services (99241-99255) are limited to initial evaluation and do not involve psychiatric treatment. Follow-up visits in the consultant's office or other outpatient facility that are initiated by the physician consultant or patient are reported using the appropriate codes for established patients, office visits (99211-99215), domiciliary, rest home (99334-99337), or home (99347-99350). If an additional request for an opinion or advice regarding the same or a new problem is received from another physician or other appropriate source and documented in the medical record, the office consultation codes may be used again. Services that constitute transfer of care (ie, are provided for the management of the patient's entire care or for the care of a specific condition or problem) are reported with the appropriate new or established patient codes for office or other outpatient visits, domiciliary, rest home services, or home services.

## Psychiatric Diagnostic or Evaluative Interview Procedures

Psychiatric diagnostic interview examination includes a history, mental status, and a disposition, and may include communication with family or other sources, ordering and medical interpretation of laboratory or other medical diagnostic studies. In certain circumstances other informants will be seen in lieu of the patient.

Interactive psychiatric diagnostic interview examination is typically furnished to children. It involves the use of physical aids and non-verbal communication to overcome barriers to therapeutic interaction between the clinician and a patient who has not yet developed, or has lost, either the expressive language communication skills to explain his/her symptoms and response to treatment, or the receptive communication skills to understand the clinician if he/she were to use ordinary adult language for communication.

**90801**   Psychiatric diagnostic interview examination

**90802**   Interactive psychiatric diagnostic interview examination using play equipment, physical devices, language interpreter, or other mechanisms of communication

## Psychiatric Therapeutic Procedures

Psychotherapy is the treatment for mental illness and behavioral disturbances in which the clinician establishes a professional contract with the patient and, through definitive therapeutic communication, attempts to alleviate the emotional disturbances, reverse or change maladaptive patterns of behavior, and encourage personality growth and development. The codes for reporting psychotherapy are divided into two broad categories: Interactive Psychotherapy; and Insight Oriented, Behavior Modifying and/or Supportive Psychotherapy.

Interactive psychotherapy is typically furnished to children. It involves the use of physical aids and non-verbal communication to overcome barriers to therapeutic interaction between the clinician and a patient who has not yet developed, or has lost, either the expressive language communication skills to explain his/her symptoms and response to treatment, or the receptive

communication skills to understand the clinician if he/she were to use ordinary adult language for communication.

Insight oriented, behavior modifying and/or supportive psychotherapy refers to the development of insight or affective understanding, the use of behavior modification techniques, the use of supportive interactions, the use of cognitive discussion of reality, or any combination of the above to provide therapeutic change.

Some patients receive psychotherapy only and others receive psychotherapy and medical evaluation and management services. These evaluation and management services involve a variety of responsibilities unique to the medical management of psychiatric patients, such as medical diagnostic evaluation (eg, evaluation of comorbid medical conditions, drug interactions, and physical examinations), drug management when indicated, physician orders, interpretation of laboratory or other medical diagnostic studies and observations.

In reporting psychotherapy, the appropriate code is chosen on the basis of the type of psychotherapy (interactive using non-verbal techniques versus insight oriented, behavior modifying and/or supportive using verbal techniques), the place of service (office versus inpatient), the face-to-face time spent with the patient during psychotherapy, and whether evaluation and management services are furnished on the same date of service as psychotherapy. Face-to-face time when providing psychotherapy with medical evaluation and management services includes time spent providing both psychotherapy and evaluation and management services (ie, 90809, 90811, 90813, 90815, 90817, 90819, 90822, 90824, 90827, 90829).

To report medical evaluation and management services furnished on a day when psychotherapy is not provided, select the appropriate code from the **Evaluation and Management Services Guidelines.**

## Office or Other Outpatient Facility

### Insight Oriented, Behavior Modifying and/or Supportive Psychotherapy

**90804**   Individual psychotherapy, insight oriented, behavior modifying and/or supportive, in an office or outpatient facility, approximately 20 to 30 minutes face-to-face with the patient;

**90805**       with medical evaluation and management services

**90806**   Individual psychotherapy, insight oriented, behavior modifying and/or supportive, in an office or outpatient facility, approximately 45 to 50 minutes face-to-face with the patient;

**90807**       with medical evaluation and management services

**Medicine**

**90808**  Individual psychotherapy, insight oriented, behavior modifying and/or supportive, in an office or outpatient facility, approximately 75 to 80 minutes face-to-face with the patient;

**90809**     with medical evaluation and management services

### Interactive Psychotherapy

**90810**  Individual psychotherapy, interactive, using play equipment, physical devices, language interpreter, or other mechanisms of non-verbal communication, in an office or outpatient facility, approximately 20 to 30 minutes face-to-face with the patient;

**90811**     with medical evaluation and management services

**90812**  Individual psychotherapy, interactive, using play equipment, physical devices, language interpreter, or other mechanisms of non-verbal communication, in an office or outpatient facility, approximately 45 to 50 minutes face-to-face with the patient;

**90813**     with medical evaluation and management services

**90814**  Individual psychotherapy, interactive, using play equipment, physical devices, language interpreter, or other mechanisms of non-verbal communication, in an office or outpatient facility, approximately 75 to 80 minutes face-to-face with the patient;

**90815**     with medical evaluation and management services

## Inpatient Hospital, Partial Hospital or Residential Care Facility

### Insight Oriented, Behavior Modifying and/ or Supportive Psychotherapy

**90816**  Individual psychotherapy, insight oriented, behavior modifying and/or supportive, in an inpatient hospital, partial hospital or residential care setting, approximately 20 to 30 minutes face-to-face with the patient;

**90817**     with medical evaluation and management services

**90818**  Individual psychotherapy, insight oriented, behavior modifying and/or supportive, in an inpatient hospital, partial hospital or residential care setting, approximately 45 to 50 minutes face-to-face with the patient;

**90819**     with medical evaluation and management services

**90821**  Individual psychotherapy, insight oriented, behavior modifying and/or supportive, in an inpatient hospital, partial hospital or residential care setting, approximately 75 to 80 minutes face-to-face with the patient;

**90822**     with medical evaluation and management services

### Interactive Psychotherapy

**90823**  Individual psychotherapy, interactive, using play equipment, physical devices, language interpreter, or other mechanisms of non-verbal communication, in an inpatient hospital, partial hospital or residential care setting, approximately 20 to 30 minutes face-to-face with the patient;

**90824**     with medical evaluation and management services

**90826**  Individual psychotherapy, interactive, using play equipment, physical devices, language interpreter, or other mechanisms of non-verbal communication, in an inpatient hospital, partial hospital or residential care setting, approximately 45 to 50 minutes face-to-face with the patient;

**90827**     with medical evaluation and management services

**90828**  Individual psychotherapy, interactive, using play equipment, physical devices, language interpreter, or other mechanisms of non-verbal communication, in an inpatient hospital, partial hospital or residential care setting, approximately 75 to 80 minutes face-to-face with the patient;

**90829**     with medical evaluation and management services

## Other Psychotherapy

**90845**  Psychoanalysis

**90846**  Family psychotherapy (without the patient present)

**90847**  Family psychotherapy (conjoint psychotherapy) (with patient present)

**90849**  Multiple-family group psychotherapy

**90853**  Group psychotherapy (other than of a multiple-family group)

**90857**  Interactive group psychotherapy

## Other Psychiatric Services or Procedures

(For analysis/programming of neurostimulators used for vagus nerve stimulation therapy, see 95970, 95974, 95975)

**90862**  Pharmacologic management, including prescription, use, and review of medication with no more than minimal medical psychotherapy

**90865**  Narcosynthesis for psychiatric diagnostic and therapeutic purposes (eg, sodium amobarbital (Amytal) interview)

▲ **90867**  Therapeutic repetitive transcranial magnetic stimulation (TMS) treatment; initial, including cortical mapping, motor threshold determination, delivery and management

(Report only once per course of treatment)

▶(Do not report 90867 in conjunction with 95928, 95929, 90868, 90869)◀

▲ **90868**     subsequent delivery and management, per session

● **90869**     subsequent motor threshold re-determination with delivery and management

▶(Do not report 90869 in conjunction with 90867, 90868)◀

▶(If a significant, separately identifiable Evaluation and Management, medication management, psychotherapy or psychotherapy with evaluation and management service is performed, the appropriate E/M, psychotherapy, psychotherapy with E/M service or 90862 may be reported in addition to 90867-90869. Evaluation and management activities directly related to cortical mapping, motor threshold determination, delivery and management of TMS are not separately reported.)◀

**90870**     Electroconvulsive therapy (includes necessary monitoring)

**90875**     Individual psychophysiological therapy incorporating biofeedback training by any modality (face-to-face with the patient), with psychotherapy (eg, insight oriented, behavior modifying or supportive psychotherapy); approximately 20-30 minutes

**90876**          approximately 45-50 minutes

**90880**     Hypnotherapy

**90882**     Environmental intervention for medical management purposes on a psychiatric patient's behalf with agencies, employers, or institutions

**90885**     Psychiatric evaluation of hospital records, other psychiatric reports, psychometric and/or projective tests, and other accumulated data for medical diagnostic purposes

**90887**     Interpretation or explanation of results of psychiatric, other medical examinations and procedures, or other accumulated data to family or other responsible persons, or advising them how to assist patient

**90889**     Preparation of report of patient's psychiatric status, history, treatment, or progress (other than for legal or consultative purposes) for other physicians, agencies, or insurance carriers

**90899**     Unlisted psychiatric service or procedure

# Biofeedback

(For psychophysiological therapy incorporating biofeedback training, see 90875, 90876)

**90901**     Biofeedback training by any modality

**90911**     Biofeedback training, perineal muscles, anorectal or urethral sphincter, including EMG and/or manometry

(For testing of rectal sensation, tone and compliance, use 91120)

(For incontinence treatment by pulsed magnetic neuromodulation, use 53899)

# Dialysis

(90918, 90922 have been deleted. To report ESRD-related services for patients younger than 2 years of age, see 90951-90953, 90963, 90967)

(90919, 90923 have been deleted. To report ESRD-related services for patients between 2 and 11 years of age, see 90954-90956, 90964, 90968)

(90920, 90924 have been deleted. To report ESRD-related services for patients between 12 and 19 years of age, see 90957-90959, 90965, 90969)

(90921, 90925 have been deleted. To report ESRD-related services for patients 20 years of age and older, see 90960-90962, 90966, 90970)

# Hemodialysis

Codes 90935, 90937 are reported to describe the hemodialysis procedure with all evaluation and management services related to the patient's renal disease on the day of the hemodialysis procedure. These codes are used for inpatient ESRD and non-ESRD procedures or for outpatient non-ESRD dialysis services. Code 90935 is reported if only one evaluation of the patient is required related to that hemodialysis procedure. Code 90937 is reported when patient re-evaluation(s) is required during a hemodialysis procedure. Use modifier 25 with Evaluation and Management codes for separately identifiable services unrelated to the dialysis procedure or renal failure which cannot be rendered during the dialysis session.

(For home visit hemodialysis services performed by a non-physician health care professional, use 99512)

(For cannula declotting, see 36831, 36833, 36860, 36861)

(For declotting of implanted vascular access device or catheter by thrombolytic agent, use 36593)

(For collection of blood specimen from a partially or completely implantable venous access device, use 36591)

(For prolonged physician attendance, see 99354-99360)

**90935**     Hemodialysis procedure with single physician evaluation

**90937**     Hemodialysis procedure requiring repeated evaluation(s) with or without substantial revision of dialysis prescription

**90940**     Hemodialysis access flow study to determine blood flow in grafts and arteriovenous fistulae by an indicator method

(For duplex scan of hemodialysis access, use 93990)

**Medicine**

# Miscellaneous Dialysis Procedures

Codes 90945, 90947 describe dialysis procedures other than hemodialysis (eg, peritoneal dialysis, hemofiltration or continuous renal replacement therapies), and all evaluation and management services related to the patient's renal disease on the day of the procedure. Code 90945 is reported if only one evaluation of the patient is required related to that procedure. Code 90947 is reported when patient re-evaluation(s) is required during a procedure. Utilize modifier 25 with Evaluation and Management codes for separately identifiable services unrelated to the procedure or the renal failure which cannot be rendered during the dialysis session.

> (For percutaneous insertion of intraperitoneal tunneled catheter, use 49418. For open insertion of tunneled intraperitoneal catheter, use 49421)

> (For prolonged physician attendance, see 99354-99360)

**90945**  Dialysis procedure other than hemodialysis (eg, peritoneal dialysis, hemofiltration, or other continuous renal replacement therapies), with single physician evaluation

> (For home infusion of peritoneal dialysis, use 99601, 99602)

**90947**  Dialysis procedure other than hemodialysis (eg, peritoneal dialysis, hemofiltration, or other continuous renal replacement therapies) requiring repeated physician evaluations, with or without substantial revision of dialysis prescription

# End-Stage Renal Disease Services

Codes 90951-90962 are reported **once** per month to distinguish age-specific services related to the patient's end-stage renal disease (ESRD) performed in an outpatient setting with three levels of service based on the number of face-to-face visits. ESRD-related physician services include establishment of a dialyzing cycle, outpatient evaluation and management of the dialysis visits, telephone calls, and patient management during the dialysis provided during a full month. In the circumstances where the patient has had a complete assessment visit during the month and services are provided over a period of less than a month, 90951-90962 may be used according to the number of visits performed.

Codes 90963-90966 are reported once per month for a full month of service to distinguish age-specific services for end-stage renal disease (ESRD) services for home dialysis patients.

For ESRD and non-ESRD dialysis services performed in an inpatient setting, and for non-ESRD dialysis services performed in an outpatient setting, see 90935-90937 and 90945-90947.

Evaluation and Management services unrelated to ESRD services that cannot be performed during the dialysis session may be reported separately.

Codes 90967-90970 are reported to distinguish age-specific services for end-stage renal disease (ESRD) services for less than a full month of service, per day, for services provided under the following circumstances: home dialysis patients less than a full month, transient patients, partial month where there was one or more face-to-face visits without the complete assessment, the patient was hospitalized before a complete assessment was furnished, dialysis was stopped due to recovery or death, or the patient received a kidney transplant. For reporting purposes, each month is considered 30 days.

*Examples:*

ESRD-related services:

ESRD-related services are initiated on July 1 for a 57-year-old male. On July 11, he is admitted to the hospital as an inpatient and is discharged on July 27. He has had a complete assessment and the physician has performed two face-to-face visits prior to admission. Another face-to-face visit occurs after discharge during the month.

In this example, 90961 is reported for the three face-to-face outpatient visits. Report inpatient E/M services as appropriate. Dialysis procedures rendered during the hospitalization (July 11-27) should be reported as appropriate (90935-90937, 90945-90947).

If the patient did not have a complete assessment during the month or was a transient or dialysis was stopped due to recovery or death, 90970 would be used to report each day outside the inpatient hospitalization as described in the home dialysis example below.

ESRD-related services for the home dialysis patient:

Home ESRD-related services are initiated on July 1 for a 57-year-old male. On July 11, he is admitted to the hospital as an inpatient and is discharged on July 27.

In this example, 90970 should be reported for each day outside of the inpatient hospitalization (30 days/month less 17 days/hospitalization = 13 days). Report inpatient E/M services as appropriate. Dialysis procedures rendered during the hospitalization (July 11-27) should be reported as appropriate (90935-90937, 90945-90947).

**90951**  End-stage renal disease (ESRD) related services monthly, for patients younger than 2 years of age to include monitoring for the adequacy of nutrition, assessment of growth and development, and counseling of parents; with 4 or more face-to-face physician visits per month

**90952**  with 2-3 face-to-face physician visits per month

**90953**  with 1 face-to-face physician visit per month

**90954**  End-stage renal disease (ESRD) related services monthly, for patients 2-11 years of age to include monitoring for the adequacy of nutrition, assessment of growth and development, and counseling of parents; with 4 or more face-to-face physician visits per month

**90955**  with 2-3 face-to-face physician visits per month

| | |
|---|---|
| **90956** | with 1 face-to-face physician visit per month |
| **90957** | End-stage renal disease (ESRD) related services monthly, for patients 12-19 years of age to include monitoring for the adequacy of nutrition, assessment of growth and development, and counseling of parents; with 4 or more face-to-face physician visits per month |
| **90958** | with 2-3 face-to-face physician visits per month |
| **90959** | with 1 face-to-face physician visit per month |
| **90960** | End-stage renal disease (ESRD) related services monthly, for patients 20 years of age and older; with 4 or more face-to-face physician visits per month |
| **90961** | with 2-3 face-to-face physician visits per month |
| **90962** | with 1 face-to-face physician visit per month |
| **90963** | End-stage renal disease (ESRD) related services for home dialysis per full month, for patients younger than 2 years of age to include monitoring for the adequacy of nutrition, assessment of growth and development, and counseling of parents |
| **90964** | End-stage renal disease (ESRD) related services for home dialysis per full month, for patients 2-11 years of age to include monitoring for the adequacy of nutrition, assessment of growth and development, and counseling of parents |
| **90965** | End-stage renal disease (ESRD) related services for home dialysis per full month, for patients 12-19 years of age to include monitoring for the adequacy of nutrition, assessment of growth and development, and counseling of parents |
| **90966** | End-stage renal disease (ESRD) related services for home dialysis per full month, for patients 20 years of age and older |
| **90967** | End-stage renal disease (ESRD) related services for dialysis less than a full month of service, per day; for patients younger than 2 years of age |
| **90968** | for patients 2-11 years of age |
| **90969** | for patients 12-19 years of age |
| **90970** | for patients 20 years of age and older |

## Other Dialysis Procedures

| | |
|---|---|
| **90989** | Dialysis training, patient, including helper where applicable, any mode, completed course |
| **90993** | Dialysis training, patient, including helper where applicable, any mode, course not completed, per training session |
| **90997** | Hemoperfusion (eg, with activated charcoal or resin) |
| **90999** | Unlisted dialysis procedure, inpatient or outpatient |

# Gastroenterology

(For duodenal intubation and aspiration, see 43756, 43757)

(For gastrointestinal radiologic procedures, see 74210-74363)

(For esophagoscopy procedures, see 43200-43228; upper GI endoscopy 43234-43259; endoscopy, small intestine and stomal 44360-44393; proctosigmoidoscopy 45300-45321; sigmoidoscopy 45330-45339; colonoscopy 45355-45385; anoscopy 46600-46615)

(91000 has been deleted)

▲ **91010** Esophageal motility (manometric study of the esophagus and/or gastroesophageal junction) study with interpretation and report;

►(91011, 91012 have been deleted. To report esophageal motility studies with stimulant or perfusion, use 91013 in conjunction with 91010)◄

+▲ **91013** with stimulation or perfusion (eg, stimulant, acid or alkali perfusion) (List separately in addition to code for primary procedure)

(Use 91013 in conjunction with 91010)

(Do not report 91013 more than once per session)

►(To report esophageal motility studies with high resolution esophageal pressure topography, use 0240T and with stimulant or perfusion, use 0241T)◄

**91020** Gastric motility (manometric) studies

**91022** Duodenal motility (manometric) study

(If gastrointestinal endoscopy is performed, use 43235)

(If fluoroscopy is performed, use 76000)

(If gastric motility study is performed, use 91020)

(Do not report 91020, 91022 in conjunction with 0242T)

**91030** Esophagus, acid perfusion (Bernstein) test for esophagitis

**91034** Esophagus, gastroesophageal reflux test; with nasal catheter pH electrode(s) placement, recording, analysis and interpretation

**91035** with mucosal attached telemetry pH electrode placement, recording, analysis and interpretation

**91037** Esophageal function test, gastroesophageal reflux test with nasal catheter intraluminal impedance electrode(s) placement, recording, analysis and interpretation;

**91038** prolonged (greater than 1 hour, up to 24 hours)

**91040** Esophageal balloon distension provocation study

(For balloon dilatation with endoscopy, see 43220, 43249, 43456, or 43458)

(91052, 91055 have been deleted. To report, see 43754, 43755)

**Medicine**

**91065** Breath hydrogen test (eg, for detection of lactase deficiency, fructose intolerance, bacterial overgrowth, or oro-cecal gastrointestinal transit)

(For H. pylori breath test analysis, use 83013 for non-radioactive (C-13) isotope or 78268 for radioactive (C-14) isotope)

(91100 has been deleted)

(To report placement of an esophageal tamponade tube for management of variceal bleeding, use 43460. To report placement of a long intestinal Miller-Abbott tube, use 44500)

(91105 has been deleted. To report, use 43753)

(For cholangiography, see 47500, 74320)

►(For abdominal paracentesis, see 49082, 49083, 49084; with instillation of medication, see 96440, 96446)◄

(For peritoneoscopy, use 49320; with biopsy, use 49321)

(For peritoneoscopy and guided transhepatic cholangiography, use 47560; with biopsy, use 47561)

(For splenoportography, see 38200, 75810)

**91110** Gastrointestinal tract imaging, intraluminal (eg, capsule endoscopy), esophagus through ileum, with physician interpretation and report

(Visualization of the colon is not reported separately)

(Append modifier 52 if the ileum is not visualized)

**91111** Gastrointestinal tract imaging, intraluminal (eg, capsule endoscopy), esophagus with physician interpretation and report

(Do not report 91111 in conjunction with 91110)

(For measurement of gastrointestinal tract transit times or pressure using wireless capsule, use 0242T)

**91117** Colon motility (manometric) study, minimum 6 hours continuous recording (including provocation tests, eg, meal, intracolonic balloon distension, pharmacologic agents, if performed), with interpretation and report

(For wireless capsule pressure measurements, use 0242T)

(Do not report 91117 in conjunction with 91120, 91122)

**91120** Rectal sensation, tone, and compliance test (ie, response to graded balloon distention)

(For biofeedback training, use 90911)

(For anorectal manometry, use 91122)

**91122** Anorectal manometry

(Do not report 91120, 91122 in conjunction with 91117)

(91123 has been deleted)

# Gastric Physiology

**91132** Electrogastrography, diagnostic, transcutaneous;

**91133** with provocative testing

# Other Procedures

**91299** Unlisted diagnostic gastroenterology procedure

# Ophthalmology

(For surgical procedures, see **Surgery,** Eye and Ocular Adnexa, 65091 et seq)

### Definitions

*Intermediate ophthalmological services* describes an evaluation of a new or existing condition complicated with a new diagnostic or management problem not necessarily relating to the primary diagnosis, including history, general medical observation, external ocular and adnexal examination and other diagnostic procedures as indicated; may include the use of mydriasis for ophthalmoscopy.

*For example:*

a. Review of history, external examination, ophthalmoscopy, biomicroscopy for an acute complicated condition (eg, iritis) not requiring comprehensive ophthalmological services.

b. Review of interval history, external examination, ophthalmoscopy, biomicroscopy and tonometry in established patient with known cataract not requiring comprehensive ophthalmological services.

*Comprehensive ophthalmological services* describes a general evaluation of the complete visual system. The comprehensive services constitute a single service entity but need not be performed at one session. The service includes history, general medical observation, external and ophthalmoscopic examinations, gross visual fields and basic sensorimotor examination. It often includes, as indicated: biomicroscopy, examination with cycloplegia or mydriasis and tonometry. It always includes initiation of diagnostic and treatment programs.

Intermediate and comprehensive ophthalmological services constitute integrated services in which medical decision making cannot be separated from the examining techniques used. Itemization of service components, such as slit lamp examination, keratometry, routine ophthalmoscopy, retinoscopy, tonometry, or motor evaluation is not applicable.

*For example:*

The comprehensive services required for diagnosis and treatment of a patient with symptoms indicating possible disease of the visual system, such as glaucoma, cataract or retinal disease, or to rule out disease of the visual system, new or established patient.

*Initiation of diagnostic and treatment program* includes the prescription of medication, and arranging for special ophthalmological diagnostic or treatment services, consultations, laboratory procedures and radiological services.

Medicine

*Special ophthalmological services* describes services in which a special evaluation of part of the visual system is made, which goes beyond the services included under general ophthalmological services, or in which special treatment is given. Special ophthalmological services may be reported in addition to the general ophthalmological services or evaluation and management services.

*For example:*

Fluorescein angioscopy, quantitative visual field examination, refraction or extended color vision examination (such as Nagel's anomaloscope) should be separately reported.

Prescription of lenses, when required, is included in 92015. It includes specification of lens type (monofocal, bifocal, other), lens power, axis, prism, absorptive factor, impact resistance, and other factors.

Interpretation and report by the physician is an integral part of special ophthalmological services where indicated. Technical procedures (which may or may not be performed by the physician personally) are often part of the service, but should not be mistaken to constitute the service itself.

# General Ophthalmological Services

## New Patient

Solely for the purposes of distinguishing between new and established patients, **professional services** are those face-to-face services rendered by a physician and reported by a specific code(s). A new patient is one who has not received any professional services from the physician or another physician of the same specialty who belongs to the same group practice within the past three years.

**92002**   Ophthalmological services: medical examination and evaluation with initiation of diagnostic and treatment program; intermediate, new patient

**92004**   comprehensive, new patient, 1 or more visits

## Established Patient

Solely for the purposes of distinguishing between new and established patients, **professional services** are those face-to-face services rendered by a physician and reported by a specific code(s). An established patient is one who has received professional services from the physician or another physician of the same specialty who belongs to the same group practice within the past three years.

**92012**   Ophthalmological services: medical examination and evaluation, with initiation or continuation of diagnostic and treatment program; intermediate, established patient

**92014**   comprehensive, established patient, 1 or more visits

(For surgical procedures, see **Surgery,** Eye and Ocular Adnexa, 65091 et seq)

# Special Ophthalmological Services

**92015**   Determination of refractive state

**92018**   Ophthalmological examination and evaluation, under general anesthesia, with or without manipulation of globe for passive range of motion or other manipulation to facilitate diagnostic examination; complete

**92019**   limited

**92020**   Gonioscopy (separate procedure)

(For gonioscopy under general anesthesia, use 92018)

**92025**   Computerized corneal topography, unilateral or bilateral, with interpretation and report

(Do not report 92025 in conjunction with 65710-65771)

(92025 is not used for manual keratoscopy, which is part of a single system Evaluation and Management or ophthalmological service)

**92060**   Sensorimotor examination with multiple measurements of ocular deviation (eg, restrictive or paretic muscle with diplopia) with interpretation and report (separate procedure)

**92065**   Orthoptic and/or pleoptic training, with continuing medical direction and evaluation

▶(92070 has been deleted. To report, see 92071, 92072)◀

● **92071**   Fitting of contact lens for treatment of ocular surface disease

▶(Do not report 92071 in conjunction with 92072)◀

▶(Report supply of lens separately with 99070 or appropriate supply code)◀

● **92072**   Fitting of contact lens for management of keratoconus, initial fitting

▶(For subsequent fittings, report using Evaluation and Management services or General Ophthalmological Services )◀

▶(Do not report 92072 in conjunction with 92071)◀

▶(Report supply of lens separately with 99070 or appropriate supply code)◀

**92081**   Visual field examination, unilateral or bilateral, with interpretation and report; limited examination (eg, tangent screen, Autoplot, arc perimeter, or single stimulus level automated test, such as Octopus 3 or 7 equivalent)

**92082**   intermediate examination (eg, at least 2 isopters on Goldmann perimeter, or semiquantitative, automated suprathreshold screening program, Humphrey suprathreshold automatic diagnostic test, Octopus program 33)

**92083**   extended examination (eg, Goldmann visual fields with at least 3 isopters plotted and static determination within the central 30°, or quantitative, automated threshold perimetry, Octopus program G-1, 32 or 42, Humphrey visual field analyzer full threshold programs 30-2, 24-2, or 30/60-2)

**Medicine**

(Gross visual field testing (eg, confrontation testing) is a part of general ophthalmological services and is not reported separately)

**92100** Serial tonometry (separate procedure) with multiple measurements of intraocular pressure over an extended time period with interpretation and report, same day (eg, diurnal curve or medical treatment of acute elevation of intraocular pressure)

▶(92120, 92130 have been deleted)◀

▶(Ocular blood flow measurements are reported with 0198T. Single-episode tonometry is a component of general ophthalmological service or E/M service)◀

**92132** Scanning computerized ophthalmic diagnostic imaging, anterior segment, with interpretation and report, unilateral or bilateral

**92133** Scanning computerized ophthalmic diagnostic imaging, posterior segment, with interpretation and report, unilateral or bilateral; optic nerve

**92134** retina

(Do not report 92133 and 92134 at the same patient encounter)

(92135 has been deleted)

(For scanning computerized ophthalmic diagnostic imaging of the optic nerve and retina, see 92133, 92134)

**92136** Ophthalmic biometry by partial coherence interferometry with intraocular lens power calculation

**92140** Provocative tests for glaucoma, with interpretation and report, without tonography

## Ophthalmoscopy

Routine ophthalmoscopy is part of general and special ophthalmologic services whenever indicated. It is a non-itemized service and is not reported separately.

**92225** Ophthalmoscopy, extended, with retinal drawing (eg, for retinal detachment, melanoma), with interpretation and report; initial

**92226** subsequent

**92227** Remote imaging for detection of retinal disease (eg, retinopathy in a patient with diabetes) with analysis and report under physician supervision, unilateral or bilateral

(Do not report 92227 in conjunction with 92002-92014, 92133, 92134, 92250, 92228 or with the evaluation and management of the single organ system, the eye, 99201-99350)

**92228** Remote imaging for monitoring and management of active retinal disease (eg, diabetic retinopathy) with physician review, interpretation and report, unilateral or bilateral

(Do not report 92228 in conjunction with 92002-92014, 92133, 92134, 92250, 92227 or with the evaluation and management of the single organ system, the eye, 99201-99350)

**92230** Fluorescein angioscopy with interpretation and report

**92235** Fluorescein angiography (includes multiframe imaging) with interpretation and report

**92240** Indocyanine-green angiography (includes multiframe imaging) with interpretation and report

**92250** Fundus photography with interpretation and report

**92260** Ophthalmodynamometry

(For ophthalmoscopy under general anesthesia, use 92018)

## Other Specialized Services

▶For prescription, fitting, and/or medical supervision of ocular prosthetic (artificial eye) adaptation by a physician, see Evaluation and Management services including Office or Other Outpatient services (99201-99215), Office or Other Outpatient Consultations (99241-99245) or General Ophthalmological service codes 92002-92014.◀

**92265** Needle oculoelectromyography, 1 or more extraocular muscles, 1 or both eyes, with interpretation and report

**92270** Electro-oculography with interpretation and report

**92275** Electroretinography with interpretation and report

(For electronystagmography for vestibular function studies, see 92541 et seq)

(For ophthalmic echography (diagnostic ultrasound), see 76511-76529)

**92283** Color vision examination, extended, eg, anomaloscope or equivalent

(Color vision testing with pseudoisochromatic plates [such as HRR or Ishihara] is not reported separately. It is included in the appropriate general or ophthalmological service, or 99172)

**92284** Dark adaptation examination with interpretation and report

**92285** External ocular photography with interpretation and report for documentation of medical progress (eg, close-up photography, slit lamp photography, goniophotography, stereo-photography)

**92286** Special anterior segment photography with interpretation and report; with specular endothelial microscopy and cell count

**92287** with fluorescein angiography

## Contact Lens Services

The prescription of contact lens includes specification of optical and physical characteristics (such as power, size, curvature, flexibility, gas-permeability). It is NOT a part of the general ophthalmological services.

The fitting of contact lens includes instruction and training of the wearer and incidental revision of the lens during the training period.

⊙=Moderate sedation  ✚=Add-on code  ✗=FDA approval pending  #=Resequenced code  ○=Recycled/reinstated code

Follow-up of successfully fitted extended wear lenses is reported as part of a general ophthalmological service (92012 et seq).

The supply of contact lenses may be reported as part of the service of fitting. It may also be reported separately by using the appropriate supply codes.

▶(For therapeutic or surgical use of contact lens, see 68340, 92071, 92072)◀

**92310** Prescription of optical and physical characteristics of and fitting of contact lens, with medical supervision of adaptation; corneal lens, both eyes, except for aphakia

(For prescription and fitting of 1 eye, add modifier 52)

**92311** corneal lens for aphakia, 1 eye

**92312** corneal lens for aphakia, both eyes

**92313** corneoscleral lens

**92314** Prescription of optical and physical characteristics of contact lens, with medical supervision of adaptation and direction of fitting by independent technician; corneal lens, both eyes except for aphakia

(For prescription and fitting of 1 eye, add modifier 52)

**92315** corneal lens for aphakia, 1 eye

**92316** corneal lens for aphakia, both eyes

**92317** corneoscleral lens

**92325** Modification of contact lens (separate procedure), with medical supervision of adaptation

**92326** Replacement of contact lens

## Spectacle Services (Including Prosthesis for Aphakia)

Prescription of lenses, when required, is included in 92015 Determination of refractive state. It includes specification of lens type (monofocal, bifocal, other), lens power, axis, prism, absorptive factor, impact resistance, and other factors.

Fitting of spectacles is a separate service; when provided by the physician, it is reported as indicated by 92340-92371.

Fitting includes measurement of anatomical facial characteristics, the writing of laboratory specifications, and the final adjustment of the spectacles to the visual axes and anatomical topography. Presence of physician is not required.

Supply of materials is a separate service component; it is not part of the service of fitting spectacles.

**92340** Fitting of spectacles, except for aphakia; monofocal

**92341** bifocal

**92342** multifocal, other than bifocal

**92352** Fitting of spectacle prosthesis for aphakia; monofocal

**92353** multifocal

**92354** Fitting of spectacle mounted low vision aid; single element system

**92355** telescopic or other compound lens system

**92358** Prosthesis service for aphakia, temporary (disposable or loan, including materials)

**92370** Repair and refitting spectacles; except for aphakia

**92371** spectacle prosthesis for aphakia

## Other Procedures

**92499** Unlisted ophthalmological service or procedure

# Special Otorhinolaryngologic Services

Diagnostic or treatment procedures that are reported as evaluation and management services (eg, otoscopy, anterior rhinoscopy, tuning fork test, removal of non-impacted cerumen) are not reported separately.

Special otorhinolaryngologic services are those diagnostic and treatment services not included in an Evaluation and Management service. These services are reported separately, using codes 92502-92700.

Code 92506 is used to report evaluation of speech production, receptive language, and expressive language abilities. Tests may examine speech sound production, articulatory movements of oral musculature, the patient's ability to understand the meaning and intent of written and verbal expressions, and the appropriate formulation and utterance of expressive thought. In contrast, 92626 and 92627 are reported for an evaluation of auditory rehabilitation status determining the patient's ability to use residual hearing in order to identify the acoustic characteristics of sounds associated with speech communication.

(For laryngoscopy with stroboscopy, use 31579)

**92502** Otolaryngologic examination under general anesthesia

**92504** Binocular microscopy (separate diagnostic procedure)

**92506** Evaluation of speech, language, voice, communication, and/or auditory processing

**92507** Treatment of speech, language, voice, communication, and/or auditory processing disorder; individual

**92508** group, 2 or more individuals

(For auditory rehabilitation, prelingual hearing loss, use 92630)

(For auditory rehabilitation, postlingual hearing loss, use 92633)

(For cochlear implant programming, see 92601-92604)

**92511** Nasopharyngoscopy with endoscope (separate procedure)

**Medicine**

92512    Nasal function studies (eg, rhinomanometry)

92516    Facial nerve function studies (eg, electroneuronography)

92520    Laryngeal function studies (ie, aerodynamic testing and acoustic testing)

(For performance of a single test, use modifier 52)

(To report flexible fiberoptic laryngeal evaluation of swallowing and laryngeal sensory testing, see 92611-92617)

(To report other testing of laryngeal function (eg, electroglottography), use 92700)

92526    Treatment of swallowing dysfunction and/or oral function for feeding

## Vestibular Function Tests, Without Electrical Recording

92531    Spontaneous nystagmus, including gaze

92532    Positional nystagmus test

(Do not report 92531, 92532 with evaluation and management services)

92533    Caloric vestibular test, each irrigation (binaural, bithermal stimulation constitutes 4 tests)

92534    Optokinetic nystagmus test

## Vestibular Function Tests, With Recording (eg, ENG)

92540    Basic vestibular evaluation, includes spontaneous nystagmus test with eccentric gaze fixation nystagmus, with recording, positional nystagmus test, minimum of 4 positions, with recording, optokinetic nystagmus test, bidirectional foveal and peripheral stimulation, with recording, and oscillating tracking test, with recording

(Do not report 92540 in conjunction with 92541, 92542, 92544, or 92545)

92541    Spontaneous nystagmus test, including gaze and fixation nystagmus, with recording

(Do not report 92541 in conjunction with 92540 or the set of 92542, 92544, 92545)

92542    Positional nystagmus test, minimum of 4 positions, with recording

(Do not report 92542 in conjunction with 92540 or the set of 92541, 92544, and 92545)

92543    Caloric vestibular test, each irrigation (binaural, bithermal stimulation constitutes 4 tests), with recording

92544    Optokinetic nystagmus test, bidirectional, foveal or peripheral stimulation, with recording

(Do not report 92544 in conjunction with 92540 or the set of 92541, 92542, and 92545)

92545    Oscillating tracking test, with recording

(Do not report 92545 in conjunction with 92540 or the set of 92541, 92542, and 92544)

92546    Sinusoidal vertical axis rotational testing

+ 92547    Use of vertical electrodes (List separately in addition to code for primary procedure)

(Use 92547 in conjunction with 92540-92546)

(For unlisted vestibular tests, use 92700)

92548    Computerized dynamic posturography

## Audiologic Function Tests

The audiometric tests listed below require the use of calibrated electronic equipment, recording of results and a report with interpretation. Hearing tests (such as whispered voice, tuning fork) that are otorhinolaryngologic Evaluation and Management services are not reported separately. All services include testing of both ears. Use modifier 52 if a test is applied to one ear instead of two ears. All codes (except 92559) apply to testing of individuals. For testing of groups, use 92559 and specify test(s) used.

(For evaluation of speech, language and/or hearing problems through observation and assessment of performance, use 92506)

92550    Tympanometry and reflex threshold measurements

(Do not report 92550 in conjunction with 92567, 92568)

92551    Screening test, pure tone, air only

92552    Pure tone audiometry (threshold); air only

92553        air and bone

92555    Speech audiometry threshold;

92556        with speech recognition

92557    Comprehensive audiometry threshold evaluation and speech recognition (92553 and 92556 combined)

(For hearing aid evaluation and selection, see 92590-92595)

(For automated audiometry, see 0208T-0212T)

▶ 92558    Code is out of numerical sequence. See 92550-92597◀

92559    Audiometric testing of groups

92560    Bekesy audiometry; screening

92561        diagnostic

92562    Loudness balance test, alternate binaural or monaural

92563    Tone decay test

92564    Short increment sensitivity index (SISI)

92565    Stenger test, pure tone

92567    Tympanometry (impedance testing)

Medicine

**92568**　Acoustic reflex testing, threshold

(92569 has been deleted. For acoustic reflex decay testing performed in conjunction with tympanometry, use 92570)

**92570**　Acoustic immittance testing, includes tympanometry (impedance testing), acoustic reflex threshold testing, and acoustic reflex decay testing

(Do not report 92570 in conjunction with 92567, 92568)

**92571**　Filtered speech test

**92572**　Staggered spondaic word test

**92575**　Sensorineural acuity level test

**92576**　Synthetic sentence identification test

**92577**　Stenger test, speech

**92579**　Visual reinforcement audiometry (VRA)

**92582**　Conditioning play audiometry

**92583**　Select picture audiometry

**92584**　Electrocochleography

**92585**　Auditory evoked potentials for evoked response audiometry and/or testing of the central nervous system; comprehensive

**92586**　　limited

#● **92558**　Evoked otoacoustic emissions, screening (qualitative measurement of distortion product or transient evoked otoacoustic emissions), automated analysis

▲ **92587**　Distortion product evoked otoacoustic emissions; limited evaluation (to confirm the presence or absence of hearing disorder, 3-6 frequencies) or transient evoked otoacoustic emissions, with interpretation and report

▲ **92588**　　comprehensive diagnostic evaluation (quantitative analysis of outer hair cell function by cochlear mapping, minimum of 12 frequencies), with interpretation and report

(For central auditory function evaluation, see 92620, 92621)

**92590**　Hearing aid examination and selection; monaural

**92591**　　binaural

**92592**　Hearing aid check; monaural

**92593**　　binaural

**92594**　Electroacoustic evaluation for hearing aid; monaural

**92595**　　binaural

**92596**　Ear protector attenuation measurements

**92597**　Evaluation for use and/or fitting of voice prosthetic device to supplement oral speech

(To report augmentative and alternative communication device services, see 92605, 92607, 92608)

# Evaluative and Therapeutic Services

Codes 92601 and 92603 describe post-operative analysis and fitting of previously placed external devices, connection to the cochlear implant, and programming of the stimulator. Codes 92602 and 92604 describe subsequent sessions for measurements and adjustment of the external transmitter and re-programming of the internal stimulator.

(For placement of cochlear implant, use 69930)

**92601**　Diagnostic analysis of cochlear implant, patient younger than 7 years of age; with programming

**92602**　　subsequent reprogramming

(Do not report 92602 in addition to 92601)

(For aural rehabilitation services following cochlear implant, including evaluation of rehabilitation status, see 92626-92627, 92630-92633)

**92603**　Diagnostic analysis of cochlear implant, age 7 years or older; with programming

**92604**　　subsequent reprogramming

(Do not report 92604 in addition to 92603)

▲ **92605**　Evaluation for prescription of non-speech-generating augmentative and alternative communication device, face-to-face with the patient; first hour

#+● **92618**　　each additional 30 minutes (List separately in addition to code for primary procedure)

►(Use 92618 in conjunction with 92605)◄

**92606**　Therapeutic service(s) for the use of non-speech-generating device, including programming and modification

**92607**　Evaluation for prescription for speech-generating augmentative and alternative communication device, face-to-face with the patient; first hour

(For evaluation for prescription of a non-speech-generating device, use 92605)

+ **92608**　　each additional 30 minutes (List separately in addition to code for primary procedure)

(Use 92608 in conjunction with 92607)

**92609**　Therapeutic services for the use of speech-generating device, including programming and modification

(For therapeutic service(s) for the use of a non-speech-generating device, use 92606)

**92610**　Evaluation of oral and pharyngeal swallowing function

(For motion fluoroscopic evaluation of swallowing function, use 92611)

(For flexible endoscopic examination, use 92612-92617)

**92611**　Motion fluoroscopic evaluation of swallowing function by cine or video recording

(For radiological supervision and interpretation, use 74230)

**Medicine**

(For evaluation of oral and pharyngeal swallowing function, use 92610)

(For flexible fiberoptic diagnostic laryngoscopy, use 31575. Do not report 31575 in conjunction with 92612-92617)

**92612** Flexible fiberoptic endoscopic evaluation of swallowing by cine or video recording;

(If flexible fiberoptic or endoscopic evaluation of swallowing is performed without cine or video recording, use 92700)

**92613** physician interpretation and report only

(To report an evaluation of oral and pharyngeal swallowing function, use 92610)

(To report motion fluoroscopic evaluation of swallowing function, use 92611)

**92614** Flexible fiberoptic endoscopic evaluation, laryngeal sensory testing by cine or video recording;

(If flexible fiberoptic or endoscopic evaluation of swallowing is performed without cine or video recording, use 92700)

**92615** physician interpretation and report only

**92616** Flexible fiberoptic endoscopic evaluation of swallowing and laryngeal sensory testing by cine or video recording;

(If flexible fiberoptic or endoscopic evaluation of swallowing is performed without cine or video recording, use 92700)

**92617** physician interpretation and report only

▶ **92618** Code is out of numerical sequence. See 92601-92633◀

**92620** Evaluation of central auditory function, with report; initial 60 minutes

+▲ **92621** each additional 15 minutes (List separately in addition to code for primary procedure)

▶(Use 92621 in conjunction with 92620)◀

(Do not report 92620, 92621 in conjunction with 92506)

**92625** Assessment of tinnitus (includes pitch, loudness matching, and masking)

(Do not report 92625 in conjunction with 92562)

(For unilateral assessment, use modifier 52)

**92626** Evaluation of auditory rehabilitation status; first hour

+ **92627** each additional 15 minutes (List separately in addition to code for primary procedure)

(Use 92627 in conjunction with 92626)

(When reporting 92626, 92627, use the face-to-face time with the patient or family)

**92630** Auditory rehabilitation; prelingual hearing loss

**92633** postlingual hearing loss

## Special Diagnostic Procedures

**92640** Diagnostic analysis with programming of auditory brainstem implant, per hour

(Report nonprogramming services separately [eg, cardiac monitoring])

## Other Procedures

**92700** Unlisted otorhinolaryngological service or procedure

# Cardiovascular

## Therapeutic Services and Procedures

(For nonsurgical septal reduction therapy [eg, alcohol ablation], use 93799)

**92950** Cardiopulmonary resuscitation (eg, in cardiac arrest)

(See also critical care services, 99291, 99292)

⊙ **92953** Temporary transcutaneous pacing

(For physician direction of ambulance or rescue personnel outside the hospital, use 99288)

⊙ **92960** Cardioversion, elective, electrical conversion of arrhythmia; external

⊙ **92961** internal (separate procedure)

(Do not report 92961 in conjunction with 93282-93284, 93287, 93289, 93295, 93296, 93618-93624, 93631, 93640-93642, 93650-93652, 93662)

**92970** Cardioassist-method of circulatory assist; internal

**92971** external

(For balloon atrial-septostomy, use 92992)

(For placement of catheters for use in circulatory assist devices such as intra-aortic balloon pump, use 33970)

⊙+ **92973** Percutaneous transluminal coronary thrombectomy (List separately in addition to code for primary procedure)

(Use 92973 in conjunction with 92980, 92982)

⊙+ **92974** Transcatheter placement of radiation delivery device for subsequent coronary intravascular brachytherapy (List separately in addition to code for primary procedure)

(Use 92974 in conjunction with 92980, 92982, 92995, 93454-93461)

(For intravascular radioelement application, see 77785-77787)

⊙ **92975** Thrombolysis, coronary; by intracoronary infusion, including selective coronary angiography

**92977**    by intravenous infusion

(For thrombolysis of vessels other than coronary, see 37201, 75896)

(For cerebral thrombolysis, use 37195)

⊙+ **92978**  Intravascular ultrasound (coronary vessel or graft) during diagnostic evaluation and/or therapeutic intervention including imaging supervision, interpretation and report; initial vessel (List separately in addition to code for primary procedure)

(Use 92978 in conjunction with 92975, 92980, 92982, 92995, 93454-93461, 93530-93533)

⊙+ **92979**    each additional vessel (List separately in addition to code for primary procedure)

(Use 92979 in conjunction with 92978)

(Intravascular ultrasound services include all transducer manipulations and repositioning within the specific vessel being examined, both before and after therapeutic intervention [eg, stent placement])

(For intravascular spectroscopy, use 0205T)

⊙ **92980**  Transcatheter placement of an intracoronary stent(s), percutaneous, with or without other therapeutic intervention, any method; single vessel

⊙+ **92981**    each additional vessel (List separately in addition to code for primary procedure)

(Use 92981 in conjunction with 92980)

(Codes 92980, 92981 are used to report coronary artery stenting. Coronary angioplasty [92982, 92984] or atherectomy [92995, 92996], in the same artery, is considered part of the stenting procedure and is not reported separately. Codes 92973 [percutaneous transluminal coronary thombectomy] and 92974 [coronary brachytherapy] are add-on codes for reporting procedures performed in addition to coronary stenting, atherectomy, and angioplasty and are not included in the "therapeutic interventions" in 92980). Codes 92978 and 92979 are add-on codes for reporting intravascular ultrasound procedures performed in addition to coronary and bypass graft diagnostic and interventional services.

(To report additional vessels treated by angioplasty or atherectomy only during the same session, see 92984, 92996)

(To report transcatheter placement of radiation delivery device for coronary intravascular brachytherapy, use 92974)

(For intravascular radioelement application, see 77785-77787)

⊙ **92982**  Percutaneous transluminal coronary balloon angioplasty; single vessel

⊙+ **92984**    each additional vessel (List separately in addition to code for primary procedure)

(Use 92984 in conjunction with 92980, 92982, 92995)

(For stent placement following completion of angioplasty or atherectomy, see 92980, 92981)

(To report transcatheter placement of radiation delivery device for coronary intravascular brachytherapy, use 92974)

(For intravascular radioelement application, see 77785-77787)

⊙ **92986**  Percutaneous balloon valvuloplasty; aortic valve

⊙ **92987**    mitral valve

**92990**    pulmonary valve

**92992**  Atrial septectomy or septostomy; transvenous method, balloon (eg, Rashkind type) (includes cardiac catheterization)

**92993**    blade method (Park septostomy) (includes cardiac catheterization)

⊙ **92995**  Percutaneous transluminal coronary atherectomy, by mechanical or other method, with or without balloon angioplasty; single vessel

⊙+ **92996**    each additional vessel (List separately in addition to code for primary procedure)

(Use 92996 in conjunction with 92980, 92982, 92995)

(For stent placement following completion of angioplasty or atherectomy, see 92980, 92981)

(To report additional vessels treated by angioplasty only during the same session, use 92984)

**92997**  Percutaneous transluminal pulmonary artery balloon angioplasty; single vessel

+ **92998**    each additional vessel (List separately in addition to code for primary procedure)

(Use 92998 in conjunction with 92997)

# Cardiography

Codes 93040-93042 are appropriate when an order for the test is triggered by an event, the rhythm strip is used to help diagnose the presence or absence of an arrhythmia, and a report is generated. There must be a specific order for an electrocardiogram or rhythm strip followed by a separate, signed, written, and retrievable report. It is not appropriate to use these codes for reviewing the telemetry monitor strips taken from a monitoring system. The need for an electrocardiogram or rhythm strip should be supported by documentation in the patient medical record.

(For echocardiography, see 93303-93350)

(For electrocardiogram, 64 leads or greater, with graphic presentation and analysis, see 0178T-0180T)

(For acoustic cardiography services, see 0223T-0225T)

**93000**  Electrocardiogram, routine ECG with at least 12 leads; with interpretation and report

**93005**    tracing only, without interpretation and report

**Medicine**

**93010**  interpretation and report only

(For ECG monitoring, see 99354-99360)

(93012, 93014 have been deleted. To report telephonic transmission of post-symptom electrocardiogram rhythm strips, see 93268-93272)

**93015**  Cardiovascular stress test using maximal or submaximal treadmill or bicycle exercise, continuous electrocardiographic monitoring, and/or pharmacological stress; with physician supervision, with interpretation and report

**93016**  physician supervision only, without interpretation and report

**93017**  tracing only, without interpretation and report

**93018**  interpretation and report only

**93024**  Ergonovine provocation test

**93025**  Microvolt T-wave alternans for assessment of ventricular arrhythmias

**93040**  Rhythm ECG, 1-3 leads; with interpretation and report

**93041**  tracing only without interpretation and report

**93042**  interpretation and report only

## Cardiovascular Monitoring Services

Cardiovascular monitoring services are diagnostic medical procedures using in-person and remote technology to assess cardiovascular rhythm (ECG) data. Holter monitors (93224-93227) include up to 48 hours of continuous recording. Mobile cardiac telemetry monitors (93228, 93229) have the capability of transmitting a tracing at any time, always have internal ECG analysis algorithms designed to detect major arrhythmias, and transmit to an attended surveillance center. Event monitors (93268-93272) record segments of ECGs with recording initiation triggered either by patient activation or by an internal automatic, pre-programmed detection algorithm (or both) and transmit the recorded electrocardiographic data when requested (but cannot transmit immediately based upon the patient or algorithmic activation rhythm) and require attended surveillance.

*Attended surveillance:* is the immediate availability of a remote technician to respond to rhythm or device alert transmissions from a patient, either from an implanted or wearable monitoring or therapy device, as they are generated and transmitted to the remote surveillance location or center.

*Electrocardiographic rhythm derived elements:* elements derived from recordings of the electrical activation of the heart including, but not limited to heart rhythm, rate, ST analysis, heart rate variability, T-wave alternans.

*Mobile cardiovascular telemetry (MCT):* continuously records the electrocardiographic rhythm from external electrodes placed on the patient"s body. Segments of the ECG data are automatically (without patient intervention) transmitted to a remote surveillance location by cellular or landline telephone signal. The segments of the rhythm, selected for transmission, are triggered automatically (MCT device algorithm) by rapid and slow heart rates or by the patient during a symptomatic episode. There is continuous real time data analysis by preprogrammed algorithms in the device and attended surveillance of the transmitted rhythm segments by a surveillance center technician to evaluate any arrhythmias and to determine signal quality. The surveillance center technician reviews the data and notifies the physician depending on the prescribed criteria.

ECG rhythm derived elements are distinct from physiologic data, even when the same device is capable of producing both. Implantable cardiovascular monitor (ICM) device services are always separately reported from implantable cardioverter-defibrillator (ICD) service.

**93224**  External electrocardiographic recording up to 48 hours by continuous rhythm recording and storage; includes recording, scanning analysis with report, physician review and interpretation

**93225**  recording (includes connection, recording, and disconnection)

**93226**  scanning analysis with report

**93227**  physician review and interpretation

(For less than 12 hours of continuous recording, use modifier 52)

**93228**  External mobile cardiovascular telemetry with electrocardiographic recording, concurrent computerized real time data analysis and greater than 24 hours of accessible ECG data storage (retrievable with query) with ECG triggered and patient selected events transmitted to a remote attended surveillance center for up to 30 days; physician review and interpretation with report

(Report 93228 only once per 30 days)

(Do not report 93228 in conjunction with 93224, 93227)

**93229**  technical support for connection and patient instructions for use, attended surveillance, analysis and physician prescribed transmission of daily and emergent data reports

(Report 93229 only once per 30 days)

(Do not report 93229 in conjunction with 93224, 93226)

(For external cardiovascular monitors that do not perform automatic ECG triggered transmissions to an attended surveillance center, see 93224-93227, 93268-93272)

(93230-93237 have been deleted. To report external electrocardiographic rhythm derived monitoring for up to 48 hours, see 93224-93227)

**93268**    External patient and, when performed, auto activated electrocardiographic rhythm derived event recording with symptom-related memory loop with remote download capability up to 30 days, 24-hour attended monitoring; includes transmission, physician review and interpretation

**93270**        recording (includes connection, recording, and disconnection)

**93271**        transmission and analysis

**93272**        physician review and interpretation

(For implanted patient activated cardiac event recording, see 33282, 93285, 93291, 93298)

**93278**    Signal-averaged electrocardiography (SAECG), with or without ECG

(For interpretation and report only, use 93278 with modifier 26)

(For unlisted cardiographic procedure, use 93799)

# Implantable and Wearable Cardiac Device Evaluations

Cardiac device evaluation services are diagnostic medical procedures using in-person and remote technology to assess device therapy and cardiovascular physiologic data. Codes 93279-93299 describe this technology and technical/professional physician and service center practice. Codes 93279-93292 are reported per procedure. Codes 93293-93296 are reported no more than **once** every 90 days. Do not report 93293-93296 if the monitoring period is less than 30 days. Codes 93297, 93298 are reported no more than **once** up to every 30 days. Do not report 93297-93299 if the monitoring period is less than 10 days.

A service center may report 93296 or 93299 during a period in which a physician performs an in-person interrogation device evaluation. A physician may not report an in-person and remote interrogation of the same device during the same period. Report only remote services when an in-person interrogation device evaluation is performed during a period of remote interrogation device evaluation. A period is established by the initiation of the remote monitoring or the 91st day of a pacemaker or implantable cardioverter-defibrillator (ICD) monitoring or the 31st day of an implantable loop recorder (ILR) or implantable cardiovascular monitor (ICM) monitoring and extends for the subsequent 90 or 30 days, respectively, for which remote monitoring is occurring. Programming device evaluations and in-person interrogation device evaluations may not be reported on the same date by the same physician. Programming device evaluations and remote interrogation device evaluations may both be reported during the remote interrogation device evaluation period.

For monitoring by wearable devices, see 93224-93272.

ECG rhythm derived elements are distinct from physiologic data, even when the same device is capable of producing both. ICM device services are always separately reported from ICD services. When ILR data is derived from an ICD or pacemaker, do not report ILR services with pacemaker or ICD services.

Do not report 93268-93272 when performing 93279-93289, 93291-93296 or 93298-93299. Do not report 93040-93042 when performing 93279-93289, 93291-93296, or 93298-93299.

The pacemaker and ICD interrogation device evaluations, peri-procedural device evaluations and programming, and programming device evaluations may not be reported in conjunction with pacemaker or ICD device and/or lead insertion or revision services by the same physician.

The following definitions and instructions apply to codes 93279-93299:

*Attended surveillance:* the immediate availability of a remote technician to respond to rhythm or device alert transmissions from a patient, either from an implanted or wearable monitoring or therapy device, as they are generated and transmitted to the remote surveillance location or center.

*Device, single lead:* a pacemaker or implantable cardioverter-defibrillator with pacing and sensing function in only one chamber of the heart.

*Device, dual lead:* a pacemaker or implantable cardioverter-defibrillator with pacing and sensing function in only two chambers of the heart.

*Device, multiple lead:* a pacemaker or implantable cardioverter-defibrillator with pacing and sensing function in three or more chambers of the heart.

*Electrocardiographic rhythm derived elements:* elements derived from recordings of the electrical activation of the heart including, but not limited to heart rhythm, rate, ST analysis, heart rate variability, T-wave alternans.

*Implantable cardiovascular monitor (ICM):* an implantable cardiovascular device used to assist the physician in the management of non-rhythm related cardiac conditions such as heart failure. The device collects longitudinal physiologic cardiovascular data elements from one or more internal sensors (such as right ventricular pressure, left atrial pressure or an index of lung water) and/or external sensors (such as blood pressure or body weight) for patient assessment and management. The data are stored and transmitted to the physician by either local telemetry or remotely to an Internet based file server or surveillance technician. The function of the ICM may be an additional function of an implantable cardiac device (eg, implantable cardioverter-defibrillator) or a function of a stand-alone device. When ICM functionality is included in an ICD device or

*Medicine*

pacemaker, the ICM data and the ICD or pacemaker, heart rhythm data such as sensing, pacing and tachycardia detection therapy are distinct and therefore, the monitoring processes are distinct.

*Implantable cardioverter-defibrillator (ICD):* an implantable device that provides high-energy and low-energy stimulation to one or more chambers of the heart to terminate rapid heart rhythms called tachycardia or fibrillation. ICDs also have pacemaker functions to treat slow heart rhythms called bradycardia. In addition to the tachycardia and bradycardia functions, the ICD may or may not include the functionality of an implantable cardiovascular monitor or an implantable loop recorder.

*Implantable loop recorder (ILR):* an implantable device that continuously records the electrocardiographic rhythm triggered automatically by rapid and slow heart rates or by the patient during a symptomatic episode. The ILR function may be the only function of the device or it may be part of a pacemaker or implantable cardioverter-defibrillator device. The data are stored and transmitted to the physician by either local telemetry or remotely to an Internet based file server or surveillance technician. Extraction of data and compilation or report for physician interpretation is usually performed in the office setting.

*Interrogation device evaluation:* an evaluation of an implantable device such as a cardiac pacemaker, implantable cardioverter-defibrillator, implantable cardiovascular monitor, or implantable loop recorder. Using an office, hospital, or emergency room instrument or via a remote interrogation system, stored and measured information about the lead(s) when present, sensor(s) when present, battery and the implanted device function, as well as data collected about the patient's heart rhythm and heart rate is retrieved. The retrieved information is evaluated to determine the current programming of the device and to evaluate certain aspects of the device function such as battery voltage, lead impedance, tachycardia detection settings, and rhythm treatment settings.

The components that must be evaluated for the various types of implantable cardiac devices are listed below. (The required components for both remote and in-person interrogations are the same.)

*Pacemaker:* Programmed parameters, lead(s), battery, capture and sensing function and heart rhythm.

*Implantable cardioverter-defibrillator:* Programmed parameters, lead(s), battery, capture and sensing function, presence or absence of therapy for ventricular tachyarrhythmias and underlying heart rhythm.

*Implantable cardiovascular monitor:* Programmed parameters and analysis of at least one recorded physiologic cardiovascular data element from either internal or external sensors.

*Implantable loop recorder:* Programmed parameters and the heart rate and rhythm during recorded episodes from both patient initiated and device algorithm detected events, when present.

*Interrogation device evaluation (remote):* a procedure performed for patients with pacemakers, implantable cardioverter-defibrillators or implantable loop recorders using data obtained remotely. All device functions, including the programmed parameters, lead(s), battery, capture and sensing function, presence or absence of therapy for ventricular tachyarrhythmias (for ICDs) and underlying heart rhythm are evaluated.

The components that must be evaluated for the various types of implantable cardiac devices are listed below. (The required components for both remote and in person interrogations are the same.)

*Pacemaker:* Programmed parameters, lead(s), battery, capture and sensing function, and heart rhythm.

*Implantable cardioverter-defibrillator:* Programmed parameters, lead(s), battery, capture and sensing function, presence or absence of therapy for ventricular tachyarrhythmias, and underlying heart rhythm.

*Implantable cardiovascular monitor:* Programmed parameters and analysis of at least one recorded physiologic cardiovascular data element from either internal or external sensors.

*Implantable loop recorder:* Programmed parameters and the heart rate and rhythm during recorded episodes from both patient-initiated and device algorithm detected events, when present.

*Pacemaker:* an implantable device that provides low energy localized stimulation to one or more chambers of the heart to initiate contraction in that chamber.

*Peri-procedural device evaluation and programming:* an evaluation of an implantable device system (either a pacemaker or implantable cardioverter defibrillator) to adjust the device to settings appropriate for the patient prior to a surgery, procedure, or test. The device system data are interrogated to evaluate the lead(s), sensor(s), and battery in addition to review of stored information, including patient and system measurements. The device is programmed to settings appropriate for the surgery, procedure, or test, as required. A second evaluation and programming are performed after the surgery, procedure, or test to provide settings appropriate to the post procedural situation, as required. If one provider performs both the pre- and post-evaluation and programming service, the appropriate code, either 93286 or 93287, would be reported two times. If one provider performs the pre-surgical service and a separate provider performs the post-surgical service, each reports either 93286 or 93287 only one time.

*Physiologic cardiovascular data elements:* data elements from one or more internal sensors (such as right ventricular pressure, left atrial pressure or an index of lung water) and/or external sensors (such as blood pressure or body weight) for patient assessement and management. It does not include ECG rhythm derived data elements.

*Programming device evaluation (in person):* a procedure performed for patients with a pacemaker, implantable cardioverter-defibrillator, or implantable loop recorder. All device functions, including the battery, programmable settings and lead(s), when present, are evaluated. To assess capture thresholds, iterative adjustments (eg, progressive changes in pacing output of a pacing lead) of the programmable parameters are conducted. The iterative adjustments provide information that permits the operator to assess and select the most appropriate final program parameters to provide for consistent delivery of the appropriate therapy and to verify the function of the device. The final program parameters may or may not change after evaluation.

The programming device evaluation includes all of the components of the interrogation device evaluation (remote) or the interrogation device evaluation (in person), and it includes the selection of patient specific programmed parameters depending on the type of device.

The components that must be evaluated for the various types of programming device evaluations are listed below. (See also required interrogation device evaluation [remote and in person] components above.)

*Pacemaker:* Programmed parameters, lead(s), battery, capture and sensing function, and heart rhythm. Often, but not always, the sensor rate response, lower and upper heart rates, AV intervals, pacing voltage and pulse duration, sensing value, and diagnostics will be adjusted during a programming evaluation.

*Implantable cardioverter-defibrillator:* Programmed parameters, lead(s), battery, capture and sensing function, presence or absence of therapy for ventricular tachyarrhythmias and underlying heart rhythm. Often, but not always, the sensor rate response, lower and upper heart rates, AV intervals, pacing voltage and pulse duration, sensing value, and diagnostics will be adjusted during a programming evaluation. In addition, ventricular tachycardia detection and therapies are sometimes altered depending on the interrogated data, patient's rhythm, symptoms, and condition.

*Implantable loop recorder:* Programmed parameters and the heart rhythm during recorded episodes from both patient initiated and device algorithm detected events. Often, but not always, the tachycardia and bradycardia detection criteria will be adjusted during a programming evaluation.

*Transtelephonic rhythm strip pacemaker evaluation:* service of transmission of an electrocardiographic rhythm strip over the telephone by the patient using a transmitter and recorded by a receiving location using a receiver/recorder (also commonly known as transtelephonic pacemaker monitoring). The electrocardiographic rhythm strip is recorded both with and without a magnet applied over the pacemaker. The rhythm strip is evaluated for heart rate and rhythm, atrial and ventricular capture (if observed) and atrial and ventricular sensing (if observed). In addition, the battery status of the pacemaker is determined by measurement of the paced rate on the electrocardiographic rhythm strip recorded with the magnet applied.

93279   Programming device evaluation (in person) with iterative adjustment of the implantable device to test the function of the device and select optimal permanent programmed values with physician analysis, review and report; single lead pacemaker system

(Do not report 93279 in conjunction with 93286, 93288)

93280      dual lead pacemaker system

(Do not report 93280 in conjunction with 93286, 93288)

93281      multiple lead pacemaker system

(Do not report 93281 in conjunction with 93286, 93288)

93282      single lead implantable cardioverter-defibrillator system

(Do not report 93282 in conjunction with 93287, 93289, 93745)

93283      dual lead implantable cardioverter-defibrillator system

(Do not report 93283 in conjunction with 93287, 93289)

93284      multiple lead implantable cardioverter-defibrillator system

(Do not report 93284 in conjunction with 93287, 93289)

93285      implantable loop recorder system

(Do not report 93285 in conjunction with 33282, 93279-93284, 93291)

93286   Peri-procedural device evaluation (in person) and programming of device system parameters before or after a surgery, procedure, or test with physician analysis, review and report; single, dual, or multiple lead pacemaker system

(Report 93286 once before and once after surgery, procedure, or test, when device evaluation and programming is performed before and after surgery, procedure, or test)

(Do not report 93286 in conjunction with 93279-93281, 93288)

**93287**  single, dual, or multiple lead implantable cardioverter-defibrillator system

(Report 93287 once before and once after surgery, procedure, or test, when device evaluation and programming is performed before and after surgery, procedure, or test)

(Do not report 93287 in conjunction with 93282-93284, 93289)

**93288**  Interrogation device evaluation (in person) with physician analysis, review and report, includes connection, recording and disconnection per patient encounter; single, dual, or multiple lead pacemaker system

(Do not report 93288 in conjunction with 93279-93281, 93286, 93294, 93296)

**93289**  single, dual, or multiple lead implantable cardioverter-defibrillator system, including analysis of heart rhythm derived data elements

(For monitoring physiologic cardiovascular data elements derived from an ICD, use 93290)

(Do not report 93289 in conjunction with 93282-93284, 93287, 93295, 93296)

**93290**  implantable cardiovascular monitor system, including analysis of 1 or more recorded physiologic cardiovascular data elements from all internal and external sensors

(For heart rhythm derived data elements, use 93289)

(Do not report 93290 in conjunction with 93297, 93299)

**93291**  implantable loop recorder system, including heart rhythm derived data analysis

(Do not report 93291 in conjunction with 33282, 93288-93290, 93298, 93299)

**93292**  wearable defibrillator system

(Do not report 93292 in conjunction with 93745)

**93293**  Transtelephonic rhythm strip pacemaker evaluation(s) single, dual, or multiple lead pacemaker system, includes recording with and without magnet application with physician analysis, review and report(s), up to 90 days

(Do not report 93293 in conjunction with 93294)

(For in person evaluation, see 93040, 93041, 93042)

(Report 93293 only once per 90 days)

**93294**  Interrogation device evaluation(s) (remote), up to 90 days; single, dual, or multiple lead pacemaker system with interim physician analysis, review(s) and report(s)

(Do not report 93294 in conjunction with 93288, 93293)

(Report 93294 only once per 90 days)

**93295**  single, dual, or multiple lead implantable cardioverter-defibrillator system with interim physician analysis, review(s) and report(s)

(For remote monitoring of physiologic cardiovascular data elements derived from an ICD, use 93297)

(Do not report 93295 in conjunction with 93289)

(Report 93295 only once per 90 days)

**93296**  single, dual, or multiple lead pacemaker system or implantable cardioverter-defibrillator system, remote data acquisition(s), receipt of transmissions and technician review, technical support and distribution of results

(Do not report 93296 in conjunction with 93288, 93289, 93299)

(Report 93296 only once per 90 days)

**93297**  Interrogation device evaluation(s), (remote) up to 30 days; implantable cardiovascular monitor system, including analysis of 1 or more recorded physiologic cardiovascular data elements from all internal and external sensors, physician analysis, review(s) and report(s)

(For heart rhythm derived data elements, use 93295)

(Do not report 93297 in conjunction with 93290, 93298)

(Report 93297 only once per 30 days)

**93298**  implantable loop recorder system, including analysis of recorded heart rhythm data, physician analysis, review(s) and report(s)

(Do not report 93298 in conjunction with 33282, 93291, 93297)

(Report 93298 only once per 30 days)

**93299**  implantable cardiovascular monitor system or implantable loop recorder system, remote data acquisition(s), receipt of transmissions and technician review, technical support and distribution of results

(Do not report 93299 in conjunction with 93290, 93291, 93296)

(Report 93299 only once per 30 days)

# Echocardiography

Echocardiography includes obtaining ultrasonic signals from the heart and great vessels, with real time image and/or Doppler ultrasonic signal documentation, with interpretation and report. When interpretation is performed separately, use modifier 26.

A complete transthoracic echocardiogram without spectral or color flow Doppler (93307) is a comprehensive procedure that includes 2-dimensional and, when performed, selected M-mode examination of the left and right atria, left and right ventricles, the aortic, mitral, and tricuspid valves, the pericardium, and adjacent portions of the aorta. Multiple views are required to obtain a complete functional and anatomic evaluation, and appropriate measurements are obtained and recorded. Despite significant effort, identification and measurement of some structures may not always be possible. In such instances, the reason that an element could not be visualized must be documented. Additional structures that may be visualized (eg, pulmonary veins, pulmonary artery, pulmonic valve, inferior vena cava) would be included as part of the service.

A complete transthoracic echocardiogram with spectral and color flow Doppler (93306) is a comprehensive procedure that includes spectral Doppler and color flow Doppler in addition to the 2-dimensional and selected M-mode examinations, when performed. Spectral Doppler (93320, 93321) and color flow Doppler (93325) provide information regarding intracardiac blood flow and hemodynamics.

A follow-up or limited echocardiographic study (93308) is an examination that does not evaluate or document the attempt to evaluate all the structures that comprise the complete echocardiographic exam. This is typically limited to, or performed in follow-up of a focused clinical concern.

In stress echocardiography, echocardiographic images are recorded from multiple cardiac windows before, after, and in some protocols, during stress. The stress is achieved by (1) walking on a treadmill; (2) using a bicycle (supine or upright); or (3) the administration of pharmacological agents that either simulate exercise (by increasing heart rate, blood pressure, or myocardial contractility) or alter coronary flow (vasodilation). The patient's ECG, heart rate, and blood pressure are monitored at baseline, throughout the procedure and during recovery. Reports are prepared to evaluate (1) the duration of stress, the reason for stopping, and the hemodynamic response to stress; (2) the electrocardiographic response to stress; and (3) the echocardiographic response to stress.

►When a stress echocardiogram is performed with a complete cardiovascular stress test (continuous electrocardiographic monitoring, physician supervision, interpretation and report), use 93351. When only the professional components of a complete stress test and a stress echocardiogram are provided (eg, in a facility setting) by the same physician, use 93351 with modifier 26. When all professional services of a stress test are not performed by the same physician performing the stress echocardiogram, use 93350 in conjunction with the appropriate codes (93016-93018) for the components of the cardiovascular stress test that are provided.◄

When left ventricular endocardial borders cannot be adequately identified by standard echocardiographic imaging, echocardiographic contrast may be infused intravenously both at rest and with stress to achieve that purpose. Code 93352 is used to report the administration of echocardiographic contrast agent in conjunction with the stress echocardiography codes (93350 or 93351). Supply of contrast agent and/or drugs used for pharmacological stress is reported separately in addition to the procedure code.

Report of an echocardiographic study, whether complete or limited, includes an interpretation of all obtained information, documentation of all clinically relevant findings including quantitative measurements obtained, plus a description of any recognized abnormalities. Pertinent images, videotape, and/or digital data are archived for permanent storage and are available for subsequent review. Use of echocardiography not meeting these criteria is not separately reportable.

Use of ultrasound, without thorough evaluation of organ(s) or anatomic region, image documentation and final, written report, is not separately reportable.

(For fetal echocardiography, see 76825-76828)

**93303** Transthoracic echocardiography for congenital cardiac anomalies; complete

**93304**      follow-up or limited study

**93306** Echocardiography, transthoracic, real-time with image documentation (2D), includes M-mode recording, when performed, complete, with spectral Doppler echocardiography, and with color flow Doppler echocardiography

(For transthoracic echocardiography without spectral and color Doppler, use 93307)

**93307** Echocardiography, transthoracic, real-time with image documentation (2D), includes M-mode recording, when performed, complete, without spectral or color Doppler echocardiography

(Do not report 93307 in conjunction with 93320, 93321, 93325)

**93308** Echocardiography, transthoracic, real-time with image documentation (2D), includes M-mode recording, when performed, follow-up or limited study

⊙ **93312** Echocardiography, transesophageal, real-time with image documentation (2D) (with or without M-mode recording); including probe placement, image acquisition, interpretation and report

⊙ **93313**      placement of transesophageal probe only

⊙ **93314**      image acquisition, interpretation and report only

⊙ **93315** Transesophageal echocardiography for congenital cardiac anomalies; including probe placement, image acquisition, interpretation and report

⊙ **93316**      placement of transesophageal probe only

⊙ **93317**      image acquisition, interpretation and report only

⊙ **93318** Echocardiography, transesophageal (TEE) for monitoring purposes, including probe placement, real time 2-dimensional image acquisition and interpretation leading to ongoing (continuous) assessment of (dynamically changing) cardiac pumping function and to therapeutic measures on an immediate time basis

+ **93320** Doppler echocardiography, pulsed wave and/or continuous wave with spectral display (List separately in addition to codes for echocardiographic imaging); complete

(Use 93320 in conjunction with 93303, 93304, 93312, 93314, 93315, 93317, 93350, 93351)

Medicine

codes from the Radiology section and the Vascular Injection Procedures section.

When cardiac catheterization is combined with pharmacologic agent administration with the specific purpose of repeating hemodynamic measurements to evaluate hemodynamic response, use 93463 in conjunction with 93451-93453 and 93456-93461. Do not report 93463 for intracoronary administration of pharmacologic agents during percutaneous coronary interventional procedures, during intracoronary assessment of coronary pressure, flow or resistance, or during intracoronary imaging procedures. Do not report 93463 in conjunction with 92975, 92977, 92980, 92982, or 92995.

When cardiac catheterization is combined with exercise (eg, walking or arm or leg ergometry protocol) with the specific purpose of repeating hemodynamic measurements to evaluate hemodynamic response, report 93464 in conjunction with 93451-93453, 93456-93461, and 93530-93533.

Contrast injection to image the access site(s) for the specific purpose of placing a closure device is inherent to the catheterization procedure and not separately reportable. Closure device placement at the vascular access site is inherent to the catheterization procedure and not separately reportable.

Modifier 51 should not be appended to 93451, 93456, 93503.

►Please see the cardiac catheterization table located following 93572.◄

⊙⃠ **93451**   Right heart catheterization including measurement(s) of oxygen saturation and cardiac output, when performed

    (Do not report 93451 in conjunction with 93453, 93456, 93457, 93460, 93461)

⊙ **93452**   Left heart catheterization including intraprocedural injection(s) for left ventriculography, imaging supervision and interpretation, when performed

    (Do not report 93452 in conjunction with 93453, 93458-93461)

⊙ **93453**   Combined right and left heart catheterization including intraprocedural injection(s) for left ventriculography, imaging supervision and interpretation, when performed

    (Do not report 93453 in conjunction with 93451, 93452, 93456-93461)

⊙ **93454**   Catheter placement in coronary artery(s) for coronary angiography, including intraprocedural injection(s) for coronary angiography, imaging supervision and interpretation;

⊙ **93455**     with catheter placement(s) in bypass graft(s) (internal mammary, free arterial, venous grafts) including intraprocedural injection(s) for bypass graft angiography

⊙⃠ **93456**     with right heart catheterization

⊙ **93457**     with catheter placement(s) in bypass graft(s) (internal mammary, free arterial, venous grafts) including intraprocedural injection(s) for bypass graft angiography and right heart catheterization

⊙ **93458**     with left heart catheterization including intraprocedural injection(s) for left ventriculography, when performed

⊙ **93459**     with left heart catheterization including intraprocedural injection(s) for left ventriculography, when performed, catheter placement(s) in bypass graft(s) (internal mammary, free arterial, venous grafts) with bypass graft angiography

⊙ **93460**     with right and left heart catheterization including intraprocedural injection(s) for left ventriculography, when performed

⊙ **93461**     with right and left heart catheterization including intraprocedural injection(s) for left ventriculography, when performed, catheter placement(s) in bypass graft(s) (internal mammary, free arterial, venous grafts) with bypass graft angiography

⊙+ **93462**   Left heart catheterization by transseptal puncture through intact septum or by transapical puncture (List separately in addition to code for primary procedure)

    (Use 93462 in conjunction with 93452, 93453, 93458-93461, 93651, 93652)

⊙+ **93463**   Pharmacologic agent administration (eg, inhaled nitric oxide, intravenous infusion of nitroprusside, dobutamine, milrinone, or other agent) including assessing hemodynamic measurements before, during, after and repeat pharmacologic agent administration, when performed (List separately in addition to code for primary procedure)

    (Use 93463 in conjunction with 93451-93453, 93456-93461, 93530-93533)

    (Report 93463 only once per catheterization procedure)

    (Do not report 93463 for pharmacologic agent administration in conjunction with coronary interventional procedure codes 92975, 92977, 92980, 92982, 92995)

⊙+ **93464**   Physiologic exercise study (eg, bicycle or arm ergometry) including assessing hemodynamic measurements before and after (List separately in addition to code for primary procedure)

    (Use 93464 in conjunction with 93451-93453, 93456-93461, 93530-93533)

    (Report 93464 only once per catheterization procedure)

    (For pharmacologic agent administration, use 93463)

    (For bundle of His recording, use 93600)

⃠ **93503**   Insertion and placement of flow directed catheter (eg, Swan-Ganz) for monitoring purposes

    (For subsequent monitoring, see 99356-99357)

⊙ **93505**   Endomyocardial biopsy

**Medicine**

(To report transcatheter placement of radiation delivery device for coronary intravascular brachytherapy, use 92974)

(For intravascular radioelement application, see 77785-77787)

(93501, 93508-93529 have been deleted. To report, see 93451-93461)

⊙ **93530**   Right heart catheterization, for congenital cardiac anomalies

**93531**   Combined right heart catheterization and retrograde left heart catheterization, for congenital cardiac anomalies

**93532**   Combined right heart catheterization and transseptal left heart catheterization through intact septum with or without retrograde left heart catheterization, for congenital cardiac anomalies

**93533**   Combined right heart catheterization and transseptal left heart catheterization through existing septal opening, with or without retrograde left heart catheterization, for congenital cardiac anomalies

## Injection Procedures

All injection codes include radiological supervision, interpretation, and report. Cardiac catheterization codes (93452-93461), other than those for congenital heart disease, include contrast injection(s) for imaging typically performed during these procedures (see Cardiac Catheterization above). Do not report 93563-93565 in conjunction with 93452-93461. When injection procedures for right ventricular, right atrial, aortic, or pulmonary angiography are performed in conjunction with cardiac catheterization, these services are reported separately (93566-93568). When right ventricular or right atrial angiography is performed at the time of heart catheterization, use 93566 with the appropriate catheterization code (93451, 93453, 93456, 93457, 93460, or 93461). Use 93567 when supravalvular ascending aortography is performed at the time of heart catheterization. Use 93568 with the appropriate right heart catheterization code when pulmonary angiography is performed. Separately reported injection procedures do not include introduction of catheters but do include repositioning of catheters when necessary and use of automatic power injectors, when performed.

When contrast injection(s) are performed in conjunction with cardiac catheterization for congenital cardiac anomalies (93530-93533), see 93563-93568. Injection procedure codes 93563-93568 include imaging supervision, interpretation, and report.

Injection procedures 93563-93568 represent separate identifiable services and may be coded in conjunction with one another when appropriate. The technical details of angiography, supervision of filming and processing, interpretation, and report are included.

(93539-93545 have been deleted. To report, see 93451-93461, 93563-93568)

(93555, 93556 have been deleted. See introductory guidelines for Cardiac Catheterization and Injection Procedures)

⊙▲ **93561**   Indicator dilution studies such as dye or thermodilution, including arterial and/or venous catheterization; with cardiac output measurement (separate procedure)

⊙▲ **93562**   subsequent measurement of cardiac output

►(Do not report 93561, 93562 in conjunction with 93451-93462)◄

(For radioisotope method of cardiac output, see 78472, 78473, or 78481)

⊙+ **93563**   Injection procedure during cardiac catheterization including imaging supervision, interpretation, and report; for selective coronary angiography during congenital heart catheterization (List separately in addition to code for primary procedure)

⊙+ **93564**   for selective opacification of aortocoronary venous or arterial bypass graft(s) (eg, aortocoronary saphenous vein, free radial artery, or free mammary artery graft) to one or more coronary arteries and in situ arterial conduits (eg, internal mammary), whether native or used for bypass to one or more coronary arteries during congenital heart catheterization, when performed (List separately in addition to code for primary procedure)

⊙+ **93565**   for selective left ventricular or left atrial angiography (List separately in addition to code for primary procedure)

(Do not report 93563-93565 in conjunction with 93452-93461)

(Use 93563-93565 in conjunction with 93530-93533)

⊙+ **93566**   for selective right ventricular or right atrial angiography (List separately in addition to code for primary procedure)

⊙+ **93567**   for supravalvular aortography (List separately in addition to code for primary procedure)

⊙+ **93568**   for pulmonary angiography (List separately in addition to code for primary procedure)

(Use 93566-93568 in conjunction with 93530-93533, 93451-93461)

⊙+ **93571**   Intravascular Doppler velocity and/or pressure derived coronary flow reserve measurement (coronary vessel or graft) during coronary angiography including pharmacologically induced stress; initial vessel (List separately in addition to code for primary procedure)

⊙+ **93572**   each additional vessel (List separately in addition to code for primary procedure)

(Intravascular distal coronary blood flow velocity measurements include all Doppler transducer manipulations and repositioning within the specific vessel being examined, during coronary angiography or therapeutic intervention [eg, angioplasty])

(For unlisted cardiac catheterization procedure, use 93799)

▶Table of Catheterization Codes

| CPT Code | Code Descriptor | Catheter Placement Type | | | | Add-on Procedures (Can Be Reported Separately) | | | | | |
|---|---|---|---|---|---|---|---|---|---|---|---|
| | | RHC | LHC | Coronary Artery Placement | Bypass Graft(s) | With Transseptal or Transapical Puncture 93462 | With Pharmacological Study 93463 | With Exercise Study 93464 | Injection Procedure for Selective Right Ventricular or Right Atrial Angiography 93566 | Injection Procedure for Supravalvular Aortography 93567 | Injection Procedure for Pulmonary Angiography 93568 |
| 93451 | **Right heart catheterization including measurement(s) of oxygen saturation and cardiac output, when performed** | X | | | | | X | X | X | | X |
| 93452 | **Left heart catheterization including intraprocedural injection(s) for left ventriculography, imaging supervision and interpretation, when performed** | | X | | | X | X | X | | X | |
| 93453 | **Combined right and left heart catheterization including injection(s) for left ventriculography, imaging supervision and interpretation, when performed** | X | X | | | X | X | X | X | X | X |
| 93454 | **Catheter placement in coronary artery(s) for coronary angiography, including intraprocedural injection(s) for coronary angiography, imaging supervision and interpretation;** | | | X | | | | | | X | |
| 93455 | Catheter placement in coronary artery(s) for coronary angiography, including intraprocedural injection(s) for coronary angiography, imaging supervision and interpretation; **with catheter placement(s) in bypass graft(s) (internal mammary, free arterial venous grafts) including intraprocedural injection(s) for bypass graft angiography**▶◀ | | | X | X | | | | | X | |

▲=Revised code   ●=New code   ▶◀=Contains new or revised text   ⊘=Modifier 51 exempt

Medicine

**Medicine**

▶Table of Catheterization Codes, *continued*

| CPT Code | Code Descriptor | Catheter Placement Type | | | | Add-on Procedures (Can Be Reported Separately) | | | | | |
|---|---|---|---|---|---|---|---|---|---|---|---|
| | | RHC | LHC | Coronary Artery Placement | Bypass Graft(s) | With Transseptal or Transapical Puncture 93462 | With Pharmacological Study 93463 | With Exercise Study 93464 | Injection Procedure for Selective Right Ventricular or Right Atrial Angiography 93566 | Injection Procedure for Supravalvular Aortography 93567 | Injection Procedure for Pulmonary Angiography 93568 |
| 93456 | Catheter placement in coronary artery(s) for coronary angiography, including intraprocedural injection(s) for coronary angiography, imaging supervision and interpretation; **with right heart catheterization** | X | | X | | | X | X | X | X | X |
| 93457 | Catheter placement in coronary artery(s) for coronary angiography, including intraprocedural injection(s) for coronary angiography, imaging supervision and interpretation; **with catheter placement(s) in bypass graft(s) (internal mammary, free arterial, venous grafts) including intraprocedural injection(s) for bypass graft angiography and right heart catheterization** | X | | X | X | | X | X | X | X | X |
| 93458 | Catheter placement in coronary artery(s) for coronary angiography, including intraprocedural injection(s) for coronary angiography, imaging supervision and interpretation; **with left heart catheterization including intraprocedural injection(s) for left ventriculography, when performed ▼** | | X | X | | X | X | X | | X | |

⊙=Moderate sedation  ✚=Add-on code  ✗=FDA approval pending  #=Resequenced code  ○=Recycled/reinstated code

▶Table of Catheterization Codes, *continued*

| CPT Code | Code Descriptor | Catheter Placement Type | | | | Add-on Procedures (Can Be Reported Separately) | | | | | |
|---|---|---|---|---|---|---|---|---|---|---|---|
| | | RHC | LHC | Coronary Artery Placement | Bypass Graft(s) | With Transseptal or Transapical Puncture 93462 | With Pharmacological Study 93463 | With Exercise Study 93464 | Injection Procedure for Selective Right Ventricular or Right Atrial Angiography 93566 | Injection Procedure for Supravalvular Aortography 93567 | Injection Procedure for Pulmonary Angiography 93568 |
| 93459 | Catheter placement in coronary artery(s) for coronary angiography, including intraprocedural injection(s) for coronary angiography, imaging supervision and interpretation; **with left heart catheterization including intraprocedural injection(s) for left ventriculography, when performed, catheter placement(s) in bypass graft(s) (internal mammary, free arterial, venous grafts) with bypass graft angiography** | | X | X | X | X | X | X | | X | |
| 93460 | Catheter placement in coronary artery(s) for coronary angiography, including intraprocedural injection(s) for coronary angiography, imaging supervision and interpretation; **with right and left heart catheterization including intraprocedural injection(s) for left ventriculography, when performed** | X | X | X | | X | X | X | X | X | X |
| 93461 | Catheter placement in coronary artery(s) for coronary angiography, including intraprocedural injection(s) for coronary angiography, imaging supervision and interpretation; **with right and left heart catheterization including intraprocedural injection(s) for left ventriculography, when performed, catheter placement(s) in bypass graft(s) (internal mammary, free arterial, venous grafts) with bypass graft angiography**▲ | X | X | X | X | X | X | X | X | X | X |

▲=Revised code    ●=New code    ▶◀=Contains new or revised text    ⊘=Modifier 51 exempt

**Medicine**

# Repair of Septal Defect

**93580**   Percutaneous transcatheter closure of congenital interatrial communication (ie, Fontan fenestration, atrial septal defect) with implant

(Percutaneous transcatheter closure of atrial septal defect includes a right heart catheterization procedure. Code 93580 includes injection of contrast for atrial and ventricular angiograms. Codes 93451-93453, 93455-93461, 93530-93533, 93564-93566 should not be reported separately in addition to code 93580)

**93581**   Percutaneous transcatheter closure of a congenital ventricular septal defect with implant

(Percutaneous transcatheter closure of ventricular septal defect includes a right heart catheterization procedure. Code 93581 includes injection of contrast for atrial and ventricular angiograms. Codes 93451-93453, 93455-93461, 93530-93533, 93564-93566 should not be reported separately in addition to code 93581)

(For echocardiographic services performed in addition to 93580, 93581, see 93303-93317, 93662 as appropriate)

# Intracardiac Electrophysiological Procedures/Studies

Intracardiac electrophysiologic studies (EPS) are an invasive diagnostic medical procedure which include the insertion and repositioning of electrode catheters, recording of electrograms before and during pacing or programmed stimulation of multiple locations in the heart, analysis of recorded information, and report of the procedure. Electrophysiologic studies are most often performed with two or more electrode catheters. In many circumstances, patients with arrhythmias are evaluated and treated at the same encounter. In this situation, a diagnostic *electrophysiologic study* is performed, induced tachycardia(s) are *mapped*, and on the basis of the diagnostic and mapping information, the tissue is *ablated*. Electrophysiologic study(ies), mapping, and ablation represent distinctly different procedures, requiring individual reporting whether performed on the same or subsequent dates.

## Definitions

**Arrhythmia Induction:** In most electrophysiologic studies, an attempt is made to induce arrhythmia(s) from single or multiple sites within the heart. Arrhythmia induction is achieved by performing pacing at different rates, programmed stimulation (introduction of critically timed electrical impulses), and other techniques. Because arrhythmia induction occurs via the same catheter(s) inserted for the electrophysiologic study(ies), catheter insertion and temporary pacemaker codes are not additionally reported. Codes 93600-93603, 93610-93612 and 93618 are used to describe unusual situations where there may be recording, pacing or an attempt at arrhythmia induction from only one site in the heart. Code 93619 describes only evaluation of the sinus node,

atrioventricular node and His-Purkinje conduction system, without arrhythmia induction. Codes 93620-93624 and 93640-93642 all include recording, pacing and attempted arrhythmia induction from one or more site(s) in the heart.

**Mapping:** Mapping is a distinct procedure performed in addition to a diagnostic electrophysiologic procedure and should be separately reported using 93609 or 93613. Do not report standard mapping (93609) in addition to 3D mapping (93613). When a tachycardia is induced, the site of tachycardia origination or its electrical path through the heart is often defined by mapping. Mapping creates a multidimensional depiction of a tachycardia by recording multiple electrograms obtained sequentially or simultaneously from multiple catheter sites in the heart. Depending upon the technique, certain types of mapping catheters may be repositioned from point-to-point within the heart, allowing sequential recording from the various sites to construct maps. Other types of mapping catheters allow mapping without a point-to-point technique by allowing simultaneous recording from many electrodes on the same catheter and computer-assisted three dimensional reconstruction of the tachycardia activation sequence.

**Ablation:** Once the part of the heart involved in the tachycardia is localized, the tachycardia may be treated by ablation (the delivery of a radiofrequency energy to the area to selectively destroy cardiac tissue). Ablation procedures (93651-93652) may be performed: independently on a date subsequent to a diagnostic electrophysiologic study and mapping; or, at the time a diagnostic electrophysiologic study, tachycardia(s) induction and mapping is performed. When an electrophysiologic study, mapping, and ablation are performed on the same date, each procedure should be separately reported. In reporting catheter ablation, 93651 and/or 93652 should be reported once to describe ablation of cardiac arrhythmias, regardless of the number of arrhythmias ablated.

Modifier 51 should not be appended to 93600-93603, 93610, 93612, 93615-93618, 93631.

⊘ **93600**   Bundle of His recording

⊘ **93602**   Intra-atrial recording

⊘ **93603**   Right ventricular recording

⊙+ **93609**   Intraventricular and/or intra-atrial mapping of tachycardia site(s) with catheter manipulation to record from multiple sites to identify origin of tachycardia (List separately in addition to code for primary procedure)

(Use 93609 in conjunction with 93620, 93651, 93652)

(Do not report 93609 in addition to 93613)

⊘ **93610**   Intra-atrial pacing

⊘ **93612**   Intraventricular pacing

(Do not report 93612 in conjunction with 93620-93622)

⊙+ **93613** Intracardiac electrophysiologic 3-dimensional mapping (List separately in addition to code for primary procedure)

(Use 93613 in conjunction with 93620, 93651, 93652)

(Do not report 93613 in addition to 93609)

⊙⊘ **93615** Esophageal recording of atrial electrogram with or without ventricular electrogram(s)

⊙⊘ **93616**      with pacing

⊙⊘ **93618** Induction of arrhythmia by electrical pacing

(For intracardiac phonocardiogram, use 93799)

⊙ **93619** Comprehensive electrophysiologic evaluation with right atrial pacing and recording, right ventricular pacing and recording, His bundle recording, including insertion and repositioning of multiple electrode catheters, without induction or attempted induction of arrhythmia

(Do not report 93619 in conjunction with 93600, 93602, 93610, 93612, 93618, or 93620-93622)

⊙ **93620** Comprehensive electrophysiologic evaluation including insertion and repositioning of multiple electrode catheters with induction or attempted induction of arrhythmia; with right atrial pacing and recording, right ventricular pacing and recording, His bundle recording

(Do not report 93620 in conjunction with 93600, 93602, 93610, 93612, 93618 or 93619)

⊙+ **93621**      with left atrial pacing and recording from coronary sinus or left atrium (List separately in addition to code for primary procedure)

(Use 93621 in conjunction with 93620)

⊙+ **93622**      with left ventricular pacing and recording (List separately in addition to code for primary procedure)

(Use 93622 in conjunction with 93620)

+ **93623** Programmed stimulation and pacing after intravenous drug infusion (List separately in addition to code for primary procedure)

(Use 93623 in conjunction with 93619, 93620)

⊙ **93624** Electrophysiologic follow-up study with pacing and recording to test effectiveness of therapy, including induction or attempted induction of arrhythmia

⊘ **93631** Intra-operative epicardial and endocardial pacing and mapping to localize the site of tachycardia or zone of slow conduction for surgical correction

(For operative ablation of an arrhythmogenic focus or pathway by a separate provider, see 33250-33261)

⊙ **93640** Electrophysiologic evaluation of single or dual chamber pacing cardioverter-defibrillator leads including defibrillation threshold evaluation (induction of arrhythmia, evaluation of sensing and pacing for arrhythmia termination) at time of initial implantation or replacement

⊙ **93641**      with testing of single or dual chamber pacing cardioverter-defibrillator pulse generator

(For subsequent or periodic electronic analysis and/or reprogramming of single or dual chamber pacing cardioverter-defibrillators, see 93282, 93283, 93289, 93292, 93295, 93642)

⊙ **93642** Electrophysiologic evaluation of single or dual chamber pacing cardioverter-defibrillator (includes defibrillation threshold evaluation, induction of arrhythmia, evaluation of sensing and pacing for arrhythmia termination, and programming or reprogramming of sensing or therapeutic parameters)

⊙ **93650** Intracardiac catheter ablation of atrioventricular node function, atrioventricular conduction for creation of complete heart block, with or without temporary pacemaker placement

⊙ **93651** Intracardiac catheter ablation of arrhythmogenic focus; for treatment of supraventricular tachycardia by ablation of fast or slow atrioventricular pathways, accessory atrioventricular connections or other atrial foci, singly or in combination

⊙ **93652**      for treatment of ventricular tachycardia

**93660** Evaluation of cardiovascular function with tilt table evaluation, with continuous ECG monitoring and intermittent blood pressure monitoring, with or without pharmacological intervention

(For testing of autonomic nervous system function, see 95921-95923)

+ **93662** Intracardiac echocardiography during therapeutic/diagnostic intervention, including imaging supervision and interpretation (List separately in addition to code for primary procedure)

(Use 93662 in conjunction with 92987, 93453, 93460-93462, 93532, 93580, 93581, 93621, 93622, 93651, or 93652, as appropriate)

(Do not report 92961 in addition to 93662)

# Peripheral Arterial Disease Rehabilitation

Peripheral arterial disease (PAD) rehabilitative physical exercise consists of a series of sessions, lasting 45-60 minutes per session, involving use of either a motorized treadmill or a track to permit each patient to achieve symptom-limited claudication. Each session is supervised by an exercise physiologist or nurse. The supervising provider monitors the individual patient's claudication threshold and other cardiovascular limitations for adjustment of workload. During this supervised rehabilitation program, the development of new arrhythmias, symptoms that might suggest angina or the continued inability of the patient to progress to an adequate level of exercise may require physician review and examination of the patient. These physician services would be separately reported with an appropriate level E/M service code.

**93668** Peripheral arterial disease (PAD) rehabilitation, per session

---

**Medicine**

# Noninvasive Physiologic Studies and Procedures

(For arterial cannulization and recording of direct arterial pressure, use 36620)

(For radiographic injection procedures, see 36000-36299)

(For vascular cannulization for hemodialysis, see 36800-36821)

(For chemotherapy for malignant disease, see 96409-96549)

(For penile plethysmography, use 54240)

**93701**   Bioimpedance-derived physiologic cardiovascular analysis

(For left ventricular filling pressure indirect measurement by computerized calibration of the arterial waveform response to Valsalva, use 93799)

▶(93720-93722 have been deleted. To report, use 94726)◀

**93724**   Electronic analysis of antitachycardia pacemaker system (includes electrocardiographic recording, programming of device, induction and termination of tachycardia via implanted pacemaker, and interpretation of recordings)

(93727 has been deleted. For programming of implantable loop recorder, use 93285. For interrogation of implantable loop recorder, see 93291, 93298)

(93731, 93732 have been deleted. For interrogation of dual lead pacemaker, see 93288, 93294. For programming of dual chamber pacemaker, use 93280)

(93733 has been deleted. For transtelephonic rhythm strip pacemaker, single and dual, or multiple lead pacemaker evaluation, use 93293)

(93734, 93735 have been deleted. For interrogation of single lead pacemaker, see 93288, 93294. For programming of single lead pacemaker, use 93279)

(93736 has been deleted. For transtelephonic rhythm strip pacemaker, single and dual, or multiple lead pacemaker evaluation, use 93293)

**93740**   Temperature gradient studies

(93741, 93742 have been deleted. For interrogation of single implantable cardioverter-defibrillator [ICD], see 93289, 93295. For programming of single ICD, use 93282. For interrogation of wearable cardioverter-defibrillator, use 93292)

(93743, 93744 have been deleted. For interrogation of dual implantable cardioverter-defibrillator [ICD], see 93289, 93295. For programming of dual ICD, use 93283)

**93745**   Initial set-up and programming by a physician of wearable cardioverter-defibrillator includes initial programming of system, establishing baseline electronic ECG, transmission of data to data repository, patient instruction in wearing system and patient reporting of problems or events

(Do not report 93745 in conjunction with 93282, 93292)

**93750**   Interrogation of ventricular assist device (VAD), in person, with physician analysis of device parameters (eg, drivelines, alarms, power surges), review of device function (eg, flow and volume status, septum status, recovery), with programming, if performed, and report

(Do not report 93750 in conjunction with 33975, 33976, 33979, 33981-33983)

(93760, 93762 have been deleted)

**93770**   Determination of venous pressure

(For central venous cannulization see 36555-36556, 36500)

**93784**   Ambulatory blood pressure monitoring, utilizing a system such as magnetic tape and/or computer disk, for 24 hours or longer; including recording, scanning analysis, interpretation and report

**93786**       recording only

**93788**       scanning analysis with report

**93790**       physician review with interpretation and report

## Other Procedures

**93797**   Physician services for outpatient cardiac rehabilitation; without continuous ECG monitoring (per session)

**93798**       with continuous ECG monitoring (per session)

**93799**   Unlisted cardiovascular service or procedure

# Noninvasive Vascular Diagnostic Studies

Vascular studies include patient care required to perform the studies, supervision of the studies and interpretation of study results with copies for patient records of hard copy output with analysis of all data, including bidirectional vascular flow or imaging when provided.

The use of a simple hand-held or other Doppler device that does not produce hard copy output, or that produces a record that does not permit analysis of bidirectional vascular flow, is considered to be part of the physical examination of the vascular system and is not separately reported. The Ankle-Brachial Index (or ABI) is reportable with 93922 or 93923 as long as simultaneous Doppler recording and analysis of bidirectional blood flow, volume plethysmography, or transcutaneous oxygen tension measurements are also performed.

*Duplex scan* (eg, 93880, 93882) describes an ultrasonic scanning procedure for characterizing the pattern and direction of blood flow in arteries or veins with the production of real-time images integrating B-mode two-dimensional vascular structure, Doppler spectral analysis, and color flow Doppler imaging.

Medicine

►*Physiologic studies* Noninvasive physiologic studies are performed using equipment separate and distinct from the duplex ultrasound imager. Codes 93922, 93923, 93924, and 93965 describe the evaluation of non-imaging physiologic recordings of pressures with Doppler analysis of bi-directional blood flow, plethysmography, and/or oxygen tension measurements appropriate for the anatomic area studied.◄

Limited studies for lower extremity require either:

(1) ankle/brachial indices at distal posterior tibial and anterior tibial/dorsalis pedis arteries plus bidirectional Doppler waveform recording and analysis at 1-2 levels; or (2) ankle/brachial indices at distal posterior tibial and anterior tibial/dorsalis pedis arteries plus volume plethysmography at 1-2 levels; or (3) ankle/brachial indices at distal posterior tibial and anterior tibial/dorsalis pedis arteries with transcutaneous oxygen tension measurements at 1-2 levels. Potential levels include high thigh, low thigh, calf, ankle, metatarsal and toes.

Limited studies for upper extremity require either:

(1) Doppler-determined systolic pressures and bidirectional Doppler waveform recording and analysis at 1-2 levels; or (2) Doppler-determined systolic pressures and volume plethysmography at 1-2 levels; or (3) Doppler-determined systolic pressures and transcutaneous oxygen tension measurements at 1-2 levels. Potential levels include arm, forearm, wrist, and digits.

Complete studies for lower extremity require either:

(1) ankle/brachial indices at distal posterior tibial and anterior tibial/dorsalis pedis arteries plus bidirectional Doppler waveform recording and analysis at 3 or more levels; or (2) ankle/brachial indices at distal posterior tibial and anterior tibial/dorsalis pedis arteries plus volume plethysmography at 3 or more levels; or (3) ankle/brachial indices at distal posterior tibial and anterior tibial/dorsalis pedis arteries with transcutaneous oxygen tension measurements at 3 or more levels. Alternatively, a complete study may be reported with measurements at a single level if provocative functional maneuvers (eg, measurements with postural provocative tests, or measurements with reactive hyperemia) are performed.

Complete studies for upper extremity require either:

(1) Doppler-determined systolic pressures and bidirectional Doppler waveform recording and analysis at 3 or more levels; or (2) Doppler-determined systolic pressures and volume plethysmography at 3 or more levels; or (3) Doppler-determined systolic pressures and transcutaneous oxygen tension measurements at 3 or more levels. Potential levels include arm, forearm, wrist, and digits. Alternatively, a complete study may be reported with measurements at a single level if provocative functional maneuvers (eg, measurements with postural provocative tests, or measurements with cold stress) are performed.

## Cerebrovascular Arterial Studies

A complete transcranial Doppler (TCD) study (93886) includes ultrasound evaluation of the right and left anterior circulation territories and the posterior circulation territory (to include vertebral arteries and basilar artery). In a limited TCD study (93888) there is ultrasound evaluation of two or fewer of these territories. For TCD, ultrasound evaluation is a reasonable and concerted attempt to identify arterial signals through an acoustic window.

►(93875 has been deleted)◄

**93880**    Duplex scan of extracranial arteries; complete bilateral study

**93882**      unilateral or limited study

(To report common carotid intima-media thickness (IMT) study for evaluation of atherosclerotic burden or coronary heart disease risk factor assessment, use Category III code 0126T)

**93886**    Transcranial Doppler study of the intracranial arteries; complete study

**93888**      limited study

**93890**      vasoreactivity study

**93892**      emboli detection without intravenous microbubble injection

**93893**      emboli detection with intravenous microbubble injection

(Do not report 93890-93893 in conjunction with 93888)

## Extremity Arterial Studies (Including Digits)

**93922**    Limited bilateral noninvasive physiologic studies of upper or lower extremity arteries, (eg, for lower extremity: ankle/brachial indices at distal posterior tibial and anterior tibial/dorsalis pedis arteries plus bidirectional, Doppler waveform recording and analysis at 1-2 levels, or ankle/brachial indices at distal posterior tibial and anterior tibial/dorsalis pedis arteries plus volume plethysmography at 1-2 levels, or ankle/brachial indices at distal posterior tibial and anterior tibial/dorsalis pedis arteries with, transcutaneous oxygen tension measurement at 1-2 levels)

(When only 1 arm or leg is available for study, report 93922 with modifier 52 for a unilateral study when recording 1-2 levels. Report 93922 when recording 3 or more levels or performing provocative functional maneuvers)

(Report 93922 only once in the upper extremity(s) and/or once in the lower extremity(s). When both the upper and lower extremities are evaluated in the same setting, 93922 may be reported twice by adding modifier 59 to the second procedure)

**Medicine**

▶(For transcutaneous oxyhemoglobin measurement in a lower extremity wound by near infrared spectroscopy, use 0286T)◀

93923   Complete bilateral noninvasive physiologic studies of upper or lower extremity arteries, 3 or more levels (eg, for lower extremity: ankle/brachial indices at distal posterior tibial and anterior tibial/dorsalis pedis arteries plus segmental blood pressure measurements with bidirectional Doppler waveform recording and analysis, at 3 or more levels, or ankle/brachial indices at distal posterior tibial and anterior tibial/dorsalis pedis arteries plus segmental volume plethysmography at 3 or more levels, or ankle/brachial indices at distal posterior tibial and anterior tibial/dorsalis pedis arteries plus segmental transcutaneous oxygen tension measurements at 3 or more levels), or single level study with provocative functional maneuvers (eg, measurements with postural provocative tests, or measurements with reactive hyperemia)

(When only 1 arm or leg is available for study, report 93922 for a unilateral study when recording 3 or more levels or when performing provocative functional maneuvers)

(Report 93923 only once in the upper extremity(s) and/or once in the lower extremity(s). When both the upper and lower extremities are evaluated in the same setting, 93923 may be reported twice by adding modifier 59 to the second procedure)

▶(For transcutaneous oxyhemoglobin measurement in a lower extremity wound by near infrared spectroscopy, use 0286T)◀

93924   Noninvasive physiologic studies of lower extremity arteries, at rest and following treadmill stress testing, (ie, bidirectional Doppler waveform or volume plethysmography recording and analysis at rest with ankle/brachial indices immediately after and at timed intervals following performance of a standardized protocol on a motorized treadmill plus recording of time of onset of claudication or other symptoms, maximal walking time, and time to recovery) complete bilateral study

(Do not report 93924 in conjunction with 93922, 93923)

93925   Duplex scan of lower extremity arteries or arterial bypass grafts; complete bilateral study

93926   unilateral or limited study

93930   Duplex scan of upper extremity arteries or arterial bypass grafts; complete bilateral study

93931   unilateral or limited study

## Extremity Venous Studies (Including Digits)

93965   Noninvasive physiologic studies of extremity veins, complete bilateral study (eg, Doppler waveform analysis with responses to compression and other maneuvers, phleborheography, impedance plethysmography)

93970   Duplex scan of extremity veins including responses to compression and other maneuvers; complete bilateral study

93971   unilateral or limited study

## Visceral and Penile Vascular Studies

93975   Duplex scan of arterial inflow and venous outflow of abdominal, pelvic, scrotal contents and/or retroperitoneal organs; complete study

93976   limited study

93978   Duplex scan of aorta, inferior vena cava, iliac vasculature, or bypass grafts; complete study

93979   unilateral or limited study

93980   Duplex scan of arterial inflow and venous outflow of penile vessels; complete study

93981   follow-up or limited study

93982   Noninvasive physiologic study of implanted wireless pressure sensor in aneurysmal sac following endovascular repair, complete study including recording, analysis of pressure and waveform tracings, interpretation and report

(Do not report 93982 in conjunction with 34806)

## Extremity Arterial-Venous Studies

93990   Duplex scan of hemodialysis access (including arterial inflow, body of access and venous outflow)

(For measurement of hemodialysis access flow using indicator dilution methods, use 90940)

## ▶Other Noninvasive Vascular Diagnostic Studies◀

● 93998   Unlisted noninvasive vascular diagnostic study

# Pulmonary

## Ventilator Management

94002   Ventilation assist and management, initiation of pressure or volume preset ventilators for assisted or controlled breathing; hospital inpatient/observation, initial day

94003   hospital inpatient/observation, each subsequent day

94004   nursing facility, per day

(Do not report 94002-94004 in conjunction with Evaluation and Management services 99201-99499)

Medicine

**94005** Home ventilator management care plan oversight of a patient (patient not present) in home, domiciliary or rest home (eg, assisted living) requiring review of status, review of laboratories and other studies and revision of orders and respiratory care plan (as appropriate), within a calendar month, 30 minutes or more

(Do not report 94005 in conjunction with 99339, 99340, 99374-99378)

(Ventilator management care plan oversight is reported separately from home or domiciliary, rest home [eg, assisted living] services. A physician may report 94005, when performed, including when a different physician reports 99339, 99340, 99374-99378 for the same 30 days)

# ►Pulmonary Diagnostic Testing and Therapies◄

►Codes 94010-94799 include laboratory procedure(s) and interpretation of test results. If a separate identifiable Evaluation and Management service is performed, the appropriate E/M service code may be reported in addition to 94010-94799.

Spirometry (94010) measures expiratory airflow and volumes and forms the basis of most pulmonary function testing. When spirometry is performed before and after administration of a bronchodilator, report 94060. Measurement of vital capacity (94150) is a component of spirometry and is only reported when performed alone. The flow-volume loop (94375) is used to identify patterns of inspiratory and/or expiratory obstruction in central or peripheral airways. Spirometry (94010, 94060) includes maximal breathing capacity (94200) and flow-volume loop (94375), when performed.

Measurement of lung volumes may be performed using plethysmography, helium dilution or nitrogen washout. Plethysmography (94726) is utilized to determine total lung capacity, residual volume, functional residual capacity, and airway resistance. Nitrogen washout or helium dilution (94727) may be used to measure lung volumes, distribution of ventilation and closing volume. Impulse oscillometry (94728) assesses airway resistance and may be reported in addition to gas dilution techniques. Spirometry (94010, 94060) and bronchial provocation (94070) are not included in 94726 and 94727 and may be reported separately.

Diffusing capacity (94729) is most commonly performed in conjunction with lung volumes or spirometry and is an add-on code to 94726-94728, 94010, 94060, 94070, and 94375.

Pulmonary function tests (94011-94013) are reported for measurements in infants and young children through 2 years of age.

Pulmonary function testing measurements are reported as actual values and as a percent of predicted values by age, gender, height, and race.◄

**94010** Spirometry, including graphic record, total and timed vital capacity, expiratory flow rate measurement(s), with or without maximal voluntary ventilation

►(Do not report 94010 in conjunction with 94150, 94200, 94375, 94728)◄

**94011** Measurement of spirometric forced expiratory flows in an infant or child through 2 years of age

**94012** Measurement of spirometric forced expiratory flows, before and after bronchodilator, in an infant or child through 2 years of age

**94013** Measurement of lung volumes (ie, functional residual capacity [FRC], forced vital capacity [FVC], and expiratory reserve volume [ERV]) in an infant or child through 2 years of age

**94014** Patient-initiated spirometric recording per 30-day period of time; includes reinforced education, transmission of spirometric tracing, data capture, analysis of transmitted data, periodic recalibration and physician review and interpretation

**94015** recording (includes hook-up, reinforced education, data transmission, data capture, trend analysis, and periodic recalibration)

**94016** physician review and interpretation only

**94060** Bronchodilation responsiveness, spirometry as in 94010, pre- and post-bronchodilator administration

►(Do not report 94060 in conjunction with 94150, 94200, 94375, 94728)◄

(Report bronchodilator supply separately with 99070 or appropriate supply code)

(For prolonged exercise test for bronchospasm with pre- and post-spirometry, use 94620)

**94070** Bronchospasm provocation evaluation, multiple spirometric determinations as in 94010, with administered agents (eg, antigen[s], cold air, methacholine)

(Report antigen[s] administration separately with 99070 or appropriate supply code)

**94150** Vital capacity, total (separate procedure)

►(Do not report 94150 in conjunction with 94010, 94060, 94728. To report thoracic gas volumes, see 94726, 94727)◄

**94200** Maximum breathing capacity, maximal voluntary ventilation

►(Do not report 94200 in conjunction with 94010, 94060)◄

►(94240 has been deleted. To report thoracic gas volumes, see 94726, 94727)◄

**94250** Expired gas collection, quantitative, single procedure (separate procedure)

►(94260 has been deleted. To report thoracic gas volumes, see 94726, 94727)◄

**Medicine**

► (94350 has been deleted. To report, see 94726, 94727) ◄

► (94360 has been deleted. To report, see 94726, 94728) ◄

► (94370 has been deleted. To report, see 94726, 94727) ◄

**94375** Respiratory flow volume loop

► (Do not report 94375 in conjunction with 94010, 94060, 94728) ◄

**94400** Breathing response to $CO_2$ ($CO_2$ response curve)

**94450** Breathing response to hypoxia (hypoxia response curve)

(For high altitude simulation test [HAST], see 94452, 94453)

**94452** High altitude simulation test (HAST), with physician interpretation and report

(For obtaining arterial blood gases, use 36600)

(Do not report 94452 in conjunction with 94453, 94760, 94761)

**94453** with supplemental oxygen titration

(For obtaining arterial blood gases, use 36600)

(Do not report 94453 in conjunction with 94452, 94760, 94761)

⊘ **94610** Intrapulmonary surfactant administration by a physician through endotracheal tube

(Do not report 94610 in conjunction with 99468-99472)

(For endotracheal intubation, use 31500)

(Report 94610 once per dosing episode)

**94620** Pulmonary stress testing; simple (eg, 6-minute walk test, prolonged exercise test for bronchospasm with pre- and post-spirometry and oximetry)

**94621** complex (including measurements of $CO_2$ production, $O_2$ uptake, and electrocardiographic recordings)

**94640** Pressurized or nonpressurized inhalation treatment for acute airway obstruction or for sputum induction for diagnostic purposes (eg, with an aerosol generator, nebulizer, metered dose inhaler or intermittent positive pressure breathing [IPPB] device)

(For more than 1 inhalation treatment performed on the same date, append modifier 76)

(For continuous inhalation treatment of 1 hour or more, see 94644, 94645)

**94642** Aerosol inhalation of pentamidine for pneumocystis carinii pneumonia treatment or prophylaxis

**94644** Continuous inhalation treatment with aerosol medication for acute airway obstruction; first hour

(For services of less than 1 hour, use 94640)

+ **94645** each additional hour (List separately in addition to code for primary procedure)

(Use 94645 in conjunction with 94644)

**94660** Continuous positive airway pressure ventilation (CPAP), initiation and management

**94662** Continuous negative pressure ventilation (CNP), initiation and management

**94664** Demonstration and/or evaluation of patient utilization of an aerosol generator, nebulizer, metered dose inhaler or IPPB device

(94664 can be reported 1 time only per day of service)

**94667** Manipulation chest wall, such as cupping, percussing, and vibration to facilitate lung function; initial demonstration and/or evaluation

**94668** subsequent

**94680** Oxygen uptake, expired gas analysis; rest and exercise, direct, simple

**94681** including $CO_2$ output, percentage oxygen extracted

**94690** rest, indirect (separate procedure)

(For single arterial puncture, use 36600)

► (94720, 94725 have been deleted. To report, see 94729) ◄

● **94726** Plethysmography for determination of lung volumes and, when performed, airway resistance

► (Do not report 94726 in conjunction with 94727, 94728) ◄

● **94727** Gas dilution or washout for determination of lung volumes and, when performed, distribution of ventilation and closing volumes

► (Do not report 94727 in conjunction with 94726) ◄

● **94728** Airway resistance by impulse oscillometry

► (Do not report 94728 in conjunction with 94010, 94060, 94070, 94375, 94726) ◄

+ ● **94729** Diffusing capacity (eg, carbon monoxide, membrane) (List separately in addition to code for primary procedure)

► (Report 94729 in conjunction with 94010, 94060, 94070, 94375, 94726-94728) ◄

**94750** Pulmonary compliance study (eg, plethysmography, volume and pressure measurements)

**94760** Noninvasive ear or pulse oximetry for oxygen saturation; single determination

(For blood gases, see 82803-82810)

**94761** multiple determinations (eg, during exercise)

**94762** by continuous overnight monitoring (separate procedure)

(For other in vivo laboratory procedures, see 88720-88741)

**94770** Carbon dioxide, expired gas determination by infrared analyzer

(For bronchoscopy, see 31622-31656)

(For placement of flow directed catheter, use 93503)

(For venipuncture, use 36410)

(For central venous catheter placement, see 36555-36556)

(For arterial puncture, use 36600)

(For arterial catheterization, use 36620)

(For thoracentesis, use 32421)

(For phlebotomy, therapeutic, use 99195)

(For lung biopsy, needle, use 32405)

(For intubation, orotracheal or nasotracheal, use 31500)

**94772** Circadian respiratory pattern recording (pediatric pneumogram), 12-24 hour continuous recording, infant

(Separate procedure codes for electromyograms, EEG, ECG, and recordings of respiration are excluded when 94772 is reported)

**94774** Pediatric home apnea monitoring event recording including respiratory rate, pattern and heart rate per 30-day period of time; includes monitor attachment, download of data, physician review, interpretation, and preparation of a report

(Do not report 94774 in conjunction with 94775-94777 during the same reporting period)

**94775** monitor attachment only (includes hook-up, initiation of recording and disconnection)

**94776** monitoring, download of information, receipt of transmission(s) and analyses by computer only

**94777** physician review, interpretation and preparation of report only

(When oxygen saturation monitoring is used in addition to heart rate and respiratory monitoring, it is not reported separately)

(Do not report 94774-94777 in conjunction with 93224-93272)

(Do not report apnea recording device separately)

(For sleep study, see 95805-95811)

● **94780** Car seat/bed testing for airway integrity, neonate, with continual nursing observation and continuous recording of pulse oximetry, heart rate and respiratory rate, with interpretation and report; 60 minutes

▶(Do not report 94780 for less than 60 minutes)◀

▶(Do not report 94780 in conjunction with 93040-93042, 94760, 94761, 99468-99472, 99477-99480)◀

+● **94781** each additional full 30 minutes (List separately in addition to code for primary procedure)

▶(Use 94781 in conjunction with 94780)◀

**94799** Unlisted pulmonary service or procedure

# Allergy and Clinical Immunology

### Definitions

*Immunotherapy (desensitization, hyposensitization)* is the parenteral administration of allergenic extracts as antigens at periodic intervals, usually on an increasing dosage scale to a dosage which is maintained as maintenance therapy. Indications for immunotherapy are determined by appropriate diagnostic procedures coordinated with clinical judgment and knowledge of the natural history of allergic diseases.

*Other therapy:* for medical conferences on the use of mechanical and electronic devices (precipitators, air conditioners, air filters, humidifiers, dehumidifiers), climatotherapy, physical therapy, occupational and recreational therapy, see **Evaluation and Management** section.

Do not report Evaluation and Management (E/M) services for test interpretation and report. If a significant separately identifiable E/M service is performed, the appropriate E/M service code should be reported using modifier 25.

## Allergy Testing

(For allergy laboratory tests, see 86000-86999)

(For therapy for severe or intractable allergic disease, see 96365-96368, 96372, 96374, 96375)

**95004** Percutaneous tests (scratch, puncture, prick) with allergenic extracts, immediate type reaction, including test interpretation and report by a physician, specify number of tests

**95010** Percutaneous tests (scratch, puncture, prick) sequential and incremental, with drugs, biologicals or venoms, immediate type reaction, including test interpretation and report by a physician, specify number of tests

**95012** Nitric oxide expired gas determination

**95015** Intracutaneous (intradermal) tests, sequential and incremental, with drugs, biologicals, or venoms, immediate type reaction, including test interpretation and report by a physician, specify number of tests

**95024** Intracutaneous (intradermal) tests with allergenic extracts, immediate type reaction, including test interpretation and report by a physician, specify number of tests

**95027** Intracutaneous (intradermal) tests, sequential and incremental, with allergenic extracts for airborne allergens, immediate type reaction, including test interpretation and report by a physician, specify number of tests

**95028** Intracutaneous (intradermal) tests with allergenic extracts, delayed type reaction, including reading, specify number of tests

| | |
|---|---|
| **95044** | Patch or application test(s) (specify number of tests) |
| **95052** | Photo patch test(s) (specify number of tests) |
| **95056** | Photo tests |
| **95060** | Ophthalmic mucous membrane tests |
| **95065** | Direct nasal mucous membrane test |
| **95070** | Inhalation bronchial challenge testing (not including necessary pulmonary function tests); with histamine, methacholine, or similar compounds |
| **95071** | with antigens or gases, specify |

(For pulmonary function tests, see 94060, 94070)

| | |
|---|---|
| **95075** | Ingestion challenge test (sequential and incremental ingestion of test items, eg, food, drug or other substance such as metabisulfite) |

## Allergen Immunotherapy

Codes 95115-95199 include the professional services necessary for allergen immunotherapy. Office visit codes may be used in addition to allergen immunotherapy if other identifiable services are provided at that time.

| | |
|---|---|
| **95115** | Professional services for allergen immunotherapy not including provision of allergenic extracts; single injection |
| **95117** | 2 or more injections |
| **95120** | Professional services for allergen immunotherapy in prescribing physicians office or institution, including provision of allergenic extract; single injection |
| **95125** | 2 or more injections |
| **95130** | single stinging insect venom |
| **95131** | 2 stinging insect venoms |
| **95132** | 3 stinging insect venoms |
| **95133** | 4 stinging insect venoms |
| **95134** | 5 stinging insect venoms |
| **95144** | Professional services for the supervision of preparation and provision of antigens for allergen immunotherapy, single dose vial(s) (specify number of vials) |

(A single dose vial contains a single dose of antigen administered in 1 injection)

| | |
|---|---|
| **95145** | Professional services for the supervision of preparation and provision of antigens for allergen immunotherapy (specify number of doses); single stinging insect venom |
| **95146** | 2 single stinging insect venoms |
| **95147** | 3 single stinging insect venoms |
| **95148** | 4 single stinging insect venoms |
| **95149** | 5 single stinging insect venoms |
| **95165** | Professional services for the supervision of preparation and provision of antigens for allergen immunotherapy; single or multiple antigens (specify number of doses) |
| **95170** | whole body extract of biting insect or other arthropod (specify number of doses) |

(For allergy immunotherapy reporting, a dose is the amount of antigen[s] administered in a single injection from a multiple dose vial)

| | |
|---|---|
| **95180** | Rapid desensitization procedure, each hour (eg, insulin, penicillin, equine serum) |
| **95199** | Unlisted allergy/clinical immunologic service or procedure |

(For skin testing of bacterial, viral, fungal extracts, see 86485-86580, 95028)

(For special reports on allergy patients, use 99080)

(For testing procedures such as radioallergosorbent testing [RAST], rat mast cell technique [RMCT], mast cell degranulation test [MCDT], lymphocytic transformation test [LTT], leukocyte histamine release [LHR], migration inhibitory factor test [MIF], transfer factor test [TFT], nitroblue tetrazolium dye test [NTD], see Immunology section in **Pathology** or use 95199)

## Endocrinology

| | |
|---|---|
| **95250** | Ambulatory continuous glucose monitoring of interstitial tissue fluid via a subcutaneous sensor for a minimum of 72 hours; sensor placement, hook-up, calibration of monitor, patient training, removal of sensor, and printout of recording |

(Do not report 95250 more than once per month)

(Do not report 95250 in conjunction with 99091)

| | |
|---|---|
| **95251** | interpretation and report |

(Do not report 95251 more than once per month)

(Do not report 95251 in conjunction with 99091)

## Neurology and Neuromuscular Procedures

Neurologic services are typically consultative, and any of the levels of consultation (99241-99255) may be appropriate.

In addition, services and skills outlined under **Evaluation and Management** levels of service appropriate to neurologic illnesses should be reported similarly.

The EEG, autonomic function, evoked potential, reflex tests, EMG, NCV, and MEG services (95812-95829 and 95860-95967) include recording, interpretation by a physician, and report. For interpretation only, use modifier 26. For EMG guidance, see 95873, 95874.

Codes 95812-95822, 95920, 95950-95953 and 95956 use recording time as a basis for code use. Recording time is when the recording is underway and data is being collected. Recording time excludes set up and take down time. Codes 95961-95962 use physician time as a basis for code use.

**Medicine**

(Do not report codes 95860-95875 in addition to 96000-96004)

## ►Sleep Medicine Testing◄

►Sleep medicine services include procedures that evaluate adult and pediatric patients for a variety of sleep disorders. Sleep medicine testing services are diagnostic procedures using in-laboratory and portable technology to assess physiologic data and therapy.◄

All sleep services (95800-95811) include recording, interpretation and report. (Report with modifier 52 if less than 6 hours of recording for 95800, 95801 and 95806-95811, and if less than four nap opportunities are recorded for 95805.)

### Definitions

For purposes of CPT reporting of sleep medicine testing services, the following definitions apply:

*Actigraphy:* the use of a portable, non-invasive, device that continuously records gross motor movement over an extended period of time. The periods of activity and rest are indirect parameters for estimates of the periods of wakefulness and sleep of an individual.

*Attended:* a technologist or qualified health care professional is physically present (ie, sufficient proximity such that the qualified health care professional can physically respond to emergencies, to other appropriate patient needs or to technical problems at the bedside) throughout the recording session.

*Electrooculogram (EOG):* a recording of electrical activity indicative of eye movement.

*Maintenance of wakefulness test (MWT):* a standardized objective test used to determine a person's ability to stay awake. MWT requires sleep staging of the trials that are performed at defined intervals and is attended by a qualified health care professional.

*Multiple sleep latency test (MSLT):* a standardized objective test of the tendency to fall asleep. MSLT requires sleep staging of the nap opportunities that are performed at defined intervals and is attended by a technologist or qualified health care professional.

*Peripheral arterial tonometry (PAT):* a plethysmography technique that continuously measures pulsatile volume changes in a digit. This reflects the relative change of blood volume as an indirect measure of sympathetic nervous system activity which is used in respiratory analysis.

*Physiological measurements of sleep as used in 95805:* the parameters measured are a frontal, central and occipital lead of EEG (3 leads), submental EMG lead and a left and right EOG. These parameters are used together for staging sleep.

*Polysomnography:* a sleep test involving the continuous, simultaneous, recording of physiological parameters for a period of at least 6 hours that is performed in a sleep laboratory and attended by a technologist or qualified health care professional. The parameters measured are a frontal, central and occipital lead of EEG (3 leads), submental EMG lead and a left and right EOG, (from which sleep is staged), plus four or more additional parameters. The additional parameters typically required in polysomnography are listed below:

A. Electrocardiogram (ECG)

B. Nasal and/or oral airflow

C. Respiratory effort

D. Oxyhemoglobin saturation, SpO2

E. Bilateral anterior tibialis EMG

*Positive airway pressure (PAP):* a device used to treat sleep-related breathing disorders with the use of non-invasive delivery of positive pressure to the airway. Examples include but are not limited to: CPAP (continuous positive airway pressure), bilevel PAP, AutoPAP (autotitrating or adjusting PAP), ASV (adaptive-servo ventilation).

*Remote:* the site of service is distant from the monitoring center. Neither a technologist nor a qualified health care professional is physically present at the testing site.

*Respiratory airflow (ventilation):* the movement of air during inhaled and exhaled breaths. This is typically assessed using thermistor and nasal pressure sensors.

*Respiratory analysis:* generation of derived parameters that describe components of respiration obtained by using direct or indirect parameters, eg, by airflow or peripheral arterial tone.

*Respiratory effort:* contraction of the diaphragmatic and/or intercostal muscles to cause (or attempt to cause) respiratory airflow. This is typically measured using transducers that estimate motion of the thorax and abdomen such as respiratory inductive plethysmography, transducers that estimate pressures generated by breathing muscles such as esophageal monometry, or by contraction of breathing muscles, such as diaphragmatic/intercostal EMG.

*Respiratory (thoracoabdominal) movement:* movement of the chest and abdomen during respiratory effort.

*Sleep latency:* the length of time it takes to transition from wakefulness to sleep. In the sleep laboratory it is the time from "lights out" to the first epoch scored as any stage of sleep.

*Sleep staging:* the delineation of the distinct sleep levels through the simultaneous evaluation of physiologic measures including a frontal, central and occipital lead of EEG (3 leads), submental EMG lead and a left and right EOG.

*Sleep testing (or sleep study):* the continuous, simultaneous monitoring of physiological parameters during sleep (eg, polysomnography, EEG).

**Medicine**

*Total sleep time:* a derived parameter obtained by sleep staging or may be estimated indirectly using actigraphy or other methods.

*Unattended:* a technologist or qualified health care professional is not physically present with the patient during the recording session.◄

(Report with modifier 52 if less than 6 hours of recording or in other cases of reduced services as appropriate)

(For unattended sleep study, use 95806)

**95800** Code is out of numerical sequence. See 95803-95811

**95801** Code is out of numerical sequence. See 95800-95811

**95803** Actigraphy testing, recording, analysis, interpretation, and report (minimum of 72 hours to 14 consecutive days of recording)

(Do not report 95803 more than once in any 14 day period)

(Do not report 95803 in conjunction with 95806-95811)

**95805** Multiple sleep latency or maintenance of wakefulness testing, recording, analysis and interpretation of physiological measurements of sleep during multiple trials to assess sleepiness

**95806** Sleep study, unattended, simultaneous recording of, heart rate, oxygen saturation, respiratory airflow, and respiratory effort (eg, thoracoabdominal movement)

(Do not report 95806 in conjunction with 93041-93227, 93228, 93229, 93268-93272, 95800, 95801)

(For unattended sleep study that measures heart rate, oxygen saturation, respiratory analysis, and sleep time, use 95800)

(For unattended sleep study that measures a minimum heart rate, oxygen saturation, and respiratory analysis, use 95801)

\# **95800** Sleep study, unattended, simultaneous recording; heart rate, oxygen saturation, respiratory analysis (eg, by airflow or peripheral arterial tone), and sleep time

(Do not report 95800 in conjunction with 93041-93227, 93228, 93229, 93268-93272, 95801, 95803, 95806)

(For unattended sleep study that measures a minimum of heart rate, oxygen saturation, and respiratory analysis, use 95801)

\# **95801** minimum of heart rate, oxygen saturation, and respiratory analysis (eg, by airflow or peripheral arterial tone)

(Do not report 95801 in conjunction with 93041-93227, 93228, 93229, 93268-93272, 95800, 95806)

(For unattended sleep study that measures heart rate, oxygen saturation, respiratory analysis and sleep time, use 95800)

**95807** Sleep study, simultaneous recording of ventilation, respiratory effort, ECG or heart rate, and oxygen saturation, attended by a technologist

**95808** Polysomnography; sleep staging with 1-3 additional parameters of sleep, attended by a technologist

**95810** sleep staging with 4 or more additional parameters of sleep, attended by a technologist

**95811** sleep staging with 4 or more additional parameters of sleep, with initiation of continuous positive airway pressure therapy or bilevel ventilation, attended by a technologist

# Routine Electroencephalography (EEG)

EEG codes 95812-95822 include hyperventilation and/or photic stimulation when appropriate. Routine EEG codes 95816-95822 include 20 to 40 minutes of recording. Extended EEG codes 95812-95813 include reporting times longer than 40 minutes.

**95812** Electroencephalogram (EEG) extended monitoring; 41-60 minutes

**95813** greater than 1 hour

**95816** Electroencephalogram (EEG); including recording awake and drowsy

**95819** including recording awake and asleep

**95822** recording in coma or sleep only

**95824** cerebral death evaluation only

**95827** all night recording

(For 24-hour EEG monitoring, see 95950-95953 or 95956)

(For EEG during nonintracranial surgery, use 95955)

(For Wada test, use 95958)

(For digital analysis of EEG, use 95957)

**95829** Electrocorticogram at surgery (separate procedure)

**95830** Insertion by physician of sphenoidal electrodes for electroencephalographic (EEG) recording

# Muscle and Range of Motion Testing

**95831** Muscle testing, manual (separate procedure) with report; extremity (excluding hand) or trunk

**95832** hand, with or without comparison with normal side

**95833** total evaluation of body, excluding hands

**95834** total evaluation of body, including hands

**95851** Range of motion measurements and report (separate procedure); each extremity (excluding hand) or each trunk section (spine)

**95852** hand, with or without comparison with normal side

**95857** Cholinesterase inhibitor challenge test for myasthenia gravis

# Electromyography

►Needle electromyographic (EMG) procedures include the interpretation of electrical waveforms measured by equipment that produces both visible and audible components of electrical signals recorded from the muscle(s) studied by the needle electrode.

Use 95870 or 95885 when four or fewer muscles are tested in an extremity. Use 95860-95864 or 95886 when five or more muscles are tested in an extremity.

Use EMG codes (95860-95864 and 95867-95870) when no nerve conduction studies (95900-95904) are performed on that day. Use 95885, 95886 and 95887 for EMG services when nerve conduction studies (95900-95904) are performed in conjunction with EMG on the same day.

Report either 95885 or 95886 once per extremity. Codes 95885 and 95886 can be reported together up to a combined total of four units of service per patient when all four extremities are tested.◄

**95860**    Needle electromyography; 1 extremity with or without related paraspinal areas

**95861**      2 extremities with or without related paraspinal areas

(For dynamic electromyography performed during motion analysis studies, see 96002-96003)

**95863**      3 extremities with or without related paraspinal areas

**95864**      4 extremities with or without related paraspinal areas

**95865**      larynx

(Do not report modifier 50 in conjunction with 95865)

(For unilateral procedure, report modifier 52 in conjunction with 95865)

**95866**      hemidiaphragm

**95867**      cranial nerve supplied muscle(s), unilateral

**95868**      cranial nerve supplied muscles, bilateral

**95869**      thoracic paraspinal muscles (excluding T1 or T12)

**95870**      limited study of muscles in 1 extremity or non-limb (axial) muscles (unilateral or bilateral), other than thoracic paraspinal, cranial nerve supplied muscles, or sphincters

(To report a complete study of the extremities, see 95860-95864)

(For anal or urethral sphincter, detrusor, urethra, perineum musculature, see 51785-51792)

(For eye muscles, use 92265)

**95872**    Needle electromyography using single fiber electrode, with quantitative measurement of jitter, blocking and/or fiber density, any/all sites of each muscle studied

#+● **95885**    Needle electromyography, each extremity, with related paraspinal areas, when performed, done with nerve conduction, amplitude and latency/velocity study; limited (List separately in addition to code for primary procedure)

#+● **95886**      complete, five or more muscles studied, innervated by three or more nerves or four or more spinal levels (List separately in addition to code for primary procedure)

►(Use 95885, 95886 in conjunction with 95900-95904)◄

►(Do not report 95885, 95886 in conjunction with 95860-95864, 95870, 95905)◄

#+● **95887**    Needle electromyography, non-extremity (cranial nerve supplied or axial) muscle(s) done with nerve conduction, amplitude and latency/velocity study (List separately in addition to code for primary procedure)

►(Use 95887 in conjunction with 95900-95904)◄

►(Do not report 95887 in conjunction with 95867-95870, 95905)◄

# Guidance for Chemodenervation and Ischemic Muscle Testing

+ **95873**    Electrical stimulation for guidance in conjunction with chemodenervation (List separately in addition to code for primary procedure)

+ **95874**    Needle electromyography for guidance in conjunction with chemodenervation (List separately in addition to code for primary procedure)

(Use 95873, 95874 in conjunction with 64612-64614)

(Do not report 95874 in conjunction with 95873)

(Do not report 95873, 95874 in conjunction with 95860-95870)

**95875**    Ischemic limb exercise test with serial specimen(s) acquisition for muscle(s) metabolite(s)

(For listing of nerves considered for separate study, see **Appendix J**)

**95885**    Code is out of numerical sequence. See 95860-95887

**95886**    Code is out of numerical sequence. See 95860-95887

**95887**    Code is out of numerical sequence. See 95860-95887

# Nerve Conduction Tests

The following applies to nerve conduction tests (95900-95904): Codes 95900-95904 describe nerve conduction tests when performed with individually placed stimulating, recording, and ground electrodes. The stimulating, recording, and ground electrode placement and the test design must be individualized to the patient's unique anatomy. Nerves tested must be limited to the specific nerves and conduction studies needed for the particular clinical question being investigated. The stimulating electrode must be placed directly over the nerve to be tested, and stimulation parameters properly adjusted to avoid stimulating other nerves or nerve branches. In most motor nerve conduction studies, and in some sensory and mixed nerve conduction studies, both proximal and distal stimulation will be used. Motor nerve conduction study recordings must be made from electrodes placed directly over the motor point of the specific muscle to be tested. Sensory nerve conduction study recordings must be made from electrodes placed directly over the specific nerve to be tested. Waveforms must be reviewed on site in real time, and the technique (stimulus site, recording site, ground site, filter settings) must be adjusted, as appropriate, as the test proceeds in order to minimize artifact, and to minimize the chances of unintended stimulation of adjacent nerves and the unintended recording from adjacent muscles or nerves. Reports must be prepared on site by the examiner, and consist of the work product of the interpretation of numerous test results, using well-established techniques to assess the amplitude, latency, and configuration of waveforms elicited by stimulation at each site of each nerve tested. This includes the calculation of nerve conduction velocities, sometimes including specialized F-wave indices, along with comparison to normal values, summarization of clinical and electrodiagnostic data, and physician or other qualified health care professional interpretation.

Code 95905 describes nerve conduction tests when performed with preconfigured electrodes customized to a specific anatomic site.

⊘ **95900**   Nerve conduction, amplitude and latency/velocity study, each nerve; motor, without F-wave study

⊘ **95903**      motor, with F-wave study

⊘ **95904**      sensory

(Report 95900, 95903, and/or 95904 only once when multiple sites on the same nerve are stimulated or recorded)

▶(Use 95885-95887 in conjunction with 95900-95904 when performing electromyography with nerve conduction studies)◀

⊘ **95905**   Motor and/or sensory nerve conduction, using preconfigured electrode array(s), amplitude and latency/velocity study, each limb, includes F-wave study when performed, with interpretation and report

(Report 95905 only once per limb studied)

▶(Do not report 95905 in conjunction with 95885, 95886, 95900-95904, 95934-95936)◀

## Intraoperative Neurophysiology

+ **95920**   Intraoperative neurophysiology testing, per hour (List separately in addition to code for primary procedure)

(Use 95920 in conjunction with the study performed, 92585, 95822, 95860, 95861, 95867, 95868, 95870, 95900, 95904, 95925-95937)

(Code 95920 describes ongoing electrophysiologic testing and monitoring performed during surgical procedures. Code 95920 is reported per hour of service, and includes only the ongoing electrophysiologic monitoring time distinct from performance of specific type[s] of baseline electrophysiologic study[s] [95860, 95861, 95867, 95868, 95870, 95900, 95904, 95928, 95929, 95933-95937] or interpretation of specific type[s] of baseline electrophysiologic study[s] [92585, 95822, 95870, 95925-95928, 95929, 95930]. The time spent performing or interpreting the baseline electrophysiologic study[s] should not be counted as intraoperative monitoring, but represents separately reportable procedures. Code 95920 should be used once per hour even if multiple electrophysiologic studies are performed. Do not report 95920 if recording lasts 30 minutes or less. The baseline electrophysiologic study[s] should be used once per operative session. For procedures that last beyond midnight, report services using the day on which the monitoring began and using the total hours monitored)

(For time spent waiting on standby before monitoring, use 99360)

(For electrocorticography, use 95829)

(For intraoperative EEG during nonintracranial surgery, use 95955)

(For intraoperative functional cortical or subcortical mapping, see 95961-95962)

(For intraoperative neurostimulator programming and analysis, see 95970-95975)

## Autonomic Function Tests

**95921**   Testing of autonomic nervous system function; cardiovagal innervation (parasympathetic function), including 2 or more of the following: heart rate response to deep breathing with recorded R-R interval, Valsalva ratio, and 30:15 ratio

**95922**      vasomotor adrenergic innervation (sympathetic adrenergic function), including beat-to-beat blood pressure and R-R interval changes during Valsalva maneuver and at least 5 minutes of passive tilt

**95923**      sudomotor, including 1 or more of the following: quantitative sudomotor axon reflex test (QSART), silastic sweat imprint, thermoregulatory sweat test, and changes in sympathetic skin potential

## Evoked Potentials and Reflex Tests

**95925**   Short-latency somatosensory evoked potential study, stimulation of any/all peripheral nerves or skin sites, recording from the central nervous system; in upper limbs

▶(Do not report 95925 in conjunction with 95926)◀

**95926**      in lower limbs

▶(Do not report 95926 in conjunction with 95925)◀

#● **95938**      in upper and lower limbs

▶(Do not report 95938 in conjunction with 95925, 95926)◀

**95927**  in the trunk or head

(To report a unilateral study, use modifier 52)

(For auditory evoked potentials, use 92585)

**95928**  Central motor evoked potential study (transcranial motor stimulation); upper limbs

►(Do not report 95928 in conjunction with 95929)◄

**95929**  lower limbs

►(Do not report 95929 in conjunction with 95928)◄

#● **95939**  in upper and lower limbs

►(Do not report 95939 in conjunction with 95928, 95929)◄

**95930**  Visual evoked potential (VEP) testing central nervous system, checkerboard or flash

**95933**  Orbicularis oculi (blink) reflex, by electrodiagnostic testing

**95934**  H-reflex, amplitude and latency study; record gastrocnemius/soleus muscle

**95936**  record muscle other than gastrocnemius/soleus muscle

(To report a bilateral study, use modifier 50)

**95937**  Neuromuscular junction testing (repetitive stimulation, paired stimuli), each nerve, any 1 method

► **95938**  Code is out of numerical sequence. See 95925-95939◄

► **95939**  Code is out of numerical sequence. See 95925-95939◄

# Special EEG Tests

Codes 95950-95953 and 95956 are used per 24 hours of recording. For recording more than 12 hours, do not use modifier 52. For recording 12 hours or less, use modifier 52. Codes 95951 and 95956 are used for recordings in which interpretations can be made throughout the recording time, with interventions to alter or end the recording or to alter the patient care during the recordings as needed.

Codes 95961 and 95962 use physician time as a basis for unit of service. Report for each hour of physician attendance. Report 95961 for the first hour of physician attendance. Use modifier 52 with 95961 for 30 minutes or less. Report 95962 for each additional hour of physician attendance.

**95950**  Monitoring for identification and lateralization of cerebral seizure focus, electroencephalographic (eg, 8 channel EEG) recording and interpretation, each 24 hours

**95951**  Monitoring for localization of cerebral seizure focus by cable or radio, 16 or more channel telemetry, combined electroencephalographic (EEG) and video recording and interpretation (eg, for presurgical localization), each 24 hours

**95953**  Monitoring for localization of cerebral seizure focus by computerized portable 16 or more channel EEG, electroencephalographic (EEG) recording and interpretation, each 24 hours, unattended

**95954**  Pharmacological or physical activation requiring physician attendance during EEG recording of activation phase (eg, thiopental activation test)

**95955**  Electroencephalogram (EEG) during nonintracranial surgery (eg, carotid surgery)

**95956**  Monitoring for localization of cerebral seizure focus by cable or radio, 16 or more channel telemetry, electroencephalographic (EEG) recording and interpretation, each 24 hours, attended by a technologist or nurse

**95957**  Digital analysis of electroencephalogram (EEG) (eg, for epileptic spike analysis)

**95958**  Wada activation test for hemispheric function, including electroencephalographic (EEG) monitoring

**95961**  Functional cortical and subcortical mapping by stimulation and/or recording of electrodes on brain surface, or of depth electrodes, to provoke seizures or identify vital brain structures; initial hour of physician attendance

+ **95962**  each additional hour of physician attendance (List separately in addition to code for primary procedure)

(Use 95962 in conjunction with 95961)

**95965**  Magnetoencephalography (MEG), recording and analysis; for spontaneous brain magnetic activity (eg, epileptic cerebral cortex localization)

**95966**  for evoked magnetic fields, single modality (eg, sensory, motor, language, or visual cortex localization)

+ **95967**  for evoked magnetic fields, each additional modality (eg, sensory, motor, language, or visual cortex localization) (List separately in addition to code for primary procedure)

(Use 95967 in conjunction with 95966)

(For electroencephalography performed in addition to magnetoencephalography, see 95812-95827)

(For somatosensory evoked potentials, auditory evoked potentials, and visual evoked potentials performed in addition to magnetic evoked field responses, see 92585, 95925, 95926, and/or 95930)

(For computerized tomography performed in addition to magnetoencephalography, see 70450-70470, 70496)

(For magnetic resonance imaging performed in addition to magnetoencephalography, see 70551-70553)

# Neurostimulators, Analysis-Programming

►Simple intraoperative or subsequent programming of the neurostimulator pulse generator/transmitter (95971) includes changes to three or fewer of the following parameters: rate, pulse amplitude, pulse duration, pulse frequency, eight or more electrode contacts, cycling, stimulation train duration, train spacing, number of programs, number of channels, alternating electrode

**Medicine**

polarities, dose time (stimulation parameters changing in time periods of minutes including dose lockout times), more than one clinical feature (eg, rigidity, dyskinesia, tremor). Complex intraoperative or subsequent programming (95972-95979) includes changes to more than three of the above.◄

Code 95970 describes subsequent electronic analysis of a previously-implanted simple or complex brain, spinal cord, or peripheral neurostimulator pulse generator system, without reprogramming. Code 95971 describes intraoperative or subsequent electronic analysis of an implanted simple spinal cord, or peripheral (ie, peripheral nerve, autonomic nerve, neuromuscular) neurostimulator pulse generator system, with programming. Codes 95972 and 95973 describe intraoperative (at initial insertion/ revision) or subsequent electronic analysis of an implanted complex spinal cord or peripheral (except cranial nerve) neurostimulator pulse generator system, with programming. Codes 95974 and 95975 describe intraoperative (at initial insertion/revision) or subsequent electronic analysis of an implanted complex cranial nerve neurostimulator pulse generator system, with programming. Codes 95978 and 95979 describe initial or subsequent electronic analysis of an implanted brain neurostimulator pulse generator system, with programming.

Code 95980 describes intraoperative electronic analysis of an implanted gastric neurostimulator pulse generator system, with programming; code 95981 describes subsequent analysis of the device; code 95982 describes subsequent analysis and reprogramming. For electronic analysis and reprogramming of gastric neurostimulator, lesser curvature, see 95980-95982.

►For 95972, 95974 and 95978, use modifier 52 if less than 31 minutes in duration.◄

►(For electronic analysis and reprogramming of a peripheral subcutaneous field stimulation pulse generator, use 0285T)◄

(For insertion of neurostimulator pulse generator, see 61885, 63685, 64590)

(For revision or removal of neurostimulator pulse generator or receiver, see 61888, 63688, 64595)

►(For implantation of neurostimulator electrodes, see 43647, 43881, 61850-61875, 63650-63655, 64553-64580. For revision or removal of neurostimulator electrodes, see 43648, 43882, 61880, 63661-63664, 64585)◄

▲ 95970 Electronic analysis of implanted neurostimulator pulse generator system (eg, rate, pulse amplitude, pulse duration, configuration of wave form, battery status, electrode selectability, output modulation, cycling, impedance and patient compliance measurements); simple or complex brain, spinal cord, or peripheral (ie, cranial nerve, peripheral nerve, sacral nerve, neuromuscular) neurostimulator pulse generator/ transmitter, without reprogramming

▲ 95971 simple spinal cord, or peripheral (ie, peripheral nerve, sacral nerve, neuromuscular) neurostimulator pulse generator/transmitter, with intraoperative or subsequent programming

▲ 95972 complex spinal cord, or peripheral (ie, peripheral nerve, sacral nerve, neuromuscular) (except cranial nerve) neurostimulator pulse generator/transmitter, with intraoperative or subsequent programming, first hour

+▲ 95973 complex spinal cord, or peripheral (ie, peripheral nerve, sacral nerve, neuromuscular) (except cranial nerve) neurostimulator pulse generator/transmitter, with intraoperative or subsequent programming, each additional 30 minutes after first hour (List separately in addition to code for primary procedure)

(Use 95973 in conjunction with 95972)

▲ 95974 complex cranial nerve neurostimulator pulse generator/transmitter, with intraoperative or subsequent programming, with or without nerve interface testing, first hour

+▲ 95975 complex cranial nerve neurostimulator pulse generator/transmitter, with intraoperative or subsequent programming, each additional 30 minutes after first hour (List separately in addition to code for primary procedure)

(Use 95975 in conjunction with 95974)

(For electronic analysis programming of gastric neurostimulator, lesser curvature, use Category III code 0162T)

95978 Electronic analysis of implanted neurostimulator pulse generator system (eg, rate, pulse amplitude and duration, battery status, electrode selectability and polarity, impedance and patient compliance measurements), complex deep brain neurostimulator pulse generator/ transmitter, with initial or subsequent programming; first hour

+ 95979 each additional 30 minutes after first hour (List separately in addition to code for primary procedure)

(Use 95979 in conjunction with 95978)

95980 Electronic analysis of implanted neurostimulator pulse generator system (eg, rate, pulse amplitude and duration, configuration of wave form, battery status, electrode selectability, output modulation, cycling, impedance and patient measurements) gastric neurostimulator pulse generator/transmitter; intraoperative, with programming

95981 subsequent, without reprogramming

95982 subsequent, with reprogramming

## Other Procedures

▲ 95990 Refilling and maintenance of implantable pump or reservoir for drug delivery, spinal (intrathecal, epidural) or brain (intraventricular), includes electronic analysis of pump, when performed;

▲ 95991 requiring physician's skill

►(Do not report 95990, 95991 in conjunction with 62367-62370. For analysis and/or reprogramming of implantable infusion pump, see 62367-62370)◄

►(For refill and maintenance of implanted infusion pump or reservoir for systemic drug therapy [eg, chemotherapy], use 96522)◄

⊘ **95992**  Canalith repositioning procedure(s) (eg, Epley maneuver, Semont maneuver), per day

(Do not report 95992 in conjunction with 92531, 92532)

**95999**  Unlisted neurological or neuromuscular diagnostic procedure

## Motion Analysis

Codes 96000-96004 describe services performed as part of a major therapeutic or diagnostic decision making process. Motion analysis is performed in a dedicated motion analysis laboratory (ie, a facility capable of performing videotaping from the front, back and both sides, computerized 3D kinematics, 3D kinetics, and dynamic electromyography). Code 96000 may include 3D kinetics and stride characteristics. Codes 96002-96003 describe dynamic electromyography.

Code 96004 should only be reported once regardless of the number of study(ies) reviewed/interpreted.

(For performance of needle electromyography procedures, see 95860-95875)

(For gait training, use 97116)

**96000**  Comprehensive computer-based motion analysis by video-taping and 3D kinematics;

**96001**  with dynamic plantar pressure measurements during walking

**96002**  Dynamic surface electromyography, during walking or other functional activities, 1-12 muscles

**96003**  Dynamic fine wire electromyography, during walking or other functional activities, 1 muscle

(Do not report 96002, 96003 in conjunction with 95860-95864, 95869-95872)

**96004**  Physician review and interpretation of comprehensive computer-based motion analysis, dynamic plantar pressure measurements, dynamic surface electromyography during walking or other functional activities, and dynamic fine wire electromyography, with written report

## Functional Brain Mapping

Code 96020 includes selection and administration of testing of language, memory, cognition, movement, sensation, and other neurological functions when conducted in association with functional neuroimaging, monitoring of performance of this testing, and determination of validity of neurofunctional testing relative to separately interpreted functional magnetic resonance images.

**96020**  Neurofunctional testing selection and administration during noninvasive imaging functional brain mapping, with test administered entirely by a physician or psychologist, with review of test results and report

(For functional magnetic resonance imaging [fMRI], brain, use 70555)

(Do not report 96020 in conjunction with 96101-96103, 96116-96120)

(Do not report 96020 in conjunction with 70554)

(Evaluation and Management services codes should not be reported on the same day as 96020)

# Medical Genetics and Genetic Counseling Services

These services are provided by trained genetic counselors and may include obtaining a structured family genetic history, pedigree construction, analysis for genetic risk assessment, and counseling of the patient and family. These activities may be provided during one or more sessions and may include review of medical data and family information, face-to-face interviews, and counseling services.

Code 96040 is reported for each 30-minute increment of face-to-face time. Do not report 96040 for 15 minutes or less of face-to-face time. Report 96040 once for 16 to 30 minutes of face-to-face time.

**96040**  Medical genetics and genetic counseling services, each 30 minutes face-to-face with patient/family

(For genetic counseling and education provided by a physician to an individual, see the appropriate Evaluation and Management codes)

(For genetic counseling and education provided by a physician to a group, use 99078)

(For education regarding genetic risks by a nonphysician to a group, see 98961, 98962)

(For genetic counseling and/or risk factor reduction intervention provided by a physician to patient(s) without symptoms or established disease, see 99401-99412)

# Central Nervous System Assessments/Tests (eg, Neuro-Cognitive, Mental Status, Speech Testing)

The following codes are used to report the services provided during testing of the cognitive function of the central nervous system. The testing of cognitive processes, visual motor responses, and abstractive abilities is accomplished by the combination of several types of

**Medicine**

testing procedures. It is expected that the administration of these tests will generate material that will be formulated into a report. A minimum of 31 minutes must be provided to report any per hour code. Services 96101, 96116, 96118 and 96125 report time as face-to-face time with the patient and the time spent interpreting and preparing the report.

(For development of cognitive skills, see 97532, 97533)

(For mini-mental status examination performed by a physician, see **Evaluation and Management** services codes)

96101 Psychological testing (includes psychodiagnostic assessment of emotionality, intellectual abilities, personality and psychopathology, eg, MMPI, Rorschach, WAIS), per hour of the psychologist's or physician's time, both face-to-face time administering tests to the patient and time interpreting these test results and preparing the report

(96101 is also used in those circumstances when additional time is necessary to integrate other sources of clinical data, including previously completed and reported technician- and computer-administered tests)

(Do not report 96101 for the interpretation and report of 96102, 96103)

96102 Psychological testing (includes psychodiagnostic assessment of emotionality, intellectual abilities, personality and psychopathology, eg, MMPI and WAIS), with qualified health care professional interpretation and report, administered by technician, per hour of technician time, face-to-face

96103 Psychological testing (includes psychodiagnostic assessment of emotionality, intellectual abilities, personality and psychopathology, eg, MMPI), administered by a computer, with qualified health care professional interpretation and report

96105 Assessment of aphasia (includes assessment of expressive and receptive speech and language function, language comprehension, speech production ability, reading, spelling, writing, eg, by Boston Diagnostic Aphasia Examination) with interpretation and report, per hour

▲ 96110 Developmental screening, with interpretation and report, per standardized instrument form

▲ 96111 Developmental testing, (includes assessment of motor, language, social, adaptive, and/or cognitive functioning by standardized developmental instruments) with interpretation and report

96116 Neurobehavioral status exam (clinical assessment of thinking, reasoning and judgment, eg, acquired knowledge, attention, language, memory, planning and problem solving, and visual spatial abilities), per hour of the psychologist's or physician's time, both face-to-face time with the patient and time interpreting test results and preparing the report

96118 Neuropsychological testing (eg, Halstead-Reitan Neuropsychological Battery, Wechsler Memory Scales and Wisconsin Card Sorting Test), per hour of the psychologist's or physician's time, both face-to-face time administering tests to the patient and time interpreting these test results and preparing the report

(96118 is also used in those circumstances when additional time is necessary to integrate other sources of clinical data, including previously completed and reported technician- and computer-administered tests)

(Do not report 96118 for the interpretation and report of 96119 or 96120)

96119 Neuropsychological testing (eg, Halstead-Reitan Neuropsychological Battery, Wechsler Memory Scales and Wisconsin Card Sorting Test), with qualified health care professional interpretation and report, administered by technician, per hour of technician time, face-to-face

96120 Neuropsychological testing (eg, Wisconsin Card Sorting Test), administered by a computer, with qualified health care professional interpretation and report

96125 Standardized cognitive performance testing (eg, Ross Information Processing Assessment) per hour of a qualified health care professional's time, both face-to-face time administering tests to the patient and time interpreting these test results and preparing the report

(For psychological and neuropsychological testing by a physician or psychologist, see 96101-96103, 96118-96120)

# Health and Behavior Assessment/Intervention

Health and behavior assessment procedures are used to identify the psychological, behavioral, emotional, cognitive, and social factors important to the prevention, treatment, or management of physical health problems.

The focus of the assessment is not on mental health but on the biopsychosocial factors important to physical health problems and treatments. The focus of the intervention is to improve the patient's health and well-being utilizing cognitive, behavioral, social, and/or psychophysiological procedures designed to ameliorate specific disease-related problems.

Codes 96150-96155 describe services offered to patients who present with primary physical illnesses, diagnoses, or symptoms and may benefit from assessments and interventions that focus on the biopsychosocial factors related to the patient's health status. These services do not represent preventive medicine counseling and risk factor reduction interventions.

For patients that require psychiatric services (90801-90899) as well as health and behavior assessment/intervention (96150-96155), report the predominant

Medicine

service performed. Do not report 96150-96155 in conjunction with 90801-90899 on the same date.

Evaluation and Management services codes (including Counseling Risk Factor Reduction and Behavior Change Intervention [99401-99412]), should not be reported on the same day.

(For health and behavior assessment and/or intervention performed by a physician, see **Evaluation and Management** or **Preventive Medicine** services codes)

**96150**   Health and behavior assessment (eg, health-focused clinical interview, behavioral observations, psychophysiological monitoring, health-oriented questionnaires), each 15 minutes face-to-face with the patient; initial assessment

**96151**   re-assessment

**96152**   Health and behavior intervention, each 15 minutes, face-to-face; individual

**96153**   group (2 or more patients)

**96154**   family (with the patient present)

**96155**   family (without the patient present)

# Hydration, Therapeutic, Prophylactic, Diagnostic Injections and Infusions, and Chemotherapy and Other Highly Complex Drug or Highly Complex Biologic Agent Administration

Physician work related to hydration, injection, and infusion services predominantly involves affirmation of treatment plan and direct supervision of staff.

►Codes 96360-96379, 96401, 96402, 96409-96425, 96521-96523 are not intended to be reported by the physician in the facility setting. If a significant, separately identifiable office or other outpatient Evaluation and Management service is performed, the appropriate E/M service (99201-99215, 99241-99245, 99354-99355) should be reported using modifier 25 in addition to 96360-96549. For same day E/M service, a different diagnosis is not required.◄

If performed to facilitate the infusion or injection, the following services are included and are not reported separately:

a. Use of local anesthesia

b. IV start

c. Access to indwelling IV, subcutaneous catheter or port

d. Flush at conclusion of infusion

e. Standard tubing, syringes, and supplies

(For declotting a catheter or port, use 36593)

When multiple drugs are administered, report the service(s) and the specific materials or drugs for each.

►When administering multiple infusions, injections or combinations, only one "initial" service code should be reported for a given date, unless protocol requires that two separate IV sites must be used. Do not report a second initial service on the same date due to an intravenous line requiring a re-start, an IV rate not being able to be reached without two lines, or for accessing a port of a multi-lumen catheter. If an injection or infusion is of a subsequent or concurrent nature, even if it is the first such service within that group of services, then a subsequent or concurrent code from the appropriate section should be reported (eg, the first IV push given subsequent to an initial one-hour infusion is reported using a subsequent IV push code).

*Initial infusion:* For physician reporting, an initial infusion is the *key or primary reason for the encounter* reported irrespective of the temporal order in which the infusion(s) or injection(s) are administered. For facility reporting, an initial infusion is based using the hierarchy. For both physician and facility reporting, only one *initial* service code (eg, 96365) should be reported unless the protocol or patient condition requires that two separate IV sites must be utilized. The difference in time and effort in providing this second IV site access is also reported using the *initial* service code with modifier 59 appended (eg, 96365, 96365-59).

*Sequential infusion:* A sequential infusion is an infusion or IV push of a new substance or drug following a primary or initial service. All sequential services require that there be a new substance or drug, except that facilities may report a sequential intravenous push of the same drug using 96376.

*Concurrent infusion:* A concurrent infusion is an infusion of a new substance or drug infused at the same time as another substance or drug. A concurrent infusion service is not time based and is only reported once per day regardless of whether an additional new drug or substance is administered concurrently. Hydration may not be reported concurrently with any other service. A separate subsequent concurrent administration of another new drug or substance (the third substance or drug) is not reported.◄

In order to determine which service should be reported as the initial service when there is more than one type of service, hierarchies have been created. These vary by whether the physician or a facility is reporting. The order of selection for physicians is based upon the physician knowledge of the clinical condition(s) and treatment(s). The hierarchy that facilities are to use is based upon a structural algorithm. When these codes are reported by

**Medicine**

the physician, the "initial" code that best describes the key or primary reason for the encounter should always be reported irrespective of the order in which the infusions or injections occur.

When these codes are reported *by the facility*, the following instructions apply. The initial code should be selected using a hierarchy whereby chemotherapy services are primary to therapeutic, prophylactic, and diagnostic services which are primary to hydration services. Infusions are primary to pushes, which are primary to injections. This hierarchy is to be followed by facilities and supersedes parenthetical instructions for add-on codes that suggest an add-on of a higher hierarchical position may be reported in conjunction with a base code of a lower position. (For example, the hierarchy would not permit reporting 96376 with 96360, as 96376 is a higher order code. IV push is primary to hydration.)

►When reporting multiple infusions of the same drug/substance on the same date of service, the initial code should be selected. The second and subsequent infusion(s) should be reported based on the individual time(s) of each additional infusion(s) of the same drug/substance using the appropriate add-on code.

*Example:* In the outpatient observation setting, a patient receives one-hour intravenous infusions of the same antibiotic every 8 hours on the same date of service through the same IV access. The hierarchy for facility reporting permits the reporting of code 96365 for the first one-hour dose administered. Add-on 96366 would be reported twice (once for the second and third one-hour infusions of the same drug).

When reporting codes for which infusion time is a factor, use the actual time over which the infusion is administered. Intravenous or intra-arterial push is defined as: (a) an injection in which the health care professional who administers the drug/substance is continuously present to administer the injection and observe the patient, or (b) an infusion of 15 minutes or less. If intravenous hydration (96360, 96361) is given from 11 PM to 2 AM, 96360 would be reported once and 96361 twice. However, if instead of a continuous infusion, a medication was given by intravenous push at 10 PM and 2 AM, as the service was not continuous, both administrations would be reported as an initial service (96374). For continuous services that last beyond midnight, use the date in which the service began and report the total units of time provided continuously. A "keep open" infusion of any type is not separately reported.◄

## Hydration

Codes 96360-96361 are intended to report a hydration IV infusion to consist of a pre-packaged fluid and electrolytes (eg, normal saline, D5-1/2 normal saline+30mEq KCl/liter), but are not used to report infusion of drugs or other substances. Hydration IV

infusions typically require direct physician supervision for purposes of consent, safety oversight, or intraservice supervision of staff. Typically such infusions require little special handling to prepare or dispose of, and staff that administer these do not typically require advanced practice training. After initial set-up, infusion typically entails little patient risk and thus little monitoring. These codes are not intended to be reported by the physician in the facility setting.

►Some chemotherapeutic agents and other therapeutic agents require pre- and/or post-hydration to be given in order to avoid specific toxicities. A minimum time duration of 31 minutes of hydration infusion is required to report the service. However, the hydration codes 96360 or 96361 are not used when the purpose of the intravenous fluid is to "keep open" an IV line prior or subsequent to a therapeutic infusion, or as a free-flowing IV during chemotherapy or other therapeutic infusion.◄

**96360**      Intravenous infusion, hydration; initial, 31 minutes to 1 hour

(Do not report 96360 if performed as a concurrent infusion service)

(Do not report intravenous infusion for hydration of 30 minutes or less)

**+ 96361**      each additional hour (List separately in addition to code for primary procedure)

(Use 96361 in conjunction with 96360)

(Report 96361 for hydration infusion intervals of greater than 30 minutes beyond 1 hour increments)

(Report 96361 to identify hydration if provided as a secondary or subsequent service after a different initial service [96360, 96365, 96374, 96409, 96413] is administered through the same IV access)

## Therapeutic, Prophylactic, and Diagnostic Injections and Infusions (Excludes Chemotherapy and Other Highly Complex Drug or Highly Complex Biologic Agent Administration)

A therapeutic, prophylactic, or diagnostic IV infusion or injection (other than hydration) is for the administration of substances/drugs. When fluids are used to administer the drug(s), the administration of the fluid is considered incidental hydration and is not separately reportable. These services typically require direct physician supervision for any or all purposes of patient assessment, provision of consent, safety oversight, and intra-service supervision of staff. Typically, such infusions require special consideration to prepare, dose or dispose of, require practice training and competency for staff who administer the infusions, and require periodic patient assessment with vital sign monitoring during the infusion. These codes are not intended to be reported by the physician in the facility setting.

See codes 96401-96549 for the administration of chemotherapy or other highly complex drug or highly complex biologic agent services. These highly complex services require advanced practice training and competency for staff who provide these services; special considerations for preparation, dosage or disposal; and commonly, these services entail significant patient risk and frequent monitoring. Examples are frequent changes in the infusion rate, prolonged presence of nurse administering the solution for patient monitoring and infusion adjustments, and frequent conferring with the physician about these issues.

(Do not report 96365-96379 with codes for which IV push or infusion is an inherent part of the procedure [eg, administration of contrast material for a diagnostic imaging study])

96365 Intravenous infusion, for therapy, prophylaxis, or diagnosis (specify substance or drug); initial, up to 1 hour

+ 96366 each additional hour (List separately in addition to code for primary procedure)

(Report 96366 in conjunction with 96365, 96367)

(Report 96366 for additional hour[s] of sequential infusion)

(Report 96366 for infusion intervals of greater than 30 minutes beyond 1 hour increments)

►(Report 96366 in conjunction with 96365 to identify each second and subsequent infusions of the same drug/substance)◄

+▲ 96367 additional sequential infusion of a new drug/substance, up to 1 hour (List separately in addition to code for primary procedure)

►(Report 96367 in conjunction with 96365, 96374, 96409, 96413 to identify the infusion of a new drug/substance provided as a secondary or subsequent service after a different initial service is administered through the same IV access. Report 96367 only once per sequential infusion of same infusate mix)◄

+ 96368 concurrent infusion (List separately in addition to code for primary procedure)

►(Report 96368 only once per date of service)◄

(Report 96368 in conjunction with 96365, 96366, 96413, 96415, 96416)

96369 Subcutaneous infusion for therapy or prophylaxis (specify substance or drug); initial, up to 1 hour, including pump set-up and establishment of subcutaneous infusion site(s)

(For infusions of 15 minutes or less, use 96372)

+ 96370 each additional hour (List separately in addition to code for primary procedure)

(Use 96370 in conjunction with 96369)

(Use 96370 for infusion intervals of greater than 30 minutes beyond 1 hour increments)

+ 96371 additional pump set-up with establishment of new subcutaneous infusion site(s) (List separately in addition to code for primary procedure)

(Use 96371 in conjunction with 96369)

(Use 96369, 96371 only once per encounter)

96372 Therapeutic, prophylactic, or diagnostic injection (specify substance or drug); subcutaneous or intramuscular

(For administration of vaccines/toxoids, see 96365, 96366, 90471, 90472)

(Report 96372 for non-antineoplastic hormonal therapy injections)

(Report 96401 for anti-neoplastic nonhormonal injection therapy)

(Report 96402 for anti-neoplastic hormonal injection therapy)

(Physicians do not report 96372 for injections given without direct physician supervision. To report, use 99211. Hospitals may report 96372 when the physician is not present)

(96372 does not include injections for allergen immunotherapy. For allergen immunotherapy injections, see 95115-95117)

96373 intra-arterial

96374 intravenous push, single or initial substance/drug

+ 96375 each additional sequential intravenous push of a new substance/drug (List separately in addition to code for primary procedure)

(Use 96375 in conjunction with 96365, 96374, 96409, 96413)

(Report 96375 to identify intravenous push of a new substance/drug if provided as a secondary or subsequent service after a different initial service is administered through the same IV access)

+ 96376 each additional sequential intravenous push of the same substance/drug provided in a facility (List separately in addition to code for primary procedure)

(Do not report 96376 for a push performed within 30 minutes of a reported push of the same substance or drug)

(96376 may be reported by facilities only)

►(Report 96376 in conjunction with 96365, 96374, 96409, 96413)◄

96379 Unlisted therapeutic, prophylactic, or diagnostic intravenous or intra-arterial injection or infusion

(For allergy immunology, see 95004 et seq)

**Medicine**

# Chemotherapy and Other Highly Complex Drug or Highly Complex Biologic Agent Administration

Chemotherapy administration codes 96401-96549 apply to parenteral administration of non-radionuclide anti-neoplastic drugs; and also to anti-neoplastic agents provided for treatment of noncancer diagnoses (eg, cyclophosphamide for auto-immune conditions) or to substances such as certain monoclonal antibody agents, and other biologic response modifiers. The highly complex infusion of chemotherapy or other drug or biologic agents requires physician work and/or clinical staff monitoring well beyond that of therapeutic drug agents (96360-96379) because the incidence of severe adverse patient reactions are typically greater. These services can be provided by any physician. Chemotherapy services are typically highly complex and require direct physician supervision for any or all purposes of patient assessment, provision of consent, safety oversight, and intraservice supervision of staff. Typically, such chemotherapy services require advanced practice training and competency for staff who provide these services; special considerations for preparation, dosage, or disposal; and commonly, these services entail significant patient risk and frequent monitoring. Examples are frequent changes in the infusion rate, prolonged presence of the nurse administering the solution for patient monitoring and infusion adjustments, and frequent conferring with the physician about these issues. When performed to facilitate the infusion of injection, preparation of chemotherapy agent(s), highly complex agent(s), or other highly complex drugs is included and is not reported separately. To report infusions that do not require this level of complexity, see 96360-96379. Codes 96401-96402, 96409-96425, 96521-96523 are not intended to be reported by the physician in the facility setting.

The term "chemotherapy" in 96401-96549 includes other highly complex drugs or highly complex biologic agents.

Report separate codes for each parenteral method of administration employed when chemotherapy is administered by different techniques. The administration of medications (eg, antibiotics, steroidal agents, antiemetics, narcotics, analgesics) administered independently or sequentially as supportive management of chemotherapy administration, should be separately reported using 96360, 96361, 96365, 96379 as appropriate.

Report both the specific service as well as code(s) for the specific substance(s) or drug(s) provided. The fluid used to administer the drug(s) is considered incidental hydration and is not separately reportable.

Regional (isolation) chemotherapy perfusion should be reported using the codes for arterial infusion (96420-96425). Placement of the intra-arterial catheter should be reported using the appropriate code from the **Cardiovascular Surgery** section. Placement of arterial and venous cannula(s) for extracorporeal circulation via a membrane oxygenator perfusion pump should be reported using 36823. Code 36823 includes dose calculation and administration of the chemotherapy agent by injection into the perfusate. Do not report 96409-96425 in conjunction with 36823.

(For home infusion services, see 99601-99602)

# Injection and Intravenous Infusion Chemotherapy and Other Highly Complex Drug or Highly Complex Biologic Agent Administration

Intravenous or intra-arterial push is defined as: (a) an injection in which the healthcare professional who administers the substance/drug is continuously present to administer the injection and observe the patient, or (b) an infusion of 15 minutes or less.

**96401** Chemotherapy administration, subcutaneous or intramuscular; non-hormonal anti-neoplastic

**96402** hormonal anti-neoplastic

**96405** Chemotherapy administration; intralesional, up to and including 7 lesions

**96406** intralesional, more than 7 lesions

**96409** intravenous, push technique, single or initial substance/drug

**+ 96411** intravenous, push technique, each additional substance/drug (List separately in addition to code for primary procedure)

(Use 96411 in conjunction with 96409, 96413)

**96413** Chemotherapy administration, intravenous infusion technique; up to 1 hour, single or initial substance/drug

(Report 96361 to identify hydration if administered as a secondary or subsequent service in association with 96413 through the same IV access)

(Report 96366, 96367, 96375 to identify therapeutic, prophylactic, or diagnostic drug infusion or injection, if administered as a secondary or subsequent service in association with 96413 through the same IV access)

**+ 96415** each additional hour (List separately in addition to code for primary procedure)

(Use 96415 in conjunction with 96413)

(Report 96415 for infusion intervals of greater than 30 minutes beyond 1-hour increments)

**96416** initiation of prolonged chemotherapy infusion (more than 8 hours), requiring use of a portable or implantable pump

(For refilling and maintenance of a portable pump or an implantable infusion pump or reservoir for drug delivery, see 96521-96523)

**+ 96417**    each additional sequential infusion (different substance/drug), up to 1 hour (List separately in addition to code for primary procedure)

(Use 96417 in conjunction with 96413)

(Report only once per sequential infusion. Report 96415 for additional hour(s) of sequential infusion)

## Intra-Arterial Chemotherapy and Other Highly Complex Drug or Highly Complex Biologic Agent Administration

**96420**    Chemotherapy administration, intra-arterial; push technique

**96422**    infusion technique, up to 1 hour

**+ 96423**    infusion technique, each additional hour (List separately in addition to code for primary procedure)

(Use 96423 in conjunction with 96422)

(Report 96423 for infusion intervals of greater than 30 minutes beyond 1-hour increments)

(For regional chemotherapy perfusion via membrane oxygenator perfusion pump to an extremity, use 36823)

**96425**    infusion technique, initiation of prolonged infusion (more than 8 hours), requiring the use of a portable or implantable pump

(For refilling and maintenance of a portable pump or an implantable infusion pump or reservoir for drug delivery, see 96521-96523)

## Other Injection and Infusion Services

Code 96523 does not require direct physician supervision. Codes 96521-96523 may be reported when these devices are used for therapeutic drugs other than chemotherapy.

(For collection of blood specimen from a completely implantable venous access device, use 36591)

**96440**    Chemotherapy administration into pleural cavity, requiring and including thoracentesis

(96445 has been deleted. To report intraperitoneal chemotherapy administration, use 96446)

**96446**    Chemotherapy administration into the peritoneal cavity via indwelling port or catheter

**96450**    Chemotherapy administration, into CNS (eg, intrathecal), requiring and including spinal puncture

(For intravesical (bladder) chemotherapy administration, use 51720)

(For insertion of subarachnoid catheter and reservoir for infusion of drug, see 62350, 62351, 62360-62362; for insertion of intraventricular catheter and reservoir, see 61210, 61215)

**96521**    Refilling and maintenance of portable pump

**96522**    Refilling and maintenance of implantable pump or reservoir for drug delivery, systemic (eg, intravenous, intra-arterial)

(For refilling and maintenance of an implantable infusion pump for spinal or brain drug infusion, use 95990-95991)

**96523**    Irrigation of implanted venous access device for drug delivery systems

(Do not report 96523 in conjunction with other services. To report collection of blood specimen, use 36591)

**96542**    Chemotherapy injection, subarachnoid or intraventricular via subcutaneous reservoir, single or multiple agents

(For radioactive isotope therapy, use 79005)

**96549**    Unlisted chemotherapy procedure

# Photodynamic Therapy

(To report ocular photodynamic therapy, use 67221)

**96567**    Photodynamic therapy by external application of light to destroy premalignant and/or malignant lesions of the skin and adjacent mucosa (eg, lip) by activation of photosensitive drug(s), each phototherapy exposure session

**+ 96570**    Photodynamic therapy by endoscopic application of light to ablate abnormal tissue via activation of photosensitive drug(s); first 30 minutes (List separately in addition to code for endoscopy or bronchoscopy procedures of lung and gastrointestinal tract)

(Report 96570 with modifier 52 for service of less than 23 minutes with report)

**+ 96571**    each additional 15 minutes (List separately in addition to code for endoscopy or bronchoscopy procedures of lung and gastrointestinal tract)

(For 23-37 minutes of service, use 96570. For 38-52 minutes of service, use 96570 in conjunction with 96571)

(96570, 96571 are to be used in addition to bronchoscopy, endoscopy codes)

(Use 96570, 96571 in conjunction with 31641, 43228 as appropriate)

# Special Dermatological Procedures

Dermatologic services are typically consultative, and any of the five levels of consultation (99241-99255) may be appropriate.

In addition, services and skills outlined under **Evaluation and Management** levels of service appropriate to dermatologic illnesses should be coded similarly.

(For intralesional injections, see 11900, 11901)

(For Tzanck smear, see 88160-88161)

**Medicine**

**96900** Actinotherapy (ultraviolet light)

►(For rhinophototherapy, intranasal application of ultraviolet and visible light, use 30999)◄

**96902** Microscopic examination of hairs plucked or clipped by the examiner (excluding hair collected by the patient) to determine telogen and anagen counts, or structural hair shaft abnormality

**96904** Whole body integumentary photography, for monitoring of high risk patients with dysplastic nevus syndrome or a history of dysplastic nevi, or patients with a personal or familial history of melanoma

**96910** Photochemotherapy; tar and ultraviolet B (Goeckerman treatment) or petrolatum and ultraviolet B

**96912** psoralens and ultraviolet A (PUVA)

**96913** Photochemotherapy (Goeckerman and/or PUVA) for severe photoresponsive dermatoses requiring at least 4-8 hours of care under direct supervision of the physician (includes application of medication and dressings)

**96920** Laser treatment for inflammatory skin disease (psoriasis); total area less than 250 sq cm

**96921** 250 sq cm to 500 sq cm

**96922** over 500 sq cm

(For laser destruction of premalignant lesions, see 17000-17004)

(For laser destruction of cutaneous vascular proliferative lesions, see 17106-17108)

(For laser destruction of benign lesions, see 17110-17111)

(For laser destruction of malignant lesions, see 17260-17286)

**96999** Unlisted special dermatological service or procedure

# Physical Medicine and Rehabilitation

Codes 97001-97755 should be used to report each distinct procedure performed. Do not append modifier 51 to 97001-97755.

The work of the qualified healthcare professional consists of face-to-face time with the patient (and caregiver, if applicable) delivering skilled services. For the purpose of determining the total time of a service, incremental intervals of treatment at the same visit may be accumulated.

(For muscle testing, range of joint motion, electromyography, see 95831 et seq)

(For biofeedback training by EMG, use 90901)

(For transcutaneous nerve stimulation (TNS), use 64550)

**97001** Physical therapy evaluation

**97002** Physical therapy re-evaluation

**97003** Occupational therapy evaluation

**97004** Occupational therapy re-evaluation

**97005** Athletic training evaluation

**97006** Athletic training re-evaluation

# Modalities

Any physical agent applied to produce therapeutic changes to biologic tissue; includes but not limited to thermal, acoustic, light, mechanical, or electric energy.

## Supervised

The application of a modality that does not require direct (one-on-one) patient contact by the provider.

**97010** Application of a modality to 1 or more areas; hot or cold packs

**97012** traction, mechanical

**97014** electrical stimulation (unattended)

(For acupuncture with electrical stimulation, see 97813, 97814)

**97016** vasopneumatic devices

**97018** paraffin bath

**97022** whirlpool

**97024** diathermy (eg, microwave)

**97026** infrared

**97028** ultraviolet

## Constant Attendance

The application of a modality that requires direct (one-on-one) patient contact by the provider.

**97032** Application of a modality to 1 or more areas; electrical stimulation (manual), each 15 minutes

►(For transcutaneous electrical modulation pain reprocessing [TEMPR/scrambler therapy], use 0278T)◄

**97033** iontophoresis, each 15 minutes

**97034** contrast baths, each 15 minutes

**97035** ultrasound, each 15 minutes

**97036** Hubbard tank, each 15 minutes

**97039** Unlisted modality (specify type and time if constant attendance)

Medicine

# Therapeutic Procedures

A manner of effecting change through the application of clinical skills and/or services that attempt to improve function.

Physician or therapist required to have direct (one-on-one) patient contact.

**97110**   Therapeutic procedure, 1 or more areas, each 15 minutes; therapeutic exercises to develop strength and endurance, range of motion and flexibility

**97112**   neuromuscular reeducation of movement, balance, coordination, kinesthetic sense, posture, and/or proprioception for sitting and/or standing activities

**97113**   aquatic therapy with therapeutic exercises

**97116**   gait training (includes stair climbing)

(Use 96000-96003 to report comprehensive gait and motion analysis procedures)

**97124**   massage, including effleurage, petrissage and/or tapotement (stroking, compression, percussion)

(For myofascial release, use 97140)

**97139**   Unlisted therapeutic procedure (specify)

**97140**   Manual therapy techniques (eg, mobilization/manipulation, manual lymphatic drainage, manual traction), 1 or more regions, each 15 minutes

►(Do not report 97140 in conjunction with 29581-29584)◄

**97150**   Therapeutic procedure(s), group (2 or more individuals)

(Report 97150 for each member of group)

(Group therapy procedures involve constant attendance of the physician or therapist, but by definition do not require one-on-one patient contact by the physician or therapist)

(For manipulation under general anesthesia, see appropriate anatomic section in **Musculoskeletal System**)

(For osteopathic manipulative treatment [OMT], see 98925-98929)

**97530**   Therapeutic activities, direct (one-on-one) patient contact by the provider (use of dynamic activities to improve functional performance), each 15 minutes

**97532**   Development of cognitive skills to improve attention, memory, problem solving (includes compensatory training), direct (one-on-one) patient contact by the provider, each 15 minutes

**97533**   Sensory integrative techniques to enhance sensory processing and promote adaptive responses to environmental demands, direct (one-on-one) patient contact by the provider, each 15 minutes

**97535**   Self-care/home management training (eg, activities of daily living (ADL) and compensatory training, meal preparation, safety procedures, and instructions in use of assistive technology devices/adaptive equipment) direct one-on-one contact by provider, each 15 minutes

**97537**   Community/work reintegration training (eg, shopping, transportation, money management, avocational activities and/or work environment/modification analysis, work task analysis, use of assistive technology device/adaptive equipment), direct one-on-one contact by provider, each 15 minutes

(For wheelchair management/propulsion training, use 97542)

**97542**   Wheelchair management (eg, assessment, fitting, training), each 15 minutes

**97545**   Work hardening/conditioning; initial 2 hours

+ **97546**   each additional hour (List separately in addition to code for primary procedure)

(Use 97546 in conjunction with 97545)

# Active Wound Care Management

Active wound care procedures are performed to remove devitalized and/or necrotic tissue and promote healing. Provider is required to have direct (one-on-one) patient contact.

(Do not report 97597-97602 in conjunction with 11042-11047 for the same wound)

(For debridement of burn wounds, see 16020-16030)

**97597**   Debridement (eg, high pressure waterjet with/without suction, sharp selective debridement with scissors, scalpel and forceps), open wound, (eg, fibrin, devitalized epidermis and/or dermis, exudate, debris, biofilm), including topical application(s), wound assessment, use of a whirlpool, when performed and instruction(s) for ongoing care, per session, total wound(s) surface area; first 20 sq cm or less

+ **97598**   each additional 20 sq cm, or part thereof (List separately in addition to code for primary procedure)

(Use 97598 in conjunction with 97597)

**97602**   Removal of devitalized tissue from wound(s), non-selective debridement, without anesthesia (eg, wet-to-moist dressings, enzymatic, abrasion), including topical application(s), wound assessment, and instruction(s) for ongoing care, per session

**97605**   Negative pressure wound therapy (eg, vacuum assisted drainage collection), including topical application(s), wound assessment, and instruction(s) for ongoing care, per session; total wound(s) surface area less than or equal to 50 square centimeters

**97606**   total wound(s) surface area greater than 50 square centimeters

**Medicine**

## Tests and Measurements

Requires direct one-on-one patient contact.

> (For muscle testing, manual or electrical, joint range of motion, electromyography or nerve velocity determination, see 95831-95904)

**97750** Physical performance test or measurement (eg, musculoskeletal, functional capacity), with written report, each 15 minutes

**97755** Assistive technology assessment (eg, to restore, augment or compensate for existing function, optimize functional tasks and/or maximize environmental accessibility), direct one-on-one contact by provider, with written report, each 15 minutes

> (To report augmentative and alternative communication devices, see 92605, 92607)

## Orthotic Management and Prosthetic Management

**97760** Orthotic(s) management and training (including assessment and fitting when not otherwise reported), upper extremity(s), lower extremity(s) and/or trunk, each 15 minutes

> (Code 97760 should not be reported with 97116 for the same extremity)

**97761** Prosthetic training, upper and/or lower extremity(s), each 15 minutes

**97762** Checkout for orthotic/prosthetic use, established patient, each 15 minutes

## Other Procedures

> (For extracorporeal shock wave musculoskeletal therapy, see Category III codes 0019T, 0101T, 0102T)

**97799** Unlisted physical medicine/rehabilitation service or procedure

## Medical Nutrition Therapy

**97802** Medical nutrition therapy; initial assessment and intervention, individual, face-to-face with the patient, each 15 minutes

**97803** re-assessment and intervention, individual, face-to-face with the patient, each 15 minutes

**97804** group (2 or more individual(s)), each 30 minutes

> (For medical nutrition therapy assessment and/or intervention performed by a physician, see **Evaluation and Management** or **Preventive Medicine** service codes)

## Acupuncture

Acupuncture is reported based on 15-minute increments of personal (face-to-face) contact with the patient, not the duration of acupuncture needle(s) placement.

If no electrical stimulation is used during a 15-minute increment, use 97810, 97811. If electrical stimulation of any needle is used during a 15-minute increment, use 97813, 97814.

Only one code may be reported for each 15-minute increment. Use either 97810 or 97813 for the initial 15-minute increment. Only one initial code is reported per day.

Evaluation and Management services may be reported separately, using modifier 25, if the patient's condition requires a significant separately identifiable E/M service, above and beyond the usual preservice and postservice work associated with the acupuncture services. The time of the E/M service is not included in the time of the acupuncture service.

**97810** Acupuncture, 1 or more needles; without electrical stimulation, initial 15 minutes of personal one-on-one contact with the patient

> (Do not report 97810 in conjunction with 97813)

**✛ 97811** without electrical stimulation, each additional 15 minutes of personal one-on-one contact with the patient, with re-insertion of needle(s) (List separately in addition to code for primary procedure)

> (Use 97811 in conjunction with 97810, 97813)

**97813** with electrical stimulation, initial 15 minutes of personal one-on-one contact with the patient

> (Do not report 97813 in conjunction with 97810)

**✛ 97814** with electrical stimulation, each additional 15 minutes of personal one-on-one contact with the patient, with re-insertion of needle(s) (List separately in addition to code for primary procedure)

> (Use 97814 in conjunction with 97810, 97813)

## Osteopathic Manipulative Treatment

Osteopathic manipulative treatment (OMT) is a form of manual treatment applied by a physician to eliminate or alleviate somatic dysfunction and related disorders. This treatment may be accomplished by a variety of techniques.

Evaluation and Management services may be reported separately if, using modifier 25, the patient's condition requires a significant separately identifiable E/M service, above and beyond the usual preservice and postservice

**Medicine**

work associated with the procedure. The E/M service may be caused or prompted by the same symptoms or condition for which the OMT service was provided. As such, different diagnoses are not required for the reporting of the OMT and E/M service on the same date.

Body regions referred to are: head region; cervical region; thoracic region; lumbar region; sacral region; pelvic region; lower extremities; upper extremities; rib cage region; abdomen and viscera region.

**98925**　Osteopathic manipulative treatment (OMT); 1-2 body regions involved

**98926**　　　3-4 body regions involved

**98927**　　　5-6 body regions involved

**98928**　　　7-8 body regions involved

**98929**　　　9-10 body regions involved

# Chiropractic Manipulative Treatment

Chiropractic manipulative treatment (CMT) is a form of manual treatment to influence joint and neurophysiological function. This treatment may be accomplished using a variety of techniques.

The chiropractic manipulative treatment codes include a pre-manipulation patient assessment. Additional Evaluation and Management services may be reported separately using modifier 25, if the patient's condition requires a significant separately identifiable E/M service, above and beyond the usual preservice and postservice work associated with the procedure. The E/M service may be caused or prompted by the same symptoms or condition for which the CMT service was provided. As such, different diagnoses are not required for the reporting of the CMT and E/M service on the same date.

For purposes of CMT, the five spinal regions referred to are: cervical region (includes atlanto-occipital joint); thoracic region (includes costovertebral and costotransverse joints); lumbar region; sacral region; and pelvic (sacro-iliac joint) region. The five extraspinal regions referred to are: head (including temporomandibular joint, excluding atlanto-occipital) region; lower extremities; upper extremities; rib cage (excluding costotransverse and costovertebral joints) and abdomen.

**98940**　Chiropractic manipulative treatment (CMT); spinal, 1-2 regions

**98941**　　　spinal, 3-4 regions

**98942**　　　spinal, 5 regions

**98943**　　　extraspinal, 1 or more regions

# Education and Training for Patient Self-Management

The following codes are used to report educational and training services prescribed by a physician and provided by a qualified, nonphysician healthcare professional using a standardized curriculum to an individual or a group of patients for the treatment of established illness(s)/disease(s) or to delay comorbidity(s). Education and training for patient self-management may be reported with these codes only when using a standardized curriculum as described below. This curriculum may be modified as necessary for the clinical needs, cultural norms and health literacy of the individual patient(s).

The purpose of the educational and training services is to teach the patient (may include caregiver[s]) how to effectively self-manage the patient's illness(s)/disease(s) or delay disease comorbidity(s) in conjunction with the patient's professional healthcare team. Education and training related to subsequent reinforcement or due to changes in the patient's condition or treatment plan are reported in the same manner as the original education and training. The type of education and training provided for the patient's clinical condition will be identified by the appropriate diagnosis code(s) reported.

The qualifications of the nonphysician healthcare professionals and the content of the educational and training program must be consistent with guidelines or standards established or recognized by a physician society, nonphysician healthcare professional society/association, or other appropriate source.

(For counseling and education provided by a physician to an individual, see the appropriate Evaluation and Management codes)

(For counseling and education provided by a physician to a group, use 99078)

(For counseling and/or risk factor reduction intervention provided by a physician to patient(s) without symptoms or established disease, see 99401-99412)

(For medical nutrition therapy, see 97802-97804)

(For health and behavior assessment/intervention that is not part of a standardized curriculum, see 96150-96155)

(For education provided as genetic counseling services, use 96040. For education to a group regarding genetic risks, see 98961, 98962)

**98960**　Education and training for patient self-management by a qualified, nonphysician health care professional using a standardized curriculum, face-to-face with the patient (could include caregiver/family) each 30 minutes; individual patient

**98961**　　　2-4 patients

**98962**　　　5-8 patients

Medicine

# Non-Face-to-Face Nonphysician Services

## Telephone Services

Telephone services are non-face-to-face assessment and management services provided by a qualified health care professional to a patient using the telephone. These codes are used to report episodes of care by the qualified health care professional initiated by an established patient or guardian of an established patient. If the telephone service ends with a decision to see the patient within 24 hours or the next available urgent visit appointment, the code is not reported; rather the encounter is considered part of the preservice work of the subsequent assessment and management service, procedure and visit. Likewise, if the telephone call refers to a service performed and reported by the qualified health care professional within the previous seven days (either qualified health care professional requested or unsolicited patient follow-up) or within the postoperative period of the previously completed procedure, then the service(s) are considered part of that previous service or procedure. (Do not report 98966-98969 if reporting 98966-98969 performed in the previous seven days.)

(For telephone services provided by a physician, see 99441-99443)

**98966**    Telephone assessment and management service provided by a qualified nonphysician health care professional to an established patient, parent, or guardian not originating from a related assessment and management service provided within the previous 7 days nor leading to an assessment and management service or procedure within the next 24 hours or soonest available appointment; 5-10 minutes of medical discussion

**98967**        11-20 minutes of medical discussion

**98968**        21-30 minutes of medical discussion

## On-line Medical Evaluation

An on-line electronic medical evaluation is a non-face-to-face assessment and management service by a qualified health care professional to a patient using Internet resources in response to a patient's on-line inquiry. Reportable services involve the qualified health care professional's personal timely response to the patient's inquiry and must involve permanent storage (electronic or hard copy) of the encounter. This service is reported only once for the same episode of care during a seven-day period, although multiple qualified healthcare professionals could report their exchange with the same patient. If the on-line medical evaluation refers to an assessment and management service previously performed and reported by the qualified health care professional within the previous seven days (either qualified health care professional requested or unsolicited patient follow-up) or within the postoperative period of the previously

completed procedure, then the service(s) are considered covered by the previous assessment and management office service or procedure. A reportable service encompasses the sum of communication (eg, related telephone calls, prescription provision, laboratory orders) pertaining to the on-line patient encounter.

(For an on-line medical evaluation provided by a physician, use 99444)

**98969**    Online assessment and management service provided by a qualified nonphysician health care professional to an established patient, guardian, or health care provider not originating from a related assessment and management service provided within the previous 7 days, using the Internet or similar electronic communications network

(Do not report 98969 when using 99339-99340, 99374-99380 for the same communication[s])

(Do not report 98969 for anticoagulation management when reporting 99363, 99364)

# Special Services, Procedures and Reports

The procedures with code numbers 99000 through 99091 provide the reporting physician or other qualified healthcare professional with the means of identifying the completion of special reports and services that are an adjunct to the basic services rendered. The specific number assigned indicates the special circumstances under which a basic procedure is performed.

Code 99091 should be reported no more than once in a 30-day period to include the physician or health care provider time involved with data accession, review and interpretation, modification of care plan as necessary (including communication to patient and/or caregiver), and associated documentation.

If the services described by 99091 are provided on the same day the patient presents for an E/M service, these services should be considered part of the E/M service and not separately reported.

Do not report 99091 if it occurs within 30 days of care plan oversight services 99374-99380. Do not report 99091 if other more specific CPT codes exist (eg, 93227, 93272 for cardiographic services; 95250 for continuous glucose monitoring). Do not report 99091 for transfer and interpretation of data from hospital or clinical laboratory computers.

►Codes 99050-99060 are reported in addition to an associated basic service. Do not append modifier 51 to 99050-99060. Typically only a single adjunct code from among 99050-99060 would be reported per patient encounter. However, there may be circumstances in which reporting multiple adjunct codes per patient encounter may be appropriate.◄

Medicine

## Miscellaneous Services

**99000**   Handling and/or conveyance of specimen for transfer from the physician's office to a laboratory

**99001**   Handling and/or conveyance of specimen for transfer from the patient in other than a physician's office to a laboratory (distance may be indicated)

**99002**   Handling, conveyance, and/or any other service in connection with the implementation of an order involving devices (eg, designing, fitting, packaging, handling, delivery or mailing) when devices such as orthotics, protectives, prosthetics are fabricated by an outside laboratory or shop but which items have been designed, and are to be fitted and adjusted by the attending physician

(For routine collection of venous blood, use 36415)

**99024**   Postoperative follow-up visit, normally included in the surgical package, to indicate that an evaluation and management service was performed during a postoperative period for a reason(s) related to the original procedure

(As a component of a surgical "package," see **Surgery Guidelines**)

**99026**   Hospital mandated on call service; in-hospital, each hour

**99027**        out-of-hospital, each hour

(For physician standby services requiring prolonged physician attendance, use 99360, as appropriate. Time spent performing separately reportable procedure(s) or service(s) should not be included in the time reported as mandated on call service)

**99050**   Services provided in the office at times other than regularly scheduled office hours, or days when the office is normally closed (eg, holidays, Saturday or Sunday), in addition to basic service

**99051**   Service(s) provided in the office during regularly scheduled evening, weekend, or holiday office hours, in addition to basic service

**99053**   Service(s) provided between 10:00 PM and 8:00 AM at 24-hour facility, in addition to basic service

**99056**   Service(s) typically provided in the office, provided out of the office at request of patient, in addition to basic service

**99058**   Service(s) provided on an emergency basis in the office, which disrupts other scheduled office services, in addition to basic service

**99060**   Service(s) provided on an emergency basis, out of the office, which disrupts other scheduled office services, in addition to basic service

**99070**   Supplies and materials (except spectacles), provided by the physician over and above those usually included with the office visit or other services rendered (list drugs, trays, supplies, or materials provided)

(For supply of spectacles, use the appropriate supply codes)

**99071**   Educational supplies, such as books, tapes, and pamphlets, provided by the physician for the patient's education at cost to physician

**99075**   Medical testimony

**99078**   Physician educational services rendered to patients in a group setting (eg, prenatal, obesity, or diabetic instructions)

**99080**   Special reports such as insurance forms, more than the information conveyed in the usual medical communications or standard reporting form

(Do not report 99080 in conjunction with 99455, 99456 for the completion of Workmen's Compensation forms)

**99082**   Unusual travel (eg, transportation and escort of patient)

**99090**   Analysis of clinical data stored in computers (eg, ECGs, blood pressures, hematologic data)

►(For physician/qualified health care professional collection and interpretation of physiologic data stored/transmitted by patient/caregiver, see 99091)◄

►(Do not report 99090 if other more specific CPT codes exist, eg, 93227, 93272, 0206T for cardiographic services; 95250 for continuous glucose monitoring; 97750 for musculoskeletal function testing)◄

**99091**   Collection and interpretation of physiologic data (eg, ECG, blood pressure, glucose monitoring) digitally stored and/or transmitted by the patient and/or caregiver to the physician or other qualified health care professional, requiring a minimum of 30 minutes of time

# Qualifying Circumstances for Anesthesia

(For explanation of these services, see **Anesthesia Guidelines**)

**+ 99100**   Anesthesia for patient of extreme age, younger than 1 year and older than 70 (List separately in addition to code for primary anesthesia procedure)

(For procedure performed on infants younger than 1 year of age at time of surgery, see 00326, 00561, 00834, 00836)

**+ 99116**   Anesthesia complicated by utilization of total body hypothermia (List separately in addition to code for primary anesthesia procedure)

**+ 99135**   Anesthesia complicated by utilization of controlled hypotension (List separately in addition to code for primary anesthesia procedure)

**+ 99140**   Anesthesia complicated by emergency conditions (specify) (List separately in addition to code for primary anesthesia procedure)

(An emergency is defined as existing when delay in treatment of the patient would lead to a significant increase in the threat to life or body part.)

# Moderate (Conscious) Sedation

Moderate (conscious) sedation is a drug induced depression of consciousness during which patients respond purposefully to verbal commands, either alone or accompanied by light tactile stimulation. No interventions are required to maintain a patent airway, and spontaneous ventilation is adequate. Cardiovascular function is usually maintained.

Moderate sedation does not include minimal sedation (anxiolysis), deep sedation or monitored anesthesia care (00100-01999).

When providing moderate sedation, the following services are included and NOT reported separately:

- Assessment of the patient (not included in intraservice time);

- Establishment of IV access and fluids to maintain patency, when performed;

- Administration of agent(s);

- Maintenance of sedation;

- Monitoring of oxygen saturation, heart rate and blood pressure; and

- Recovery (not included in intraservice time).

Intraservice time starts with the administration of the sedation agent(s), requires continuous face-to-face attendance, and ends at the conclusion of personal contact by the physician providing the sedation.

Do not report 99143-99150 in conjunction with 94760-94762.

Do not report 99143-99145 in conjunction with codes listed in Appendix G. Do not report 99148-99150 in conjunction with codes listed in Appendix G when performed in the nonfacility setting.

When a second physician other than the healthcare professional performing the diagnostic or therapeutic services provides moderate sedation in the facility setting (eg, hospital, outpatient hospital/ambulatory surgery center, skilled nursing facility) for the procedures listed in Appendix G, the second physician reports 99148-99150. However, for the circumstance in which these services are performed by the second physician in the nonfacility setting (eg, physician office, freestanding imaging center), codes 99148-99150 are not reported.

⊘ **99143**  Moderate sedation services (other than those services described by codes 00100-01999) provided by the same physician performing the diagnostic or therapeutic service that the sedation supports, requiring the presence of an independent trained observer to assist in the monitoring of the patient's level of consciousness and physiological status; younger than 5 years of age, first 30 minutes intra-service time

⊘ **99144**  age 5 years or older, first 30 minutes intra-service time

+ **99145**  each additional 15 minutes intra-service time (List separately in addition to code for primary service)

(Use 99145 in conjunction with 99143, 99144)

**99148**  Moderate sedation services (other than those services described by codes 00100-01999), provided by a physician other than the health care professional performing the diagnostic or therapeutic service that the sedation supports; younger than 5 years of age, first 30 minutes intra-service time

**99149**  age 5 years or older, first 30 minutes intra-service time

+ **99150**  each additional 15 minutes intra-service time (List separately in addition to code for primary service)

(Use 99150 in conjunction with 99148, 99149)

# Other Services and Procedures

**99170**  Anogenital examination with colposcopic magnification in childhood for suspected trauma

(For conscious sedation, use 99143-99150)

**99172**  Visual function screening, automated or semi-automated bilateral quantitative determination of visual acuity, ocular alignment, color vision by pseudoisochromatic plates, and field of vision (may include all or some screening of the determination[s] for contrast sensitivity, vision under glare)

(This service must employ graduated visual acuity stimuli that allow a quantitative determination of visual acuity [eg, Snellen chart]. This service may not be used in addition to a general ophthalmological service or an E/M service)

(Do not report 99172 in conjunction with 99173)

**99173**  Screening test of visual acuity, quantitative, bilateral

(The screening test used must employ graduated visual acuity stimuli that allow a quantitative estimate of visual acuity [eg, Snellen chart]. Other identifiable services unrelated to this screening test provided at the same time may be reported separately [eg, preventive medicine services]. When acuity is measured as part of a general ophthalmological service or of an E/M service of the eye, it is a diagnostic examination and not a screening test.)

(Do not report 99173 in conjunction with 99172)

**99174**  Ocular photoscreening with interpretation and report, bilateral

(Do not report 99174 in conjunction with 92002-92014, 99172, 99173)

**99175**  Ipecac or similar administration for individual emesis and continued observation until stomach adequately emptied of poison

Medicine

(For diagnostic intubation, see 43754, 43755)

(For gastric lavage for diagnostic purposes, see 43754, 43755)

**99183**   Physician attendance and supervision of hyperbaric oxygen therapy, per session

(Evaluation and Management services and/or procedures [eg, wound debridement] provided in a hyperbaric oxygen treatment facility in conjunction with a hyperbaric oxygen therapy session should be reported separately)

(99185, 99186 have been deleted)

**99190**   Assembly and operation of pump with oxygenator or heat exchanger (with or without ECG and/or pressure monitoring); each hour

**99191**   45 minutes

**99192**   30 minutes

**99195**   Phlebotomy, therapeutic (separate procedure)

**99199**   Unlisted special service, procedure or report

# Home Health Procedures/Services

These codes are used by non-physician health care professionals. Physicians should utilize the home visit codes 99341-99350 and utilize CPT codes other than 99500-99600 for any additional procedure/service provided to a patient living in a residence.

The following codes are used to report services provided in a patient's residence (including assisted living apartments, group homes, nontraditional private homes, custodial care facilities, or schools).

Health care professionals who are authorized to use Evaluation and Management (E/M) Home Visit codes (99341-99350) may report 99500-99600 in addition to 99341-99350 if both services are performed. E/M services may be reported separately, using modifier 25, if the patient's condition requires a significant separately identifiable E/M service, above and beyond the home health service(s)/procedure(s) codes 99500-99600.

**99500**   Home visit for prenatal monitoring and assessment to include fetal heart rate, non-stress test, uterine monitoring, and gestational diabetes monitoring

**99501**   Home visit for postnatal assessment and follow-up care

**99502**   Home visit for newborn care and assessment

**99503**   Home visit for respiratory therapy care (eg, bronchodilator, oxygen therapy, respiratory assessment, apnea evaluation)

**99504**   Home visit for mechanical ventilation care

**99505**   Home visit for stoma care and maintenance including colostomy and cystostomy

**99506**   Home visit for intramuscular injections

**99507**   Home visit for care and maintenance of catheter(s) (eg, urinary, drainage, and enteral)

**99509**   Home visit for assistance with activities of daily living and personal care

(To report self-care/home management training, see 97535)

(To report home medical nutrition assessment and intervention services, see 97802-97804)

(To report home speech therapy services, see 92507-92508)

**99510**   Home visit for individual, family, or marriage counseling

**99511**   Home visit for fecal impaction management and enema administration

**99512**   Home visit for hemodialysis

(For home infusion of peritoneal dialysis, use 99601, 99602)

**99600**   Unlisted home visit service or procedure

# Home Infusion Procedures/Services

**99601**   Home infusion/specialty drug administration, per visit (up to 2 hours);

+ **99602**   each additional hour (List separately in addition to code for primary procedure)

(Use 99602 in conjunction with 99601)

# Medication Therapy Management Services

Medication therapy management service(s) (MTMS) describe face-to-face patient assessment and intervention as appropriate, by a pharmacist, upon request. MTMS is provided to optimize the response to medications or to manage treatment-related medication interactions or complications.

MTMS includes the following documented elements: review of the pertinent patient history, medication profile (prescription and nonprescription), and recommendations for improving health outcomes and treatment compliance. These codes are not to be used to describe the provision of product-specific information at the point of dispensing or any other routine dispensing-related activities.

**99605**   Medication therapy management service(s) provided by a pharmacist, individual, face-to-face with patient, with assessment and intervention if provided; initial 15 minutes, new patient

**99606**   initial 15 minutes, established patient

+ **99607**   each additional 15 minutes (List separately in addition to code for primary service)

(Use 99607 in conjunction with 99605, 99606)

**Medicine**

# Notes

⊙=Moderate sedation  ✚=Add-on code  ✗=FDA approval pending  #=Resequenced code  ○=Recycled/reinstated code

Medicine

# Category II Codes

The following section of *Current Procedural Terminology* (CPT) contains a set of supplemental tracking codes that can be used for performance measurement. It is anticipated that the use of Category II codes for performance measurement will decrease the need for record abstraction and chart review, and thereby minimize administrative burden on physicians, other health care professionals, hospitals, and entities seeking to measure the quality of patient care. These codes are intended to facilitate data collection about the quality of care rendered by coding certain services and test results that support nationally established performance measures and that have an evidence base as contributing to quality patient care.

The use of these codes is optional. The codes are not required for correct coding and may not be used as a substitute for Category I codes.

These codes describe clinical components that may be typically included in evaluation and management services or clinical services and, therefore, do not have a relative value associated with them. Category II codes may also describe results from clinical laboratory or radiology tests and other procedures, identified processes intended to address patient safety practices, or services reflecting compliance with state or federal law.

Category II codes described in this section make use of alphabetical characters as the 5th character in the string (ie, 4 digits followed by the letter **F**). These digits are not intended to reflect the placement of the code in the regular (Category I) part of the CPT codebook. To promote understanding of these codes and their associated measures, users are referred to the Alphabetical Clinical Topics Listing, which contains information about performance measurement exclusion modifiers, measures, and the measure's source.

Cross-references to the measures associated with each Category II code and their source are included for reference in the Alphabetical Clinical Topics Listing. In addition, acronyms for the related diseases or clinical condition(s) have been added at the end of each code descriptor to identify the topic or clinical category in which that code is included. A complete listing of the diseases/clinical conditions, and their acronyms are provided in alphabetical order in the Alphabetical Clinical Topics Listing. The Alphabetical Clinical Topics Listing can be accessed on the Web site at www.ama-assn. org, under the Category II link. Users should review the complete measure(s) associated with each code prior to implementation.

Category II codes are reviewed by the Performance Measures Advisory Group (PMAG), an advisory body to the CPT Editorial Panel and the CPT/HCPAC Advisory Committee. The PMAG is comprised of performance measurement experts representing the Agency for Healthcare Research and Quality (AHRQ), the American Medical Association (AMA), the Centers for Medicare and Medicaid Services (CMS), The Joint Commission (TJC), and the Physician Consortium for Performance Improvement® (PCPI). The PMAG may seek additional expertise and/or input from other national health care organizations, as necessary, for the development of tracking codes. These may include national medical specialty societies, other national health care professional associations, accrediting bodies, and federal regulatory agencies.

The most current listing of Category II codes, including guidelines, Code Change Proposal forms, and release and implementation dates for Category II codes may be accessed at http://www.ama-assn.org/go/cpt.

> (For blood pressure measured, use 2000F)

> (For tobacco use cessation intervention, pharmacologic therapy, use 4001F)

The superscripted numbers included at the end of each code descriptor direct users to the footnotes. The following information identifies the name and web address of the measure developers that are associated with these footnotes:

**Footnotes**

[1]Physician Consortium for Performance Improvement®(PCPI), www.physicianconsortium.org.

[2]National Committee on Quality Assurance (NCQA), Health Employer Data Information Set (HEDIS®), www.ncqa.org.

[3]Joint Commission on Accreditation of Healthcare Organizations (JCAHO), ORYX Initiative Performance Measures, www.jcaho.org/pms.

[4]National Diabetes Quality Improvement Alliance (NDQIA), www.nationaldiabetesalliance.org.

[5]Joint measure from The Physician Consortium for Performance Improvement, www.physician consortium.org and National Committee on Quality Assurance (NCQA), www.ncqa.org.

[6]The Society of Thoracic Surgeons at www.sts.org and National Quality Forum, www.qualityforum.org.

[7]Ingenix, www.ingenix.com.

[8]American Academy of Neurology, www.aan.com/go/practice/quality/measurements or quality@aan.com.

►[9]College of American Pathologists (CAP), www.cap.org/apps/docs/advocacy/pathology performance measurement.pdf◄

# Modifiers

The following performance measurement modifiers may be used for Category II codes to indicate that a service specified in the associated measure(s) was considered but, due to either medical, patient, or system circumstance(s) documented in the medical record, the service was not provided. These modifiers serve as denominator exclusions from the performance measure. The user should note that not all listed measures provide for exclusions (see Alphabetical Clinical Topics Listing for more discussion regarding exclusion criteria).

Category II modifiers should only be reported with Category II codes—they should not be reported with Category I or Category III codes. In addition, the modifiers in the Category II section should only be used where specified in the guidelines, reporting instructions, parenthetic notes, or code descriptor language listed in the Category II section (code listing and the Alphabetical Clinical Topics Listing).

**1P**  Performance Measure Exclusion Modifier due to Medical Reasons

Reasons include:

- Not indicated (absence of organ/limb, already received/performed, other)
- Contraindicated (patient allergic history, potential adverse drug interaction, other)
- Other medical reasons

**2P**  Performance Measure Exclusion Modifier due to Patient Reasons

Reasons include:

- Patient declined
- Economic, social, or religious reasons
- Other patient reasons

**3P**  Performance Measure Exclusion Modifier due to System Reasons

Reasons include:

- Resources to perform the services not available
- Insurance coverage/payor-related limitations
- Other reasons attributable to health care delivery system

Modifier 8P is intended to be used as a "reporting modifier" to allow the reporting of circumstances when an action described in a measure's numerator is not performed and the reason is not otherwise specified.

**8P**  Performance measure reporting modifier–action not performed, reason not otherwise specified

# Composite Codes

Composite codes combine several measures grouped within a single code descriptor to facilitate reporting for a clinical condition when all components are met. If only some of the components are met or if services are provided in addition to those included in the composite code, they may be reported individually using the corresponding CPT Category II codes for those services.

**0001F**  Heart failure assessed (includes assessment of all the following components) (CAD)[1]:

Blood pressure measured (2000F)[1]

Level of activity assessed (1003F)[1]

Clinical symptoms of volume overload (excess) assessed (1004F)[1]

Weight, recorded (2001F)[1]

Clinical signs of volume overload (excess) assessed (2002F)[1]

(To report blood pressure measured, use 2000F)

**0005F**  Osteoarthritis assessed (OA)[1]

Includes assessment of all the following components:

Osteoarthritis symptoms and functional status assessed (1006F)[1]

Use of anti-inflammatory or over-the-counter (OTC) analgesic medications assessed (1007F)[1]

Initial examination of the involved joint(s) (includes visual inspection, palpation, range of motion) (2004F)[1]

(To report tobacco use cessation intervention, use 4001F)

**0012F**  Community-acquired bacterial pneumonia assessment (includes all of the following components) (CAP)[1]:

Co-morbid conditions assessed (1026F)[1]

Vital signs recorded (2010F)[1]

Mental status assessed (2014F)[1]

Hydration status assessed (2018F)[1]

**0014F**  Comprehensive preoperative assessment performed for cataract surgery with intraocular lens (IOL) placement (includes assessment of all of the following components) (EC)[5]:

Dilated fundus evaluation performed within 12 months prior to cataract surgery (2020F)[5]

Pre-surgical (cataract) axial length, corneal power measurement and method of intraocular lens power calculation documented (must be performed within 12 months prior to surgery) (3073F)[5]

Preoperative assessment of functional or medical indication(s) for surgery prior to the cataract surgery with intraocular lens placement (must be performed within 12 months prior to cataract surgery) (3325F)[5]

**0015F**    Melanoma follow up completed (includes assessment of all of the following components) (ML)[5]:

         History obtained regarding new or changing moles (1050F)[5]

         Complete physical skin exam performed (2029F)[5]

         Patient counseled to perform a monthly self skin examination (5005F)[5]

# Patient Management

Patient management codes describe utilization measures or measures of patient care provided for specific clinical purposes (eg, prenatal care, pre- and post-surgical care).

**0500F**    Initial prenatal care visit (report at first prenatal encounter with health care professional providing obstetrical care. Report also date of visit and, in a separate field, the date of the last menstrual period [LMP]) (Prenatal)[2]

**0501F**    Prenatal flow sheet documented in medical record by first prenatal visit (documentation includes at minimum blood pressure, weight, urine protein, uterine size, fetal heart tones, and estimated date of delivery). Report also: date of visit and, in a separate field, the date of the last menstrual period [LMP] (Note: If reporting 0501F Prenatal flow sheet, it is not necessary to report 0500F Initial prenatal care visit) (Prenatal)[1]

**0502F**    Subsequent prenatal care visit (Prenatal)[2]

         [Excludes: patients who are seen for a condition unrelated to pregnancy or prenatal care (eg, an upper respiratory infection; patients seen for consultation only, not for continuing care)]

**0503F**    Postpartum care visit (Prenatal)[2]

**0505F**    Hemodialysis plan of care documented (ESRD, P-ESRD)[1]

**0507F**    Peritoneal dialysis plan of care documented (ESRD)[1]

**0509F**    Urinary incontinence plan of care documented (GER)[5]

**0513F**    Elevated blood pressure plan of care documented (CKD)[1]

**0514F**    Plan of care for elevated hemoglobin level documented for patient receiving Erythropoiesis-Stimulating Agent therapy (ESA) (CKD)[1]

**0516F**    Anemia plan of care documented (ESRD)[1]

**0517F**    Glaucoma plan of care documented (EC)[5]

**0518F**    Falls plan of care documented (GER)[5]

**0519F**    Planned chemotherapy regimen, including at a minimum: drug(s) prescribed, dose, and duration, documented prior to initiation of a new treatment regimen (ONC)[1]

**0520F**    Radiation dose limits to normal tissues established prior to the initiation of a course of 3D conformal radiation for a minimum of 2 tissue/organ (ONC)[1]

**0521F**    Plan of care to address pain documented (COA)[2] (ONC)[1]

**0525F**    Initial visit for episode (BkP)[2]

**0526F**    Subsequent visit for episode (BkP)[2]

**0528F**    Recommended follow-up interval for repeat colonoscopy of at least 10 years documented in colonoscopy report (End/Polyp)[5]

**0529F**    Interval of 3 or more years since patient's last colonoscopy, documented (End/Polyp)[5]

**0535F**    Dyspnea management plan of care, documented (Pall Cr)[5]

**0540F**    Glucorticoid Management Plan Documented (RA)[5]

**0545F**    Plan for follow-up care for major depressive disorder, documented (MDD ADOL)[1]

● **0550F**    Cytopathology report on routine nongynecologic specimen finalized within two working days of accession date (PATH)[9]

● **0551F**    Cytopathology report on nongynecologic specimen with documentation that the specimen was non-routine (PATH)[9]

● **0555F**    Symptom management plan of care documented (HF)[1]

● **0556F**    Plan of care to achieve lipid control documented (CAD)[1]

● **0557F**    Plan of care to manage anginal symptoms documented (CAD)[1]

**0575F**    HIV RNA control plan of care, documented (HIV)[5]

# Patient History

Patient history codes describe measures for select aspects of patient history or review of systems.

**1000F**    Tobacco use assessed (CAD, CAP, COPD, PV)[1] (DM)[4]

**1002F**    Anginal symptoms and level of activity assessed (NMA – No Measure Associated)

**1003F**    Level of activity assessed (NMA – No Measure Associated)

**1004F**    Clinical symptoms of volume overload (excess) assessed (NMA – No Measure Associated)

**1005F**    Asthma symptoms evaluated (includes physician documentation of numeric frequency of symptoms or patient completion of an asthma assessment tool/survey/questionnaire) (NMA – No Measure Associated)

**1006F**    Osteoarthritis symptoms and functional status assessed (may include the use of a standardized scale or the completion of an assessment questionnaire, such as the SF-36, AAOS Hip & Knee Questionnaire) (OA)[1]

         [Instructions: Report when osteoarthritis is addressed during the patient encounter]

**1007F**    Use of anti-inflammatory or analgesic over-the-counter (OTC) medications for symptom relief assessed (OA)[1]

**1008F**    Gastrointestinal and renal risk factors assessed for patients on prescribed or OTC non-steroidal anti-inflammatory drug (NSAID) (OA)[1]

● **1010F**    Severity of angina assessed by level of activity (CAD)[1]

**Category II Codes**

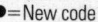

● **1011F** Angina present (CAD)[1]

● **1012F** Angina absent (CAD)[1]

**1015F** Chronic obstructive pulmonary disease (COPD) symptoms assessed (Includes assessment of at least 1 of the following: dyspnea, cough/sputum, wheezing), or respiratory symptom assessment tool completed (COPD)[1]

**1018F** Dyspnea assessed, not present (COPD)[1]

**1019F** Dyspnea assessed, present (COPD)[1]

**1022F** Pneumococcus immunization status assessed (CAP, COPD)[1]

**1026F** Co-morbid conditions assessed (eg, includes assessment for presence or absence of: malignancy, liver disease, congestive heart failure, cerebrovascular disease, renal disease, chronic obstructive pulmonary disease, asthma, diabetes, other co-morbid conditions) (CAP)[1]

**1030F** Influenza immunization status assessed (CAP)[1]

● **1031F** Smoking status and exposure to second hand smoke in the home assessed (Asthma)[1]

● **1032F** Current tobacco smoker OR currently exposed to secondhand smoke (Asthma)[1]

● **1033F** Current tobacco non-smoker AND not currently exposed to secondhand smoke[1]

**1034F** Current tobacco smoker (CAD, CAP, COPD, PV)[1] (DM)[4]

**1035F** Current smokeless tobacco user (eg, chew, snuff) (PV)[1]

**1036F** Current tobacco non-user (CAD, CAP, COPD, PV)[1] (DM)[4]

**1038F** Persistent asthma (mild, moderate or severe) (Asthma)[1]

**1039F** Intermittent asthma (Asthma)[1]

**1040F** DSM-IV™ criteria for major depressive disorder documented at the initial evaluation (MDD, MDD ADOL)[1]

**1050F** History obtained regarding new or changing moles (ML)[5]

**1055F** Visual functional status assessed (EC)[5]

**1060F** Documentation of permanent OR persistent OR paroxysmal atrial fibrillation (STR)[5]

**1061F** Documentation of absence of permanent AND persistent AND paroxysmal atrial fibrillation (STR)[5]

**1065F** Ischemic stroke symptom onset of less than 3 hours prior to arrival (STR)[5]

**1066F** Ischemic stroke symptom onset greater than or equal to 3 hours prior to arrival (STR)[5]

**1070F** Alarm symptoms (involuntary weight loss, dysphagia, or gastrointestinal bleeding) assessed; none present (GERD)[5]

**1071F** 1 or more present (GERD)[5]

(1080F has been deleted. To report Surrogate decision maker or advance care plan documented in the medical record, report code 1123F or 1124F.)

**1090F** Presence or absence of urinary incontinence assessed (GER)[5]

**1091F** Urinary incontinence characterized (eg, frequency, volume, timing, type of symptoms, how bothersome) (GER)[5]

**1100F** Patient screened for future fall risk; documentation of 2 or more falls in the past year or any fall with injury in the past year (GER)[5]

**1101F** documentation of no falls in the past year or only 1 fall without injury in the past year (GER)[5]

**1110F** Patient discharged from an inpatient facility (eg, hospital, skilled nursing facility, or rehabilitation facility) within the last 60 days (GER)[5]

**1111F** Discharge medications reconciled with the current medication list in outpatient medical record (COA)[2] (GER)[5]

**1116F** Auricular or periauricular pain assessed (AOE)[1]

**1118F** GERD symptoms assessed after 12 months of therapy (GERD)[5]

**1119F** Initial evaluation for condition (HEP C)[1](EPI)[8]

**1121F** Subsequent evaluation for condition (HEP C)[1](EPI)[8]

**1123F** Advance Care Planning discussed and documented advance care plan or surrogate decision maker documented in the medical record (DEM)[1] (GER, Pall Cr)[5]

**1124F** Advance Care Planning discussed and documented in the medical record, patient did not wish or was not able to name a surrogate decision maker or provide an advance care plan (DEM)[1] (GER, Pall Cr)[5]

**1125F** Pain severity quantified; pain present (COA)[2] (ONC)[1]

**1126F** no pain present (COA)[2] (ONC)[1]

○ **1127F** New episode for condition (NMA-No Measure Associated)

○ **1128F** Subsequent episode for condition (NMA-No Measure Associated)

**1130F** Back pain and function assessed, including all of the following: Pain assessment AND functional status AND patient history, including notation of presence or absence of "red flags" (warning signs) AND assessment of prior treatment and response, AND employment status (BkP)[2]

**1134F** Episode of back pain lasting 6 weeks or less (BkP)[2]

**1135F** Episode of back pain lasting longer than 6 weeks (BkP)[2]

**1136F** Episode of back pain lasting 12 weeks or less (BkP)[2]

**1137F** Episode of back pain lasting longer than 12 weeks (BkP)[2]

**1150F** Documentation that a patient has a substantial risk of death within 1 year (Pall Cr)[5]

**1151F** Documentation that a patient does not have a substantial risk of death within one year (Pall Cr)[5]

**1152F** Documentation of advanced disease diagnosis, goals of care prioritize comfort (Pall Cr)[5]

**1153F** Documentation of advanced disease diagnosis, goals of care do not prioritize comfort (Pall Cr)[5]

**Category II Codes**

**1157F** Advance care plan or similar legal document present in the medical record (COA)[2]

**1158F** Advance care planning discussion documented in the medical record (COA)[2]

**1159F** Medication list documented in medical record (COA)[2]

**1160F** Review of all medications by a prescribing practitioner or clinical pharmacist (such as, prescriptions, OTCs, herbal therapies and supplements) documented in the medical record (COA)[2]

**1170F** Functional status assessed (COA)[2] (RA)[5]

● **1175F** Functional status for dementia assessed and results reviewed (DEM)[1]

**1180F** All specified thromboembolic risk factors assessed (AFIB)[1]

● **1181F** Neuropsychiatric symptoms assessed and results reviewed (DEM)[1]

● **1182F** Neuropsychiatric symptoms, one or more present (DEM)[1]

● **1183F** Neuropsychiatric symptoms, absent (DEM)[1]

**1200F** Seizure type(s) and current seizure frequency(ies) documented (EPI)[8]

**1205F** Etiology of epilepsy or epilepsy syndrome(s) reviewed and documented (EPI)[8]

**1220F** Patient screened for depression (SUD)[5]

**1400F** Parkinson's disease diagnosis reviewed (Prkns)[8]

● **1450F** Symptoms improved or remained consistent with treatment goals since last assessment (HF)[1]

● **1451F** Symptoms demonstrated clinically important deterioration since last assessment (HF)[1]

● **1460F** Qualifying cardiac event/diagnosis in previous 12 months (CAD)[1]

● **1461F** No qualifying cardiac event/diagnosis in previous 12 months (CAD)[1]

● **1490F** Dementia severity classified, mild (DEM)[1]

● **1491F** Dementia severity classified, moderate (DEM)

● **1493F** Dementia severity classified, severe (DEM)[1]

● **1494F** Cognition assessed and reviewed (DEM)[1]

# Physical Examination

Physical examination codes describe aspects of physical examination or clinical assessment.

**2000F** Blood pressure measured (CKD)[1](DM)[2,4]

**2001F** Weight recorded (PAG)[1]

**2002F** Clinical signs of volume overload (excess) assessed (NMA – No Measure Associated)

**2004F** Initial examination of the involved joint(s) (includes visual inspection, palpation, range of motion) (OA)[1]

[Instructions: Report only for initial osteoarthritis visit or for visits for new joint involvement]

**2010F** Vital signs (temperature, pulse, respiratory rate, and blood pressure) documented and reviewed (CAP)[1] (EM)[5]

**2014F** Mental status assessed (CAP)[1] (EM)[5]

● **2015F** Asthma impairment assessed (Asthma)[1]

● **2016F** Asthma risk assessed (Asthma)[1]

**2018F** Hydration status assessed (normal/mildly dehydrated/ severely dehydrated) (CAP)[1]

**2019F** Dilated macular exam performed, including documentation of the presence or absence of macular thickening or hemorrhage AND the level of macular degeneration severity (EC)[5]

**2020F** Dilated fundus evaluation performed within 12 months prior to cataract surgery (EC)[5]

**2021F** Dilated macular or fundus exam performed, including documentation of the presence or absence of macular edema AND level of severity of retinopathy (EC)[5]

**2022F** Dilated retinal eye exam with interpretation by an ophthalmologist or optometrist documented and reviewed (DM)[2,4]

**2024F** 7 standard field stereoscopic photos with interpretation by an ophthalmologist or optometrist documented and reviewed (DM)[2,4]

**2026F** Eye imaging validated to match diagnosis from 7 standard field stereoscopic photos results documented and reviewed (DM)[2,4]

**2027F** Optic nerve head evaluation performed (EC)[5]

**2028F** Foot examination performed (includes examination through visual inspection, sensory exam with monofilament, and pulse exam – report when any of the 3 components are completed) (DM)[4]

**2029F** Complete physical skin exam performed (ML)[5]

**2030F** Hydration status documented, normally hydrated (PAG)[1]

**2031F** Hydration status documented, dehydrated (PAG)[1]

**2035F** Tympanic membrane mobility assessed with pneumatic otoscopy or tympanometry (OME)[1]

**2040F** Physical examination on the date of the initial visit for low back pain performed, in accordance with specifications (BkP)[2]

**2044F** Documentation of mental health assessment prior to intervention (back surgery or epidural steroid injection) or for back pain episode lasting longer than 6 weeks (BkP)[2]

**2050F** Wound characteristics including size AND nature of wound base tissue AND amount of drainage prior to debridement documented (CWC)[5]

**2060F** Patient interviewed directly by evaluating clinician on or before date of diagnosis of major depressive disorder (MDD ADOL)[1]

**Category II Codes**

# Diagnostic/Screening Processes or Results

Diagnostic/screening processes or results codes describe results of tests ordered (clinical laboratory tests, radiological or other procedural examinations, and conclusions of medical decision-making).

(To report blood pressure use the corresponding systolic codes [3074F, 3075F, 3077F] and diastolic codes [3078F, 3079F, 3080F])

**3006F**   Chest X-ray results documented and reviewed (CAP)[1]

**3008F**   Body Mass Index (BMI), documented (PV)[1]

**3011F**   Lipid panel results documented and reviewed (must include total cholesterol, HDL-C, triglycerides and calculated LDL-C) (CAD)[1]

**3014F**   Screening mammography results documented and reviewed (PV)[1,2]

**3015F**   Cervical cancer screening results documented and reviewed (PV)[1]

**3016F**   Patient screened for unhealthy alcohol use using a systematic screening method (PV)[1]

**3017F**   Colorectal cancer screening results documented and reviewed (PV)[1,2]

**3018F**   Pre-procedure risk assessment AND depth of insertion AND quality of the bowel prep AND complete description of polyp(s) found, including location of each polyp, size, number and gross morphology AND recommendations for follow-up in final colonoscopy report documented (End/Polyp)[5]

● **3019F**   Left ventricular ejection fraction (LVEF) assessment planned post discharge (HF)[1]

**3020F**   Left ventricular function (LVF) assessment (eg, echocardiography, nuclear test, or ventriculography) documented in the medical record (Includes quantitative or qualitative assessment results) (NMA – No Measure Associated)

**3021F**   Left ventricular ejection fraction (LVEF) less than 40% or documentation of moderately or severely depressed left ventricular systolic function (CAD, HF)[1]

**3022F**   Left ventricular ejection fraction (LVEF) greater than or equal to 40% or documentation as normal or mildly depressed left ventricular systolic function (CAD, HF)[1]

**3023F**   Spirometry results documented and reviewed (COPD)[1]

**3025F**   Spirometry test results demonstrate $FEV_1/FVC$ less than 70% with COPD symptoms (eg, dyspnea, cough/sputum, wheezing) (CAP, COPD)[1]

**3027F**   Spirometry test results demonstrate $FEV_1/FVC$ greater than or equal to 70% or patient does not have COPD symptoms (COPD)[1]

**3028F**   Oxygen saturation results documented and reviewed (includes assessment through pulse oximetry or arterial blood gas measurement) (CAP, COPD)[1] (EM)[5]

**3035F**   Oxygen saturation less than or equal to 88% or a $PaO_2$ less than or equal to 55 mm Hg (COPD)[1].

**3037F**   Oxygen saturation greater than 88% or $PaO_2$ greater than 55 mm Hg (COPD)[1]

**3038F**   Pulmonary function test performed within 12 months prior to surgery (Lung/Esop Cx)[6]

**3040F**   Functional expiratory volume ($FEV_1$) less than 40% of predicted value (COPD)[1]

**3042F**   Functional expiratory volume ($FEV_1$) greater than or equal to 40% of predicted value (COPD)[1]

**3044F**   Most recent hemoglobin A1c (HbA1c) level less than 7.0% (DM)[2,4]

**3045F**   Most recent hemoglobin A1c (HbA1c) level 7.0–9.0% (DM)[2,4]

**3046F**   Most recent hemoglobin A1c level greater than 9.0% (DM)[4]

(To report most recent hemoglobin A1c level less than or equal to 9.0%, see codes 3044F-3045F)

**3048F**   Most recent LDL-C less than 100 mg/dL (CAD)[1] (DM)[4]

**3049F**   Most recent LDL-C 100-129 mg/dL (CAD)[1] (DM)[4]

**3050F**   Most recent LDL-C greater than or equal to 130 mg/dL (CAD)[1] (DM)[4]

● **3055F**   Left ventricular ejection fraction (LVEF) less than or equal to 35% (HF)[1]

● **3056F**   Left ventricular ejection fraction (LVEF) greater than 35% or no LVEF result available (HF)[1]

**3060F**   Positive microalbuminuria test result documented and reviewed (DM)[2,4]

**3061F**   Negative microalbuminuria test result documented and reviewed (DM)[2,4]

**3062F**   Positive macroalbuminuria test result documented and reviewed (DM)[2,4]

**3066F**   Documentation of treatment for nephropathy (eg, patient receiving dialysis, patient being treated for ESRD, CRF, ARF, or renal insufficiency, any visit to a nephrologist) (DM)[2,4]

**3072F**   Low risk for retinopathy (no evidence of retinopathy in the prior year) (DM)[2,4]

**3073F**   Pre-surgical (cataract) axial length, corneal power measurement and method of intraocular lens power calculation documented within 12 months prior to surgery (EC)[5]

**3074F**   Most recent systolic blood pressure less than 130 mm Hg (DM)[2,4] (HTN, CKD, CAD)[1]

**3075F**   Most recent systolic blood pressure 130 - 139 mm Hg (DM)[2,4] (HTN, CKD, CAD)[1]

( To report most recent systolic blood pressure less than 140 mm Hg, see codes 3074F-3075F)

**3077F**   Most recent systolic blood pressure greater than or equal to 140 mm Hg (HTN, CKD, CAD)[1] (DM)[2,4]

Category II Codes

**3078F**    Most recent diastolic blood pressure less than 80 mm Hg (HTN, CKD, CAD)[1] (DM)[2,4]

**3079F**    Most recent diastolic blood pressure 80-89 mm Hg (HTN, CKD, CAD)[1] (DM)[2,4]

**3080F**    Most recent diastolic blood pressure greater than or equal to 90 mm Hg (HTN, CKD, CAD)[1] (DM)[2,4]

**3082F**    Kt/V less than 1.2 (Clearance of urea [Kt]/volume [V]) (ESRD, P-ESRD)[1]

**3083F**    Kt/V equal to or greater than 1.2 and less than 1.7 (Clearance of urea [Kt]/volume [V]) (ESRD, P-ESRD)[1]

**3084F**    Kt/V greater than or equal to 1.7 (Clearance of urea [Kt]/volume [V]) (ESRD, P-ESRD)[1]

**3085F**    Suicide risk assessed (MDD, MDD ADOL)[1]

**3088F**    Major depressive disorder, mild (MDD)[1]

**3089F**    Major depressive disorder, moderate (MDD)[1]

**3090F**    Major depressive disorder, severe without psychotic features (MDD)[1]

**3091F**    Major depressive disorder, severe with psychotic features (MDD)[1]

**3092F**    Major depressive disorder, in remission (MDD)[1]

**3093F**    Documentation of new diagnosis of initial or recurrent episode of major depressive disorder (MDD)[1]

**3095F**    Central dual-energy X-ray absorptiometry (DXA) results documented (OP)[5]

**3096F**    Central dual-energy X-ray absorptiometry (DXA) ordered (OP)[5]

**3100F**    Carotid imaging study report (includes direct or indirect reference to measurements of distal internal carotid diameter as the denominator for stenosis measurement) (STR, RAD)[5]

**3110F**    Documentation in final CT or MRI report of presence or absence of hemorrhage and mass lesion and acute infarction (STR)[5]

▲ **3111F**    CT or MRI of the brain performed in the hospital within 24 hours of arrival OR performed in an outpatient imaging center, to confirm initial diagnosis of stroke, TIA or intracranial hemorrhage (STR)[5]

▲ **3112F**    CT or MRI of the brain performed greater than 24 hours after arrival to the hospital OR performed in an outpatient imaging center for purpose other than confirmation of initial diagnosis of stroke, TIA, or intracranial hemorrhage (STR)[5]

● **3115F**    Quantitative results of an evaluation of current level of activity and clinical symptoms (HF)[1]

● **3117F**    Heart Failure disease specific structured assessment tool completed (HF)[1]

● **3118F**    New York Heart Association (NYHA) Class documented (HF)[1]

● **3119F**    No Evaluation of level of activity or clinical symptoms (HF)[1]

**3120F**    12-Lead ECG Performed (EM)[5]

● **3125F**    Esophageal biopsy report with statement about dysplasia (present, absent, or indefinite) (PATH)[9]

**3130F**    Upper gastrointestinal endoscopy performed (GERD)[5]

**3132F**    Documentation of referral for upper gastrointestinal endoscopy (GERD)[5]

**3140F**    Upper gastrointestinal endoscopy report indicates suspicion of Barrett's esophagus (GERD)[5]

**3141F**    Upper gastrointestinal endoscopy report indicates no suspicion of Barrett's esophagus (GERD)[5]

**3142F**    Barium swallow test ordered (GERD)[1]

     (To report documentation of barium swallow study, use code 3142F)

**3150F**    Forceps esophageal biopsy performed (GERD)[5]

**3155F**    Cytogenetic testing performed on bone marrow at time of diagnosis or prior to initiating treatment (HEM)[1]

**3160F**    Documentation of iron stores prior to initiating erythropoietin therapy (HEM)[1]

**3170F**    Flow cytometry studies performed at time of diagnosis or prior to initiating treatment (HEM)[1]

**3200F**    Barium swallow test not ordered (GERD)[5]

**3210F**    Group A Strep Test Performed (PHAR)[2]

**3215F**    Patient has documented immunity to Hepatitis A (HEP-C)[1]

**3216F**    Patient has documented immunity to Hepatitis B (HEP-C)[1]

     (3217F has been deleted)

**3218F**    RNA testing for Hepatitis C documented as performed within 6 months prior to initiation of antiviral treatment for Hepatitis C (HEP-C)[1]

     (3219F has been deleted)

**3220F**    Hepatitis C quantitative RNA testing documented as performed at 12 weeks from initiation of antiviral treatment (HEP-C)[1]

**3230F**    Documentation that hearing test was performed within 6 months prior to tympanostomy tube insertion (OME)[1]

**3250F**    Specimen site other than anatomic location of primary tumor (PATH)[1]

**3260F**    pT category (primary tumor), pN category (regional lymph nodes), and histologic grade documented in pathology report (PATH)[1]

**3265F**    Ribonucleic acid (RNA) testing for Hepatitis C viremia ordered or results documented (HEP C)[1]

**3266F**    Hepatitis C genotype testing documented as performed prior to initiation of antiviral treatment for Hepatitis C (HEP C)[1]

● **3267F**    Pathology report includes pT category, pN category, Gleason score, and statement about margin status (PATH)[9]

**Category II Codes**

**3268F** Prostate-specific antigen (PSA), AND primary tumor (T) stage, AND Gleason score documented prior to initiation of treatment (PRCA)[1]

**3269F** Bone scan performed prior to initiation of treatment or at any time since diagnosis of prostate cancer (PRCA)[1]

**3270F** Bone scan not performed prior to initiation of treatment nor at any time since diagnosis of prostate cancer (PRCA)[1]

**3271F** Low risk of recurrence, prostate cancer (PRCA)[1]

**3272F** Intermediate risk of recurrence, prostate cancer (PRCA)[1]

**3273F** High risk of recurrence, prostate cancer (PRCA)[1]

**3274F** Prostate cancer risk of recurrence not determined or neither low, intermediate nor high (PRCA)[1]

**3278F** Serum levels of calcium, phosphorus, intact Parathyroid Hormone (PTH) and lipid profile ordered (CKD)[1]

**3279F** Hemoglobin level greater than or equal to 13 g/dL (CKD, ESRD)[1]

**3280F** Hemoglobin level 11 g/dL to 12.9 g/dL (CKD, ESRD)[1]

**3281F** Hemoglobin level less than 11 g/dL (CKD, ESRD)[1]

**3284F** Intraocular pressure (IOP) reduced by a value of greater than or equal to 15% from the pre-intervention level (EC)[5]

**3285F** Intraocular pressure (IOP) reduced by a value less than 15% from the pre-intervention level (EC)[5]

**3288F** Falls risk assessment documented (GER)[5]

**3290F** Patient is D (Rh) negative and unsensitized (Pre-Cr)[1]

**3291F** Patient is D (Rh) positive or sensitized (Pre-Cr)[1]

**3292F** HIV testing ordered or documented and reviewed during the first or second prenatal visit (Pre-Cr)[1]

**3293F** ABO and Rh blood typing documented as performed (Pre-Cr)[7]

**3294F** Group B Streptococcus (GBS) screening documented as performed during week 35-37 gestation (Pre-Cr)[7]

**3300F** American Joint Committee on Cancer (AJCC) stage documented and reviewed (ONC)[1]

**3301F** Cancer stage documented in medical record as metastatic and reviewed (ONC)[1]

(Codes 3302F-3312F have been deleted)

(To report measures for cancer staging, see 3321F-3390F)

**3315F** Estrogen receptor (ER) or progesterone receptor (PR) positive breast cancer (ONC)[1]

**3316F** Estrogen receptor (ER) and progesterone receptor (PR) negative breast cancer (ONC)[1]

**3317F** Pathology report confirming malignancy documented in the medical record and reviewed prior to the initiation of chemotherapy (ONC)[1]

**3318F** Pathology report confirming malignancy documented in the medical record and reviewed prior to the initiation of radiation therapy (ONC)[1]

**3319F** 1 of the following diagnostic imaging studies ordered: chest x-ray, CT, Ultrasound, MRI, PET, or nuclear medicine scans (ML)[5]

**3320F** None of the following diagnostic imaging studies ordered: chest X-ray, CT, Ultrasound, MRI, PET, or nuclear medicine scans (ML)[5]

**3321F** AJCC Cancer Stage 0 or IA Melanoma, documented (ML)[5]

**3322F** Melanoma greater than AJCC Stage 0 or IA (ML)[5]

**3323F** Clinical tumor, node and metastases (TNM) staging documented and reviewed prior to surgery (Lung/Esop Cx)[6]

**3324F** MRI or CT scan ordered, reviewed or requested (EPI)[8]

**3325F** Preoperative assessment of functional or medical indication(s) for surgery prior to the cataract surgery with intraocular lens placement (must be performed within 12 months prior to cataract surgery) (EC)[5]

**3328F** Performance status documented and reviewed within 2 weeks prior to surgery (Lung/Esop Cx)[6]

**3330F** Imaging study ordered (BkP)[2]

**3331F** Imaging study not ordered (BkP)[2]

**3340F** Mammogram assessment category of "incomplete: need additional imaging evaluation" documented (RAD)[5]

**3341F** Mammogram assessment category of "negative," documented (RAD)[5]

**3342F** Mammogram assessment category of "benign," documented (RAD)[5]

**3343F** Mammogram assessment category of "probably benign," documented (RAD)[5]

**3344F** Mammogram assessment category of "suspicious," documented (RAD)[5]

**3345F** Mammogram assessment category of "highly suggestive of malignancy," documented (RAD)[5]

**3350F** Mammogram assessment category of "known biopsy proven malignancy," documented (RAD)[5]

**3351F** Negative screen for depressive symptoms as categorized by using a standardized depression screening/assessment tool (MDD)[2]

**3352F** No significant depressive symptoms as categorized by using a standardized depression assessment tool (MDD)[2]

**3353F** Mild to moderate depressive symptoms as categorized by using a standardized depression screening/assessment tool (MDD)[2]

**3354F** Clinically significant depressive symptoms as categorized by using a standardized depression screening/assessment tool (MDD)[2]

**3370F** AJCC Breast Cancer Stage 0 documented (ONC)[1]

**3372F** AJCC Breast Cancer Stage I: T1mic, T1a or T1b (tumor size ≤ 1 cm) documented (ONC)[1]

**3374F** AJCC Breast Cancer Stage I: T1c (tumor size > 1 cm to 2 cm) documented (ONC)[1]

**Category II Codes**

⊙=Moderate sedation  ✛=Add-on code  ⟋=FDA approval pending  #=Resequenced code  ○=Recycled/reinstated code

**3376F**  AJCC Breast Cancer Stage II documented (ONC)[1]

**3378F**  AJCC Breast Cancer Stage III documented (ONC)[1]

**3380F**  AJCC Breast Cancer Stage IV documented (ONC)[1]

**3382F**  AJCC colon cancer, Stage 0 documented (ONC)[1]

**3384F**  AJCC colon cancer, Stage I documented (ONC)[1]

**3386F**  AJCC colon cancer, Stage II documented (ONC)[1]

**3388F**  AJCC colon cancer, Stage III documented (ONC)[1]

**3390F**  AJCC colon cancer, Stage IV documented (ONC)[1]

● **3394F**  Quantitative HER2 immunohistochemistry (IHC) evaluation of breast cancer consistent with the scoring system defined in the ASCO/CAP guidelines (PATH)[9]

● **3395F**  Quantitative non-HER2 immunohistochemistry (IHC) evaluation of breast cancer (eg, testing for estrogen or progesterone receptors [ER/PR]) performed (PATH)[9]

**3450F**  Dyspnea screened, no dyspnea or mild dyspnea (Pall Cr)[5]

**3451F**  Dyspnea screened, moderate or severe dyspnea (Pall Cr)[5]

**3452F**  Dyspnea not screened (Pall Cr)[5]

**3455F**  TB screening performed and results interpreted within six months prior to initiation of first-time biologic disease modifying anti-rheumatic drug therapy for RA (RA)[5]

**3470F**  Rheumatoid arthritis (RA) disease activity, low (RA)[5]

**3471F**  Rheumatoid arthritis (RA) disease activity, moderate (RA)[5]

**3472F**  Rheumatoid arthritis (RA) disease activity, high (RA)[5]

**3475F**  Disease prognosis for rheumatoid arthritis assessed, poor prognosis documented (RA)[5]

**3476F**  Disease prognosis for rheumatoid arthritis assessed, good prognosis documented (RA)[5]

**3490F**  History of AIDS-defining condition (HIV)[5]

**3491F**  HIV indeterminate (infants of undetermined HIV status born of HIV-infected mothers) (HIV)[5]

**3492F**  History of nadir CD4+ cell count <350 cells/mm$^3$ (HIV)[5]

**3493F**  No history of nadir CD4+ cell count <350 cells/mm$^3$ AND no history of AIDS-defining condition (HIV)[5]

**3494F**  CD4+ cell count <200 cells/mm$^3$ (HIV)[5]

**3495F**  CD4+ cell count 200 – 499 cells/mm$^3$ (HIV)[5]

**3496F**  CD4+ cell count ≥500 cells/mm$^3$ (HIV)[5]

**3497F**  CD4+ cell percentage <15% (HIV)[5]

**3498F**  CD4+ cell percentage ≥15% (HIV)[5]

**3500F**  CD4+ cell count or CD4+ cell percentage documented as performed (HIV)[5]

**3502F**  HIV RNA viral load below limits of quantification (HIV)[5]

**3503F**  HIV RNA viral load not below limits of quantification (HIV)[5]

**3510F**  Documentation that tuberculosis (TB) screening test performed and results interpreted (HIV)[5]

**3511F**  Chlamydia and gonorrhea screenings documented as performed (HIV)[5]

**3512F**  Syphilis screening documented as performed (HIV)[5]

**3513F**  Hepatitis B screening documented as performed (HIV)[5]

**3514F**  Hepatitis C screening documented as performed (HIV)[5]

**3515F**  Patient has documented immunity to Hepatitis C (HIV)[5]

**3550F**  Low risk for thromboembolism (AFIB)[1]

**3551F**  Intermediate risk for thromboembolism (AFIB)[1]

**3552F**  High risk for thromboembolism (AFIB)[1]

**3555F**  Patient had International Normalized Ratio (INR) measurement performed (AFIB)[1]

**3570F**  Final report for bone scintigraphy study includes correlation with existing relevant imaging studies (eg, x-ray, MRI, CT) corresponding to the same anatomical region in question (NUC_MED)[1]

**3572F**  Patient considered to be potentially at risk for fracture in a weight-bearing site (NUC_MED)[1]

**3573F**  Patient not considered to be potentially at risk for fracture in a weight-bearing site (NUC_MED)[1]

**3650F**  Electroencephalogram (EEG) ordered, reviewed or requested (EPI)[8]

**3700F**  Psychiatric disorders or disturbances assessed (Prkns)[8]

**3720F**  Cognitive impairment or dysfunction assessed (Prkns)[8]

● **3725F**  Screening for depression performed (DEM)[1]

# Therapeutic, Preventive, or Other Interventions

Therapeutic, preventive, or other interventions codes describe pharmacologic, procedural, or behavioral therapies, including preventive services such as patient education and counseling.

**4000F**  Tobacco use cessation intervention, counseling (COPD, CAP, CAD, Asthma)[1](DM)[4](PV)[2]

**4001F**  Tobacco use cessation intervention, pharmacologic therapy (COPD, CAD, CAP, PV, Asthma)[1] (DM)[4](PV)[2]

▶(4002F has been deleted. To report statin therapy, use 4013F)◀

**4003F**  Patient education, written/oral, appropriate for patients with heart failure, performed (NMA – No measure Associated)[1]

▲ **4004F**  Patient screened for tobacco use AND received tobacco cessation intervention (counseling, pharmacotherapy, or both), if identified as a tobacco user (PV, CAD)[1]

**4005F**  Pharmacologic therapy (other than minerals/vitamins) for osteoporosis prescribed (OP)[5]

▶(4006F has been deleted. To report beta blocker therapy, use 4008F.)◀

---

(4007F has been deleted. To report age related eye disease study (AREDS) formulation prescribed or recommended, use code 4177F)

● **4008F** Beta blocker therapy prescribed or currently being taken (CAD,HF)[1]

**4009F** Angiotensin converting enzyme (ACE) inhibitor or angiotensin receptor blocker (ARB) therapy prescribed (CKD)[1], (DM)[2]

● **4010F** Angiotensin Converting Enzyme (ACE) Inhibitor or Angiotensin Receptor Blocker (ARB) therapy prescribed or currently being taken (CAD, HF)[1]

**4011F** Oral antiplatelet therapy prescribed (CAD)[1]

**4012F** Warfarin therapy prescribed (NMA-No Measure Associated)[1]

● **4013F** Statin therapy prescribed or currently being taken (CAD)[1]

**4014F** Written discharge instructions provided to heart failure patients discharged home (Instructions include all of the following components: activity level, diet, discharge medications, follow-up appointment, weight monitoring, what to do if symptoms worsen) (NMA-No Measure Associated)

(Excludes patients less than 18 years of age)

**4015F** Persistent asthma, preferred long term control medication or an acceptable alternative treatment, prescribed (NMA – No Measure Associated)

(Note: There are no medical exclusion criteria)

(Do not report modifier 1P with 4015F)

(To report patient reasons for not prescribing, use modifier 2P)

**4016F** Anti-inflammatory/analgesic agent prescribed (OA)[1]

(Use for prescribed or continued medication[s], including over-the-counter medication[s])

**4017F** Gastrointestinal prophylaxis for NSAID use prescribed (OA)[1]

**4018F** Therapeutic exercise for the involved joint(s) instructed or physical or occupational therapy prescribed (OA)[1]

**4019F** Documentation of receipt of counseling on exercise AND either both calcium and vitamin D use or counseling regarding both calcium and vitamin D use (OP)[5]

**4025F** Inhaled bronchodilator prescribed (COPD)[1]

**4030F** Long-term oxygen therapy prescribed (more than 15 hours per day) (COPD)[1]

**4033F** Pulmonary rehabilitation exercise training recommended (COPD)[1]

(Report 4033F with 1019F)

**4035F** Influenza immunization recommended (COPD)[1]

**4037F** Influenza immunization ordered or administered (COPD, PV, CKD, ESRD)[1]

**4040F** Pneumococcal vaccine administered or previously received (COPD)[1], (PV)[1,2]

**4041F** Documentation of order for cefazolin OR cefuroxime for antimicrobial prophylaxis (PERI 2)[5]

**4042F** Documentation that prophylactic antibiotics were neither given within 4 hours prior to surgical incision nor given intraoperatively (PERI 2)[5]

**4043F** Documentation that an order was given to discontinue prophylactic antibiotics within 48 hours of surgical end time, cardiac procedures (PERI 2)[5]

**4044F** Documentation that an order was given for venous thromboembolism (VTE) prophylaxis to be given within 24 hours prior to incision time or 24 hours after surgery end time (PERI 2)[5]

**4045F** Appropriate empiric antibiotic prescribed (CAP)[1], (EM)[5]

**4046F** Documentation that prophylactic antibiotics were given within 4 hours prior to surgical incision or given intraoperatively (PERI 2)[5]

**4047F** Documentation of order for prophylactic parenteral antibiotics to be given within 1 hour (if fluoroquinolone or vancomycin, 2 hours) prior to surgical incision (or start of procedure when no incision is required) (PERI 2)[5]

**4048F** Documentation that administration of prophylactic parenteral antibiotic was initiated within 1 hour (if fluoroquinolone or vancomycin, 2 hours) prior to surgical incision (or start of procedure when no incision is required) as ordered (PERI 2)[5]

**4049F** Documentation that order was given to discontinue prophylactic antibiotics within 24 hours of surgical end time, non-cardiac procedure (PERI 2)[5]

**4050F** Hypertension plan of care documented as appropriate (NMA – No Measure Associated)[1]

**4051F** Referred for an arteriovenous (AV) fistula (ESRD, CKD)[1]

**4052F** Hemodialysis via functioning arteriovenous (AV) fistula (ESRD)[1]

**4053F** Hemodialysis via functioning arteriovenous (AV) graft (ESRD)[1]

**4054F** Hemodialysis via catheter (ESRD)[1]

**4055F** Patient receiving peritoneal dialysis (ESRD)[1]

**4056F** Appropriate oral rehydration solution recommended (PAG)[1]

**4058F** Pediatric gastroenteritis education provided to caregiver (PAG)[1]

**4060F** Psychotherapy services provided (MDD, MDD ADOL)[1]

**4062F** Patient referral for psychotherapy documented (MDD, MDD ADOL)[1]

**4063F** Antidepressant pharmacotherapy considered and not prescribed (MDD ADOL)[1]

**4064F** Antidepressant pharmacotherapy prescribed (MDD, MDD ADOL)[1]

**Category II Codes**

**4065F**   Antipsychotic pharmacotherapy prescribed (MDD)[1]

**4066F**   Electroconvulsive therapy (ECT) provided (MDD)[1]

**4067F**   Patient referral for electroconvulsive therapy (ECT) documented (MDD)[1]

**4070F**   Deep vein thrombosis (DVT) prophylaxis received by end of hospital day 2 (STR)[5]

**4073F**   Oral antiplatelet therapy prescribed at discharge (STR)[5]

**4075F**   Anticoagulant therapy prescribed at discharge (STR)[5]

**4077F**   Documentation that tissue plasminogen activator (t-PA) administration was considered (STR)[5]

**4079F**   Documentation that rehabilitation services were considered (STR)[5]

**4084F**   Aspirin received within 24 hours before emergency department arrival or during emergency department stay (EM)[5]

● **4086F**   Aspirin or clopidogrel prescribed or currently being taken (CAD)[1]

**4090F**   Patient receiving erythropoietin therapy (HEM)[1]

**4095F**   Patient not receiving erythropoietin therapy (HEM)[1]

**4100F**   Bisphosphonate therapy, intravenous, ordered or received (HEM)[1]

**4110F**   Internal mammary artery graft performed for primary, isolated coronary artery bypass graft procedure (CABG)[6]

**4115F**   Beta blocker administered within 24 hours prior to surgical incision (CABG)[6]

**4120F**   Antibiotic prescribed or dispensed (URI, PHAR)[2], (A-BRONCH)[2]

**4124F**   Antibiotic neither prescribed nor dispensed (URI, PHAR)[2], (A-BRONCH)[2]

**4130F**   Topical preparations (including OTC) prescribed for acute otitis externa (AOE)[1]

**4131F**   Systemic antimicrobial therapy prescribed (AOE)[1]

**4132F**   Systemic antimicrobial therapy not prescribed (AOE)[1]

**4133F**   Antihistamines or decongestants prescribed or recommended (OME)[1]

**4134F**   Antihistamines or decongestants neither prescribed nor recommended (OME)[1]

**4135F**   Systemic corticosteroids prescribed (OME)[1]

**4136F**   Systemic corticosteroids not prescribed (OME)[1]

● **4140F**   Inhaled corticosteroids prescribed (Asthma)[1]

● **4144F**   Alternative long-term control medication prescribed (Asthma)[1]

● **4145F**   Two or more anti-hypertensive agents prescribed or currently being taken (CAD, HTN)

**4148F**   Hepatitis A vaccine injection administered or previously received (HEP-C)[1]

**4149F**   Hepatitis B vaccine injection administered or previously received (HEP-C, HIV)[1]

**4150F**   Patient receiving antiviral treatment for Hepatitis C (HEP-C)[1]

**4151F**   Patient not receiving antiviral treatment for Hepatitis C (HEP-C)[1]

(Code 4152F has been deleted.)

**4153F**   Combination peginterferon and ribavirin therapy prescribed (HEP-C)[1]

(Code 4154F has been deleted.)

**4155F**   Hepatitis A vaccine series previously received (HEP-C)[1]

(Code 4156F has been deleted.)

**4157F**   Hepatitis B vaccine series previously received (HEP-C)[1]

**4158F**   Patient counseled about risks of alcohol use (HEP-C)[1]

**4159F**   Counseling regarding contraception received prior to initiation of antiviral treatment (HEP-C)[1]

**4163F**   Patient counseling at a minimum on all of the following treatment options for clinically localized prostate cancer: active surveillance, AND interstitial prostate brachytherapy, AND external beam radiotherapy, AND radical prostatectomy, provided prior to initiation of treatment (PRCA)[1]

**4164F**   Adjuvant (ie, in combination with external beam radiotherapy to the prostate for prostate cancer) hormonal therapy (gonadotropin-releasing hormone [GnRH] agonist or antagonist) prescribed/administered (PRCA)[1]

**4165F**   3-dimensional conformal radiotherapy (3D-CRT) or intensity modulated radiation therapy (IMRT) received (PRCA)[1]

**4167F**   Head of bed elevation (30-45 degrees) on first ventilator day ordered (CRIT)[1]

**4168F**   Patient receiving care in the intensive care unit (ICU) and receiving mechanical ventilation, 24 hours or less (CRIT)[1]

**4169F**   Patient either not receiving care in the intensive care unit (ICU) OR not receiving mechanical ventilation OR receiving mechanical ventilation greater than 24 hours (CRIT)[1]

**4171F**   Patient receiving erythropoiesis-stimulating agents (ESA) therapy (CKD)[1]

**4172F**   Patient not receiving erythropoiesis-stimulating agents (ESA) therapy (CKD)[1]

**4174F**   Counseling about the potential impact of glaucoma on visual functioning and quality of life, and importance of treatment adherence provided to patient and/or caregiver(s) (EC)[5]

**4175F**   Best-corrected visual acuity of 20/40 or better (distance or near) achieved within the 90 days following cataract surgery (EC)[5]

**Category II Codes**

---

▲=Revised code    ●=New code    ▶ ◀=Contains new or revised text    ⊘=Modifier 51 exempt

**Category II Codes**

**4176F**   Counseling about value of protection from UV light and lack of proven efficacy of nutritional supplements in prevention or progression of cataract development provided to patient and/or caregiver(s) (NMA No Measure Associated)

**4177F**   Counseling about the benefits and/or risks of the Age-Related Eye Disease Study (AREDS) formulation for preventing progression of age-related macular degeneration (AMD) provided to patient and/or caregiver(s) (EC)[5]

**4178F**   Anti-D immune globulin received between 26 and 30 weeks gestation (Pre-Cr)[1]

**4179F**   Tamoxifen or aromatase inhibitor (AI) prescribed (ONC)[1]

**4180F**   Adjuvant chemotherapy referred, prescribed, or previously received for Stage III colon cancer (ONC)[1]

**4181F**   Conformal radiation therapy received (NMA-No Measure Assoc.)

**4182F**   Conformal radiation therapy not received (NMA-No Measure Assoc.)

**4185F**   Continuous (12-months) therapy with proton pump inhibitor (PPI) or histamine H2 receptor antagonist (H2RA) received (GERD)[5]

**4186F**   No continuous (12-months) therapy with either proton pump inhibitor (PPI) or histamine H2 receptor antagonist (H2RA) received (GERD)[5]

**4187F**   Disease modifying anti-rheumatic drug therapy prescribed or dispensed (RA)[2]

**4188F**   Appropriate angiotensin converting enzyme (ACE)/ angiotensin receptor blockers (ARB) therapeutic monitoring test ordered or performed (AM)[2]

**4189F**   Appropriate digoxin therapeutic monitoring test ordered or performed (AM)[2]

**4190F**   Appropriate diuretic therapeutic monitoring test ordered or performed (AM)[2]

**4191F**   Appropriate anticonvulsant therapeutic monitoring test ordered or performed (AM)[2]

**4192F**   Patient not receiving glucocorticoid therapy (RA)[5]

**4193F**   Patient receiving <10 mg daily prednisone (or equivalent), or RA activity is worsening, or glucocorticoid use is for less than 6 months (RA)[5]

**4194F**   Patient receiving ≥10 mg daily prednisone (or equivalent) for longer than 6 months, and improvement or no change in disease activity (RA)[5]

**4195F**   Patient receiving first-time biologic disease modifying anti-rheumatic drug therapy for rheumatoid arthritis (RA)[5]

**4196F**   Patient not receiving first-time biologic disease modifying anti-rheumatic drug therapy for rheumatoid arthritis (RA)[5]

**4200F**   External beam radiotherapy as primary therapy to prostate with or without nodal irradiation (PRCA)[1]

**4201F**   External beam radiotherapy with or without nodal irradiation as adjuvant or salvage therapy for prostate cancer patient (PRCA)[1]

**4210F**   Angiotensin converting enzyme (ACE) or angiotensin receptor blockers (ARB) medication therapy for 6 months or more (MM)[2]

**4220F**   Digoxin medication therapy for 6 months or more (MM)[2]

**4221F**   Diuretic medication therapy for 6 months or more (MM)[2]

**4230F**   Anticonvulsant medication therapy for 6 months or more (MM)[2]

**4240F**   Instruction in therapeutic exercise with follow-up by the physician provided to patients during episode of back pain lasting longer than 12 weeks (BkP)[2]

**4242F**   Counseling for supervised exercise program provided to patients during episode of back pain lasting longer than 12 weeks (BkP)[2]

**4245F**   Patient counseled during the initial visit to maintain or resume normal activities (BkP)[2]

**4248F**   Patient counseled during the initial visit for an episode of back pain against bed rest lasting 4 days or longer (BkP)[2]

**4250F**   Active warming used intraoperatively for the purpose of maintaining normothermia, OR at least 1 body temperature equal to or greater than 36 degrees Centigrade (or 96.8 degrees Fahrenheit) recorded within the 30 minutes immediately before or the 15 minutes immediately after anesthesia end time (CRIT)[1]

**4255F**   Duration of general or neuraxial anesthesia 60 minutes or longer, as documented in the anesthesia record (CRIT)[5]

**4256F**   Duration of general or neuraxial anesthesia less than 60 minutes, as documented in the anesthesia record (CRIT)[5]

**4260F**   Wound surface culture technique used (CWC)[5]

**4261F**   Technique other than surface culture of the wound exudate used (eg, Levine/deep swab technique, semi-quantitative or quantitative swab technique) OR wound surface culture technique not used (CWC)[5]

**4265F**   Use of wet to dry dressings prescribed or recommended (CWC)[5]

**4266F**   Use of wet to dry dressings neither prescribed nor recommended (CWC)[5]

**4267F**   Compression therapy prescribed (CWC)[5]

**4268F**   Patient education regarding the need for long term compression therapy including interval replacement of compression stockings received (CWC)[5]

**4269F**   Appropriate method of offloading (pressure relief) prescribed (CWC)[5]

**4270F**   Patient receiving potent antiretroviral therapy for 6 months or longer (HIV)[5]

**4271F**   Patient receiving potent antiretroviral therapy for less than 6 months or not receiving potent antiretroviral therapy (HIV)[5]

**4274F**   Influenza immunization administered or previously received (HIV)[5] (P-ESRD)[1]

►(4275F has been deleted. To report Hepatitis B vaccine injection administered or previously received, use 4149F)◄

**4276F**   Potent antiretroviral therapy prescribed (HIV)[5]

**4279F**   Pneumocystis jiroveci pneumonia prophylaxis prescribed (HIV)[5]

**4280F**   Pneumocystis jiroveci pneumonia prophylaxis prescribed within 3 months of low CD4+ cell count or percentage (HIV)[5]

**4290F**   Patient screened for injection drug use (HIV)[5]

**4293F**   Patient screened for high-risk sexual behavior (HIV)[5]

**4300F**   Patient receiving warfarin therapy for nonvalvular atrial fibrillation or atrial flutter (AFIB)[1]

**4301F**   Patient not receiving warfarin therapy for nonvalvular atrial fibrillation or atrial flutter (AFIB)[1]

**4305F**   Patient education regarding appropriate foot care AND daily inspection of the feet received (CWC)[5]

**4306F**   Patient counseled regarding psychosocial AND pharmacologic treatment options for opioid addiction (SUD)[1]

**4320F**   Patient counseled regarding psychosocial AND pharmacologic treatment options for alcohol dependence (SUD)[5]

● **4322F**   Caregiver provided with education and referred to additional resources for support (DEM)[1]

**4324F**   Patient (or caregiver) queried about Parkinson's disease medication related motor complications (Prkns)[8]

**4325F**   Medical and surgical treatment options reviewed with patient (or caregiver) (Prkns)[8]

**4326F**   Patient (or caregiver) queried about symptoms of autonomic dysfunction (Prkns)[8]

**4328F**   Patient (or caregiver) queried about sleep disturbances (Prkns)[8]

**4330F**   Counseling about epilepsy specific safety issues provided to patient (or caregiver(s)) (EPI)[8]

**4340F**   Counseling for women of childbearing potential with epilepsy (EPI)[8]

● **4350F**   Counseling provided on symptom management, end of life decisions, and palliation (DEM)[1]

**4400F**   Rehabilitative therapy options discussed with patient (or caregiver) (Prkns)[8]

● **4450F**   Self-care education provided to patient (HF)[1]

● **4470F**   Implantable cardioverter-defibrillator (ICD) counseling provided (HF)[1]

● **4480F**   Patient receiving ACE inhibitor/ARB therapy and beta-blocker therapy for 3 months or longer (HF)[1]

● **4481F**   Patient receiving ACE inhibitor/ARB therapy and beta-blocker therapy for less than 3 months or patient not receiving ACE inhibitor/ARB therapy and beta-blocker therapy (HF)[1]

● **4500F**   Referred to an outpatient cardiac rehabilitation program (CAD)[1]

● **4510F**   Previous cardiac rehabilitation for qualifying cardiac event completed (CAD)[1]

● **4525F**   Neuropsychiatric intervention ordered (DEM)[1]

● **4526F**   Neuropsychiatric intervention received (DEM)[1]

# Follow-up or Other Outcomes

Follow-up or other outcomes codes describe review and communication of test results to patients, patient satisfaction or experience with care, patient functional status, and patient morbidity and mortality.

**5005F**   Patient counseled on self-examination for new or changing moles (ML)[5]

**5010F**   Findings of dilated macular or fundus exam communicated to the physician managing the diabetes care (EC)[5]

**5015F**   Documentation of communication that a fracture occurred and that the patient was or should be tested or treated for osteoporosis (OP)[5]

**5020F**   Treatment summary report communicated to physician(s) managing continuing care and to the patient within 1 month of completing treatment (ONC)[1]

**5050F**   Treatment plan communicated to provider(s) managing continuing care within 1 month of diagnosis (ML)[5]

**5060F**   Findings from diagnostic mammogram communicated to practice managing patient's on-going care within 3 business days of exam interpretation (RAD)[5]

**5062F**   Findings from diagnostic mammogram communicated to the patient within 5 days of exam interpretation (RAD)[5]

**5100F**   Potential risk for fracture communicated to the referring physician within 24 hours of completion of the imaging study (NUC_MED)[1]

**5200F**   Consideration of referral for a neurological evaluation of appropriateness for surgical therapy for intractable epilepsy within the past 3 years (EPI)[8]

● **5250F**   Asthma discharge plan provided to patient (Asthma)[1]

**Category II Codes**

# Patient Safety

Patient safety codes that describe patient safety practices.

**6005F** Rationale (eg, severity of illness and safety) for level of care (eg, home, hospital) documented (CAP)[1]

**6010F** Dysphagia screening conducted prior to order for or receipt of any foods, fluids, or medication by mouth (STR)[5]

**6015F** Patient receiving or eligible to receive foods, fluids, or medication by mouth (STR)[5]

**6020F** NPO (nothing by mouth) ordered (STR)[5]

**6030F** All elements of maximal sterile barrier technique followed including: cap AND mask AND sterile gown AND sterile gloves AND a large sterile sheet AND hand hygiene AND 2% chlorhexidine for cutaneous antisepsis (or acceptable alternative antiseptics, per current guideline) (CRIT)[1]

**6040F** Use of appropriate radiation dose reduction devices OR manual techniques for appropriate moderation of exposure, documented (RAD)[5]

**6045F** Radiation exposure or exposure time in final report for procedure using fluoroscopy, documented (RAD)[5]

**6070F** Patient queried and counseled about anti-epileptic drug (AED) side effects (EPI)[8]

**6080F** Patient (or caregiver) queried about falls (Prkns)[8]

**6090F** Patient (or caregiver) counseled about safety issues appropriate to patient's stage of disease (Prkns)[8]

● **6100F** Timeout to verify correct patient, correct site, and correct procedure, documented (PATH)[9]

● **6101F** Safety counseling for dementia provided (DEM)[1]

● **6102F** Safety counseling for dementia ordered (DEM)[1]

● **6110F** Counseling provided regarding risks of driving and the alternatives to driving (DEM)[1]

# Structural Measures

Structural measures codes are used to identify measures that address the setting or system of the delivered care. These codes also address aspects of the capabilities of the organization or health care professional providing the care.

**7010F** Patient information entered into a recall system that includes: target date for the next exam specified AND a process to follow up with patients regarding missed or unscheduled appointments (ML)[5]

**7020F** Mammogram assessment category (eg, Mammography Quality Standards Act [MQSA], Breast Imaging Reporting and Data System [BI-RADS®], or FDA approved equivalent categories) entered into an internal database to allow for analysis of abnormal interpretation (recall) rate (RAD)[5]

**7025F** Patient information entered into a reminder system with a target due date for the next mammogram (RAD)[5]

**Category II Codes**

# Category III Codes

The following section contains a set of temporary codes for emerging technology, services, and procedures. Category III codes allow data collection for these services/procedures. Use of unlisted codes does not offer the opportunity for the collection of specific data. If a Category III code is available, this code must be reported instead of a Category I unlisted code. This is an activity that is critically important in the evaluation of health care delivery and the formation of public and private policy. The use of the codes in this section allow physicians and other qualified health care professionals, insurers, health services researchers, and health policy experts to identify emerging technology, services, and procedures for clinical efficacy, utilization and outcomes.

The inclusion of a service or procedure in this section neither implies nor endorses clinical efficacy, safety or the applicability to clinical practice. The codes in this section may not conform to the usual requirements for CPT Category I codes established by the Editorial Panel. For Category I codes, the Panel requires that the service/procedure be performed by many health care professionals in clinical practice in multiple locations and that FDA approval, as appropriate, has already been received. The nature of emerging technology, services, and procedures is such that these requirements may not be met. For these reasons, temporary codes for emerging technology, services, and procedures have been placed in a separate section of the CPT codebook and the codes are differentiated from Category I CPT codes by the use of alphanumeric characters.

▶Services/procedures described in this section make use of alphanumeric characters. These codes have an alpha character as the 5th character in the string, preceded by four digits. The digits are not intended to reflect the placement of the code in the Category I section of CPT nomenclature. Codes in this section may or may not eventually receive a Category I CPT code. In either case, in general, a given Category III code will be archived five years from the date of initial publication or extension unless a modification of the archival date is specifically noted at the time of a revision or change to a code (eg, addition of parenthetical instructions, reinstatement). Services/procedures described by Category III codes which have been archived after five years, without conversion, must be reported using the Category I unlisted code unless another specific cross reference is established at the time of archiving. New codes in this section are released semi-annually via the AMA/CPT internet site, to expedite dissemination for reporting. The full set of temporary codes for emerging technology, services, and procedures are published annually in the CPT codebook. Go to www.ama-assn.org/go/cpt for the most current listing.◀

(0016T, 0017T have been deleted)

(For destruction of localized lesion of choroid by transpupillary thermotherapy, use 67299)

(For destruction of macular drusen, photocoagulation, use 67299)

**0019T** Extracorporeal shock wave involving musculoskeletal system, not otherwise specified, low energy
Sunset January 2017

(For application of high energy extracorporeal shock wave involving musculoskeletal system not otherwise specified, use 0101T)

(For application of high energy extracorporeal shock wave involving lateral humeral epicondyle, use 0102T)

(0024T has been deleted)

(For non-surgical septal reduction therapy, use 93799)

(0026T has been deleted)

(For lipoprotein, direct measurement, intermediate density lipoproteins [IDL] [remnant lipoprotein], use 84999)

(0027T has been deleted)

(For endoscopic lysis of epidural adhesions with direct visualization using mechnical means or solution injection [eg, normal saline], use 64999)

(0028T has been deleted)

(For dual energy x-ray absorptiometry [DXA] body composition study, use 76499)

(0029T has been deleted)

(For pulsed magnetic neuromodulation incontinence treatment, use 53899)

**0030T** Antiprothrombin (phospholipid cofactor) antibody, each Ig class
Sunset January 2013

(0031T, 0032T have been deleted)

(For speculoscopy, including sampling, use 58999)

(0041T has been deleted)

(For urinalysis infectious agent detection, semi-quantitative analysis of volatile compounds, use 81099)

**0042T** Cerebral perfusion analysis using computed tomography with contrast administration, including post-processing of parametric maps with determination of cerebral blood flow, cerebral blood volume, and mean transit time
Sunset January 2014

(0043T has been deleted)

(For carbon monoxide, expired gas analysis [eg, $ETCO_c$/hemolysis breath test], use 84999)

---

▲=Revised code   ●=New code   ▶◀=Contains new or revised text   ⊘=Modifier 51 exempt

(0046T, 0047T have been deleted)

(For mammary duct[s] catheter lavage, use 19499)

**0048T**   Implantation of a ventricular assist device, extracorporeal, percutaneous transseptal access, single or dual cannulation
Sunset January 2014

(0049T has been deleted)

(For prolonged extracorporeal percutaneous transseptal ventricular assist device, use 33999)

**0050T**   Removal of a ventricular assist device, extracorporeal, percutaneous transseptal access, single or dual cannulation
Sunset January 2014

(For replacement of a ventricular assist device, extracorporeal, percutaneous transseptal access, use 33999)

**0051T**   Implantation of a total replacement heart system (artificial heart) with recipient cardiectomy
Sunset January 2014

(For implantation of heart assist or ventricular assist device, see 33975, 33976)

**0052T**   Replacement or repair of thoracic unit of a total replacement heart system (artificial heart)
Sunset January 2014

(For replacement or repair of other implantable components in a total replacement heart system (artificial heart), use 0053T)

**0053T**   Replacement or repair of implantable component or components of total replacement heart system (artificial heart), excluding thoracic unit
Sunset January 2014

(For replacement or repair of a thoracic unit of a total replacement heart system (artificial heart), use 0052T)

**+ 0054T**   Computer-assisted musculoskeletal surgical navigational orthopedic procedure, with image-guidance based on fluoroscopic images (List separately in addition to code for primary procedure)
Sunset January 2014

**+ 0055T**   Computer-assisted musculoskeletal surgical navigational orthopedic procedure, with image-guidance based on CT/MRI images (List separately in addition to code for primary procedure)
Sunset January 2014

(When CT and MRI are both performed, report 0055T only once)

(0056T has been deleted. To report, use 20985)

**0058T**   Cryopreservation; reproductive tissue, ovarian
Sunset January 2016

**0059T**       oocyte(s)
Sunset January 2016

(For cryopreservation of embryo(s), sperm and testicular reproductive tissue, see 89258, 89259, 89335)

(0060T has been deleted)

(For electrical impedance breast scan, use 76499)

(0061T has been deleted)

(For destruction/reduction of malignant breast tumor, microwave phased array thermotherapy, use 19499)

(0062T, 0063T have been deleted)

(For percutaneous intradiscal annuloplasty, any method other than electrothermal, use 22899)

(For intradiscal electrothermal annuloplasty, see 22526, 22527)

(0064T has been deleted. To report, use 94799)

(0066T has been deleted)

(To report CT colon, screening, use 74263)

(0067T has been deleted)

(To report CT colon, diagnostic, see 74261-74262)

(0068T-0070T have been deleted)

(For acoustic heart sound recording and computer analysis, use 93799)

**0071T**   Focused ultrasound ablation of uterine leiomyomata, including MR guidance; total leiomyomata volume less than 200 cc of tissue
Sunset January 2015

**0072T**       total leiomyomata volume greater or equal to 200 cc of tissue
Sunset January 2015

(Do not report 0071T, 0072T in conjunction with 51702 or 77022)

**0073T**   Compensator-based beam modulation treatment delivery of inverse planned treatment using 3 or more high resolution (milled or cast) compensator convergent beam modulated fields, per treatment session
Sunset January 2015

(For treatment planning, use 77301)

(Do not report 0073T in conjunction with 77401-77416, 77418)

**0075T**   Transcatheter placement of extracranial vertebral or intrathoracic carotid artery stent(s), including radiologic supervision and interpretation, percutaneous; initial vessel
Sunset January 2015

**+ 0076T**       each additional vessel (List separately in addition to code for primary procedure)
Sunset January 2015

(Use 0076T in conjunction with 0075T)

(When the ipsilateral extracranial vertebral or intrathoracic carotid arteriogram (including imaging and selective catheterization) confirms the need for stenting, then 0075T and 0076T include all ipsilateral extracranial vertebral or intrathoracic selective carotid catheterization, all diagnostic imaging for ipsilateral extracranial vertebral or intrathoracic carotid artery stenting, and all related radiologic supervision and interpretation. If stenting is not indicated, then the appropriate codes for selective catheterization and imaging should be reported in lieu of code 0075T or 0076T.)

(0077T has been deleted. To report, see 61107, 61210)

(0078T-0081T should be reported in accordance with the Endovascular Abdominal Aneurysm Repair guidelines established for 34800-34826)

**0078T** Endovascular repair using prosthesis of abdominal aortic aneurysm, pseudoaneurysm or dissection, abdominal aorta involving visceral branches (superior mesenteric, celiac and/or renal artery[s])
Sunset January 2015

(Do not report 0078T in conjunction with 34800-34805, 35081, 35102, 35452, 35472)

(Report 0078T in conjunction with 37205-37208, 37220-37223, only when these procedures are performed outside the target zone of the endoprosthesis)

**+ 0079T** Placement of visceral extension prosthesis for endovascular repair of abdominal aortic aneurysm involving visceral vessels, each visceral branch (List separately in addition to code for primary procedure)
Sunset January 2015

(Use 0079T in conjunction with 0078T)

**▲ 0080T** Endovascular repair using prosthesis of abdominal aortic aneurysm, pseudoaneurysm or dissection, abdominal aorta involving visceral vessels (superior mesenteric, celiac and/or renal artery[s]), radiological supervision and interpretation
Sunset January 2017

(Do not report 0080T in conjunction with 34800-34805, 35081, 35102, 35452, 35472)

(Report 0080T in conjunction with 37205-37208, 37220-37223, only when these procedures are performed outside the target zone of the endoprosthesis)

**+ 0081T** Placement of visceral extension prosthesis for endovascular repair of abdominal aortic aneurysm involving visceral vessels, each visceral branch, radiological supervision and interpretation (List separately in addition to code for primary procedure)
Sunset January 2015

(Use 0081T in conjunction with 0080T)

(0084T has been deleted. To report, use 53855)

**0085T** Breath test for heart transplant rejection
Sunset January 2016

(0086T has been deleted. To report use, 93799)

(0087T has been deleted. To report, use 89398)

(0088T has been deleted. To report, use 41530)

(0089T has been deleted. For actigraphy testing, use 95803)

(0090T has been deleted. To report total disc cervical arthroplasty, use 22856)

(To report total disc lumbar arthroplasty, use 22857)

**+ 0092T** Total disc arthroplasty (artificial disc), anterior approach, including discectomy with end plate preparation (includes osteophytectomy for nerve root or spinal cord decompression and microdissection), each additional interspace, cervical (List separately in addition to code for primary procedure)
Sunset January 2014

(Use 0092T in conjunction with 22856)

(Do not report 0092T in conjunction with 22851 when performed at the same level)

(0093T has been deleted. To report removal of total disc cervical arthroplasty, use 22864)

(To report removal of total disc lumbar arthroplasty, use 22865)

**+ 0095T** Removal of total disc arthroplasty (artificial disc), anterior approach, each additional interspace, cervical (List separately in addition to code for primary procedure)
Sunset January 2014

(Use 0095T in conjunction with 22864)

(0096T has been deleted. To report revision of total disc cervical arthroplasty, use 22861)

(To report revision of total disc lumbar arthroplasty, use 22862)

**+ 0098T** Revision including replacement of total disc arthroplasty (artificial disc), anterior approach, each additional interspace, cervical (List separately in addition to code for primary procedure)
Sunset January 2014

(Use 0098T in conjunction with 22861)

(Do not report 0098T in conjunction with 0095T)

(Do not report 0098T in conjunction with 22851 when performed at the same level)

(For decompression, see 63001-63048)

**0099T** Implantation of intrastromal corneal ring segments
Sunset January 2016

**0100T** Placement of a subconjunctival retinal prosthesis receiver and pulse generator, and implantation of intra-ocular retinal electrode array, with vitrectomy
Sunset January 2016

---

▲=Revised code   ●=New code   ► ◄=Contains new or revised text   ⊘=Modifier 51 exempt

**0101T**  Extracorporeal shock wave involving musculoskeletal system, not otherwise specified, high energy
Sunset January 2016

(For application of low energy musculoskeletal system extracorporeal shock wave, use 0019T)

**0102T**  Extracorporeal shock wave, high energy, performed by a physician, requiring anesthesia other than local, involving lateral humeral epicondyle
Sunset January 2016

(For application of low energy musculoskeletal system extracorporeal shock wave, use 0019T)

**0103T**  Holotranscobalamin, quantitative
Sunset January 2016

(0104T, 0105T have been deleted)

(For inert gas rebreathing for cardiac output measurement during rest, use 93799)

(For inert gas rebreathing for cardiac output measurement during exercise, use 93799)

**0106T**  Quantitative sensory testing (QST), testing and interpretation per extremity; using touch pressure stimuli to assess large diameter sensation
Sunset January 2016

**0107T**  using vibration stimuli to assess large diameter fiber sensation
Sunset January 2016

**0108T**  using cooling stimuli to assess small nerve fiber sensation and hyperalgesia
Sunset January 2016

**0109T**  using heat-pain stimuli to assess small nerve fiber sensation and hyperalgesia
Sunset January 2016

**0110T**  using other stimuli to assess sensation
Sunset January 2016

**0111T**  Long-chain (C20-22) omega-3 fatty acids in red blood cell (RBC) membranes
Sunset January 2016

(For very long chain fatty acids, use 82726)

**0123T**  Fistulization of sclera for glaucoma, through ciliary body
Sunset January 2016

**0124T**  Conjunctival incision with posterior extrascleral placement of pharmacological agent (does not include supply of medication)
Sunset January 2014

(For suprachoroidal delivery of pharmacologic agent, use 0186T)

**0126T**  Common carotid intima-media thickness (IMT) study for evaluation of atherosclerotic burden or coronary heart disease risk factor assessment
Sunset January 2016

(0130T has been deleted)

(For validated, statistically reliable, randomized, controlled, single-patient clinical investigation of FDA approved chronic care drugs, provided by a pharmacist, interpretation and report to the prescribing health care professional, use 99199)

(0137T has been deleted. For transperineal stereotactic template guided saturation prostate biopsies, use 55706)

(0140T has been deleted. To report, use 83987)

►(0141T-0143T have been deleted)◄

►(To report pancreatic islet cell transplantation, use 48999)◄

(0144T-0151T have been deleted. To report, see 75571-75574)

►(0155T, 0156T have been deleted)◄

►(For laparoscopic implantation, replacement, revision, or removal of gastric stimulation electrodes, lesser curvature, use 43659)◄

►(0157T, 0158T have been deleted)◄

►(For open implantation, replacement, revision, or removal of gastric stimulation electrodes, lesser curvature, use 43999)◄

**+ 0159T**  Computer-aided detection, including computer algorithm analysis of MRI image data for lesion detection/characterization, pharmacokinetic analysis, with further physician review for interpretation, breast MRI (List separately in addition to code for primary procedure)
Sunset January 2017

(Use 0159T in conjunction with 77058, 77059)

(Do not report 0159T in conjunction with 76376, 76377)

►(0160T, 0161T have been deleted. To report, see 90867, 90869)◄

(0162T has been deleted. To report, see 95980-95982)

**+ 0163T**  Total disc arthroplasty (artificial disc), anterior approach, including discectomy to prepare interspace (other than for decompression), each additional interspace, lumbar (List separately in addition to code for primary procedure)
Sunset January 2014

(Use 0163T in conjunction with 22857)

**+ 0164T**  Removal of total disc arthroplasty, (artificial disc), anterior approach, each additional interspace, lumbar (List separately in addition to code for primary procedure)
Sunset January 2014

(Use 0164T in conjunction with 22865)

**+ 0165T**  Revision including replacement of total disc arthroplasty (artificial disc), anterior approach, each additional interspace, lumbar (List separately in addition to code for primary procedure)
Sunset January 2014

(Use 0165T in conjunction with 22862)

(Do not report 0163T-0165T in conjunction with 22851, 49010, when performed at the same level)

*Category III Codes*

(For decompression, see 63001-63048)

►(0166T, 0167T have been deleted)◄

►(For transmyocardial transcatheter closure of ventricular septal defect, with implant, including cardiopulmonary bypass if performed, use 33999)◄

►(0168T has been deleted)◄

►(For rhinophototherapy, intranasal application of ultraviolet and visible light, use 30999)◄

**0169T**   Stereotactic placement of infusion catheter(s) in the brain for delivery of therapeutic agent(s), including computerized stereotactic planning and burr hole(s)
Sunset January 2017

(Do not report code 0169T in conjunction with 20660, 61107, 61781, 61782, 61783)

(0170T has been deleted. To report, use 46707)

**0171T**   Insertion of posterior spinous process distraction device (including necessary removal of bone or ligament for insertion and imaging guidance), lumbar; single level
Sunset January 2013

**+ 0172T**      each additional level (List separately in addition to code for primary procedure)
Sunset January 2013

(Use 0172T in conjunction with 0171T)

**+ 0173T**   Monitoring of intraocular pressure during vitrectomy surgery (List separately in addition to code for primary procedure)
Sunset January 2013

(Use 0173T in conjunction with 67036, 67039-67043, 67108, 67112, 67113)

**+ 0174T**   Computer-aided detection (CAD) (computer algorithm analysis of digital image data for lesion detection) with further physician review for interpretation and report, with or without digitization of film radiographic images, chest radiograph(s), performed concurrent with primary interpretation (List separately in addition to code for primary procedure)
Sunset January 2013

(Use 0174T in conjunction with 71010, 71020, 71021, 71022, 71030)

**0175T**   Computer-aided detection (CAD) (computer algorithm analysis of digital image data for lesion detection) with further physician review for interpretation and report, with or without digitization of film radiographic images, chest radiograph(s), performed remote from primary interpretation
Sunset January 2013

(Do not report 0175T in conjunction with 71010, 71020, 71021, 71022, 71030)

(0176T, 0177T have been deleted. To report, see 66174, 66175)

**0178T**   Electrocardiogram, 64 leads or greater, with graphic presentation and analysis; with interpretation and report
Sunset January 2013

**0179T**      tracing and graphics only, without interpretation and report
Sunset January 2013

**0180T**      interpretation and report only
Sunset January 2013

(For electrocardiogram, routine, with at least 12 leads separately performed, see 93000-93010)

**0181T**   Corneal hysteresis determination, by air impulse stimulation, bilateral, with interpretation and report
Sunset January 2013

**0182T**   High dose rate electronic brachytherapy, per fraction
Sunset January 2013

(Do not report 0182T in conjunction with 77761-77763, 77776-77778, 77785-77787, 77789)

**0183T**   Low frequency, non-contact, non-thermal ultrasound, including topical application(s), when performed, wound assessment, and instruction(s) for ongoing care, per day
Sunset January 2017

**0184T**   Excision of rectal tumor, transanal endoscopic microsurgical approach (ie, TEMS), including muscularis propria (ie, full thickness)
Sunset January 2014

(For non-endoscopic excision of rectal tumor, see 45160, 45171, 45172)

(Do not report 0184T in conjunction with 45300-45327, 69990)

**0185T**   Multivariate analysis of patient-specific findings with quantifiable computer probability assessment, including report
Sunset January 2014

(Do not report 0185T in conjunction with 99090)

**0186T**   Suprachoroidal delivery of pharmacologic agent (does not include supply of medication)
Sunset January 2014

(0187T has been deleted. To report, use 92132)

# Remote Real-Time Interactive Videoconferenced Critical Care Services

Remote real-time interactive video-conferenced critical care is the direct delivery by a physician(s) of medical care for a critically ill or critically injured patient from an off-site location. Remote real-time interactive video-conferenced critical care is intended to supplement on-site critical care services at times when a critically ill or injured patient requires additional critical care resources than are available on-site. (For definitions of critical illness or injury and critical care services, see **Critical Care Services** section).

Category III Codes

In order to report remote real-time interactive video-conferenced critical care, the physician(s) in the remote location must have real-time access to the patient's medical record including progress notes, nursing notes, current medications, vital signs, clinical laboratory test results, other diagnostic test results, and radiographic images. The physician must have real-time capability to enter electronic orders; document the remote care services provided in the hospital medical record; videoconference with the on-site health care team in the patient room; assess patients in their individual rooms, using high fidelity audio and video capabilities, including clear observation of the patient, monitors, ventilators, and infusion pumps; and speak to patients and family members.

The review and/or interpretation of all diagnostic information is included in reporting remote real-time interactive video-conferenced critical care when performed during the critical period by the physician(s) providing remote real-time interactive video-conferenced critical care and should not be reported separately.

The remote real-time interactive video-conferenced critical care codes 0188T and 0189T are used to report the total duration of time spent by a physician providing remote real-time interactive video-conferenced critical care services to a critically ill or critically injured patient, even if the time spent by the physician on that date is not continuous. For any given period of time spent providing remote real-time interactive video-conferenced critical care services, the physician must devote his or her full attention to the patient and, therefore, cannot provide services to any other patient during the same period of time.

Time spent with the individual patient should be recorded in the patient's record. The time that can be reported as remote real-time interactive video-conferenced critical care is the time spent engaged in work directly related to the individual patient's care. For example, time spent reviewing test results or imaging studies, discussing the critically ill patient's care with other medical staff or documenting remote real-time interactive video-conferenced critical care services in the medical record would be reported as remote real-time interactive video-conferenced critical care, even though it does not occur at the bedside. Also, when the patient is unable or lacks capacity to participate in discussions, time spent from the remote site with family members or surrogate decision makers obtaining a medical history, reviewing the patient's condition or prognosis, or discussing treatment or limitation(s) of treatment may be reported as remote real-time interactive video-conferenced critical care, provided that the conversation bears directly on the management of the patient.

Time spent in activities that occur away from the bedside when the physician does not have the real-time capabilities described above may not be reported as remote real-time interactive video-conferenced critical

care because the physician is not immediately available to the patient. Time spent in activities that do not directly contribute to the treatment of the patient may not be reported as remote real-time interactive video-conferenced critical care, even if they are performed in the remote site (eg, participation in administrative meetings or telephone calls to discuss other patients). Only one physician may report either Critical Care Services (99291, 99292) or remote real-time interactive video-conferenced Critical Care for the same period of time. Do not report remote real-time interactive video-conferenced critical care if another physician reports Pediatric or Neonatal Critical Care or Intensive Care services (99468-99476).

Code 0188T is used to report the first 30 to 74 minutes of remote real-time interactive video-conferenced, critical care on a given date. It should be used only once per date even if the time spent by the physician is not continuous on that date. Remote real-time interactive video-conferenced, critical care of less than 30 minutes total duration on a given date should not be reported.

Code 0189T is used to report additional block(s) of time, of up to 30 minutes each, beyond the first 74 minutes (see table below).

The following examples illustrate the correct reporting of remote critical care services:

| Total Duration of Critical Care | Codes |
|---|---|
| less than 30 minutes (less than 1/2 hour) | do not report |
| 30-74 minutes (1/2 hr. - 1 hr. 14 min.) | 0188T X 1 |
| 75-104 minutes (1 hr. 15 min. - 1 hr. 44 min.) | 0188T X 1 AND 0189T X 1 |
| 105-134 minutes (1 hr. 45 min. - 2 hr. 14 min.) | 0188T X 1 AND 0189T X 2 |

**0188T**   Remote real-time interactive video-conferenced critical care, evaluation and management of the critically ill or critically injured patient; first 30-74 minutes
Sunset January 2014

**+ 0189T**   each additional 30 minutes (List separately in addition to code for primary service)
Sunset January 2014

(Use 0189T in conjunction with 0188T)

**+ 0190T**   Placement of intraocular radiation source applicator (List separately in addition to primary procedure)
Sunset January 2014

(Use 0190T in conjunction with 67036)

(For application of the source by radiation oncologist, see Clinical Brachytherapy section)

**0191T**   Insertion of anterior segment aqueous drainage device, without extraocular reservoir; internal approach, into the trabecular meshwork
Sunset January 2014

Category III Codes

**# 0253T**     internal approach, into the suprachoroidal space
Sunset January 2016

**0192T**     external approach
Sunset January 2014

(0193T has been deleted. To report, use 53860)

(0194T has been deleted. To report procalcitonin, use 84145)

**0195T**     Arthrodesis, pre-sacral interbody technique, including instrumentation, imaging (when performed), and discectomy to prepare interspace, lumbar; single interspace
Sunset January 2014

**+ 0196T**     each additional interspace (List separately in addition to code for primary procedure)
Sunset January 2014

(Use 0196T in conjunction with 0195T)

(Do not report 0195T, 0196T in conjunction with 22558, 22845, 22851, 76000, 76380, 76496, 76497)

**0197T**     Intra-fraction localization and tracking of target or patient motion during delivery of radiation therapy (eg, 3D positional tracking, gating, 3D surface tracking), each fraction of treatment
Sunset January 2015

**0198T**     Measurement of ocular blood flow by repetitive intraocular pressure sampling, with interpretation and report
Sunset January 2015

**0199T**     Physiologic recording of tremor using accelerometer(s) and/or gyroscope(s) (including frequency and amplitude), including interpretation and report
Sunset January 2015

**⊙ 0200T**     Percutaneous sacral augmentation (sacroplasty), unilateral injection(s), including the use of a balloon or mechanical device, when used, 1 or more needles
Sunset January 2015

**⊙ 0201T**     Percutaneous sacral augmentation (sacroplasty), bilateral injections, including the use of a balloon or mechanical device, when used, 2 or more needles
Sunset January 2015

(For radiological supervision and interpretation, see 72291, 72292)

(If bone biopsy is performed, see 20220, 20225)

**0202T**     Posterior vertebral joint(s) arthroplasty (eg, facet joint[s] replacement), including facetectomy, laminectomy, foraminotomy, and vertebral column fixation, injection of bone cement, when performed, including fluoroscopy, single level, lumbar spine
Sunset January 2015

(Do not report 0202T in conjunction with 22521, 22524, 22840, 22851, 22857, 63005, 63012, 63017, 63030, 63042, 63047, 63056 at the same level)

(0203T has been deleted. To report, use 95800)

(0204T has been deleted. To report, use 95801)

**+ 0205T**     Intravascular catheter-based coronary vessel or graft spectroscopy (eg, infrared) during diagnostic evaluation and/or therapeutic intervention including imaging supervision, interpretation, and report, each vessel (List separately in addition to code for primary procedure)
Sunset January 2015

(Use 0205T in conjunction with 92980, 92982, 92995, 93452-93462, 93530-93533, 93563, 93564)

**0206T**     Algorithmic analysis, remote, of electrocardiographic-derived data with computer probability assessment, including report
Sunset January 2015

(When a 12-lead ECG is performed, 93000-93010 may be reported, as appropriate)

**0207T**     Evacuation of meibomian glands, automated, using heat and intermittent pressure, unilateral
Sunset January 2015

**0208T**     Pure tone audiometry (threshold), automated; air only
Sunset January 2016

**0209T**     air and bone
Sunset January 2016

**0210T**     Speech audiometry threshold, automated;
Sunset January 2016

**0211T**     with speech recognition
Sunset January 2016

**0212T**     Comprehensive audiometry threshold evaluation and speech recognition (0209T, 0211T combined), automated
Sunset January 2016

(For audiometric testing using audiometers performed manually by a qualified health care professional, see 92551-92557)

**0213T**     Injection(s), diagnostic or therapeutic agent, paravertebral facet (zygapophyseal) joint (or nerves innervating that joint) with ultrasound guidance, cervical or thoracic; single level
Sunset January 2016

(To report bilateral procedure, use 0213T with modifier 50)

**+ 0214T**     second level (List separately in addition to code for primary procedure)
Sunset January 2016

(To report bilateral procedure, use 0214T with modifier 50)

**+ 0215T**     third and any additional level(s) (List separately in addition to code for primary procedure)
Sunset January 2016

(Do not report 0215T more than once per day)

(Use 0214T, 0215T in conjunction with 0213T)

(To report bilateral procedure, use 0215T with modifier 50)

**Category III Codes**

**0216T**  Injection(s), diagnostic or therapeutic agent, paravertebral facet (zygapophyseal) joint (or nerves innervating that joint) with ultrasound guidance, lumbar or sacral; single level
Sunset January 2016

(To report bilateral procedure, use 0216T with modifier 50)

**+ 0217T**  second level (List separately in addition to code for primary procedure)
Sunset January 2016

(To report bilateral procedure, use 0217T with modifier 50)

**+ 0218T**  third and any additional level(s) (List separately in addition to code for primary procedure)
Sunset January 2016

(Do not report 0218T more than once per day)

(Use 0217T, 0218T in conjunction with 0216T)

(If injection(s) are performed using fluoroscopy or CT, see 64490-64495)

(To report bilateral procedure, use 0218T with modifier 50)

**0219T**  Placement of a posterior intrafacet implant(s), unilateral or bilateral, including imaging and placement of bone graft(s) or synthetic device(s), single level; cervical
Sunset January 2016

**0220T**  thoracic
Sunset January 2016

**0221T**  lumbar
Sunset January 2016

(Do not report 0219T-0221T in conjunction with any radiological service)

(Do not report 0219T-0221T in conjunction with 20930, 20931, 22600-22614, 22840, 22851 at the same level)

**+ 0222T**  each additional vertebral segment (List separately in addition to code for primary procedure)
Sunset January 2016

(Use 0222T in conjunction with 0219T-0221T)

(For posterior or posterolateral arthrodesis technique, see 22600-22614)

Acoustic cardiography codes 0223T-0225T describe the evaluation and optimization of physiologic data including systolic and diastolic heart sounds and their temporal relationships to the electrocardiogram (ECG).

Codes 0224T and 0225T also include interrogation and limited reprogramming of a cardiac pacing device to ensure hemodynamic optimization (heart rate parameter and/or automated timing modes, including explicit changes of AV/VV intervals) and facilitate device parameter optimization. Do not report 0224T or 0225T in conjunction with 93288 or 93289.

Acoustic cardiography services include a rhythm strip ECG. Do not report 93040-93042 in conjunction with 0223T-0225T.

For complete programming services as a separate procedure, see 93280, 93281, 93283, and 93284.

**0223T**  Acoustic cardiography, including automated analysis of combined acoustic and electrical intervals; single, with interpretation and report
Sunset January 2016

**0224T**  multiple, including serial trended analysis and limited reprogramming of device parameter, AV or VV delays only, with interpretation and report
Sunset January 2016

**0225T**  multiple, including serial trended analysis and limited reprogramming of device parameter, AV and VV delays, with interpretation and report
Sunset January 2016

**0226T**  Anoscopy, high resolution (HRA) (with magnification and chemical agent enhancement); diagnostic, including collection of specimen(s) by brushing or washing when performed
Sunset January 2016

**0227T**  with biopsy(ies)
Sunset January 2016

**0228T**  Injection(s), anesthetic agent and/or steroid, transforaminal epidural, with ultrasound guidance, cervical or thoracic; single level
Sunset January 2016

**+ 0229T**  each additional level (List separately in addition to code for primary procedure)
Sunset January 2016

(Use 0229T in conjunction with 0228T)

**0230T**  Injection(s), anesthetic agent and/or steroid, transforaminal epidural, with ultrasound guidance, lumbar or sacral; single level
Sunset January 2016

**+ 0231T**  each additional level (List separately in addition to code for primary procedure)
Sunset January 2016

(Use 0231T in conjunction with 0230T)

(For transforaminal epidural injections performed under fluoroscopy or CT, see 64479–64484)

(Do not report 0228T-0231T in conjunction with 76942, 76998, 76999)

**0232T**  Injection(s), platelet rich plasma, any site, including image guidance, harvesting and preparation when performed
Sunset January 2016

(Do not report 0232T in conjunction with 20550, 20551, 20600-20610, 20926, 76942, 77002, 77012, 77021, 86965)

Category III Codes

**0233T**     Skin advanced glycation endproducts (AGE) measurement by multi-wavelength fluorescent spectroscopy
Sunset January 2016

## Atherectomy (Open or Percutaneous) for Supra-Inguinal Arteries

Codes 0234T-0238T describe atherectomy performed by any method (eg, directional, rotational, laser) in arteries above the inguinal ligaments. These codes are structured differently than the codes describing atherectomy performed below the inguinal ligaments (37225, 37227, 37229, 37231, 37233, 37235).

These supra-inguinal atherectomy codes all include the surgical work of performing the atherectomy plus the radiological supervision and interpretation of the atherectomy. Unlike the atherectomy codes for infra-inguinal arteries, this set of Category III codes does not include accessing and selectively catheterizing the vessel, traversing the lesion, embolic protection if used, other intervention used to treat the same or other vessels, or closure of the arteriotomy by any method. These codes describe endovascular procedures performed percutaneously and/or through an open surgical exposure.

**0234T**     Transluminal peripheral atherectomy, open or percutaneous, including radiological supervision and interpretation; renal artery
Sunset January 2016

**0235T**         visceral artery (except renal), each vessel
Sunset January 2016

**0236T**         abdominal aorta
Sunset January 2016

**0237T**         brachiocephalic trunk and branches, each vessel
Sunset January 2016

**0238T**         iliac artery, each vessel
Sunset January 2016

**0239T**     Bioimpedance spectroscopy (BIS), measuring 100 frequencies or greater, direct measurement of extracellular fluid differences between the limbs
Sunset January 2016

▲ **0240T**     Esophageal motility (manometric study of the esophagus and/or gastroesophageal junction) study with interpretation and report; with high resolution esophageal pressure topography
Sunset January 2016

►(Do not report 0240T in conjunction with 91010 or 91013)◄

+▲ **0241T**         with stimulation or perfusion during high resolution esophageal pressure topography study (eg, stimulant, acid or alkali perfusion) (List separately in addition to code for primary procedure)
Sunset January 2016

(Use 0241T in conjunction with 0240T)

►(Do not report 0241T in conjunction with 91010 or 91013)◄

►(Do not report 0241T more than once per session)◄

►(To report esophageal motility studies without high resolution esophageal pressure topography, use 91010 and with stimulant or perfusion, use 91013)◄

**0242T**     Gastrointestinal tract transit and pressure measurement, stomach through colon, wireless capsule, with interpretation and report
Sunset January 2016

(Do not report 0242T in conjunction with 91020, 91022)

**0243T**     Intermittent measurement of wheeze rate for bronchodilator or bronchial-challenge diagnostic evaluation(s), with interpretation and report
Sunset January 2016

(Use 0243T once per 24 hour period)

(Do not report 0243T in conjunction with 0244T for the same 24 hour period)

**0244T**     Continuous measurement of wheeze rate during treatment assessment or during sleep for documentation of nocturnal wheeze and cough for diagnostic evaluation 3 to 24 hours, with interpretation and report
Sunset January 2016

**0245T**     Open treatment of rib fracture requiring internal fixation, unilateral; 1-2 ribs
Sunset January 2016

**0246T**         3-4 ribs
Sunset January 2016

**0247T**         5-6 ribs
Sunset January 2016

**0248T**         7 or more ribs
Sunset January 2016

**0249T**     Ligation, hemorrhoidal vascular bundle(s), including ultrasound guidance
Sunset January 2016

(Do not report 0249T in conjunction with 46020, 46221, 46250-46262, 46600, 46945, 46946, 76872, 76942, 76998)

⊙+ **0250T**     Airway sizing and insertion of bronchial valve(s), each lobe (List separately in addition to code for primary procedure)
Sunset January 2016

(Use 0250T in conjunction with 31622, 31634)

⊙ **0251T**     Bronchoscopy, rigid or flexible, including fluoroscopic guidance, when performed; with removal of bronchial valve(s), initial lobe
Sunset January 2016

(Do not report 0251T in conjunction with 31622-31626, 31628-31631, 31634-31636, 31638-31646)

**Category III Codes**

---

⊙✚ **0252T**    with removal of bronchial valve(s), each additional lobe (List separately in addition to code for primary procedure)
Sunset January 2016

(Use 0252T in conjunction with 0251T)

**0253T**    Code is out of numerical sequence. See 0188T-0259T

**0254T**    Endovascular repair of iliac artery bifurcation (eg, aneurysm, pseudoaneurysm, arteriovenous malformation, trauma) using bifurcated endoprosthesis from the common iliac artery into both the external and internal iliac artery, unilateral;
Sunset January 2016

**0255T**    radiological supervision and interpretation
Sunset January 2016

**0256T**    Implantation of catheter-delivered prosthetic aortic heart valve; endovascular approach
Sunset January 2016

(Code 0256T does not include cardiac catheterization [93451–93572] when performed at the time of the procedure for diagnostic purposes prior to aortic valve placement. Code 0256T includes all other catheterization[s], temporary pacing, intraprocedural contrast injection[s], fluoroscopic radiological supervision and interpretation, and imaging guidance, which are not reported separately when performed to complete the aortic valve procedure)

**0257T**    open thoracic approach (eg, transapical, transventricular)
Sunset January 2016

(Code 0257T does not include cardiac catheterization [93451–93572] when performed at the time of the procedure for diagnostic purposes prior to aortic valve placement. Code 0257T includes all other catheterization[s], temporary pacing, intraprocedural contrast injection[s], all fluoroscopic radiological supervision and interpretation, and imaging guidance, which are not reported separately when performed to complete the aortic valve procedure)

(Report transthoracic cardiac exposure separately with 0258T, 0259T)

(Do not report 0256T, 0257T in conjunction with 33210, 33211, 92986, 93503)

(When prior diagnostic cardiac catheterization has been performed, do not report 0256T, 0257T in conjunction with 93451-93464, 93530-93533, 93561-93568)

**0258T**    Transthoracic cardiac exposure (eg, sternotomy, thoracotomy, subxiphoid) for catheter-delivered aortic valve replacement; without cardiopulmonary bypass
Sunset January 2016

**0259T**    with cardiopulmonary bypass
Sunset January 2016

(For implantation of catheter-delivered prosthetic aortic heart valve post cardiac exposure, use 0257T)

(Do not report 0258T, 0259T in conjunction with 32100, 32551, 33210-33211, 33310, 33315, 33400-33413, 39010)

(Report 1 aortic valve placement procedure per session)

● **0260T**    Total body systemic hypothermia, per day, in the neonate 28 days of age or younger
Sunset January 2017

● **0261T**    Selective head hypothermia, per day, in the neonate 28 days of age or younger
Sunset January 2017

● **0262T**    Implantation of catheter-delivered prosthetic pulmonary valve, endovascular approach
Sunset January 2017

▶(0262T includes all congenital cardiac catheterization[s], intraprocedural contrast injection[s], fluoroscopic radiological supervision and interpretation, and imaging guidance performed to complete the pulmonary valve procedure. Do not report 0262T in conjunction with 76000, 76001, 93530, 93563, 93566-93568)◀

▶(0262T includes percutaneous balloon angioplasty/ valvuloplasty of the pulmonary valve/conduit. Do not report 0262T in conjunction with 92990)◀

▶(0262T includes stent deployment within the pulmonary conduit. Do not report 37205, 37206, 75960 for stent placement within the pulmonary conduit. Report 92980, 92981, 37205, 37206, 75960 separately when cardiovascular stent placement is performed at a site separate from the prosthetic valve delivery site. Report 92997, 92998 separately when pulmonary artery angioplasty is performed at a site separate from the prosthetic valve delivery site)◀

● **0263T**    Intramuscular autologous bone marrow cell therapy, with preparation of harvested cells, multiple injections, one leg, including ultrasound guidance, if performed; complete procedure including unilateral or bilateral bone marrow harvest
Sunset January 2017

▶(Do not report 0263T in conjunction with 38204-38242, 76942, 93925, 93926)◀

● **0264T**    complete procedure excluding bone marrow harvest
Sunset January 2017

▶(Do not report 0264T in conjunction with 38204-38242, 76942, 93925, 93926, 0265T)◀

● **0265T**    unilateral or bilateral bone marrow harvest only for intramuscular autologous bone marrow cell therapy
Sunset January 2017

▶(Do not report 0265T in conjunction with 38204-38242, 0264T. For complete procedure, use 0263T)◀

● **0266T**    Implantation or replacement of carotid sinus baroreflex activation device; total system (includes generator placement, unilateral or bilateral lead placement, intra-operative interrogation, programming, and repositioning, when performed)
Sunset January 2017

● **0267T**　　lead only, unilateral (includes intra-operative interrogation, programming, and repositioning, when performed)
Sunset January 2017

►(For bilateral lead implantation or replacement, use 0267T with modifier 50)◄

● **0268T**　　pulse generator only (includes intra-operative interrogation, programming, and repositioning, when performed)
Sunset January 2017

►(Do not report 0267T, 0268T in conjunction with 0266T, 0269T-0273T)◄

● **0269T**　Revision or removal of carotid sinus baroreflex activation device; total system (includes generator placement, unilateral or bilateral lead placement, intra-operative interrogation, programming, and repositioning, when performed)
Sunset January 2017

►(Do not report 0269T in conjunction with 0266T-0268T, 0270T-0273T)◄

● **0270T**　　lead only, unilateral (includes intra-operative interrogation, programming, and repositioning, when performed)
Sunset January 2017

►(Do not report 0270T in conjunction with 0266T-0269T, 0271T-0273T)◄

►(For bilateral lead removal, use 0270T with modifier 50)◄

►(For removal of total carotid sinus baroreflex activation device, use 0269T)◄

● **0271T**　　pulse generator only (includes intra-operative interrogation, programming, and repositioning, when performed)
Sunset January 2017

►(Do not report 0271T in conjunction with 0266T-0270T, 0272T, 0273T)◄

►(For removal and replacement, see 0266T, 0267T, 0268T)◄

● **0272T**　Interrogation device evaluation (in person), carotid sinus baroreflex activation system, including telemetric iterative communication with the implantable device to monitor device diagnostics and programmed therapy values, with interpretation and report (eg, battery status, lead impedance, pulse amplitude, pulse width, therapy frequency, pathway mode, burst mode, therapy start/stop times each day);
Sunset January 2017

►(Do not report 0272T in conjunction with 0266T-0271T, 0273T)◄

● **0273T**　　with programming
Sunset January 2017

►(Do not report 0273T in conjunction with 0266T-0272T)◄

● **0274T**　Percutaneous laminotomy/laminectomy (interlaminar approach) for decompression of neural elements, (with or without ligamentous resection, discectomy, facetectomy and/or foraminotomy), any method, under indirect image guidance (eg, fluoroscopic, CT), with or without the use of an endoscope, single or multiple levels, unilateral or bilateral; cervical or thoracic
Sunset January 2017

● **0275T**　　lumbar
Sunset January 2017

►(For laminotomy/hemilaminectomy performed using an open and endoscopically-assisted approach, see 63020-63035)◄

►(For percutaneous decompression of the nucleus pulposus of intervertebral disc utilizing needle based technique, use 62287)◄

⊙● **0276T**　Bronchoscopy, rigid or flexible, including fluoroscopic guidance, when performed; with bronchial thermoplasty, 1 lobe
Sunset January 2017

⊙● **0277T**　　with bronchial thermoplasty, 2 or more lobes
Sunset January 2017

● **0278T**　Transcutaneous electrical modulation pain reprocessing (eg, scrambler therapy), each treatment session (includes placement of electrodes)
Sunset January 2017

● **0279T**　Cell enumeration using immunologic selection and identification in fluid specimen (eg, circulating tumor cells in blood);
Sunset January 2017

● **0280T**　　interpretation and report

►(Use 0280T in conjunction with 0279T)◄

►(For flow cytometric immunophenotyping, see 88184-88189. For flow cytometric quantitation, see 86355-86357, 86359-86361, 86367)◄

● **0281T**　Percutaneous transcatheter closure of the left atrial appendage with implant, including fluoroscopy, transseptal puncture, catheter placement(s), left atrial angiography, left atrial appendage angiography, radiological supervision and interpretation
Sunset January 2017

►(Do not report 0281T in conjunction with 93462 [left heart catheterization by transseptal puncture])◄

►(Report cardiac catheterization procedures [93451-93461, 93530-93533] separately for indications distinct from the left atrial appendage closure procedure)◄

►(For left ventriculography performed by transseptal approach for indications distinct from the left atrial appendage closure procedure, use 93565)◄

**Category III Codes**

►(Do not report 0281T in conjunction with 93452, 93453, 93458-93461, 93531-93533 unless catheterization of the left ventricle is performed by a non-transseptal approach for indications distinct from the left atrial appendage closure procedure)◄

►(Do not report 0281T in conjunction with 93451, 93453, 93456, 93460, 93461, 93530-93533 unless complete right heart catheterization is performed for indications distinct from the left atrial appendage closure procedure)◄

⊙● **0282T**   Percutaneous or open implantation of neurostimulator electrode array(s), subcutaneous (peripheral subcutaneous field stimulation), including imaging guidance, when performed, cervical, thoracic or lumbar; for trial, including removal at the conclusion of trial period
Sunset January 2017

⊙● **0283T**       permanent, with implantation of a pulse generator
Sunset January 2017

⊙● **0284T**   Revision or removal of pulse generator or electrodes, including imaging guidance, when performed, including addition of new electrodes, when performed
Sunset January 2017

● **0285T**   Electronic analysis of implanted peripheral subcutaneous field stimulation pulse generator, with reprogramming when performed
Sunset January 2017

►(Do not report 0282T-0285T in conjunction with 64550-64595, 77002, 77003, 95970-95973)◄

● **0286T**   Near-infrared spectroscopy studies of lower extremity wounds (eg, for oxyhemoglobin measurement)
Sunset January 2017

● **0287T**   Near-infrared guidance for vascular access requiring real-time digital visualization of subcutaneous vasculature for evaluation of potential access sites and vessel patency
Sunset January 2017

● **0288T**   Anoscopy, with delivery of thermal energy to the muscle of the anal canal (eg, for fecal incontinence)
Sunset January 2017

►(Do not report 0288T in conjunction with 46600-46615)◄

+● **0289T**   Corneal incisions in the donor cornea created using a laser, in preparation for penetrating or lamellar keratoplasty (List separately in addition to code for primary procedure)
Sunset January 2017

►(Use 0289T in conjunction with 65710, 65730, 65750, 65755)◄

+● **0290T**   Corneal incisions in the recipient cornea created using a laser, in preparation for penetrating or lamellar keratoplasty (List separately in addition to code for primary procedure)
Sunset January 2017

►(Use 0290T in conjunction with 65710, 65730, 65750, 65755)◄

**Category III Codes**

# Appendix A

## Modifiers

This list includes all of the modifiers applicable to *CPT 2012* codes.

A modifier provides the means to report or indicate that a service or procedure that has been performed has been altered by some specific circumstance but not changed in its definition or code. Modifiers also enable health care professionals to effectively respond to payment policy requirements established by other entities.

(Modifier 21 has been deleted. To report prolonged physician services, see 99354-99357)

**22 Increased Procedural Services:** When the work required to provide a service is substantially greater than typically required, it may be identified by adding modifier 22 to the usual procedure code. Documentation must support the substantial additional work and the reason for the additional work (ie, increased intensity, time, technical difficulty of procedure, severity of patient's condition, physical and mental effort required). **Note:** This modifier should not be appended to an E/M service.

➔ *CPT Assistant* Jan 09:8, Apr 09:8, Jun 09:8,10 *CPT Changes: An Insider's View* 2008

**23 Unusual Anesthesia:** Occasionally, a procedure, which usually requires either no anesthesia or local anesthesia, because of unusual circumstances must be done under general anesthesia. This circumstance may be reported by adding modifier 23 to the procedure code of the basic service.

**24 Unrelated Evaluation and Management Service by the Same Physician During a Postoperative Period:** The physician may need to indicate that an evaluation and management service was performed during a postoperative period for a reason(s) unrelated to the original procedure. This circumstance may be reported by adding modifier 24 to the appropriate level of E/M service.

**25 Significant, Separately Identifiable Evaluation and Management Service by the Same Physician on the Same Day of the Procedure or Other Service:** It may be necessary to indicate that on the day a procedure or service identified by a CPT code was performed, the patient's condition required a significant, separately identifiable E/M service above and beyond the other service provided or beyond the usual preoperative and postoperative care associated with the procedure that was performed. A significant, separately identifiable E/M service is defined or substantiated by documentation that satisfies the relevant criteria for the respective E/M service to be reported (see **Evaluation and Management Services Guidelines** for instructions on determining level of E/M service). The E/M service may be prompted by the symptom or condition for which the procedure and/or service was provided. As such, different diagnoses are not required for reporting of the E/M services on the same date. This circumstance may be reported by adding modifier 25 to the appropriate level of E/M service. **Note:** This modifier is not used to report an E/M service that resulted in a decision to perform surgery. See modifier 57. For significant, separately identifiable non-E/M services, see modifier 59.

➔ *CPT Assistant* Feb 09:22, Mar 09:3, Apr 09:4; Jun 09:11 *CPT Changes: An Insider's View* 2008

**26 Professional Component:** Certain procedures are a combination of a physician component and a technical component. When the physician component is reported separately, the service may be identified by adding modifier 26 to the usual procedure number.

➔ *CPT Assistant* Jan 09:7, Apr 09:4, May 09:7

**32 Mandated Services:** Services related to *mandated* consultation and/or related services (eg, third party payer, governmental, legislative or regulatory requirement) may be identified by adding modifier 32 to the basic procedure.

**33 ▶Preventive Services:** When the primary purpose of the service is the delivery of an evidence based service in accordance with a US Preventive Services Task Force A or B rating in effect and other preventive services identified in preventive services mandates (legislative or regulatory), the service may be identified by adding 33 to the procedure. For separately reported services specifically identified as preventive, the modifier should not be used.◀

➔ *CPT Changes: An Insider's View* 2012

**47 Anesthesia by Surgeon:** Regional or general anesthesia provided by the surgeon may be reported by adding modifier 47 to the basic service. (This does not include local anesthesia.) **Note:** Modifier 47 would not be used as a modifier for the anesthesia procedures.

**50 Bilateral Procedure:** Unless otherwise identified in the listings, bilateral procedures that are performed at the same session, should be identified by adding modifier 50 to the appropriate 5 digit code.

➔ *CPT Assistant* Apr 09:9, *CPT Changes: An Insider's View* 2011

**51 Multiple Procedures:** When multiple procedures, other than E/M services, Physical Medicine and Rehabilitation services or provision of supplies (eg, vaccines), are performed at the same session by the same provider, the primary procedure or service may be reported as listed. The additional procedure(s) or service(s) may be identified by appending modifier 51 to the additional procedure or service code(s). **Note:** This modifier should not be appended to designated "add-on" codes (see Appendix D).

➔ *CPT Assistant* Feb 09:6, Mar 09:10, Apr 09:8 *CPT Changes: An Insider's View* 2008

**52 Reduced Services:** Under certain circumstances a service or procedure is partially reduced or eliminated at the physician's discretion. Under these circumstances the service provided can be identified by its usual procedure number and the addition of modifier 52, signifying that the service is reduced. This provides a means of reporting reduced services without disturbing the identification of the basic service. **Note:** For hospital outpatient reporting of a previously scheduled procedure/service that is partially reduced or cancelled as a result of extenuating circumstances or those that threaten the well-being of the patient prior to or after administration of anesthesia, see modifiers 73 and 74 (see modifiers approved for ASC hospital outpatient use).

➔ *CPT Assistant* Mar 09:11, Apr 09:5, May 09:8, Jun 09:10

**53 Discontinued Procedure:** Under certain circumstances, the physician may elect to terminate a surgical or diagnostic procedure. Due to extenuating circumstances or those that threaten the well being of the patient, it may be necessary to indicate that a surgical or diagnostic procedure was started but discontinued. This circumstance may be reported by adding modifier 53 to the code reported by the physician for the discontinued procedure. **Note:** This modifier is not used to report the elective cancellation of a procedure prior to the patient's anesthesia induction and/or surgical preparation in the operating suite. For outpatient hospital/ambulatory surgery center (ASC) reporting of a previously scheduled procedure/service that is partially reduced or cancelled as a result of extenuating circumstances or those that threaten the well being of the patient prior to or after administration of anesthesia, see modifiers 73 and 74 (see modifiers approved for ASC hospital outpatient use).

**54 Surgical Care Only:** When 1 physician performs a surgical procedure and another provides preoperative and/or postoperative management, surgical services may be identified by adding modifier 54 to the usual procedure number.

**55 Postoperative Management Only:** When 1 physician performed the postoperative management and another physician performed the surgical procedure, the postoperative component may be identified by adding modifier 55 to the usual procedure number.

**56 Preoperative Management Only:** When 1 physician performed the preoperative care and evaluation and another physician performed the surgical procedure, the preoperative component may be identified by adding modifier 56 to the usual procedure number.

**57 Decision for Surgery:** An evaluation and management service that resulted in the initial decision to perform the surgery may be identified by adding modifier 57 to the appropriate level of E/M service.

➔ *CPT Assistant* May 09:9

**58 Staged or Related Procedure or Service by the Same Physician During the Postoperative Period:** It may be necessary to indicate that the performance of a procedure or service during the postoperative period was: (a) planned or anticipated (staged); (b) more extensive than the original procedure; or (c) for therapy following a surgical procedure. This circumstance may be reported by adding modifier 58 to the staged or related procedure. **Note:** For treatment of a problem that requires a return to the operating/procedure room (eg, unanticipated clinical condition), see modifier 78.

➔ *CPT Changes: An Insider's View* 2008

**59 Distinct Procedural Service:** Under certain circumstances, it may be necessary to indicate that a procedure or service was distinct or independent from other non-E/M services performed on the same day. Modifier 59 is used to identify procedures/services, other than E/M services, that are not normally reported together, but are appropriate under the circumstances. Documentation must support a different session, different procedure or surgery, different site or organ system, separate incision/excision, separate lesion, or separate injury (or area of injury in extensive injuries) not ordinarily encountered or performed on the same day by the same individual. However, when another already established modifier is appropriate it should be used rather than modifier 59. Only if no more descriptive modifier is available, and the use of modifier 59 best explains the circumstances, should modifier 59 be used. **Note:** Modifier 59 should not be appended to an E/M service. To report a separate and distinct E/M service with a non-E/M service performed on the same date, see modifier 25.

➔ *CPT Assistant* Feb 09:17, Apr 09:4,8, May 09:6, Jun 09:8 *CPT Changes: An Insider's View* 2008

**62 Two Surgeons:** When 2 surgeons work together as primary surgeons performing distinct part(s) of a procedure, each surgeon should report his/her distinct operative work by adding modifier 62 to the procedure code and any associated add-on code(s) for that procedure as long as both surgeons continue to work together as primary surgeons. Each surgeon should report the co-surgery once using the same procedure code. If additional procedure(s) (including add-on procedure(s) are performed during the same surgical session, separate code(s) may also be reported with modifier 62 added. **Note:** If a co-surgeon acts as an assistant in the performance of additional procedure(s) during the same surgical session, those services may be reported using separate procedure code(s) with modifier 80 or modifier 82 added, as appropriate.

**63 Procedure Performed on Infants less than 4 kg:** Procedures performed on neonates and infants up to a present body weight of 4 kg may involve significantly increased complexity and physician work commonly associated with these patients. This circumstance may be reported by adding modifier 63 to the procedure number. **Note:** Unless otherwise designated, this modifier may only be appended to procedures/services listed in the 20005-69990 code series. Modifier 63 should not be appended to any CPT codes listed in the **Evaluation and Management Services, Anesthesia, Radiology, Pathology/Laboratory, or Medicine** sections.

**66 Surgical Team:** Under some circumstances, highly complex procedures (requiring the concomitant services of several physicians, often of different specialties, plus other highly skilled, specially trained personnel, various types of complex equipment) are carried out under the "surgical team" concept. Such circumstances may be identified by each participating physician with the addition of modifier 66 to the basic procedure number used for reporting services.

**76 Repeat Procedure or Service by Same Physician or Other Qualified Health Care Professional:** It may be necessary to indicate that a procedure or service was repeated by the same physician or other qualified health care professional subsequent to the original procedure or service. This circumstance may be reported by adding modifier 76 to the repeated procedure or service. **Note:** This modifier should not be appended to an E/M service.

➔ *CPT Assistant* Feb 09:6 *CPT Changes: An Insider's View* 2008, 2011

**77** **Repeat Procedure by Another Physician or Other Qualified Health Care Professional:** It may be necessary to indicate that a basic procedure or service was repeated by another physician or other qualified health care professional subsequent to the original procedure or service. This circumstance may be reported by adding modifier 77 to the repeated procedure or service. **Note:** This modifier should not be appended to an E/M service.

➔ *CPT Changes: An Insider's View* 2008, 2011

**78** **Unplanned Return to the Operating/Procedure Room by the Same Physician or Other Qualified Health Care Professional Following Initial Procedure for a Related Procedure During the Postoperative Period:** It may be necessary to indicate that another procedure was performed during the postoperative period of the initial procedure (unplanned procedure following initial procedure). When this procedure is related to the first, and requires the use of an operating/procedure room, it may be reported by adding modifier 78 to the related procedure. (For repeat procedures, see modifier 76.)

➔ *CPT Changes: An Insider's View* 2008, 2011

**79** **Unrelated Procedure or Service by the Same Physician During the Postoperative Period:** The physician may need to indicate that the performance of a procedure or service during the postoperative period was unrelated to the original procedure. This circumstance may be reported by using modifier 79. (For repeat procedures on the same day, see modifier 76.)

**80** **Assistant Surgeon:** Surgical assistant services may be identified by adding modifier 80 to the usual procedure number(s).

**81** **Minimum Assistant Surgeon:** Minimum surgical assistant services are identified by adding modifier 81 to the usual procedure number.

**82** **Assistant Surgeon (when qualified resident surgeon not available):** The unavailability of a qualified resident surgeon is a prerequisite for use of modifier 82 appended to the usual procedure code number(s).

**90** **Reference (Outside) Laboratory:** When laboratory procedures are performed by a party other than the treating or reporting physician, the procedure may be identified by adding modifier 90 to the usual procedure number.

**91** **Repeat Clinical Diagnostic Laboratory Test:** In the course of treatment of the patient, it may be necessary to repeat the same laboratory test on the same day to obtain subsequent (multiple) test results. Under these circumstances, the laboratory test performed can be identified by its usual procedure number and the addition of modifier 91. **Note:** This modifier may not be used when

tests are rerun to confirm initial results; due to testing problems with specimens or equipment; or for any other reason when a normal, one-time, reportable result is all that is required. This modifier may not be used when other code(s) describe a series of test results (eg, glucose tolerance tests, evocative/suppression testing). This modifier may only be used for laboratory test(s) performed more than once on the same day on the same patient.

➔ *CPT Assistant* May 09:6

**92** ▶**Alternative Laboratory Platform Testing:** When laboratory testing is being performed using a kit or transportable instrument that wholly or in part consists of a single use, disposable analytical chamber, the service may be identified by adding modifier 92 to the usual laboratory procedure code (HIV testing 86701-86703, and 87389). The test does not require permanent dedicated space, hence by its design may be hand carried or transported to the vicinity of the patient for immediate testing at that site, although location of the testing is not in itself determinative of the use of this modifier.◀

➔ *CPT Changes: An Insider's View* 2008, 2012

**99** **Multiple Modifiers:** Under certain circumstances 2 or more modifiers may be necessary to completely delineate a service. In such situations modifier 99 should be added to the basic procedure, and other applicable modifiers may be listed as part of the description of the service.

## Anesthesia Physical Status Modifiers

The Physical Status modifiers are consistent with the American Society of Anesthesiologists ranking of patient physical status, and distinguishing various levels of complexity of the anesthesia service provided. All anesthesia services are reported by use of the anesthesia five-digit procedure code (00100-01999) with the appropriate physical status modifier appended.

Example: 00100-P1

Under certain circumstances, when another established modifier(s) is appropriate, it should be used in addition to the physical status modifier.

Example: 00100-P4-53

**Physical Status Modifier P1:** A normal healthy patient

**Physical Status Modifier P2:** A patient with mild systemic disease

**Physical Status Modifier P3:** A patient with severe systemic disease

**Physical Status Modifier P4:** A patient with severe systemic disease that is a constant threat to life

**Physical Status Modifier P5:** A moribund patient who is not expected to survive without the operation

**Physical Status Modifier P6:** A declared brain-dead patient whose organs are being removed for donor purposes

# Modifiers Approved for Ambulatory Surgery Center (ASC) Hospital Outpatient Use

## CPT Level I Modifiers

**25  Significant, Separately Identifiable Evaluation and Management Service by the Same Physician on the Same Day of the Procedure or Other Service:** It may be necessary to indicate that on the day a procedure or service identified by a CPT code was performed, the patient's condition required a significant, separately identifiable E/M service above and beyond the other service provided or beyond the usual preoperative and postoperative care associated with the procedure that was performed. A significant, separately identifiable E/M service is defined or substantiated by documentation that satisfies the relevant criteria for the respective E/M service to be reported (see **Evaluation and Management Services Guidelines** for instructions on determining level of E/M service). The E/M service may be prompted by the symptom or condition for which the procedure and/or service was provided. As such, different diagnoses are not required for reporting of the E/M services on the same date. This circumstance may be reported by adding modifier 25 to the appropriate level of E/M service. **Note:** This modifier is not used to report an E/M service that resulted in a decision to perform surgery. See modifier 57. For significant, separately identifiable non-E/M services, see modifier 59.

**27  Multiple Outpatient Hospital E/M Encounters on the Same Date:** For hospital outpatient reporting purposes, utilization of hospital resources related to separate and distinct E/M encounters performed in multiple outpatient hospital settings on the same date may be reported by adding modifier 27 to each appropriate level outpatient and/or emergency department E/M code(s). This modifier provides a means of reporting circumstances involving evaluation and management services provided by physician(s) in more than one (multiple) outpatient hospital setting(s) (eg, hospital emergency department, clinic). **Note:** This modifier is not to be used for physician reporting of multiple E/M services performed by the same physician on the same date. For physician reporting of all outpatient evaluation and management services provided by the same physician on the same date and performed in multiple outpatient setting(s) (eg, hospital emergency department, clinic), see **Evaluation and Management, Emergency Department, or Preventive Medicine Services** codes.

**50  Bilateral Procedure:** Unless otherwise identified in the listings, bilateral procedures that are performed at the same session, should be identified by adding modifier 50 to the appropriate 5 digit code.

**52  Reduced Services:** Under certain circumstances a service or procedure is partially reduced or eliminated at the physician's discretion. Under these circumstances the service provided can be identified by its usual procedure number and the addition of modifier 52, signifying that the service is reduced. This provides a means of reporting reduced services without disturbing the identification of the basic service. **Note:** For hospital outpatient reporting of a previously scheduled procedure/service that is partially reduced or cancelled as a result of extenuating circumstances or those that threaten the well-being of the patient prior to or after administration of anesthesia, see modifiers 73 and 74 (see modifiers approved for ASC hospital outpatient use).

**58  Staged or Related Procedure or Service by the Same Physician During the Postoperative Period:** It may be necessary to indicate that the performance of a procedure or service during the postoperative period was: (a) planned or anticipated (staged); (b) more extensive than the original procedure; or (c) for therapy following a surgical procedure. This circumstance may be reported by adding modifier 58 to the staged or related procedure. **Note:** For treatment of a problem that requires a return to the operating/procedure room (eg, unanticipated clinical condition), see modifier 78.

**59  Distinct Procedural Service:** Under certain circumstances, it may be necessary to indicate that a procedure or service was distinct or independent from other non-E/M services performed on the same day. Modifier 59 is used to identify procedures/services, other than E/M services, that are not normally reported together, but are appropriate under the circumstances. Documentation must support a different session, different procedure or surgery, different site or organ system, separate incision/excision, separate lesion, or separate injury (or area of injury in extensive injuries) not ordinarily encountered or performed on the same day by the same individual. However, when another already established modifier is appropriate it should be used rather than modifier 59. Only if no more descriptive modifier is available, and the use of modifier 59 best explains the circumstances, should modifier 59 be used. **Note:** Modifier 59 should not be appended to an E/M service. To report a separate and distinct E/M service with a non-E/M service performed on the same date, see modifier 25.

**73  Discontinued Out-Patient Hospital/Ambulatory Surgery Center (ASC) Procedure Prior to the Administration of Anesthesia:** Due to extenuating circumstances or those that threaten the well being of the patient, the physician may cancel a surgical or diagnostic procedure subsequent to the patient's surgical preparation (including sedation when provided, and being taken to the room where the procedure is to be performed), but prior to the administration of anesthesia (local, regional block(s) or general). Under these circumstances, the intended service that is prepared for but cancelled can be reported by its usual procedure number and the addition of modifier 73. **Note:** The elective cancellation of a service prior to the administration of anesthesia and/or surgical preparation of the patient should not be reported. For physician reporting of a discontinued procedure, see modifier 53.

**74  Discontinued Out-Patient Hospital/Ambulatory Surgery Center (ASC) Procedure After Administration of Anesthesia:** Due to extenuating circumstances or those that threaten the well being of the patient, the physician may terminate a surgical or diagnostic procedure after the administration of anesthesia (local, regional block(s), general) or after the procedure was started (incision made, intubation started, scope inserted, etc). Under these circumstances, the procedure started but terminated can be reported by its usual procedure number and the addition of modifier 74. **Note:** The elective cancellation of a service prior to the administration of anesthesia and/or surgical preparation of the patient should not be reported. For physician reporting of a discontinued procedure, see modifier 53.

**76 Repeat Procedure or Service by Same Physician or Other Qualified Health Care Professional:** It may be necessary to indicate that a procedure or service was repeated by the same physician or other qualified health care professional subsequent to the original procedure or service. This circumstance may be reported by adding modifier 76 to the repeated procedure or service. **Note:** This modifier should not be appended to an E/M service.

**77 Repeat Procedure by Another Physician or Other Qualified Health Care Professional:** It may be necessary to indicate that a basic procedure or service was repeated by another physician or other qualified health care professional subsequent to the original procedure or service. This circumstance may be reported by adding modifier 77 to the repeated procedure or service. **Note:** This modifier should not be appended to an E/M service.

**78 Unplanned Return to the Operating/Procedure Room by the Same Physician or Other Qualified Health Care Professional Following Initial Procedure for a Related Procedure During the Postoperative Period:** It may be necessary to indicate that another procedure was performed during the postoperative period of the initial procedure (unplanned procedure following initial procedure). When this procedure is related to the first, and requires the use of an operating/procedure room, it may be reported by adding modifier 78 to the related procedure. (For repeat procedures, see modifier 76.)

**79 Unrelated Procedure or Service by the Same Physician During the Postoperative Period:** The physician may need to indicate that the performance of a procedure or service during the postoperative period was unrelated to the original procedure. This circumstance may be reported by using modifier 79. (For repeat procedures on the same day, see modifier 76.)

**91 Repeat Clinical Diagnostic Laboratory Test:** In the course of treatment of the patient, it may be necessary to repeat the same laboratory test on the same day to obtain subsequent (multiple) test results. Under these circumstances, the laboratory test performed can be identified by its usual procedure number and the addition of modifier 91. **Note:** This modifier may not be used when tests are rerun to confirm initial results; due to testing problems with specimens or equipment; or for any other reason when a normal, one-time, reportable result is all that is required. This modifier may not be used when other code(s) describe a series of test results (eg, glucose tolerance tests, evocative/suppression testing). This modifier may only be used for laboratory test(s) performed more than once on the same day on the same patient.

## Level II (HCPCS/National) Modifiers

**E1** Upper left, eyelid

**E2** Lower left, eyelid

**E3** Upper right, eyelid

**E4** Lower right, eyelid

**F1** Left hand, second digit

**F2** Left hand, third digit

**F3** Left hand, fourth digit

**F4** Left hand, fifth digit

**F5** Right hand, thumb

**F6** Right hand, second digit

**F7** Right hand, third digit

**F8** Right hand, fourth digit

**F9** Right hand, fifth digit

**FA** Left hand, thumb

**GG** Performance and payment of a screening mammogram and diagnostic mammogram on the same patient, same day

**GH** Diagnostic mammogram converted from screening mammogram on same day

**LC** Left circumflex coronary artery

**LD** Left anterior descending coronary artery

**LT** Left side (used to identify procedures performed on the left side of the body)

**QM** Ambulance service provided under arrangement by a provider of services

**QN** Ambulance service furnished directly by a provider of services

**RC** Right coronary artery

**RT** Right side (used to identify procedures performed on the right side of the body)

**T1** Left foot, second digit

**T2** Left foot, third digit

**T3** Left foot, fourth digit

**T4** Left foot, fifth digit

**T5** Right foot, great toe

**T6** Right foot, second digit

**T7** Right foot, third digit

**T8** Right foot, fourth digit

**T9** Right foot, fifth digit

**TA** Left foot, great toe

# Appendix B

## Summary of Additions, Deletions, and Revisions

Appendix B shows the actual changes that were made to the code descriptors. New codes appear with a bullet ( ● ) and are indicated as "Code Added." Revised codes are preceded with a triangle ( ▲ ). The symbol ○ precedes codes that are recycled or reinstated. Within revised codes, the deleted language appears with a ~~strikethrough~~, while new text appears <u>underlined</u>. Codes with which conscious sedation would not be separately reported when performed at the same session by the same provider are denoted with the bullseye ( ⊙ ). The symbol ⋌ is used to identify codes for vaccines that are pending FDA approval (see **Appendix K**). The symbol # is used to identify codes that have been resequenced (see **Appendix N**). CPT add-on codes are annotated by the symbol ✛ (see **Appendix D**). The symbol ⊘ is used to identify codes that are exempt from the use of modifier 51 (see **Appendix E**).

## Evaluation and Management

▲ 99218    **Initial observation care,** per day, for the evaluation and management of a patient which requires these 3 key components:

A detailed or comprehensive history;

A detailed or comprehensive examination; and

Medical decision making that is straightforward or of low complexity.

Counseling and/or coordination of care with other providers or agencies are provided consistent with the nature of the problem(s) and the patient's and/or family's needs.

Usually, the problem(s) requiring admission to "observation status" are of low severity. <u>Physicians typically spend 30 minutes at the bedside and on the patient's hospital floor or unit.</u>;

▲ 99219    **Initial observation care,** per day, for the evaluation and management of a patient, which requires these 3 key components:

A comprehensive history;

A comprehensive examination; and

Medical decision making of moderate complexity.

Counseling and/or coordination of care with other providers or agencies are provided consistent with the nature of the problem(s) and the patient's and/or family's needs.

Usually, the problem(s) requiring admission to "observation status" are of moderate severity. <u>Physicians typically spend 50 minutes at the bedside and on the patient's hospital floor or unit.</u>;

▲ 99220    **Initial observation care,** per day, for the evaluation and management of a patient which requires these 3 key components:

A comprehensive history;

A comprehensive examination; and

Medical decision making of high complexity.

Counseling and/or coordination of care with other providers or agencies are provided consistent with the nature of the problem(s) and the patient's and/or family's needs.

Usually, the problem(s) requiring admission to "observation status" are of high severity. <u>Physicians typically spend 70 minutes at the bedside and on the patient's hospital floor or unit.</u>;

✛▲ 99354    Prolonged ~~physician~~ service in the office or other outpatient setting requiring direct ~~(face-to-face)~~ patient contact beyond the usual service; first hour (List separately in addition to code for office or other outpatient **Evaluation and Management** service)

✛▲ 99355    each additional 30 minutes (List separately in addition to code for prolonged ~~physician~~ service)

✛▲ 99356    Prolonged ~~physician~~ service in the inpatient <u>or observation</u> setting, requiring unit/floor time beyond the usual service; first hour (List separately in addition to code for inpatient **Evaluation and Management** service)

✛▲ 99357    each additional 30 minutes (List separately in addition to code for prolonged ~~physician~~ service)

▲ 99358    **Prolonged evaluation and management service** before and/or after direct ~~(face-to-face)~~ patient care; first hour

✛▲ 99359    each additional 30 minutes (List separately in addition to code for prolonged ~~physician~~ service)

## Surgery

~~11975~~    ~~Insertion, implantable contraceptive capsules;~~

~~11977~~    ~~Removal with reinsertion, implantable contraceptive capsules;~~

▲ 15150    Tissue cultured ~~epidermal~~<u>skin</u> autograft, trunk, arms, legs; first 25 sq cm or less

✛▲ 15151    additional 1 sq cm to 75 sq cm (List separately in addition to code for primary procedure)

✛▲ 15152    each additional 100 sq cm, or each additional 1% of body area of infants and children, or part thereof (List separately in addition to code for primary procedure)

▲ 15155    Tissue cultured ~~epidermal~~<u>skin</u> autograft, face, scalp, eyelids, mouth, neck, ears, orbits, genitalia, hands, feet, and/or multiple digits; first 25 sq cm or less

✛▲ 15156    additional 1 sq cm to 75 sq cm (List separately in addition to code for primary procedure)

✛▲ 15157    each additional 100 sq cm, or each additional 1% of body area of infants and children, or part thereof (List separately in addition to code for primary procedure)

~~15170~~    ~~Acellular dermal replacement, trunk, arms, legs; first 100 sq cm or less, or 1% of body area of infants and children~~

~~15171~~    ~~each additional 100 sq cm, or each additional 1% of body area of infants and children, or part thereof (List separately in addition to code for primary procedure)~~

~~15175~~    ~~Acellular dermal replacement, face, scalp, eyelids, mouth, neck, ears, orbits, genitalia, hands, feet, and/or multiple digits; first 100 sq cm or less, or 1% of body area of infants and children~~

~~15176~~    ~~each additional 100 sq cm, or each additional 1% of body area of infants and children, or part thereof (List separately in addition to code for primary procedure)~~

● 15271    Code added

+ ● **15272** Code added

● **15273** Code added

+ ● **15274** Code added

● **15275** Code added

+ ● **15276** Code added

● **15277** Code added

+ ● **15278** Code added

**15300** ~~Allograft skin for temporary wound closure, trunk, arms, legs; first 100 sq cm or less, or 1% of body area of infants and children~~

**15301** ~~each additional 100 sq cm, or each additional 1% of body area of infants and children, or part thereof (List separately in addition to code for primary procedure)~~

**15320** ~~Allograft skin for temporary wound closure, face, scalp, eyelids, mouth, neck, ears, orbits, genitalia, hands, feet, and/or multiple digits; first 100 sq cm or less, or 1% of body area of infants and children~~

**15321** ~~each additional 100 sq cm, or each additional 1% of body area of infants and children, or part thereof (List separately in addition to code for primary procedure)~~

**15330** ~~Acellular dermal allograft, trunk, arms, legs; first 100 sq cm or less, or 1% of body area of infants and children~~

**15331** ~~each additional 100 sq cm, or each additional 1% of body area of infants and children, or part thereof (List separately in addition to code for primary procedure)~~

**15335** ~~Acellular dermal allograft, face, scalp, eyelids, mouth, neck, ears, orbits, genitalia, hands, feet, and/or multiple digits; first 100 sq cm or less, or 1% of body area of infants and children~~

**15336** ~~each additional 100 sq cm, or each additional 1% of body area of infants and children, or part thereof (List separately in addition to code for primary procedure)~~

**15340** ~~Tissue cultured allogeneic skin substitute; first 25 sq cm or less~~

**15341** ~~each additional 25 sq cm, or part thereof (List separately in addition to code for primary procedure)~~

**15360** ~~Tissue cultured allogeneic dermal substitute, trunk, arms, legs; first 100 sq cm or less, or 1% of body area of infants and children~~

**15361** ~~each additional 100 sq cm, or each additional 1% of body area of infants and children, or part thereof (List separately in addition to code for primary procedure)~~

**15365** ~~Tissue cultured allogeneic dermal substitute, face, scalp, eyelids, mouth, neck, ears, orbits, genitalia, hands, feet, and/or multiple digits; first 100 sq cm or less, or 1% of body area of infants and children~~

**15366** ~~each additional 100 sq cm, or each additional 1% of body area of infants and children, or part thereof (List separately in addition to code for primary procedure)~~

**15400** ~~Xenograft, skin (dermal), for temporary wound closure, trunk, arms, legs; first 100 sq cm or less, or 1% of body area of infants and children~~

**15401** ~~each additional 100 sq cm, or each additional 1% of body area of infants and children, or part thereof (List separately in addition to code for primary procedure)~~

**15420** ~~Xenograft skin (dermal), for temporary wound closure, face, scalp, eyelids, mouth, neck, ears, orbits, genitalia, hands, feet, and/or multiple digits; first 100 sq cm or less, or 1% of body area of infants and children~~

**15421** ~~each additional 100 sq cm, or each additional 1% of body area of infants and children, or part thereof (List separately in addition to code for primary procedure)~~

**15430** ~~Acellular xenograft implant; first 100 sq cm or less, or 1% of body area of infants and children~~

**15431** ~~each additional 100 sq cm, or each additional 1% of body area of infants and children, or part thereof (List separately in addition to code for primary procedure)~~

+ ● **15777** Code added

● **20527** Code added

⊙ ▲ **22520** Percutaneous vertebroplasty (bone biopsy included when performed), 1 vertebral body, unilateral or bilateral injection; thoracic

⊙ ▲ **22521** lumbar

+ ▲ **22522** each additional thoracic or lumbar vertebral body (List separately in addition to code for primary procedure)

▲ **22610** thoracic (with ~~or without~~ lateral transverse technique, when performed)

▲ **22612** lumbar (with ~~or without~~ lateral transverse technique, when performed)

● **22633** Code added

+ ● **22634** Code added

● **26341** Code added

▲ **27096** Injection procedure for sacroiliac joint, anesthetic/steroid, with image guidance (fluoroscopy or CT) including arthrography when performed;

▲ **29581** Application of multi-layer ~~venous wound~~ compression system; ~~below knee;~~ leg (below knee), including ankle and foot

● **29582** Code added

● **29583** Code added

● **29584** Code added

+ ▲ **29826** decompression of subacromial space with partial acromioplasty, with coracoacromial ~~without~~ ligament (ie, arch) release, when performed (List separately in addition to code for primary procedure)

▲ **29880** with meniscectomy (medial AND lateral, including any meniscal shaving) including debridement/shaving of articular cartilage (chondroplasty), same or separate compartment(s), when performed

▲ **29881** with meniscectomy (medial OR lateral, including any meniscal shaving) including debridement/shaving of articular cartilage (chondroplasty), same or separate compartment(s), when performed

**32095** ~~Thoracotomy, limited, for biopsy of lung or pleura;~~

● **32096** Code added

● **32097** Code added

● **32098** Code added

▲ **32100** Thoracotomy~~, major~~; with exploration ~~and biopsy~~

▲ **32110** with control of traumatic hemorrhage and/or repair of lung tear

▲ **32120** for postoperative complications

▲ **32124** with open intrapleural pneumonolysis

▲ 32140 with cyst(s) removal, ~~with or without a~~includes pleural procedure_ when performed

▲ 32141 with ~~excision~~resection-plication of bullae, ~~with or without~~includes any pleural procedure_ when performed

▲ 32150 with removal of intrapleural foreign body or fibrin deposit

▲ 32151 with removal of intrapulmonary foreign body

▲ 32160 with cardiac massage

~~32402~~ ~~open~~

⊙▲ 32405 Biopsy, lung or mediastinum, percutaneous needle;

▲ 32440 Removal of lung, ~~total~~ pneumonectomy;

▲ 32442 with resection of segment of trachea followed by broncho-tracheal anastomosis (sleeve pneumonectomy)

▲ 32445 extrapleural

▲ 32480 Removal of lung, other than ~~total~~ pneumonectomy; single lobe (lobectomy)

▲ 32482 2 lobes (bilobectomy)

▲ 32484 single segment (segmentectomy)

▲ 32486 with circumferential resection of segment of bronchus followed by broncho-bronchial anastomosis (sleeve lobectomy)

▲ 32488 with all remaining lung following previous removal of a portion of lung (completion pneumonectomy)

▲ 32491 ~~excision~~with resection-plication of emphysematous lung(s) (bullous or non-bullous) for lung volume reduction, sternal split or transthoracic approach, ~~with or without~~includes any pleural procedure, when performed

~~32500~~ ~~wedge resection, single or multiple~~

● 32505 Code added

+● 32506 Code added

+● 32507 Code added

▲ 32601 Thoracoscopy, diagnostic (separate procedure); lungs ~~and,~~ pericardial sac, mediastinal or pleural space, without biopsy

~~32602~~ ~~lungs and pleural space, with biopsy~~

~~32603~~ ~~pericardial sac, without biopsy~~

~~32605~~ ~~mediastinal space, without biopsy~~

● 32607 Code added

● 32608 Code added

● 32609 Code added

▲ 32655 with ~~excision~~resection-plication of bullae, ~~including~~includes any pleural procedure when performed

~~32657~~ ~~with wedge resection of lung, single or multiple~~

~~32660~~ ~~with total pericardiectomy~~

▲ 32663 with lobectomy, ~~total or segmental~~ (single lobe)

● 32666 Code added

+● 32667 Code added

+● 32668 Code added

● 32669 Code added

● 32670 Code added

● 32671 Code added

● 32672 Code added

● 32673 Code added

+● 32674 Code added

▲ 33050 ~~Excision~~Resection of pericardial cyst or tumor;

⊙▲ 33206 Insertion of new or replacement of permanent pacemaker with transvenous electrode(s); atrial

⊙▲ 33207 ventricular

⊙▲ 33208 atrial and ventricular

⊙▲ 33212 Insertion ~~or replacement~~ of pacemaker pulse generator only; ~~single chamber, atrial or ventricular~~with existing single lead

⊙▲ 33213 with existing dual ~~chamber~~leads

⊙#● 33221 Code added

⊙▲ 33218 Repair of single transvenous electrode ~~for a single chamber~~, permanent pacemaker or ~~single chamber~~ pacing cardioverter-defibrillator;

⊙▲ 33220 Repair of 2 transvenous electrodes for ~~a dual chamber~~ permanent pacemaker or ~~dual chamber~~ pacing cardioverter-defibrillator;

▲ 33224 Insertion of pacing electrode, cardiac venous system, for left ventricular pacing, with attachment to previously placed pacemaker or pacing cardioverter-defibrillator pulse generator (including revision of pocket, removal, insertion, and/or replacement of existing generator);

+▲ 33225 Insertion of pacing electrode, cardiac venous system, for left ventricular pacing, at time of insertion of pacing cardioverter-defibrillator or pacemaker pulse generator (including upgrade to dual chamber system and pocket revision) (List separately in addition to code for primary procedure);

▲ 33226 Repositioning of previously implanted cardiac venous system (left ventricular) electrode (including removal, insertion and/or replacement of existing generator);

▲ 33233 Removal of permanent pacemaker pulse generator only;

⊙#● 33227 Code added

⊙#● 33228 Code added

⊙#● 33229 Code added

⊙▲ 33240 Insertion of ~~single or dual chamber~~ pacing cardioverter-defibrillator pulse generator only; with existing single lead

⊙#● 33230 Code added

⊙#● 33231 Code added

⊙▲ 33241 ~~Subcutaneous removal~~Removal of ~~single or dual chamber~~ pacing cardioverter-defibrillator pulse generator only;

⊙#● 33262 Code added

⊙#● 33263 Code added

⊙#● 33264 Code added

⊙▲ 33249 Insertion or ~~repositioning~~replacement of ~~electrode~~permanent pacing cardioverter-defibrillator system with transvenous lead(s) ~~for~~, single or dual chamber ~~pacing cardioverter-defibrillator and insertion of pulse generator~~;

▲ 33960 Prolonged extracorporeal circulation for cardiopulmonary insufficiency; initial ~~24 hours~~day

▲ 33961 each ~~additional 24 hours (List separately in addition to code for primary procedure)~~subsequent day

~~35459~~ ~~tibioperoneal trunk and branches~~

~~35548~~ ~~aortoiliofemoral, unilateral~~

| | |
|---|---|
| 35549 | ~~aortoiliofemoral, bilateral~~ |
| 35551 | ~~aortofemoral-popliteal~~ |
| 35651 | ~~aortofemoral-popliteal~~ |
| ⊙▲ 36200 | Introduction of catheter, aorta; |
| ⊙▲ 36245 | Selective catheter placement, arterial system; each first order abdominal, pelvic, or lower extremity artery branch, within a vascular family |
| ⊙▲ 36246 | initial second order abdominal, pelvic, or lower extremity artery branch, within a vascular family |
| ⊙▲ 36247 | initial third order or more selective abdominal, pelvic, or lower extremity artery branch, within a vascular family |
| ⊙+▲ 36248 | additional second order, third order, and beyond, abdominal, pelvic, or lower extremity artery branch, within a vascular family (List in addition to code for initial second or third order vessel as appropriate) |
| ⊙● 36251 | Code added |
| ⊙● 36252 | Code added |
| ⊙● 36253 | Code added |
| ⊙● 36254 | Code added |
| ⊙● 37191 | Code added |
| ⊙● 37192 | Code added |
| ⊙● 37193 | Code added |
| ● 37619 | Code added |
| 37620 | ~~Interruption, partial or complete, of inferior vena cava by suture, ligation, plication, clip, extravascular, intravascular (umbrella device);~~ |
| ▲ 38208 | thawing of previously frozen harvest, without washing, per donor |
| ▲ 38209 | thawing of previously frozen harvest, with washing, per donor |
| ▲ 38230 | Bone marrow harvesting for transplantation; allogeneic |
| ● 38232 | Code added |
| +▲ 38746 | Thoracic lymphadenectomy, ~~regional~~ by thoracotomy, ~~including~~ mediastinal and ~~peritracheal nodes~~ regional lymphadenectomy (List separately in addition to code for primary procedure); |
| ▲ 38792 | radioactive tracer for identification of sentinel node |
| ▲ 39200 | ~~Excision~~ Resection of mediastinal cyst; |
| ▲ 39220 | ~~Excision~~ Resection of mediastinal tumor; |
| ▲ 39400 | Mediastinoscopy, ~~with or without biopsy~~ includes biopsy(ies), when performed; |
| ⊙▲ 47000 | Biopsy of liver, needle; percutaneous |
| 49080 | ~~Peritoneocentesis, abdominal paracentesis, or peritoneal lavage (diagnostic or therapeutic); initial~~ |
| 49081 | ~~subsequent~~ |
| ● 49082 | Code added |
| ● 49083 | Code added |
| ● 49084 | Code added |
| 49420 | ~~Insertion of intraperitoneal cannula or catheter for drainage or dialysis; temporary~~ |
| ▲ 62287 | Decompression procedure, percutaneous, of nucleus pulposus of intervertebral disc, any method, ~~single~~ utilizing needle based technique to remove disc material under fluoroscopic imaging or ~~multiple levels~~ other form of indirect visualization, ~~lumbar (eg~~ with the use of an endoscope, ~~manual~~ with discography and/or ~~automated percutaneous discectomy~~ epidural injection(s) at the treated level(s), when performed, ~~percutaneous laser discectomy)~~ single or multiple levels, lumbar; |
| ▲ 62310 | Injection, ~~single (not via indwelling catheter), not including neurolytic substances, with or without contrast (for either localization or epidurography)~~ (s), of diagnostic or therapeutic substance(s) (including anesthetic, antispasmodic, opioid, steroid, other solution), not including neurolytic substances, including needle or catheter placement, includes contrast for localization when performed, epidural or subarachnoid; cervical or thoracic |
| ▲ 62311 | lumbar, or sacral (caudal) |
| ▲ 62318 | Injection(s), including indwelling catheter placement, continuous infusion or intermittent bolus, ~~not including neurolytic substances, with or without contrast (for either localization or epidurography)~~, of diagnostic or therapeutic substance(s) (including anesthetic, antispasmodic, opioid, steroid, other solution), not including neurolytic substances, includes contrast for localization when performed, epidural or subarachnoid; cervical or thoracic |
| ▲ 62319 | lumbar, or sacral (caudal) |
| ▲ 62367 | Electronic analysis of programmable, implanted pump for intrathecal or epidural drug infusion (includes evaluation of reservoir status, alarm status, drug prescription status); without reprogramming or refill |
| ● 62369 | Code added |
| ● 62370 | Code added |
| ▲ 63020 | Laminotomy (hemilaminectomy), with decompression of nerve root(s), including partial facetectomy, foraminotomy and/or excision of herniated intervertebral disc, ~~including open and endoscopically-assisted approaches~~; 1 interspace, cervical |
| ▲ 63030 | 1 interspace, lumbar |
| +▲ 63035 | each additional interspace, cervical or lumbar (List separately in addition to code for primary procedure) |
| ▲ 64553 | Percutaneous implantation of neurostimulator electrodes array; cranial nerve |
| ▲ 64555 | peripheral nerve (excludes sacral nerve) |
| 64560 | ~~autonomic nerve~~ |
| ▲ 64561 | sacral nerve (transforaminal placement) |
| ▲ 64565 | neuromuscular |
| ▲ 64575 | Incision for implantation of neurostimulator electrodes array; peripheral nerve (excludes sacral nerve) |
| 64577 | ~~autonomic nerve~~ |
| ▲ 64580 | neuromuscular |
| ▲ 64581 | sacral nerve (transforaminal placement) |
| ▲ 64585 | Revision or removal of peripheral neurostimulator electrodes array; |
| 64622 | ~~Destruction by neurolytic agent, paravertebral facet joint nerve; lumbar or sacral, single level~~ |
| 64623 | ~~lumbar or sacral, each additional level (List separately in addition to code for primary procedure)~~ |
| 64626 | ~~cervical or thoracic, single level~~ |

64627    ~~cervical or thoracic, each additional level (List separately in addition to code for primary procedure)~~

#● 64633    Code added

+#● 64634    Code added

#● 64635    Code added

+#● 64636    Code added

69802    ~~with mastoidectomy~~

## Radiology

▲ 70355    Orthopantogram (eg, panoramic x-ray);

71090    ~~Insertion pacemaker, fluoroscopy and radiography, radiological supervision and interpretation;~~

▲ 72114    complete, including bending views, minimum of 6 views

▲ 72120    bending views only, 2 or 3 views

73542    ~~Radiological examination, sacroiliac joint arthrography, radiological supervision and interpretation;~~

● 74174    Code added

75722    ~~Angiography, renal, unilateral, selective (including flush aortogram), radiological supervision and interpretation;~~

75724    ~~Angiography, renal, bilateral, selective (including flush aortogram), radiological supervision and interpretation;~~

75940    ~~Percutaneous placement of IVC filter, radiological supervision and interpretation;~~

▲ 75962    Transluminal balloon angioplasty, peripheral artery other than ~~cervical carotid, renal,~~ or other visceral artery, iliac or lower extremity, radiological supervision and interpretation;

+▲ 75964    Transluminal balloon angioplasty, each additional peripheral artery other ~~than cervical carotid;~~than  renal, or other visceral artery, iliac ~~and~~or lower extremity, radiological supervision and interpretation (List separately in addition to code for primary procedure);

▲ 77003    Fluoroscopic guidance and localization of needle or catheter tip for spine or paraspinous diagnostic or therapeutic injection procedures (epidural, ~~subarachnoid,~~ or ~~sacroiliac joint~~subarachnoid), ~~including neurolytic agent destruction;~~

77079    ~~appendicular skeleton (peripheral) (eg, radius, wrist, heel)~~

77083    ~~Radiographic absorptiometry (eg, photodensitometry, radiogrammetry), 1 or more sites;~~

#● 77424    Code added

#● 77425    Code added

● 77469    Code added

▲ 77470    Special treatment procedure (eg, total body irradiation, hemibody radiation, per oral~~, endocavitary~~ or ~~intraoperative cone~~endocavitary irradiation);

78220    ~~Liver function study with hepatobiliary agents, with serial images;~~

78223    ~~Hepatobiliary ductal system imaging, including gallbladder, with or without pharmacologic intervention, with or without quantitative measurement of gallbladder function;~~

● 78226    Code added

● 78227    Code added

● 78579    Code added

▲ 78580    Pulmonary perfusion imaging (eg, particulate);

● 78582    Code added

● 78597    Code added

● 78598    Code added

78584    ~~Pulmonary perfusion imaging, particulate, with ventilation; single breath~~

78585    ~~Pulmonary perfusion imaging, particulate, with ventilation; rebreathing and washout, with or without single breath~~

78586    ~~Pulmonary ventilation imaging, aerosol; single projection~~

78587    ~~multiple projections (eg, anterior, posterior, lateral views)~~

78588    ~~Pulmonary perfusion imaging, particulate, with ventilation imaging, aerosol, 1 or multiple projections;~~

78591    ~~Pulmonary ventilation imaging, gaseous, single breath, single projection;~~

78593    ~~Pulmonary ventilation imaging, gaseous, with rebreathing and washout with or without single breath; single projection~~

78594    ~~multiple projections (eg, anterior, posterior, lateral views)~~

78596    ~~Pulmonary quantitative differential function (ventilation/perfusion) study;~~

## Pathology and Laboratory

● 81200    Code added

● 81205    Code added

● 81206    Code added

● 81207    Code added

● 81208    Code added

● 81209    Code added

● 81210    Code added

● 81211    Code added

● 81212    Code added

● 81213    Code added

● 81214    Code added

● 81215    Code added

● 81216    Code added

● 81217    Code added

● 81220    Code added

● 81221    Code added

● 81222    Code added

● 81223    Code added

● 81224    Code added

● 81225    Code added

● 81226    Code added

● 81227    Code added

● 81228    Code added

● 81229    Code added

● 81240    Code added

● 81241    Code added

● 81242    Code added

● 81243    Code added

● 81244    Code added

● 81245    Code added

● 81250    Code added

● 81251    Code added

● 81255    Code added

● 81256    Code added

● 81257    Code added

● 81260    Code added

● 81261    Code added

● 81262    Code added

● 81263    Code added

● 81264    Code added

● 81265    Code added

✚● 81266    Code added

● 81267    Code added

● 81268    Code added

● 81270    Code added

● 81275    Code added

● 81280    Code added

● 81281    Code added

● 81282    Code added

● 81290    Code added

● 81291    Code added

● 81292    Code added

● 81293    Code added

● 81294    Code added

● 81295    Code added

● 81296    Code added

● 81297    Code added

● 81298    Code added

● 81299    Code added

● 81300    Code added

● 81301    Code added

● 81302    Code added

● 81303    Code added

● 81304    Code added

● 81310    Code added

● 81315    Code added

● 81316    Code added

● 81317    Code added

● 81318    Code added

● 81319    Code added

● 81330    Code added

● 81331    Code added

● 81332    Code added

● 81340    Code added

● 81341    Code added

● 81342    Code added

● 81350    Code added

● 81355    Code added

● 81370    Code added

● 81371    Code added

● 81372    Code added

● 81373    Code added

● 81374    Code added

● 81375    Code added

● 81376    Code added

● 81377    Code added

● 81378    Code added

● 81379    Code added

● 81380    Code added

● 81381    Code added

● 81382    Code added

● 81383    Code added

● 81400    Code added

● 81401    Code added

● 81402    Code added

● 81403    Code added

● 81404    Code added

● 81405    Code added

● 81406    Code added

● 81407    Code added

● 81408    Code added

● 86386    Code added

▲ 86703    HIV-1 and HIV-2, single ~~assay~~<u>result</u>

● 87389    Code added

88107    ~~smears and simple filter preparation with interpretation~~

▲ 88312    Special stain<u>s including interpretation and report</u>; Group I for microorganisms (eg, ~~Gridley,~~ acid fast, methenamine silver)~~, including interpretation and report, each~~

▲ 88313    Group II, all other (eg, iron, trichrome), except ~~immunocytochemistry and immunoperoxidase~~<u>stain for microorganisms,</u> stains <u>for enzyme constituents, ~~including interpretation~~<u>or immunocytochemistry</u> and ~~report, each~~<u>immunohistochemistry</u>

✚▲ 88314    histochemical staining ~~with~~ <u>on</u> frozen ~~section(s), including interpretation and report~~<u>tissue block</u> (List separately in addition to code for primary procedure)

88318    ~~Determinative histochemistry to identify chemical components (eg, copper, zinc);~~

▲ 88319    <u>Group III, for enzyme constituents</u>

# Medicine

▲ **90460** Immunization administration through 18 years of age via any route of administration, with counseling by physician or other qualified health care professional; first ~~or only~~ component of each vaccine~~/~~ or toxoid ~~component~~administered

✚▲ **90461** each additional vaccine~~/~~ or toxoid component administered (List separately in addition to code for primary procedure)

**90470** ~~H1N1 immunization administration (intramuscular, intranasal), including counseling when performed;~~

▲ **90581** Anthrax vaccine, for subcutaneous or intramuscular use;

✗▲ **90644** Meningococcal conjugate vaccine, serogroups C & Y and Hemophilus influenza B vaccine~~, tetanus toxoid conjugate (Hib-MenCY-TT)~~ (Hib-MenCY), 4 dose schedule, when administered to children 2-15 months of age, for intramuscular use;

● **90654** Code added

**90663** ~~Influenza virus vaccine, pandemic formulation, H1N1;~~

▲ **90867** Therapeutic repetitive transcranial magnetic stimulation (TMS) treatment; ~~planning~~initial, including cortical mapping, motor threshold determination, delivery and management

▲ **90868** subsequent delivery and management, per session

● **90869** Code added

▲ **91010** Esophageal motility (manometric study of the esophagus and/or gastroesophageal junction) study with interpretation and report~~; 2-dimensional data;~~

**91012** ~~with acid perfusion studies~~

✚▲ **91013** with stimulation or perfusion ~~during 2-dimensional data study~~ (eg, stimulant, acid or alkali perfusion) (List separately in addition to code for primary procedure)

**92070** ~~Fitting of contact lens for treatment of disease, including supply of lens;~~

● **92071** Code added

● **92072** Code added

**92120** ~~Tonography for measurement of aqueous humor outflow facility; with interpretation and report;~~

**92130** ~~Tonography with water provocation;~~

#● **92558** Code added

▲ **92587** ~~Evoked~~Distortion product evoked otoacoustic emissions; limited evaluation (~~single stimulus level~~to confirm the presence or absence of hearing disorder, ~~either~~3-6 frequencies) or transient ~~or distortion products)~~evoked otoacoustic emissions, with interpretation and report

▲ **92588** comprehensive ~~or~~diagnostic evaluation (~~comparison~~quantitative analysis of ~~transient and/or distortion product otoacoustic emissions at multiple levels and~~outer hair cell function by cochlear mapping, minimum of 12 frequencies), with interpretation and report

▲ **92605** Evaluation for prescription of non-speech-generating augmentative and alternative communication device, face-to-face with the patient; first hour

✚#● **92618** Code added

✚▲ **92621** each additional 15 minutes (List separately in addition to code for primary procedure)

▲ **93561** Indicator dilution studies such as dye or ~~thermal dilution~~thermodilution, including arterial and/or venous catheterization; with cardiac output measurement (separate procedure)

▲ **93562** subsequent measurement of cardiac output

**93720** ~~Plethysmography, total body; with interpretation and report~~

**93721** ~~tracing only, without interpretation and report~~

**93722** ~~interpretation and report only~~

**93875** ~~Noninvasive physiologic studies of extracranial arteries, complete bilateral study (eg, periorbital flow direction with arterial compression, ocular pneumoplethysmography, Doppler ultrasound spectral analysis);~~

● **93998** Code added

**94240** ~~Functional residual capacity or residual volume: helium method, nitrogen open circuit method, or other method;~~

**94260** ~~Thoracic gas volume;~~

**94350** ~~Determination of maldistribution of inspired gas: multiple breath nitrogen washout curve including alveolar nitrogen or helium equilibration time;~~

**94360** ~~Determination of resistance to airflow, oscillatory or plethysmographic methods;~~

**94370** ~~Determination of airway closing volume, single breath tests;~~

**94720** ~~Carbon monoxide diffusing capacity (eg, single breath, steady state);~~

**94725** ~~Membrane diffusion capacity;~~

● **94726** Code added

● **94727** Code added

● **94728** Code added

✚● **94729** Code added

● **94780** Code added

✚● **94781** Code added

✚#● **95885** Code added

✚#● **95886** Code added

✚#● **95887** Code added

#● **95938** Code added

#● **95939** Code added

▲ **95970** Electronic analysis of implanted neurostimulator pulse generator system (eg, rate, pulse amplitude ~~and~~, pulse duration, configuration of wave form, battery status, electrode selectability, output modulation, cycling, impedance and patient compliance measurements); simple or complex brain, spinal cord, or peripheral (ie, cranial nerve, peripheral nerve, ~~autonomic~~sacral nerve, neuromuscular) neurostimulator pulse generator/transmitter, without reprogramming

▲ **95971** simple spinal cord, or peripheral (ie, peripheral nerve, ~~autonomic~~sacral nerve, neuromuscular) neurostimulator pulse generator/transmitter, with intraoperative or subsequent programming

▲ **95972** complex spinal cord, or peripheral (ie, peripheral nerve, autonomic nerve, sacral nerve, neuromuscular) (except cranial nerve) neurostimulator pulse generator/transmitter, with intraoperative or subsequent programming, first hour

+▲ 95973  complex spinal cord, or peripheral (ie, peripheral nerve, autonomic nerve, sacral nerve, neuromuscular) (except cranial nerve) neurostimulator pulse generator/transmitter, with intraoperative or subsequent programming, each additional 30 minutes after first hour (List separately in addition to code for primary procedure)

▲ 95974  complex cranial nerve neurostimulator pulse generator/transmitter, with intraoperative or subsequent programming, with or without nerve interface testing, first hour

+▲ 95975  complex cranial nerve neurostimulator pulse generator/transmitter, with intraoperative or subsequent programming, each additional 30 minutes after first hour (List separately in addition to code for primary procedure)

▲ 95990  Refilling and maintenance of implantable pump or reservoir for drug delivery, spinal (intrathecal, epidural) or brain (intraventricular), includes electronic analysis of pump, when performed;

▲ 95991  administered byrequiring physician's skill

▲ 96110  Developmental testingscreening, with interpretation and report, per standardized instrument form; limited (eg, Developmental Screening Test II, Early Language Milestone Screen), with interpretation and report

▲ 96111  Developmental testing, (includes assessment of motor, language, social, adaptive, and/or cognitive functioning by standardized developmental instruments) with interpretation and report; extended (includes assessment of motor, language, social, adaptive and/or cognitive functioning by standardized developmental instruments) with interpretation and report

+▲ 96367  additional sequential infusion of a new drug/substance, up to 1 hour (List separately in addition to code for primary procedure)

## Category II Codes

● 0550F  Code added
● 0551F  Code added
● 0555F  Code added
● 0556F  Code added
● 0557F  Code added
● 1010F  Code added
● 1011F  Code added
● 1012F  Code added
● 1031F  Code added
● 1032F  Code added
● 1033F  Code added
1128F  Subsequent episode for condition (ML)[5];
▲ 1127F  New episode for condition (NMA-No Measure Associated);
▲ 1128F  Subsequent episode for condition (NMA-No Measure Associated);
● 1175F  Code added
● 1181F  Code added
● 1182F  Code added
● 1183F  Code added

● 1450F  Code added
● 1451F  Code added
● 1460F  Code added
● 1461F  Code added
● 1490F  Code added
● 1491F  Code added
● 1493F  Code added
● 1494F  Code added
● 2015F  Code added
● 2016F  Code added
● 3019F  Code added
● 3055F  Code added
● 3056F  Code added
▲ 3111F  CT or MRI of the brain performed in the hospital within 24 hours of arrival OR performed in an outpatient imaging center, to confirm initial diagnosis of stroke, TIA or intracranial hemorrhage (STR)[5];
▲ 3112F  CT or MRI of the brain performed greater than 24 hours after arrival to the hospital OR performed in an outpatient imaging center for purpose other than confirmation of initial diagnosis of stroke, TIA, or intracranial hemorrhage (STR)[5];
● 3115F  Code added
● 3117F  Code added
● 3118F  Code added
● 3119F  Code added
● 3125F  Code added
● 3267F  Code added
● 3394F  Code added
● 3395F  Code added
● 3725F  Code added
▲ 4004F  Patient screened for tobacco use AND received tobacco cessation intervention (counseling, pharmacotherapy, or both), if identified as a tobacco user (PV)(PV, CAD)[1];
● 4008F  Code added
● 4010F  Code added
● 4013F  Code added
● 4086F  Code added
● 4140F  Code added
● 4144F  Code added
● 4145F  Code added
4275F  Hepatitis B vaccine injection administered or previously received (HIV)[5];
● 4322F  Code added
● 4350F  Code added
● 4450F  Code added
● 4470F  Code added
● 4480F  Code added
● 4481F  Code added

● 4500F    Code added

● 4510F    Code added

● 4525F    Code added

● 4526F    Code added

● 5250F    Code added

● 6100F    Code added

● 6101F    Code added

● 6102F    Code added

● 6110F    Code added

## Category III Codes

▲ 0080T    Endovascular repair using prosthesis of abdominal aortic aneurysm, pseudoaneurysm or dissection, abdominal aorta involving visceral vessels (superior mesenteric, celiac and/or renal), using fenestrated modular bifurcated prosthesis (2 docking limbs artery[s]), radiological supervision and interpretation;

0143T    Laparoscopy, surgical, pancreatic islet cell transplantation through portal vein;

0155T    Laparoscopy, surgical; implantation or replacement of gastric stimulation electrodes, lesser curvature (ie, morbid obesity)

0156T    revision or removal of gastric stimulation electrodes, lesser curvature (ie, morbid obesity)

0157T    Laparotomy, implantation or replacement of gastric stimulation electrodes, lesser curvature (ie, morbid obesity);

0158T    Laparotomy, revision or removal of gastric stimulation electrodes, lesser curvature (ie, morbid obesity);

0161T    Therapeutic repetitive transcranial magnetic stimulation treatment delivery and management, per session;

0166T    Transmyocardial transcatheter closure of ventricular septal defect, with implant; without cardiopulmonary bypass

0167T    with cardiopulmonary bypass

0168T    Rhinophototherapy, intranasal application of ultraviolet and visible light, bilateral;

▲ 0240T    Esophageal motility (manometric study of the esophagus and/or gastroesophageal junction) study with interpretation and report; with 3-dimensional high resolution esophageal pressure topography

+▲ 0241T    with stimulation or perfusion during 3-dimensional high resolution esophageal pressure topography study; (eg, stimulant, acid or alkali perfusion) (List separately in addition to code for primary procedure)

● 0260T    Code added

● 0261T    Code added

● 0262T    Code added

● 0263T    Code added

● 0264T    Code added

● 0265T    Code added

● 0266T    Code added

● 0267T    Code added

● 0268T    Code added

● 0269T    Code added

● 0270T    Code added

● 0271T    Code added

● 0272T    Code added

● 0273T    Code added

● 0274T    Code added

● 0275T    Code added

⊙ ● 0276T    Code added

⊙ ● 0277T    Code added

● 0278T    Code added

● 0279T    Code added

● 0280T    Code added

● 0281T    Code added

⊙ ● 0282T    Code added

⊙ ● 0283T    Code added

⊙ ● 0284T    Code added

● 0285T    Code added

● 0286T    Code added

● 0287T    Code added

● 0288T    Code added

+● 0289T    Code added

+● 0290T    Code added

# Appendix C

## Clinical Examples

As described in *CPT 2012*, clinical examples of the CPT codes for Evaluation and Management (E/M) services are intended to be an important element of the coding system. The clinical examples, when used with the E/M descriptors contained in the full text of *CPT*, provide a comprehensive and powerful tool for physicians to report the services provided to their patients.

The American Medical Association is pleased to provide you with these clinical examples for *CPT 2012*. The clinical examples that are provided in this supplement are limited to Office or Other Outpatient Services, Hospital Inpatient Services, Consultations, Critical Care, Prolonged Services and Care Plan Oversight.

These clinical examples do not encompass the entire scope of medical practice. Inclusion or exclusion of any particular specialty group does not infer any judgment of importance or lack thereof; nor does it limit the applicability of the example to any particular specialty.

Of utmost importance is that these clinical examples are just that: examples. A particular patient encounter, depending on the specific circumstances, must be judged by the services provided by the physician for that particular patient. Simply because the patient's complaints, symptoms, or diagnoses match those of a particular clinical example, does not automatically assign that patient encounter to that particular level of service. The three components (history, examination, and medical decision making) must be met and documented in the medical record to report a particular level of service.

## Office or Other Outpatient Service

### New Patient

99201 Initial office visit for a 50-year-old male from out-of-town who needs a prescription refill for a nonsteroidal anti-inflammatory drug. (Anesthesiology)

Initial office visit for a 40-year-old female, new patient, requesting information about local pain clinics. (Anesthesiology/Pain Medicine)

Initial office visit for a 10-year-old girl for determination of visual acuity as part of a summer camp physical (does not include determination of refractive error). (Ophthalmology)

Initial office visit for an out-of-town patient requiring topical refill. (Dermatology)

Initial office visit for a 65-year-old male for reassurance about an isolated seborrheic keratosis on upper back. (Plastic Surgery)

Initial office visit for an out-of-state visitor who needs refill of topical steroid to treat lichen planus. (Dermatology)

Initial office visit for an 86-year-old male, out-of-town visitor, who needs prescription refilled for an anal skin preparation that he forgot. (General Surgery/Colon & Rectal Surgery)

Initial office visit for a patient with alveolar osteitis for repacking. (Oral & Maxillofacial Surgery)

Initial office visit for a patient with a pedunculated lesion of the neck, which is unsightly. (Dermatology)

Initial office visit for a 10-year-old male, for limited subungual hematoma not requiring drainage. (Internal Medicine)

Initial office visit with an out-of-town visitor who needs a prescription refilled because she forgot her hay fever medication. (Allergy & Immunology/Internal Medicine)

Initial office visit with a 9-month-old female with diaper rash. (Pediatrics)

Initial office visit with a 10-year-old male with severe rash and itching for the past 24 hours, positive history for contact with poison oak 48 hours prior to the visit. (Family Medicine)

Initial office visit with a 5-year-old female to remove sutures from simple wound placed by another physician. (Plastic Surgery)

Initial office visit for a 22-year-old male with a small area of sunburn requiring first aid. (Dermatology/Family Medicine/Internal Medicine)

Initial office visit for the evaluation and management of a contusion of a finger. (Orthopaedic Surgery)

99202 Initial office visit for a 13-year-old patient with comedopapular acne of the face unresponsive to over-the-counter medications. (Family Medicine)

Initial office visit for a patient with a clinically benign lesion or nodule of the lower leg which has been present for many years. (Dermatology)

Initial office visit for a patient with a circumscribed patch of dermatitis of the leg. (Dermatology)

Initial office visit for a patient with papulosquamous eruption of elbows. (Dermatology)

Initial office visit for a 9-year-old patient with erythematous grouped, vesicular eruption of the lip of three day's duration. (Pediatrics)

Initial office visit for an 18-year-old male referred by an orthodontist for advice regarding removal of four wisdom teeth. (Oral & Maxillofacial Surgery)

Initial office visit for a 14-year-old male, who was referred by his orthodontist, for advice on the exposure of impacted maxillary cuspids. (Oral & Maxillofacial Surgery)

Initial office visit for a patient presenting with itching patches on the wrists and ankles. (Dermatology)

Initial office visit for a 30-year-old male for evaluation and discussion of treatment of rhinophyma. (Plastic Surgery)

Initial office visit for a 16-year-old male with severe cystic acne, new patient. (Dermatology)

Initial office evaluation for gradual hearing loss, 58-year-old male, history and physical examination, with interpretation of complete audiogram, air bone, etc. (Otolaryngology)

Initial evaluation and management of recurrent urinary infection in female. (Internal Medicine)

Initial office visit with a 10-year-old girl with history of chronic otitis media and a draining ear. (Pediatrics)

Initial office visit for a 10-year-old female with acute maxillary sinusitis. (Family Medicine)

Initial office visit for a patient with recurring episodes of herpes simplex who has developed a clustering of vesicles on the upper lip. (Internal Medicine)

Initial office visit for a 25-year-old patient with a single season allergic rhinitis. (Allergy & Immunology)

**99203** Initial office visit of a 76-year-old male with a stasis ulcer of three month's duration. (Dermatology)

Initial office visit for a 30-year-old female with pain in the lateral aspect of the forearm. (Physical Medicine & Rehabilitation)

Initial office visit for a 15-year-old patient with a four-year history of moderate comedopapular acne of the face, chest, and back with early scarring. Discussion of use of systemic medication. (Dermatology)

Initial office visit for a patient with papulosquamous eruption of the elbow with pitting of nails and itchy scalp. (Dermatology)

Initial office visit for a 57-year-old female who complains of painful parotid swelling for one week's duration. (Oral & Maxillofacial Surgery)

Initial office visit for a patient with an ulcerated non-healing lesion or nodule on the tip of the nose. (Dermatology)

Initial office visit for a patient with dermatitis of the antecubital and popliteal fossae. (Dermatology)

Initial office visit for a 22-year-old female with irregular menses. (Family Medicine)

Initial office visit for a 50-year-old female with dyspepsia and nausea. (Family Medicine)

Initial office visit for a 53-year-old laborer with degenerative joint disease of the knee with no prior treatment. (Orthopaedic Surgery)

Initial office visit for a 60-year-old male with Dupuytren's contracture of one hand with multiple digit involvement. (Orthopaedic Surgery)

Initial office visit for a 33-year-old male with painless gross hematuria without cystoscopy. (Internal Medicine)

Initial office visit for a 55-year-old female with chronic blepharitis. There is a history of use of many medications. (Ophthalmology)

Initial office visit for an 18-year-old female with a two-day history of acute conjunctivitis. Extensive history of possible exposures, prior normal ocular history, and medication use is obtained. (Ophthalmology)

Initial office visit for a 14-year-old male with unilateral anterior knee pain. (Physical Medicine & Rehabilitation)

Initial office visit of an adult who presents with symptoms of an upper-respiratory infection that has progressed to unilateral purulent nasal discharge and discomfort in the right maxillary teeth. (Otolaryngology, Head & Neck Surgery)

Initial office visit of a 40-year-old female with symptoms of atopic allergies including eye and sinus congestion, often associated with infections. She would like to be tested for allergies. (Otolaryngology, Head & Neck Surgery)

Initial office visit of a 65-year-old with nasal stuffiness. (Otolaryngology, Head & Neck Surgery)

Initial office visit for initial evaluation of a 48-year-old man with recurrent low back pain radiating to the leg. (General Surgery)

Initial office visit for evaluation, diagnosis, and management of painless gross hematuria in a new patient, without cystoscopy. (Internal Medicine)

Initial office visit with couple for counseling concerning voluntary vasectomy for sterility. Spent 30 minutes discussing procedure, risks and benefits, and answering questions. (Urology)

Initial office visit of a 49-year-old male with nasal obstruction. Detailed exam with topical anesthesia. (Plastic Surgery)

Initial office visit for evaluation of a 13-year-old female with progressive scoliosis. (Physical Medicine & Rehabilitation)

Initial office visit for a 21-year-old female desiring counseling and evaluation of initiation of contraception. (Family Practice/Internal Medicine/Obstetrics & Gynecology)

Initial office visit for a 49-year-old male presenting with painless blood per rectum associated with bowel movement. (Colon & Rectal Surgery)

Initial office visit for a 19-year-old football player with three-day-old acute knee injury; now with swelling and pain. (Orthopaedic Surgery)

**99204**   Initial office visit for a 13-year-old female with progressive scoliosis. (Orthopaedic Surgery)

Initial office visit for a 34-year-old female with primary infertility for evaluation and counseling. (Obstetrics & Gynecology)

Initial office visit for a 6-year-old male with multiple upper respiratory infections. (Allergy & Immunology)

Initial office visit for a patient with generalized dermatitis of 80 percent of the body surface area. (Dermatology)

Initial office visit for an adolescent who was referred by school counselor because of repeated skipping school. (Psychiatry)

Initial office visit for a 50-year-old machinist with a generalized eruption. (Dermatology)

Initial office visit for a 45-year-old female who has been abstinent from alcohol and benzodiazepines for three months but complains of headaches, insomnia, and anxiety. (Psychiatry)

Initial office visit for a 60-year-old male with recent change in bowel habits, weight loss, and abdominal pain. (Abdominal Surgery/General Surgery)

Initial office visit for a 50-year-old male with an aortic aneurysm who is considering surgery. (General Surgery)

Initial office visit for a 17-year-old female with depression. (Internal Medicine)

Initial office visit of a 40-year-old with chronic draining ear, imbalance, and probable cholesteatoma. (Otolaryngology, Head & Neck Surgery)

Initial office visit for initial evaluation of a 63-year-old male with chest pain on exertion. (Cardiology/Internal Medicine)

Initial office visit for evaluation of a 70-year-old patient with recent onset of episodic confusion. (Internal Medicine)

Initial office visit for a 7-year-old female with juvenile diabetes mellitus, new to area, past history of hospitalization times three. (Pediatrics)

Initial office visit of a 50-year-old female with progressive solid food dysphagia. (Gastroenterology)

Initial office visit for a 34-year-old patient with primary infertility, including counseling. (Obstetrics & Gynecology)

Initial office visit for evaluation of a 70-year-old female with polyarthralgia. (Rheumatology)

Initial office visit for a patient with papulosquamous eruption involving 60 percent of the cutaneous surface with joint pain. Combinations of topical and systemic treatments discussed. (Dermatology)

**99205**   Initial office visit for a patient with disseminated lupus erythematosus with kidney disease, edema, purpura, and scarring lesions on the extremities plus cardiac symptoms. (Dermatology/General Surgery/Internal Medicine)

Initial office visit for a 25-year-old female with systemic lupus erythematosus, fever, seizures, and profound thrombocytopenia. (Rheumatology/Allergy & Immunology)

Initial office visit for an adult with multiple cutaneous blisters, denuded secondarily infected ulcerations, oral lesions, weight loss, and increasing weakness refractory to high dose corticosteroid. Initiation of new immunosuppressive therapy. (Dermatology)

Initial office visit for a 28-year-old male with systemic vasculitis and compromised circulation to the limbs. (Rheumatology)

Initial office visit for a 41-year-old female new to the area requesting rheumatologic care, on disability due to scleroderma and recent hospitalization for malignant hypertension. (Rheumatology)

Initial office visit for a 52-year-old female with acute four extremity weakness and shortness of breath one week post-flu vaccination. (Physical Medicine & Rehabilitation)

Initial office visit for a 60-year-old male with previous back surgery; now presents with back and pelvic pain, two-month history of bilateral progressive calf and thigh tightness and weakness when walking, causing several falls. (Orthopaedic Surgery)

Initial office visit for an adolescent referred from emergency room after making suicide gesture. (Psychiatry)

Initial office visit for a 49-year-old female with a history of headaches and dependence on opioids. She reports weight loss, progressive headache, and depression. (Psychiatry)

Initial office visit for a 50-year-old female with symptoms of rash, swellings, recurrent arthritic complaints, and diarrhea and lymphadenopathy. Patient has had a 25 lb weight loss and was recently camping in the Amazon. (Allergy & Immunology)

Initial office visit for a 34-year-old uremic Type I diabetic patient referred for ESRD modality assessment and planning. (Nephrology)

Initial office visit for a 75-year-old female with neck and bilateral shoulder pain, brisk deep tendon reflexes, and stress incontinence. (Physical Medicine & Rehabilitation)

Initial office visit for an 8-year-old male with cerebral palsy and spastic quadriparesis. (Physical Medicine & Rehabilitation)

Initial office visit for a 73-year-old male with known prostate malignancy, who presents with severe back pain and a recent onset of lower extremity weakness. (Physical Medicine & Rehabilitation)

Initial office visit for a 38-year-old male with paranoid delusions and a history of alcohol abuse. (Psychiatry)

Initial office visit for a 12-week-old with bilateral hip dislocations and bilateral club feet. (Orthopaedic Surgery)

Initial office visit for a 29-year-old female with acute orbital congestion, eyelid retraction, and bilateral visual loss from optic neuropathy. (Ophthalmology)

Initial office visit for a 70-year-old diabetic patient with progressive visual field loss, advanced optic disc cupping and neovascularization of retina. (Ophthalmology)

Initial office visit for a newly diagnosed Type I diabetic patient. (Endocrinology)

Initial office evaluation of a 65-year-old female with exertional chest pain, intermittent claudication, syncope and a murmur of aortic stenosis. (Cardiology)

Initial office visit for a 73-year-old male with an unexplained 20 lb weight loss. (Hematology/Oncology)

Initial office evaluation, patient with systemic lupus erythematosus, fever, seizures and profound thrombocytopenia. (Allergy & Immunology/Internal Medicine/Rheumatology)

Initial office evaluation and management of patient with systemic vasculitis and compromised circulation to the limbs. (Rheumatology)

Initial office visit for a 24-year-old homosexual male who has a fever, a cough, and shortness of breath. (Infectious Disease)

Initial outpatient evaluation of a 69-year-old male with severe chronic obstructive pulmonary disease, congestive heart failure, and hypertension. (Family Medicine)

Initial office visit for a 17-year-old female, who is having school problems and has told a friend that she is considering suicide. The patient and her family are consulted in regard to treatment options. (Psychiatry)

Initial office visit for a female with severe hirsutism, amenorrhea, weight loss and a desire to have children. (Endocrinology/Obstetrics & Gynecology)

Initial office visit for a 42-year-old male on hypertensive medication, newly arrived to the area, with diastolic blood pressure of 110, history of recurrent calculi, episodic headaches, intermittent chest pain and orthopnea. (Internal Medicine)

## Established Patient

**99211**  Office visit for an 82-year-old female, established patient, for a monthly B12 injection with documented Vitamin B12 deficiency. (Geriatrics/Internal Medicine/Family Medicine)

Office visit for a 50-year-old male, established patient, for removal of uncomplicated facial sutures. (Plastic Surgery)

Office visit for an established patient who lost prescription for lichen planus. Returned for new copy. (Dermatology)

Office visit for an established patient undergoing orthodontics who complains of a wire which is irritating his/her cheek and asks you to check it. (Oral & Maxillofacial Surgery)

Office visit for a 50-year-old female, established patient, seen for her gold injection by the nurse. (Rheumatology)

Office visit for a 73-year-old female, established patient, with pernicious anemia for weekly B12 injection. (Gastroenterology)

Office visit for an established patient for dressing change on a skin biopsy. (Dermatology)

Office visit for a 19-year-old, established patient, for removal of sutures from a 2 cm laceration of forehead, which you placed four days ago in ER. (Plastic Surgery)

Office visit of a 20-year-old female, established patient, who receives an allergy vaccine injection and is observed for a reaction by the nurse. (Otolaryngology, Head & Neck Surgery)

Office visit for a 45-year-old male, established patient, with chronic renal failure for the administration of erythropoietin. (Nephrology)

Office visit for an established patient, a Peace Corps enlistee, who requests documentation that third molars have been removed. (Oral & Maxillofacial Surgery)

Office visit for a 69-year-old female, established patient, for partial removal of antibiotic gauze from an infected wound site. (Plastic Surgery)

Office visit for a 9-year-old, established patient, successfully treated for impetigo, requiring release to return to school. (Dermatology/Pediatrics)

Office visit for an established patient requesting a return-to-work certificate for resolving contact dermatitis. (Dermatology)

Office visit for an established patient who is performing glucose monitoring and wants to check accuracy of machine with lab blood glucose by technician who checks accuracy and function of patient machine. (Endocrinology)

Follow-up office visit for a 65-year-old female with a chronic indwelling percutaneous nephrostomy catheter seen for routine pericatheter skin care and dressing change. (Interventional Radiology)

Outpatient visit with 19-year-old male, established patient, for supervised drug screen. (Addiction Medicine)

Office visit with 12-year-old male, established patient, for cursory check of hematoma one day after venipuncture. (Internal Medicine)

Office visit with 31-year-old female, established patient, for return to work certificate. (Anesthesiology)

Office visit for a 42-year-old, established patient, to read tuberculin test results. (Allergy & Immunology)

Office visit for 14-year-old, established patient, to re-dress an abrasion. (Orthopaedic Surgery)

Office visit for a 45-year-old female, established patient, for a blood pressure check. (Obstetrics & Gynecology)

Office visit for a 23-year-old, established patient, for instruction in use of peak flow meter. (Allergy & Immunology)

Office visit for prescription refill for a 35-year-old female, established patient, with schizophrenia who is stable but has run out of neuroleptic and is scheduled to be seen in a week. (Psychiatry)

**99212** Office visit for an 11-year-old, established patient, seen in follow-up for mild comedonal acne of the cheeks on topical desquamating agents. (Dermatology/Family Medicine/Pediatrics)

Office visit for a 10-year-old female, established patient, who has been swimming in a lake, now presents with a one-day history of left ear pain with purulent drainage. (Family Medicine)

Office visit for a child, established patient, with chronic secretory otitis media. (Otolaryngology, Head & Neck Surgery)

Office visit for an established patient seen in follow-up of clearing patch of localized contact dermatitis. (Family Medicine/Dermatology)

Office visit for an established patient returning for evaluation of response to treatment of lichen planus on wrists and ankles. (Dermatology)

Office visit for an established patient with tinea pedis being treated with topical therapy. (Dermatology)

Office visit for an established patient with localized erythematous plaque of psoriasis with topical hydration. (Dermatology)

Office visit for a 50-year-old male, established patient, recently seen for acute neck pain, diagnosis of spondylosis, responding to physical therapy and intermittent cervical traction. Returns for evaluation for return to work. (Neurology)

Office visit for an established patient with recurring episodes of herpes simplex who has developed a clustering of vesicles on the upper lip. (Oral & Maxillofacial Surgery)

Evaluation of a 50-year-old male, established patient, who has experienced a recurrence of knee pain after he discontinued NSAID. (Anesthesiology/Pain Medicine)

Office visit for an established patient with an irritated skin tag for reassurance. (Dermatology)

Office visit for a 40-year-old, established patient, who has experienced a systemic allergic reaction following administration of immunotherapy. The dose must be readjusted. (Allergy & Immunology)

Office visit for a 33-year-old, established patient, for contusion and abrasion of lower extremity. (Orthopaedic Surgery)

Office visit for a 22-year-old male, established patient, one month after I & D of "wrestler's ear". (Plastic Surgery)

Office visit for a 21-year-old, established patient, who is seen in follow-up after antibiotic therapy for acute bacterial tonsillitis. (Otolaryngology, Head & Neck Surgery)

Office visit for a 4-year-old, established patient, with tympanostomy tubes, check-up. (Otolaryngology, Head & Neck Surgery)

Office visit for an established patient who has had needle aspiration of a peritonsillar abscess. (Otolaryngology, Head & Neck Surgery)

Follow-up office examination for evaluation and treatment of acute draining ear in a 5-year-old with tympanotomy tubes. (Otolaryngology, Head & Neck Surgery)

Office visit, established patient, 6-year-old with sore throat and headache. (Family Medicine/Pediatrics)

Office evaluation for possible purulent bacterial conjunctivitis with one- to two-day history of redness and discharge, 16-year-old female, established patient. (Pediatrics/Internal Medicine/Family Medicine)

Office visit for a 65-year-old female, established patient, returns for three-week follow-up for resolving severe ankle sprain. (Orthopaedic Surgery)

Office visit, sore throat, fever, and fatigue in a 19-year-old college student, established patient. (Internal Medicine)

Office visit with a 33-year-old female, established patient, recently started on treatment for hemorrhoidal complaints, for re-evaluation. (Colon & Rectal Surgery)

Office visit with a 36-year-old male, established patient, for follow-up on effectiveness of medicine management of oral candidiasis. (Oral & Maxillofacial Surgery)

Office visit for a 27-year-old female, established patient, with complaints of vaginal itching. (Obstetrics & Gynecology)

Office visit for a 65-year-old, established patient, with eruptions on both arms from poison oak exposure. (Allergy & Immunology/Internal Medicine)

**99213** Office visit for an established patient with new lesions of lichen planus in spite of topical therapies. (Dermatology)

Office visit for the quarterly follow-up of a 45-year-old male with stable chronic asthma requiring regular drug therapy. (Allergy & Immunology)

Office visit for a 13-year-old, established patient, with comedopapular acne of the face which has shown poor response to topical medication. Discussion of use of systemic medication. (Dermatology)

Office visit for a 62-year-old female, established patient, for follow-up for stable cirrhosis of the liver. (Internal Medicine/Family Medicine)

Office visit for a 3-year-old, established patient, with atopic dermatitis and food hypersensitivity for quarterly follow-up evaluation. The patient is on topical lotions and steroid creams as well as oral antihistamines. (Allergy & Immunology)

Office visit for an 80-year-old female, established patient, to evaluate medical management of osteoarthritis of the temporomandibular joint. (Rheumatology)

Office visit for a 70-year-old female, established patient, one year post excision of basal cell carcinoma of nose with nasolabial flap. Now presents with new suspicious recurrent lesion and suspicious lesion of the back. (Plastic Surgery)

Office visit for a 68-year-old female, established patient, with polymyalgia rheumatic, maintained on chronic low-dose corticosteroid, with no new complaints. (Rheumatology)

Office visit for a 3-year-old female, established patient, for earache and dyshidrosis of feet. (Pediatrics/Family Medicine)

Office visit for an established patient for 18-months post-operative follow-up of TMJ repair. (Oral & Maxillofacial Surgery)

Office visit for a 45-year-old male, established patient, being re-evaluated for recurrent acute prostatitis. (Urology)

Office visit for a 43-year-old male, established patient, with known reflex sympathetic dystrophy. (Anesthesiology)

Office visit for an established patient with an evenly pigmented superficial nodule of leg which is symptomatic. (Dermatology)

Office visit for an established patient with psoriasis involvement of the elbows, pitting of the nails, and itchy scalp. (Dermatology)

Office visit for a 27-year-old male, established patient, with deep follicular and perifollicular inflammation unable to tolerate systemic antibiotics due to GI upset, requires change of systemic medication. (Dermatology)

Office visit for a 16-year-old male, established patient, who is on medication for exercise-induced bronchospasm. (Allergy & Immunology)

Office visit for a 60-year-old, established patient, with chronic essential hypertension on multiple drug regimen, for blood pressure check. (Family Medicine)

Office visit for a 20-year-old male, established patient, for removal of sutures in hand. (Family Medicine)

Office visit for a 58-year-old female, established patient, with unilateral painful bunion. (Orthopaedic Surgery)

Office visit for a 45-year-old female, established patient, with known osteoarthritis and painful swollen knees. (Rheumatology)

Office visit for a 25-year-old female, established patient, complaining of bleeding and heavy menses. (Obstetrics & Gynecology)

Office visit for a 55-year-old male, established patient, with hypertension managed by a beta blocker/thiazide regime; now experiencing mild fatigue. (Nephrology)

Office visit for a 65-year-old female, established patient, with primary glaucoma for interval determination of intraocular pressure and possible adjustment of medication. (Ophthalmology)

Office visit for a 56-year-old male, established patient, with stable exertional angina who complains of new onset of calf pain while walking. (Cardiology)

Office visit for a 63-year-old female, established patient, with rheumatoid arthritis on auranofin and ibuprofen, seen for routine follow-up visit. (Rheumatology)

Office visit for an established patient with Graves' disease, three months post I-131 therapy, who presents with lassitude and malaise. (Endocrinology)

Office visit for the quarterly follow-up of a 63-year-old male, established patient, with chronic myofascial pain syndrome, effectively managed by doxepin, who presents with new onset urinary hesitancy. (Pain Medicine)

Office visit for the biannual follow-up of an established patient with migraine variant having infrequent, intermittent, moderate to severe headaches with nausea and vomiting, which are sometimes effectively managed by ergotamine tartrate and an antiemetic, but occasionally requiring visits to an emergency department. (Pain Medicine)

Office visit for an established patient after discharge from a pain rehabilitation program to review and adjust medication dosage. (Pain Medicine)

Office visit with 55-year-old male, established patient, for management of hypertension, mild fatigue, on beta blocker/thiazide regimen. (Family Medicine/Internal Medicine)

Outpatient visit with 37-year-old male, established patient, who is three years post total colectomy for chronic ulcerative colitis, presents for increased irritation at his stoma. (General Surgery)

Office visit for a 70-year-old diabetic hypertensive established patient with recent change in insulin requirement. (Internal Medicine/Nephrology)

Office visit with 80-year-old female, established patient, for follow-up osteoporosis, status-post compression fractures. (Rheumatology)

Office visit for an established patient with stable cirrhosis of the liver. (Gastroenterology)

Routine, follow-up office evaluation at a three-month interval for a 77-year-old female, established patient, with nodular small cleaved-cell lymphoma. (Hematology/Oncology)

Quarterly follow-up office visit for a 45-year-old male, established patient, with stable chronic asthma, on steroid and bronchodilator therapy. (Pulmonary Medicine)

Office visit for a 50-year-old female, established patient, with insulin-dependent diabetes mellitus and stable coronary artery disease, for monitoring. (Family Medicine/Internal Medicine)

**99214** Office visit for an established patient now presenting with generalized dermatitis of 80% of the body surface area. (Dermatology)

Office visit for a 32-year-old female, established patient, with new onset right lower quadrant pain. (Family Medicine)

Office visit for reassessment and reassurance/counseling of a 40-year-old female, established patient, who is experiencing increased symptoms while on a pain management treatment program. (Pain Medicine)

Office visit for a 30-year-old, established patient, under management for intractable low back pain, who now presents with new onset right posterior thigh pain. (Pain Medicine)

Office visit for an established patient with frequent intermittent, moderate to severe headaches requiring beta blocker or tricyclic antidepressant prophylaxis, as well as four symptomatic treatments, but who is still experiencing headaches at a frequency of several times a month that are unresponsive to treatment. (Pain Medicine)

Office visit for an established patient with psoriasis with extensive involvement of scalp, trunk, palms, and soles with joint pain. Combinations of topical and systemic treatments discussed and instituted. (Dermatology)

Office visit for a 55-year-old male, established patient, with increasing night pain, limp, and progressive varus of both knees. (Orthopaedic Surgery)

Follow-up visit for a 15-year-old withdrawn patient with four-year history of papulocystic acne of the face, chest, and back with early scarring and poor response to past treatment. Discussion of use of systemic medication. (Dermatology)

Office visit for a 28-year-old male, established patient, with regional enteritis, diarrhea, and low-grade fever. (Internal Medicine)

Office visit for a 25-year-old female, established patient, following recent arthrogram and MR imaging for TMJ pain. (Oral & Maxillofacial Surgery)

Office visit for a 32-year-old female, established patient, with large obstructing stone in left mid-ureter, to discuss management options including urethroscopy with extraction or ESWL. (Urology)

Evaluation for a 28-year-old male, established patient, with new onset of low back pain. (Anesthesiology/Pain Medicine)

Office visit for a 28-year-old female, established patient, with right lower quadrant abdominal pain, fever, and anorexia. (Internal Medicine/Family Medicine)

Office visit for a 45-year-old male, established patient, four months follow-up of L4-5 discectomy, with persistent incapacitating low back and leg pain. (Orthopaedic Surgery)

Outpatient visit for a 77-year-old male, established patient, with hypertension, presenting with a three-month history of episodic substernal chest pain on exertion. (Cardiology)

Office visit for a 25-year-old female, established patient, for evaluation of progressive saddle nose deformity of unknown etiology. (Plastic Surgery)

Office visit for a 65-year-old male, established patient, with BPH and severe bladder outlet obstruction, to discuss management options such as TURP. (Urology)

Office visit for an adult diabetic established patient with a past history of recurrent sinusitis who presents with a one-week history of double vision. (Otolaryngology, Head & Neck Surgery)

Office visit for an established patient with lichen planus and 60% of the cutaneous surface involved, not responsive to systemic steroids, as well as developing symptoms of progressive heartburn and paranoid ideation. (Dermatology)

Office visit for a 52-year-old male, established patient, with a 12-year history of bipolar disorder responding to lithium carbonate and brief psychotherapy. Psychotherapy and prescription provided. (Psychiatry)

Office visit for a 63-year-old female, established patient, with a history of familial polyposis, status post-colectomy with sphincter sparing procedure, who now presents with rectal bleeding and increase in stooling frequency. (General Surgery)

Office visit for a 68-year-old male, established patient, with the sudden onset of multiple flashes and floaters in the right eye due to a posterior vitreous detachment. (Ophthalmology)

Office visit for a 55-year-old female, established patient, on cyclosporin for treatment of resistant, small vessel vasculitis. (Rheumatology)

Follow-up office visit for a 55-year-old male, two months after iliac angioplasty with new onset of contralateral extremity claudication. (Interventional Radiology)

Office visit for a 68-year-old male, established patient, with stable angina, two months post myocardial infarction, who is not tolerating one of his medications. (Cardiology)

Weekly office visit for 5FU therapy for an ambulatory established patient with metastatic colon cancer and increasing shortness of breath. (Hematology/Oncology)

Follow-up office visit for a 60-year-old male, established patient, whose post-traumatic seizures have disappeared on medication and who now raises the question of stopping the medication. (Neurology)

Office evaluation on new onset RLQ pain in a 32-year-old female, established patient. (Urology/General Surgery/Internal Medicine/Family Medicine)

Office evaluation of 28-year-old, established patient, with regional enteritis, diarrhea, and low-grade fever. (Family Medicine/Internal Medicine)

Office visit with 50-year-old female, established patient, diabetic, blood sugar controlled by diet. She now complains of frequency of urination and weight loss, blood sugar of 320, and negative ketones on dipstick. (Internal Medicine)

Follow-up office visit for a 45-year-old, established patient, with rheumatoid arthritis on gold, methotrexate, or immunosuppressive therapy. (Rheumatology)

Office visit for a 60-year-old male, established patient, two years post-removal of intracranial meningioma, now with new headaches and visual disturbance. (Neurosurgery)

Office visit for a 68-year-old female, established patient, for routine review and follow-up of non-insulin dependent diabetes, obesity, hypertension, and congestive heart failure. Complains of vision difficulties and admits dietary noncompliance. Patient is counseled concerning diet and current medications adjusted. (Family Medicine)

**99215** Office visit for an established patient who developed persistent cough, rectal bleeding, weakness, and diarrhea plus pustular infection on skin. Patient on immunosuppressive therapy. (Dermatology)

Office visit for an established patient with disseminated lupus erythematosus, extensive edema of extremities, kidney disease, and weakness requiring monitored course on azathioprene, corticosteroid, and complicated by acute depression. (Dermatology/Internal Medicine/Rheumatology)

Office visit for an established patient with progressive dermatomyositis and recent onset of fever, nasal speech, and regurgitation of fluids through the nose. (Dermatology)

Office visit for a 28-year-old female, established patient, who is abstinent from previous cocaine dependence, but reports progressive panic attacks and chest pains. (Psychiatry)

Office visit for an established adolescent patient with history of bipolar disorder treated with lithium; seen on urgent basis at family's request because of severe depressive symptoms. (Psychiatry)

Office visit for an established patient having acute migraine with new onset neurological symptoms and whose headaches are unresponsive to previous attempts at management with a combination of preventive and abortive medication. (Pain Medicine)

Office visit for an established patient with exfoliative lichen planus with daily fever spikes, disorientation, and shortness of breath. (Dermatology)

Office visit for a 25-year-old, established patient, two years post-burn with bilateral ectropion, hypertrophic facial burn scars, near absence of left breast, and burn syndactyly of both hands. Discussion of treatment options following examination. (Plastic Surgery)

Office visit for a 6-year-old, established patient, to review newly diagnosed immune deficiency with recommendations for therapy including IV immunoglobulin and chronic antibiotics. (Allergy & Immunology)

Office visit for a 36-year-old, established patient, three-month status post-transplant, with new onset of peripheral edema, increased blood pressure, and progressive fatigue. (Nephrology)

Office visit for an established patient with Kaposi's sarcoma who presents with fever and widespread vesicles. (Dermatology)

Office visit for a 27-year-old female, established patient, with bipolar disorder who was stable on lithium carbonate and monthly supportive psychotherapy but now has developed symptoms of hypomania. (Psychiatry)

Office visit for a 25-year-old male, established patient with a history of schizophrenia who has been seen bi-monthly but is complaining of auditory hallucinations. (Psychiatry)

Office visit for a 62-year-old male, established patient, three years postoperative abdominal perineal resection, now with a rising carcinoembryonic antigen, weight loss, and pelvic pain. (Abdominal Surgery)

Office visit for a 42-year-old male, established patient, nine months postoperative emergency vena cava shunt for variceal bleeding, now presents with complaints of one episode of "dark" bowel movement, weight gain, tightness in abdomen, whites of eyes seem yellow, and occasional drowsiness after eating hamburgers. (Abdominal Surgery)

Office visit for a 68-year-old male, established patient, with biopsy-proven rectal carcinoma, for evaluation and discussion of treatment options. (General Surgery)

Office visit for a 60-year-old, established patient, with diabetic nephropathy with increasing edema and dyspnea. (Endocrinology)

Office visit with 30-year-old male, established patient for three-month history of fatigue, weight loss, intermittent fever, and presenting with diffuse adenopathy and splenomegaly. (Family Medicine)

Office visit for restaging of an established patient with new lymphadenopathy one year post-therapy for lymphoma. (Hematology/Oncology)

Office visit for evaluation of recent onset syncopal attacks in a 70-year-old female, established patient. (Internal Medicine)

Follow-up visit, 40-year-old mother of three, established patient, with acute rheumatoid arthritis, anatomical Stage 3, ARA function Class 3 rheumatoid arthritis, and deteriorating function. (Rheumatology)

Follow-up office visit for a 65-year-old male, established patient, with a fever of recent onset while on outpatient antibiotic therapy for endocarditis. (Infectious Disease)

Office visit for a 75-year-old, established patient, with ALS (amyotrophic lateral sclerosis), who is no longer able to swallow. (Neurology)

Office visit for a 70-year-old female, established patient, with diabetes mellitus and hypertension, presenting with a two-month history of increasing confusion, agitation and short-term memory loss. (Family Medicine/Internal Medicine)

# Hospital Inpatient Services

## Initial Hospital Care

### New or Established Patient

99221    Initial hospital visit following admission for a 42-year-old male for observation following an uncomplicated mandible fracture. (Plastic Surgery/Oral & Maxillofacial Surgery)

Initial hospital visit for a 40-year-old patient with a thrombosed synthetic arteriovenous conduit. (Nephrology)

Initial hospital visit for a healthy 24-year-old male with an acute onset of low back pain following a lifting injury. (Internal Medicine/Anesthesiology/Pain Medicine)

Initial hospital visit for a 69-year-old female with controlled hypertension, scheduled for surgery. (Internal Medicine/Cardiology)

Initial hospital visit for a 24-year-old healthy female with benign tumor of palate. (Oral & Maxillofacial Surgery)

Initial hospital visit for a 14-year-old female with infectious mononucleosis and dehydration. (Internal Medicine)

Initial hospital visit for a 62-year-old female with stable rheumatoid arthritis, admitted for total joint replacement. (Rheumatology)

Initial hospital visit for a 12-year-old patient with a laceration of the upper eyelid, involving the lid margin and superior canaliculus, admitted prior to surgery for IV antibiotic therapy. (Plastic Surgery)

Initial hospital visit for a 69-year-old female with controlled hypertension, scheduled for surgery. (Cardiology)

Hospital admission, examination, and initiation of treatment program for a 67-year-old male with uncomplicated pneumonia who requires IV antibiotic therapy. (Internal Medicine)

Hospital admission for an 18-month-old with 10% dehydration. (Pediatrics)

Hospital admission for a 12-year-old with a laceration of the upper eyelid involving the lid margin and superior canaliculus, admitted prior to surgery for IV antibiotic therapy. (Ophthalmology)

Hospital admission for a 32-year-old female with severe flank pain, hematuria and presumed diagnosis of ureteral calculus as determined by Emergency Department physician. (Urology)

Initial hospital visit for a patient with several large venous stasis ulcers not responding to outpatient therapy. (Dermatology)

Initial hospital visit for 21-year-old pregnant patient (nine-weeks gestation) with hyperemesis gravidarum. (Obstetrics & Gynecology)

Initial hospital visit for a 73-year-old female with acute pyelonephritis who is otherwise generally healthy. (Geriatrics)

Initial hospital visit for 62-year-old patient with cellulitis of the foot requiring bedrest and intravenous antibiotics. (Orthopaedic Surgery)

99222    Initial hospital visit for a 50-year-old patient with lower quadrant abdominal pain and increased temperature, but without septic picture. (General Surgery/Abdominal Surgery/Colon & Rectal Surgery)

Initial hospital visit for airway management, due to a benign laryngeal mass. (Otolaryngology, Head & Neck Surgery)

Initial hospital visit for a 66-year-old female with an L-2 vertebral compression fracture with acute onset of paralytic ileus; seen in the office two days previously. (Orthopaedic Surgery)

Initial hospital visit and evaluation of a 15-year-old male admitted with peritonsillar abscess or cellulitis requiring intravenous antibiotic therapy. (Otolaryngology, Head & Neck Surgery)

Initial hospital visit for a 42-year-old male with vertebral compression fracture following a motor vehicle accident. (Orthopaedic Surgery)

Initial hospital visit for a patient with generalized atopic dermatitis and secondary infection. (Dermatology)

Initial hospital visit for a 3-year-old patient with high temperature, limp, and painful hip motion of 18 hours' duration. (Pediatrics/Orthopaedic Surgery)

Initial hospital visit for a young adult, presenting with an acute asthma attack unresponsive to outpatient therapy. (Allergy & Immunology)

Initial hospital visit for an 18-year-old male who has suppurative sialoadenitis and dehydration. (Oral & Maxillofacial Surgery)

Initial hospital visit for a 65-year-old female for acute onset of thrombotic cerebrovascular accident with contralateral paralysis and aphasia. (Neurology)

Initial hospital visit for a 50-year-old male chronic paraplegic patient with pain and spasm below the lesion. (Anesthesiology)

Partial hospital admission for an adolescent patient from chaotic blended family, transferred from inpatient setting, for continued treatment to control symptomatic expressions of hostility and depression. (Psychiatry)

Initial hospital visit for a 15-year-old male with acute status asthmaticus, unresponsive to outpatient therapy. (Internal Medicine)

Initial hospital visit for a 61-year-old male with history of previous myocardial infarction, who now complains of chest pain. (Internal Medicine)

Initial hospital visit of a 15-year-old on medications for a sore throat over the last two weeks. The sore throat has worsened and patient now has dysphagia. The exam shows large necrotic tonsils with an adequate airway and small palpable nodes. The initial mono test was negative. (Otolaryngology, Head & Neck Surgery)

Initial hospital evaluation of a 23-year-old allergy patient admitted with eyelid edema and pain on fifth day of oral antibiotic therapy. (Otolaryngology, Head & Neck Surgery)

Hospital admission, young adult patient, failed previous therapy and now presents in acute asthmatic attack. (Family Medicine/Allergy & Immunology)

Hospital admission of a 62-year-old smoker, established patient, with bronchitis in acute respiratory distress. (Internal Medicine/Pulmonary Medicine)

Hospital admission, examination, and initiation of a treatment program for a 65-year-old female with new onset of right-sided paralysis and aphasia. (Neurology)

Hospital admission, examination, and initiation of treatment program for a 66-year-old chronic hemodialysis patient with fever and a new pulmonary infiltrate. (Nephrology)

Hospital admission for an 8-year-old febrile patient with chronic sinusitis and severe headache, unresponsive to oral antibiotics. (Allergy & Immunology)

Hospital admission for a 40-year-old male with submaxillary cellulitis and trismus from infected lower molar. (Oral & Maxillofacial Surgery)

**99223** Initial hospital visit for a 45-year-old female, who has a history of rheumatic fever as a child and now has anemia, fever, and congestive heart failure. (Cardiology)

Initial hospital visit for a 50-year-old male with acute chest pain and diagnostic electrocardiographic changes of an acute anterior myocardial infarction. (Cardiology/Family Medicine/Internal Medicine)

Initial hospital visit of a 75-year-old with progressive stridor and dysphagia with history of cancer of the larynx treated by radiation therapy in the past. Exam shows a large recurrent tumor of the glottis with a mass in the neck. (Otolaryngology, Head & Neck Surgery)

Initial hospital visit for a 70-year-old male admitted with chest pain, complete heart block, and congestive heart failure. (Cardiology)

Initial hospital visit for an 82-year-old male who presents with syncope, chest pain, and ventricular arrhythmias. (Cardiology)

Initial hospital visit for a 75-year-old male with history of arteriosclerotic coronary vascular disease, who is severely dehydrated, disoriented, and experiencing auditory hallucinations. (Psychiatry)

Initial hospital visit for a 70-year-old male with alcohol and sedative-hypnotic dependence, admitted by family for severe withdrawal, hypertension, and diabetes mellitus. (Psychiatry)

Initial hospital visit for a persistently suicidal latency-aged child whose parents have requested admission to provide safety during evaluation, but are anxious about separation from her. (Psychiatry)

Initial psychiatric visit for an adolescent patient without previous psychiatric history, who was transferred from the medical ICU after a significant overdose. (Psychiatry)

Initial hospital visit for a 35-year-old female with severe systemic lupus erythematosus on corticosteroid and cyclophosphamide, with new onset of fever, chills, rash, and chest pain. (Rheumatology)

Initial hospital visit for a 52-year-old male with known rheumatic heart disease who presents with anasarca, hypertension, and history of alcohol abuse. (Cardiology)

Initial hospital visit for a 55-year-old female with a history of congenital heart disease; now presents with cyanosis. (Cardiology)

Initial hospital visit for a psychotic, hostile, violently combative adolescent, involuntarily committed, for seclusion and restraint in order to provide for safety on unit. (Psychiatry)

Initial hospital visit for a now subdued and sullen teenage male with six-month history of declining school performance, increasing self-endangerment, and resistance of parental expectations, including running away past weekend after physical fight with father. (Psychiatry)

Initial partial hospital admission for a 17-year-old female with history of borderline mental retardation who has developed auditory hallucinations. Parents are known to abuse alcohol, and Child Protective Services is investigating allegations of sexual abuse of a younger sibling. (Psychiatry)

Initial hospital visit of a 67-year-old male admitted with a large neck mass, dysphagia, and history of myocardial infarction three months before. (Otolaryngology, Head & Neck Surgery)

Initial hospital visit for a patient with suspected cerebrospinal fluid rhinorrhea which developed two weeks after head injury. (Otolaryngology, Head & Neck Surgery)

Initial hospital visit for a 25-year-old female with history of poly-substance abuse and psychiatric disorder. The patient appears to be psychotic with markedly elevated vital signs. (Psychiatry)

Initial hospital visit for a 70-year-old male with cutaneous T-cell lymphoma who has developed fever and lymphadenopathy. (Internal Medicine)

Initial hospital visit for a 62-year-old female with known coronary artery disease, for evaluation of increasing edema, dyspnea on exertion, confusion, and sudden onset of fever with productive cough. (Internal Medicine)

Initial hospital visit for a 3-year-old female with 36-hour history of sore throat and high fever; now with sudden onset of lethargy, irritability, photophobia, and nuchal rigidity. (Pediatrics)

Initial hospital visit for a 26-year-old female for evaluation of severe facial fractures (LeFort's II/III). (Plastic Surgery)

Initial hospital visit for a 55-year-old female for bilateral mandibular fractures resulting in flail mandible and airway obstruction. (Plastic Surgery)

Initial hospital visit for a 71-year-old patient with a red painful eye four days following uncomplicated cataract surgery due to endophthalmitis. (Ophthalmology)

Initial hospital visit for a 45-year-old patient involved in a motor vehicle accident who suffered a perforating corneoscleral laceration with loss of vision. (Ophthalmology)

Initial hospital visit for a 58-year-old male who has Ludwig's angina and progressive airway compromise. (Oral & Maxillofacial Surgery)

Initial hospital visit for a patient with generalized systemic sclerosis, receiving immunosuppressive therapy because of recent onset of cough, fever, and inability to swallow. (Dermatology)

Initial hospital visit for an 82-year-old male who presents with syncope, chest pain, and ventricular arrhythmias. (Cardiology)

Initial hospital visit for a 62-year-old male with history of previous myocardial infarction, comes in with recurrent, sustained ventricular tachycardia. (Cardiology)

Initial hospital visit for a chronic dialysis patient with infected PTFE fistula, septicemia, and shock. (Nephrology)

Initial hospital visit for a 1-year-old male, victim of child abuse, with central nervous system depression, skull fracture, and retinal hemorrhage. (Family Medicine/ Neurology)

Initial hospital visit for a 25-year-old female with recent C4-5 quadriplegia, admitted for rehabilitation. (Physical Medicine & Rehabilitation)

Initial hospital visit for an 18-year-old male, post-traumatic brain injury with multiple impairment. (Physical Medicine & Rehabilitation)

Initial partial hospital admission for 16-year-old male, sullen and subdued, with six-month history of declining school performance, increasing self-endangerment, and resistance to parental expectations. (Psychiatry)

Initial hospital visit for a 16-year-old primigravida at 32-weeks gestation with severe hypertension (200/110), thrombocytopenia, and headache. (Obstetrics & Gynecology)

Initial hospital visit for a 49-year-old male with cirrhosis of liver with hematemesis, hepatic encephalopathy, and fever. (Gastroenterology)

Initial hospital visit for a 55-year-old female in chronic pain who has attempted suicide. (Psychiatry)

Initial hospital visit for a 70-year-old male, with multiple organ system disease, admitted with history of being aneuric and septic for 24 hours prior to admission. (Urology)

Initial hospital visit for a 3-year-old female with 36-hour history of sore throat and high fever, now with sudden onset of lethargy, irritability, photophobia, and nuchal rigidity. (Internal Medicine)

Initial hospital visit for a 78-year-old male, transfers from nursing home with dysuria and pyuria, increasing confusion, and high fever. (Internal Medicine)

Initial hospital visit for a 1-day-old male with cyanosis, respiratory distress, and tachypnea. (Cardiology)

Initial hospital visit for a 3-year-old female with recurrent tachycardia and syncope. (Cardiology)

Initial hospital visit for a thyrotoxic patient who presents with fever, atrial fibrillation, and delirium. (Endocrinology)

Initial hospital visit for a 50-year-old Type I diabetic who presents with diabetic ketoacidosis with fever and obtundation. (Endocrinology)

Initial hospital visit for a 40-year-old female with anatomical stage 3, ARA functional class 3 rheumatoid arthritis on methotrexate, corticosteroid, and nonsteroidal anti-inflammatory drugs. Patient presents with severe arthritis flare, new oral ulcers, abdominal pain, and leukopenia. (Rheumatology)

Initial hospital exam of a pediatric patient with high fever and proptosis. (Otolaryngology, Head & Neck Surgery)

Initial hospital visit for a 25-year-old patient admitted for the first time to the rehab unit, with recent C4-C5 quadriplegia. (Physical Medicine & Rehabilitation)

Hospital admission, examination, and initiation of treatment program for a previously unknown 58-year-old male who presents with acute chest pain. (Cardiology)

Hospital admission, examination, and initiation of induction chemotherapy for a 42-year-old patient with newly diagnosed acute myelogenous leukemia. (Hematology/Oncology)

Hospital admission following a motor vehicle accident of a 24-year-old male with fracture dislocation of C5-C6; neurologically intact. (Neurosurgery)

Hospital admission for a 78-year-old female with left lower lobe pneumonia and a history of coronary artery disease, congestive heart failure, osteoarthritis and gout. (Family Medicine)

Hospital admission, examination, and initiation of treatment program for a 65-year-old immunosuppressed male with confusion, fever, and a headache. (Infectious Disease)

Hospital admission for a 9-year-old with vomiting, dehydration, fever, tachypnea, and an admitting diagnosis of diabetic ketoacidosis. (Pediatrics)

Initial hospital visit for a 65-year-old male who presents with acute myocardial infarction, oliguria, hypotension, and altered state of consciousness. (Cardiology)

Initial hospital visit for a hostile/resistant adolescent patient who is severely depressed and involved in poly-substance abuse. Patient is experiencing significant conflict in his chaotic family situation and was suspended from school following an attack on a teacher with a baseball bat. (Psychiatry)

Initial hospital visit for 89-year-old female with fulminant hepatic failure and encephalopathy. (Gastroenterology)

Initial hospital visit for a 42-year-old female with rapidly progressing scleroderma, malignant hypertension, digital infarcts, and oligurea. (Rheumatology)

# Subsequent Hospital Care

**99231**   Subsequent hospital visit for a 65-year-old female, post-open reduction and internal fixation of a fracture. (Physical Medicine & Rehabilitation)

Subsequent hospital visit for a 33-year-old patient with pelvic pain who is responding to pain medication and observation. (Obstetrics & Gynecology)

Subsequent hospital visit for a 21-year-old female with hyperemesis who has responded well to intravenous fluids. (Obstetrics & Gynecology)

Subsequent hospital visit to re-evaluate postoperative pain and titrate patient-controlled analgesia for a 27-year-old female. (Anesthesiology)

Follow-up hospital visit for a 35-year-old female, status post-epidural analgesia. (Anesthesiology/Pain Medicine)

Subsequent hospital visit for a 56-year-old male, post-gastrectomy, for maintenance of analgesia using an intravenous dilaudid infusion. (Anesthesiology)

Subsequent hospital visit for a 4-year-old on day three receiving medication for uncomplicated pneumonia. (Allergy & Immunology)

Subsequent hospital visit for a 30-year-old female with urticaria which has stabilized with medication. (Allergy & Immunology)

Subsequent hospital visit for a 76-year-old male with venous stasis ulcers. (Dermatology)

Subsequent hospital visit for a 24-year-old female with otitis externa, seen two days before in consultation, now to have otic wick removal. (Otolaryngology, Head & Neck Surgery)

Subsequent hospital visit for a 27-year-old with acute labyrinthitis. (Otolaryngology, Head & Neck Surgery)

Subsequent hospital visit for a 10-year-old male admitted for lobar pneumonia with vomiting and dehydration; is becoming afebrile and tolerating oral fluids. (Family Medicine/Pediatrics)

Subsequent hospital visit for a 62-year-old patient with resolving cellulitis of the foot. (Orthopaedic Surgery)

Subsequent hospital visit for a 25-year-old male admitted for supra-ventricular tachycardia and converted on medical therapy. (Cardiology)

Subsequent hospital visit for a 27-year-old male two days after open reduction and internal fixation for malar complex fracture. (Plastic Surgery)

Subsequent hospital visit for a 76-year-old male with venous stasis ulcers. (Geriatrics)

Subsequent hospital visit for a 67-year-old female admitted three days ago with bleeding gastric ulcer; now stable. (Gastroenterology)

Subsequent hospital visit for stable 33-year-old male, status post-lower gastrointestinal bleeding. (General Surgery/Gastroenterology)

Subsequent hospital visit for a 29-year-old auto mechanic with effort thrombosis of left upper extremity. (General Surgery)

Subsequent hospital visit for a 14-year-old female in middle phase of inpatient treatment, who is now behaviorally stable and making satisfactory progress in treatment. (Psychiatry)

Subsequent hospital visit for an 18-year-old male with uncomplicated asthma who is clinically stable. (Allergy & Immunology)

Subsequent hospital visit for a 55-year-old male with rheumatoid arthritis, two days following an uncomplicated total joint replacement. (Rheumatology)

Subsequent hospital visit for a 60-year-old dialysis patient with an access infection, now afebrile on antibiotic. (Nephrology)

Subsequent hospital visit for a 36-year-old female with stable post-rhinoplasty epistaxis. (Plastic Surgery)

Subsequent hospital visit for a 66-year-old female with L-2 vertebral compression fracture with resolving ileus. (Orthopaedic Surgery)

Subsequent hospital visit for a patient with peritonsillar abscess. (Otolaryngology, Head & Neck Surgery)

Subsequent hospital visit for an 18-year-old female responding to intravenous antibiotic therapy for ear or sinus infection. (Otolaryngology, Head & Neck Surgery)

Subsequent hospital visit for a 70-year-old male admitted with congestive heart failure who has responded to therapy. (Cardiology)

Follow-up hospital visit for a 32-year-old female with left ureteral calculus; being followed in anticipation of spontaneous passage. (Urology)

Subsequent hospital visit for a 4-year-old female, admitted for acute gastroenteritis and dehydration, requiring IV hydration; now stable. (Family Medicine)

Subsequent hospital visit for a 50-year-old Type II diabetic who is clinically stable and without complications requiring regulation of a single dose of insulin daily. (Endocrinology)

Subsequent hospital visit to reassesses the status of a 65-year-old patient post-open reduction and internal fixation of hip fracture, on the rehab unit. (Physical Medicine & Rehabilitation)

Subsequent hospital visit for a 78-year-old male with cholangiocarcinoma managed by biliary drainage. (Interventional Radiology)

Subsequent hospital visit for a 50-year-old male with uncomplicated myocardial infarction who is clinically stable and without chest pain. (Family Medicine/ Cardiology/Internal Medicine)

Subsequent hospital visit for a stable 72-year-old lung cancer patient undergoing a five-day course of infusion chemotherapy. (Hematology/Oncology)

Subsequent hospital visit, two days post admission for a 65-year-old male with a CVA (cerebral vascular accident) and left hemiparesis, who is clinically stable. (Neurology/ Physical Medicine and Rehabilitation)

Subsequent hospital visit for now stable, 33-year-old male, status post lower gastrointestinal bleeding. (General Surgery)

Subsequent visit on third day of hospitalization for a 60-year-old female recovering from an uncomplicated pneumonia. (Infectious Disease/Internal Medicine/ Pulmonary Medicine)

Subsequent hospital visit for a 3-year-old patient in traction for a congenital dislocation of the hip. (Orthopaedic Surgery)

Subsequent hospital visit for a 4-year-old female, admitted for acute gastroenteritis and dehydration, requiring IV hydration; now stable. (Family Medicine/ Internal Medicine)

Subsequent hospital visit for 50-year-old female with resolving uncomplicated acute pancreatitis. (Gastroenterology)

**99232** Subsequent hospital visit for a patient with venous stasis ulcers who developed fever and red streaks adjacent to the ulcer. (Dermatology/Internal Medicine/Family Medicine)

Subsequent hospital visit for a 66-year-old male for dressing changes and observation. Patient has had a myocutaneous flap to close a pharyngeal fistula and now has a low-grade fever. (Plastic Surgery)

Subsequent hospital visit for a 54-year-old female admitted for myocardial infarction, but who is now having frequent premature ventricular contractions. (Internal Medicine)

Subsequent hospital visit for an 80-year-old patient with a pelvic rim fracture, inability to walk, and severe pain; now 36 hours post-injury, experiencing urinary retention. (Orthopaedic Surgery)

Subsequent hospital visit for a 17-year-old female with fever, pharyngitis, and airway obstruction, who after 48 hours develops a maculopapular rash. (Pediatrics/Family Medicine)

Follow-up hospital visit for a 32-year-old patient admitted the previous day for corneal ulcer. (Dermatology)

Follow-up visit for a 67-year-old male with congestive heart failure who has responded to antibiotics and diuretics, and has now developed a monoarthropathy. (Internal Medicine)

Follow-up hospital visit for a 58-year-old male receiving continuous opioids who is experiencing severe nausea and vomiting. (Pain Medicine)

Subsequent hospital visit for a patient after an auto accident who is slow to respond to ambulation training. (Physical Medicine & Rehabilitation)

Subsequent hospital visit for a 14-year-old with unstable bronchial asthma complicated by pneumonia. (Allergy & Immunology)

Subsequent hospital visit for a 50-year-old diabetic, hypertensive male with back pain not responding to conservative inpatient management with continued radiation of pain to the lower left extremity. (Orthopaedic Surgery)

Subsequent hospital visit for a 37-year-old female on day five of antibiotics for bacterial endocarditis, who still has low-grade fever. (Cardiology)

Subsequent hospital visit for a 54-year-old patient, post MI (myocardial infarction), who is out of the CCU (coronary care unit) but is now having frequent premature ventricular contractions on telemetry. (Cardiology/Internal Medicine)

Subsequent hospital visit for a patient with neutropenia, a fever responding to antibiotics, and continued slow gastrointestinal bleeding on platelet support. (Hematology/Oncology)

Subsequent hospital visit for a 50-year-old male admitted two days ago for sub-acute renal allograft rejection. (Nephrology)

Subsequent hospital visit for a 35-year-old drug addict, not responding to initial antibiotic therapy for pyelonephritis. (Urology)

Subsequent hospital visit of an 81-year-old male with abdominal distention, nausea, and vomiting. (General Surgery)

Subsequent hospital care for a 62-year-old female with congestive heart failure, who remains dyspneic and febrile. (Internal Medicine)

Subsequent hospital visit for a 73-year-old female with recently diagnosed lung cancer, who complains of unsteady gait. (Pulmonary Medicine)

Subsequent hospital visit for a 20-month-old male with bacterial meningitis treated one week with antibiotic therapy; has now developed a temperature of 101 degrees. (Pediatrics)

Subsequent hospital visit for 13-year-old male admitted with left lower quadrant abdominal pain and fever, not responding to therapy. (General Surgery)

Subsequent hospital visit for a 65-year-old male with hemiplegia and painful paretic shoulder. (Physical Medicine & Rehabilitation)

**99233**    Subsequent hospital visit for a 38-year-old male, quadriplegic with acute autonomic hyperreflexia, who is not responsive to initial care. (Physical Medicine & Rehabilitation)

Follow-up hospital visit for a teenage female who continues to experience severely disruptive, violent and life-threatening symptoms in a complicated multi-system illness. Family/social circumstances also a contributing factor. (Psychiatry)

Subsequent hospital visit for a 42-year-old female with progressive systemic sclerosis (scleroderma), renal failure on dialysis, congestive heart failure, cardiac arrhythmias, and digital ulcers. (Allergy & Immunology)

Subsequent hospital visit for a 50-year-old diabetic, hypertensive male with nonresponding back pain and radiating pain to the lower left extremity, who develops chest pain, cough, and bloody sputum. (Orthopaedic Surgery)

Subsequent hospital visit for a 64-year-old female, status post-abdominal aortic aneurysm resection, with non-responsive coagulopathy, who has now developed lower GI bleeding. (Abdominal Surgery/Colon & Rectal Surgery/General Surgery)

Follow-up hospital care of a patient with pansinusitis infection complicated by a brain abscess and asthma; no response to current treatment. (Otolaryngology, Head & Neck Surgery)

Subsequent hospital visit for a patient with a laryngeal neoplasm who develops airway compromise, suspected metastasis. (Otolaryngology, Head & Neck Surgery)

Subsequent hospital visit for a 49-year-old male with significant rectal bleeding, etiology undetermined, not responding to treatment. (Abdominal Surgery/General Surgery/Colon & Rectal Surgery)

Subsequent hospital visit for a 50-year-old male, post-aortocoronary bypass surgery; now develops hypotension and oliguria. (Cardiology)

Subsequent hospital visit for an adolescent patient who is violent, unsafe, and noncompliant, with multiple expectations for participation in treatment plan and behavior on the treatment unit. (Psychiatry)

Subsequent hospital visit for an 18-year-old male being treated for presumed PCP psychosis. Patient is still moderately symptomatic with auditory hallucinations and is insisting on signing out against medical advice. (Psychiatry)

Subsequent hospital visit for an 8-year-old female with caustic ingestion, who now has fever, dyspnea, and dropping hemoglobin. (Gastroenterology)

Follow-up hospital visit for a chronic renal failure patient on dialysis who develops chest pain and shortness of breath and a new onset pericardial friction rub. (Nephrology)

Subsequent hospital visit for a 44-year-old patient with electrical burns to the left arm with ascending infection. (Orthopaedic Surgery)

Subsequent hospital visit for a patient with systemic sclerosis who has aspirated and is short of breath. (Dermatology)

Subsequent hospital visit for a 65-year-old female, status postoperative resection of abdominal aortic aneurysm, with suspected ischemic bowel. (General Surgery)

Subsequent hospital visit for a 50-year-old male, post-aortocoronary bypass surgery, now develops hypotension and oliguria. (Cardiology)

Subsequent hospital visit for a 65-year-old male, following an acute myocardial infarction, who complains of shortness of breath and new chest pain. (Cardiology)

Subsequent hospital visit for a 65-year-old female with rheumatoid arthritis (stage 3, class 3) admitted for urosepsis. On the third hospital day, chest pain, dyspnea and fever develop. (Rheumatology)

Follow-up hospital care of a pediatric case with stridor, laryngomalacia, established tracheostomy, complicated by multiple medical problems in PICU. (Otolaryngology, Head & Neck Surgery)

Subsequent hospital visit for a 60-year-old female, four days post uncomplicated inferior myocardial infarction who has developed severe chest pain, dyspnea, diaphoresis, and nausea. (Family Medicine)

Subsequent hospital visit for a patient with AML (acute myelogenous leukemia), fever, elevated white count and uric acid undergoing induction chemotherapy. (Hematology/Oncology)

Subsequent hospital visit for a 38-year-old quadriplegic male with acute autonomic hyperreflexia, who is not responsive to initial care. (Physical Medicine & Rehabilitation)

Subsequent hospital visit for a 65-year-old female postoperative resection of abdominal aortic aneurysm, with suspected ischemic bowel. (General Surgery)

Subsequent hospital visit for a 60-year-old female with persistent leukocytosis and a fever seven days after a sigmoid colon resection for carcinoma. (Infectious Disease)

Subsequent hospital visit for a chronic renal failure patient on dialysis, who develops chest pain, shortness of breath, and new onset of pericardial friction rub. (Nephrology)

Subsequent hospital visit for a 65-year-old male with acute myocardial infarction who now demonstrates complete heart block and congestive heart failure. (Cardiology)

Subsequent hospital visit for a 25-year-old female with hypertension and systemic lupus erythematosus, admitted for fever and respiratory distress. On the third hospital day, the patient presented with purpuric skin lesions and acute renal failure. (Allergy & Immunology)

Subsequent hospital visit for a 55-year-old male with severe chronic obstructive pulmonary disease and bronchospasm; initially admitted for acute respiratory distress requiring ventilatory support in the ICU. The patient was stabilized, extubated, and transferred to the floor, but has now developed acute fever, dyspnea, left lower lobe rhonchi, and laboratory evidence of carbon dioxide retention and hypoxemia. (Family Medicine/ Internal Medicine)

Subsequent hospital visit for 46-year-old female, known liver cirrhosis patient, with recent upper gastrointestinal hemorrhage from varices; now with worsening ascites and encephalopathy. (Gastroenterology)

Subsequent hospital visit for 62-year-old female admitted with acute subarachnoid hemorrhage, negative cerebral arteriogram, increased lethargy, and hemiparesis with fever. (Neurosurgery)

# Consultations

## Office or Other Outpatient Consultations

### New or Established Patient

**99241**  Initial office consultation for a 40-year-old female in pain from blister on lip following a cold. (Oral & Maxillofacial Surgery)

Initial office consultation for a 62-year-old construction worker with olecranon bursitis. (Orthopaedic Surgery)

Office consultation with 25-year-old postpartum female with severe symptomatic hemorrhoids. (Colon & Rectal Surgery)

Office consultation with 58-year-old male, referred for follow-up of creatinine level and evaluation of obstructive uropathy, relieved two months ago. (Nephrology)

Office consultation for 30-year-old female tennis player with sprain or contusion of the forearm. (Orthopaedic Surgery)

Office consultation for a 45-year-old male, requested by his internist, with asymptomatic torus palatinus requiring no further treatment. (Oral & Maxillofacial Surgery)

**99242**  Initial office consultation for a 20-year-old male with acute upper respiratory tract symptoms. (Allergy & Immunology)

Initial office consultation for a 29-year-old soccer player with painful proximal thigh/groin injury. (Orthopaedic Surgery)

Initial office consultation for a 66-year-old female with wrist and hand pain, numbness of finger tips, suspected median nerve compression by carpal tunnel syndrome. (Plastic Surgery)

Initial office consultation for a patient with a solitary lesion of discoid lupus erythematosus on left cheek to rule out malignancy or self-induced lesion. (Dermatology)

Office consultation for management of systolic hypertension in a 70-year-old male scheduled for elective prostate resection. (Geriatrics)

Office consultation with 27-year-old female, with old amputation, for evaluation of existing above-knee prosthesis. (Physical Medicine & Rehabilitation)

Office consultation with 66-year-old female with wrist and hand pain, and finger numbness, secondary to suspected carpal tunnel syndrome. (Orthopaedic Surgery)

Office consultation for 61-year-old female, recently on antibiotic therapy, now with diarrhea and leukocytosis. (Abdominal Surgery)

Office consultation for a patient with papulosquamous eruption of elbow with pitting of nails and itchy scalp. (Dermatology)

Office consultation for a 30-year-old female with single season allergic rhinitis. (Allergy & Immunology)

**99243** Initial office consultation for a 60-year-old male with avascular necrosis of the left femoral head with increasing pain. (Orthopaedic Surgery)

Office consultation for a 31-year-old woman complaining of palpitations and chest pains. Her internist had described a mild systolic click. (Cardiology)

Office consultation for a 65-year-old female with persistent bronchitis. (Infectious Disease)

Office consultation for a 65-year-old man with chronic low-back pain radiating to the leg. (Neurosurgery)

Office consultation for 23-year-old female with Crohn's disease not responding to therapy. (Abdominal Surgery/Colon & Rectal Surgery)

Office consultation for 25-year-old patient with symptomatic knee pain and swelling, with torn anterior cruciate ligament and/or torn meniscus. (Orthopaedic Surgery)

Office consultation for a 67-year-old patient with osteoporosis and mandibular atrophy with regard to reconstructive alternatives. (Oral & Maxillofacial Surgery)

Office consultation for 39-year-old patient referred at a perimenopausal age for irregular menses and menopausal symptoms. (Obstetrics & Gynecology)

**99244** Initial office consultation for a 28-year-old male, HIV+, with a recent change in visual acuity. (Ophthalmology)

Initial office consultation for a 15-year-old male with failing grades, suspected drug abuse. (Pediatrics)

Initial office consultation for a 36-year-old factory worker, status four months post-occupational low back injury and requires management of intractable low back pain. (Pain Medicine)

Initial office consultation for a 45-year-old female with a history of chronic arthralgia of TMJ and associated myalgia and sudden progressive symptomatology over last two to three months. (Oral & Maxillofacial Surgery)

Initial office consultation for evaluation of a 70-year-old male with appetite loss and diminished energy. (Psychiatry)

Initial office consultation for an elementary school-aged patient, referred by pediatrician, with multiple systematic complaints and recent onset of behavioral discontrol. (Psychiatry)

Initial office consultation for a 23-year-old female with developmental facial skeletal anomaly and subsequent abnormal relationship of jaw(s) to cranial base. (Oral & Maxillofacial Surgery)

Initial office consultation for a 45-year-old myopic patient with a one-week history of floaters and a partial retinal detachment. (Ophthalmology)

Initial office consultation for a 65-year-old female with moderate dementia, mild unsteadiness, back pain fatigue on ambulation, intermittent urinary incontinence. (Neurosurgery)

Initial office consultation for a 33-year-old female referred by endocrinologist with amenorrhea and galactorrhea, for evaluation of pituitary tumor. (Neurosurgery)

Initial office consultation for a 34-year-old male with new onset nephrotic syndrome. (Nephrology)

Initial office consultation for a 39-year-old female with intractable chest wall pain secondary to metastatic breast cancer. (Anesthesiology/Pain Medicine)

Initial office consultation for a patient with multiple giant tumors of jaws. (Oral & Maxillofacial Surgery)

Initial office consultation for a patient with a failed total hip replacement with loosening and pain upon walking. (Orthopaedic Surgery)

Initial office consultation for a 60-year-old female with three-year history of intermittent tic-like unilateral facial pain; now constant pain for six weeks without relief by adequate carbamazepine dosage. (Neurosurgery)

Initial office consultation for a 45-year-old male heavy construction worker with prior lumbar disc surgery two years earlier; now gradually recurring low back and unilateral leg pain for three months, unable to work for two weeks. (Neurosurgery)

Initial office consultation of a patient who presents with a 30-year history of smoking and right neck mass. (Otolaryngology, Head & Neck Surgery)

Office consultation with 38-year-old female, with inflammatory bowel disease, who now presents with right lower quadrant pain and suspected intra-abdominal abscess. (General Surgery/Colon & Rectal Surgery)

Office consultation with 72-year-old male with esophageal carcinoma, symptoms of dysphagia and reflux. (Thoracic Surgery)

Office consultation for discussion of treatment options for a 40-year-old female with a 2 cm adenocarcinoma of the breast. (Radiation Oncology)

Office consultation for young patient referred by pediatrician because of patient's short attention span, easy distractibility, and hyperactivity. (Psychiatry)

Office consultation for 66-year-old female, history of colon resection for adenocarcinoma six years earlier, now with severe mid-back pain; X-rays showing osteoporosis and multiple vertebral compression fractures. (Neurosurgery)

Office consultation for a patient with chronic pelvic inflammatory disease who now has left lower quadrant pain with a palpable pelvic mass. (Obstetrics & Gynecology)

Office consultation for a patient with long-standing psoriasis with acute onset of erythroderma, pustular lesions, chills, and fever. Combinations of topical and systemic treatments discussed and instituted. (Dermatology)

**99245**   Initial office consultation for a 35-year-old multiple-trauma male patient with complex pelvic fractures, for evaluation and formulation of management plan. (Orthopaedic Surgery)

Initial emergency room consultation for 10-year-old male in status epilepticus, recent closed head injury, information about medication not available. (Neurosurgery)

Initial emergency room consultation for a 23-year-old patient with severe abdominal pain, guarding, febrile, and unstable vital signs. (Obstetrics & Gynecology)

Office consultation for a 67-year-old female longstanding uncontrolled diabetic who presents with retinopathy, nephropathy, and a foot ulcer. (Endocrinology)

Office consultation for a 37-year-old male for initial evaluation and management of Cushing's disease. (Endocrinology)

Office consultation for a 60-year-old male who presents with thyrotoxicosis, exophthalmos, frequent premature ventricular contractions, and congestive heart failure. (Endocrinology)

Initial office consultation for a 36-year-old patient, one year status post occupational herniated cervical disk treated by laminectomy, requiring management of multiple sites of intractable pain, depression, and narcotic dependence. (Pain Medicine)

Office consultation for a 58-year-old man with a history of MI and CHF who complains of the recent onset of rest angina and shortness of breath. The patient has a systolic blood pressure of 90 mmHG and is in Class IV heart failure. (Cardiology)

Emergency department consultation for a 1-year-old with a three-day history of fever with increasing respiratory distress who is thought to have cardiac tamponade by the ER physician. (Cardiology)

Office consultation in the emergency department for a 25-year-old male with severe, acute, closed head injury. (Neurosurgery)

Office consultation for a 23-year-old female with Stage II A Hodgkins disease with positive supraclavicular and mediastinal nodes. (Radiation Oncology)

Office consultation for a 27-year-old juvenile diabetic patient with severe diabetic retinopathy, gastric atony, nephrotic syndrome and progressive renal failure, now with a serum creatinine of 2.7, and a blood pressure of 170/114. (Nephrology)

Office consultation for independent medical evaluation of a patient with a history of complicated low back and neck problems with previous multiple failed back surgeries. (Orthopaedic Surgery)

Office consultation for an adolescent referred by pediatrician for recent onset of violent and self-injurious behavior. (Psychiatry)

Office consultation for a 6-year-old male for evaluation of severe muscle and joint pain and a diffuse rash. Patient was feeling well until 4-6 weeks earlier, when he developed arthralgia, myalgias, and a fever of 102 degrees for one week. (Rheumatology)

# Inpatient Consultations

## New or Established Patient

**99251**   Initial hospital consultation for a 27-year-old female with fractured incisor post-intubation. (Oral & Maxillofacial Surgery)

Initial hospital consultation for an orthopaedic patient on IV antibiotics who has developed an apparent candida infection of the oral cavity. (Oral & Maxillofacial Surgery)

Initial inpatient consultation for a 30-year-old female complaining of vaginal itching, post orthopaedic surgery. (Obstetrics & Gynecology)

Initial inpatient consultation for a 36-year-old male on orthopaedic service with complaint of localized dental pain. (Oral & Maxillofacial Surgery)

**99252**   Initial hospital consultation for a 45-year-old male, previously abstinent alcoholic, who relapsed and was admitted for management of gastritis. The patient readily accepts the need for further treatment. (Addiction Medicine)

Initial hospital consultation for a 35-year-old dialysis patient with episodic oral ulcerations. (Oral & Maxillofacial Surgery)

Initial inpatient preoperative consultation for a 43-year-old female with cholecystitis and well-controlled hypertension. (Cardiology)

Initial inpatient consultation for recommendation of antibiotic prophylaxis for a patient with a synthetic heart valve who will undergo urologic surgery. (Internal Medicine)

Initial inpatient consultation for possible drug induced skin eruption in 50-year-old male. (Dermatology)

Preoperative inpatient consultation for evaluation of hypertension in a 60-year-old male who will undergo a cholecystectomy. Patient had a normal annual check-up in your office four months ago. (Internal Medicine)

Initial inpatient consultation for 66-year-old patient with wrist and hand pain and finger numbness, secondary to carpal tunnel syndrome. (Orthopaedic Surgery/Plastic Surgery)

Initial inpatient consultation for a 66-year-old male smoker referred for pain management immediately status post-biliary tract surgery done via sub-costal incision. (Anesthesiology/Pain Medicine)

**99253** Initial hospital consultation for a 50-year-old female with incapacitating knee pain due to generalized rheumatoid arthritis. (Orthopaedic Surgery)

Initial hospital consultation for a 60-year-old male with avascular necrosis of the left femoral heel with increasing pain. (Orthopaedic Surgery)

Initial hospital consultation for a 45-year-old female with compound mandibular fracture and concurrent head, abdominal and/or orthopaedic injuries. (Oral & Maxillofacial Surgery)

Initial hospital consultation for a 22-year-old female, paraplegic, to evaluate wrist and hand pain. (Orthopaedic Surgery)

Initial hospital consultation for a 40-year-old male with 10-day history of incapacitating unilateral sciatica, unable to walk now, not improved by bed rest. (Neurosurgery)

Initial hospital consultation, requested by pediatrician, for treatment recommendations for a patient admitted with persistent inability to walk following soft tissue injury to ankle. (Physiatry)

Initial hospital consultation for a 27-year-old previously healthy male who vomited during IV sedation and may have aspirated gastric contents. (Anesthesiology)

Initial hospital consultation for a 33-year-old female, post-abdominal surgery, who now has a fever. (Internal Medicine)

Initial inpatient consultation for a 57-year-old male, post lower endoscopy, for evaluation of abdominal pain and fever. (General Surgery)

Initial inpatient consultation for rehabilitation of a 73-year-old female one week after surgical management of a hip fracture. (Physical Medicine & Rehabilitation)

Initial inpatient consultation for diagnosis/management of fever following abdominal surgery. (Internal Medicine)

Initial inpatient consultation for a 35-year-old female with a fever and pulmonary infiltrate following cesarean section. (Pulmonary Medicine)

Initial inpatient consultation for a 42-year-old non-diabetic patient, postoperative cholecystectomy, now with an acute urinary tract infection. (Nephrology)

Initial inpatient consultation for 53-year-old female with moderate uncomplicated pancreatitis. (Gastroenterology)

Initial inpatient consultation for 45-year-old patient with chronic neck pain with radicular pain of the left arm. (Orthopaedic Surgery)

Initial inpatient consultation for 8-year-old patient with new onset of seizures who has a normal examination and previous history. (Neurology)

**99254** Initial hospital consultation for a 15-year-old patient with painless swelling of proximal humerus with lytic lesion by X-ray. (Orthopaedic Surgery)

Initial hospital consultation for evaluation of a 29-year-old female with a diffusely positive medical review of systems and history of multiple surgeries. (Psychiatry)

Initial hospital consultation for a 70-year-old diabetic female with gangrene of the foot. (Orthopaedic Surgery)

Initial inpatient consultation for a 47-year-old female with progressive pulmonary infiltrate, hypoxemia, and diminished urine output. (Anesthesiology)

Initial hospital consultation for a 13-month-old with spasmodic cough, respiratory distress, and fever. (Allergy & Immunology)

Initial hospital consultation for a patient with failed total hip replacement with loosening and pain upon walking. (Orthopaedic Surgery)

Initial hospital consultation for a 62-year-old female with metastatic breast cancer to the femoral neck and thoracic vertebra. (Orthopaedic Surgery)

Initial hospital consultation for a 39-year-old female with nephrolithiasis requiring extensive opioid analgesics, whose vital signs are now elevated. She initially denied any drug use, but today gives history of multiple substance abuse, including opioids and prior treatment for a personality disorder. (Psychiatry)

Initial hospital consultation for a 70-year-old female without previous psychiatric history, who is now experiencing nocturnal confusion and visual hallucinations following hip replacement surgery. (Psychiatry)

Initial inpatient consultation for evaluation of a 63-year-old in the ICU with diabetes and chronic renal failure who develops acute respiratory distress syndrome 36 hours after a mitral valve replacement. (Anesthesiology)

Initial inpatient consultation for a 66-year-old female with enlarged supraclavicular lymph nodes, found on biopsy to be malignant. (Hematology/Oncology)

Initial inpatient consultation for a 43-year-old female for evaluation of sudden painful visual loss, optic neuritis, and episodic paresthesia. (Ophthalmology)

Initial inpatient consultation for evaluation of a 71-year-old male with hyponatremia (serum sodium 114) who was admitted to the hospital with pneumonia. (Nephrology)

Initial inpatient consultation for a 72-year-old male with emergency admission for possible bowel obstruction. (Internal Medicine/General Surgery)

Initial inpatient consultation for a 35-year-old female with fever, swollen joints, and rash of one-week duration. (Rheumatology)

**99255** Initial inpatient consultation for a 76-year-old female with massive, life-threatening gastrointestinal hemorrhage and chest pain. (Gastroenterology)

Initial inpatient consultation for a 75-year-old female, admitted to intensive care with acute respiratory distress syndrome, who is hypersensitive, has a moderate metabolic acidosis, and a rising serum creatinine. (Nephrology)

Initial hospital consultation for patient with a history of complicated low back pain and neck problems with previous multiple failed back surgeries. (Orthopaedic Surgery/Neurosurgery)

Initial hospital consultation for a 66-year-old female, two days post-abdominal aneurysm repair, with oliguria and hypertension of one-day duration. (Nephrology/Internal Medicine)

Initial hospital consultation for a patient with shotgun wound to face with massive facial trauma and airway obstruction. (Oral & Maxillofacial Surgery)

Initial hospital consultation for patient with severe pancreatitis complicated by respiratory insufficiency, acute renal failure, and abscess formation. (General Surgery/Colon & Rectal Surgery)

Initial hospital consultation for a 35-year-old multiple-trauma male patient with complex pelvic fractures to evaluate and formulate management plan. (Orthopaedic Surgery)

Initial inpatient consultation for adolescent patient with fractured femur and pelvis who pulled out IVs and disconnected traction in attempt to elope from hospital. (Psychiatry)

Initial hospital consultation for a 16-year-old primigravida at 32-weeks gestation requested by a family practitioner for evaluation of severe hypertension, thrombocytopenia, and headache. (Obstetrics & Gynecology)

Initial hospital consultation for a 58-year-old insulin-dependent diabetic with multiple antibiotic allergies, now with multiple fascial plane abscesses and airway obstruction. (Oral & Maxillofacial Surgery)

Initial inpatient consultation for a 55-year-old male with known cirrhosis and ascites, now with jaundice, encephalopathy, and massive hematemesis. (Gastroenterology)

Initial hospital consultation for a 25-year-old male, seen in emergency room with severe, closed head injury. (Neurosurgery)

Initial hospital consultation for a 2-day-old male with single ventricle physiology and subaortic obstruction. Family counseling following evaluation for multiple, staged surgical procedures. (Thoracic Surgery)

Initial hospital consultation for a 45-year-old male admitted with subarachnoid hemorrhage and intracranial aneurysm on angiogram. (Neurosurgery)

Initial inpatient consultation for myxedematous patient who is hypoventilating and obtunded. (Endocrinology)

Initial hospital consultation for a 45-year-old patient with widely metastatic lung carcinoma, intractable back pain, and a history that includes substance dependence, NSAID allergy, and two prior laminectomies with fusion for low back pain. (Pain Medicine)

Initial hospital consultation for evaluation of treatment options in a 50-year-old patient with cirrhosis, known peptic ulcer disease, hypotension, encephalopathy, and massive acute upper gastrointestinal bleeding which cannot be localized by endoscopy. (Interventional Radiology)

Initial inpatient consultation in the ICU for a 70-year-old male who experienced a cardiac arrest during surgery and was resuscitated. (Cardiology)

Initial inpatient consultation for a patient with severe pancreatitis complicated by respiratory insufficiency, acute renal failure, and abscess formation. (Gastroenterology)

Initial inpatient consultation for a 70-year-old cirrhotic male admitted with ascites, jaundice, encephalopathy, and massive hematemesis. (Gastroenterology)

Initial inpatient consultation in the ICU for a 51-year-old patient who is on a ventilator and has a fever two weeks after a renal transplantation. (Infectious Disease)

Initial inpatient consultation for evaluation and formulation of plan for management of multiple-trauma patient with complex pelvic fracture, 35-year-old male. (General Surgery/Orthopaedic Surgery)

Initial inpatient consultation for a 50-year-old male with a history of previous myocardial infarction, now with acute pulmonary edema and hypotension. (Cardiology)

Initial inpatient consultation for 45-year-old male with recent, acute subarachnoid hemorrhage, hesitant speech, mildly confused, drowsy. High risk group for HIV+ status. (Neurosurgery)

Initial inpatient consultation for 36-year-old female referred by her internist to evaluate a patient being followed for abdominal pain and fever. The patient has developed diffuse abdominal pain, guarding, rigidity and increased fever. (Obstetrics & Gynecology)

# Emergency Department Services

## New or Established Patient

**99281** Emergency department visit for a patient for removal of sutures from a well-healed, uncomplicated laceration. (Emergency Medicine)

Emergency department visit for a patient for tetanus toxoid immunization. (Emergency Medicine)

Emergency department visit for a patient with several uncomplicated insect bites. (Emergency Medicine)

**99282**  Emergency department visit for a 20-year-old student who presents with a painful sunburn with blister formation on the back. (Emergency Medicine)

Emergency department visit for a child presenting with impetigo localized to the face. (Emergency Medicine)

Emergency department visit for a patient with a minor traumatic injury of an extremity with localized pain, swelling, and bruising. (Emergency Medicine)

Emergency department visit for an otherwise healthy patient whose chief complaint is a red, swollen cystic lesion on his/her back. (Emergency Medicine)

Emergency department visit for a patient presenting with a rash on both legs after exposure to poison ivy. (Emergency Medicine)

Emergency department visit for a young adult patient with infected sclera and purulent discharge from both eyes without pain, visual disturbance or history of foreign body in either eye. (Emergency Medicine)

**99283**  Emergency department visit for a sexually active female complaining of vaginal discharge who is afebrile and denies experiencing abdominal or back pain. (Emergency Medicine)

Emergency department visit for a well-appearing 8-year-old who has a fever, diarrhea, and abdominal cramps, is tolerating oral fluids and is not vomiting. (Emergency Medicine)

Emergency department visit for a patient with an inversion ankle injury, who is unable to bear weight on the injured foot and ankle. (Emergency Medicine)

Emergency department visit for a patient who has a complaint of acute pain associated with a suspected foreign body in the painful eye. (Emergency Medicine)

Emergency department visit for a healthy, young adult patient who sustained a blunt head injury with local swelling and bruising without subsequent confusion, loss of consciousness or memory deficit. (Emergency Medicine)

**99284**  Emergency department visit for a 4-year-old who fell off a bike sustaining a head injury with brief loss of consciousness. (Emergency Medicine)

Emergency department visit for an elderly female who has fallen and is now complaining of pain in her right hip and is unable to walk. (Emergency Medicine)

Emergency department visit for a patient with flank pain and hematuria. (Emergency Medicine)

Emergency department visit for a female presenting with lower abdominal pain and a vaginal discharge. (Emergency Medicine)

**99285**  Emergency department visit for a patient with a complicated overdose requiring aggressive management to prevent side effects from the ingested materials. (Emergency Medicine)

Emergency department visit for a patient with a new onset of rapid heart rate requiring IV drugs. (Emergency Medicine)

Emergency department visit for a patient exhibiting active, upper gastrointestinal bleeding. (Emergency Medicine)

Emergency department visit for a previously healthy young adult patient who is injured in an automobile accident and is brought to the emergency department immobilized and has symptoms compatible with intra-abdominal injuries or multiple extremity injuries. (Emergency Medicine)

Emergency department visit for a patient with an acute onset of chest pain compatible with symptoms of cardiac ischemia and/or pulmonary embolus. (Emergency Medicine)

Emergency department visit for a patient who presents with a sudden onset of "the worst headache of her life," and complains of a stiff neck, nausea, and inability to concentrate. (Emergency Medicine)

Emergency department visit for a patient with a new onset of a cerebral vascular accident. (Emergency Medicine)

Emergency department visit for acute febrile illness in an adult, associated with shortness of breath and an altered level of alertness. (Emergency Medicine)

# Critical Care Services

**99291**  First hour of critical care of a 65-year-old male with septic shock following relief of ureteral obstruction caused by a stone.

First hour of critical care of a 15-year-old with acute respiratory failure from asthma.

First hour of critical care of a 45-year-old who sustained a liver laceration, cerebral hematoma, flailed chest, and pulmonary contusion after being struck by an automobile.

First hour of critical care of a 65-year-old female who, following a hysterectomy, suffered a cardiac arrest associated with a pulmonary embolus.

First hour of critical care of a 6-month-old with hypovolemic shock secondary to diarrhea and dehydration.

First hour of critical care of a 3-year-old with respiratory failure secondary to pneumocystis carinii pneumonia.

# Prolonged Services

## Prolonged Physician Service With Direct (Face-to-Face) Patient Contact

### Office or Other Outpatient

**99354** A 20-year-old female with history of asthma presents with acute bronchospasm and moderate respiratory distress. Initial evaluation shows respiratory rate 30, labored breathing and wheezing heard in all lung fields. Office treatment is initiated which includes intermittent bronchial dilation and subcutaneous epinephrine. Requires intermittent physician face-to-face time with patient over a period of 2-3 hours. (Family Medicine/Internal Medicine)

**99355** A 20-year-old female with history of asthma presents with acute bronchospasm and moderate respiratory distress. Initial evaluation shows respiratory rate 30, labored breathing and wheezing heard in all lung fields. Office treatment is initiated which includes intermittent bronchial dilation and subcutaneous epinephrine. Requires intermittent physician face-to-face time with patient over a period of 2-3 hours. (Family Medicine/Internal Medicine)

### Inpatient

**99356** A 34-year-old primigravida presents to hospital in early labor. Admission history and physical reveals severe preeclampsia. Physician supervises management of preeclampsia, IV magnesium initiation and maintenance, labor augmentation with pitocin, and close maternal-fetal monitoring. Physician face-to-face involvement includes 40 minutes of continuous bedside care until the patient is stable, then is intermittent over several hours until the delivery. (Family Medicine/Internal Medicine/Obstetrics & Gynecology)

## Prolonged Physician Service Without Direct Patient (Face-to-Face) Contact

**99358** An 85-year-old new patient with multiple complicated medical problems has moved to the area to live closer to her daughter. She is brought to the primary care office by her daughter and has been seen and examined by the physician. The physician indicated that past medical records would be obtained from the patient's prior physicians' and that he will communicate further with the daughter upon review of them.

**99359** An 85-year-old new patient with multiple complicated medical problems has moved to the area to live closer to her daughter. She is brought to the primary care office by her daughter and has been seen and examined by the physician. The physician indicated that past medical records would be obtained from the patient's prior physicians' and that he will communicate further with the daughter upon review of them.

# Physician Standby Services

**99360** A 24-year-old patient is admitted to OB unit attempting VBAC. Fetal monitoring shows increasing fetal distress. Patient's blood pressure is rising and labor progressing slowly. A primary care physician is requested by the OB/GYN to standby in the unit for possible cesarean delivery and neonatal resuscitation. (Family Medicine/Internal Medicine)

# Care Plan Oversight Services

**99375** First month of care plan oversight for terminal care of a 58-year-old female with advanced intraabdominal ovarian cancer. Care plan includes home oxygen, diuretics IV for edema and ascites control, and pain control management involving IV morphine infusion when progressive ileus occurred. Physician phone contacts with nurse, family, and MSW. Discussion with MSW concerning plans to withdraw supportive measures per patient wishes. Documentation includes review and modification of care plan and certifications from nursing, MSW, pharmacy, and DME. (Family Medicine/Internal Medicine)

# Appendix D

## Summary of CPT Add-on Codes

This listing is a summary of CPT add-on codes for *CPT 2012*. The codes listed below are identified in *CPT 2012* with a ✚ symbol.

| | | | | | | |
|---|---|---|---|---|---|---|
| 01953 | 15261 | 22527 | 32668 | 35685 | 49327 | 63091 |
| 01968 | 15272 | 22534 | 32674 | 35686 | 49412 | 63103 |
| 01969 | 15274 | 22552 | 33141 | 35697 | 49435 | 63295 |
| 11001 | 15276 | 22585 | 33225 | 35700 | 49568 | 63308 |
| 11008 | 15278 | 22614 | 33257 | 36148 | 49905 | 63621 |
| 11045 | 15777 | 22632 | 33258 | 36218 | 51797 | 64480 |
| 11046 | 15787 | 22634 | 33259 | 36248 | 56606 | 64484 |
| 11047 | 15847 | 22840 | 33508 | 36476 | 57267 | 64491 |
| 11101 | 16036 | 22841 | 33517 | 36479 | 58110 | 64492 |
| 11201 | 17003 | 22842 | 33518 | 37185 | 58611 | 64494 |
| 11732 | 17312 | 22843 | 33519 | 37186 | 59525 | 64495 |
| 11922 | 17314 | 22844 | 33521 | 37206 | 60512 | 64634 |
| 13102 | 17315 | 22845 | 33522 | 37208 | 61316 | 64636 |
| 13122 | 19001 | 22846 | 33523 | 37222 | 61517 | 64727 |
| 13133 | 19126 | 22847 | 33530 | 37223 | 61609 | 64778 |
| 13153 | 19291 | 22848 | 33572 | 37232 | 61610 | 64783 |
| 14302 | 19295 | 22851 | 33768 | 37233 | 61611 | 64787 |
| 15003 | 19297 | 26125 | 33884 | 37234 | 61612 | 64832 |
| 15005 | 20930 | 26861 | 33924 | 37235 | 61641 | 64837 |
| 15101 | 20931 | 26863 | 34806 | 37250 | 61642 | 64859 |
| 15111 | 20936 | 27358 | 34808 | 37251 | 61781 | 64872 |
| 15116 | 20937 | 27692 | 34813 | 38102 | 61782 | 64874 |
| 15121 | 20938 | 29826 | 34826 | 38746 | 61783 | 64876 |
| 15131 | 20985 | 31620 | 35306 | 38747 | 61797 | 64901 |
| 15136 | 22103 | 31627 | 35390 | 38900 | 61799 | 64902 |
| 15151 | 22116 | 31632 | 35400 | 43273 | 61800 | 65757 |
| 15152 | 22208 | 31633 | 35500 | 43283 | 61864 | 66990 |
| 15156 | 22216 | 31637 | 35572 | 43338 | 61868 | 67225 |
| 15157 | 22226 | 32501 | 35600 | 43635 | 62148 | 67320 |
| 15201 | 22328 | 32506 | 35681 | 44015 | 62160 | 67331 |
| 15221 | 22522 | 32507 | 35682 | 44121 | 63035 | 67332 |
| 15241 | 22525 | 32667 | 35683 | 44128 | 63043 | 67334 |
| | | | | 44139 | 63044 | 67335 |
| | | | | 44203 | 63048 | 67340 |
| | | | | 44213 | 63057 | 69990 |
| | | | | 44701 | 63066 | 74301 |
| | | | | 44955 | 63076 | 75565 |
| | | | | 47001 | 63078 | 75774 |
| | | | | 47550 | 63082 | 75946 |
| | | | | 48400 | 63086 | 75964 |
| | | | | 49326 | 63088 | 75968 |

| | | | |
|---|---|---|---|
| 76125 | 92984 | 96366 | 0163T |
| 76802 | 92996 | 96367 | 0164T |
| 76810 | 92998 | 96368 | 0165T |
| 76812 | 93320 | 96370 | 0172T |
| 76814 | 93321 | 96371 | 0173T |
| 76937 | 93325 | 96375 | 0174T |
| 77001 | 93352 | 96376 | 0189T |
| 77051 | 93462 | 96411 | 0190T |
| 77052 | 93463 | 96415 | 0196T |
| 78020 | 93464 | 96417 | 0205T |
| 78496 | 93563 | 96423 | 0214T |
| 78730 | 93564 | 96570 | 0215T |
| 81266 | 93565 | 96571 | 0217T |
| 82952 | 93566 | 97546 | 0218T |
| 83901 | 93567 | 97598 | 0222T |
| 86826 | 93568 | 97811 | 0229T |
| 87187 | 93571 | 97814 | 0231T |
| 87503 | 93572 | 99100 | 0241T |
| 87904 | 93609 | 99116 | 0250T |
| 88155 | 93613 | 99135 | 0252T |
| 88177 | 93621 | 99140 | 0289T |
| 88185 | 93622 | 99145 | 0290T |
| 88311 | 93623 | 99150 | |
| 88314 | 93662 | 99292 | |
| 88332 | 94645 | 99354 | |
| 88334 | 94729 | 99355 | |
| 88388 | 94781 | 99356 | |
| 90461 | 95873 | 99357 | |
| 90472 | 95874 | 99359 | |
| 90474 | 95885 | 99467 | |
| 91013 | 95886 | 99602 | |
| 92547 | 95887 | 99607 | |
| 92608 | 95915 | 0054T | |
| 92618 | 95916 | 0055T | |
| 92621 | 95920 | 0076T | |
| 92627 | 95962 | 0079T | |
| 92973 | 95967 | 0081T | |
| 92974 | 95973 | 0092T | |
| 92978 | 95975 | 0095T | |
| 92979 | 95979 | 0098T | |
| 92981 | 96361 | 0159T | |

# Appendix E

## Summary of CPT Codes Exempt from Modifier 51

This listing is a summary of CPT codes that are exempt from the use of modifier 51. Procedures on this list are typically performed with another procedure but may be a stand alone procedure and not always be performed with other specified procedures. For add-on codes see Appendix D. This is not an exhaustive list of procedures that are typically exempt from multiple procedure reductions. The codes listed below are identified in *CPT 2012* with a ⊘ symbol.

17004

20697

20974

20975

31500

36620

44500

61107

93503

93600

93602

93603

93610

93612

93615

93616

93618

93631

94610

95900

95903

95904

95905

95992

99143

99144

# Appendix F

## Summary of CPT Codes Exempt from Modifier 63

The listing is a summary of CPT codes that are exempt from the use of modifier 63. The codes listed below are additionally identified in *CPT 2012* with the parenthetical instruction "(Do not report modifier 63 in conjunction with…)"

| | | |
|---|---|---|
| 30540 | 36415 | 49496 |
| 30545 | 36420 | 49600 |
| 31520 | 36450 | 49605 |
| 33401 | 36460 | 49606 |
| 33403 | 36510 | 49610 |
| 33470 | 36660 | 49611 |
| 33472 | 39503 | 53025 |
| 33502 | 43313 | 54000 |
| 33503 | 43314 | 54150 |
| 33505 | 43520 | 54160 |
| 33506 | 43831 | 63700 |
| 33610 | 44055 | 63702 |
| 33611 | 44126 | 63704 |
| 33619 | 44127 | 63706 |
| 33647 | 44128 | 65820 |
| 33670 | 46070 | |
| 33690 | 46705 | |
| 33694 | 46715 | |
| 33730 | 46716 | |
| 33732 | 46730 | |
| 33735 | 46735 | |
| 33736 | 46740 | |
| 33750 | 46742 | |
| 33755 | 46744 | |
| 33762 | 47700 | |
| 33778 | 47701 | |
| 33786 | 49215 | |
| 33922 | 49491 | |
| 33960 | 49492 | |
| 33961 | 49495 | |

# Appendix G

## Summary of CPT Codes That Include Moderate (Conscious) Sedation

The following list of procedures includes conscious sedation as an inherent part of providing the procedure. These codes are identified in the CPT codebook with a ⊙ symbol.

Since these services include moderate sedation, it is not appropriate for the same physician to report both the service and the sedation codes 99143-99145. It is expected that if conscious sedation is provided to the patient as part of one of these services, it is provided by the same physician who is providing the service.

In the unusual event when a second physician other than the health care professional performing the diagnostic or therapeutic services provides moderate sedation in the facility setting (eg, hospital, outpatient hospital/ ambulatory surgery center, skilled nursing facility) for the procedures listed in Appendix G, the second physician can report 99148-99150. However, for the circumstance in which these services are performed by the second physician in the nonfacility setting (eg, physician office, freestanding imaging center), codes 99148-99150 would not be reported. Moderate sedation does not include minimal sedation (anxiolysis), deep sedation, or monitored anesthesia care (00100-01999).

The inclusion of a procedure on this list does not prevent separate reporting of an associated anesthesia procedure/ service (CPT codes 00100-01999) when performed by a physician other than the health care professional performing the diagnostic or therapeutic procedure. In such cases the person providing anesthesia services shall be present for the purpose of continuously monitoring the patient and shall not act as a surgical assistant. When clinical conditions of the patient require such anesthesia services, or in the circumstances when the patient does not require sedation, the operating physician is not required to report the procedure as a reduced service using modifier 52.

| | | | |
|---|---|---|---|
| 19298 | 31620 | 31628 | 31725 |
| 20982 | 31622 | 31629 | 32201 |
| 22520 | 31623 | 31634 | 32405 |
| 22521 | 31624 | 31635 | 32550 |
| 22526 | 31625 | 31645 | 32551 |
| 22527 | 31626 | 31646 | 32553 |
| 31615 | 31627 | 31656 | 33010 |

| | | |
|---|---|---|
| 33011 | 36248 | 37223 |
| 33206 | 36251 | 37224 |
| 33207 | 36252 | 37225 |
| 33208 | 36253 | 37226 |
| 33210 | 36254 | 37227 |
| 33211 | 36481 | 37228 |
| 33212 | 36555 | 37229 |
| 33213 | 36557 | 37230 |
| 33214 | 36558 | 37231 |
| 33216 | 36560 | 37232 |
| 33217 | 36561 | 37233 |
| 33218 | 36563 | 37234 |
| 33220 | 36565 | 37235 |
| 33221 | 36566 | 43200 |
| 33222 | 36568 | 43201 |
| 33223 | 36570 | 43202 |
| 33227 | 36571 | 43204 |
| 33228 | 36576 | 43205 |
| 33229 | 36578 | 43215 |
| 33230 | 36581 | 43216 |
| 33231 | 36582 | 43217 |
| 33233 | 36583 | 43219 |
| 33234 | 36585 | 43220 |
| 33235 | 36590 | 43226 |
| 33240 | 36870 | 43227 |
| 33241 | 37183 | 43228 |
| 33244 | 37184 | 43231 |
| 33249 | 37185 | 43232 |
| 33262 | 37186 | 43234 |
| 33263 | 37187 | 43235 |
| 33264 | 37188 | 43236 |
| 35471 | 37191 | 43237 |
| 35472 | 37192 | 43238 |
| 35475 | 37193 | 43239 |
| 35476 | 37203 | 43240 |
| 36147 | 37210 | 43241 |
| 36148 | 37215 | 43242 |
| 36200 | 37216 | 43243 |
| 36245 | 37220 | 43244 |
| 36246 | 37221 | 43245 |
| 36247 | 37222 | 43246 |

| | | | | |
|---|---|---|---|---|
| 43247 | 44383 | 45384 | 92973 | 93566 |
| 43248 | 44385 | 45385 | 92974 | 93567 |
| 43249 | 44386 | 45386 | 92975 | 93568 |
| 43250 | 44388 | 45387 | 92978 | 93571 |
| 43251 | 44389 | 45391 | 92979 | 93572 |
| 43255 | 44390 | 45392 | 92980 | 93609 |
| 43256 | 44391 | 47000 | 92981 | 93613 |
| 43257 | 44392 | 47011 | 92982 | 93615 |
| 43258 | 44393 | 47382 | 92984 | 93616 |
| 43259 | 44394 | 47525 | 92986 | 93618 |
| 43260 | 44397 | 48511 | 92987 | 93619 |
| 43261 | 44500 | 49021 | 92995 | 93620 |
| 43262 | 44901 | 49041 | 92996 | 93621 |
| 43263 | 45303 | 49061 | 93312 | 93622 |
| 43264 | 45305 | 49411 | 93313 | 93624 |
| 43265 | 45307 | 49418 | 93314 | 93640 |
| 43267 | 45308 | 49440 | 93315 | 93641 |
| 43268 | 45309 | 49441 | 93316 | 93642 |
| 43269 | 45315 | 49442 | 93317 | 93650 |
| 43271 | 45317 | 49446 | 93318 | 93651 |
| 43272 | 45320 | 50021 | 93451 | 93652 |
| 43273 | 45321 | 50200 | 93452 | 94011 |
| 43453 | 45327 | 50382 | 93453 | 94012 |
| 43456 | 45332 | 50384 | 93454 | 94013 |
| 43458 | 45333 | 50385 | 93455 | 0200T |
| 44360 | 45334 | 50386 | 93456 | 0201T |
| 44361 | 45335 | 50387 | 93457 | 0250T |
| 44363 | 45337 | 50592 | 93458 | 0251T |
| 44364 | 45338 | 50593 | 93459 | 0252T |
| 44365 | 45339 | 57155 | 93460 | 0276T |
| 44366 | 45340 | 58823 | 93461 | 0277T |
| 44369 | 45341 | 66720 | 93462 | 0282T |
| 44370 | 45342 | 69300 | 93463 | 0283T |
| 44372 | 45345 | 77371 | 93464 | 0284T |
| 44373 | 45355 | 77600 | 93505 | |
| 44376 | 45378 | 77605 | 93530 | |
| 44377 | 45379 | 77610 | 93561 | |
| 44378 | 45380 | 77615 | 93562 | |
| 44379 | 45381 | 92953 | 93563 | |
| 44380 | 45382 | 92960 | 93564 | |
| 44382 | 45383 | 92961 | 93565 | |

# Appendix H

## Alphabetical Clinical Topics Listing (AKA – Alphabetical Listing)

**The Alphabetical Clinical Topics Listing** (formerly Appendix H) has been removed from the CPT codebook. Since this document is a dynamic and rapidly expanding source of information to link *CPT* Category II codes, clinical conditions, and measure abstracts, the Alphabetical Listing is now solely accessed on the AMA web site at www.ama-assn.org/go/cpt.

In addition, new codes for the publication cycle (ie, **the Update to the List of Category II Codes**) will continue to be located on the AMA web site prior to publication in the next edition of the CPT codebook (subsequent to its listing to the Web).

# Appendix I

## Genetic Testing Code Modifiers

This listing of modifiers is intended for reporting with molecular laboratory procedures related to genetic testing. Genetic testing modifiers should be used in conjunction with CPT and HCPCS codes to provide diagnostic granularity of service to enable providers to submit complete and precise genetic testing information without altering test descriptors. These two-character modifiers are categorized by mutation. The first (numeric) character indicates the disease category and the second (alpha) character denotes gene type. Introductory guidelines in the molecular diagnostic and molecular cytogenetic code sections of the CPT codebook provide further guidance in interpretation and application of genetic testing modifiers.

## Neoplasia (Solid Tumor, Excluding Sarcoma and Lymphoma)

| | |
|---|---|
| 0A | BRCA1 (hereditary breast/ovarian cancer) |
| 0B | BRCA2 (hereditary breast cancer) |
| 0C | Neurofibromin (neurofibromatosis, type 1) |
| 0D | Merlin (neurofibromatosis, type 2) |
| 0E | c-RET (multiple endocrine neoplasia, types 2A/B, familial medullary thyroid carcinoma) |
| 0F | VHL (Von Hippel Lindau disease, renal carcinoma) |
| 0G | SDHD (hereditary paraganglioma) |
| 0H | SDHB (hereditary paraganglioma) |
| 0I | ERRB2, commonly called Her-2/neu |
| 0J | MLH1 (HNPCC, mismatch repair genes) |
| 0K | MSH2, MSH6, or PMS2 (HNPCC, mismatch repair genes) |
| 0L | APC (hereditary polyposis coli) |
| 0M | Rb (retinoblastoma) |
| 0N | TP53, commonly called p53 |
| 0O | PTEN (Cowden's syndrome) |
| 0P | KIT, also called CD117 (gastrointestinal stromal tumor) |
| 0Z | Solid tumor gene, not otherwise specified |

## Neoplasia (Sarcoma)

| | |
|---|---|
| 1A | WT1 or WT2 (Wilm's tumor) |
| 1B | PAX3, PAX7, or FOXO1A (alveolar rhabdomyosarcoma) |
| 1C | FLI1, ERG, ETV1, or EWSR1 (Ewing's sarcoma, desmoplastic round cell) |
| 1D | DDIT3 or FUS (myxoid liposarcoma) |
| 1E | NR4A3, RBF56, or TCF12 (myxoid chondrosarcoma) |
| 1F | SSX1, SSX2, or SYT (synovial sarcoma) |
| 1G | MYCN (neuroblastoma) |
| 1H | COL1A1 or PDGFB (dermatofibrosarcoma protruberans) |
| 1I | TFE3 or ASPSCR1 (alveolar soft parts sarcoma) |
| 1J | JAZF1 or JJAZ1 (endometrial stromal sarcoma) |
| 1Z | Sarcoma gene, not otherwise specified |

## Neoplasia (Lymphoid/Hematopoietic)

| | |
|---|---|
| 2A | RUNX1 or CBFA2T1, commonly called AML1 or ETO, genes associated with t(8;21) AML1—also ETO (acute myelogenous leukemia) |
| 2B | BCR or ABL1, genes associated with t(9;22) (chronic myelogenous or acute leukemia) BCR—also ABL (chronic myeloid, acute lymphoid leukemia) |
| 2C | PBX1 or TCF3, genes associated with t(1;19) (acute lymphoblastic leukemia) CGF1 |
| 2D | CBFB or MYH11, genes associated with inv 16 (acute myelogenous leukemia) CBF beta (leukemia) |
| 2E | MLL (acute leukemia) |
| 2F | PML or RARA, genes associated with t(15;17) (acute promyelocytic leukemia) PML/RAR alpha (promyelocytic leukemia) |
| 2G | ETV6, commonly called TEL, gene associated with t(12;21) (acute leukemia) TEL (Leukemia) |
| 2H | BCL2 (B cell lymphoma, follicle center cell origin) bcl-2 (Lymphoma) |
| 2I | CCND1, commonly called BCL1, cyclin D1 (Mantle cell lymphoma, myeloma) bcl-1 (lymphoma) |
| 2J | MYC (Burkitt lymphoma) c-myc (lymphoma) |
| 2K | IgH (lymphoma/leukemia) |
| 2L | IGK (lymphoma/leukemia) |
| 2M | TRB, T cell receptor beta (lymphoma/leukemia) |
| 2N | TRG, T cell receptor gamma (lymphoma/leukemia) |

| | |
|---|---|
| 2O | SIL or TAL1 (T cell leukemia) |
| 2T | BCL6 (B cell lymphoma) |
| 2Q | API1 or MALT1 (MALT lymphoma) |
| 2R | NPM or ALK, genes associated with t(2;5) (anaplastic large cell lymphoma) |
| 2S | FLT3 (Acute myelogenous leukemia) |
| 2Z | Lymphoid/hematopoietic neoplasia, not otherwise specified |

## Non-Neoplastic Hematology/Coagulation

| | |
|---|---|
| 3A | F5, commonly called Factor V (Leiden, others) (hypercoagulable state) |
| 3B | FACC (Fanconi anemia) |
| 3C | FACD (Fanconi anemia) |
| 3D | HBB, beta globin (thalassemia, sickle cell anemia, other hemoglobinopathies) |
| 3E | HBA, commonly called alpha globin (thalassemia) |
| 3F | MTHFR (elevated homocystinemia) |
| 3G | F2, commonly called prothrombin (20210, others) (hypercoagulable state) prothrombin (factor II, 20210A) (hypercoagulable state) |
| 3H | F8, commonly called factor VIII (hemophilia A/VWF) |
| 3I | F9, commonly called factor IX (hemophilia B) |
| 3K | F13, commonly called factor XIII (bleeding or hypercoagulable state) beta globin |
| 3Z | Non-neoplastic hematology/coagulation, not otherwise specified |

## Histocompatiblity/Blood Typing/Identity/Microsatellite

| | |
|---|---|
| ▲4A | HLA-A* |
| ▲4B | HLA-B* |
| ▲4C | HLA-C* |
| | (Modifier 4D has been deleted) |
| ▲4E | HLA-DRB all |
| # ●4P | HLA-DRB1* |
| # ●4Q | HLA-DRB3* |
| # ●4R | HLA-DRB4* |
| # ●4S | HLA-DRB5* |
| # ●4T | HLA-DQA1* |

| | |
|---|---|
| ▲4F | HLA-DQB1* |
| #●4U | HLA-DPA1* |
| ▲4G | HLA-DPB1* |
| 4H | Kell |
| 4I | Fingerprint for engraftment (post allogeneic progenitor cell transplant) |
| 4J | Fingerprint for donor allelotype (allogeneic transplant) |
| 4K | Fingerprint for recipient allelotype (allogeneic transplant) |
| 4L | Fingerprint for leukocyte chimerism (allogeneic solid organ transplant) |
| 4M | Fingerprint for maternal versus fetal origin |
| 4N | Microsatellite instability |
| 4O | Microsatellite loss (loss of heterozygosity) |
| # 4P | Modifier is out of numerical sequence. See Modifier 4A-4Z |
| # 4Q | Modifier is out of numerical sequence. See Modifier 4A-4Z |
| # 4R | Modifier is out of numerical sequence. See Modifier 4A-4Z |
| # 4S | Modifier is out of numerical sequence. See Modifier 4A-4Z |
| # 4T | Modifier is out of numerical sequence. See Modifier 4A-4Z |
| # 4U | Modifier is out of numerical sequence. See Modifier 4A-4Z |
| ▲4Z | Histocompatiblity/typing, not otherwise specified |

## Neurologic, Non-Neoplastic

| | |
|---|---|
| 5A | ASPA, commonly called Aspartoacylase A (Canavan disease) |
| 5B | FMR-1 (fragile X, FRAXA, syndrome) |
| 5C | FRDA, commonly called Frataxin (Freidreich ataxia) |
| 5D | HD, commonly called Huntington (Huntington's disease) |
| 5E | GABRA5, NIPA1, UBE3A, or ANCR GABRA (Prader Willi-Angelman syndrome) |
| 5F | GJB2, commonly called Connexin-26 (hereditary hearing loss) Connexin-32 (GJB2) (hereditary deafness) |
| 5G | GJB1, commonly called Connexin-32 (X-linked Charcot-Marie-Tooth disease) |
| 5H | SNRPN (Prader Willi-Angelman syndrome) |

5I   SCA1, commonly called Ataxin-1 (spinocerebellar ataxia, type 1)

5J   SCA2, commonly called Ataxin-2 (spinocerebellar ataxia, type 2)

5K   MJD, commonly called Ataxin-3 (spinocerebellar ataxia, type 3, Machado-Joseph disease)

5L   CACNA1A (spinocerebellar ataxia, type 6)

5M   ATXN7 Ataxin-7 (spinocerebellar ataxia, type 7)

5N   PMP-22 (Charcot-Marie-Tooth disease, type 1A)

5O   MECP2 (Rett syndrome)

5Z   Neurologic, non-neoplastic, not otherwise specified

## Muscular, Non-Neoplastic

6A   DMD, commonly called dystrophin (Duchenne/Becker muscular dystrophy)

6B   DMPK (myotonic dystrophy, type 1)

6C   ZNF-9 (myotonic dystrophy, type 2)

6D   SMN1/SMN2 (autosomal recessive spinal muscular atrophy)

6E   MTTK, commonly called tRNAlys (myotonic epilepsy, MERRF)

6F   MTTL1, commonly called tRNAleu (mitochondrial encephalomyopathy, MELAS)

6Z   Muscular, not otherwise specified

## Metabolic, Other

7A   APOE, commonly called apolipoprotein E (cardiovascular disease or Alzheimer's disease)

7B   NPC1 or NPC2, commonly called sphingomyelin phosphodiesterase (Nieman-Pick disease)

7C   GBA, commonly called acid beta glucosidase (Gaucher disease)

7D   HFE (hemochromatosis)

7E   HEXA, commonly called hexosaminidase A (Tay-Sachs disease)

7F   ACADM (medium chain acyl CoA dehydrogenase deficiency)

7Z   Metabolic, other, not otherwise specified

## Metabolic, Transport

8A   CFTR (cystic fibrosis)

8B   PRSS1 (hereditary pancreatitis)

8C   Long QT syndrome, KCN (Jervell and Lange-Nielsen syndromes, types 1, 2, 5, and 6) and SCN (Brugada syndrome, SIDS and type 3)

8Z   Metabolic, transport, not otherwise specified

## Metabolic-Pharmacogenetics

9A   TPMT, commonly called (thiopurine methyltransferase) (patients on antimetabolite therapy)

9B   CYP2 genes, commonly called cytochrome p450 (drug metabolism)

9C   ABCB1, commonly called MDR1 or p-glycoprotein (drug transport)

9D   NAT2 (drug metabolism)

9L   Metabolic-pharmacogenetics, not otherwise specified

## Dysmorphology

9M   FGFR1 (Pfeiffer and Kallman syndromes)

9N   FGFR2 (Crouzon, Jackson-Weiss, Apert, Saethre-Chotzen syndromes)

9O   FGFR3 (achondroplasia, hypochondroplasia, thanatophoric dysplasia, types I and II, Crouzon syndrome with acanthosis nigricans, Muencke syndromes)

9P   TWIST (Saethre-Chotzen syndrome)

9Q   DGCR, commonly called CATCH-22 (DiGeorge and 22q11 deletion syndromes)

9Z   Dysmorphology, not otherwise specified

# Appendix J

## Electrodiagnostic Medicine Listing of Sensory, Motor, and Mixed Nerves

This summary assigns each sensory, motor, and mixed nerve with its appropriate nerve conduction study code in order to enhance accurate reporting of codes 95900, 95903, and 95904. Each nerve constitutes one unit of service.

### Motor Nerves Assigned to Codes 95900 and 95903

I. Upper extremity, cervical plexus, and brachial plexus motor nerves
  A. Axillary motor nerve to the deltoid
  B. Long thoracic motor nerve to the serratus anterior
  C. Median nerve
    1. Median motor nerve to the abductor pollicis brevis
    2. Median motor nerve, anterior interosseous branch, to the flexor pollicis longus
    3. Median motor nerve, anterior interosseous branch, to the pronator quadratus
    4. Median motor nerve to the first lumbrical
    5. Median motor nerve to the second lumbrical
  D. Musculocutaneous motor nerve to the biceps brachii
  E. Radial nerve
    1. Radial motor nerve to the extensor carpi ulnaris
    2. Radial motor nerve to the extensor digitorum communis
    3. Radial motor nerve to the extensor indicis proprius
    4. Radial motor nerve to the brachioradialis
  F. Suprascapular nerve
    1. Suprascapular motor nerve to the supraspinatus
    2. Suprascapular motor nerve to the infraspinatus
  G. Thoracodorsal motor nerve to the latissimus dorsi

H. Ulnar nerve
    1. Ulnar motor nerve to the abductor digiti minimi
    2. Ulnar motor nerve to the palmar interosseous
    3. Ulnar motor nerve to the first dorsal interosseous
    4. Ulnar motor nerve to the flexor carpi ulnaris
  I. Other
II. Lower extremity motor nerves
  A. Femoral motor nerve to the quadriceps
    1. Femoral motor nerve to vastus medialis
    2. Femoral motor nerve to vastus lateralis
    3. Femoral motor nerve to vastus intermedialis
    4. Femoral motor nerve to rectus femoris
  B. Ilioinguinal motor nerve
  C. Peroneal (fibular) nerve
    1. Peroneal motor nerve to the extensor digitorum brevis
    2. Peroneal motor nerve to the peroneus brevis
    3. Peroneal motor nerve to the peroneus longus
    4. Peroneal motor nerve to the tibialis anterior
  D. Plantar motor nerve
  E. Sciatic nerve
  F. Tibial nerve
    1. Tibial motor nerve, inferior calcaneal branch, to the abductor digiti minimi
    2. Tibial motor nerve, medial plantar branch, to the abductor hallucis
    3. Tibial motor nerve, lateral plantar branch, to the flexor digiti minimi brevis
  G. Other
III. Cranial nerves and trunk
  A. Cranial nerve VII (facial motor nerve)
    1. Facial nerve to the frontalis
    2. Facial nerve to the nasalis
    3. Facial nerve to the orbicularis oculi
    4. Facial nerve to the orbicularis oris
  B. Cranial nerve XI (spinal accessory motor nerve)
  C. Cranial nerve XII (hypoglossal motor nerve)
  D. Intercostal motor nerve
  E. Phrenic motor nerve to the diaphragm
  F. Recurrent laryngeal nerve
  G. Other
IV. Nerve Roots
  A. Cervical nerve root stimulation
    1. Cervical level 5 (CT)
    2. Cervical level 6 (C6)
    3. Cervical level 7 (C7)
    4. Cervical level 8 (C8)

B. Thoracic nerve root stimulation
  1. Thoracic level 1 (T1)
  2. Thoracic level 2 (T2)
  3. Thoracic level 3 (T3)
  4. Thoracic level 4 (T4)
  5. Thoracic level 5 (T5)
  6. Thoracic level 6 (T6)
  7. Thoracic level 7 (T7)
  8. Thoracic level 8 (T8)
  9. Thoracic level 9 (T9)
 10. Thoracic level 10 (T10)
 11. Thoracic level 11 (T11)
 12. Thoracic level 12 (T12)
C. Lumbar nerve root stimulation
  1. Lumbar level 1 (L1)
  2. Lumbar level 2 (L2)
  3. Lumbar level 3 (L3)
  4. Lumbar level 4 (L4)
  5. Lumbar level 5 (L5)
D. Sacral nerve root stimulation
  1. Sacral level 1 (S1)
  2. Sacral level 2 (S2)
  3. Sacral level 3 (S3)
  4. Sacral level 4 (S4)

## Sensory and Mixed Nerves Assigned to Code 95904

I. Upper extremity sensory and mixed nerves
  A. Lateral antebrachial cutaneous sensory nerve
  B. Medial antebrachial cutaneous sensory nerve
  C. Medial brachial cutaneous sensory nerve
  D. Median nerve
    1. Median sensory nerve to the first digit
    2. Median sensory nerve to the second digit
    3. Median sensory nerve to the third digit
    4. Median sensory nerve to the fourth digit
    5. Median palmar cutaneous sensory nerve
    6. Median palmar mixed nerve
  E. Posterior antebrachial cutaneous sensory nerve
  F. Radial sensory nerve
    1. Radial sensory nerve to the base of the thumb
    2. Radial sensory nerve to digit 1
  G. Ulnar nerve
    1. Ulnar dorsal cutaneous sensory nerve
    2. Ulnar sensory nerve to the fourth digit
    3. Ulnar sensory nerve to the fifth digit
    4. Ulnar palmar mixed nerve
  H. Intercostal sensory nerve
  I. Other

II. Lower extremity sensory and mixed nerves
  A. Lateral femoral cutaneous sensory nerve
  B. Medial calcaneal sensory nerve
  C. Medial femoral cutaneous sensory nerve
  D. Peroneal nerve
    1. Deep peroneal sensory nerve
    2. Superficial peroneal sensory nerve, medial dorsal cutaneous branch
    3. Superficial peroneal sensory nerve, intermediate dorsal cutaneous branch
  E. Posterior femoral cutaneous sensory nerve
  F. Saphenous nerve
    1. Saphenous sensory nerve (distal technique)
    2. Saphenous sensory nerve (proximal technique)
  G. Sural nerve
    1. Sural sensory nerve, lateral dorsal cutaneous branch
    2. Sural sensory nerve
  H. Tibial sensory nerve (digital nerve to toe 1)
  I. Tibial sensory nerve (medial plantar nerve)
  J. Tibial sensory nerve (lateral plantar nerve)
  K. Other

III. Head and trunk sensory nerves
  A. Dorsal nerve of the penis
  B. Greater auricular nerve
  C. Ophthalmic branch of the trigeminal nerve
  D. Pudendal sensory nerve
  E. Suprascapular sensory nerves
  F. Other

The following table provides a reasonable maximum number of studies performed per diagnostic category necessary for a physician to arrive at a diagnosis in 90% of patients with that final diagnosis. The numbers in each column represent the number of studies recommended. The appropriate number of studies to be performed is based upon the physician's discretion.

| Indication | Needle EMG (95860-95864, 95867-95870) | Nerve Conduction Studies (95900, 95903, 95904) | | Other EMG Studies (95934, 95936, 95937) | |
|---|---|---|---|---|---|
| | | Motor NCS With and/or Without F wave | Sensory NCS | H-Reflex | Neuromuscular Junction Testing (Repetitive Stimulation) |
| Carpal Tunnel (Unilateral) | 1 | 3 | 4 | — | — |
| Carpal Tunnel (Bilateral) | 2 | 4 | 6 | — | — |
| Radiculopathy | 2 | 3 | 2 | 2 | — |
| Mononeuropathy | 1 | 3 | 3 | 2 | — |
| Polyneuropathy/Mononeuropathy Multiplex | 3 | 4 | 4 | 2 | — |
| Myopathy | 2 | 2 | 2 | — | 2 |
| Motor Neuronopathy (eg, ALS) | 4 | 4 | 2 | — | 2 |
| Plexopathy | 2 | 4 | 6 | 2 | — |
| Neuromuscular Junction | 2 | 2 | 2 | — | 3 |
| Tarsal Tunnel Syndrome (Unilateral) | 1 | 4 | 4 | — | — |
| Tarsal Tunnel Syndrome (Bilateral) | 2 | 5 | 6 | — | — |
| Weakness, Fatigue, Cramps, or Twitching (Focal) | 2 | 3 | 4 | — | 2 |
| Weakness, Fatigue, Cramps, or Twitching (General) | 4 | 4 | 4 | — | 2 |
| Pain, Numbness, or Tingling (Unilateral) | 1 | 3 | 4 | 2 | — |
| Pain, Numbness, or Tingling (Bilateral) | 2 | 4 | 6 | 2 | — |

# Appendix K

## Product Pending FDA Approval

Some vaccine products have been assigned a CPT Category I code in anticipation of future approval from the Food and Drug Administration (FDA). Following is a list of the vaccine product codes pending FDA approval status that are identified in the CPT codebook with the (✗) symbol. Upon revision of the approval status by the FDA, notation of this revision will be provided via the AMA CPT "Category I Vaccine Codes" Internet listing (www.ama-assn.org/ama/pub/category/10902.html) and in subsequent publications of the CPT codebook.

90644

90661

90664

90666

90667

90668

# Appendix L

## Vascular Families

Assignment of branches to first, second, and third order in this table makes the assumption that the starting point is catheterization of the aorta. This categorization would not be accurate, for instance, if a femoral or carotid artery were catheterized directly in an antegrade direction. Arteries highlighted in bold are those more commonly reported during arteriographic procedures.

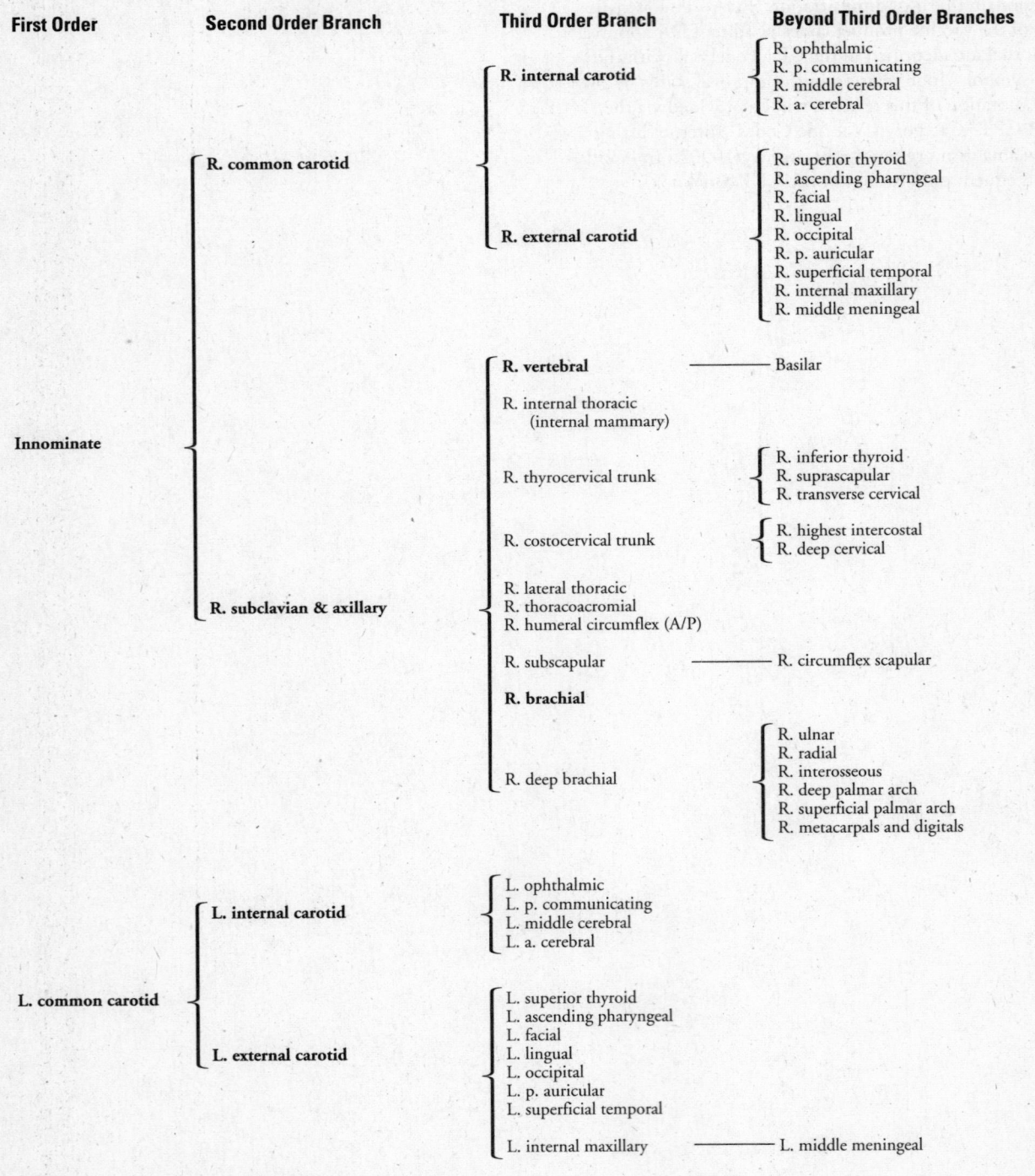

| First Order | Second Order Branch | Third Order Branch | Beyond Third Order Branches |
|---|---|---|---|
| | **R. common carotid** | **R. internal carotid** | R. ophthalmic<br>R. p. communicating<br>R. middle cerebral<br>R. a. cerebral |
| | | **R. external carotid** | R. superior thyroid<br>R. ascending pharyngeal<br>R. facial<br>R. lingual<br>R. occipital<br>R. p. auricular<br>R. superficial temporal<br>R. internal maxillary<br>R. middle meningeal |
| **Innominate** | | **R. vertebral** | Basilar |
| | | R. internal thoracic (internal mammary) | |
| | | R. thyrocervical trunk | R. inferior thyroid<br>R. suprascapular<br>R. transverse cervical |
| | | R. costocervical trunk | R. highest intercostal<br>R. deep cervical |
| | **R. subclavian & axillary** | R. lateral thoracic<br>R. thoracoacromial<br>R. humeral circumflex (A/P) | |
| | | R. subscapular | R. circumflex scapular |
| | | **R. brachial** | |
| | | R. deep brachial | R. ulnar<br>R. radial<br>R. interosseous<br>R. deep palmar arch<br>R. superficial palmar arch<br>R. metacarpals and digitals |
| **L. common carotid** | **L. internal carotid** | L. ophthalmic<br>L. p. communicating<br>L. middle cerebral<br>L. a. cerebral | |
| | **L. external carotid** | L. superior thyroid<br>L. ascending pharyngeal<br>L. facial<br>L. lingual<br>L. occipital<br>L. p. auricular<br>L. superficial temporal | |
| | | L. internal maxillary | L. middle meningeal |

R = right, L = left, A = anterior, P = posterior

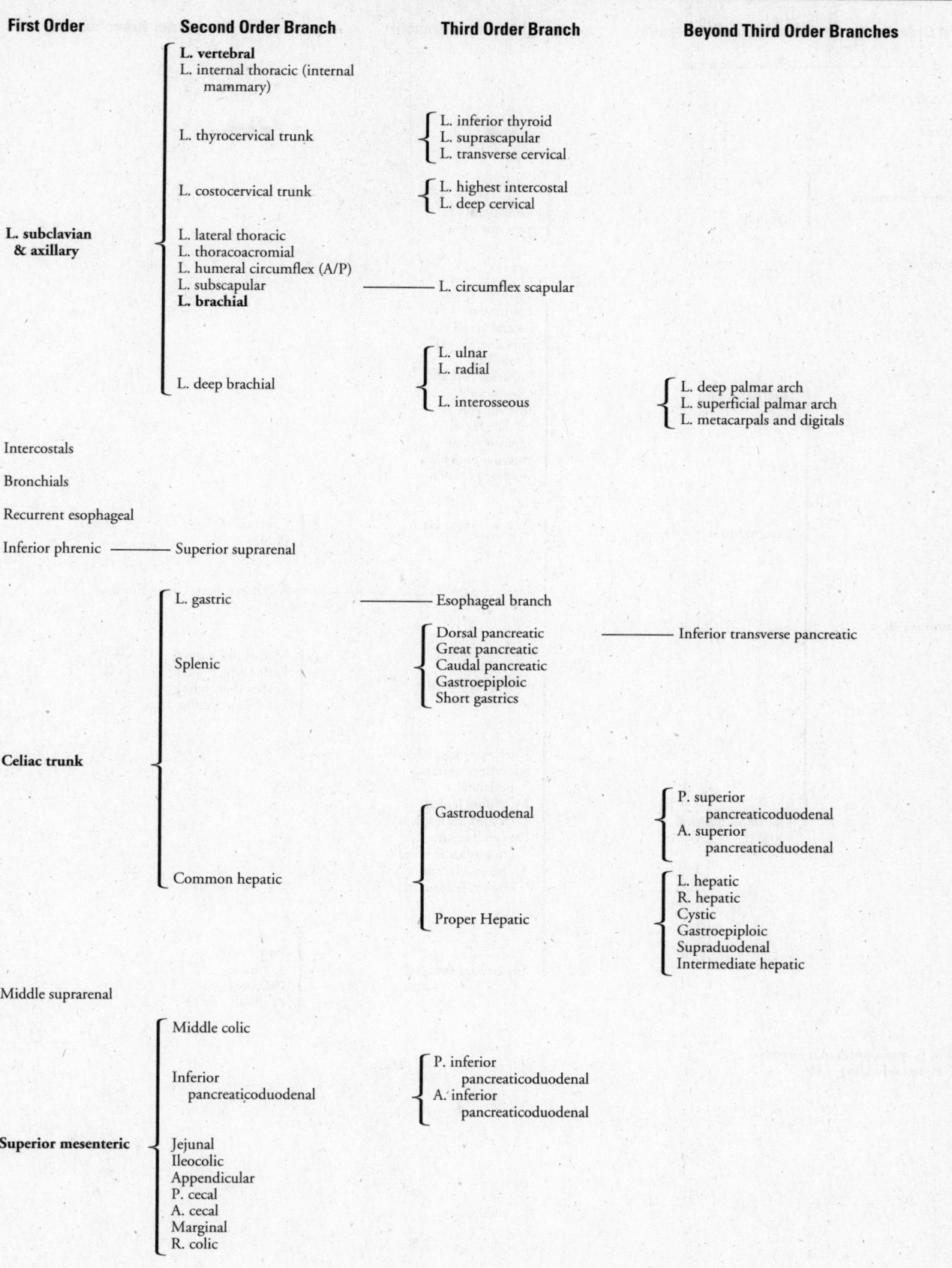

| First Order | Second Order Branch | Third Order Branch | Beyond Third Order Branches |
|---|---|---|---|
| **L. subclavian & axillary** | **L. vertebral** | | |
| | L. internal thoracic (internal mammary) | | |
| | L. thyrocervical trunk | L. inferior thyroid<br>L. suprascapular<br>L. transverse cervical | |
| | L. costocervical trunk | L. highest intercostal<br>L. deep cervical | |
| | L. lateral thoracic<br>L. thoracoacromial<br>L. humeral circumflex (A/P)<br>L. subscapular<br>**L. brachial** | L. circumflex scapular | |
| | L. deep brachial | L. ulnar<br>L. radial<br>L. interosseous | L. deep palmar arch<br>L. superficial palmar arch<br>L. metacarpals and digitals |
| Intercostals | | | |
| Bronchials | | | |
| Recurrent esophageal | | | |
| Inferior phrenic | Superior suprarenal | | |
| **Celiac trunk** | L. gastric | Esophageal branch | |
| | Splenic | Dorsal pancreatic<br>Great pancreatic<br>Caudal pancreatic<br>Gastroepiploic<br>Short gastrics | Inferior transverse pancreatic |
| | Common hepatic | Gastroduodenal | P. superior pancreaticoduodenal<br>A. superior pancreaticoduodenal |
| | | Proper Hepatic | L. hepatic<br>R. hepatic<br>Cystic<br>Gastroepiploic<br>Supraduodenal<br>Intermediate hepatic |
| Middle suprarenal | | | |
| **Superior mesenteric** | Middle colic | | |
| | Inferior pancreaticoduodenal | P. inferior pancreaticoduodenal<br>A. inferior pancreaticoduodenal | |
| | Jejunal<br>Ileocolic<br>Appendicular<br>P. cecal<br>A. cecal<br>Marginal<br>R. colic | | |

R = right, L = left, A = anterior, P = posterior

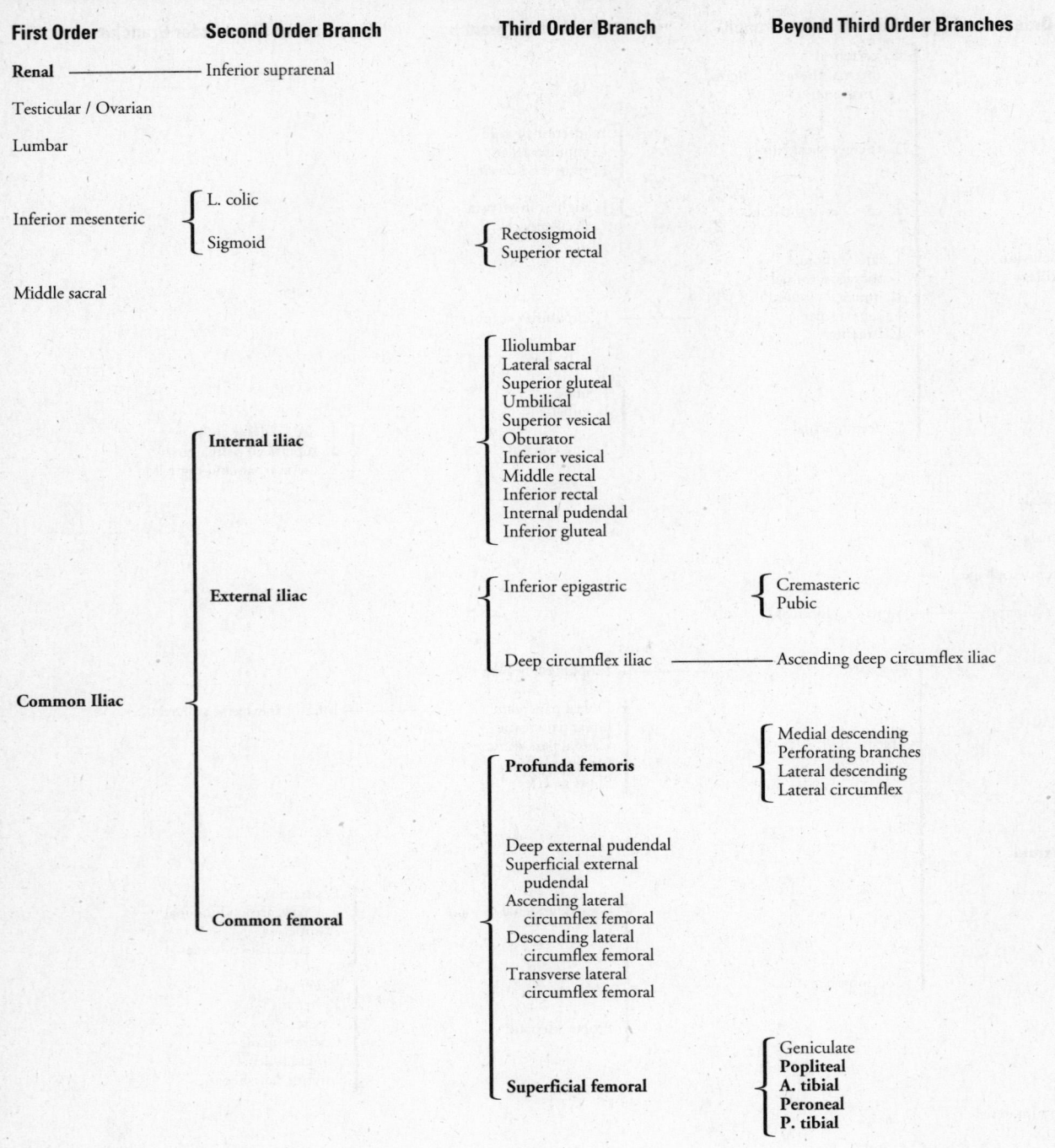

| First Order | Second Order Branch | Third Order Branch | Beyond Third Order Branches |
|---|---|---|---|
| **Renal** ———————— | Inferior suprarenal | | |
| Testicular / Ovarian | | | |
| Lumbar | | | |
| Inferior mesenteric | { L. colic / Sigmoid | { Rectosigmoid / Superior rectal | |
| Middle sacral | | | |
| **Common Iliac** | **Internal iliac** | { Iliolumbar / Lateral sacral / Superior gluteal / Umbilical / Superior vesical / Obturator / Inferior vesical / Middle rectal / Inferior rectal / Internal pudendal / Inferior gluteal | |
| | **External iliac** | { Inferior epigastric | { Cremasteric / Pubic |
| | | Deep circumflex iliac ——— | Ascending deep circumflex iliac |
| | **Common femoral** | **Profunda femoris** | { Medial descending / Perforating branches / Lateral descending / Lateral circumflex |
| | | { Deep external pudendal / Superficial external pudendal / Ascending lateral circumflex femoral / Descending lateral circumflex femoral / Transverse lateral circumflex femoral | |
| | | **Superficial femoral** | { Geniculate / **Popliteal** / **A. tibial** / **Peroneal** / **P. tibial** |

**R. & L. main pulmonary arteries**
**(venous selective)**

***Reference:*** Kadir S. *Atlas of Normal and Variant Angiographic Anatomy.* Philadephia, Pa: WB Saunders Co; 1991.
R = right, L = left, A = anterior, P = posterior

# Appendix M

## Deleted CPT Codes

This listing is a summary of crosswalked deleted and renumbered codes and descriptors with the associated *CPT Assistant* references for the deleted codes. This listing includes codes deleted and renumbered from 2007 to 2009. Additional codes will not be added, since the principle of deleting and renumbering is no longer being utilized in the CPT code set.

| Current Code(s) | Deleted/Former Code | Year Code Deleted | Citations Referencing Former Code— Applicable to Current Code(s) |
|---|---|---|---|
| 89240 | 0058T | 2009 | Jun 04:8 CPT Changes: An Insider's View 2004 |
| 89240 | 0059T | 2009 | CPT Changes: An Insider's View 2004 |
| 41530 | 0088T | 2009 | May 05:7, Sep 05:9 CPT Changes: An Insider's View 2005 |
| 95803 | 0089T | 2009 | Jun 05:6, Feb 06:1 CPT Changes: An Insider's View 2006 |
| 22856 | 0090T | 2009 | Jun 05:6, Feb 06:1 CPT Changes: An Insider's View 2006, 2007 |
| 22864 | 0093T | 2009 | Jun 05:6, Feb 06:1 CPT Changes: An Insider's View 2006, 2007 |
| 22861 | 0096T | 2009 | Jun 05:6, Feb 06:1 CPT Changes: An Insider's View 2006, 2007 |
| 55706 | 0137T | 2009 | CPT Changes: An Insider's View 2006 |
| 95980-95982 | 0162T | 2009 | CPT Changes: An Insider's View 2007 |
| 1123F, 1124F | 1080F | 2009 | CPT Changes: An Insider's View 2008 |
| 0054T, 0055T | 20986 | 2009 | CPT Changes: An Insider's View 2008 |
| 0054T, 0055T | 20987 | 2009 | CPT Changes: An Insider's View 2008 |
| 4177F | 4007F | 2009 | CPT Changes: An Insider's View 2008 |
| 52214 | 52606 | 2009 | Apr 01:4 |
| 52601 | 52612 | 2009 | Apr 01:4 |
| 52601 | 52614 | 2009 | Apr 01:4 |
| 52630 | 52620 | 2009 | Apr 01:4 |
| 61796-61800, 63620, 63621 | 61793 | 2009 | Nov 97:23, May 03:19, Apr 04:15, Jan 06:46 |
| 77785, 77786 | 77781 | 2009 | Winter 90:10, Winter 91:23, Mar 99:3, Feb 02:7, Mar 02:2, Sep 05:1, Nov 05:15 |
| 77785-77787 | 77782 | 2009 | Winter 90:10, Winter 91:23, Mar 99:3, Feb 02:7, Mar 02:2, Sep 05:1, Nov 05:15 |
| 77785-77787 | 77783 | 2009 | Winter 90:10, Winter 91:23, Mar 99:3, Feb 02:7, Mar 02:2, Sep 05:1, Nov 05:15 |
| 77785-77787 | 77784 | 2009 | Winter 90:10, Winter 91:23, Mar 99:3, Feb 02:7, Mar 02:2, Sep 05:1, Nov 05:15 |
| 88720 | 88400 | 2009 | Aug 05:9 |
| 96360 | 90760 | 2009 | Nov 05:1, Jul 06:4, Sep 06:14, Dec 06:14 CPT Changes: An Insider's View 2006, 2008 |
| 96361 | 90761 | 2009 | Nov 05:1, Jul 06:4, Sep 06:14, Dec 06:14, Mar 07:10 CPT Changes: An Insider's View 2006, 2007 |
| 96365 | 90765 | 2009 | Nov 05:1, Sep 06:14, Nov 06:22, Dec 06:14 CPT Changes: An Insider's View 2006 |
| 96366 | 90766 | 2009 | Nov 05:1, Sep 06:14, Dec 06:14, Mar 07:10 CPT Changes: An Insider's View 2006, 2007 |
| 96367 | 90767 | 2009 | Nov 05:1, Sep 06:14, Nov 06:22, Dec 06:14 CPT Changes: An Insider's View 2006 |
| 96368 | 90768 | 2009 | Nov 05:1, Aug 06:11, Sep 06:14, Nov 06:22, Dec 06:14 CPT Changes: An Insider's View 2006 |
| 96369 | 90769 | 2009 | CPT Changes: An Insider's View 2008 |
| 96370 | 90770 | 2009 | CPT Changes: An Insider's View 2008 |
| 96371 | 90771 | 2009 | CPT Changes: An Insider's View 2008 |
| 96372 | 90772 | 2009 | Nov 05:1, Sep 06:14, Dec 06:14 CPT Changes: An Insider's View 2006 |
| 96373 | 90773 | 2009 | Nov 05:1, Sep 06:14, Dec 06:14 CPT Changes: An Insider's View 2006 |

CPT

| Current Code(s) | Deleted/Former Code | Year Code Deleted | Citations Referencing Former Code—Applicable to Current Code(s) |
|---|---|---|---|
| 96374 | 90774 | 2009 | Nov 05:1, Sep 06:14, Dec 06:14 CPT Changes: An Insider's View 2006 |
| 96375 | 90775 | 2009 | Nov 05:1, Sep 06:14, Dec 06:14 CPT Changes: An Insider's View 2006 |
| 96376 | 90776 | 2009 | CPT Changes: An Insider's View 2008 |
| 96379 | 90779 | 2009 | Nov 05:1, Sep 06:14, Dec 06:14 CPT Changes: An Insider's View 2006 |
| 90951-90953, 90963, 90967 | 90918 | 2009 | Fall 93:5, May 96:4, May 02:17, Jan 03:22 |
| 90954-90956, 90964, 90968 | 90919 | 2009 | Fall 93:5, May 96:5, May 02:17, Jan 03:22 |
| 90957-90959, 90965, 90969 | 90920 | 2009 | Fall 93:5, May 96:5, May 02:17, Jan 03:22 |
| 90960-90962, 90966, 90970 | 90921 | 2009 | Fall 93:5, May 96:5, May 02:17, Jan 03:22 |
| 90951-90953, 90963, 90967 | 90922 | 2009 | Fall 93:5, May 96:5, May 02:17, Jan 03:22 |
| 90954-90956, 90964, 90968 | 90923 | 2009 | May 96:5, May 02:17, Jan 03:22 |
| 90957-90959, 90965, 90969 | 90924 | 2009 | May 96:5, May 02:17, Jan 03:22 |
| 90960-90962, 90966, 90970 | 90925 | 2009 | May 96:5, May 02:17, Jan 03:22 |
| 93285, 93291, 93298 | 93727 | 2009 | Nov 99:50, Jul 00:5, CPT Changes: An Insider's View 2000 |
| 93280, 93288, 93294 | 93731 | 2009 | Summer 94:23, Feb 98:11 |
| 93280, 93288, 93294 | 93732 | 2009 | Summer 94:23, Feb 98:11, Mar 00:10 |
| 93293 | 93733 | 2009 | Summer 94:23 |
| 93279, 93288, 93294 | 93734 | 2009 | Summer 94:23, Feb 98:11 |
| 93279, 93288, 93294 | 93735 | 2009 | Summer 94:23, Feb 98:11 |
| 93293 | 93736 | 2009 | Summer 94:23 |
| 93282, 93289, 93292, 93295 | 93741 | 2009 | Nov 99:50-51, Jul 00:5, Nov 00:9, Sep 05:8 CPT Changes: An Insider's View 2000, 2005 |
| 93282, 93289, 93292, 93295 | 93742 | 2009 | Nov 99:50-51, Jul 00:5, Nov 00:9 CPT Changes: An Insider's View 2000, 2005 |
| 93283, 93289, 93295 | 93743 | 2009 | Nov 99:50-51, Jul 00:5, Nov 00:9, Sep 05:8 CPT Changes: An Insider's View 2000 |
| 93283, 93289, 93295 | 93744 | 2009 | Nov 99:50-51, Jul 00:5, Nov 00:9 CPT Changes: An Insider's View 2000 |
| 99466 | 99289 | 2009 | May 05:1, Jul 06:4 CPT Changes: An Insider's View 2002, 2003 |
| 99467 | 99290 | 2009 | CPT Changes: An Insider's View 2002 |
| 99471 | 99293 | 2009 | Feb 03:15, Oct 03:2, Aug 04:7, 10, May 05:1, Nov 05:10, Jul 06:4, Apr 07:3 CPT Changes: An Insider's View 2003, 2004, 2005 |
| 99472 | 99294 | 2009 | Feb 03:15, Oct 03:2, Aug 04:7, Nov 05:10, Jul 06:4, Apr 07:3 CPT Changes: An Insider's View 2003, 2004, 2005 |
| 99468 | 99295 | 2009 | Summer 93:1, Nov 97:4-5, Mar 98:11, Nov 99:5-6, Dec 00:14, Feb 03:15, Oct 03:1, May 05:1, Nov 05:10, CPT Changes: An Insider's View 2000, 2003, 2004, 2005 |
| 99469 | 99296 | 2009 | Summer 93:1, Nov 97:4-5, Mar 98:11, Nov 99:5-6, Dec 00:14, Feb 03:15, Oct 03:1, Nov 05:10, CPT Changes: An Insider's View 2000, 2003, 2004, 2005, 2008 |

| Current Code(s) | Deleted/Former Code | Year Code Deleted | Citations Referencing Former Code—Applicable to Current Code(s) |
|---|---|---|---|
| 99478 | 99298 | 2009 | Nov 98:2-3, Nov 99: 5-6, Aug 00:4, Dec 00:15, Oct 03:2, May 05:1, Nov 05:10; CPT Changes: An Insider's View 2000, 2003 |
| 99479 | 99299 | 2009 | Oct 03:2, Nov 05:10; CPT Changes: An Insider's View 2003 |
| 99480 | 99300 | 2009 | CPT Changes: An Insider's View 2006 |
| 99460 | 99431 | 2009 | Apr 97:10, Nov 97:9, Sep 98:5, Apr 04:14, May 05:1 |
| 99461 | 99432 | 2009 | Sep 98:5, May 99:11, Apr 04:14 |
| 99462 | 99433 | 2009 | Sep 98:5, Apr 03:27 |
| 99463 | 99435 | 2009 | Sep 98:5, Apr 04:14 |
| 99464 | 99436 | 2009 | Nov 97:9-10, Sep 98:5, Nov 99:5-6, Aug 00:3, Aug 04:9, Nov 05:15 |
| 99465 | 99440 | 2009 | Summer 93:3, Mar 96:10, Nov 97:9, Sep 98:5, Nov 99:5-6, Aug 00:3, Oct 03:3, Aug 04:9, Apr 07:3 |
| 20985-20987 | 0054T | 2008 | May 04:14, Jun 04:8 CPT Changes: An Insider's View 2004 |
| 20985-20987 | 0055T | 2008 | May 04:14, Jun 04:8 CPT Changes: An Insider's View 2004, 2005 |
| 20985-20987 | 0056T | 2008 | May 04:14, Jun 04:8 CPT Changes: An Insider's View 2004 |
| 99174 | 0065T | 2008 | Mar 05:1, 3-4 CPT Changes: An Insider's View 2005 |
| 99444 | 0074T | 2008 | May 05:7, Sep 05:6 CPT Changes: An Insider's View 2005 |
| 99605-99607 | 0115T | 2008 | CPT Changes: An Insider's View 2006 |
| 99605-99607 | 0116T | 2008 | CPT Changes: An Insider's View 2006 |
| 99605-99607 | 0117T | 2008 | CPT Changes: An Insider's View 2006 |
| 50593 | 0135T | 2008 | CPT Changes: An Insider's View 2006, Clinical Examples in Radiology Winter 06:18 |
| 34806 | 0153T | 2008 | CPT Changes: An Insider's View 2007, Clinical Examples in Radiology Winter 06:19 |
| 93982 | 0154T | 2008 | CPT Changes: An Insider's View 2007, Clinical Examples in Radiology Winter 06:19 |
| 01935, 01936 | 01905 | 2008 | Mar 06:15 CPT Changes: An Insider's View 2002 |
| 24357-24359 | 24350 | 2008 | |
| 24357-24359 | 24351 | 2008 | |
| 24357-24359 | 24352 | 2008 | |
| 24357-24359 | 24354 | 2008 | |
| 24357-24359 | 24356 | 2008 | |
| 3044F-3045F | 3047F | 2008 | CPT Changes: An Insider's View 2007 |
| 3074F-3075F | 3076F | 2008 | CPT Changes: An Insider's View 2007 |
| 32421 | 32000 | 2008 | Spring 91:4, Winter 92:20 |
| 32422 | 32002 | 2008 | Nov 03:14 |
| 32560 | 32005 | 2008 | |
| 32550 | 32019 | 2008 | CPT Changes: An Insider's View 2005 |
| 32551 | 32020 | 2008 | Fall 92:13, Nov 03:14 |
| 36591 | 36540 | 2008 | Jan 02:11, Nov 02:3, Apr 03:26, Nov 05:1 CPT Changes: An Insider's View 2001, 2003 |
| 36593 | 36550 | 2008 | Nov 99:20, Nov 05:1 CPT Changes: An Insider's View 2000 |
| 49203-49205, 58957, 58958 | 49200 | 2008 | CPT Changes: An Insider's View 2003 |
| 49203-49205, 58957, 58958 | 49201 | 2008 | |
| 51100 | 51000 | 2008 | Nov 99:32-33, Aug 00:3, Oct 03:2 |
| 51101 | 51005 | 2008 | |
| 51102 | 51010 | 2008 | |
| 60300 | 60001 | 2008 | |
| 67041, 67042, 67043 | 67038 | 2008 | Aug 03:15, Sep 05:12 |

| Current Code(s) | Deleted/Former Code | Year Code Deleted | Citations Referencing Former Code— Applicable to Current Code(s) |
|---|---|---|---|
| 75557-75564 | 75552 | 2008 | Fall 95:2 |
| 75557-75564 | 75553 | 2008 | Fall 95:2 |
| 75557-75564 | 75554 | 2008 | Fall 95:2 |
| 75557-75564 | 75555 | 2008 | Fall 95:2 |
| 75557-75564 | 75556 | 2008 | Fall 95:2 |
| 78610 | 78615 | 2008 | CPT Changes: An Insider's View 2002 |
| 86356, 86486 | 86586 | 2008 | Jul 98:11 |
| 99366-99368 | 99361 | 2008 | May 05:1 |
| 99366-99368 | 99362 | 2008 | |
| 99441-99443 | 99371 | 2008 | Spring 94:34, May 00:11, May 05:1, Nov 05:10 |
| 99441-99443 | 99372 | 2008 | Spring 94:34, May 00:11, Nov 05:10 |
| 99441-99443 | 99373 | 2008 | Spring 94:34, May 00:11, Nov 05:10 |
| 0160T, 0161T | 0018T | 2007 | CPT Changes: An Insider's View 2002 |
| 96904 | 0044T | 2007 | CPT Changes: An Insider's View 2003, 2004 |
| 96904 | 0045T | 2007 | Jul 04:7 CPT Changes: An Insider's View 2004 |
| 77371-77373 | 0082T | 2007 | CPT Changes: An Insider's View 2005 |
| 77371-77373 | 0083T | 2007 | CPT Changes: An Insider's View 2005 |
| 22857 | 0091T | 2007 | CPT Changes: An Insider's View 2006 |
| 22865 | 0094T | 2007 | CPT Changes: An Insider's View 2006 |
| 22862 | 0097T | 2007 | CPT Changes: An Insider's View 2006 |
| 19105 | 0120T | 2007 | CPT Changes: An Insider's View 2006 |
| 15002, 15004 | 15000 | 2007 | Fall 93:7, Apr 97:4, Aug 97:6, Sep 97:2, Nov 98:5, Jan 99:4, Apr 99:10, May 99:10, Nov 02:7, Aug 03:14 CPT Changes: An Insider's View 2001, 2006 |
| 15003, 15005 | 15001 | 2007 | Nov 98:5-6, Jan 99:4, May 99:10, Aug 03:14 |
| 15830, 15847, 17999 | 15831 | 2007 | May 01:11 CPT Changes: An Insider's View 2007 |
| 17311 | 17304 | 2007 | Winter 94:19, Mar 99:11, Jun 99:10, Nov 02:7, Nov 03:15, Feb 04:11, Jul 04:2 CPT Changes: An Insider's View 2003 |
| 17312, 17314 | 17305 | 2007 | Winter 94:19, Mar 99:11, Jun 99:10, Nov 02:7, Feb 04:11, Jul 04:3 |
| 17312, 17314 | 17306 | 2007 | Winter 94:19, Mar 99:11, Jun 99:10, Nov 02:7, Feb 04:11, Jul 04:4 |
| 17312, 17314 | 17307 | 2007 | Winter 94:19, Mar 99:11, Jun 99:10, Nov 02:7, Nov 03:15, Feb 04:11, Jul 04:4 |
| 17315 | 17310 | 2007 | Winter 94:19, Mar 99:11, Jun 99:10, Nov 02:7, Feb 04:11, May 04:14, Jul 04:4 CPT Changes: An Insider's View 2003 |
| 19300 | 19140 | 2007 | Feb 96:9, Apr 05:13 |
| 19301 | 19160 | 2007 | Apr 05:7 CPT Changes: An Insider's View 2005 |
| 19302 | 19162 | 2007 | Jun 00:11, Apr 05:7 |
| 19303 | 19180 | 2007 | Apr 05:7 |
| 19304 | 19182 | 2007 | Apr 05:7 |
| 19305 | 19200 | 2007 | Apr 05:7 |
| 19306 | 19220 | 2007 | Apr 05:7 |
| 19307 | 19240 | 2007 | Apr 05:7 |
| 25606 | 25611 | 2007 | Fall 93:23, Oct 99:5 |
| 25607-25609 | 25620 | 2007 | |
| 26390 | 26504 | 2007 | |
| 27325 | 27315 | 2007 | |
| 27326 | 27320 | 2007 | |

| Current Code(s) | Deleted/Former Code | Year Code Deleted | Citations Referencing Former Code— Applicable to Current Code(s) |
|---|---|---|---|
| 28055 | 28030 | 2007 | |
| 33254-33256 | 33253 | 2007 | |
| 35302-35306 | 35381 | 2007 | |
| 35506 | 35507 | 2007 | |
| 35537, 35538 | 35541 | 2007 | |
| 35539, 35540 | 35546 | 2007 | |
| 35637, 35638 | 35641 | 2007 | Dec 01:7 |
| 44799 | 44152 | 2007 | |
| 44799 | 44153 | 2007 | |
| 47719 | 47716 | 2007 | |
| 48105 | 48005 | 2007 | |
| 48548 | 48180 | 2007 | |
| 49402 | 49085 | 2007 | |
| 54150 | 54152 | 2007 | Sep 96:11, Dec 96:10, May 98:11, Apr 03:27 CPT Changes: An Insider's View 2007 |
| 54865 | 54820 | 2007 | Oct 01:8 |
| 55875 | 55859 | 2007 | Apr 04:6 |
| 56442 | 56720 | 2007 | |
| 57558 | 57820 | 2007 | |
| 67346 | 67350 | 2007 | |
| 77001 | 75998 | 2007 | Dec 04:12-13 CPT Changes: An Insider's View 2004 Clinical Examples in Radiology Inaugural 04:1-2, Winter 05:9 |
| 77002 | 76003 | 2007 | Fall 93:14, Jul 01:7 CPT Changes: An Insider's View 2001 Clinical Examples in Radiology Spring 05:5-6 |
| 77003 | 76005 | 2007 | Nov 99:32, 34, 41, Jan 00:2, Feb 00:6, Aug 00:8, Sep 02:11, Sep 04:5 CPT Changes: An Insider's View 2000 |
| 77071 | 76006 | 2007 | Nov 98:21 CPT Changes: An Insider's View 2003 |
| 72291 | 76012 | 2007 | Mar 01:2 CPT Changes: An Insider's View 2001, 2006 |
| 72292 | 76013 | 2007 | Mar 01:2 CPT Changes: An Insider's View 2001 |
| 77072 | 76020 | 2007 | |
| 77073 | 76040 | 2007 | |
| 77074 | 76061 | 2007 | |
| 77075 | 76062 | 2007 | |
| 77076 | 76065 | 2007 | |
| 77077 | 76066 | 2007 | CPT Changes: An Insider's View 2002 |
| 77078 | 76070 | 2007 | Nov 97:24 CPT Changes: An Insider's View 2002, 2003 |
| 77079 | 76071 | 2007 | CPT Changes: An Insider's View 2003 |
| 77080 | 76075 | 2007 | Nov 97:24, Jun 03:11 CPT Changes: An Insider's View 2005 |
| 77081 | 76076 | 2007 | Nov 97:24 |
| 77082 | 76077 | 2007 | CPT Changes: An Insider's View 2005 |
| 77083 | 76078 | 2007 | Nov 97:24 CPT Changes: An Insider's View 2002 |
| 77051 | 76082 | 2007 | CPT Changes: An Insider's View 2004 |
| 77052 | 76083 | 2007 | CPT Changes: An Insider's View 2004 |
| 77053 | 76086 | 2007 | |
| 77054 | 76088 | 2007 | |
| 77055 | 76090 | 2007 | Jul 96:6, Jun 99:10 CPT Changes: An Insider's View 2004 |
| 77056 | 76091 | 2007 | Jul 96:6 CPT Changes: An Insider's View 2004 |

| Current Code(s) | Deleted/Former Code | Year Code Deleted | Citations Referencing Former Code— Applicable to Current Code(s) |
|---|---|---|---|
| 77057 | 76092 | 2007 | Jul 96:6, Jun 99:10 CPT Changes: An Insider's View 2004 |
| 77058 | 76093 | 2007 | |
| 77059 | 76094 | 2007 | |
| 77031 | 76095 | 2007 | Apr 96:9, Nov 97:24, Jan 01:9 CPT Changes: An Insider's View 2001 |
| 77032 | 76096 | 2007 | Jan 01:10 CPT Changes: An Insider's View 2001 |
| 77011 | 76355 | 2007 | CPT Changes: An Insider's View 2002, 2003 |
| 77012 | 76360 | 2007 | Fall 93:12, Fall 94:2, Jan 01:9-10, Mar 05:2 CPT Changes: An Insider's View 2001, 2002, 2003 |
| 77013 | 76362 | 2007 | Oct 02:4 CPT Changes: An Insider's View 2002, 2004 |
| 77014 | 76370 | 2007 | Fall 91:12 CPT Changes: An Insider's View 2002, 2003 |
| 77021 | 76393 | 2007 | Jan 01:10, Mar 05:2 CPT Changes: An Insider's View 2001, 2002 |
| 77022 | 76394 | 2007 | Oct 02:4, Mar 05:5 CPT Changes: An Insider's View 2002, 2004 |
| 77084 | 76400 | 2007 | |
| 76775, 76776 | 76778 | 2007 | CPT Changes: An Insider's View 2002 |
| 76998 | 76986 | 2007 | CPT Changes: An Insider's View 2001 |
| 78707-78709 | 78704 | 2007 | |
| 78701-78709 | 78715 | 2007 | |
| 78761 | 78760 | 2007 | |
| 92700 | 92573 | 2007 | |
| 94002, 94004 | 94656 | 2007 | Fall 92:30, Spring 95:4, Summer 95:4, Feb 96:9, Aug 00:2, Oct 03:2 |
| 94003, 94004 | 94657 | 2007 | Fall 92:30, Spring 95:4, Summer 95:4, Feb 96:9, Aug 00:2, Oct 03:2 |

# Appendix N

## Summary of Resequenced CPT Codes

This is a summary of CPT codes that do not apear in numeric sequence in the listing of CPT codes. Rather than deleting and renumbering, resequencing allows existing codes to be relocated to an appropriate location for the code concept, regardless of the numeric sequence. The codes listed below are identified in *CPT 2012* with a # symbol for location of the resequenced number within the family of related concepts. Numerically placed references (eg, **Code is out of numerical sequence. See...**) are used as navigational alerts to direct the user to the location of out-of-sequence code.

| | | |
|---|---|---|
| 11045 | 33221 | 92558 |
| 11046 | 33227 | 92618 |
| 11047 | 33228 | 95800 |
| 21552 | 33229 | 95801 |
| 21554 | 33230 | 95885 |
| 23071 | 33231 | 95886 |
| 23073 | 33262 | 95887 |
| 24071 | 33263 | 95938 |
| 24073 | 33264 | 95939 |
| 25071 | 46220 | 99224 |
| 25073 | 46320 | 99225 |
| 26111 | 46945 | 99226 |
| 26113 | 46946 | 0253T |
| 27043 | 46947 | |
| 27045 | 51797 | |
| 27059 | 64633 | |
| 27329 | 64634 | |
| 27337 | 64635 | |
| 27339 | 64636 | |
| 27632 | 77424 | |
| 27634 | 77425 | |
| 28039 | 80104 | |
| 28041 | 82652 | |
| 29914 | 87906 | |
| 29915 | 88177 | |
| 29916 | 90665 | |

# Notes

# Index

## Instructions for the Use of the CPT Index

### Main Terms

The index is organized by main terms. Each main term can stand alone, or be followed by up to three modifying terms. There are four primary classes of main entries:

1. Procedure or service.
   For example: Endoscopy; Anastomosis; Splint

2. Organ or other anatomic site.
   For example: Tibia; Colon; Salivary Gland

3. Condition.
   For example: Abscess; Entropion; Tetralogy of Fallot

4. Synonyms, Eponyms, and Abbreviations.
   For example: EEG; Bricker Operation; Clagett Procedure

### Modifying Terms

A main term may be followed by a series of up to three indented terms that modify the main term. When modifying terms appear, one should review the list, as these subterms do have an effect on the selection of the appropriate code for the procedure.

### Code Ranges

Whenever more than one code applies to a given index entry, a code range is listed. If several non-sequential codes apply, they will be separated by a comma. For example:

Esophagus
   Reconstruction . . . . . . . . 43300, 43310, 43313

If two or more sequential codes apply, they will be separated by a hyphen. For example:

Debridement
   Burns . . . . . . . . . . .01951-01953, 16020-16030

## Conventions

As a space saving convention, certain words infer some meaning. This convention is primarily used when a procedure or service is listed as a subterm. For example:

Knee
   Incision (of)

In this example, the word in parentheses (of) does not appear in the index, but it is inferred. As another example:

Pancreas
   Anesthesia (for procedures on)

In this example, as there is no such entity as pancreas anesthesia, the words in parentheses are inferred. That is, anesthesia for procedures on the pancreas.

**The alphabetic index is NOT a substitute for the main text of the CPT codebook. Even if only one code appears, the user must refer to the main text to ensure that the code selection is accurate.**

# A

Appendix
  Incision and Drainage . . . . . . . . . . . . . 44900
    Open . . . . . . . . . . . . . . . . . . . . . . 44900
    Percutaneous . . . . . . . . . . . . . . . . . 44901
Arm, Lower . . . . . . . . . . . . . . . . . . . . . . . . 25028
  Excision . . . . . . . . . . . . . . . . . . . . . . . 25145
  Incision and Drainage . . . . . . . . . . . . 25035
Arm, Upper
  Incision and Drainage . . . . . . . . 23930-23935
Auditory Canal, External . . . . . . . . . . . . . 69020
Bartholin's Gland
  Incision and Drainage . . . . . . . . . . . . . 56420
Bladder
  Incision and Drainage . . . . . . . . . . . . . 51080
Brain
  Drainage . . . . . . . . . . . . . . . . . 61150-61151
  Excision . . . . . . . . . . . . . . . 61514, 61522
  Incision and Drainage . . . . . . . . 61320-61321
Breast
  Incision and Drainage . . . . . . . . . . . 19020
Carpals
  Incision, Deep . . . . . . . . . . . . . . . . . 25035
Clavicle
  Sequestrectomy . . . . . . . . . . . . . . . . . 23170
Drainage
  with X-ray . . . . . . . . . . . . . . . . . . . . . 75989
Ear, External
  Complicated . . . . . . . . . . . . . . . . . . 69005
  Simple . . . . . . . . . . . . . . . . . . . . . . 69000
Elbow
  Incision and Drainage . . . . . . . . 23930-23935
Epididymis
  Incision and Drainage . . . . . . . . . . . . 54700
Excision
  Olecranon Process . . . . . . . . . . . . . . 24138
  Radius . . . . . . . . . . . . . . . . . . . . . . . 24136
  Ulna . . . . . . . . . . . . . . . . . . . . . . . . . 24138
Eyelid
  Incision and Drainage . . . . . . . . . . . . 67700
Facial Bones
  Excision . . . . . . . . . . . . . . . . . . . . . 21026
Finger . . . . . . . . . . . . . . . . . . 26010-26011
  Incision and Drainage . . . . . . . . . . . . 26034
Foot
  Incision . . . . . . . . . . . . . . . . . . . . . . 28005
Gums
  Incision and Drainage . . . . . . . . . . . . 41800
Hand
  Incision and Drainage . . . . . . . . . . . . 26034
Hematoma
  Incision and Drainage . . . . . . . . . . . . 27603
Hip
  Incision and Drainage . . . . . . . 26990-26992
Humeral Head . . . . . . . . . . . . . . . . . . . 23174
Humerus
  Excision . . . . . . . . . . . . . . . . . . . . . 24134
  Incision and Drainage . . . . . . . . . . . . 23935
Kidney
  Incision and Drainage . . . . . . . . . . . . 50020
    Open . . . . . . . . . . . . . . . . . . . . . . 50020
    Percutaneous . . . . . . . . . . . . . . . . . 50021
Leg, Lower
  Incision and Drainage . . . . . . . . . . . . 27603
Liver . . . . . . . . . . . . . . . . . . . . . . . . . . 47010
  Drainage
    Open . . . . . . . . . . . . . . . . . . . . . . 47010
  Injection . . . . . . . . . . . . . . . . . . . . . 47015
  Repair . . . . . . . . . . . . . . . . . . . . . . . 47300
Localization
  Nuclear Medicine . . . . . . . . . . . 78806-78807
Lung
  Percutaneous Drainage . . . . . . . 32200-32201

Lymph Node
  Incision and Drainage . . . . . . . . 38300-38305
Lymphocele Drainage . . . . . . . . . . . . . . . 49062
Mandible
  Excision . . . . . . . . . . . . . . . . . . . . . 21025
Mouth
  Incision and Drainage . . . . . . . . 40800-40801,
                        41005-41009, 41015-41018
Nasal Septum
  Incision and Drainage . . . . . . . . . . . . 30020
Neck
  Incision and Drainage . . . . . . . . 21501-21502
Ovarian
  Incision and Drainage . . . . . . . . 58820-58822
    Abdominal Approach . . . . . . . . . . . . 58822
    Vaginal Approach . . . . . . . . . . . . . . 58820
Ovary
  Drainage
    Percutaneous . . . . . . . . . . . . . . . . . 58823
Palate
  Incision and Drainage . . . . . . . . . . . . 42000
Paraurethral Gland
  Incision and Drainage . . . . . . . . . . . . 53060
Parotid Gland Drainage . . . . . . . . . 42300-42305
Pelvic
  Drainage
    Percutaneous . . . . . . . . . . . . . . . . . 58823
Pelvis
  Incision and Drainage . . . 26990-26992, 45000
Pericolic
  Drainage
    Percutaneous . . . . . . . . . . . . . . . . . 58823
Perineum
  Incision and Drainage . . . . . . . . . . . . 56405
Perirenal or Renal
  Drainage . . . . . . . . . . . . . . . . . 50020-50021
    Percutaneous . . . . . . . . . . . . . . . . . 50021
Peritoneum
  Incision and Drainage
    Open . . . . . . . . . . . . . . . . . . . . . . 49020
    Percutaneous . . . . . . . . . . . . . . . . . 49021
Prostate
  Incision and Drainage . . . . . . . . 55720-55725
  Transurethral Drainage . . . . . . . . . . . . 52700
Radius
  Incision, Deep . . . . . . . . . . . . . . . . . 25035
Rectum
  Incision and Drainage . . . . . . . . 45005-45020,
                                      46040, 46060
Retroperitoneal . . . . . . . . . . . . . . . 49060-49061
  Drainage
    Open . . . . . . . . . . . . . . . . . . . . . . 49060
    Percutaneous . . . . . . . . . . . . . . . . . 49061
Salivary Gland
  Drainage . . . . . . . . . . . . . . . . . 42300-42320
Scapula
  Sequestrectomy . . . . . . . . . . . . . . . . . 23172
Scrotum
  Incision and Drainage . . . . . . . . 54700, 55100
Shoulder
  Drainage . . . . . . . . . . . . . . . . . . . . . 23030
Skene's Gland
  Incision and Drainage . . . . . . . . . . . . 53060
Skin
  Incision and Drainage . . . . . . . . 10060-10061
  Puncture Aspiration . . . . . . . . . . . . . . 10160
Soft Tissue
  Incision and Drainage . . . . . . . . . . . . 20005
Spine
  Incision and Drainage . . . . . . . . 22010-22015
Subdiaphragmatic . . . . . . . . . . . . . 49040-49041
Sublingual Gland
  Drainage . . . . . . . . . . . . . . . . . 42310-42320

Submaxillary Gland
  Drainage . . . . . . . . . . . . . . . . . 42310-42320
Subphrenic . . . . . . . . . . . . . . . . . 49040-49041
Testis
  Incision and Drainage . . . . . . . . . . . . 54700
Thoracostomy . . . . . . . . . . . . . . . . . . . 32551
Thorax
  Incision and Drainage . . . . . . . . 21501-21502
Throat
  Incision and Drainage . . . . . . . . 42700-42725
Tongue
  Incision and Drainage . . . . . . . . 41000-41006
Tonsil
  Incision and Drainage . . . . . . . . . . . . 42700
Ulna
  Incision, Deep . . . . . . . . . . . . . . . . . 25035
Urethra
  Incision and Drainage . . . . . . . . . . . . 53040
Uvula
  Incision and Drainage . . . . . . . . . . . . 42000
Vagina
  Incision and Drainage . . . . . . . . . . . . 57010
Vulva
  Incision and Drainage . . . . . . . . . . . . 56405
Wrist
  Excision . . . . . . . . . . . . . . . . . . . . . 25145
  Incision and Drainage . . . . . . . . 25028, 25035
X-ray . . . . . . . . . . . . . . . . . . . . . . . . . . 76080

## Abscess, Nasal
See Nose, Abscess

## Abscess, Parotid Gland
See Parotid Gland, Abscess

## Absorptiometry
Dual Energy . . . . . . . . . . . . . . . . . . . 3095F-3096F
  Bone
    Appendicular . . . . . . . . . . . . . . . . . 77081
    Axial Skeleton . . . . . . . . . . . . . . . . 77080
    Vertebral . . . . . . . . . . . . . . . . . . . 77082
Dual Photon
  Bone . . . . . . . . . . . . . . . . . . . . . . . 78351
Single Photon
  Bone . . . . . . . . . . . . . . . . . . . . . . . 78350

## Absorption Spectrophotometry, Atomic
See Atomic Absorption Spectroscopy

## Accessory Nerve, Spinal
See Nerves, Spinal Accessory

## Accessory, Toes
See Polydactyly, Toes

## ACE
See Angiotensin Converting Enzyme (ACE),
Performance Measures

## Acetabuloplasty . . . . . 27120-27122, 29915

## Acetabulum
Fracture
  Closed Treatment . . . . . . . . . . . . 27220-27222
  Open Treatment . . . . . . . . . . . . . 27226-27228
  with Manipulation . . . . . . . . . . . . . . . 27222
  without Manipulation . . . . . . . . . . . . . 27220
Reconstruction . . . . . . . . . . . . . . . . . . 27120
  with Resection, Femoral Head . . . . . . . . 27122
Tumor
  Excision . . . . . . . . . . . . . . . . . . . . . 27076

## Acetaldehyde
Blood . . . . . . . . . . . . . . . . . . . . . . . . . 82000

## ADH
*See* Antidiuretic Hormone

## Adhesions
Epidural..........................62263-62264
Eye
   Corneovitreal.....................65880
   Incision
      Anterior Segment...........65860-65870
      Posterior Segment..............65875
Intermarginal
   Construction.....................67880
      Transposition of Tarsal Plate........67882
Intestinal
   Enterolysis......................44005
   Laparoscopic.....................44180
Intracranial
   Lysis...........................62161
Intrauterine
   Lysis...........................58559
Labial
   Lysis...........................56441
Lungs
   Lysis...........................32124
Pelvic
   Lysis............58660, 58662, 58740
Penile
   Lysis
      Post-circumcision...............54162
Preputial
   Lysis...........................54450
Urethral
   Lysis...........................53500

## Adipectomy
*See* Lipectomy

## ADL
*See* Activities of Daily Living

## Administration
Immunization
   Each Additional
      Vaccine/Toxoid..............90472, 90474
         with Counseling...................90461
      One Vaccine/Toxoid..........90471, 90473
         with Counseling...................90460
Occlusive Substance.....................31634
Pharmacologic Agent....................93463

## ADP
*See* Adenosine Diphosphate

## ADP Phosphocreatine Phosphotransferase
*See* CPK

## Adrenal Cortex Hormone
*See* Corticosteroids

## Adrenal Gland
Biopsy..........................60540-60545
Excision
   Laparoscopy.....................60650
   Retroperitoneal Tumor..............60545
Exploration.....................60540-60545
Nuclear Medicine
   Imaging.........................78075

## Adrenal Medulla
*See* Medulla

## Adrenalectomy ..................60540
Anesthesia........................00866
Laparoscopic.......................50545

## Adrenalin
*See* Catecholamines
Blood...........................82383
Urine...........................82384

## Adrenaline-Noradrenaline
Testing........................82382-82384

## Adrenocorticotropic Hormone (ACTH)............80400-80406, 80412,
                        80418, 82024
Blood or Urine......................82024
Stimulation Panel................80400-80406

## Adrenogenital Syndrome .................56805, 57335

## Adult T Cell Leukemia Lymphoma Virus I
*See* HTLV I

## Advanced Life Support
*See* Emergency Department Services
Physician Direction....................99288

## Advancement
Genioglossus.......................21199
Tendon
   Foot............................28238

## Advancement Flap
*See* Skin, Adjacent Tissue Transfer

## Aerosol Inhalation
*See* Pulmonology, Therapeutic
Pentamidine........................94642

## AFB
*See* Acid Fast Bacilli (AFB)

## Afferent Nerve
*See* Sensory Nerve

## AFP
*See* Alpha-Fetoprotein

## After Hours Medical Services .......................99050

## Agents, Anticoagulant
*See* Clotting Inhibitors

## Agglutinin
Cold...........................86156-86157
Febrile...........................86000

## Aggregation
Platelet...........................85576

## AHG
*See* Clotting Factor

## AICD (Pacing Cardioverter-Defibrillator)
*See* Defibrillator, Heart; Pacemaker, Heart

## Aid, Hearing
*See* Hearing Aid

## AIDS Antibodies
*See* Antibody, HIV

## AIDS Virus
*See* HIV-1

## Akin Operation
*See* Bunion Repair

## ALA
*See* Aminolevulinic Acid (ALA)

## Alanine 2 Oxoglutarate Aminotransferase
*See* Transaminase, Glutamic Pyruvic

## Alanine Amino (ALT) ...........84460

## Alanine Transaminase
*See* Transaminase, Glutamic Pyruvic

## Albarran Test
*See* Water Load Test

## Albumin
Ischemia modified.....................82045
Serum, Plasma or Whole Blood ..........82040
Urine........................82042-82044

## Alcohol
Breath...........................82075
Ethyl
   Blood...........................82055
   Urine...........................82055
Ethylene Glycol......................82693

## Alcohol Dehydrogenase
*See* Antidiuretic Hormone

## Alcohol, Isopropyl
*See* Isopropyl Alcohol

## Alcohol, Methyl
*See* Methanol

## Aldolase
Blood...........................82085

## Aldosterone
Blood...........................82088
Suppression Evaluation................80408
Urine...........................82088

## Alimentary Canal
*See* Gastrointestinal Tract

## Alkaline Phosphatase ....84075-84080
Leukocyte.........................85540
WBC...........................85540

## Alkaloids
*See* Specific Drug
Urine...........................82101

## Allergen Bronchial Provocation Tests
*See* Allergy Tests; Bronchial Challenge Test

## Allergen Challenge, Endobronchial
*See* Bronchial Challenge Test

## Allergen Immunotherapy
Allergen
   Prescription/Supply/Injection ... 95120-95125
   with Extract Supply.................95144
      Injection..................95115-95117
Antigens...........................95144
IgE...........................86003-86005
IgG...........................86001
Insect Venom
   Prescription/Supply...........95145-95149
   Prescription/Supply/Injection ... 95130-95134
Prescription/Supply..................95165
   Insect, Whole Body.................95170
Rapid Desensitization..................95180

## ANA
*See* Antinuclear Antibodies (ANA)

## Anabolic Steroid
*See* Androstenedione

## Anal Abscess
*See* Abscess, Anal

## Anal Bleeding
*See* Anus, Hemorrhage

## Anal Fistula
*See* Fistula, Anal

## Anal Fistulectomy
*See* Excision, Fistula, Anal

## Anal Fistulotomy
*See* Fistulotomy, Anal

## Anal Sphincter
Dilation . . . . . . . . . . . . . . . . . . . . . . . 45905
Incision . . . . . . . . . . . . . . . . . . . . . . . 46080

## Anal Ulceration
*See* Anus, Fissure

## Analgesia
*See* Anesthesia; Sedation

## Analgesic Cutaneous Electrostimulation
*See* Application, Neurostimulation

## Analysis
Computer Data . . . . . . . . . . . . . . . . . . 99090
   Cardiovascular Monitoring . . . . . . . . . 93290,
                              93297, 93299
   Device Evaluation and Programming
     Cardioverter-Defibrillator . . . 93282-93284,
                93287, 93289-93290, 93292,
                            93295-93297
     Loop Recorder . . . . . . . . . . 93285, 93291,
                            93298-93299
     Pacemaker . . . . . . . . . . . . . . 93279-93281,
                            93293-93294
   Electrocardiograph
     Data Analysis . . . . . . . . . . . . . . . . . 0206T
     Multivariate Probability Assessment . . . 0185T
     Pacemaker . . . . . . . . . . . 93288, 93293-93294
   Electroencephalogram
     Digital . . . . . . . . . . . . . . . . . . . . . . 95957
   Electronic
     Drug Infusion Pump . . . . . . . . . . 62367-62370
     Pacing Cardioverter-Defibrillator
      Data Analysis . . . . . . . 93289, 93295-93296
      Initial Evaluation . . . . . . . . . . . . . . . 93640
       *See* Pacemaker, Heart
     Pulse Generator
      Neurostimulator . . . . . . . . . . . 95970-95982
   Physiologic Data, Remote . . . . . . . . . . . . . 99091
   Protein
     Tissue
      Western Blot . . . . . . . . . . . . . . . . . 88372
   Semen . . . . . . . . . . . . . . . . . . . 89320-89322
     Sperm Isolation . . . . . . . . . . . . . 89260-89261

## Analysis, Spectrum
*See* Spectrophotometry

## Anaspadias
*See* Epispadias

## Anastomosis
Arteriovenous Fistula
   Direct . . . . . . . . . . . . . . . . . . . . . . . 36821
   with Bypass Graft . . . . . . . . . . . . . . . . 35686
   with Graft . . . . . . . . . . . 36825-36830, 36832
Artery
   to Aorta . . . . . . . . . . . . . . . . . . . . . . 33606
   to Artery
     Cranial . . . . . . . . . . . . . . . . . . . . . 61711
Bile Duct
   to Bile Duct . . . . . . . . . . . . . . . . . . . 47800
   to Intestines . . . . . . . . . . . . . . 47760, 47780
Bile Duct to Gastrointestinal . . . . . . . . . . . 47785
Broncho-Bronchial . . . . . . . . . . . . . . . . . 32486
Caval to Mesenteric . . . . . . . . . . . . . . . . 37160
Cavopulmonary . . . . . . . . . . . . . . . 33622, 33768
Colorectal . . . . . . . . . . . . . . . . . . . . . . 44620
Epididymis
   to Vas Deferens
     Bilateral . . . . . . . . . . . . . . . . . . . . 54901
     Unilateral . . . . . . . . . . . . . . . . . . . 54900
Excision
   Trachea . . . . . . . . . . . . . . . . . 31780-31781
Fallopian Tube . . . . . . . . . . . . . . . . . . . 58750
Gallbladder to Intestines . . . . . . . . . 47720-47740
Hepatic Duct to Intestines . . . . . . . . 47765, 47802
Ileo-Anal . . . . . . . . . . . . . . . . . . . . . . 45113
Intestine to Intestine . . . . . . . . . . . . . . . 44130
Intestines
   Colo-anal . . . . . . . . . . . . . . . . . . . . . 45119
   Cystectomy . . . . . . . . . . . . . . . . . . . . 51590
   Enterocystoplasty . . . . . . . . . . . . . . . . 51960
   Ileoanal . . . . . . . . . . . . . . . . . 44157-44158
   Resection
     Laparoscopic . . . . . . . . . . . . . 44202-44205
Intrahepatic Portosystemic . . . . . . . . 37182-37183
Jejunum . . . . . . . . . . . . . . . . . . . . . . 43825
Microvascular
   Free Transfer
     Jejunum . . . . . . . . . . . . . . . . . . . . 43496
Nerve
   Facial to Hypoglossal . . . . . . . . . . . . . . 64868
   Facial to Phrenic . . . . . . . . . . . . . . . . 64870
Oviduct . . . . . . . . . . . . . . . . . . . . . . . 58750
Pancreas to Intestines . . . . . . 48520-48540, 48548
Portocaval . . . . . . . . . . . . . . . . . . . . . 37140
Pulmonary . . . . . . . . . . . . . . . . . . . . . 33606
Renoportal . . . . . . . . . . . . . . . . . . . . . 37145
Splenorenal . . . . . . . . . . . . . . . . 37180-37181
Stomach . . . . . . . . . . . . . . . . . . . . . . 43825
   to Duodenum . . . . . . . . . . . . . . 43810, 43855
     Revision . . . . . . . . . . . . . . . . . . . . 43850
   to Jejunum . . . . . . . . . . . 43820, 43860-43865
Tubotubal . . . . . . . . . . . . . . . . . . . . . 58750
Ureter
   to Bladder . . . . . . . . . . . . . . . . 50780-50785
   to Colon . . . . . . . . . . . . . . . . . 50810-50815
     Removal . . . . . . . . . . . . . . . . . . . . 50830
   to Intestine . . . . . . . . . . . 50800, 50820-50825
     Removal . . . . . . . . . . . . . . . . . . . . 50830
   to Kidney . . . . . . . . . . . . . . . . 50727-50750
   to Ureter . . . . . . . . . . . . 50727, 50760-50770
Vein
   Saphenopopliteal . . . . . . . . . . . . . . . . 34530
Vein to Vein . . . . . . . . 37140-37160, 37182-37183

## Anastomosis of Lacrimal Sac to Conjunctival Sac
*See* Conjunctivorhinostomy

## Anastomosis of Pancreas
*See* Pancreas, Anastomosis

## Anastomosis, Aorta-Pulmonary Artery
*See* Aorta, Anastomosis, to Pulmonary Artery

## Anastomosis, Bladder, to Intestine
*See* Enterocystoplasty

## Anastomosis, Hepatic Duct
*See* Hepatic Duct, Anastomosis

## Anderson Tibial
Lengthening . . . . . . . . . . . . . . 27715
*See* Ankle; Tibia, Osteoplasty, Lengthening

## Androstanediol
Glucuronide . . . . . . . . . . . . . . . . . . . 82154

## Androstanolone
*See* Dihydrotestosterone

## Androstenedione
Blood or Urine . . . . . . . . . . . . . . . . . . 82157

## Androstenolone
*See* Dehydroepiandrosterone

## Androsterone
Blood or Urine . . . . . . . . . . . . . . . . . . 82160

## Anesthesia
*See* Analgesia
Abbe-Estlander Procedure . . . . . . . . . . . . . 00102
Abdomen
   Abdominal Wall . . . . . . . . . . . . . 00700, 00730,
              00800-00802, 00820, 00836
     Halsted Repair . . . . . . . . . . . . 00750-00756
     Blood Vessels . . . . . . . . . 00770, 00880-00882
     Endoscopy . . . . . . . . . . . . . 00740, 00810
     Extraperitoneal . . . . . . . . . . . . . 00860-00862,
               00866-00868, 00870
     Hernia Repair . . . . . . . . . . . . . . 00830-00836
      Halsted Repair . . . . . . . . . . . 00750-00756
     Intraperitoneal . . . . . . . . . . . . 00790-00797,
                 00840-00842
Abdominoperineal Resection . . . . . . . . . . . 00844
Abortion
   Incomplete . . . . . . . . . . . . . . . . . . . . 01965
   Induced . . . . . . . . . . . . . . . . . . . . . . 01966
Achilles Tendon Repair . . . . . . . . . . . . . . 01472
Acromioclavicular Joint . . . . . . . . . . . . . . 01620
Adrenalectomy . . . . . . . . . . . . . . . . . . . 00866
Amniocentesis . . . . . . . . . . . . . . . . . . . 00842
Aneurysm
   Axillary-Brachial . . . . . . . . . . . . . . . . . 01652
   Knee . . . . . . . . . . . . . . . . . . . . . . . . 01444
   Popliteal Artery . . . . . . . . . . . . . . . . . 01444
Angiography . . . . . . . . . . . . . . . . . . . . 01920
Ankle . . . . . . . . . . 00400, 01462-01522
Anorectal Procedure . . . . . . . . . . . . . . . . 00902
Anus . . . . . . . . . . . . . . . . . . . . . . . . . 00902
Arm
   Lower . . . . . 00400, 01810-01820, 01830-01860
   Upper . . . . . . . . . . . . . 00400, 01710-01782
Arrhythmias . . . . . . . . . . . . . . . . . . . . 00410
Arteriography . . . . . . . . . . . . . . . . . . . 01916
Arteriovenous Fistula . . . . . . . . . . . . . . . 01432
Arthroplasty
   Hip . . . . . . . . . . . . . . . . . . . . 01214-01215
   Knee . . . . . . . . . . . . . . . . . . . . . . . 01402
Arthroscopic Procedures
   Ankle . . . . . . . . . . . . . . . . . . . . . . . 01464
   Elbow . . . . . . . . . . . . . . . . . . . 01732-01740

**Anorectal Exam (Surgical)** ....45990

**Anorectal Myectomy**
See Myomectomy, Anorectal

**Anorectovaginoplasty** ....46744-46746

**Anoscopy**
Ablation
    Polyp.........................46615
    Tumor........................46615
Biopsy.............................46606
with Delivery of Thermal Energy.........0288T
Dilation............................46604
Exploration.........................46600
Hemorrhage........................46614
High Resolution Anoscopy (HRA)
    Diagnostic....................0226T
    with Biopsy(ies)................0227T
Removal
    Foreign Body..................46608
    Polyp....................46610-46612
    Tumor....................46610-46612

**Antebrachium**
See Forearm

**Antecedent, Plasma Thromboplastin**
See Plasma Thromboplastin, Antecedent

**Antepartum Care**
Cesarean Delivery .................59510
    Previous..................59610, 59618
Vaginal Delivery................59425-59426

**Anterior Ramus of Thoracic Nerve**
See Intercostal Nerve

**Anthrax Vaccine**
See Vaccines

**Anthrogon**
See Follicle Stimulating Hormone (FSH)

**Anti Australia Antigens**
See Antibody, Hepatitis B

**Anti D Immunoglobulin**
See Immune Globulins, Rho (D)

**Anti-Human Globulin Consumption Test**
See Coombs Test

**Anti-Phospholipid Antibody**
See Antibody, Phospholipid

**Antiactivator, Plasmin**
See Alpha-2 Antiplasmin

**Antibiotic Administration**
Injection .....................96372-96379
Prescribed or Dispensed ..........4120F-4124F

**Antibiotic Sensitivity**.....87181-87184, 87188
Enzyme Detection ..................87185
Minimum Bactericidal Concentration......87187
Minimum Inhibitory Concentration........87186

**Antibodies, Thyroid-Stimulating**
See Immunoglobulin, Thyroid Stimulating

**Antibodies, Viral**
See Viral Antibodies

**Antibody**
See Antibody Identification; Microsomal Antibody
Actinomyces.......................86602
Adenovirus........................86603
Antinuclear...................86038-86039
Antiphosphatidylserine (Phospholipid).....86148
Antiprothrombin......................0030T
Antistreptolysin O .............86060-86063
Aspergillus........................86606
Bacterium.........................86609
Bartonella........................86611
Beta 2 Glycoprotein I.................86146
Blastomyces.......................86612
Blood Crossmatch .............86920-86923
Bordetella.........................86615
Borrelia....................86618-86619
Brucella..........................86622
Campylobacter......................86625
Candida...........................86628
Cardiolipin........................86147
Chlamydia.................86631-86632
Coccidioides.......................86635
Coxiella Burnetii....................86638
Cryptococcus......................86641
Cyclic Citrullinated Peptide (CCP).........86200
Cytomegalovirus..............86644-86645
Cytotoxic Screen.............86807-86808
Deoxyribonuclease..................86215
Deoxyribonucleic Acid (DNA) ......86225-86226
Diphtheria........................86648
Ehrlichia..........................86666
Encephalitis.................86651-86654
Enterovirus........................86658
Epstein-Barr Virus...........86663-86665
Fluorescent..................86255-86256
Francisella Tularensis................86668
Fungus...........................86671
Giardia Lamblia ....................86674
Growth Hormone....................86277
Helicobacter Pylori..................86677
Helminth..........................86682
Hemophilus Influenza ...............86684
Hepatitis
    Delta Agent....................86692
Hepatitis A .................86708-86709
Hepatitis B
    Core ........................86704
    IgM.........................86705
    Surface......................86706
Hepatitis Be ......................86707
Hepatitis C .................86803-86804
Herpes Simplex .............86694-86696
Heterophile.................86308-86310
Histoplasma.......................86698
HIV ..............86689, 86701-86703
HIV-1 ....................86701, 86703
HIV-2.....................86702-86703
HTLV-I ...................86687, 86689
HTLV-II ..........................86688
Influenza Virus.....................86710
Insulin............................86337
Intrinsic Factor.....................86340
Islet Cell..........................86341
Legionella.........................86713
Leishmania........................86717
Leptospira.........................86720
Listeria Monocytogenes ..............86723
Lyme Disease ......................86617
Lymphocytic Choriomeningitis ........86727
Lymphogranuloma Venereum ...........86729
Microsomal .......................86376
Mucormycosis .....................86732

Mumps ..........................86735
Mycoplasma.......................86738
Neisseria Meningitidis ...............86741
Nocardia..........................86744
Nuclear Antigen....................86235
Other Virus........................86790
Parvovirus.........................86747
Phospholipid...............85597, 86147
    Neutralization .............85597-85598
Phospholipid Cofactor ...............0030T
Plasmodium.......................86750
Platelet.........85597-85598, 86022-86023
Protozoa..........................86753
Red Blood Cell .............86850-86870
Respiratory Syncytial Virus ...........86756
Rickettsia.........................86757
Rotavirus..........................86759
Rubella...........................86762
Rubeola...........................86765
Salmonella........................86768
Shigella...........................86771
Sperm ...........................89325
Streptokinase......................86590
Tetanus...........................86774
Thyroglobulin......................86800
Toxoplasma. .............86777-86778
Treponema Pallidum ................86780
Trichinella.........................86784
Varicella-Zoster....................86787
West Nile Virus .............86788-86789
White Blood Cell ...................86021
Yersinia...........................86793

**Antibody Identification**
Leukocyte Antibodies ...............86021
Platelet....................86022-86023
Red Blood Cell
    Pretreatment .............86970-86972
Serum
    Pretreatment .............86975-86978

**Antibody Neutralization Test**
See Neutralization Test

**Antibody Receptor**
See FC Receptor

**Antibody Screening** .......86807-86808

**Anticoagulant**
See Clotting Inhibitors

**Anticoagulant Management** ..............99363-99364

**Antidiabetic Hormone**
See Glucagon

**Antidiuretic Hormone Measurement**
Vasopressin ......................84588

**AntiDNA Autoantibody**
See Antinuclear Antibodies (ANA)

**Antigen**
Allergen Immunotherapy...............95144
Carcinoembryonic ..................82378
Prostate Specific ...............84152-84153

**Antigen Bronchial Provocation Tests**
See Bronchial Challenge Test

## Antigen Detection

Direct Fluorescence . . . . . . . 87265-87272, 87276,
87278, 87280, 87285-87290
  Bordetella . . . . . . . . . . . . . . . . . . . . . 87265
  Chlamydia Trachomatis . . . . . . . . . . . . . 87270
  Cryptosporidium . . . . . . . . . . . . . . . . 87272
  Cytomegalovirus . . . . . . . . . . . . . . . . 87271
  Enterovirus . . . . . . . . . . . . . . . . . . . 87267
  Giardia . . . . . . . . . . . . . . . . . . . . . . 87269
  Influenza A . . . . . . . . . . . . . . . . . . . . 87276
  Legionella Pneumophila . . . . . . . . . . . . 87278
  Not Otherwise Specified . . . . . . . . . . . . 87299
  Respiratory Syncytial Virus . . . . . . . . . . 87280
  Treponema Pallidum . . . . . . . . . . . . . . 87285
  Varicella-Zoster . . . . . . . . . . . . . . . . . 87290
Enzyme Immunoassay . . . . . . . . . . . 87301-87451
  Adenovirus . . . . . . . . . . . . . . . . . . . . 87301
  Aspergillus . . . . . . . . . . . . . . . . . . . . 87305
  Chlamydia Trachomatis . . . . . . . . . . . . . 87320
  Clostridium Difficile . . . . . . . . . . . . . . 87324
  Cryptococcus Neoformans . . . . . . . . . . . 87327
  Cryptosporidium . . . . . . . . . . . . . . . . 87328
  Cytomegalovirus . . . . . . . . . . . . . . . . 87332
  Entamoeba Histolytica Dispar Group . . . . 87336
  Entamoeba Histolytica Group . . . . . . . . 87337
  Escherichia coli 0157 . . . . . . . . . . . . . 87335
  Giardia . . . . . . . . . . . . . . . . . . . . . . 87329
  Helicobacter Pylori . . . . . . . . 87338-87339
  Hepatitis B Surface Antigen
  (HBsAg) . . . . . . . . . . . . . . . . . . . . . 87340
  Hepatitis B Surface Antigen
  (HBsAg) Neutralization . . . . . . . . . . . . 87341
  Hepatitis Be Antigen (HBeAg) . . . . . . . . 87350
  Hepatitis Delta Agent . . . . . . . . . . . . . 87380
  Histoplasma capsulatum . . . . . . . . . . . 87385
  HIV-1 . . . . . . . . . . . . . . . . . . . . . . . 87390
  HIV-2 . . . . . . . . . . . . . . . . . . . . . . . 87391
  Influenza A . . . . . . . . . . . . . . . . . . . . 87400
  Influenza B . . . . . . . . . . . . . . . . . . . : 87400
  Multiple Step Method . . . . . . . . 87301-87449
    Polyvalent . . . . . . . . . . . . . . . . . . 87451
  Not Otherwise Specified . . . . . 87449, 87451
  Respiratory Syncytial Virus . . . . . . . . . . 87420
  Rotavirus . . . . . . . . . . . . . . . . . . . . . 87425
  Shigella-like Toxin . . . . . . . . . . . . . . . 87427
  Single Step Method . . . . . . . . . . . . . . . 87450
  Streptococcus, Group A . . . . . . . . . . . . 87430
Immunoassay
  Direct Optical
    Clostridium Difficile Toxin A . . . . . . . . 87803
    Influenza . . . . . . . . . . . . . . . . . . . 87804
    Respiratory Syncytial Virus . . . . . . . . 87807
    Streptococcus, Group B . . . . . . . . . . 87802
    Trichomonas Vaginalis . . . . . . . . . . . 87808
Immunofluorescence . . . . . . . . . . . 87260-87300
  Adenovirus . . . . . . . . . . . . . . . . . . . . 87260
  Herpes Simplex . . . . . . . . . . 87273-87274
  Influenza B . . . . . . . . . . . . . . . . . . . . 87275
  Legionella Micdadei . . . . . . . . . . . . . . 87277
  Not Otherwise Specified . . . . . . . . . . . . 87299
  Parainfluenza Virus . . . . . . . . . . . . . . . 87279
  Pneumocystis Carinii . . . . . . . . . . . . . . 87281
  Polyvalent . . . . . . . . . . . . . . . . . . . . 87300
  Rubeola . . . . . . . . . . . . . . . . . . . . . 87283

## Antigen, Australia
*See* Hepatitis Antigen, B Surface

## Antigen, CD4
*See* CD4

## Antigen, CD8
*See* CD8

## Antigens, CD142
*See* Thromboplastin

## Antigens, CD143
*See* Angiotensin Converting Enzyme (ACE)

## Antigens, E
*See* Hepatitis Antigen, Be

## Antigens, Hepatitis
*See* Hepatitis Antigen

## Antigens, Hepatitis B
*See* Hepatitis Antigen, B

## Antihemophilic Factor B
*See* Christmas Factor

## Antihemophilic Factor C
*See* Plasma Thromboplastin, Antecedent

## Antihemophilic Globulin
(AHG) . . . . . . . . . . . . . . . . . . . . . . 85240

## Antihuman Globulin . . . . . . 86880-86886

## Antimony . . . . . . . . . . . . . . . . . . . . 83015

## Antinuclear Antibodies
(ANA) . . . . . . . . . . . . . . . . . . . 86038-86039

## Antiplasmin, Alpha-2 . . . . . . . . . . 85410

## Antiplatelet Therapy
*See* Performance Measures

## Antiprotease, Alpha 1
*See* Alpha-1 Antitrypsin

## Antiprothrombin Antibody . . . . . 0030T

## Antistreptococcal Antibody . . . 86215

## Antistreptokinase Titer . . . . . . . 86590

## Antistreptolysin O . . . . . . . . 86060-86063

## Antithrombin III . . . . . . . . . . 85300-85301

## Antithrombin VI
*See* Fibrin Degradation Products

## Antitoxin Assay . . . . . . . . . . . . . . . 87230

## Antiviral Antibody
*See* Viral Antibodies

## Antrostomy
Sinus
  Maxillary . . . . . . . . . . . . . . . . . 31256-31267

## Antrotomy
Sinus
  Maxillary . . . . . . . . . . . . . . . . . 31020-31032
  Transmastoid . . . . . . . . . . . . . . . . . . 69501

## Antrum of Highmore
*See* Sinus, Maxillary

## Antrum Puncture
Sinus
  Maxillary . . . . . . . . . . . . . . . . . . . . . 31000
  Sphenoid . . . . . . . . . . . . . . . . . . . . . 31002

## Anus
*See* Hemorrhoids; Rectum
Ablation . . . . . . . . . . . . . . . . . . . . . . . 46615
Abscess
  Incision and Drainage . . . . . . . . 46045-46050
Anal Canal
  Delivery of Thermal Energy . . . . . . . . . . 0288T

Biofeedback . . . . . . . . . . . . . . . . . . . . . 90911
Biopsy
  Endoscopy . . . . . . . . . . . . . . . . . . . . 46606
Crypt
  Excision . . . . . . . . . . . . . . . . . . . . . 46999
Dilation
  Endoscopy . . . . . . . . . . . . . . . . . . . . 46604
Endoscopy
  Biopsy . . . . . . . . . . . . . . . . . . . . . . 46606
  Dilation . . . . . . . . . . . . . . . . . . . . . 46604
  Exploration . . . . . . . . . . . . . . . . . . . 46600
  Hemorrhage . . . . . . . . . . . . . . . . . . . 46614
  High Resolution Anoscopy
  (HRA) . . . . . . . . . . . . . . . . . . . 0226T-0227T
  Removal
    Foreign Body . . . . . . . . . . . . . . . . . 46608
    Polyp . . . . . . . . . . . . . . . . 46610, 46612
    Tumor . . . . . . . . . . . . . . . . 46610, 46612
Excision
  Tag . . . . . . . . . . . . . . . . . . 46220, 46230
Exploration
  Endoscopy . . . . . . . . . . . . . . . . . . . . 46600
  Surgical . . . . . . . . . . . . . . . . . . . . . 45990
Fissure
  Destruction . . . . . . . . . . . . . . 46940-46942
  Excision . . . . . . . . . . . . . . . . . . . . . 46200
Fistula
  Excision . . . . . . . . . . . . . . . . 46270-46285
  Repair . . . . . . . . . . . . . . . . . . . . . . 46706
Hemorrhage
  Endoscopic Control . . . . . . . . . . . . . . 46614
Hemorrhoids
  Clot Excision . . . . . . . . . . . . . . . . . . 46320
  Destruction . . . . . . . . . . . . . . . . . . . 46930
  Excision . . . . . . . . . . . . . . . . 46250-46262
  Injection . . . . . . . . . . . . . . . . . . . . . 46500
  Ligation . . . . . . . . 0249T, 46221, 46945-46946
  Stapling . . . . . . . . . . . . . . . . . . . . . 46947
  Suture . . . . . . . . . . . . . . . . . 46945-46946
Imperforated
  Repair . . . . . . . . . . . . . . . . . 46715-46742
Incision
  Septum . . . . . . . . . . . . . . . . . . . . . . 46070
  Sphincterotomy . . . . . . . . . . . . . . . . . 46200
Lesion
  Destruction . . . . . . . . . . 46900-46917, 46924
  Excision . . . . . . . . . . . . . . . . 45108, 46922
Manometry . . . . . . . . . . . . . . . . . . . . . 91122
Placement
  Seton . . . . . . . . . . . . . . . . . . . . . . . 46020
Reconstruction . . . . . . . . . . . . . . . . . . . 46742
  Congenital Absence . . . . . . . . . . 46730-46740
  Sphincter . . . . 46750-46751, 46760-46762
  with Graft . . . . . . . . . . . . . . . . . . . . 46753
  with Implant . . . . . . . . . . . . . . . . . . 46762
Removal
  Foreign Body . . . . . . . . . . . . . . . . . . 46608
  Seton . . . . . . . . . . . . . . . . . . . . . . . 46030
  Suture . . . . . . . . . . . . . . . . . . . . . . 46754
  Wire . . . . . . . . . . . . . . . . . . . . . . . . 46754
Repair
  Anovaginal Fistula . . . . . . . . . . . 46715-46716
  Cloacal Anomaly . . . . . . . . . . . . . . . . 46748
  Fistula . . . . . . . . . . . . . . . . . . . . . . 46706
  Stricture . . . . . . . . . . . . . . . . 46700-46705
Sphincter
  Chemodenervation . . . . . . . . . . . . . . . 46505
  Electromyography . . . . . . . . . . . 51784-51785
  Needle . . . . . . . . . . . . . . . . . . . . . . 51785
  Sphincterotomy . . . . . . . . . . . . . . . . . 46200
Unlisted Services and Procedures . . . . . . . . 46999

## Aorta

Abdominal
Aneurysm....... 0078T, 0079T, 0080T, 0081T, 34800-34805, 34825-34832, 35081-35103, 75952-75953
Thromboendarterectomy............ 35331
Anastomosis
to Pulmonary Artery................. 33606
Angiogram
Radiologic Injection................. 93567
See Cardiac Catheterization, Injection
Angioplasty........................... 35452
Aortography ............... 75600-75630
Ascending
Graft........................... 33864
Balloon....................... 33967, 33970
Catheterization
Catheter........................ 36200
Intracatheter/Needle.............. 36160
Circulation Assist................ 33967, 33970
Conduit to Heart..................... 33404
Excision
Coarctation.................. 33840-33851
Insertion
Balloon Device.................. 33967
Graft................. 33330-33335, 33864
Intracatheter/Needle.............. 36160
Removal
Balloon Assist Device......... 33968, 33971
Repair............ 33320-33322, 33802-33803
Coarctation.................. 33840-33851
Graft...................... 33860-33877
Ascending....................... 33864
Hypoplastic or Interrupted
Aortic Arch............... 33852-33853
Sinus of Valsalva............. 33702-33720
Suspension........................... 33800
Suture...................... 33320-33322
Thoracic
Repair...................... 75956-75959
Endovascular ............. 33880-33891
Translocation
Aortic Root.................. 33782-33783
Valve
Implantation.................0256T-0257T
Incision......................... 33415
Repair...................... 33400-33403
Left Ventricle................. 33414
Supravalvular Stenosis............ 33417
Replacement .... 0258T-0259T, 33405-33413
X-ray with Contrast.............. 75600-75630

## Aorta-Pulmonary ART Transposition

See Transposition, Great Arteries

## Aortic Sinus

See Sinus of Valsalva

## Aortic Stenosis

Repair............................. 33415
Nikaidoh Procedure........... 33782-33783
Supravalvular....................... 33417

## Aortic Valve

See Heart, Aortic Valve

## Aortic Valve Replacement

See Replacement, Aortic Valve

## Aortocoronary Bypass

See Coronary Artery Bypass Graft (CABG)

## Aortocoronary Bypass for Heart Revascularization

See Artery, Coronary, Bypass

## Aortography ... 75600-75605, 75630, 93567

See Angiography
Serial............................. 75625
with Iliofemoral Artery................. 75630

## Aortoiliac

Embolectomy.................. 34151-34201
Thrombectomy................. 34151-34201

## Aortopexy.......................... 33800

## Aortoplasty

Supravalvular Stenosis................. 33417

## AP

See Voiding Pressure Studies

## Apert-Gallais Syndrome

See Adrenogenital Syndrome

## Aphasia Testing ............... 96105

See Neurology, Diagnostic

## Apheresis

Therapeutic.................. 36511-36516

## Apical-Aortic Conduit.......... 33404

## Apicectomy

with Mastoidectomy.................. 69605
Petrous......................... 69530

## Apoaminotransferase, Aspartate

See Transaminase, Glutamic Oxaloacetic

## Apolipoprotein

Blood or Urine ...................... 82172

## Appendectomy ......... 44950-44960

Laparoscopic ....................... 44970

## Appendiceal Abscess

See Abscess, Appendix

## Appendico-Vesicostomy

Cutaneous........................... 50845

## Appendix

Abscess
Incision and Drainage
Open......................... 44900
Percutaneous................. 44901
Excision....................... 44950-44960

## Application

Allergy Tests....................... 95044
Bone Fixation Device
Multiplane...................... 20692
Stereotactic Computer
Assisted.................. 20696-20697
Uniplane...................... 20690
Caliper.......................... 20660
Cranial Tongs...................... 20660
Fixation Device
Shoulder........................ 23700
Halo
Cranial........................ 20661
Thin Skull Osteology............. 20664
Femoral........................ 20663
Maxillofacial Fixation ........... 21100
Pelvic......................... 20662
Interdental Fixation Device............. 21110
Intervertebral Device.................. 22851
Neurostimulation.............. 64550, 64566

Radioelement.................. 77761-77778
Surface....................... 77789
with Ultrasound.................. 76965
Stereotactic Frame.................... 20660
Headframe...................... 61800
Strapping
Multi-layer Compression System
Arm..................... 29583-29584
Leg..................... 29581-29582

## Application of External Fixation Device

See Fixation Device, Application, External

## APPT

See Thromboplastin, Partial, Time

## Aquatic Therapy

See Physical Medicine/Therapy/Occupational Therapy

## Aqueous Shunt

to Extraocular Reservoir ............. 66180
Revision..................... 66185

## Arch Ligament

See Coracoacromial Ligament

## Arch, Zygomatic

See Zygomatic Arch

## Arm

See Radius; Ulna; Wrist
Lower
Abscess......................... 25028
Amputation ............. 24900-24920, 25900-25905, 25915
Cineplasty.................... 24940
Revision ................. 25907-25909
Angiography..................... 73206
Artery
Ligation..................... 37618
Biopsy...................... 25065-25066
Bursa
Incision and Drainage............ 25031
Bypass Graft...................... 35903
Cast............................ 29075
CT Scan .................. 73200-73206
Decompression ............. 25020-25025
Exploration
Blood Vessel.................. 35860
Fasciotomy........... 24495, 25020-25025
Hematoma...................... 25028
Lesion, Tendon Sheath
Excision...................... 25110
Magnetic Resonance Imaging
(MRI)........... 73218-73220, 73223
Reconstruction
Ulna........................ 25337
Removal
Foreign Body.................. 25248
Repair
Blood Vessel with Other Graft...... 35266
Blood Vessel with Vein Graft........ 35236
Decompression................. 24495
Muscle............. 25260-25263, 25270
Secondary.................. 25265
Secondary
Muscle ................. 25272-25274
Tendon................. 25272-25274
Tendon ........... 25260-25263, 25270, 25280-25295, 25310-25316
Secondary................. 25265
Tendon Sheath................. 25275

Carotid
- Aneurysm . . . . . . . 35001-35002, 61697-61705
  - Vascular Malformation or Carotid
  - Cavernous Fistula . . . . . . . . . . 61705-61710
- Angiography . . . . . . . . . . . . . . . . . . 75660-75680
- Bypass Graft . . . . . . . . . 33891, 35501-35510,
  - 35601-35606, 35642
- Catheterization . . . . . . . . . . . . . . . . . . . . . 36100
- Decompression . . . . . . . . . . . . . 61590-61591,
  - 61595-61596
- Embolectomy . . . . . . . . . . . . . . . . . . . . . . 34001
- Exploration . . . . . . . . . . . . . . . . . . . . . . . 35701
- Ligation . . . . . . . . 37600-37606, 61611-61612
- Stenosis
  - Imaging Study Measurement . . . . . . . 3100F
- Thrombectomy . . . . . . . . . . . . . . . . . . . . . 34001
- Thromboendarterectomy . . . . . . . 35301, 35390
- Transection . . . . . . . . . . . . . . . . . . 61611-61612
- Transposition . . . . . . . . . . . . . . . . . . . . . . 33889

Carotid, Common
- Intima-Media Thickness (IMT) Study . . . . 0126T

Celiac
- Aneurysm . . . . . . . . . . . . . . . . . 35121-35122
- Bypass Graft . . . . . . . . . . . . . . 35531, 35631
- Embolectomy . . . . . . . . . . . . . . . . . . . . . . 34151
- Thrombectomy . . . . . . . . . . . . . . . . . . . . . 34151
- Thromboendarterectomy . . . . . . . . . . . . 35341

Chest
- Ligation . . . . . . . . . . . . . . . . . . . . . . . . . 37616

Coronary
- Angiography . . . . . . . . . . . . . . . . . . . . . . . 93556
- Atherectomy . . . . . . . . . . . . . . . . . 92995-92996
- Bypass . . . . . . . . . . . . . . . . . . . . 33517-33519
  - Arterial . . . . . . . . . . . . . . . . . . 33533-33536
- Bypass Venous Graft . . . . 33510-33517, 35523
  - Internal Mammary Artery Graft . . . . . . 4110F
- Graft . . . . . . . . . . . . . . . . . . . . . . 33503-33505
- Ligation . . . . . . . . . . . . . . . . . . . . . . . . . 33502
- Repair . . . . . . . . . . . . . . . . . . . . . 33500-33507
- Thrombectomy
  - Percutaneous . . . . . . . . . . . . . . . . . . . . 92973

Digital
- Sympathectomy . . . . . . . . . . . . . . . . . . . . 64820

Ethmoidal
- Ligation . . . . . . . . . . . . . . . . . . . . . . . . . 30915

Extra Corporeal Circulation
- for Regional Chemotherapy of
  - Extremity . . . . . . . . . . . . . . . . . . . . . . . . 36823

Extremities
- Vascular Studies . . . . . . . . . . . . . 93922-93923

Extremity
- Bypass Graft Revision . . . . . . . . . 35879-35884
- Catheterization . . . . . . . . . . . . . . . . . . . . 36140
- Ligation . . . . . . . . . . . . . . . . . . . . . . . . . 37618

Femoral
- Aneurysm . . . . . . . . . . . . . . . . . 35141-35142
- Angioplasty . . . . . . . . . . . . . . . . . . . . . . . 37224
- Atherectomy . . . . . . . . . . . . . . . . . 37225, 37227
- Bypass Graft . . . . . 35521, 35533, 35556-35558,
  - 35566, 35621, 35646-35647,
  - 35654-35661, 35666, 35700
- Bypass Graft Revision . . . . . . . . 35883-35884
- Bypass In-Situ . . . . . . . . . . . . . . 35583-35585
- Embolectomy . . . . . . . . . . . . . . . . . . . . . . 34201
- Exploration . . . . . . . . . . . . . . . . . . . . . . . 35721
- Exposure . . . . . . . . . . . . . . . . . . . . 34812-34813
- Thrombectomy . . . . . . . . . . . . . . . . . . . . . 34201
- Thromboendarterectomy . . . . . . . 35371-35372

Great Vessel
- Repair . . . . . . . . . . . . . . . . . . . . . 33770-33781

Head
- Angiography . . . . . . . . . . . . . . . . . . . . . . . 75650

Hepatic
- Aneurysm . . . . . . . . . . . . . . . . . 35121-35122

Iliac
- Aneurysm . . . . . . . . . . . . . 35131-35132, 75954
- Angioplasty . . . . . . . . . . . . . . . . . . . . . . . 37222
- Bypass Graft . . . . 35563, 35632-35634, 35663
- Embolectomy . . . . . . . . . . . . . . . . 34151-34201
- Endoprosthesis . . . . . . . . . . . . . . . 0254T-0255T
- Exposure . . . . . . . . . . . . . . . . . . . . 34820, 34833
- Occlusion Device . . . . . . . . . . . . . . . . . . . 34808
- Revascularization . . . . . . . . . . . . . . . . . . . 37222
- Thrombectomy . . . . . . . . . . . . . . . 34151-34201
- Thromboendarterectomy . . . . . . . . . . . 35351,
  - 35361-35363
- Tube Endoprosthesis . . . . . . . . . . 34900, 75954

Ilio-celiac
- Bypass Graft . . . . . . . . . . . . . . . . . . . . . . 35632

Iliofemoral
- Bypass Graft . . . . . . . . . . . . . . . . . . . . . . 35565
- Thromboendarterectomy . . . . . . . 35355, 35363
- X-ray with Contrast . . . . . . . . . . . . . . . . . 75630

Ilio-mesenteric
- Bypass Graft . . . . . . . . . . . . . . . . . . . . . . 35633

Iliorenal
- Bypass Graft . . . . . . . . . . . . . . . . . . . . . . 35634

Innominate
- Aneurysm . . . . . . . . . . . . . . . . . 35021-35022
- Embolectomy . . . . . . . . . . . . . . . . 34001-34101
- Thrombectomy . . . . . . . . . . . . . . . 34001-34101
- Thromboendarterectomy . . . . . . . . . . . . 35311

Leg
- Angiography . . . . . . . . . . . . . . . . . 75710-75716
- Catheterization . . . . . . . . . . . . . . . 36245-36248

Mammary
- Angiography . . . . . . . . . . . . . . . . . . . . . . . 75756

Maxillary
- Ligation . . . . . . . . . . . . . . . . . . . . . . . . . 30920

Mesenteric
- Aneurysm . . . . . . . . . . . . . . . . . 35121-35122
- Bypass Graft . . . . . . . . . . . . . . 35531, 35631
- Embolectomy . . . . . . . . . . . . . . . . . . . . . . 34151
- Thrombectomy . . . . . . . . . . . . . . . . . . . . . 34151
- Thromboendarterectomy . . . . . . . . . . . . 35341

Middle Cerebral Artery, Fetal
- Vascular Studies . . . . . . . . . . . . . . . . . . . 76821

Neck
- Angiography . . . . . . . . . . . . . . . . . . . . . . . 75650
- Ligation . . . . . . . . . . . . . . . . . . . . . . . . . 37615

Nose
- Incision . . . . . . . . . . . . . . . . . . . . . 30915-30920

Other Angiography . . . . . . . . . . . . . . . . . . . 75774

Other Artery
- Exploration . . . . . . . . . . . . . . . . . . . . . . . 35761

Pelvic
- Angiography . . . . . . . . . . . . . . . . . . . . . . . 75736
- Catheterization . . . . . . . . . . . . . . . 36245-36248

Peripheral Arterial Rehabilitation . . . . . . . . 93668

Peroneal
- Bypass Graft . . . . . . 35566-35571, 35666-35671
- Bypass In-Situ . . . . . . . . . . . . . . 35585-35587
- Embolectomy . . . . . . . . . . . . . . . . . . . . . . 34203
- Thrombectomy . . . . . . . . . . . . . . . . . . . . . 34203
- Thromboendarterectomy . . . . . . . 35305-35306

Popliteal
- Aneurysm . . . . . . . . . . . . . . . . . 35151-35152
- Angioplasty . . . . . . . . . . . . . . . . . . . . . . . 37224
- Atherectomy . . . . . . . . . . . . . . . . . 37225, 37227
- Bypass Graft . . . . . . 35556-35556, 35571,
  - 35623, 35656, 35671, 35700
- Bypass In-Situ . . . . . . . . . . . . . . 35583, 35587
- Embolectomy . . . . . . . . . . . . . . . . . . . . . . 34203
- Exploration . . . . . . . . . . . . . . . . . . . . . . . 35741

Thrombectomy . . . . . . . . . . . . . . . . . . . . . 34203
Thromboendarterectomy . . . . . . . . . . . . . 35303

Pulmonary
- Anastomosis . . . . . . . . . . . . . . . . . . . . . . 33606
- Angiography . . . . . . . . . . . . . . . . . 75741-75746
- Banding . . . . . . . . . . . . . . . . . . . . . . . . . 33620
- Repair . . . . . . . . . . . . . . . 33690, 33925-33926

Radial
- Aneurysm . . . . . . . . . . . . . . . . . . . . . . . . 35045
- Embolectomy . . . . . . . . . . . . . . . . . . . . . . 34111
- Sympathectomy . . . . . . . . . . . . . . . . . . . . 64821
- Thrombectomy . . . . . . . . . . . . . . . . . . . . . 34111

Rehabilitation . . . . . . . . . . . . . . . . . . . . . . . 93668

Reimplantation
- Carotid . . . . . . . . . . . 35691, 35694-35695
- Subclavian . . . . . . . . . . . . . . . . . 35693-35695
- Vertebral . . . . . . . . . . . . . . . . . . . 35691-35693
- Visceral . . . . . . . . . . . . . . . . . . . . . . . . . 35697

Renal
- Aneurysm . . . . . . . . . . . . . . . . . 35121-35122
- Angiography . . . . . . . . . . . . . . . . . 36251-36254
- Angioplasty . . . . . . . . . . . . . . . . . . . . . . . 35450
- Bypass Graft . . . . . . . . . 35535-35536, 35560,
  - 35631-35636
- Catheterization . . . . . . . . . . . . . . . 36251-36254
- Embolectomy . . . . . . . . . . . . . . . . . . . . . . 34151
- Thrombectomy . . . . . . . . . . . . . . . . . . . . . 34151
- Thromboendarterectomy . . . . . . . . . . . . 35341

Repair
- Aneurysm . . . . . . . . . . . . . . . . . 61697-61708
- Angioplasty
  - Radiological Supervision . . . . . 75962-75968

Revision
- Hemodialysis Graft or Fistula
  - with Thrombectomy . . . . . . . . . . . . . 36833
  - without Thrombectomy . . . . . . . . . . . 36832

Spine
- Angiography . . . . . . . . . . . . . . . . . . . . . . . 75705

Splenic
- Aneurysm . . . . . . . . . . . . . . . . . 35111-35112
- Bypass Graft . . . . . . . . . . . . . . 35536, 35636

Subclavian
- Aneurysm . . . . . . . 35001-35002, 35021-35022
- Angioplasty . . . . . . . . . . . . . . . . . . . . . . . 35458
- Bypass Graft . . . . . . . . 35506, 35511-35516,
  - 35606-35616, 35645
- Embolectomy . . . . . . . . . . . . . . . . 34001-34101
- Thrombectomy . . . . . . . . . . . . . . . 34001-34101
- Thromboendarterectomy . . . . . . . 35301, 35311
- Transposition . . . . . . . . . . . . . . . . . . . . . . 33889
- Unlisted Services and Procedures . . . . . . 37799

Superficial Femoral
- Thromboendarterectomy . . . . . . . . . . . . 35302

Superficial Palmar Arch
- Sympathectomy . . . . . . . . . . . . . . . . . . . . 64823

Temporal
- Biopsy . . . . . . . . . . . . . . . . . . . . . . . . . . 37609
- Ligation . . . . . . . . . . . . . . . . . . . . . . . . . 37609

Thoracic
- Catheterization . . . . . . . . 33621, 36215-36218

Thrombectomy . . . . . . . . . . . . . . . . . 37184-37186
- Hemodialysis Graft or Fistula . . . . . . . . 36831
- Other than Hemodialysis Graft or
  - Fistula . . . . . . . . . . . . . . . . . . . 35875, 36870

Tibial
- Bypass Graft . . . . . . . . . 35566-35571, 35623,
  - 35666-35671
- Bypass In-Situ . . . . . . . . . . . . . . 35585-35587
- Embolectomy . . . . . . . . . . . . . . . . . . . . . . 34203
- Thrombectomy . . . . . . . . . . . . . . . . . . . . . 34203
- Thromboendarterectomy . . . . . . . 35305-35306

Shoulder . . . . . . . . . . . . . . . 29806-29828
  Biceps Tenodesis . . . . . . . . . . . . . 29828
Subtalar Joint
  with Acetabuloplasty . . . . . . . . . . . . 29915
  Arthrodesis . . . . . . . . . . . . . . . . . 29907
  Debridement . . . . . . . . . . . . . . . . 29906
  with Labral Repair . . . . . . . . . . . . . 29916
  Removal of Loose or Foreign Body . . . . 29904
  Synovectomy . . . . . . . . . . . . . . . . 29905
Temporomandibular Joint . . . . . . . . . . 29804
Wrist . . . . . . . . . . . . . . . . . 29843-29848
Unlisted Services and Procedures . . . . . . . 29999

## Arthroscopy of Ankle
*See* Ankle, Arthroscopy

## Arthrotomy
Acromioclavicular Joint . . . . . . . . . . . . . 23044
Ankle . . . . . . . . . . . 27610-27612, 27620
Ankle Joint . . . . . . . . . . . . . 27625-27626
Carpometacarpal Joint . . . . . . . . . . . . 26070
  with Biopsy, Synovium
    with Synovial Biopsy . . . . . . . . . . . 26100
Elbow . . . . . . . . . . . . . . . . . . . . . 24000
  Capsular Release . . . . . . . . . . . . . . 24006
  with Joint Exploration . . . . . . . . . . . 24101
  with Synovectomy . . . . . . . . . . . . . 24102
  with Synovial Biopsy . . . . . . . . . . . . 24100
Finger Joint . . . . . . . . . . . . . . . . . . 26075
  Interphalangeal
    with Synovial Biopsy . . . . . . . . . . . 26110
  Metacarpophalangeal
    with Biopsy, Synovium . . . . . . . . . . 26105
Glenohumeral Joint . . . . . . . . . . . . . . 23040
Hip . . . . . . . . . . . . . . . . . . . . . . 27033
  for Infection
    with Drainage . . . . . . . . . . . . . . . 27030
    with Synovectomy . . . . . . . . . . . . 27054
Interphalangeal Joint . . . . . . . . . 26080, 26110
  Toe . . . . . . . . . . . . . . . . 28024, 28054
Intertarsal Joint . . . . . . . . . . . . 28020, 28050
Knee . . . . . . . 27310, 27330-27335, 27403, 29868
Metacarpophalangeal Joint . . . . . . . 26075, 26105
Metatarsophalangeal Joint . . . . . . . 28022, 28052
Shoulder . . . . . . . . . . . . . 23044, 23105-23107
Shoulder Joint . . . . . . . . . . . . . 23100-23101
  Exploration and/or Removal of Loose
  or Foreign Body . . . . . . . . . . . . . . 23107
Sternoclavicular Joint . . . . . . . . . . . . . 23044
Tarsometatarsal Joint . . . . . . . . . . 28020, 28050
Temporomandibular Joint . . . . . . . . . . . 21010
with Biopsy
  Acromioclavicular Joint . . . . . . . . . . . 23101
  Glenohumeral Joint . . . . . . . . . . . . . 23100
  Hip Joint . . . . . . . . . . . . . . . . . . 27052
  Knee Joint . . . . . . . . . . . . . . . . . 27330
  Sacroiliac Joint
    Hip Joint . . . . . . . . . . . . . . . . . 27050
  Sternoclavicular Joint . . . . . . . . . . . . 23101
with Synovectomy
  Glenohumeral Joint . . . . . . . . . . . . . 23105
  Sternoclavicular Joint . . . . . . . . . . . . 23106
Wrist . . . . . . . . . . . . . 25040, 25100-25107

## Arthrotomy for Removal of Prosthesis of Ankle
*See* Ankle, Removal, Implant

## Arthrotomy for Removal of Prosthesis of Hip
*See* Hip, Removal, Prosthesis

## Arthrotomy for Removal of Prosthesis of Wrist
*See* Prosthesis, Wrist, Removal

## Articular Ligament
*See* Ligament

## Artificial Abortion
*See* Abortion

## Artificial Cardiac Pacemaker
*See* Heart, Pacemaker

## Artificial Eye
*See* Prosthesis

## Artificial Genitourinary Sphincter
*See* Prosthesis, Urethral Sphincter

## Artificial Insemination . . . . . . . . 58976
*See* In Vitro Fertilization
Intra-Cervical . . . . . . . . . . . . . . . . . 58321
Intra-Uterine . . . . . . . . . . . . . . . . . 58322
Sperm Washing . . . . . . . . . . . . . . . . 58323

## Artificial Knee Joints
*See* Prosthesis, Knee

## Artificial Penis
*See* Penile Prosthesis

## Artificial Pneumothorax
*See* Pneumothorax, Therapeutic

## Arytenoid
Excision
  Endoscopic . . . . . . . . . . . . 31560-31561

## Arytenoid Cartilage
Excision . . . . . . . . . . . . . . . . . . . . 31400
Repair . . . . . . . . . . . . . . . . . . . . . 31400

## Arytenoidectomy . . . . . . . . . . . . 31400
Endoscopic . . . . . . . . . . . . . . . . . . 31560

## Arytenoidopexy . . . . . . . . . . . . . 31400

## Ascorbic Acid
Blood . . . . . . . . . . . . . . . . . . . . . . 82180

## ASPA . . . . . . . . . . . . . . . . . . . . 81200

## Aspartate Aminotransferase
*See* Transaminase, Glutamic Oxaloacetic

## Aspergillus
Antibody . . . . . . . . . . . . . . . . . . . . 86606
Antigen Detection
  Enzyme Immunoassay . . . . . . . . . . . . 87305

## Aspiration
*See* Puncture Aspiration
Amniotic Fluid
  Diagnostic . . . . . . . . . . . . . . . . . 59000
  Therapeutic . . . . . . . . . . . . . . . . . 59001
Bladder . . . . . . . . . . . . . . . 51100-51102
Bone Marrow . . . . . . . . . . . . . . . . . 38220
Brain Lesion
  Stereotactic . . . . . . . . . . . . 61750-61751
Breast
  Metallic Localization Clip Placement . . . 19295
Bronchi
  Endoscopy . . . . . . . . . . . . . 31645-31646
Bursa . . . . . . . . . . . . . . . . 20600-20610
Catheter
  Nasotracheal . . . . . . . . . . . . . . . . 31720
  Tracheobronchial . . . . . . . . . . . . . . 31725
Cyst
  Bone . . . . . . . . . . . . . . . . . . . . 20615

Kidney . . . . . . . . . . . . . . . . . . . . . 50390
Pelvis . . . . . . . . . . . . . . . . . . . . . 50390
Spinal Cord . . . . . . . . . . . . . . . . . . 62268
Thyroid . . . . . . . . . . . . . . . . . . . . 60300
Disc . . . . . . . . . . . . . . . . . . . . . . 62267
Duodenal . . . . . . . . . . . . . . 43756-43757
Fetal Fluid . . . . . . . . . . . . . . . . . . . 59074
Ganglion Cyst . . . . . . . . . . . . . . . . . 20612
Hydrocele
  Tunica Vaginalis . . . . . . . . . . . . . . . 55000
Joint . . . . . . . . . . . . . . . . 20600-20610
Laryngoscopy
  Direct . . . . . . . . . . . . . . . . . . . . 31515
Lens Material . . . . . . . . . . . . . . . . . 66840
Liver . . . . . . . . . . . . . . . . . . . . . . 47015
Lung . . . . . . . . . . . . . . . . . . . . . . 32420
Orbital Contents . . . . . . . . . . . . . . . . 67415
Pelvis
  Endoscopy . . . . . . . . . . . . . . . . . 49322
Pericardium . . . . . . . . . . . . . 33010-33011
Pleural Cavity . . . . . . . . . . . . 32421-32422
Puncture
  Cyst
    Breast . . . . . . . . . . . . . 19000-19001
Spinal Cord
  Stereotaxis . . . . . . . . . . . . . . . . . 63615
  Sub . . . . . . . . . . . . . . . . . . . Stomach
  Diagnostic . . . . . . . . . . . . . 43754-43755
  Therapeutic . . . . . . . . . . . . . . . . . 43753
Syrinx
  Spinal Cord . . . . . . . . . . . . . . . . . 62268
Thyroid . . . . . . . . . . . . . . . . . . . . 60300
Trachea
  Nasotracheal . . . . . . . . . . . . . . . . 31720
  Puncture . . . . . . . . . . . . . . . . . . 31612
Tunica Vaginalis
  Hydrocele . . . . . . . . . . . . . . . . . . 55000
Vitreous . . . . . . . . . . . . . . . . . . . . 67015

## Aspiration Lipectomies
*See* Liposuction

## Aspiration of Bone Marrow from Donor for Transplant
*See* Bone Marrow, Harvesting

## Aspiration, Chest
*See* Thoracentesis

## Aspiration, Lung Puncture
*See* Pneumocentesis

## Aspiration, Nail
*See* Evacuation, Hematoma, Subungual

## Aspiration, Spinal Puncture
*See* Spinal Tap

## Assay Tobramycin
*See* Tobramycin

## Assay, Very Long Chain Fatty Acids
*See* Fatty Acid, Very Long Chain

## Assisted Circulation
*See* Circulation Assist

## AST
*See* Transaminase, Glutamic Oxaloacetic

## Astragalectomy . . . . . . . . . . . . . 28130

## Astragalus
*See* Talus

## Asymmetry, Face
*See* Hemifacial Microsomia

Gross Exam.................... 88000-88016
Organ ........................... 88037
Regional ........................ 88036
Unlisted Services and Procedures ........ 88099

**Autotransfusion**
Blood.......................... 86890-86891

**Autotransplant**
See Autograft

**Autotransplantation**
Renal............................ 50380

**AV Fistula**
See Arteriovenous Fistula

**AV Shunt**
See Arteriovenous Shunt

**Avulsion**
Nails ........................ 11730-11732
Nerve ........................ 64732-64772

**Axillary Arteries**
See Artery, Axillary

**Axillary Nerve**
Injection
    Anesthetic ...................... 64417

**Axis, Dens**
See Odontoid Process

# B

**B Antibodies, Hepatitis**
See Antibody, Hepatitis B

**B Antigens, Hepatitis**
See Hepatitis Antigen, B

**B Complex Vitamins**
B-12 Absorption : .............. 78270-78272

**B-Cells**
Count............................ 86355

**B-DNA**
See Deoxyribonucleic Acid

**b-Hexosaminidase** ............. 83080

**B-1 Vitamin**
See Thiamine

**B-6 Vitamin**
See Vitamin, B-6

**B-12 Vitamin**
See Cyanocobalamin

**Bacillus Calmette Guerin Vaccine**
See BCG Vaccine

**Back/Flank**
Biopsy........................ 21920-21925
Repair
    Hernia........................ 49540
Tumor
    Excision ................... 21930-21933
    Radical Resection ........... 21935-21936
Wound Exploration
    Penetrating.................... 20102

**Backbone**
See Spine

**Bacteria Culture**
Additional Methods.................... 87077
Aerobic......................... 87040-87071
Anaerobic...................... 87073-87076
Blood............................ 87040
Other Source .................. 87070-87075
Screening ........................ 87081
Stool ........................ 87045-87046
Urine ........................ 87086-87088

**Bacterial Endotoxins**............87176

**Bacterial Overgrowth Breath Test**.............................91065

**Bactericidal Titer, Serum**......87197

**Bacterium**
Antibody........................... 86609

**BAER**
See Evoked Potential, Auditory Brainstem

**Baker Tube**
Intestine Decompression............... 44021

**Baker's Cyst** .........................27345

**Balanoplasty**
See Penis, Repair

**Balkan Grippe**
See Q Fever

**Balloon Angioplasties, Coronary**
See Percutaneous Transluminal Angioplasty

**Balloon Angioplasty**
See Angioplasty

**Balloon Assisted Device**
Aorta......................... 33967-33974

**Band, Pulmonary Artery**
See Banding, Artery, Pulmonary

**Banding**
Artery
    Fistula........................ 37607
    Pulmonary ..................... 33690
    Application..................... 33620
    Removal ...................... 33622

**Bank, Blood**
See Blood Banking

**Bankart Procedure**
See Capsulorrhaphy, Anterior

**Barany Caloric Test**
See Caloric Vestibular Test

**Barbiturates**
Blood or Urine .................... 82205

**Bardenheuer Operation**
See Ligation, Artery, Chest

**Bariatric Surgery** ........ 43644-43645,
    43770-43775, 43842-43848, 43886-43888

**Barium** ........................83015

**Barium Enema** ............ 74270-74280

**Barker Operation**
See Talus, Excision

**Baroreflex Activation Device**
Implantation/Replacement .....0266T-0268T
Interrogation Evaluation .......0272T-0273T
Revision/Removal ............0269T-0271T

**Barr Bodies**....................88130

**Barr Procedure**
See Tendon, Transfer, Leg, Lower

**Bartholin's Gland**
Abscess
    Incision and Drainage .............. 56420
Cyst
    Repair...................... 56440
Excision........................ 56740
Marsupialization ................. 56440

**Bartonella**
Antibody......................... 86611

**Bartonella Detection**...... 87470-87472

**Basic Life Services** ............99450

**Basic Proteins, Myelin**
See Myelin Basic Protein

**Basilar Arteries**
See Artery, Basilar

**Batch-Spittler-McFaddin Operation**
See Disarticulation, Knee

**BCG Vaccine**............... 90585-90586
See Vaccines

**BCKDHB** ........................81205

**BCR/ABL1** ................. 81206-81208

**Be Antigens, Hepatitis**
See Hepatitis Antigen, Be

**Bed Sores**
See Debridement; Pressure Ulcer (Decubitus); Skin Graft and Flap

**Bed Testing** ............... 94780, 94781

**Bekesy Audiometry**
See Audiometry, Bekesy

**Belsey IV Procedure**
See Fundoplasty

**Bender-Gestalt Test** ...... 96101-96103

**Benedict Test for Urea**
See Urinalysis, Qualitative

**Benign Cystic Mucinous Tumor**
See Ganglion

**Benign Neoplasm of Cranial Nerves**
See Cranial Nerve

**Bennett Fracture**
See Phalanx; Thumb, Fracture

**Bennett Procedure**
See Repair, Leg, Upper, Muscle; Revision

**Benzidine Test**
See Blood, Feces

**Benzodiazepine**
Assay ........................... 80154

Epididymis . . . . . . . . . . . . . . . . . . . . . 54800, 54865
Esophagus
    Endoscopy . . . . . . . . . . . . . . . . . . . . . 43202
    Forceps . . . . . . . . . . . . . . . . . . . . . . . . . 3150F
Eye Muscle . . . . . . . . . . . . . . . . . . . . . . . . . 67346
Eyelid . . . . . . . . . . . . . . . . . . . . . . . . . . . . 67810
Forearm
    Soft Tissue . . . . . . . . . . . . . . . 25065-25066
Gallbladder
    Endoscopy . . . . . . . . . . . . . . . . . . . . . 43261
Gastrointestinal, Upper
    Endoscopy . . . . . . . . . . . . . . . . . . . . . 43239
Hand Joint
    Synovium . . . . . . . . . . . . . . . . . . . . . . 26100
Heart . . . . . . . . . . . . . . . . . . . . . . . . . . . . . 93505
Hip . . . . . . . . . . . . . . . . . . . . . . . . 27040-27041
    Joint . . . . . . . . . . . . . . . . . . . . . . . . . . 27052
Hypopharynx . . . . . . . . . . . . . . . . . . . . . . . 42802
Ileum
    Endoscopy . . . . . . . . . . . . . . . . . . . . . 44382
Interphalangeal Joint
    Finger . . . . . . . . . . . . . . . . . . . . . . . . . 26110
    Toe . . . . . . . . . . . . . . . . . . . . . . . . . . . 28054
Intertarsal Joint
    Toe . . . . . . . . . . . . . . . . . . . . . . . . . . . 28050
Intestines, Small . . . . . . . . . . . . . 44020, 44100
    Endoscopy . . . . . . . . . . . . . . . 44361, 44377
Kidney . . . . . . . . . . . . . . . . . . . . . 50200-50205
    Endoscopic . . . . . . . . . . . . . . . . 50555-50557,
                  50574-50576, 52354
Knee . . . . . . . . . . . . . . . . . . . . . . . 27323-27324
    Synovium . . . . . . . . . . . . . . . . . . . . . . 27330
Knee Joint
    Synovium . . . . . . . . . . . . . . . . . . . . . . 27330
Lacrimal Gland . . . . . . . . . . . . . . . . . . . . . 68510
Lacrimal Sac . . . . . . . . . . . . . . . . . . . . . . . 68525
Larynx
    Endoscopy . . . . . . . . . . . . . . . 31510, 31576
Leg
    Lower . . . . . . . . . . . . . . . . . . . 27613-27614
    Upper . . . . . . . . . . . . . . . . . . . 27323-27324
Lip . . . . . . . . . . . . . . . . . . . . . . . . . . . . . . 40490
Liver . . . . . . . . . . . . . . . . . 47000-47001, 47100
Lung
    Needle . . . . . . . . . . . . . . . . . . . . . . . . 32405
    Thoracoscopy . . . . . . . . . . . . . . 32607-32608
    Thoracotomy . . . . . . . . . . . . . . 32096-32097
Lymph Nodes . . . . . . . . . . . . . . . . 38500-38530
    Injection Procedure
        Radioactive Tracer . . . . . . . . . . . . . 38792
    Laparoscopic . . . . . . . . . . . . . . 38570-38572
    Needle . . . . . . . . . . . . . . . . . . . . . . . . 38505
    Open . . . . . . . . . . . . . . 38500, 38510-38530
        Superficial . . . . . . . . . . . . . . . . . . . 38500
Mediastinum . . . . . . . . . . . . . . . . . . . . . . . 39400
    Needle . . . . . . . . . . . . . . . . . . . . . . . . 32405
Metacarpophalangeal Joint . . . . . . . . . . . . 26105
Metatarsophalangeal Joint . . . . . . . . . . . . 28052
Mouth . . . . . . . . . . . . . . . . . . . . 40808, 41108
Muscle . . . . . . . . . . . . . . . . . . . . 20200-20206
Nail . . . . . . . . . . . . . . . . . . . . . . . . . . . . . 11755
Nasopharynx . . . . . . . . . . . . . . . . 42804-42806
Neck . . . . . . . . . . . . . . . . . . . . . . . . . . . . 21550
Nerve . . . . . . . . . . . . . . . . . . . . . . . . . . . . 64795
Nose
    Endoscopic . . . . . . . . . . . . . . . . . . . . . 31237
    Intranasal . . . . . . . . . . . . . . . . . . . . . . 30100
Oocyte Polar Body . . . . . . . . . . . . 89290-89291
Orbit . . . . . . . . . . . . . . . . . . . . . . . . . . . . 61332
    Exploration . . . . . . . . . . . . . . . 67400, 67450
    Fine Needle Aspiration . . . . . . . . . . . . 67415
Oropharynx . . . . . . . . . . . . . . . . . . . . . . . 42800
Ovary . . . . . . . . . . . . . . . . . . . . . . . . . . . . 58900

Palate . . . . . . . . . . . . . . . . . . . . . . . . . . . 42100
Pancreas . . . . . . . . . . . . . . . . . . . . . . . . . 48100
Pelvis . . . . . . . . . . . . . . . . . . . . . 27040-27041
Penis . . . . . . . . . . . . . . . . . . . . . . . . . . . . 54100
    Deep Structures . . . . . . . . . . . . . . . . . 54105
Percutaneous Needle
    Spinal Cord . . . . . . . . . . . . . . . . . . . . 62269
Perineum . . . . . . . . . . . . . . . . . . . 56605-56606
Peritoneum
    Endoscopic . . . . . . . . . . . . . . . . . . . . . 47561
Pharynx . . . . . . . . . . . . . . . . . . . . 42800-42806
Pleura
    Needle . . . . . . . . . . . . . . . . . . . . . . . . 32400
    Thoracoscopy . . . . . . . . . . . . . . . . . . . 32609
    Thoracotomy . . . . . . . . . . . . . 32098, 32400
Prostate . . . . . . . . . . . . . . . . . . . . 55700-55706
Rectum . . . . . . . . . . . . . . . . . . . . . . . . . . 45100
Retroperitoneal Area . . . . . . . . . . . . . . . . 49010
Sacroiliac Joint . . . . . . . . . . . . . . . . . . . . 27050
Salivary Gland . . . . . . . . . . . . . . . . . . . . . 42405
Shoulder
    Deep . . . . . . . . . . . . . . . . . . . . . . . . . 23066
    Soft Tissue . . . . . . . . . . . . . . . . . . . . . 23065
Shoulder Joint . . . . . . . . . . . . . . . 23100-23101
Sinus
    Sphenoid . . . . . . . . . . . . . . . . 31050-31051
Skin Lesion . . . . . . . . . . . . . . . . . 11100-11101
Spinal Cord . . . . . . . . . . . . . . . . . 63275-63290
    Percutaneous . . . . . . . . . . . . . . . . . . . 62269
    Stereotaxis . . . . . . . . . . . . . . . . . . . . . 63615
Stomach . . . . . . . . . . . . . . . . . . . . . . . . . 43605
Tarsometatarsal Joint
    Synovial . . . . . . . . . . . . . . . . . . . . . . . 28050
Testis . . . . . . . . . . . . . . . . . . . . . . 54500-54505
Thorax . . . . . . . . . . . . . . . . . . . . . . . . . . 21550
Throat . . . . . . . . . . . . . . . . . . . . . 42800-42806
Tongue . . . . . . . . . . . . . . . . . . . . 41100-41105
Transcatheter . . . . . . . . . . . . . . . . . . . . . 37200
Ureter . . . . . . . . . . . . . . . . . . . . . . . . . . . 52354
    Endoscopic . . . . . . 50955-50957, 50974-50976
Urethra . . . . . . . . . . . . . 52204, 52354, 53200
Uterus
    Endometrial . . . . . . . . . . . . . . . 58100-58110
    Endoscopic . . . . . . . . . . . . . . . . . . . . . 58558
Uvula . . . . . . . . . . . . . . . . . . . . . . . . . . . 42100
Vagina . . . . . . . . . . . . . 57100-57105, 57421
Vertebral Body . . . . . . . . . . . . . . . 20250-20251
Vulva . . . . . . . . . . . . . . . 56605-56606, 56821
with Arthrotomy
    Acromioclavicular Joint . . . . . . . . . . . . 23101
    Glenohumeral Joint . . . . . . . . . . . . . . 23100
    Sternoclavicular Joint . . . . . . . . . . . . 23101
with Cystourethroscopy . . . . . . . . . . . . . 52354
Wrist . . . . . . . . . . . 25065-25066, 25100-25101

## Biopsy, Skin
*See* Skin, Biopsy

## Biopsy, Vein
*See* Vein, Biopsy

## Biostatistics
*See* Biometry

## Biosterol
*See* Vitamin, A

## Biotinidase . . . . . . . . . . . . . . . . . . . . . 82261

## Birthing Room
Newborn Care . . . . . . . . . . . . . . 99460, 99463
    Attendance at Delivery . . . . . . . . . . . . 99464
    Resuscitation . . . . . . . . . . . . . . . . . . . 99465

## Bischof Procedure
*See* Laminectomy, Surgical

## Bismuth . . . . . . . . . . . . . . . . . . . . . . . 83015

## Bizzozero's Corpuscle/Cell
*See* Blood, Platelet

## Bladder
Abscess
    Incision and Drainage . . . . . . . . . . . . . 51080
Anastomosis . . . . . . . . . . . . . . . . . . . . . . 51960
Aspiration . . . . . . . . . . . . . . . . . 51100-51102
Biopsy . . . . . . . . . . . . . . . . . . . . . . . . . . 52204
Catheterization . . . . . . . . . 51045, 51701-51703
Change Tube . . . . . . . . . . . . . . . 51705-51710
Creation
    Stoma . . . . . . . . . . . . . . . . . . . . . . . . 51980
Cyst
    Urachal
        Excision . . . . . . . . . . . . . . . . . . . . . 51500
Destruction
    Endoscopic . . . . . . . . . 52214-52224, 52354
Dilation
    Ureter . . . . . . . . . 52260-52265, 52341-52342,
                        52344-52345
Diverticulum
    Excision . . . . . . . . . . . . . . . . . . . . . . . 51525
    Incision . . . . . . . . . . . . . . . . . . . . . . . 52305
    Resection . . . . . . . . . . . . . . . . . . . . . . 52305
Endoscopy . . . . . . . . . . . . . . . . . . . . . . . 52000
    Biopsy . . . . . . . . . . . . . . . . . 52204, 52354
    Catheterization . . . . . . . . . . . . 52005, 52010
    Destruction . . . . . . . . . . 52214-52224, 52400
    Dilation . . . . . . . . . . . . . . . . . 52260-52265
    Diverticulum . . . . . . . . . . . . . . . . . . . 52305
    Evacuation
        Clot . . . . . . . . . . . . . . . . . . . . . . . . 52001
    Excision
        Tumor . . . . . . . . . 52234-52240, 52355
    Exploration . . . . . . . . . . . . . . . . . . . . 52351
    Injection . . . . . . . . . . . . . . . . . . . . . . 52283
    Lithotripsy . . . . . . . . . . . . . . . . . . . . 52353
    Radiotracer . . . . . . . . . . . . . . . . . . . . 52250
    Removal
        Calculus . . . . . . . . . . . 52310-52315, 52352
        Foreign Body . . . . . . . . . . . . 52310-52315
    Sphincter Surgery . . . . . . . . . . . . . . . 52277
    Tumor
        Excision . . . . . . . . . . . . . . . . . . . . . 52355
    Ureter Surgery . . . . . . . . . . . . 52290-52300
    Urethral Syndrome . . . . . . . . . . . . . . . 52285
    with Urethrotomy . . . . . . . . . . . 52270-52276
Excision
    Partial . . . . . . . . . . . . . . . . . 51550-51565
    Total . . . . . . . 51570, 51580, 51590-51597
        with Nodes . . . . . . . . 51575, 51585, 51595
    Transurethral . . . . . . . . . . . . . . . . . . . 52640
    Tumor . . . . . . . . . . . . . . . . . 52234-52240
Incision
    Catheter . . . . . . . . . . . . . . . . . . . . . . 51045
    with Destruction . . . . . . . . . . . . 51020-51030
    with Radiotracer . . . . . . . . . . . . . . . . 51020
Incision and Drainage . . . . . . . . . . . . . . . 51040
Injection
    Radiologic . . . . . . . . . . . . . . . 51600-51610
Insertion
    Stent . . . . . . . . . . . . . . . . . . 51045, 52334
Instillation
    Drugs . . . . . . . . . . . . . . . . . . . . . . . . 51720
Irrigation . . . . . . . . . . . . . . . . . . . . . . . . 51700
Laparoscopy . . . . . . . . . . . . . . . . . . . . . . 51999
Lesion
    Destruction . . . . . . . . . . . . . . . . . . . . 51030

**Blood Cell, Red**
See Red Blood Cell (RBC)

**Blood Cell, White**
See Leukocyte

**Blood Coagulation**
Defect
  See Coagulopathy
Disorders
  See Clot
Factor
  See Clotting Factor
  Factor I
  See Fibrinogen
    Factor II
      See Prothrombin
    Factor III
      See Thromboplastin
    Factor IV
      See Calcium
    Factor VII
      See Proconvertin
    Factor VIII
      See Clotting Factor
    Factor IX
      See Christmas Factor
    Factor X
      See Stuart-Prower Factor
    Factor X, Activated
      See Thrombokinase
    Factor XI
      See Plasma Thromboplastin, Antecedent
    Factor XIII
      See Fibrin Stabilizing Factor
Test
  See Coagulation

**Blood Component Removal**
See Apheresis

**Blood Count, Complete**
See Complete Blood Count (CBC)

**Blood Flow Check, Graft** . . . . . . . . . . . . . . . 15860, 90940

**Blood Gases**
$CO_2$ . . . . . . . . . . . . . . . . . . . . . . . . . . . . . . . . 82803
$HCO_3$ . . . . . . . . . . . . . . . . . . . . . . . . . . . . . . 82803
$O_2$ Saturation . . . . . . . . . . . . . . . . . . 82805-82810
$pCO_2$ . . . . . . . . . . . . . . . . . . . . . . . . . . . . . . 82803
pH . . . . . . . . . . . . . . . . . . 82800-82803, 82930
$pO_2$ . . . . . . . . . . . . . . . . . . . . . . . . . . . . . . . . 82803

**Blood Letting**
See Phlebotomy

**Blood Lipoprotein**
See Lipoprotein

**Blood Occult**
See Occult, Blood

**Blood Pool Imaging** . . . . . . 78472-78473,
          78481-78483, 78494-78496

**Blood Pressure**
See Performance Measures
Baroreflex
  Activation Device . . . . . . . . . . . . . 0266T-0273T
Ocular
  Measurement . . . . . . . . . . . . . . . . . . . . . . 0198T
Monitoring, 24 Hour . . . . . . . . . . . . . 93784-93790
Systolic . . . . . . . . . . . . . . . . . . . . . . . 3074F-3075F
Venous . . . . . . . . . . . . . . . . . . . . . . . . . . . . 93770

**Blood Products**
Irradiation . . . . . . . . . . . . . . . . . . . . . . . . 86945
Pooling . . . . . . . . . . . . . . . . . . . . . . . . . . 86965
Splitting . . . . . . . . . . . . . . . . . . . . . . . . . 86985
Volume Reduction . . . . . . . . . . . . . . . . . . 86960

**Blood Sample**
Fetal . . . . . . . . . . . . . . . . . . . . . . . . . . . . 59030

**Blood Serum**
See Serum

**Blood Smear** . . . . . . . . . . . . . . . . . . 85060

**Blood Syndrome**
Chromosome Analysis . . . . . . . . . . . 88245-88248

**Blood Tests**
Iron Stores . . . . . . . . . . . . . . . . . . . . . . . 3160F
Kt/V . . . . . . . . . . . . . . . . . . . . . . . . 3082F-3084F
Nuclear Medicine
  Plasma Volume . . . . . . . . . . . . . 78110-78111
  Platelet Survival . . . . . . . . . . . . 78190-78191
  Red Cell Volume . . . . . . . . . . . . 78120-78121
  Whole Blood Volume . . . . . . . . . . . . 78122
Panels
  Electrolyte . . . . . . . . . . . . . . . . . . . . 80051
  General Health Panel . . . . . . . . . . . . . 80050
  Hepatic Function . . . . . . . . . . . . . . . 80076
  Hepatitis, Acute . . . . . . . . . . . . . . . . 80074
  Lipid Panel . . . . . . . . . . . . . . . . . . . . 80061
  Metabolic Panel, Basic
    Ionized Calcium . . . . . . . . . . . . . . 80047
    Total Calcium . . . . . . . . . . . . . . . 80048
    Comprehensive . . . . . . . . . . . . . . 80053
  Obstetric Panel . . . . . . . . . . . . . . . . 80055
  Renal Function . . . . . . . . . . . . . . . . . 80069
Volume Determination . . . . . . . . . . . . . . 78122

**Blood Transfusion, Autologous**
See Autotransfusion

**Blood Typing**
ABO Only . . . . . . . . . . . . . . . . . . . . . . . 86900
Antigen Screen . . . . . . . . . . . . . . . . . . . 86904
Antigen Testing, Donor Blood . . . . . . . . . . 86902
Crossmatch . . . . . . . . . . . . . . . . . 86920-86923
Other RBC Antigens . . . . . . . . . . . . . . . . 86905
Paternity Testing . . . . . . . . . . . . . . 86910-86911
Rh (D) . . . . . . . . . . . . . . . . . . . . . . . . . 86901
Rh Phenotype . . . . . . . . . . . . . . . . . . . . 86906

**Blood Urea Nitrogen** . . . . . 84520-84525

**Blood Vessels**
See Artery; Vein
Angioscopy
  Non-Coronary . . . . . . . . . . . . . . . . . . 35400
Endoscopy
  Surgical . . . . . . . . . . . . . . . . . . . . . . 37500
Excision
  Arteriovenous Malformation . . . . 63250-63252
Exploration
  Abdomen . . . . . . . . . . . . . . . . . . . . 35840
  Chest . . . . . . . . . . . . . . . . . . . . . . . 35820
  Extremity . . . . . . . . . . . . . . . . . . . . 35860
  Neck . . . . . . . . . . . . . . . . . . . . . . . 35800
Great
  Suture . . . . . . . . . . . . . . . . . . . 33320-33322
Harvest
  Endoscopic . . . . . . . . . . . . . . . . . . . 33508
  Lower Extremity Vein . . . . . . . . . . . . . 35572
  Upper Extremity Artery . . . . . . . . . . . . 35600
  Upper Extremity Vein . . . . . . . . . . . . . 35500
Kidney
  Repair . . . . . . . . . . . . . . . . . . . . . . . 50100

Repair
  Abdomen
    See Aneurysm Repair; Fistula, Repair
    with Composite Graft . . . . . . . . 35681-35683
    with Other Graft . . . . . . . . . . . . . . . 35281
    with Vein Graft . . . . . . . . . . . . . . . . 35251
  Aneurysm . . . . . . . . . . . . . . . . 61705-61708
  Arteriovenous Malformation . . . . 61680-61692,
        61705-61710, 63250-63252
  Chest
    with Composite Graft . . . . . . . . 35681-35683
    with Other Graft . . . . . . . . . . . 35271-35276
    with Vein Graft . . . . . . . . . . . . 35241-35246
  Direct . . . . . . . . . . . . . . . . . . . 35201-35226
  Finger . . . . . . . . . . . . . . . . . . . . . . . 35207
  Graft Defect . . . . . . . . . . . . . . . . . . . 35870
  Hand . . . . . . . . . . . . . . . . . . . . . . . . 35207
  Lower Extremity . . . . . . . . . . . . . . . . . 35226
    with Composite Graft . . . . . . . . 35681-35683
    with Other Graft . . . . . . . . . . . . . . . 35281
    with Vein Graft . . . . . . . . . . . . . . . . 35251
  Neck
    with Composite Graft . . . . . . . . 35681-35683
    with Other Graft . . . . . . . . . . . . . . . 35261
    with Vein Graft . . . . . . . . . . . . . . . . 35231
  Upper Extremity . . . . . . . . . . . . . . . . . 35206
    with Composite Graft . . . . . . . . 35681-35683
    with Other Graft . . . . . . . . . . . . . . . 35266
    with Vein Graft . . . . . . . . . . . . . . . . 35236
Shunt Creation
  Direct . . . . . . . . . . . . . . . . . . 36818, 36821
  Thomas Shunt . . . . . . . . . . . . . . . . . 36835
  with Bypass Graft . . . . . . . . . . . . . . . 35686
  with Graft . . . . . . . . . . . . . . . . 36825-36830
Shunt Revision
  with Graft . . . . . . . . . . . . . . . . . . . . 36832

**Blood, Occult**
See Occult Blood

**Bloom Syndrome**
Chromosome Analysis . . . . . . . . . . . 81209, 88245

**Blot Test, Ink**
See Inkblot Test

**Blotting, Western**
See Western Blot

**Blow-Out Fracture**
Orbital Floor . . . . . . . . . . . . . . . . . 21385-21395

**Blue, Dome Cyst**
See Breast, Cyst

**BMT**
See Bone Marrow, Transplantation

**Boarding Home Care** . . . . . 99324-99337

**Bodies**
Acetone
  See Acetone Body
Barr
  See Barr Bodies
Carotid
  See Carotid Body
Ciliary
  See Ciliary Body
Heinz
  See Heinz Bodies
Inclusion
  See Inclusion Bodies
Ketone
  See Ketone Body

## Body Cast
Halo . . . . . . . . . . . . . . . . . . . . . . . . . 29000
Removal . . . . . . . . . . . . 29700, 29710-29715
Repair . . . . . . . . . . . . . . . . . . . . . . . . 29720
Risser Jacket . . . . . . . . . . . . . . . 29010-29015
Turnbuckle Jacket . . . . . . . . . . . . . 29020-29025
Upper Body and Head . . . . . . . . . . . . . . . 29040
Upper Body and Legs . . . . . . . . . . . . . . . 29046
Upper Body and One Leg . . . . . . . . . . . . . 29044
Upper Body Only . . . . . . . . . . . . . . . . . 29035

## Body Fluid
Crystal Identification . . . . . . . . . . . . . . . 89060

## Body of Vertebra
*See* Vertebral Body

## Body Section
X-ray . . . . . . . . . . . . . . . . . . . . . . . . . 76100
  Motion . . . . . . . . . . . . . . . . . . . 76101-76102

## Body System, Neurologic
*See* Nervous System

## Boil
*See* Furuncle

## Boil, Vulva
*See* Abscess, Vulva

## Bone
*See* Specific Bone
Ablation
  Tumor . . . . . . . . . . . . . . . . . . . . . . 20982
Biopsy . . . . . . . . . . . . 20220-20245, 22520-22522
Carpal
  *See* Carpal Bone
Cheek
  *See* Cheekbone
CT Scan
  Density Study . . . . . . . . . . . . . . . . . 77078
Cyst
  Drainage . . . . . . . . . . . . . . . . . . . . 20615
  Injection . . . . . . . . . . . . . . . . . . . . 20615
Debridement . . . . . . . . . . . . . . . 11044, 11047
Dual Energy X-ray
Absorptiometry . . . . . . . . . . . . . 77080-77081
Excision
  Epyphyseal Bar . . . . . . . . . . . . . . . . 20150
  Facial Bones . . . . . . . . . . . . . . . . . 21026
  Mandible . . . . . . . . . . . . . . . . . . . 21025
Facial
  *See* Facial Bone
Fixation
  Caliper . . . . . . . . . . . . . . . . . . . . 20660
  Cranial Tong . . . . . . . . . . . . . . . . . 20660
  Halo . . . . . . . . . . . . 20661-20663, 21100
  Interdental . . . . . . . . . . . . . . . . . . 21110
  Multiplane . . . . . . . . . . . . . . . . . . 20692
    Stereotactic Computer
    Assisted . . . . . . . . . . . . . . 20696-20697
  Pin/Wire . . . . . . . . . . . . . . . . . . . 20650
  Skeletal
    Humeral Epicondyle
      Percutaneous . . . . . . . . . . . . . 24566
    Stereotactic Frame . . . . . . . . . . . . 20660
    Uniplane . . . . . . . . . . . . . . . . . . 20690
    Vertebral with Arthroplasty . . . . . . . . . 0202T
Fracture
  Osteoporosis Screening . . . . . . . . . . . . 5015F
Hyoid
  *See* Hyoid Bone

Insertion
  Needle . . . . . . . . . . . . . . . . . . . . 36680
  Osseointegrated Implant
    for External Speech Processor/Cochlear
    Stimulator . . . . . . . . . . . . . 69714-69718
Marrow
  Cell Therapy . . . . . . . . . . . . . 0263T-0265T
  Cytogenic Testing . . . . . . . . . . . . . . 3155F
Metatarsal
  *See* Metatarsal Bone
Nasal
  *See* Nasal Bone
Navicular
  *See* Navicular
Nuclear Medicine
  Density Study . . . . . . . . . . . 78350-78351
  Imaging . . . . . . . . . . . . . . 78300-78320
  SPECT . . . . . . . . . . . . . . . . . . 78320
  Unlisted Services and Procedures . . . . . . 78399
Osteoporosis
  Pharmacologic Therapy . . . . . . . . . . . . 4005F
Protein . . . . . . . . . . . . . . . . . . . . . 83937
Removal
  Fixation Device . . . . . . . . . . . 20670-20680
Replacement
  Osseointegrated Implant
    for External Speech Processor/Cochlear
    Stimulator . . . . . . . . . . . . . 69717-69718
Scan
  *See* Bone, Nuclear Medicine; Nuclear Medicine
  Imaging
Semilunar
  *See* Lunate
Sesamoid
  *See* Sesamoid Bone
Spur
  *See* Exostosis
Tarsal
  *See* Ankle Bone
Temporal
  *See* Temporal Bone
X-ray
  Age Study . . . . . . . . . . . . . . . . . 77072
  Dual Energy Absorptiometry . . . . 77080-77081
  Length Study . . . . . . . . . . . . . . . 77073
  Osseous Survey . . . . . . . . . . . . 77074-77077

## Bone 4-Carboxyglutamic Protein
*See* Osteocalcin

## Bone Conduction Hearing Device, Electromagnetic
Implantation/Replacement . . . . . . . . . . . . 69710
Removal/Repair . . . . . . . . . . . . . . . . . 69711

## Bone Density Study
Appendicular Skeleton . . . . . . . . . . . . . 77081
Axial Skeleton . . . . . . . . . . . . 77078, 77080
Ultrasound . . . . . . . . . . . . . . . . . . . 76977
Vertebral Fracture Assessment . . . . . . . . . 77082

## Bone Graft
Any Donor Area . . . . . . . . . . . . 20900-20902
Augmentation
  Mandibular Body . . . . . . . . . . . . . . 21127
Femur . . . . . . . . . . . . . . . . . . . . . 27170
Fracture
  Orbit . . . . . . . . . . . . . . . . . . . . 21408
Harvesting . . . . . . . . . . . . . . 20900-20902
Malar Area . . . . . . . . . . . . . . . . . . 21210
Mandible . . . . . . . . . . . . . . . . . . . 21215
Mandibular Ramus . . . . . . . . . . . . . . . 21194
Maxilla . . . . . . . . . . . . . . . . . . . . 21210

Microvascular Anastomosis
  Fibula . . . . . . . . . . . . . . . . . . . 20955
  Other . . . . . . . . . . . . . . . . . . . 20962
Nasal Area . . . . . . . . . . . . . . . . . . 21210
Nasomaxillary Complex Fracture . . . . . . . . 21348
Open Treatment
  Craniofacial Separation . . . . . . . . . . 21436
Osteocutaneous Flap . . . . . . . . . . . 20969-20973
Reconstruction
  Mandibular Rami . . . . . . . . . . . . . . 21194
  Midface . . . . . . . . . . . . . . 21145-21160
Skull . . . . . . . . . . . . . . . . . . . . . 61316
  Excision . . . . . . . . . . . . . . . . . . 62148
Spine Surgery
  Allograft
    Morselized . . . . . . . . . . . . . . . . 20930
    Structural . . . . . . . . . . . . . . . . 20931
  Autograft
    Local . . . . . . . . . . . . . . . . . . . 20936
    Morselized . . . . . . . . . . . . . . . . 20937
    Structural . . . . . . . . . . . . . . . . 20938
Vascular Pedicle . . . . . . . . . . . . . . . 25430
Vertebra . . . . . . . . . . . . . . . . . . . 0222T
  Cervical . . . . . . . . . . . . . . . . . . 0219T
  Lumbar . . . . . . . . . . . . . . . . . . 0221T
  Thoracic . . . . . . . . . . . . . . . . . . 0220T

## Bone Healing
Electrical Stimulation
  Invasive . . . . . . . . . . . . . . . . . . 20975
  Noninvasive . . . . . . . . . . . . . . . . 20974
Ultrasound Stimulation . . . . . . . . . . . . 20979

## Bone Infection
*See* Osteomyelitis

## Bone Marrow
Aspiration . . . . . . . . . . . . . . . . . . 38220
Cell Therapy . . . . . . . . . . . . . 0263T-0265T
Harvesting
  Allogeneic . . . . . . . . . . . . . . . . . 38230
  Autologous . . . . . . . . . . . . . . . . 38232
Magnetic Resonance Imaging (MRI) . . . . . . 77084
Needle Biopsy . . . . . . . . . . . . . . . . 38221
Nuclear Medicine
  Imaging . . . . . . . . . . . . . . 78102-78104
Smear . . . . . . . . . . . . . . . . . . . . 85097
T-Cell Transplantation . . . . . . . . . 38240-38242
Trocar Biopsy . . . . . . . . . . . . . . . . 38221

## Bone Plate
Mandible . . . . . . . . . . . . . . . . . . . 21244

## Bone Wedge Reversal
Osteotomy . . . . . . . . . . . . . . . . . . 21122

## Bordetella
Antibody . . . . . . . . . . . . . . . . . . . 86615
Antigen Detection
  Direct Fluorescence . . . . . . . . . . . . 87265

## Borrelia
Antibody . . . . . . . . . . . . . . . 86618-86619

## Borrelia burgdorferi ab
*See* Antibody, Lyme Disease

## Borreliosis, Lyme
*See* Lyme Disease

## Bost Fusion
*See* Arthrodesis, Wrist

## Bosworth Operation
*See* Acromioclavicular Joint, Dislocation;
Arthrodesis, Vertebrae; Fasciotomy

## CHCT
*See* Caffeine Halothane Contracture Test

## Cheek
Bone
  Excision . . . . . . . . . . . . . . . 21030, 21034
  Fracture
    Closed Treatment with
    Manipulation . . . . . . . . . . . . . . . 21355
    Open Treatment . . . . . . . . . . 21360-21366
  Reconstruction . . . . . . . . . . . . . . . . 21270
Fascia Graft . . . . . . . . . . . . . . . . . . 15840
Muscle Graft . . . . . . . . . . . . 15841-15845
Muscle Transfer . . . . . . . . . . . . . . . 15845

## Cheilectomy
Metatarsophalangeal Joint Release . . . . . . 28289

## Cheiloplasty
*See* Lip, Repair

## Cheiloschisis
*See* Cleft Lip

## Cheilotomy
*See* Incision, Lip

## Chemical Cauterization
Granulation Tissue . . . . . . . . . . . . . . . 17250

## Chemical Exfoliation . . . . . . . . . . . 17360

## Chemical Peel . . . . . . . . . . 15788-15793

## Chemiluminescent Assay . . . . . . 82397

## Chemistry Tests
Clinical
  Unlisted Services and Procedures . . . . . . 84999

## Chemocauterization
Corneal Epithelium . . . . . . . . . . . . . . . 65435
  with Chelating Agent . . . . . . . . . . . . 65436

## Chemodenervation
Anal Sphincter . . . . . . . . . . . . . . . . . 46505
Eccrine Glands
  Axillae . . . . . . . . . . . . . . . . . . . . 64650
  Other Area . . . . . . . . . . . . . . . . . 64653
Electrical Stimulation for Guidance . . . . . 95873
Extraocular Muscle . . . . . . . . . . . . . . 67345
Extremity Muscle . . . . . . . . . . . . . . . 64614
Facial Muscle . . . . . . . . . . . . . . . . . 64612
Neck Muscle . . . . . . . . . . . . . . . . . 64613
Needle Electromyography for Guidance . . . . 95874
Salivary Glands . . . . . . . . . . . . . . . . 64611
Trunk Muscle . . . . . . . . . . . . . . . . . 64614

## Chemonucleolysis . . . . . . . . . . . . . 62292

## Chemosurgery
Destruction of Benign Lesions . . . . . 17110-17111
Skin Lesion . . . . . . . . 17000-17004, 17110-17111,
                  17270, 17280

## Chemotaxis Assay . . . . . . . . . . . . 86155

## Chemotherapy
Arterial Catheterization . . . . . . . . . . . . 36640
Bladder Instillation . . . . . . . . . . . . . . . 51720
CNS . . . . . . . . . . . . . . . . . . 61517, 96450
Extracorporeal Circulation
  Extremity . . . . . . . . . . . . . . . . . . 36823
Home Infusion Procedures . . . . . . . 99601-99602
Intra-Arterial . . . . . . . . . . . . . 96420-96425
Intralesional . . . . . . . . . . . . . 96405-96406
Intramuscular . . . . . . . . . . . . . 96401-96402

Intravenous . . . . . . . . . . . . 96409-96415, 96417
  Infusion Pump . . . . . . . . . . . . . . . 96416
Kidney Instillation . . . . . . . . . . . . . . . 50391
Peritoneal Cavity . . . . . . . . . . . . . . . 96446
Pleural Cavity . . . . . . . . . . . . . . . . . 96440
Pump Services
  Implantable . . . . . . . . . . . . . . . . . 96522
  Maintenance . . . . . . . . . . . . 95990-95991
  Portable . . . . . . . . . . . . . . . . . . . 96521
Reservoir Filling . . . . . . . . . . . . . . . . 96542
Subcutaneous . . . . . . . . . . . . . 96401-96402
Unlisted Services and Procedures . . . . . . . 96549
Ureteral Instillation . . . . . . . . . . . . . . 50391

## Chest
*See* Mediastinum; Thorax
Angiography . . . . . . . . . . . . . . . . . . 71275
Artery
  Ligation . . . . . . . . . . . . . . . . . . . 37616
CT Scan . . . . . . . . . . . . . . . . 71250-71275
Exploration
  Blood Vessel . . . . . . . . . . . . . . . . 35820
Exposure
  Transthoracic Cardiac . . . . . . . . . 0258T-0259T
Magnetic Resonance Imaging
(MRI) . . . . . . . . . . . . . . . . . 71550-71552
Repair
  Blood Vessel . . . . . . . . . . . . . 35211-35216
  with Other Graft . . . . . . . . . . . 35271-35276
  with Vein Graft . . . . . . . . . . . . 35241-35246
Ultrasound . . . . . . . . . . . . . . . . . . 76604
Wound Exploration
  Penetrating . . . . . . . . . . . . . . . . . 20101
X-ray . . . . . . . . . . . . . . . . . 71010-71035
  Complete (Four Views)
    with Fluoroscopy . . . . . . . . . . . . 71034
  Partial (Two Views)
    with Fluoroscopy . . . . . . . . . . . . 71023
  Stereo . . . . . . . . . . . . . . . . . . . 71015
  with Computer-aided
  Detection . . . . . . . . . . . . . . 0174T-0175T

## Chest Cavity
Bypass Graft . . . . . . . . . . . . . . . . . 35905
Thoracoscopy
  Diagnostic . . . . . . . 32601, 32604, 32606
  Surgical . . . . . . . . . . . . . 32650-32674

## Chest Wall
*See* Pulmonology, Therapeutic
Manipulation . . . . . . . . . . . . . . 94667-94668
Reconstruction . . . . . . . . . . . . . . . . 49904
  Trauma . . . . . . . . . . . . . . . . . . . 32820
Repair . . . . . . . . . . . . . . . . . . . . . 32905
  Closure . . . . . . . . . . . . . . . . . . . 32810
  Fistula . . . . . . . . . . . . . . . . . . . . 32906
Tumor
  Excision . . . . . . . . . . . . . . . 19260-19272
Unlisted Services and Procedures . . . . . . . 32999

## Chest Wall Fistula
*See* Fistula, Chest Wall

## Chest, Funnel
*See* Pectus Excavatum

## Chevron Procedure . . . . . . . . . . . 28296

## Chiari Osteotomy of the Pelvis
*See* Osteotomy, Pelvis

## Chicken Pox Vaccine . . . . . . . . . 90716

## Child Procedure
*See* Excision, Pancreas, Partial

## Chimerism . . . . . . . . . . . . 81267, 81268

## Chin
Repair
  Augmentation . . . . . . . . . . . . . . . 21120
  Osteotomy . . . . . . . . . . . . . 21121-21123

## Chinidin
*See* Quinidine

## Chiropractic Manipulation
*See* Manipulation, Chiropractic

## Chiropractic Treatment
Spinal
  Extraspinal . . . . . . . . . . . . . 98940-98943

## Chlamydia
Antibody . . . . . . . . . . . . . . . 86631-86632
Antigen Detection
  Direct Fluorescence . . . . . . . . . . . . 87270
  Direct Optical . . . . . . . . . . . . . . . 87810
  Enzyme Immunoassay . . . . . . . . . . . 87320
Culture . . . . . . . . . . . . . . . . . . . . 87110

## Chloramphenicol . . . . . . . . . . . . . 82415

## Chloride
Blood . . . . . . . . . . . . . . . . . . . . . 82435
Other Source . . . . . . . . . . . . . . . . . 82438
Spinal Fluid . . . . . . . . . . . . . . . . . . 82438
Urine . . . . . . . . . . . . . . . . . . . . . 82436

## Chloride, Methylene
*See* Dichloromethane

## Chlorinated Hydrocarbons . . . . . . 82441

## Chlorohydrocarbon
*See* Chlorinated Hydrocarbons

## Chlorpromazine . . . . . . . . . . . . . 84022

## Choanal Atresia
Repair . . . . . . . . . . . . . . . . . 30540-30545

## Cholangiography
Injection . . . . . . . . . . . . . . . 47500-47505
Intraoperative . . . . . . . . . . . . 74300-74301
Percutaneous . . . . . . . . . . . . . . . . . 74320
  with Laparoscopy . . . . . . . . . . . 47560-47561
Postoperative . . . . . . . . . . . . . . . . . 74305
Repair
  with Bile Duct Exploration . . . . . . . . . . 47700
  with Cholecystectomy . . . 47563, 47605, 47620

## Cholangiopancreatography . . . . . 43260
*See* Bile Duct; Pancreatic Duct
Repair
  *See* Bile Duct; Pancreatic Duct
  with Biopsy . . . . . . . . . . . . . . . . . 43261
  with Surgery . . . . . . . . . 43262-43267, 43269

## Cholangiostomy
*See* Hepaticostomy

## Cholangiotomy
*See* Hepaticostomy

## Cholecalciferol
*See* Vitamin, D-3

## Cholecystectomy . . . . . . . . 47562-47564
                    47600-47620
Any Method . . . . . . . . . . . . . . 47562-47564
  with Cholangiography . . . 47563, 47605, 47620
  with Exploration Common
  Duct . . . . . . . . . . . . . . . . 47564, 47610

**Clavicula**
See Clavicle

**Claviculectomy**
Partial ............................ 23120
Total ............................... 23125

**Claw Finger Repair** ............ 26499

**Cleft Cyst, Branchial**
See Branchial Cleft, Cyst

**Cleft Foot**
Reconstruction ...................... 28360

**Cleft Hand**
Repair ............................. 26580

**Cleft Lip**
Repair ....................... 40700-40761
Rhinoplasty .................. 30460-30462

**Cleft Palate**
Repair ....................... 42200-42225
Rhinoplasty .................. 30460-30462

**Cleft, Branchial**
See Branchial Cleft

**Clinical Act of Insertion**
See Insertion

**Clinical Chemistry Test**
See Chemistry Tests, Clinical

**Clinical Investigation**
FDA-approved Drugs
  Single Patient

**Clinical Pathology**
See Pathology, Clinical

**Clitoroplasty**
Intersex State ....................... 56805

**Closed [Transurethral] Biopsy of Bladder**
See Biopsy, Bladder, Cystourethroscopy

**Clostridial Tetanus**
See Tetanus

**Clostridium Botulinum Toxin**
See Chemodenervation

**Clostridium Difficile**
Antigen Detection
  Enzyme Immunoassay ............... 87324
by Immunoassay
  with Direct Optical Observation ....... 87803

**Clostridium Tetani ab**
See Antibody, Tetanus

**Closure** ................. 12001-13160
Anal Fistula ........................ 46288
Atrioventricular Valve ................ 33600
Cystostomy ......................... 51880
Enterostomy ................... 44625-44626
  Laparoscopic ..................... 44227
Lacrimal Fistula ..................... 68770
Lacrimal Punctum
  Plug ............................ 68761
  Thermocauterization, Ligation or
  Laser Surgery .................... 68760
Left Atrial Appendage
  with Implant ...................... 0281T
Rectovaginal Fistula ........... 57300-57308
Semilunar Valve .................... 33602

Septal Defect ...................... 33615
  Ventricular ........... 33675-33677, 93581
Sternotomy ........................ 21750
Ventricular Tunnel ................. 33722

**Closure of Esophagostomy**
See Esophagostomy, Closure

**Closure of Gastrostomy**
See Gastrostomy, Closure

**Closure, Atrial Septal Defect**
See Heart, Repair, Atrial Septum

**Closure, Cranial Sutures, Premature**
See Craniosynostosis

**Closure, Fistula, Vesicouterine**
See Fistula, Vesicouterine, Closure

**Closure, Meningocele Spinal**
See Meningocele Repair

**Closure, Vagina**
See Vagina, Closure

**Clot** ...... 34401-34490, 35875-35876, 50230
See Thrombectomy; Thromboendarterectomy

**Clot Lysis Time** ................. 85175

**Clot Retraction** ............... 85170

**Clotting Disorder**
See Coagulopathy

**Clotting Factor** ........... 85210-85293

**Clotting Inhibitors** ... 85300-85305, 85307

**Clotting Operation**
See Excision, Nail Fold

**Clotting Test**
Protein C ..................... 85303, 85307
Protein S .......................... 85306

**Clotting Time**
See Coagulation Time

**Clubfoot Cast** .................. 29450
Wedging ........................... 29750

**CMG**
See Cystometrogram

**CMRI**
See Cardiac Magnetic Resonance Imaging

**CMV**
See Cytomegalovirus

**CNPB**
See Continuous Negative Pressure Breathing
(CNPB); Pulmonology, Therapeutic

**Co-Factor I, Heparin**
See Antithrombin III

**CO2**
See Carbon Dioxide

**Coagulation**
Unlisted Services and Procedures ........ 85999

**Coagulation Defect**
See Coagulopathy

**Coagulation Factor**
See Clotting Factor
Factor I
  See Fibrinogen
  See Gene Analysis
Factor II
  See Prothrombin
Factor III
  See Thromboplastin
Factor IV
  See Calcium
Factor VII
  See Proconvertin
Factor VIII
  See Clotting Factor
Factor IX
  See Christmas Factor
Factor X
  See Stuart-Prower Factor
Factor Xa
  See Thrombokinase
Factor XI
  See Plasma Thromboplastin, Antecedent
Factor XII
  See Hageman Factor
Factor XIII
  See Fibrin Stabilizing Factor

**Coagulation Time** ......... 85345-85348

**Coagulation, Blood**
See Blood Clot

**Coagulation, Light**
See Photocoagulation

**Coagulin**
See Thromboplastin

**Coagulopathy** ................... 85390
Assay ............................. 85130

**Cocaine**
Blood or Urine ...................... 82520
Screen ............................. 82486

**Coccidioides**
Antibody ........................... 86635

**Coccidioidin Test**
See Streptokinase, Antibody

**Coccidioidomycosis**
Skin Test .......................... 86490

**Coccygeal Spine Fracture**
See Coccyx, Fracture

**Coccygectomy** ....... 15920-15922, 27080

**Coccyx**
Excision ............................ 27080
Fracture
  Closed Treatment ................. 27200
  Open Treatment ................... 27202
Tumor
  Excision ......................... 49215
X-ray .............................. 72220

**Cochlear Device**
Insertion ........................... 69930
Programming .................. 92601-92604

**Codeine**
Alkaloid Screening ................... 82101

**Codeine Screen** ................. 82486

## Colonoscopy
Biopsy .......................... 45380, 45392
Collection Specimen ................... 45380
    via Colotomy ...................... 45355
Destruction
    Lesion ............................ 45383
    Tumor ............................ 45383
Dilation .............................. 45386
Hemorrhage Control ................... 45382
Injection
    Submucosal ....................... 45381
Placement
    Stent ............................. 45387
Removal
    Foreign Body ...................... 45379
    Polyp ...................... 45384-45385
    Tumor ...................... 45384-45385
Surveillance Intervals ............ 0528F-0529F
Ultrasound ..................... 45391-45392
via Stoma ...................... 44388-44390
    Biopsy ........................... 44389
    Destruction
      of Lesion ...................... 44393
      of Tumor ...................... 44393
    Exploration ....................... 44388
    Hemorrhage ...................... 44391
    Placement
      Stent ......................... 44397
    Removal
      Foreign Body .................. 44390
      Polyp .................. 44392, 44394
      Tumor ................. 44392, 44394

## Color Vision Examination ...... 92283

## Colorrhaphy .................... 44604

## Colostomy ................. 44320, 45563
Abdominal
    Establishment ..................... 50810
Colostomy .......................... 44188
Home Visit .......................... 99505
Intestine, Large
    with Suture ....................... 44605
Laparoscopic ........................ 44188
Perineal
    Establishment ..................... 50810
Revision ............................ 44340
    Paracolostomy Hernia ........ 44345-44346

## Colotomy ...................... 44025

## Colpectomy
Partial .............................. 57106
Total ............................... 57110
with Hysterectomy ........... 58275-58280
    with Repair of Enterocele ........... 58280

## Colpo-Urethrocystopexy ....... 58152,
                                 58267, 58293
Marshall-Marchetti-Krantz Procedure .... 58152,
                                 58267, 58293
Pereyra Procedure ........... 58267, 58293

## Colpoceliocentesis
See Colpocentesis

## Colpocentesis ................. 57020

## Colpocleisis ................... 57120

## Colpocleisis Complete
See Vagina, Closure

## Colpohysterectomies
See Excision, Uterus, Vaginal

## Colpoperineorrhaphy .......... 57210

## Colpopexy
Extra-Peritoneal ..................... 57282
Intra-Peritoneal ..................... 57283
Laparoscopic ........................ 57425
Open ............................... 57280

## Colpoplasty
See Repair, Vagina

## Colporrhaphy
Anterior ..................... 57240, 57289
    with Insertion of Mesh ............. 57267
    with Insertion of Prosthesis ......... 57267
Anteroposterior ............. 57260-57265
    with Enterocele Repair ............. 57265
    with Insertion of Mesh ............. 57267
    with Insertion of Prosthesis ......... 57267
Nonobstetrical ...................... 57200
Posterior ........................... 57250
    with Insertion of Mesh ............. 57267
    with Insertion of Prosthesis ......... 57267

## Colposcopy
Biopsy ....... 56821, 57421, 57454-57455, 57460
    Endometrium ...................... 58110
Cervix ................. 57421, 57452-57461
Exploration ......................... 57452
Loop Electrode Biopsy ................ 57460
Loop Electrode Conization ............. 57461
Perineum ........................... 99170
Vagina .................... 57420-57421
Vulva .............................. 56820
    Biopsy ........................... 56821

## Colpotomy
Drainage
    Abscess .......................... 57010
Exploration ......................... 57000

## Colprosterone
See Progesterone

## Column Chromatography/Mass Spectrometry .............. 82541-82544

## Columna Vertebralis
See Spine

## Combined Heart-Lung Transplantation
See Transplantation, Heart-Lung

## Combined Right and Left Heart Cardiac Catheterization
See Cardiac Catheterization, Combined Left and Right Heart

## Comedones
Removal ............................ 10040

## Commissurotomy
Right Ventricle ................. 33476-33478

## Common Sensory Nerve
Repair/Suture ....................... 64834

## Common Truncus
See Truncus Arteriosus

## Communication Device
Non-Speech-Generating .... 92605-92606, 92618
Speech-Generating ............. 92606-92609

## Community/Work Reintegration
Training ............................ 97537
    See Physical Medicine/Therapy/Occupational
Therapy

## Comparative Analysis (Short Tandem Repeat) .......... 81265, 81266

## Compatibility Test
Blood ........................ 86920, 86923

## Complement
Antigen ............................ 86160
Fixation Test ........................ 86171
Functional Activity ................... 86161
Hemolytic
    Total ............................. 86162
Total ............................... 86162

## Complete Blood Count (CBC) ..................... 85025-85027
See Blood Cell Count

## Complete Colectomy
See Colectomy, Total

## Complete Pneumonectomy
See Pneumonectomy, Completion

## Complete Transposition of Great Vessels
See Transposition, Great Arteries

## Complex, Factor IX
See Christmas Factor

## Complex, Vitamin B
See B Complex Vitamins

## Component Removal, Blood
See Apheresis

## Composite Graft .......... 15760-15770,
                                  35681-35683

## Compound B
See Corticosterone

## Compound F
See Cortisol

## Compression, Nerve, Median
See Carpal Tunnel Syndrome

## Computed Tomographic Scintigraphy
See Emission Computerized Tomography

## Computed Tomographic Angiography
See CT Scan; Specific Anatomic Site

## Computed Tomography (CT)
See CT Scan; Specific Anatomic Site

## Computer Analysis
Acoustic Recording
    Heart Sounds
Probability Assessment ............... 0185T

## Computer-Aided Detection
Chest X-ray ......................... 0152T
Lesion
    Chest Radiograph ............. 0174T-0175T
Mammography ................ 77051-77052
    Magnetic Resonance Imaging (MRI) .... 0159T

## Contralateral Ligament
Repair
    Knee....................................27405

## Contrast Aortogram
*See* Aortography

## Contrast Bath Therapy.........97034
*See* Physical Medicine/Therapy/Occupational Therapy

## Contrast Material
Injection
    via Peritoneal Catheter..............49424

## Contrast Phlebogram
*See* Venography

## Contusion
*See* Hematoma

## Converting Enzyme, Angiotensin
*See* Angiotensin Converting Enzyme (ACE)

## Coombs Test.........86880, 86885-86886

## Copper.....................82525

## Coprobilinogen
Feces....................................84577

## Coproporphyrin................84120

## Coracoacromial Ligament
Release.......................23415, 29826

## Coracoid Process Transfer.....23462

## Cord, Spermatic
*See* Spermatic Cord

## Cord, Spinal
*See* Spinal Cord

## Cord, Vocal
*See* Vocal Cords

## Cordectomy...................31300

## Cordocenteses
*See* Cordocentesis

## Cordocentesis................59012

## Cordotomy..............63194-63199

## Corectomy
*See* Excision, Iris

## Coreoplasty...................66762

## Cornea
Biopsy..................................65410
Curettage.......................65435-65436
    with Chelating Agent................65436
Epithelium
    Excision......................65435-65436
        with Chelating Agent............65436
Hysteresis Determination...............0181T
Incision
    for Keratoplasty.............0289T-0290T
Lesion
    Destruction......................65450
    Excision.........................65400
        with Graft....................65426
        without Graft.................65420
Pachymetry...........................76514
Prosthesis...........................65770
Pterygium
    Excision.........................65420

Puncture..............................65600
Relaxing Incisions.............65772-65775
Repair
    Astigmatism.................65772-65775
    Wedge Resection...................65775
    with Amniotic Membrane......65778-65780
    with Glue........................65286
    Wound
        Nonperforating..................65275
        Perforating...............65280-65285
        Tissue Glue.....................65286
Reshape
    Epikeratoplasty...................65765
    Keratomileusis....................65760
    Keratoprosthesis..................65767
Scraping
    Smear............................65430
Tattoo................................65600
Tear Osmolarity........................83861
Thickness Measurement.................76514
Transplantation
    Autograft or Homograft
        Allograft Preparation...0289T-0290T, 65757
        Endothelial.....................65756
        Lamellar........................65710
        Penetrating..............65730-65755
    for Aphakia......................65750

## Coronary
Atherectomy
    Percutaneous...............92995-92996
Thrombectomy
    Percutaneous......................92973

## Coronary Angioplasty, Transluminal Balloon
*See* Percutaneous Transluminal Angioplasty

## Coronary Artery
Insertion
    Stent......................92980-92981
Ligation...............................33502
Placement
    Radiation Delivery Device............92974
Repair.........................33500-33507

## Coronary Artery Bypass Graft (CABG).........33503-33505, 33510-33516
Arterial......................33533-33536
Arterial Graft...........................33548
    Spectroscopy
        Catheter Based...................0205T
Arterial-Venous................33517-33523
Beta Blocker Administered.............4115F
Harvest
    Upper Extremity Artery.............35600
Internal Mammary Artery Graft........4110F
Reoperation...........................33530
Venous........................33510-33516

## Coronary Endarterectomy......33572

## Coroner's Exam...............88045

## Coronoidectomy
Temporomandibular Joint..............21070

## Corpectomy................63101-63103

## Corpora Cavernosa
Corpus Spongiosum Shunt..............54430
Glans Penis Fistulization..............54435
Injection..............................54235
Irrigation
    Priapism.........................54220

Saphenous Vein Shunt.................54420
X-ray with Contrast....................74445

## Corpora Cavernosa, Plastic Induration
*See* Peyronie Disease

## Corpora Cavernosography.....74445

## Corpus Callosum
Transection...........................61541

## Corpus Vertebrae (Vertebrale)
*See* Vertebral Body

## Correction of Cleft Palate
*See* Cleft Palate, Repair

## Correction of Lid Retraction
*See* Repair, Eyelid, Retraction

## Correction of Malrotation of Duodenum
*See* Ladd Procedure

## Correction of Syndactyly
*See* Syndactyly, Repair

## Correction of Ureteropelvic Junction
*See* Pyeloplasty

## Cortex Decortication, Cerebral
*See* Decortication

## Cortical Mapping
Transection
    by Electric Stimulation.........95961-95962

## Corticoids
*See* Corticosteroids

## Corticoliberin
*See* Corticotropic Releasing Hormone (CRH)

## Corticosteroid Binding Globulin
*See* Transcortin

## Corticosteroid Binding Protein
*See* Transcortin

## Corticosteroids
Blood.................................83491
Urine.................................83491

## Corticosterone
Blood or Urine.........................82528

## Corticotropic Releasing Hormone (CRH).................................80412

## Cortisol.........80400-80406, 80418-80420, 80436, 82530
Stimulation...........................80412
Total.................................82533

## Cortisol Binding Globulin......84449

## Costectomy
*See* Resection, Ribs

## Costen Syndrome
*See* Temporomandibular Joint (TMJ)

## Costotransversectomy.........21610

## Cothromboplastin
*See* Proconvertin

Subarachnoid-Subdural . . . . . . . . . . . . . 62190
Ventriculo . . . . . . . . . . . . . . . . . . . . . . . 62220
Sigmoid Bladder . . . . . . . . . . . . . . . . . . . . . 50810
Speech Prosthesis . . . . . . . . . . . . . . . . . . . 31611
Stoma
    Bladder . . . . . . . . . . . . . . . . . . . . . . . . . 51980
    Kidney . . . . . . . . . . . . . . . . . . . . . . . . . . 50395
    Renal Pelvis . . . . . . . . . . . . . . . . . . . . . 50395
    Tympanic Membrane . . . . . . . . . 69433-69436
    Ureter . . . . . . . . . . . . . . . . . . . . . . . . . . 50860
Ventral Hernia . . . . . . . . . . . . . . . . . . . . . . 39503

## CRF
*See* Corticotropic Releasing Hormone (CRH)

## CRH
*See* Corticotropic Releasing Hormone (CRH)

## Cricoid Cartilage Split
Larynx . . . . . . . . . . . . . . . . . . . . . . . . . . . . . 31587

## Cricothyroid Membrane
Incision . . . . . . . . . . . . . . . . . . . . . . . . . . . . 31605

## Cristobalite
*See* Silica

## Critical Care Services . . . . 99291-99292
*See* Emergency Department Services;
Prolonged Attendance
Evaluation and Management . . . . . . 99291-99292
Interfacility Transport . . . . . . . . . . . . 99466-99467
Ipecac Administration for Poison . . . . . . . . 99175
Neonatal
    Initial . . . . . . . . . . . . . . . . . . . . . . . . . . 99468
    Low Birth Weight Infant . . . . . . . 99478-99479
    Subsequent . . . . . . . . . . . . . . . . . . . . . 99469
Pediatric
    Initial . . . . . . . . . . . . . . . . . . . . . 99471, 99475
    Interfacility Transport . . . . . . . . . 99466-99467
    Subsequent . . . . . . . . . . . . . . . . 99472, 99476
Remote
    Video-Conferenced Evaluation and
    Management . . . . . . . . . . . . . . . . . 0188T-0189T

## Cross Finger Flap . . . . . . . . . . . . . 15574

## Crossmatch . . . . 86825-86826, 86920-86923

## Crossmatching, Tissue
*See* Tissue, Typing

## Cruciate Ligament
Arthroscopic Repair . . . . . . . . . . . . . . 29888-29889
Repair . . . . . . . . . . . . . . . . . . . . . . . . 27407-27409
    Knee
        with Collateral Ligament . . . . . . . . . . 27409

## Cryoablation
*See* Cryosurgery

## Cryofibrinogen . . . . . . . . . . . . . . . . 82585

## Cryofixation
*See* Cryopreservation

## Cryoglobulin . . . . . . . . . . . . . . . . . . 82595

## Cryopreservation
Cells . . . . . . . . . . . . 38207-38209, 88240-88241
Embryo . . . . . . . . . . . . . . . . . . . . . . . . . . . 89258
for Transplantation . . . . . . . . 32850, 33930, 33940,
                 44132, 47133, 47140, 48550,
                 50300-50320, 50547
Freezing and Storage . . . . . . . . . . . . 38207, 88240
Sperm . . . . . . . . . . . . . . . . . . . . . . . . . . . 89259
Testes . . . . . . . . . . . . . . . . . . . . . . . . . . . 89335

Thawing
    Embryo . . . . . . . . . . . . . . . . . . . . . . . . 89352
    Oocytes . . . . . . . . . . . . . . . . . . . . . . . 89353
    Reproductive Tissue . . . . . . . . . . . . . 89354
    Sperm . . . . . . . . . . . . . . . . . . . . . . . . 89356

## Cryosurgery . . . . 17000-17286, 47371, 47381
*See* Cryotherapy; Destruction
Fibroadenoma . . . . . . . . . . . . . . . . . . . . . 0120T
    Breast . . . . . . . . . . . . . . . . . . . . . . . . . 19105
Lesion
    Kidney . . . . . . . . . . . . . . . . . . . . . . . . . 50250
    Mouth . . . . . . . . . . . . . . . . . . . . . . . . . 40820
    Penis . . . . . . . . . . . . . . . . . . . 54056, 54065
    Vagina . . . . . . . . . . . . . . . . . . 57061-57065
    Vulva . . . . . . . . . . . . . . . . . . . . 56501-56515

## Cryotherapy
Ablation
    Renal Tumor . . . . . . . . . . . . . . . . . . . . 50593
Acne . . . . . . . . . . . . . . . . . . . . . . . . . . . . 17340
Destruction
    Ciliary Body . . . . . . . . . . . . . . . . . . . . 66720
Lesion
    Cornea . . . . . . . . . . . . . . . . . . . . . . . . 65450
    Retina . . . . . . . . . . . . . . . . . . 67208, 67227
Retinal Detachment
    Prophylaxis . . . . . . . . . . . . . . . . . . . . 67141
    Repair . . . . . . . . . . . . . . . . . . 67101, 67113
Trichiasis
    Correction . . . . . . . . . . . . . . . . . . . . . . 67825

## Cryptectomy . . . . . . . . . . . . . . . . . 46999

## Cryptococcus
Antibody . . . . . . . . . . . . . . . . . . . . . . . . . 86641
Antigen Detection
    Enzyme Immunoassay . . . . . . . . . . . . . 87327

## Cryptococcus Neoformans
Antigen Detection
    Enzyme Immunoassay . . . . . . . . . . . . . 87327

## Cryptorchism
*See* Testis, Undescended

## Cryptosporidium
Antigen Detection
    Direct Fluorescence . . . . . . . . . . . . . . . 87272
    Enzyme Immunoassay . . . . . . . . . . . . . 87328

## Crystal Identification
Any Body Fluid . . . . . . . . . . . . . . . . . . . . . 89060
Tissue . . . . . . . . . . . . . . . . . . . . . . . . . . . 89060

## CSF
*See* Cerebrospinal Fluid Leak

## CT Scan
3-D Rendering . . . . . . . . . . . . . . . . . 76376-76377
Bone
    Density Study . . . . . . . . . . . . . . . . . . . 77078
Brain . . . . . . . . . . . . . . . . . . . . . . . . 70450-70470
Drainage . . . . . . . . . . . . . . . . . . . . . . . . . 75989
Follow-up Study . . . . . . . . . . . . . . . . . . . . 76380
Guidance
    Localization . . . . . . . . . . . . . . . . . . . . . 77011
    Needle Placement . . . . . . . . . . . . . . . . 77012
    Parenchymal Tissue Ablation . . . . . . . . . 77013
    Radiation Therapy . . . . . . . . . . . . . . . . 77014
    Vertebroplasty . . . . . . . . . . . . . . . . . . . 72292
    Visceral Tissue Ablation . . . . . . . . . . . . 77013
Heart
    Evaluation
        Angiography . . . . . . . . . . . . . . . . . 75574
        for Coronary Calcium . . . . . . . . . . 75571

    for Structure and
        Morphology . . . . . . . . . . . . . 75572-75573
    Hemorrhage Documented . . . . . . . . . . 3110F
    Infarction Documented . . . . . . . . . . . . 3110F
    Lesion Documented . . . . . . . . . . . . . . 3110F
Unlisted Services and Procedures . . . . . . . . 76497
with Contrast . . . . . . . . . . . . . . . . . . . . . 70460
    Abdomen . . . . . . . . . . . . . . . . . . . . . . 74160
    Arm . . . . . . . . . . . . . . . . . . . . . . . . . . 73201
    Brain . . . . . . . . . . . . . . . . . 0042T, 70460
    Cerebral Blood Flow/Volume . . . . . . . 0042T
    Ear . . . . . . . . . . . . . . . . . . . . . . . . . . 70481
    Face . . . . . . . . . . . . . . . . . . . . . . . . . 70487
    Head . . . . . . . . . . . . . . . . . . . . . . . . . 70460
    Leg . . . . . . . . . . . . . . . . . . . . . . . . . . 73701
    Maxilla . . . . . . . . . . . . . . . . . . . . . . . 70487
    Neck . . . . . . . . . . . . . . . . . . . . . . . . . 70491
    Orbit . . . . . . . . . . . . . . . . . . . . . . . . . 70481
    Pelvis . . . . . . . . . . . . . . . . . . . . . . . . 72193
    Sella Turcica . . . . . . . . . . . . . . . . . . . 70481
    Spine
        Cervical . . . . . . . . . . . . . . . . . . . . . 72126
        Lumbar . . . . . . . . . . . . . . . . . . . . . 72132
        Thoracic . . . . . . . . . . . . . . . . . . . . 72129
    Thorax . . . . . . . . . . . . . . . . . . . . . . . . 71260
without and with Contrast
    Abdomen . . . . . . . . . . 74170, 74174, 74175,
                     74178, 75635
    Arm . . . . . . . . . . . . . . . . . . . . . 73202-73206
    Brain . . . . . . . . . . . . . . . . . . . 70470, 70496
    Chest . . . . . . . . . . . . . . . . . . . . . . . . . 71275
    Ear . . . . . . . . . . . . . . . . . . . . . . . . . . 70482
    Face . . . . . . . . . . . . . . . . . . . . . . . . . 70488
    Head . . . . . . . . . . . . . . . . . . . 70470, 70496
    Leg . . . . . . . . . . . . . . . . . 73702-73706, 75635
    Maxilla . . . . . . . . . . . . . . . . . . . . . . . 70488
    Neck . . . . . . . . . . . . . . . . . . . 70492, 70498
    Orbit . . . . . . . . . . . . . . . . . . . . . . . . . 70482
    Pelvis . . . . 72191, 72194, 74174, 74176-74178
    Sella Turcica . . . . . . . . . . . . . . . . . . . 70482
    Spine
        Cervical . . . . . . . . . . . . . . . . . . . . . 72127
        Lumbar . . . . . . . . . . . . . . . . . . . . . 72133
        Thoracic . . . . . . . . . . . . . . . . . . . . 72130
    Thorax . . . . . . . . . . . . . . . . . . 71270-71275
without Contrast . . . . . . . . . . . . . . . . . . . 70450
    Abdomen . . . . . . . . . . 74150, 74176, 74178
    Arm . . . . . . . . . . . . . . . . . . . . . . . . . . 73200
    Brain . . . . . . . . . . . . . . . . . . . . . . . . . 70450
    Colon
        Colonography . . . . . . . . . . . . 74261-74263
    Ear . . . . . . . . . . . . . . . . . . . . . . . . . . 70480
    Face . . . . . . . . . . . . . . . . . . . . . . . . . 70486
    Head . . . . . . . . . . . . . . . . . . . . . . . . . 70450
    Leg . . . . . . . . . . . . . . . . . . . . . . . . . . 73700
    Maxilla . . . . . . . . . . . . . . . . . . . . . . . 70486
    Neck . . . . . . . . . . . . . . . . . . . . . . . . . 70490
    Orbit . . . . . . . . . . . . . . . . . . . . . . . . . 70480
    Pelvis . . . . . . . . . . . . . 72192, 74176, 74178
    Sella Turcica . . . . . . . . . . . . . . . . . . . 70480
    Spine
        Cervical . . . . . . . . . . . . . . . . . . . . . 72125
        Lumbar . . . . . . . . . . . . . . . . . . . . . 72131
        Thoracic . . . . . . . . . . . . . . . . . . . . 72128
    Thorax . . . . . . . . . . . . . . . . . . . . . . . . 71250

## CT Scan, Radionuclide
*See* Emission Computerized Tomography

## Cuff, Rotator
*See* Rotator Cuff

## Culdocentesis
*See* Colpocentesis

Liver ........................................ 47010
   Drainage ................................. 47010
     Open ................................. 47010
   Repair ................................... 47300
Lung
   Incision and Drainage .............. 32200
   Removal ................................. 32140
Lymph Node
   Axillary/Cervical
     Excision .................... 38550-38555
Mandible
   Excision ............. 21040, 21046-21047
Maxilla
   Excision ............. 21030, 21048-21049
Mediastinal
   Resection ............................. 39200
Metacarpal ........................ 26200-26205
Metatarsal ........................ 28104-28107
Mouth ............. 41005-41009, 41015-41018
   Incision and Drainage ........ 40800-40801
Mullerian Duct
   Excision ................................ 55680
Nose
   Excision ........................ 30124-30125
Olecranon ................................ 24120
Ovarian
   Excision ................................ 58925
   Incision and Drainage ........ 58800-58805
Pancreas ................................. 48500
   Anastomosis ................. 48520-48540
   Excision ................................ 48120
Pelvis
   Aspiration .............................. 50390
   Injection ............................... 50390
Pericardial
   Resection ............................. 33050
Phalanges
   Finger ........................ 26210-26215
   Toe .................................... 28108
Pilonidal
   Excision ....................... 11770-11772
   Incision and Drainage ........ 10080-10081
Pubis ............................. 27065-27067
Radius ................. 24120, 25120-25126
Rathke's Pouch
   *See* Craniopharyngioma
Removal
   Skin ................................... 10040
Retroperitoneal
   Destruction/Excision ........ 49203-49205
Salivary Gland Creation
   Destruction/Excision
     Drainage ........................... 42409
     Excision ........................... 42408
Scapula
   Excision ....................... 23140-23146
Seminal Vesicle
   Excision ............................... 55680
Skin
   Puncture Aspiration ................. 10160
Spinal Cord
   Aspiration .............................. 62268
   Incision and Drainage ........ 63172-63173
Sublingual Gland Drainage ............. 42409
   Excision ............................... 42408
Talus ............................. 28100-28103
Tarsal ............................. 28104-28107
Thyroglossal Duct
   Excision ....................... 60280-60281
   Incision and Drainage ............... 60000
Thyroid Gland Aspiration .............. 60300
   Excision ............................... 60200
   Injection .............................. 60300

Tibia ............................. 27635-27638
Tongue ................. 41000-41006, 41015
Ulna ............. 24120, 25120-25126
Urachal
   Bladder
     Excision ........................... 51500
Vaginal
   Excision ............................... 57135
Wrist ........................... 25130-25136
   Excision ....................... 25111-25112
Zygoma
   Excision ............................... 21030

## Cyst, Ovary
*See* Ovary, Cyst

## Cystatin C
Blood ................................... 82610

## Cystatins, Kininogen
*See* Kininogen

## Cystectomy
Complete ............................... 51570
   with Bilateral Pelvic
   Lymphadenectomy ...... 51575, 51585, 51595
   with Continent Diversion ............. 51596
   with Ureteroileal Conduit ............ 51590
   with Ureterosigmoidostomy .......... 51580
Ovarian ................................. 58925
   Laparoscopic .......................... 58661
Partial
   Complicated ........................... 51555
   Reimplantation of Ureters ........... 51565
   Simple ................................ 51550

## Cystic Hygroma
*See* Hygroma

## Cystine
Urine ................................... 82615

## Cystitis
Interstitial ...................... 52260-52265

## Cystography .................... 74430
Injection .............................. 52281
   Radiologic ............................ 51600

## Cystolithotomy ............... 51050

## Cystometrogram .......... 51725-51729

## Cystoplasty ..................... 51800

## Cystorrhaphy .............. 51860-51865

## Cystoscopy ..................... 52000

## Cystoscopy, with Biopsy
*See* Biopsy, Bladder, Cystourethroscopy

## Cystostomy
Change Tube .................... 51705-51710
Closure ................................. 51880
Home Visit ............................. 99505
with Fulguration ...................... 51020
with Insertion Radioactive Material ...... 51020
with Urethrectomy
   Female ............................... 53210
   Male ................................. 53215

## Cystotomy
Excision
   Bladder Diverticulum ................ 51525
   Bladder Tumor ....................... 51530
   Repair of Ureterocele ............... 51535
   Vesical Neck .......................... 51520

Repair Ureterocele .................... 51535
with Calculus Basket Extraction ......... 51065
with Destruction Intravesical Lesion ...... 51030
with Drainage ......................... 51040
with Fulguration ...................... 51020
with Insertion
   Radioactive Material ................ 51020
   Ureteral Catheter ................... 51045
with Removal Calculus .......... 51050, 51065

## Cystourethrogram, Retrograde
*See* Urethrocystography, Retrograde

## Cystourethropexy
*See* Vesicourethropexy

## Cystourethroplasty ....... 51800-51820
Radiofrequency Micro-Remodeling ...... 53860

## Cystourethroscopy ...... 52000, 52351,
              52601, 52647-52648, 53500
Biopsy ........................ 52204, 52354
   Brush ................................. 52007
Calibration and/or Dilation Urethral
Stricture or Stenosis ................. 52281
Catheterization
   Ejaculatory Duct ..................... 52010
   Ureteral .............................. 52005
Destruction
   Lesion ................................ 52400
Dilation
   Bladder ....................... 52260-52265
   Intra-Renal Stricture ......... 52343, 52346
   Ureter ......... 52341-52342, 52344-52345
   Urethra ............................... 52281
Evacuation
   Clot .................................. 52001
Female Urethral Syndrome .............. 52285
Incision
   Ejaculatory Duct ..................... 52402
Injection of Implant Material ........... 52327
Insertion
   Indwelling Ureteral Stent ...... 50947, 52332
   Radioactive Substance ............... 52250
   Ureteral Guide Wire ................. 52334
   Urethral Stent ....................... 52282
Lithotripsy ............................. 52353
Manipulation of Ureteral Calculus ....... 52330
Meatotomy
   Ureteral ....................... 52290-52305
Removal
   Calculus ... 52310-52315, 52320-52325, 52352
   Foreign Body ................. 52310-52315
   Urethral Stent ............... 52310-52315
Resection
   Ejaculatory Duct ..................... 52402
   External Sphincter ................... 52277
   Tumor ................................ 52355
Urethral Syndrome ..................... 52285
Vasectomy
   Transurethral ........................ 52402
Vasotomy
   Transurethral ........................ 52402
with Direct Vision Internal Urethrotomy ... 52276
with Ejaculatory Duct Catheterization .... 52010
with Fulguration ............... 52214, 52354
   Lesion ................................ 52224
   Tumor ......................... 52234-52240
with Internal Urethrotomy
   Female ............................... 52270
   Male ................................. 52275
with Steroid Injection ................. 52283
with Ureteral Catheterization .......... 52005
with Ureteral Meatotomy ........ 52290-52305

## Decortication
Lung
    Endoscopic . . . . . . . . . . . . . . . . . 32651-32652
    Partial . . . . . . . . . . . . . . . . . . . . . . . . 32225
    Total . . . . . . . . . . . . . . . . . . . . . . . . . 32220
    with Parietal Pleurectomy . . . . . . . . . . . 32320

## Decubiti
*See* Pressure Ulcer (Decubitus)

## Decubitus Ulcers
*See* Debridement; Pressure Ulcer (Decubitus);
Skin Graft and Flap

## Deetjeen's Body
*See* Blood, Platelet

## Defect, Coagulation
*See* Coagulopathy

## Defect, Heart Septal
*See* Septal Defect

## Defect, Septal Closure, Atrial
*See* Heart, Repair, Atrial Septum

## Deferens, Ductus
*See* Vas Deferens

## Defibrillation
*See* Cardioversion

## Defibrillator, Heart
*See* Pacemaker, Heart
Cardioverter-Defibrillator, Implantable System
    Data Analysis . . . . . . . . 93289, 93295-93296
    Electrode Insertion . . . . . . . . . . . 33216-33217,
                    33224-33225
    Electrode Removal . . . . . . . . . . . 33243-33244
    Evaluation of Programming . . . . . 93282-93284,
               93287, 93289, 93292,
         93295-93296, 93640-93642
    Insertion . . . . . . . . . . . . . . . . . . . . . . 33249
    Pulse Generator
        Insertion . . . . . . . . . . . 33230-33231, 33240
        Removal . . . . . . . . . . . . . . 33233, 33241
        Replacement . . . . . . . . . . . . . . 33262-33264
Repair
    Electrodes, Transvenous . . . . . . . 33218-33220
Replacement . . . . . . . . . . . . . . . . . . . . . . 33249
Repositioning
    Electrodes . . . . . . . . . . . . . . 33215, 33226
Revise Pocket Chest . . . . . . . . . . . . . . . . 33223
Wearable Device . . . . . . . . . . . . . . . . . . . 93745

## Deformity, Boutonniere
*See* Boutonniere Deformity

## Deformity, Sprengel's
*See* Sprengel's Deformity

## Degenerative, Articular Cartilage, Patella
*See* Chondromalacia Patella

## Degradation Products, Fibrin
*See* Fibrin Degradation Products

## Dehydroepiandrosterone . . . . . . .82626

## Dehydroepiandrosterone Sulfate . . . . . . . . . . . . . . . . . . . . .82627

## Dehydrogenase, 6-Phosphogluconate
*See* Phosphogluconate-6, Dehydrogenase

## Dehydrogenase, Alcohol
*See* Antidiuretic Hormone

## Dehydrogenase, Glucose-6-Phosphate
*See* Glucose-6-Phosphate, Dehydrogenase

## Dehydrogenase, Glutamate
*See* Glutamate Dehydrogenase

## Dehydrogenase, Isocitrate
*See* Isocitric Dehydrogenase

## Dehydrogenase, Lactate
*See* Lactic Dehydrogenase

## Dehydrogenase, Malate
*See* Malate Dehydrogenase

## Dehydroisoandrosterone Sulfate
*See* Dehydroepiandrosterone Sulfate

## Delay of Flap
Skin Graft . . . . . . . . . . . . . . . . . . . 15600-15630

## Deligation
Ureter . . . . . . . . . . . . . . . . . . . . . . . . 50940

## Deliveries, Abdominal
*See* Cesarean Delivery

## Delivery
*See* Cesarean Delivery; Vaginal Delivery

## Delorme Operation
*See* Pericardiectomy

## Denervation
Hip
    Femoral . . . . . . . . . . . . . . . . . . . . 27035
    Obturator . . . . . . . . . . . . . . . . . . . 27035
    Sciatic . . . . . . . . . . . . . . . . . . . . . 27035

## Denervation, Sympathetic
*See* Excision, Nerve, Sympathetic

## Denis-Browne Splint . . . . . . . . . .29590

## Dens Axis
*See* Odontoid Process

## Denver Developmental Screening Test . . . . . . . . . . . . . . . . . . . . . . . 96101-96103

## Denver Krupic Procedure
*See* Aqueous Shunt, to Extraocular Reservoir

## Denver Shunt
Patency Test . . . . . . . . . . . . . . . . . . . . . 78291

## Denver-Krupin Procedure . . . . . .66180

## Deoxycorticosterone
*See* Desoxycorticosterone

## Deoxycortisol . . . . . . . . . . . .80436, 82634

## Deoxyephedrine
*See* Methamphetamine

## Deoxyribonuclease
Antibody . . . . . . . . . . . . . . . . . . . . . . 86215

## Deoxyribonuclease I
*See* DNAse

## Deoxyribonucleic Acid
Antibody . . . . . . . . . . . . . . . . . . 86225-86226
Extraction . . . . . . . . . . . . . . . . . 83890-83891

## Depilation
*See* Removal, Hair

## Depletion
Plasma . . . . . . . . . . . . . . . . . . . . . . . 38214
Platelet . . . . . . . . . . . . . . . . . . . . . . . 38213
T-Cell . . . . . . . . . . . . . . . . . . . . . . . . 38210
Tumor Cell . . . . . . . . . . . . . . . . . . . . . 38211

## Deposit Calcium
*See* Calcium, Deposits

## Depth Electrode
Insertion . . . . . . . . . . . . . . . . . . . . . . 61760

## Derma-Fat-Fascia Graft . . . . . . . .15770

## Dermabrasion . . . . . . . . . . . . 15780-15783

## Dermatology
Actinotherapy . . . . . . . . . . . . . . . . . . . 96900
Examination of Hair
    Microscopic . . . . . . . . . . . . . . . . . . 96902
Ultraviolet A Treatment . . . . . . . . . . . . . 96912
Ultraviolet B Treatment . . . . . . . . . . . . . 96910
Ultraviolet Light Treatment . . . . . . . 96900, 96913
Unlisted Services and Procedures . . . . . . 96999

## Dermatoplasty
Septal . . . . . . . . . . . . . . . . . . . . . . . . 30620

## Dermoid
*See* Cyst, Dermoid

## Derrick-Burnet Disease
*See* Q Fever

## Descending Abdominal Aorta
*See* Aorta, Abdominal

## Desipramine
Assay . . . . . . . . . . . . . . . . . . . . . . . . 80160

## Desmotomy
*See* Ligament, Release

## Desoxycorticosterone . . . . . . . . .82633

## Desoxycortone
*See* Desoxycorticosterone

## Desoxyephedrine
*See* Methamphetamine

## Desoxynorephedrin
*See* Amphetamine

## Desoxyphenobarbital
*See* Primidone

## Desquamation
*See* Exfoliation

## Destruction
Acne . . . . . . . . . . . . . . . . . . . . . 17340-17360
    Cryotherapy . . . . . . . . . . . . . . . . . . 17340
Arrhythmogenic Focus
    Heart . . . . . . . . . . . . . . 33250-33251, 33261
Bladder . . . . . . . . . . . 51020, 52214-52224, 52354
Calculus
    Bile Duct . . . . . . . . . . . . . . . . . . . 43265
    Kidney . . . . . . . . . . . . . . . . . . . . . 50590
    Pancreatic Duct . . . . . . . . . . . . . . . 43265
Chemical Cauterization
    Granulation Tissue . . . . . . . . . . . . . . 17250
Chemosurgery . . . . . . . . . . . . . . . 17110-17111
Ciliary Body
    Cryotherapy . . . . . . . . . . . . . . . . . . 66720
    Cyclodialysis . . . . . . . . . . . . . . . . . . 66740

Patient Training
- Completed Course . . . . . . . . . . . . . . . . . 90989
- Per Session . . . . . . . . . . . . . . . . . . . . . 90993
Peritoneal . . . . . . . . . . . . . . . 90945-90947, 4055F
- Catheter Insertion . . . . . . . . . 49418-49421
- Catheter Removal . . . . . . . . . . . . . . . 49422
- Plan of Care Documented . . . . . . . . . . 0507F
Unlisted Services and Procedures . . . . . . . . 90999

## Dialysis, Extracorporeal
*See* Hemodialysis

## Diaphragm
Repair
- for Eventration . . . . . . . . . . . . . . . . . . . 39545
- Hernia . . . . . . . . . . . . . 39503, 39540-39541
- Laceration . . . . . . . . . . . . . . . . . . . . . 39501
Resection . . . . . . . . . . . . . . . . . 39560-39561
Unlisted Procedures . . . . . . . . . . . . . . . . 39599
Vagina
- Fitting . . . . . . . . . . . . . . . . . . . . . . . . . 57170

## Diaphragm Contraception
*See* Contraception, Diaphragm

## Diaphysectomy
Calcaneus . . . . . . . . . . . . . . . . . . . . . . . . 28120
Clavicle . . . . . . . . . . . . . . . . . . . . . . . . . 23180
Femur . . . . . . . . . . . . . . . . . . . . . . . . . . 27360
Fibula . . . . . . . . . . . . . . . . . . . 27360, 27641
Humerus . . . . . . . . . . . . . . . . . 23184, 24140
Metacarpal . . . . . . . . . . . . . . . . . . . . . . . 26230
Metatarsal . . . . . . . . . . . . . . . . . . . . . . . 28122
Olecranon Process . . . . . . . . . . . . . . . . . . 24147
Phalanges
- Finger . . . . . . . . . . . . . . . . . . . 26235-26236
- Toe . . . . . . . . . . . . . . . . . . . . . . . . . . 28124
Radius . . . . . . . . . . . . . . . . . . . 24145, 25151
Scapula . . . . . . . . . . . . . . . . . . . . . . . . . 23182
Talus . . . . . . . . . . . . . . . . . . . . . . . . . . . 28120
Tarsal . . . . . . . . . . . . . . . . . . . . . . . . . . 28122
Tibia . . . . . . . . . . . . . . . . . . . . 27360, 27640
Ulna . . . . . . . . . . . . . . . . . . . . 24147, 25150

## Diastase
*See* Amylase

## Diastasis
*See* Separation

## Diathermy . . . . . . . . . . . . . . . . . . . . . . . 97024
*See* Physical Medicine/Therapy/Occupational
Therapy
Destruction
- Ciliary Body . . . . . . . . . . . . . . . . . . . . . 66700
Lesion
- Retina . . . . . . . . . . . . . . . . . . . 67208, 67227
Retinal Detachment
- Prophylaxis . . . . . . . . . . . . . . . . . . . . . 67141
- Repair . . . . . . . . . . . . . . . . . . . . . . . . . 67101

## Diathermy, Surgical
*See* Electrocautery

## Dibucaine Number . . . . . . . . . . . . . . . . 82638

## Dichloride, Methylene
*See* Dichloromethane

## Dichlorides, Ethylene
*See* Dichloroethane

## Dichloroethane . . . . . . . . . . . . . . . . . . . 84600

## Dichloromethane . . . . . . . . . . . . . . . . . 84600

## Diethylamide, Lysergic Acid
*See* Lysergic Acid Diethylamide

## Diethylether . . . . . . . . . . . . . . . . . . . . . 84600

## Differential Count
*See* White Blood Cell Count

## Differentiation Reversal Factor
*See* Prothrombin

## Diffusion Test, Gel
*See* Immunodiffusion

## Digestive Tract
*See* Gastrointestinal Tract

## Digit
*See* Finger; Toe
Destruction . . . . . . . . . . . . . . . . . . . . . . . 64632
Injection . . . . . . . . . . . . . . . . . . . . . . . . . 64455
Replantation . . . . . . . . . . . . . . . 20816-20822

## Digital Artery Sympathectomy . . . . . . . . . . . . . . . . . 64820

## Digital Slit-Beam Radiograph
*See* Scanogram

## Digits
Pinch Graft . . . . . . . . . . . . . . . . . . . . . . . 15050

## Digoxin
Assay . . . . . . . . . . . . . . . . . . . . . . . . . . . 80162

## Dihydrocodeinone . . . . . . . . . . . . . . . . 82646

## Dihydrocodeinone Screen . . . . . 82486

## Dihydroepitestosterone
*See* Dihydrotestosterone

## Dihydrohydroxycodeinone
*See* Oxycodinone

## Dihydromorphinone . . . . . . . 82486, 82649

## Dihydrotestosterone . . . . . . . . . . . . 82651

## Dihydroxyethanes
*See* Ethylene Glycol

## Dihydroxyvitamin D . . . . . . . . . . . 82652

## Dilatation, Transluminal Arterial
*See* Angioplasty, Transluminal

## Dilation
*See* Dilation and Curettage
Anal
- Endoscopy . . . . . . . . . . . . . . . . . . . . . 46604
- Sphincter . . . . . . . . . . . . . . . . . . . . . . 45905
Bile Duct
- Endoscopy . . . . . . . . . . 43271, 47555-47556
- Stricture . . . . . . . . . . . . . . . . . . . . . . . 74363
Bladder
- Cystourethroscopy . . . . . . . . . . 52260-52265
Bronchi
- Endoscopy . . . . . . . . . 31630, 31636-31638
Cerebral Vessels
- Intracranial Vasospasm . . . . . . . 61640-61642
Cervix
- Canal . . . . . . . . . . . . . . . . . . . . . . . . . 57800
- Stump . . . . . . . . . . . . . . . . . . . . . . . . . 57558
Colon
- Endoscopy . . . . . . . . . . . . . . . . . . . . . 45386
Colon-Sigmoid
- Endoscopy . . . . . . . . . . . . . . . . . . . . . 45340
Esophagus . . . . . . . . . . . . . . . . 43450-43458
- Balloon . . . . . . . . . . . . . . . . . 43220, 43249
- Endoscopy . . . . . . . . . 43220-43226, 43249
- Surgical . . . . . . . . . . . . . . . . . . . . . . . . 43510

Intestines, Small
- Endoscopy . . . . . . . . . . . . . . . . . . . . . 44370
Kidney . . . . . . . . . . . . . . . . . . . . . . . . . . 50395
- Intra-Renal Stricture . . . . . . . . 52343, 52346
Lacrimal Punctum . . . . . . . . . . . . . . . . . . 68801
Larynx
- Endoscopy . . . . . . . . . . . . . . . 31528-31529
Nasolacrimal Duct
- Balloon Catheter . . . . . . . . . . . . . . . . . 68816
Nose
- Balloon . . . . . . . . . . . . . . . . . 31295-31297
Pancreatic Duct
- Endoscopy . . . . . . . . . . . . . . . . . . . . . 43271
Rectum
- Endoscopy . . . . . . . . . . . . . . . . . . . . . 45303
- Sphincter . . . . . . . . . . . . . . . . . . . . . . 45910
Salivary Duct . . . . . . . . . . . . . . . 42650-42660
Trachea
- Endoscopy . . . . . . . . 31630-31631, 31636-31638
Transluminal
- Aqueous Outflow Canal . . . . . . . 66174-66175
Ureter . . . . . . . . 50395, 52341-52342, 52344-52345
- Endoscopy . . . . . . 50553, 50572, 50953, 50972
Urethra . . . . . . . . . . . . . . . . . . . 52260-52265
- General . . . . . . . . . . . . . . . . . . . . . . . . 53665
- Suppository and/or
  Instillation . . . . . . . . . . . . . . 53660-53661
Urethral
- Stenosis . . . . . . . . . . . . . . . . . . . . . . . 52281
- Stricture . . . . . . . . . . . . . 52281, 53600-53621
Vagina . . . . . . . . . . . . . . . . . . . . . . . . . . 57400

## Dilation and Curettage . . . . . . . . . 59840
*See* Curettage; Dilation
Cervical Stump . . . . . . . . . . . . . . . . . . . . 57558
Cervix . . . . . . . . . . . . . . . . . . . 57558, 57800
Corpus Uteri . . . . . . . . . . . . . . . . . . . . . . 58120
Hysteroscopy . . . . . . . . . . . . . . . . . . . . . 58558
Postpartum . . . . . . . . . . . . . . . . . . . . . . . 59160
with Amniotic Injections . . . . . . . . . . . . . . 59851
with Vaginal Suppositories . . . . . . . . . . . . 59856

## Dilation and Evacuation . . . . . . . . . 59841
with Amniotic Injections . . . . . . . . . . . . . . 59851

## Dimethadione . . . . . . . . . . . . . . . . . . . 82654

## Dioxide, Carbon
*See* Carbon Dioxide

## Dioxide, Silicon
*See* Silica

## Dipeptidyl Peptidase A
*See* Angiotensin Converting Enzyme (ACE)

## Diphenylhydantoin
*See* Phenytoin

## Diphosphate, Adenosine
*See* Adenosine Diphosphate

## Diphtheria
*See* Vaccines
Antibody . . . . . . . . . . . . . . . . . . . . . . . . . 86648

## Dipropylacetic Acid
Assay . . . . . . . . . . . . . . . . . . . . . . . . . . . 80164

## Direct Pedicle Flap
Formation . . . . . . . . . . . . . . . . . . 15570-15576

## Disability Evaluation Services
Basic Life and/or Disability Evaluation . . . . . 99450
Work-Related or Medical Disability
Evaluation . . . . . . . . . . . . . . . . . 99455-99456

Lumbar
  Open Treatment . . . . . . . . . . . . . . . . . 22325
Thoracic
  Open Treatment . . . . . . . . . . . . . . . . . 22327
Wrist
  Closed Treatment . . . . . . . 25660, 25675, 25680
  Intercarpal . . . . . . . . . . . . . . . . . . . . 25660
    Open Treatment . . . . . . . . . . . . . . . . 25670
  Open Treatment . . . . . . . . . . . . . 25670, 25685
  Percutaneous Fixation . . . . . . . . . . . . . . 25671
  Radiocarpal . . . . . . . . . . . . . . . . . . . . 25660
    Open Treatment . . . . . . . . . . . . . . . . 25670
  Radioulnar
    Closed Treatment . . . . . . . . . . . . . . . 25675
    Open Treatment . . . . . . . . . . . . . . . . 25676
    Percutaneous Fixation . . . . . . . . . . . . . 25671
  with Fracture
    Closed Treatment . . . . . . . . . . . . . . . 25680
    Open Treatment . . . . . . . . . . . . . . . . 25685
  with Manipulation . . . . . . 25660, 25675, 25680

## Dislocation, Radiocarpal Joint
See Radiocarpal Joint, Dislocation

## Disorder
Blood Coagulation
  See Coagulopathy
Penis
  See Penis
Retinal
  See Retina

## Displacement Therapy
Nose . . . . . . . . . . . . . . . . . . . . . . . . . . . 30210

## Dissection
Hygroma, Cystic
  Axillary/Cervical . . . . . . . . . . . . . 38550-38555
Lymph Nodes . . . . . . . . . . . . . . . . . . . . . 38542

## Dissection, Neck, Radical
See Radical Neck Dissection

## Distention
See Dilation

## Diverticula, Meckel's
See Diverticulum, Meckel's

## Diverticulectomy . . . . . . . . . . . . . . . 44800
Esophagus . . . . . . . . . . . . . . . . . . . . 43130-43135

## Diverticulectomy, Meckel's
See Meckel's Diverticulum, Excision

## Diverticulum
Bladder
  See Bladder, Diverticulum
Meckel's
  Excision . . . . . . . . . . . . . . . . . . . . . . 44800
Repair
  Urethra . . . . . . . . . . . . . . . . . . . . 53400-53405

## Division
Muscle
  Foot . . . . . . . . . . . . . . . . . . . . . . . . . 28250
Plantar Fascia
  Foot . . . . . . . . . . . . . . . . . . . . . . . . . 28250

## Division, Isthmus, Horseshoe Kidney
See Symphysiotomy, Horseshoe Kidney

## Division, Scalenus Anticus Muscle
See Muscle Division, Scalenus Anticus

## DI-Amphetamine
See Amphetamine

## DMO
See Dimethadione

## DNA
Antibody . . . . . . . . . . . . . . . . . . . . 86225-86226

## DNA Endonuclease
See DNAse

## DNA Probe
See Cytogenetics Studies; Nucleic Acid Probe

## DNAse
Antibody . . . . . . . . . . . . . . . . . . . . . . . . 86215

## Domiciliary Services
See Nursing Facility Services
Assisted Living . . . . . . . . . . . . . . . . 99339-99340
Discharge Services . . . . . . . . . . . . . 99315-99316
Established Patient . . . . . . . . . . . . . 99334-99337
New Patient . . . . . . . . . . . . . . . . . . 99324-99328

## Donor Procedures
Conjunctival Graft . . . . . . . . . . . . . . . . . 68371
Heart Excision . . . . . . . . . . . . . . . . . . . . 33940
Heart/Lung Excision . . . . . . . . . . . . . . . . 33930
Liver Segment . . . . . . . . . . . . . . . 47140-47142
Stem Cells
  Donor Search . . . . . . . . . . . . . . . . . . . 38204

## Dopamine
See Catecholamines
Blood . . . . . . . . . . . . . . . . . . . . . 82383-82384
Urine . . . . . . . . . . . . . . . . . . . . . 82382, 82384

## Doppler Echocardiography . . . . . . . . 76827-76828,
                                    93306-93308, 93320-93350
Intracardiac . . . . . . . . . . . . . . . . . . . . . 93662
Transesophageal . . . . . . . . . . . . . . . . . . 93318
Transthoracic . . . . . . . . . . . . . . . . . 93303-93317

## Doppler Scan
Arterial Studies
  Extremities . . . . . . . . . . . . . . . . . 93922-93924
  Fetal
    Middle Cerebral Artery . . . . . . . . . . . . 76821
    Umbilical Artery . . . . . . . . . . . . . . . . 76820
Extremities . . . . . . . . . . . . . . . . . . . . . . 93965
Intracranial Arteries . . . . . . . . . . . . . 93886-93893

## Dorsal Vertebra
See Vertebra, Thoracic

## Dose Plan
See Dosimetry

## Dosimetry
Radiation Therapy . . . . . . . . . . . . . 77300, 77331
  Brachytherapy . . . . . . . . . . . . . . 77326-77328
  Intensity Modulation . . . . . . . . . 77301, 77338
  Teletherapy . . . . . . . . . . . . . . . 77305-77321

## Double-Stranded DNA
See Deoxyribonucleic Acid

## Doxepin
Assay . . . . . . . . . . . . . . . . . . . . . . . . . 80166

## DPH
See Phenytoin

## Drainage
See Excision; Incision; Incision and Drainage;
Paracentesis
Abdomen
  Abdomen Fluid . . . . . . . . . . . . . . 49082-49083
Abscess
  Appendix . . . . . . . . . . . . . . . . . 44900-44901
    Percutaneous . . . . . . . . . . . . . . . . . 44901
  Brain . . . . . . . . . . . . . . . . . . . 61150-61151
  Eyelid . . . . . . . . . . . . . . . . . . . . . . . 67700
  Liver . . . . . . . . . . . . . . . . . . . 47010-47011
  Ovary
    Percutaneous . . . . . . . . . . . . . . . . . 58823
  Pelvic
    Percutaneous . . . . . . . . . . . . . . . . . 58823
  Pericolic
    Percutaneous . . . . . . . . . . . . . . . . . 58823
  Perirenal or Renal . . . . . . . . . . . . 50020-50021
    Percutaneous . . . . . . . . . . . . . . . . . 50021
  Prostate . . . . . . . . . . . . . . . . . . . . . . 52700
  Retroperitoneal . . . . . . . . . . . . . . 49060-49061
  Soft Tissue
    Percutaneous . . . . . . . . . . . . . . . . . 49061
    Subfascial . . . . . . . . . . . . . . . . . . . 20005
  Subdiaphragmatic or
    Subphrenic . . . . . . . . . . . . . . . 49040-49041
    Percutaneous . . . . . . . . . . . . . 49040-49041
  with X-ray . . . . . . . . . . . . . . . . . . . . 75989
Amniotic Fluid
  Diagnostic Aspiration . . . . . . . . . . . . . . 59000
  Therapeutic Aspiration . . . . . . . . . . . . . 59001
Bile Duct
  Transhepatic . . . . . . . . . . . . . . . . . . . 75980
Brain Fluid . . . . . . . . . . . . . . . . . . . . . . 61070
Bursa . . . . . . . . . . . . . . . . . . . . . 20600-20610
Cerebrospinal Fluid . . . . . . . . . . . . . 61000-61020,
                                      61050, 61070, 62272
Cervical Fluid . . . . . . . . . . . . . . . . . . . . 61050
Cisternal Fluid . . . . . . . . . . . . . . . . . . . 61050
Cyst
  Bone . . . . . . . . . . . . . . . . . . . . . . . . 20615
  Brain . . . . . . . . . 61150-61151, 62161-62162
  Breast . . . . . . . . . . . . . . . . . . . 19000-19001
  Ganglion . . . . . . . . . . . . . . . . . . . . . . 20612
  Liver . . . . . . . . . . . . . . . . . . . 47010-47011
    Percutaneous . . . . . . . . . . . . . . . . . 47011
  Salivary Gland . . . . . . . . . . . . . . . . . . 42409
  Sublingual Gland . . . . . . . . . . . . . . . . . 42409
Extraperitoneal Lymphocele
  Laparoscopic . . . . . . . . . . . . . . . . . . . 49323
  Open . . . . . . . . . . . . . . . . . . . . . . . . 49062
Eye
  Anterior Segment
    into Suprachoroidal Space . . . . . . . . . 0253T
    into Trabecular Meshwork . . . . . 0191T-0192T
  Paracentesis
    with Aqueous Aspiration . . . . . . . . . . 65800
    with Aqueous-Release . . . . . . . . . . . . 65805
  with Removal
    Blood . . . . . . . . . . . . . . . . . . . . . . 65815
    Discission of Anterior Hyaloid
      Membrane . . . . . . . . . . . . . . . . . 65810
    Vitreous . . . . . . . . . . . . . . . . . . . . 65810
Fetal Fluid . . . . . . . . . . . . . . . . . . . . . . 59074
Ganglion Cyst . . . . . . . . . . . . . . . . . . . . 20612
Hematoma
  Brain . . . . . . . . . . . . . . . . . . . 61154-61156
  Vagina . . . . . . . . . . . . . . . . . . . 57022-57023
Hematoma, Subungual . . . . . . . . . . . . . . . 11740
Joint . . . . . . . . . . . . . . . . . . . . . . 20600-20610
Liver
  Abscess or Cyst . . . . . . . . . . . . . 47010-47011
    Percutaneous . . . . . . . . . . . . . . . . . 47011

**Dust, Angel**
*See* Phencyclidine

**Duvries Operation**
*See* Tenoplasty

**Dwyer Procedure**
*See* Osteotomy, Calcaneus

**DXA**
*See* Dual X-ray Absorptiometry (DXA)

**Dynamometry**
*See* Osteotomy, Calcaneus
Venous Studies
  *See* Osteotomy, Calcaneus
  with Ophthalmoscopy . . . . . . . . . . . . . . 92260

# E

**E Antigens**
*See* Hepatitis Antigen, Be

**E B Virus**
*See* Epstein-Barr Virus

**E Vitamin**
*See* Tocopherol

**E1**
*See* Estrone

**E2**
*See* Estradiol

**E3**
*See* Estriol

**Ear**
Collection of Blood . . . . . . . . . . . . . . 36415-36416
Drum . . . . . . . . . . . . . 69420-69421, 69433-69436,
                    69450, 69610-69620
  *See* Tympanic Membrane
External
  Abscess Incision and Drainage
    Complicated . . . . . . . . . . . . . . . . . . . 69005
    Simple . . . . . . . . . . . . . . . . . . . . . . . 69000
  Biopsy . . . . . . . . . . . . . . . . . . . . . . . . 69100
  Excision
    Partial . . . . . . . . . . . . . . . . . . . . . . . 69110
    Total . . . . . . . . . . . . . . . . . . . . . . . . 69120
  Hematoma
    Incision and Drainage . . . . . . . . 69000-69005
  Reconstruction . . . . . . . . . . . . . . . . . . 69300
  Unlisted Services and Procedures . . . . . . 69399
Inner
  CT Scan . . . . . . . . . . . . . . . . . . . 70480-70482
  Excision
    Labyrinth . . . . . . . . . . . . . . . . . 69905-69910
  Exploration
    Endolymphatic Sac . . . . . . . . . . 69805-69806
  Incision . . . . . . . . . . . . . . . . . . . . . . . 69820
    Labyrinth . . . . . . . . . . . . . . . . . . . . . 69801
    Semicircular Canal . . . . . . . . . . . . . . 69840
  Insertion
    Cochlear Device . . . . . . . . . . . . . . . . 69930
  Semicircular Canal . . . . . . . . . . . . . . . 69820
  Unlisted Services and Procedures . . . . . . 69949
Vertigo
    *See* Canalith Repositioning

Middle
  Catheterization . . . . . . . . . . . . . . . . . . 69405
  CT Scan . . . . . . . . . . . . . . . . . 70480-70482
  Exploration . . . . . . . . . . . . . . . . . . . . 69440
  Inflation
    with Catheterization . . . . . . . . . . . . . 69400
    without Catheterization . . . . . . . . . . . 69401
  Insertion
    Catheter . . . . . . . . . . . . . . . . . . . . . 69405
  Lesion
    Excision . . . . . . . . . . . . . . . . . . . . . 69540
  Reconstruction
    Tympanoplasty with Antrotomy or
    Mastoidotomy . . . . . . . . . . . . 69635-69637
    Tympanoplasty with
    Mastoidectomy . . . . . . . . . . . . 69641-69646
    Tympanoplasty without
    Mastoidectomy . . . . . . . . . . . . 69631-69633
  Removal
    Ventilating Tube . . . . . . . . . . . . . . . . 69424
  Repair
    Oval Window . . . . . . . . . . . . . . . . . . 69666
    Round Window . . . . . . . . . . . . . . . . . 69667
  Revision
    Stapes . . . . . . . . . . . . . . . . . . . . . . 69662
  Tumor
    Excision . . . . . . . . . . . . . . . . 69550-69554
  Unlisted Services and Procedures . . . . . . 69799
Outer
  CT Scan . . . . . . . . . . . . . . . . . 70480-70482

**Ear Canal**
*See* Auditory Canal

**Ear Cartilage**
Graft
  to Face . . . . . . . . . . . . . . . . . . . . . . . 21235

**Ear Lobes**
Pierce . . . . . . . . . . . . . . . . . . . . . . . . . 69090

**Ear Protector Attenuation** . . . . . . . 92596
*See* Hearing Aid Services

**Ear Wax**
*See* Cerumen

**Ear, Nose, and Throat**
*See* Hearing Aid Services; Otorhinolaryngology,
Diagnostic
Audiologic Function Tests
  Acoustic Reflex . . . . . . . . . . . . . . . . . 92568
  Acoustic Reflex Decay . . . . . . . . . . . . . 92570
  Audiometry
    Bekesy . . . . . . . . . . . . . . . . 92560-92561
    Comprehensive . . . . . . . . . . . . 0212T, 92557
    Conditioning Play . . . . . . . . . . . . . . . 92582
    Evoked Response . . . . . . . . . . 92585-92586
    Groups . . . . . . . . . . . . . . . . . . . . . . 92559
    Pure Tone . . . . . . 0208T-0209T, 92552-92553
    Select Picture . . . . . . . . . . . . . . . . . 92583
    Speech . . . . . . . 0210T-0211T, 92555-92556
  Brainstem Evoked Response . . . . 92585-92586
  Central Auditory Function . . . . . . 92620-92621
  Ear Protector Evaluation . . . . . . . . . . . 92596
  Electrocochleography . . . . . . . . . . . . . . 92584
  Filtered Speech . . . . . . . . . . . . . . . . . 92571
  Hearing Aid Evaluation . . . . . . . 92590-92595
  Loudness Balance . . . . . . . . . . . . . . . . 92562
  Screening Test . . . . . . . . . . . . . . . . . . 92551
  Sensorineural Acuity . . . . . . . . . . . . . . 92575
  Short Increment Sensitivity
  Index (SISI) . . . . . . . . . . . . . . . . . . . . 92564
  Staggered Spondaic Word Test . . . . . . . 92572
  Stenger Test . . . . . . . . . . . . . . . 92565, 92577

  Synthetic Sentence Test . . . . . . . . . . . . 92576
  Tone Decay . . . . . . . . . . . . . . . . . . . . 92563
  Tympanometry . . . . . . . . 92550, 92567, 92570
Audiometry
  Evoked Otoacoustic Emissions . . . . . . . 92558,
                         92587-92588
  Visual Reinforcement . . . . . . . . . . . . . . 92579
Binocular Microscopy . . . . . . . . . . . . . . . 92504
Diagnostic Analysis
  Auditory Brainstem Implant . . . . . . . . . 92640
Facial Nerve Function Study . . . . . . . . . . 92516
Hearing, Language and Speech
Evaluation . . . . . . . . . . . . . . . . . . . . . . 92506
Laryngeal Function Study . . . . . . . . . . . . 92520
Nasal Function Study . . . . . . . . . . . . . . . 92512
Nasopharyngoscopy . . . . . . . . . . . . . . . . 92511
Vestibular Function Tests
  Additional Electrodes . . . . . . . . . . . . . 92547
  Caloric Tests . . . . . . . . . . . . 92533, 92543
  Foveal Stimulation . . . . . . . . . . . . . . . 92540
  Nystagmus
    Optokinetic . . . . . . . . 92534, 92540, 92544
    Positional . . . . . . . . . . 92532, 92540, 92542
    Spontaneous . . . . . . . 92531, 92540-92541
  Peripheral Stimulation . . . . . . . . . . . . . 92540
  Posturography . . . . . . . . . . . . . . . . . . 92548
  Torsion Swing Test . . . . . . . . . . . . . . . 92546
  Tracking Tests . . . . . . . . . . . . . . . . . . 92545

**Ebstein Anomaly Repair** . . . . . . . 33468

**Eccrine Glands**
Chemodenervation
  Axillae . . . . . . . . . . . . . . . . . . . . . . . 64650
  Feet . . . . . . . . . . . . . . . . . . . . . . . . . 64999
  Hands . . . . . . . . . . . . . . . . . . . . . . . . 64999
  Other Area . . . . . . . . . . . . . . . . . . . . 64653

**ECG**
*See* Electrocardiography

**Echinococcosis** . . . . . . . . . . 86171, 86280

**Echocardiography**
Cardiac . . . . . . . . . . . . . . . . . . . 93320-93350
  Intracardiac . . . . . . . . . . . . . . . . . . . . 93662
  Transesophageal . . . . . . . . . . . . . . . . 93318
  Transthoracic . . . . . . . . . . . . . 93303-93317
  with Stress Test . . . . . . . . . . . 93350-93352
Doppler . . . . . . 93303-93317, 93320-93321, 93662
Fetal Heart . . . . . . . . . . . . . . . . . 76825-76826
  Doppler
    Complete . . . . . . . . . . . . . . . . . . . . 76827
    Follow-up or Repeat Study . . . . . . . . . 76828
  for Congenital Anomalies
    Transesophageal . . . . . . . . . . . 93315-93317
    Transthoracic . . . . . . . . . . . . . 93303-93304
Intracardiac . . . . . . . . . . . . . . . . . . . . . 93662
Transesophageal . . . . . . . . . . . . . . . . . . 93318
  for Congenital Anomalies . . . . . . 93315-93317
Transthoracic . . . . . . . . 93303-93318, 93350
  for Congenital Anomalies . . . . . . 93303-93304
  with Stress Test . . . . . . . . . . . 93351-93352

**Echoencephalography** . . . . . . . . 76506

**Echography**
Abdomen . . . . . . . . . . . . . . . . . . . 76700-76705
Arm
  Complete . . . . . . . . . . . . . . . . . . . . . 76881
  Limited . . . . . . . . . . . . . . . . . . . . . . 76882
Breast . . . . . . . . . . . . . . . . . . . . . . . . . 76645
Cardiac . . . . . . . . . . . 93303-93317, 93320-93321,
                 93350-93352, 93662
  Guidance . . . . . . . . . . . . . . . . . . . . . 76932
Chest . . . . . . . . . . . . . . . . . . . . . . . . . 76604

## Echotomography
*See* Echography

## ECMO
*See* Extracorporeal Membrane Oxygenation

## ECS
*See* Emission Computerized Tomography

## ECSF (Erythrocyte Colony Stimulating Factor)
*See* Erythropoietin

## ECT
*See* Emission Computerized Tomography

## Ectasia
*See* Dilation

## Ectopic Pregnancy
*See* Obstetrical Care

## Ectropion
Repair

## Education Services

## Education Supplies . . . . . . . . . . . 99071

## EEG
*See* Electroencephalography (EEG)

## Egg
*See* Ova

## Ehrlichia
Antibody. . . . . . . . . . . . . . . . . . . . . . . . . 86666

## EKG
*See* Electrocardiography

## Elastase . . . . . . . . . . . . . . . . . . . . . . . 82656

## Elbow
*See* Humerus; Radius; Ulna

## Elbow, Golfer
*See* Elbow, Tendon; Tennis Elbow

## Elbows, Tennis
*See* Elbow, Tendon; Tennis Elbow

## Electric Countershock
*See* Cardioversion

## Electric Stimulation
*See* Electrical Stimulation

## Electric Stimulation, Transcutaneous
*See* Application, Neurostimulation

## Electrical Modulation Pain Reprocessing, Transcutaneous . . . . . . . . . . . . . . . . 0278T

## Electrical Stimulation

## Electro-Hydraulic Procedure . . . 52325

## Electro-Oculography . . . . . . . . 92270

## Electroanalgesia
*See* Application, Neurostimulation

## Electrocardiography

Stent Placement . . . . . . . . . . . . . . . . . 43256
Thermal Radiation . . . . . . . . . . . . . . . 43257
Tube Placement . . . . . . . . . . . . . . . . . 43246
Ultrasound . . . . 43237-43242, 43259, 76975
Vein Ligation . . . . . . . . . . . . . . . . . . . 43244
Heart
Atria . . . . . . . . . . . . . . . . . . . 33265-33266
Ileum
via Stoma . . . . . . . . . . . . . . . . . . . . . 44383
Intestines, Small
Biopsy . . . . . . . . . . . . . . 44361, 44377
Destruction
Lesion . . . . . . . . . . . . . . . . . . . . . . 44369
Tumor . . . . . . . . . . . . . . . . . . . . . . 44369
Diagnostic . . . . . . . . . . . . . . . . . . . . 44376
Exploration . . . . . . . . . . . . . . . . . . . . 44360
Hemorrhage . . . . . . . . . . . . . . 44366, 44378
Insertion
Stent . . . . . . . . . . . . . . 44370, 44379
Tube . . . . . . . . . . . . . . . . . . . . . . . 44379
Pelvic Pouch . . . . . . . . . . . . . . . 44385-44386
Removal
Foreign Body . . . . . . . . . . . . . . . . 44363
Lesion . . . . . . . . . . . . . . . . . . . . . . 44365
Polyp . . . . . . . . . . . . . 44364-44365
Tube Placement . . . . . . . . . . . . . . . . 44372
Tube Revision . . . . . . . . . . . . . . . . . 44373
via Stoma . . . . . . . . . . . . . . . 44380-44383
Tumor . . . . . . . . . . . . . 44364-44365
Intracranial . . . . . . . . . . . . . . . . 62160-62165
Kidney
Biopsy . . . . . . . . 50555, 50574-50576, 52354
Catheterization . . . . . . . . . . . . 50553, 50572
Destruction . . . . . . . . . . 50557, 50576, 52354
Dilation of Ureter . . . . . . . . . . . . . . . . 50553
Excision
Tumor . . . . . . . . . . . . . . . . . . . . . . 52355
Exploration . . . . . . . . . . . . . . . . . . . . 52351
Lithotripsy . . . . . . . . . . . . . . . . . . . . 52353
Removal
Calculus . . . . . . . . . . . 50561, 50580, 52352
Foreign Body . . . . . . . . . . . 50561, 50580
via Incision . . . . . . . . . . . . . . . 50562-50580
via Stoma . . . . . . . . . . . . . . . . 50551-50561
Larynx
Biopsy . . . . . . . . . . . 31510, 31535-31536
Direct . . . . . . . . . . . . . . . . . . . 31515-31571
Exploration . . . . . . 31505, 31520-31526, 31575
Fiberoptic . . . . . . . . . . . . . . . . 31575-31579
Indirect . . . . . . . . . . . . . . . . . . 31505-31513
Operative . . . . . . . . . . . . . . . . 31530-31561
Removal
Foreign Body . . . . . . . . . . . . 31530-31531
Lesion . . . . . . . . . . . 31511, 31545-31546
*See* Endoscopic
Mediastinoscopy
Biopsy . . . . . . . . . . . . . . . . . . . . . . . 39400
Exploration . . . . . . . . . . . . . . . . . . . . 39400
Nose
Diagnostic . . . . . . . . . . . . . . 31231-31235
Surgical . . . . . . . . . . . . . . . . 31237-31297
Unlisted Services and Procedures . . . . . . 31299
Pancreatic Duct
Cannulation . . . . . . . . . . . . . . . . . . . . 43273
Destruction
Calculi (Stone) . . . . . . . . . . . . . . . . 43265
Tumor . . . . . . . . . . . . . . . . . . . . . . 43272
Dilation . . . . . . . . . . . . . . . . . . . . . . . 43271
Removal
Calculi (Stone) . . . . . . . . . . . . . . . . 43264
Foreign Body . . . . . . . . . . . . . . . . . 43269
Stent . . . . . . . . . . . . . . . . . . . . . . 43269
Specimen Collection . . . . . . . . . . . . . . 43260

Sphincter Pressure . . . . . . . . . . . . . . . 43263
Sphincterotomy . . . . . . . . . . . . . . . . . 43262
Tube Placement . . . . . . . . . . . . 43267-43268
Pelvis
Aspiration . . . . . . . . . . . . . . . . . . . . . 49322
Destruction of Lesion . . . . . . . . . . . . . 58662
Lysis of Adhesions . . . . . . . . . . . . . . . 58660
Oviduct Surgery . . . . . . . . . . . 58670-58671
Removal of Adnexal Structures . . . . . . . 58661
Peritoneum
Biopsy . . . . . . . . . . . . . . . . . . . . . . . 47561
Drainage
Lymphocele . . . . . . . . . . . . . 49323, 54690
Radiologic . . . . . . . . . . . . . . . . . . . 47560
Pleural Cavity
Ablation
Photodynamic Therapy . . . . . . 96570-96571
Rectum
Biopsy . . . . . . . . . . . . . . . . . . . . . . . 45305
Destruction
Tumor . . . . . . . . . . . . . . . . . . . . . . 45320
Dilation . . . . . . . . . . . . . . . . . . . . . . . 45303
Exploration . . . . . . . . . . . . . . . . . . . . 45300
Hemorrhage . . . . . . . . . . . . . . . . . . . 45317
Removal
Foreign Body . . . . . . . . . . . . . . . . . 45307
Polyp . . . . . . . . . . . . . . 45308-45315
Tumor . . . . . . . . . . . . . . 45308-45315
Volvulus . . . . . . . . . . . . . . . . . . . . . . 45321
Spleen
Removal . . . . . . . . . . . . . . . . . . . . . . 38120
Testis
Removal . . . . . . . . . . . . . . . . . . . . . . 54690
Trachea
*See* Bronchoscopy
Dilation . . . . . . . . 31630-31631, 31636-31638
via Tracheostomy . . . . . . . . . . . . . . . . 31615
Ureter
Biopsy . . . . . 50955-50957, 50974-50976, 52354
Catheterize . . . . . . . . . . . . . . 50953, 50972
Destruction . . . . . . . . . . 50957, 50976, 52354
Excision
Tumor . . . . . . . . . . . . . . . . . . . . . . 52355
Exploration . . . . . . . . . . . . . . . . . . . . 52351
Injection of Implant Material . . . . . . . . . 52327
Lithotripsy . . . . . . . . . . . . . . . . . . . . 52353
Manipulation of Ureteral Calculus . . . . . 52330
Placement
Stent . . . . . . . . . . . . . . . . . . . . . . 50947
Removal
Calculus . . . . . . . . . 50961, 50980, 52352
Foreign Body . . . . . . . . . . . 50961, 50980
Resection . . . . . . . . . . . . . . . . . . . . . 52355
via Incision . . . . . . . . . . . . . . . 50970-50980
via Stoma . . . . . . . . . . . . . . . . 50951-50961
Ureteral
Biopsy . . . . . . . . . . . . . . . . . . . . . . . 52007
Catheterization . . . . . . . . . . . . . . . . . 52005
Urethra . . . . . . . . . . . . . . . . . . . . . . . . . 52000
Biopsy . . . . . . . . . . . . . . 52204, 52354
Catheterization . . . . . . . . . . . . . . . . . 52010
Destruction . . . . . . . . . . . . . . . . . . . . 52354
Lesion . . . . . . . . . . . . . . . . . . . . . . 52400
Evacuation
Clot . . . . . . . . . . . . . . . . . . . . . . . 52001
Excision
Tumor . . . . . . . . . . . . . . . . . . . . . . 52355
Exploration . . . . . . . . . . . . . . . . . . . . 52351
Incision
Ejaculatory Duct . . . . . . . . . . . . . . . 52402
Injection of Implant Material . . . . . . . . . 51715
Lithotripsy . . . . . . . . . . . . . . . . . . . . 52353

Removal
Calculus . . . . . . . . . . . . . . . . . . . . 52352
Resection
Ejaculatory Duct . . . . . . . . . . . . . . . 52402
Vasectomy . . . . . . . . . . . . . . . . . . . . 52402
Vasotomy . . . . . . . . . . . . . . . . . . . . . 52402
Uterus
Anesthesia . . . . . . . . . . . . . . . . . . . . 00952
Hysteroscopy
Diagnostic . . . . . . . . . . . . . . . . . . . 58555
with Division/Resection Intrauterine
Septum . . . . . . . . . . . . . . . . . 58560
with Lysis of Intrauterine
Adhesions . . . . . . . . . . . . . . . . 58559
Placement
Fallopian Tube . . . . . . . . . . . . . . . . 58565
Removal
Endometrial . . . . . . . . . . . . . . . . . . 58563
Impacted Foreign Body . . . . . . . . . . . 58562
Leiomyomata . . . . . . . . . . . . . . . . . 58561
Surgical with Biopsy . . . . . . . . . . . . . . 58558
Vagina
Anesthesia . . . . . . . . . . . . . . . . . . . . 00950
Biopsy . . . . . . . . . . . . . . . . . . . . . . . 57454
Exploration . . . . . . . . . . . . . . . . . . . . 57452
Vascular
Surgical . . . . . . . . . . . . 33508, 37500-37501

## Endosteal Implant
Reconstruction
Mandible . . . . . . . . . . . . . . . . 21248-21249
Maxilla . . . . . . . . . . . . . . . . . . 21248-21249

## Endothelioma, Dural
*See* Meningioma

## Endotracheal Intubation
*See* Insertion, Endotracheal Tube

## Endotracheal Tube
Intubation . . . . . . . . . . . . . . . . . . . . . . . 31500

## Endovascular Repair . . . . . . 0078T, 0079T,
0080T, 0081T, 0255T, 33880-33891,
34800-34805, 34812-34826, 34833-34900
Angiography . . . . . . . . . . . . . . . 75952-75959
Endoprosthetic . . . . . . . . . . . . . . . . .0254T-0257T
Lower Extremity for Occlusive
Disease . . . . . . . . . . . . . . . . . . 37220-37235

## Endovascular Therapy
Ablation
Vein . . . . . . . . . . . . . . . . . . . . 36475-36479
Occlusion . . . . . . . . . . . . . . . . . . . . . . . 61623

## Enema
Home Visit for Fecal Impaction . . . . . . . . . 99511
Intussusception . . . . . . . . . . . . . . . . . . . 74283
Therapeutic
for Intussusception . . . . . . . . . . . . . . 74283

## Energies, Electromagnetic
*See* Irradiation

## ENT
*See* Ear, Nose, and Throat; Otorhinolaryngology,
Diagnostic
Therapeutic
*See* Otorhinolaryngology

## Entamoeba Histolytica
Antigen Detection
Enzyme Immunoassay . . . . . . . . 87336-87337

## Enterectomy ... 44120-44121, 44126-44128,
44137, 44202
Donor .......................... 44132-44133
with Enterostomy....................... 44125

## Enterocele
Repair...................................... 57556
   Hysterectomy
     with Colpectomy................. 58280

## Enterocystoplasty ..............51960
Camey...................................... 50825

## Enteroenterostomy
See Anastomosis, Intestines

## Enterolysis........................44005
Laparoscopic............................. 44180

## Enteropancreatostomy
See Anastomosis, Pancreas to Intestines

## Enterorrhaphy ....... 44602-44603, 44615

## Enterostomy .....................44300
Closure ......................... 44625-44626
with Enterectomy
   Intestine, Small ..................... 44125

## Enterotomy.......................44615

## Enterovirus
Antibody.................................. 86658

## Entropion
Repair........................... 67921-67924
   Excision Tarsal Wedge............... 67923
   Suture................................ 67921
   Thermocauterization ............... 67922

## Enucleation
Eye
   with Implant....................... 65103
     Muscles Attached ............... 65105
   without Implant ................... 65101
Pleural.................................... 32540

## Enucleation, Cyst, Ovarian
See Cystectomy, Ovarian

## Enucleation, Prostate
See Prostate, Enucleation

## Environmental Intervention
for Psychiatric Patients ................. 90882

## Enzyme Activity
Non-Radioactive Substrate............. 82657
Infectious Agent........................ 87905
Radioactive Substrate .................. 82658

## Enzyme, Angiotensin Converting
See Angiotensin Converting Enzyme (ACE)

## Enzyme, Angiotensin-Forming
See Renin

## EOG
See Electro-oculography

## Eosinocyte
See Eosinophils

## Eosinophils
Nasal Smear............................. 89190

## Epiandrosterone................82666

## Epicondylitides, Lateral Humeral
See Tennis Elbow

## Epicondylitis, Radiohumeral
See Tennis Elbow

## Epidemic Parotitis
See Mumps

## Epididymectomy
Bilateral .................................. 54861
Unilateral ................................ 54860

## Epididymis
Abscess
   Incision and Drainage .............. 54700
Anastomosis
   to Vas Deferens
     Bilateral ........................ 54901
     Unilateral ...................... 54900
Biopsy .......................... 54800, 54865
Epididymography ...................... 74440
Excision
   Bilateral ........................... 54861
   Unilateral ......................... 54860
Exploration
   Biopsy............................. 54865
Hematoma
   Incision and Drainage .............. 54700
Lesion
   Excision
     Local........................... 54830
     Spermatocele.................. 54840
Needle Biopsy ......................... 54800
Spermatocele
   Excision ........................... 54840
Unlisted Services and Procedures ........ 55899
X-ray with Contrast .................... 74440

## Epididymograms ................55300

## Epididymography ..............74440

## Epididymoplasty
See Repair, Epididymis

## Epididymovasostomy
Bilateral .................................. 54901
Unilateral ................................ 54900

## Epidural
Electrode
   Insertion.......................... 61531
   Removal .......................... 61535
Injection ........... 62281-62282, 62310-62319
   with Imaging Guidance ........ 64479-64484
Lysis ........................... 62263-62264

## Epidural Anesthesia
See Anesthesia, Epidural

## Epidurography .................72275

## Epigastric
Hernia Repair............................ 49572

## Epiglottidectomy ..............31420

## Epiglottis
Excision.................................. 31420

## Epikeratoplasty...............65767

## Epilation
See Removal, Hair

## Epinephrine
See Catecholamines
Blood.......................... 82383-82384
Urine..................................... 82384

## Epiphyseal Arrest
Femur .................. 20150, 27185, 27475,
27479-27485, 27742
Fibula ........20150, 27477-27485, 27730-27742
Radius..................... 20150, 25450-25455
Tibia ...20150, 27477-27485, 27730, 27734-27742
Ulna....................... 20150, 25450-25455

## Epiphyseal Separation
Radius
   Closed Treatment................. 25600
   Open Treatment ............. 25607-25609

## Epiphysiodesis
See Epiphyseal Arrest

## Epiphysis
See Bone; Specific Bone

## Epiploectomy ...................49255

## Episiotomy ....................59300

## Epispadias
Penis
   Reconstruction.................... 54385
Repair ......................... 54380-54390
   with Exstrophy of Bladder ............ 54390
   with Incontinence ............ 54380-54390

## Epistaxis .................. 30901-30906
with Nasal/Sinus Endoscopy ............ 31238

## EPO
See Erythropoietin

## Epstein-Barr Virus
Antibody....................... 86663-86665

## Equina, Cauda
See Cauda Equina

## ERCP
See Bile Duct; Cholangiopancreatography;
Pancreatic Duct

## ERG
See Electroretinography

## Ergocalciferol
See Vitamin D

## Ergocalciferols
See Vitamin D

## Ergonovine Provocation Test ...93024

## Erythrocyte
See Red Blood Cell (RBC)

## Erythrocyte ab
See Antibody, Red Blood Cell

## Erythrocyte Count
See Red Blood Cell (RBC), Count

## Erythropoietin ..................82668

## Escharotomy
Burns........................ 16035-16036

## Escherichia coli 0157
Antigen Detection
   Enzyme Immunoassay .............. 87335

## ESD
See Endoscopy, Gastrointestinal, Upper

## Esophageal Acid Infusion Test
See Acid Perfusion Test

**Esophageal Polyp**
*See* Polyp, Esophagus

**Esophageal Tumor**
*See* Tumor, Esophagus

**Esophageal Varices**
Ligation........................ 43205, 43400
Transection/Repair..................... 43401

**Esophagectomy**
Partial.......................... 43116-43124
Total.................... 43107-43113, 43124

**Esophagoenterostomy**
with Total Gastrectomy.................. 43620

**Esophagogastroduodenoscopies**
*See* Endoscopy, Gastrointestinal, Upper

**Esophagogastromyotomy**
*See* Esophagomyotomy

**Esophagogastrostomy**.......... 43320

**Esophagojejunostomy**.... 43340-43341

**Esophagomyotomy**............ 32665,
                             43330-43331
with Fundoplasty..................... 43279

**Esophagorrhaphy**
*See* Esophagus, Suture

**Esophagoscopies**
*See* Endoscopy, Esophagus

**Esophagostomy**.......... 43350-43352
Closure..................... 43420-43425

**Esophagotomy**.......... 43020, 43045

**Esophagotracheal Fistula**
*See* Fistula, Tracheoesophageal

**Esophagus**
Acid Perfusion Test .................... 91030
Acid Reflux Tests ............... 91034-91038
Balloon Distension
   Provocation Study ................... 91040
Biopsy
   Endoscopy ....................... 43202
   Forceps.......................... 3150F
Cineradiography...................... 74230
Dilation...................... 43450-43458
   Endoscopic....... 43220-43226, 43248-43249
   Surgical ......................... 43510
Endoscopy
   Biopsy........................... 43202
   Dilation................... 43220-43226
   Exploration....................... 43200
   Hemorrhage....................... 43227
   Injection.................... 43201, 43204
   Insertion Stent.................... 43219
   Needle Biopsy..................... 43232
   Removal
      Foreign Body.................... 43215
      Polyp.......... 43216-43217, 43228
      Tumor .............. 43216, 43228
   Ultrasound .............. 43231-43232
   Vein Ligation ..................... 43205
Excision
   Diverticula ............... 43130-43135
   Partial.................... 43116-43124
   Total .............. 43107-43113, 43124
Exploration
   Endoscopy ....................... 43200
Hemorrhage ......................... 43227

Incision ..................... 43020, 43045
   Muscle .......................... 43030
Injection
   Sclerosing Agent .................. 43204
   Submucosal ...................... 43201
Insertion
   Stent............................ 43219
   Tamponade....................... 43460
   Tube ........................... 43510
Lengthening ................. 43283, 43338
Lesion
   Excision .................. 43100-43101
Ligation............................ 43405
Motility Study............. 78258, 91010, 91013
   with Perfusion ................... 0241T
   with Pressure Topography ........... 0240T
   with Stimulation ................. 0241T
Needle Biopsy
   Endoscopy ....................... 43232
Nuclear Medicine
   Imaging (Motility)................. 78258
   Reflux Study..................... 78262
Reconstruction .......... 43300, 43310, 43313
   Creation
      Stoma.................. 43350-43352
   Esophagostomy ................... 43350
   Fistula........... 43305, 43312, 43314
   Gastrointestinal ............ 43360-43361
Removal
   Foreign Bodies ... 43020, 43045, 43215, 74235
   Lesion........................... 43216
   Polyp............. 43216-43217, 43228
Repair ................ 43300, 43310, 43313
   Esophagogastric Fundoplasty ........ 43325,
                        43327-43328
      Laparoscopic................... 43280
   Esophagogastrostomy ............... 43320
   Esophagojejunostomy ......... 43340-43341
   Fistula.... 43305, 43312, 43314, 43420-43425
   Muscle .................... 43330-43331
   Paraesophageal Hernia
      Laparascopic.............. 43281-43282
   Pre-existing Perforation............. 43405
   Varices ......................... 43401
   Wound .................... 43410-43415
Suture............................. 43405
   Wound .................... 43410-43415
Ultrasound
   Endoscopy ................. 43231-43232
Unlisted Services and Procedures ....... 43289,
                             43499
Vein
   Ligation ................... 43205, 43400
Video.............................. 74230
X-ray .............................. 74220

**Esophagus Neoplasm**
*See* Tumor, Esophagus

**Esophagus, Varix**
*See* Esophageal Varices

**Established Patient**
Domiciliary or Rest Home Visit..... 99334-99337
Emergency Department Services ... 99281-99285
Home Services.................. 99347-99350
Hospital Inpatient Services....... 99221-99239
Hospital Observation Services ..... 99217-99220
Inpatient Consultations.......... 99251-99255
Office and/or Other Outpatient
   Consultations.................. 99241-99245
Office Visit.................... 99211-99215
Online Medical Evaluation ....... 98969, 99444
Outpatient Visit................. 99211-99215

Telephone Services ...98966-98968, 99441-99443

**Establishment**
Colostomy
   Abdominal ....................... 50810
   Perineal ........................ 50810

**Estes Operation**
*See* Ovary, Transposition

**Estlander Procedure** ............. 40525

**Estradiol** ........................ 82670
Response .......................... 80414

**Estriol**
Blood or Urine ...................... 82677

**Estrogen**
Blood or Urine .............. 82671-82672
Receptor.......................... 84233

**Estrone**
Blood or Urine ...................... 82679

**Ethanediols**
*See* Ethylene Glycol

**Ethanol**
Blood............................. 82055
Breath............................ 82075
Urine ............................ 82055

**Ethchlorovynol**
*See* Ethchlorvynol

**Ethchlorvinol**
*See* Ethchlorvynol

**Ethchlorvynol**
Blood............................. 82690
Urine............................. 82690

**Ethmoid**
Fracture
   with Fixation ..................... 21340

**Ethmoid, Sinus**
*See* Sinus, Ethmoid

**Ethmoidectomy** ........... 31200-31205
Endoscopic..................... 31254-31255
Skull Base Surgery............. 61580-61581
with Nasal/Sinus Endoscopy ...... 31254-31255

**Ethosuccimid**
*See* Ethosuximide

**Ethosuximide** ................. 80168
Assay............................. 80168

**Ethyl Alcohol**
*See* Ethanol

**Ethylene Dichlorides**
*See* Dichloroethane

**Ethylene Glycol** ................. 82693

**Ethylmethylsuccimide**
*See* Ethosuximide

**Etiocholanalone Measurement**
*See* Etiocholanolone

**Etiocholanolone** ................ 82696

**ETOH**
*See* Alcohol, Ethyl

**Euglobulin Lysis** ............. 85360

## European Blastomycosis
*See* Cryptococcus

## Eustachian Tube
Catheterization . . . . . . . . . . . . . . . . . . . . . . . . 69405
Inflation
    Myringotomy . . . . . . . . . . . . . . . . . . . . 69420
        Anesthesia . . . . . . . . . . . . . . . . . . . . . 69421
    with Catheterization . . . . . . . . . . . . . . . 69400
    without Catheterization . . . . . . . . . . . . . 69401
Insertion
    Catheter . . . . . . . . . . . . . . . . . . . . . . . . 69405

## Eutelegenesis
*See* Artificial Insemination

## Evacuation
Cervical Pregnancy . . . . . . . . . . . . . . . . . . . . 59140
Hematoma
    Brain . . . . . . . . . . . . . . . . . . . 61312-61315
        Anesthesia . . . . . . . . . . . . . . . . . . . . . 00211
    Subungual . . . . . . . . . . . . . . . . . . . . . . . 11740
Hydatidiform Mole . . . . . . . . . . . . . . . . . . . . 59870
Meibomian Glands . . . . . . . . . . . . . . . . . . . . 0207T

## Evaluation
Aneurysm Pressure . . . . . . . . . . . . . . . . . . . . 93982
Cine . . . . . . . . . . . . . . . . . . . . . . . . . . . . . . . 74230
Treatment . . . . . . . . . . . . . . . . . . . . . . . . . . 92526
Video . . . . . . . . . . . . . . . . . . . . . . . . . . . . . . 74230

## Evaluation and Management
Assistive Technology
    Assessment . . . . . . . . . . . . . . . . . . . . . 97755
Athletic Training
    Evaluation . . . . . . . . . . . . . . . . . . . . . . 97005
    Re-evaluation . . . . . . . . . . . . . . . . . . . . 97006
Basic Life and/or Disability Evaluation
Services . . . . . . . . . . . . . . . . . . . . . . . . . . . 99450
Care Plan Oversight Services . . . . . . 99339-99340,
                              99374-99380
    Home Health Agency Care . . . . . . . . . . . 99374
    Home or Rest Home Care . . . . . . 99339-99340
    Hospice . . . . . . . . . . . . . . . . . . 99377-99378
    Nursing Facility . . . . . . . . . . . . . 99379-99380
Case Management Services . . . . . . . 99366-99368
Consultation . . . . . . . . . . . . . . . . . 99241-99255
Critical Care . . . . . . . . . . . . . . . . . 99291-99292
    Interfacility Pediatric
    Transport . . . . . . . . . . . . . . . . . 99466-99467
Domiciliary or Rest Home
    Established Patient . . . . . . . . . . . 99334-99337
    New Patient . . . . . . . . . . . . . . . . 99324-99328
Emergency Department . . . . . . . . . . 99281-99288
Health Behavior
    Assessment . . . . . . . . . . . . . . . . . . . . . 96150
    Family Intervention . . . . . . . . . . . 96154-96155
    Group Intervention . . . . . . . . . . . . . . . . 96153
    Individual Intervention . . . . . . . . . . . . . 96152
    Re-assessment . . . . . . . . . . . . . . . . . . . 96151
Home Services . . . . . . . . . . . . . . . . 99341-99350
Hospital . . . . . . . . . . . . . . . . . . . . . 99221-99233
    Discharge . . . . . . . . . . . . . . . . . . 99238-99239
Hospital Services
    Observation Care . . . . . . . . . . . 99217-99220,
              99224-99226, 99234-99236
Insurance Exam . . . . . . . . . . . . . . . 99455-99456
Internet Communication . . . . . . . . . 98969, 99444
Low Birthweight Infant . . . . . . . . . . 99478-99479
Medical
    with Individual Psychotherapy
        Hospital or Residential Care . . . . . . . 90817,
          90819, 90822, 90824, 90827, 90829
        Office or Outpatient . . . 90805, 90807, 90809

        with Individual Psychotherapy, Interactive
        Office or Outpatient . . . 90811, 90813, 90815
Medical Team Conferences . . . . . . . . 99366-99368
Neonatal Critical Care . . . . . . . . . . . 99468-99469
Newborn Care . . . . . . . . . . . . . . . . 99460-99465
Nursing Facility
    *See* Nursing Facility Services
    Annual Assessment . . . . . . . . . . . . . . . 99318
    Discharge . . . . . . . . . . . . . . . . . 99315-99316
    Initial Care . . . . . . . . . . . . . . . . 99304-99306
    Other . . . . . . . . . . . . . . . . . . . . . . . . . 99318
    Subsequent Care . . . . . . . . . . . 99307-99310
Occupation Therapy Evaluation . . . . . . . . 97003
    Re-evaluation . . . . . . . . . . . . . . . . . . . 97004
Office and Other Outpatient . . . . . . 99201-99215
Online Services . . . . . . . . . . . . . . . . 98969, 99444
Pediatric Critical Care . . . . . . . . . . . 99471-99472
Pediatric Interfacility Transport . . . . 99466-99476
Physical Therapy Evaluation . . . . . . . . . . 97001
    Re-evaluation . . . . . . . . . . . . . . . . . . . 97002
Physician Standby Services . . . . . . . . . . . 99360
Preventive Services . . . . . . . . . . . . . 99381-99429
Prolonged Services . . . . . . . . . . . . . 99354-99360
Psychiatric
    Records or Reports . . . . . . . . . . . . . . . 90885
Team Conferences . . . . . . . . . . . . . 99366-99368
Telephone Services . . . 98966-98968, 99441-99443
Unlisted Services and Procedures . . . . . . . 99499
Work-Related and/or Medical Disability
Evaluation . . . . . . . . . . . . . . . . . . . . . . . 99455

## Evaluation Studies, Drug, Pre-Clinical
*See* Drug Screen

## Evisceration
Ocular Contents
    with Implant . . . . . . . . . . . . . . . . . . . . 65093
    without Implant . . . . . . . . . . . . . . . . . . 65091

## Evisceration, Pelvic
*See* Exenteration, Pelvis

## Evocative/Suppression Test . . . . . . . . . . . . . . . . . . . . . . 80400-80440
Stimulation Panel . . . . . . . . . . . . . . . . . . . . 80410

## Evoked Potential
*See* Audiologic Function Tests
Auditory Brainstem . . . . . . . . . . . . 92585-92586
Central Motor
    Transcranial Motor
    Stimulation . . . . . . . . . . . . . . . . 95928-95929
Somatosensory Testing . . . . . . . . . 95925-95927,
                               95938-95939
Visual, CNS . . . . . . . . . . . . . . . . . . . . . . . . 95930

## Evoked Potential, Auditory
*See* Auditory Evoked Potentials

## Ewart Procedure
*See* Palate, Reconstruction, Lengthening

## Excavatum, Pectus
*See* Pectus Excavatum

## Exchange
Drainage Catheter
    Under Radiologic Guidance . . . . . . . . . . 49423
Intraocular Lens . . . . . . . . . . . . . . . . . . . . . 66986
Intravascular Catheter . . . . . . . . . . . . 37209, 75900

## Exchange Transfusion
*See* Blood, Transfusion, Exchange

## Excision
*See* Debridement; Destruction
Abscess
    Brain . . . . . . . . . . . . . . . . . . 61514, 61522
    Olecranon Process . . . . . . . . . . . . . . . . 24138
    Radius . . . . . . . . . . . . . . . . . . . . . . . . 24136
    Ulna . . . . . . . . . . . . . . . . . . . . . . . . . 24138
Acromion
    Shoulder . . . . . . . . . . . . . . . . . . . . . . 23130
Adenoids . . . . . . . . . . . . . . . . 42830-42836
Adenoma
    Thyroid Gland . . . . . . . . . . . . . . . . . . . 60200
Adrenal Gland . . . . . . . . . . . . . . . . . . . . . 60540
    Laparoscopic . . . . . . . . . . . . . . . . . . . 60650
    with Excision Retroperitoneal Tumor . . . . 60545
Alveolus . . . . . . . . . . . . . . . . . . . . . . . . . 41830
Anal Crypt . . . . . . . . . . . . . . . . . . . . . . . . 46999
Anal Fissure . . . . . . . . . . . . . . . . . . . . . . . 46200
Anal Tag . . . . . . . . . . . . . . . . . . 46220, 46230
Aorta
    Coarctation . . . . . . . . . . . . . . . . 33840-33851
Appendix . . . . . . . . . . . . . . . . . . 44950-44960
Arteriovenous Malformation
    Spinal . . . . . . . . . . . . . . . . . . . 63250-63252
Arytenoid Cartilage . . . . . . . . . . . . . . . . . 31400
    Endoscopic . . . . . . . . . . . . . . . . 31560-31561
Atrial Septum . . . . . . . . . . . . . . . . 33735-33737
Bartholin's Gland . . . . . . . . . . . . . . . . . . . 56740
Bladder
    Diverticulum . . . . . . . . . . . . . . . . . . . . 51525
    Neck . . . . . . . . . . . . . . . . . . . . . . . . . 51520
    Partial . . . . . . . . . . . . . . . . . . . 51550-51565
    Total . . . . . . . . . . . 51570, 51580, 51590-51597
        with Nodes . . . . . . . . 51575, 51585, 51595
    Transurethral . . . . . . . . . . . . . . . . . . . 52640
    Tumor . . . . . . . . . . . . . . . . . . . . . . . . 51530
Bladder Neck Contracture
    Postoperative . . . . . . . . . . . . . . . . . . . 52640
Bone
    Facial . . . . . . . . . . . . . . . . . . . . . . . . 21026
    Mandible . . . . . . . . . . . . . . . . . . . . . . 21025
    Postoperative
        Femur . . . . . . . . . . . . . . . . . . . . . . 20150
        Fibula . . . . . . . . . . . . . . . . . . . . . . 20150
        Radius . . . . . . . . . . . . . . . . . . . . . . 20150
        Tibia . . . . . . . . . . . . . . . . . . . . . . . 20150
        Ulna . . . . . . . . . . . . . . . . . . . . . . . 20150
Bone Abscess
    Facial . . . . . . . . . . . . . . . . . . . . . . . . 21026
    Mandible . . . . . . . . . . . . . . . . . . . . . . 21025
Brain
    Amygdala . . . . . . . . . . . . . . . . . . . . . . 61566
    Epileptogenic Focus . . . . . . . . . . . . . . . 61536
    Hemisphere . . . . . . . . . . . . . . . 61542-61543
    Hippocampus . . . . . . . . . . . . . . . . . . . 61566
    Other Lobe . . . . . . . . . . . 61323, 61539-61540
    Temporal Lobe . . . . . . . . . . . . . . 61537-61538
Brain Lobe
    *See* Lobectomy, Brain
Breast
    Biopsy . . . . . . . . . . . . . . . . . . . 19100-19103
    Chest Wall Tumor . . . . . . . . . . . 19260-19272
    Cyst . . . . . . . . . . . . . . . . . . . . 19120-19126
    Lactiferous Duct Fistula . . . . . . . . . . . . 19112
    Lesion . . . . . . . . . . . . . . . . . . . 19120-19126
        by Needle Localization . . . . . . . 19125-19126
    Mastectomy . . . . . . . . . . . . . . . 19300-19307
    Nipple Exploration . . . . . . . . . . . . . . . . 19110
Bulbourethral Gland . . . . . . . . . . . . . . . . . 53250
Bullae
    Lung . . . . . . . . . . . . . . . . . . . . . . . . . 32141
    Burns . . . . . . . . . . . . 01951-01953, 15002-15005

# F

## Fluoride
Blood . . . . . . . . . . . . . . . . . . . . . . . . . . 82735
Urine . . . . . . . . . . . . . . . . . . . . . . . . . . 82735

## Fluoroscopy
Bile Duct
    Calculus Removal . . . . . . . . . . . . . . . . 74327
    Guide Catheter . . . . . . . . . . . . . . 74328, 74330
Chest
    Bronchoscopy . . . . . . . . . . . . . . 31622-31646
    Complete (Four Views) . . . . . . . . . . . . . 71034
    Partial (Two Views) . . . . . . . . . . . . . . 71023
Drain Abscess . . . . . . . . . . . . . . . . . . . . . 75989
GI Tract
    Guide Intubation . . . . . . . . . . . . . . . . 74340
Hourly . . . . . . . . . . . . . . . . . . 76000-76001
Introduction
    GI Tube . . . . . . . . . . . . . . . . . . . . . . . 74340
Larynx . . . . . . . . . . . . . . . . . . . . . . . . . . 70370
Nasogastric . . . . . . . . . . . . . . . . . . . . . . 43752
Needle Biopsy . . . . . . . . . . . . . . . . . . . . 77002
Orogastric . . . . . . . . . . . . . . . . . . . . . . . 43752
Pancreatic Duct
    Guide Catheter . . . . . . . . . . . . . 74329-74330
Pharynx . . . . . . . . . . . . . . . . . . . . . . . . . 70370
Renal
    Guide Catheter . . . . . . . . . . . . . . . . . . 74475
Sacroiliac Joint
    Injection Guidance . . . . . . . . . . . . . . . 27096
Spine/Paraspinous
    Guide Catheter/Needle . . . . . . . . . . . . 77003
Unlisted Services and Procedures . . . . . . . . 76496
Ureter
    Guide Catheter . . . . . . . . . . . . . . . . . . 74480
Venous Access Device . . . . . . . . . . . 36598, 77001
Vertebra
    Osteoplasty . . . . . . . . . . . . . . . . . . . . 72291

## Flurazepam
Blood or Urine . . . . . . . . . . . . . . . . . . . . 82742

## FMR1 . . . . . . . . . . . . . . . . . . . . . 81243-81244

## FNA
See Fine Needle Aspiration

## Foam Stability Test . . . . . . . . . . . . . 83662

## Fold, Vocal
See Vocal Cords

## Foley Operation Pyeloplasty
See Pyeloplasty

## Foley Y-Pyeloplasty . . . . . . . 50400-50405

## Folic Acid . . . . . . . . . . . . . . . . . . . . . 82747
Blood . . . . . . . . . . . . . . . . . . . . . . . . . . 82746

## Follicle Stimulating Hormone (FSH) . . . . . . . . . . . . . . 80418, 80426, 83001

## Folliculin
See Estrone

## Follitropin
See Follicle Stimulating Hormone (FSH)

## Follow-up Inpatient Consultations
See Consultation, Follow-up Inpatient

## Follow-up Services
See Hospital Services; Office and/or Other
Outpatient Services
Post-Op . . . . . . . . . . . . . . . . . . . . . . . 99024

## Fontan Procedure
See Repair, Heart, Anomaly; Revision

## Food Allergy Test . . . . . . . . . . . . . . 95075
See Allergy Tests

## Foot
See Metatarsal; Tarsal
Amputation . . . . . . . . . . . . . . . . . 28800-28805
Bursa
    Incision and Drainage . . . . . . . . . . . . . 28001
Capsulotomy . . . . . . . . . . . . . . . . . 28260-28264
Cast . . . . . . . . . . . . . . . . . . . . . . . . . . . 29450
Fasciectomy . . . . . . . . . . . . . . . . . . . . . 28060
    Radical . . . . . . . . . . . . . . . . . . . 28060-28062
Fasciotomy . . . . . . . . . . . . . . . . . . . . . . 28008
    Endoscopic . . . . . . . . . . . . . . . . . . . . 29893
Incision . . . . . . . . . . . . . . . . . . . . 28002-28005
Joint
    See Talotarsal Joint; Tarsometatarsal Joint
    Magnetic Resonance Imaging
    (MRI) . . . . . . . . . . . . . . . . . . . . 73721-73723
Lesion
    Excision . . . . . . . . . . . . . . . . . 28080, 28090
Magnetic Resonance Imaging
(MRI) . . . . . . . . . . . . . . . . . . . . 73718-73720
Nerve
    Destruction
      Neurolytic . . . . . . . . . . . . . . . . . . 64632
    Excision . . . . . . . . . . . . . . . . . . . . . . 28055
    Incision . . . . . . . . . . . . . . . . . . . . . . . 28035
Neurectomy . . . . . . . . . . . . . . . . . . . . . 28055
Neuroma
    Excision . . . . . . . . . . . . . . . . . . . . . . 28080
    Injection of Anesthetic or Steroid . . . . . 64455
    Morton,Äôs
      Destruction . . . . . . . . . . . . . . . . . . 64632
      Injection . . . . . . . . . . . . . . . . . . . . 64455
Reconstruction
    Cleft Foot . . . . . . . . . . . . . . . . . . . . . 28360
Removal
    Foreign Body . . . . . . . . . . . . . . 28190-28193
Repair
    Muscle . . . . . . . . . . . . . . . . . . . . . . . 28250
    Tendon . . . . . . . . 28200-28230, 28234-28238
Replantation . . . . . . . . . . . . . . . . . . . . . 20838
Sesamoid
    Excision . . . . . . . . . . . . . . . . . . . . . . 28315
Splint . . . . . . . . . . . . . . . . . . . . . . . . . . 29590
Strapping . . . . . . . . . . . . . . . . . . 29540, 29590
Suture
    Tendon . . . . . . . . . . . . . . . . . . . 28200-28210
Tendon Sheath
    Excision . . . . . . . . . . . . . . . . . . 28086-28088
Tenotomy . . . . . . . . . . . . . . . . . . 28230, 28234
Tumor
    Excision . . . . . . . . . . . . . . . . . 28039-28045
    Radical Resection . . . . . . . . . . . 28046-28047
Unlisted Services and Procedures . . . . . . . . 28899
X-ray . . . . . . . . . . . . . . . . . . . . . 73620-73630

## Foot Abscess
See Abscess, Foot

## Foot Navicular Bone
See Navicular

## Forearm . . . . . . . . . . . . . . . . . . . . . 20805
See Arm, Lower

## Forehead
Flap . . . . . . . . . . . . . . . . . . . . . . . . . . . 15731
Reconstruction . . . . . . 21179-21180, 21182-21184
    Midface . . . . . . . . . . . . . . . . . 21159-21160
Reduction . . . . . . . . . . . . . . . . . 21137-21139

## Forehead and Orbital Rim
Reconstruction . . . . . . . . . . . . . . 21172-21180

## Foreign Body Removal
Peritoneal Cavity . . . . . . . . . . . . . . . . . . 49402
Pharynx . . . . . . . . . . . . . . . . . . . . . . . . 42809
Shoulder . . . . . . . . . . . . . . . . . . . . . . . 23331

## Forensic Exam . . . . . . . . . . . . . . . . 88040
Cytopathology . . . . . . . . . . . . . . . . . . . 88125
Phosphatase, Acid . . . . . . . . . . . . . . . . . 84061

## Foreskin of Penis
See Penis, Prepuce

## Formycin Diphosphate
See Fibrin Degradation Products

## Fournier's Gangrene
See Debridement, Skin, Subcutaneous Tissue,
Infected

## Fowler-Stephens Orchiopexy
See Orchiopexy

## Fowler-Stephens Procedure . . . . . . . . . . . . . . . . . . . . . . 54650

## Fraction, Factor IX
See Christmas Factor

## Fracture
Acetabulum
    Closed Treatment . . . . . . . . . . . 27220-27222
    Open Treatment . . . . . . . . . . . . 27226-27228
    with Manipulation . . . . . . . . . . . . . . . . 27222
    without Manipulation . . . . . . . . . . . . . 27220
Alveola
    Closed Treatment . . . . . . . . . . . . . . . . 21421
    Open Treatment . . . . . . . . . . . . 21422-21423
Alveolar Ridge
    Closed Treatment . . . . . . . . . . . . . . . . 21440
    Open Treatment . . . . . . . . . . . . . . . . . 21445
Ankle
    Bimalleolar . . . . . . . . . . . . . . . . 27808-27814
    Closed . . . . . . . . . . . . . . . . . . . 27816-27818
    Lateral . . . . . . . . . . . . . . 27786-27814, 27792
    Medial . . . . . . . . . 27760-27766, 27808-27814
    Posterior . . . . . . . . 27767-27769, 27808-27814
    Trimalleolar . . . . . . . . . . . . . . . 27816-27823
    with Manipulation . . . . . . . . . . . . . . . . 27818
    without Manipulation . . . . . . . . . . . . . 27816
Ankle Bone
    Medial . . . . . . . . . . . . . . . . . . . 27760-27762
Bennett's
    See Thumb, Fracture
Bronchi
    Endoscopy . . . . . . . . . . . . . . . . . . . . 31630
Calcaneus
    Closed Treatment . . . . . . . . . . . 28400-28405
    Open Treatment . . . . . . . . . . . . 28415-28420
    Percutaneous Fixation . . . . . . . . . . . . . 28436
    with Manipulation . . . . . . . . . . . 28405-28406
    without Manipulation . . . . . . . . . . . . . 28400
Carpal
    Closed Treatment
      with Manipulation . . . . . . . . . 25624, 25635
      without Manipulation . . . . . . . 25622, 25630
    Open Treatment . . . . . . . . . . . . 25628, 25645
Carpal Scaphoid
    Closed Treatment . . . . . . . . . . . . . . . . 25622
    Open Treatment . . . . . . . . . . . . . . . . . 25628
Cheekbone
    Open Treatment . . . . . . . . . . . . 21360-21366
    with Manipulation . . . . . . . . . . . . . . . . 21355

with Manipulation . . . . . . . . . . . . . . . 26742
Closed Treatment . . . . . . . . . . . . 26742, 28510
  Articular . . . . . . . . . . . . . . . . . . . . . . 26740
  Distal . . . . . . . . . . . . . . . . . . . . . . . . 26750
  with Manipulation . . . . . . . . . . . . . . . 26755
Distal . . . . . . . . . . . . . . . . . . . . . 26755-26756
  Closed Treatment . . . . . . . . . . . . . . . . 26750
  Finger or Thumb . . . . . . . . . . . . . . . . . 26765
  Percutaneous Fixation . . . . . . . . . . . . . 26756
Finger/Thumb
  Closed Treatment . . . . . . . . . . 26720-26725
  Shaft . . . . . . . . . . . . . . . . . 26720, 26727
  with Manipulation . . . . . . . . . 26725-26727
Great Toe . . . . . . . . . . . . . . . . . . . . . . 28490
  Closed Treatment . . . . . . . . . . . . . . . . 28495
  Distal . . . . . . . . . . . . . . . . . . . . . . . . 26765
  Open Treatment . . . . . . . . . . . . . . . . . 28505
  Percutaneous Fixation . . . . . . . . . . . . . 28496
  with Manipulation . . . . . . . . . 28495-28496
Shaft
  Closed Treatment . . . . . . . . . . . . . . . . 26725
  Open Treatment . . . . . . . . . . . . . . . . . 26735
  Percutaneous Fixation . . . . . . . . . . . . . 26727
Toe
  Closed Treatment . . . . . . . . . . . . . . . . 28515
  Open Treatment . . . . . . . . . . . . . . . . . 28525
  with Manipulation . . . . . . . . . . . . . . . 28515
  without Manipulation. . . . . . . . . . . . . . 28510
with Manipulation . . . . . . . . . . . 26742, 26755
without Manipulation . . . . . . . . . 26740, 26750
Radius
  Closed Treatment . . . . . . . . . . . 25560-25565
  Colles . . . . . . . . . . . . . . . . . . . 25600-25605
  Distal . . . . . . . . . . . . . . . . . . . 25600-25609
    Open Treatment . . . . . . . . . . . 25607-25609
    Smith . . . . . . . . . . . . . . . . . 25600-25605
  Head/Neck
    Closed Treatment . . . . . . . . . . 24650-24655
    Open Treatment . . . . . . . . . . . 24665-24666
  Open Treatment . . . . . . . 25515, 25607-25609
    Internal Fixation . . . . . . . . . . . 25607-25609
  Percutaneous Fixation . . . . . . . . . . . . . 25606
  Shaft . . . . . . . . . . . . . . 25500, 25525-25526
    Closed Treatment . . . . . . 25500-25505, 25520
    Open Treatment . . . . . . 25515, 25525-25526,
                                         25574
  with Manipulation . . . . . . . . . . . 25565, 25605
  with Radioulnar Joint
    Dislocation . . . . . . . . . . . . . . . 25525-25526
  with Ulna . . . . . . . . . . . . . . . . 25560-25565
    Open Treatment . . . . . . . . . . . 25574-25575
  without Manipulation . . . . . . . . . 25560, 25600
Rib
  Closed Treatment . . . . . . . . . . . . . . . . 21800
  External Fixation . . . . . . . . . . . . . . . . . 21810
    Internal Fixation . . . . . . . . . . . 0245T-0248T
  Open Treatment . . . . . . . . . . . . . . . . . 21805
Scaphoid
  Closed Treatment . . . . . . . . . . . . . . . . 25622
  Open Treatment . . . . . . . . . . . . . . . . . 25628
  with Dislocation
    Closed Treatment . . . . . . . . . . . . . . . 25680
    Open Treatment . . . . . . . . . . . . . . . . 25685
    with Manipulation . . . . . . . . . . . . . . . 25624
Scapula
  Closed Treatment
    with Manipulation . . . . . . . . . . . . . . . 23575
    without Manipulation. . . . . . . . . . . . . . 23570
  Open Treatment . . . . . . . . . . . . . . . . . 23585
Sesamoid
  Closed Treatment . . . . . . . . . . . . . . . . 28530
  Foot . . . . . . . . . . . . . . . . . . . 28530-28531
  Open Treatment . . . . . . . . . . . . . . . . . 28531

Skin
  Debridement . . . . . . . . . . . . . . . 11010-11012
Skull . . . . . . . . . . . . . . . . . . . . . . 62000-62010
Sternum
  Closed Treatment . . . . . . . . . . . . . . . . 21820
  Open Treatment . . . . . . . . . . . . . . . . . 21825
Talus
  Closed Treatment . . . . . . . . . . . 28430-28435
  Open Treatment . . . . . . . . . . . . . . . . . 28445
  with Manipulation . . . . . . . . . . 28435-28436
  without Manipulation . . . . . . . . . . . . . . 28430
Tarsal
  Open Treatment . . . . . . . . . . . . . . . . . 28465
  Percutaneous Fixation . . . . . . . . . . . . . 28456
  with Manipulation . . . . . . . . . . 28455-28456
Thumb
  with Dislocation . . . . . . . . . . . . 26645-26650
    Open Treatment . . . . . . . . . . . . . . . . 26665
    with Manipulation . . . . . . . . . . . . . . . 26650
Tibia . . . . . . . . . . . . . . . . . . . . . . . . . . 27759
  Arthroscopic Treatment . . . . . . . . 29855-29856
  Plateau
    Bicondylar . . . . . . . . . . . . . . . . . . . 29856
    Unicondylar . . . . . . . . . . . . . . . . . . 29855
  Bimalleolar
    Closed Treatment . . . . . . . . . . 27808-27810
    Open Treatment . . . . . . . . . . . . . . . . 27814
  Closed Treatment . . . . . . 27530-27532, 27538,
                  27750-27752, 27760-27762,
                  27808-27810, 27824-27825
  Distal . . . . . . . . . . . . . . . . . . . 27824-27828
    Articular . . . . . . . . . . . . . . . . 27826-27828
  Intercondylar . . . . . . . . . . . . . . 27538-27540
  Malleolus . . . . . . . 27760-27769, 27808-27814
  Open Treatment . . . . . . . . 27535-27536, 27540,
             27758, 27766, 27814, 27826-27828
  Percutaneous Fixation . . . . . . . . . . . . . 27756
  Plateau . . . . . . . . . . . . . . . . . 27530-27536
    Arthroscopic Treatment . . . . . . 29855-29856
  Unicondylar
    Open Treatment . . . . . . . . . . . . . . . . 27535
  Shaft . . . . . . . . . . . . . . . . . . . 27750-27759
  with Manipulation . . . . . . 27752, 27760-27762,
                                     27810
  without Manipulation . . . . . . . . 27530, 27750,
                 27760-27762, 27808, 27825
Trachea
  Endoscopy . . . . . . . . . . . . . . . . . . . . . 31630
Ulna
  *See* Elbow; Humerus; Radius
  Closed Treatment . . . . . . . . . . . 25560-25565
  Olecranon
    Closed Treatment . . . . . . . . . . 24670-24675
    Open Treatment . . . . . . . . . . . . . . . . 24685
  Open Treatment . . . . . . . . . . . . 25574-25575
  Shaft
    Closed Treatment . . . . . . . . . . 25530-25535
    Open Treatment . . . . . . . . . . . 25545, 25574
  Styloid Process
    Closed Treatment . . . . . . . . . . . . . . . 25650
    Open Treatment . . . . . . . . . . . . . . . . 25652
    Percutaneous Fixation . . . . . . . . . . . . 25651
  with Dislocation
    Closed Treatment . . . . . . . . . . . . . . . 24620
    Monteggia . . . . . . . . . . . . . . . 24620-24635
    Open Treatment . . . . . . . . . . . . . . . . 24635
  with Manipulation . . . . . . . . . . . 25535, 25565
  with Radius . . . . . . . . . . . . . . . 25560-25565
    Open Treatment . . . . . . . . . . . . . . . . 25575
  without Manipulation . . . . . . . . . 25530, 25560
Ulna and Radius
  Open Treatment . . . . . . . . . . . . 25574-25575

Vertebra
  Additional Segment
    Open Treatment . . . . . . . . . . . . . . . . 22328
  Cervical
    Open Treatment . . . . . . . . . . . . . . . . 22326
  Closed Treatment
    with Manipulation, Casting and/or
      Bracing . . . . . . . . . . . . . . . . . . . . 22315
    without Manipulation. . . . . . . . . . . . . 22310
  Lumbar
    Open Treatment . . . . . . . . . . . . . . . . 22325
  Posterior
    Open Treatment . . . . . . . . . . . 22325-22327
  Thoracic
    Open Treatment . . . . . . . . . . . . . . . . 22327
  with Shoulder Dislocation
    Closed Treatment . . . . . . . . . . . . . . . 23675
    Open Treatment . . . . . . . . . . . . . . . . 23680
  Vertebral Process
    Closed Treatment . . . . . . . . . . . . . . . 22305
  Wrist
    with Dislocation
      Closed Treatment . . . . . . . . . . . . . . 25680
      Open Treatment . . . . . . . . . . . . . . . 25685
  Zygomatic Arch
    Open Treatment . . . . . . . . . . . 21356-21366
    with Manipulation . . . . . . . . . . . . . . . 21355

## Fragile-X
Chromosome Analysis . . . . . . . . . . . . . . . 88248

## Fragility
Red Blood Cell
  Mechanical . . . . . . . . . . . . . . . . . . . . 85547
  Osmotic . . . . . . . . . . . . . . . . . 85555-85557

## Frames, Stereotactic
*See* Stereotactic Frame

## Francisella . . . . . . . . . . . . . . . . . . . . . .86000
Antibody . . . . . . . . . . . . . . . . . . . . . . . . 86668

## Fredet-Ramstedt Procedure . . . .43520

## Free E3
*See* Estriol

## Free Skin Graft
*See* Skin, Grafts, Free

## Free T4
*See* Thyroxine, Free

## Frei Disease
*See* Lymphogranuloma Venereum

## Frenectomy . . . . . . . . . . . . . . .40819, 41115

## Frenectomy, Lingual
*See* Excision, Tongue, Frenum

## Frenotomy . . . . . . . . . . . . . . . .40806, 41010

## Frenulectomy . . . . . . . . . . . . . . . . . . .40819

## Frenuloplasty . . . . . . . . . . . . . . . . . .41520

## Frenum
Lip
  Incision . . . . . . . . . . . . . . . . . . . . . . 40806
    *See* Lip

## Frenumectomy . . . . . . . . . . . . . . . . . .40819

## Frickman Operation
*See* Proctopexy

## Frontal Craniotomy . . . . . . . . . . . .61556

Sleeve........................... 43775
Total...................... 43621-43622
   with Esophagoenterostomy.......... 43620
with Gastroduodenostomy............. 43631

## Gastric Acid ............ 82930

## Gastric Analysis Test
Secretory Study.......... 43755-43757, 89135

## Gastric Electrodes
Implantation
   Laparoscopic
     Neurostimulator................... 43647
   Open
     Neurostimulator................... 43881
Removal
   Laparoscopic
     Neurostimulator................... 43648
   Open
     Neurostimulator................... 43882
Replacement
   Laparoscopic
     Neurostimulator................... 43647
   Open
     Neurostimulator................... 43881
Revision
   Laparoscopic
     Neurostimulator................... 43648
   Open
     Neurostimulator................... 43882

## Gastric Intubation
Diagnostic.................... 43754-43757
Therapeutic...................... 43753

## Gastric Lavage, Therapeutic ...43753

## Gastric Tests
Manometry...................... 91020

## Gastric Ulcer Disease
See Stomach, Ulcer

## Gastrin ................ 82938-82941

## Gastrocnemius Recession
Leg, Lower...................... 27687

## Gastroduodenostomy ......... 43810,
43850-43855

## Gastroenterology, Diagnostic
Breath Hydrogen Test ............. 91065
Colon Tests
   Motility Study .................. 91117
Esophagus Tests
   Acid Perfusion .................. 91030
   Acid Reflux............. 91034-91038
   Balloon Distension Provocation
   Study .......................... 91040
   Intubation with Specimen Collection ... 91000
   Motility Study ............. 91010, 91013
Gastric Tests
   Manometry...................... 91020
Gastroesophageal Reflux Test
   See Acid Reflux
Intestine
   Bleeding Tube .................. 91100
Manometry......................... 91020
Rectum
   Sensation, Tone, and Compliance
   Test........................... 91120
Rectum/Anus
   Manometry..................... 91122
Stomach
   Stimulation of Secretion .......... 43755

Unlisted Services and Procedures ........ 91299

## Gastroenterostomy
for Obesity ......... 43644-43645, 43842-43848

## Gastroesophageal Reflux
## Test...................... 91034-91038

## Gastrointestinal Endoscopies
See Endoscopy, Gastrointestinal

## Gastrointestinal Exam
Nuclear Medicine
   Blood Loss Study ............... 78278
   Protein Loss Study .............. 78282
   Shunt Testing................... 78291
   Unlisted Services and Procedures...... 78299

## Gastrointestinal Tract
Imaging
   Intraluminal ................. 91110-91111
Measurements
   Transit ....................... 0242T
   Pressure ...................... 0242T
Reconstruction ............ 43360-43361
Upper
   Dilation....................... 43249
X-ray ..................... 74240-74245
   Guide Dilator .................. 74360
   Guide Intubation ............... 74340
   with Contrast .............. 74246-74249

## Gastrointestinal, Upper
Biopsy
   Endoscopy ..................... 43239
Dilation
   Endoscopy ..................... 43245
   Esophagus ..................... 43248
Endoscopy
   Catheterization................. 43241
   Destruction
     Lesion ..................... 43258
   Dilation...................... 43245
   Drainage
     Pseudocyst ................. 43240
   Exploration............. 43234-43235
   Hemorrhage ................... 43255
   Inject Varices ................. 43243
   Injection ..................... 43236
   Needle Biopsy ......... 43238, 43242
   Removal
     Foreign Body................ 43247
     Lesion ..................... 43251
     Polyp ...................... 43251
     Tumor ..................... 43251
   Stent Placement................ 43256
   Suturing Esophagastric Junction..... 0008T
   Thermal Radiation .............. 43257
   Tube Placement ................ 43246
   Ultrasound ........... 43237-43238, 43242,
43259, 76975
Exploration
   Endoscopy ............. 43234-43235
Hemorrhage
   Endoscopic Control .......... 43255
Injection
   Submucosal .................. 43236
   Varices ...................... 43243
Lesion
   Destruction................... 43258
Ligation of Vein .............. 43244
Needle Biopsy
   Endoscopy ................. 43238, 43242
Removal
   Foreign Body .................. 43247

Lesion........................... 43250
Polyp...................... 43250-43251
Tumor........................... 43250
Tube Placement
   Endoscopy ..................... 43246
Ultrasound
   Endoscopy ........... 43237-43238, 43242,
43259, 76975

## Gastrojejunostomy ........ 43860-43865
Conversion from Gastostomy Tube........ 49446
Contrast Injection...................... 49465
Removal of Obstructive Material ......... 49460
Replacement of Tube.................... 49452
with Duodenal Exclusion............... 48547
with Partial Gastrectomy............... 43632
with Vagotomy........................ 43825
without Vagotomy ..................... 43820

## Gastroplasty
Laparoscopic ............. 43279, 43280, 43283
Revision
   for Obesity ....... 43644-43645, 43842-43848

## Gastroplasty with Esophagogastric
## Fundoplasty............... 43842-43843

## Gastrorrhaphy .................43840

## Gastroschises
See Gastroschisis

## Gastroschisis..................49605

## Gastrostomy
Closure ........................... 43870
Laparoscopic
   Temporary .................... 43653
Temporary........................... 43830
   Laparoscopic ................. 43653
   Neonatal ..................... 43831
with Pancreatic Drain ................. 48001
with Pyloroplasty ..................... 43640
with Vagotomy....................... 43640

## Gastrostomy Tube
Change of......................... 43760
Contrast Injection..................... 49465
Conversion to Gastro-Jejunostomy Tube ... 49446
Directed Placement
   Endoscopic ..................... 43246
Insertion ........................... 49440
Obstructive Material Removal .......... 49460
Placement
   Percutaneous
     Endoscopic ................. 43246
     Nonendoscopic.............. 49440
Replacement ....................... 49450
Repositioning ....................... 43761

## Gastrotomy........... 43500-43501, 43510

## GBA .........................81251

## GDH
See Glutamate Dehydrogenase

## Gel Diffusion...................86331

## Gel Diffusion Test
See Immunodiffusion

## Gene Analysis
ASPA ............................ 81200
BCKDHB .......................... 81205
BCR/ABL1 .................. 81206-81208
BLM............................. 81209
BRAF............................ 81210

BRCA1 . . . . . . . . . . . . . . . . . . . . . . . 81214-81215
BRCA2 . . . . . . . . . . . . . . . . . . . . . . . 81216-81217
BRCA1, BRCA2 . . . . . . . . . . . . . . . . . 81211-81213
CFTR . . . . . . . . . . . . . . . . . . . . . . . . 81220-81224
Chimerism Analysis . . . . . . . . . . . . . 81267-81268
Comparative Analysis Using Short Tandem
Repeat (STR) Markers . . . . . . . . . . . 81265-81266
CYP2C19 . . . . . . . . . . . . . . . . . . . . . . . . . . 81225
CYP2D6 . . . . . . . . . . . . . . . . . . . . . . . . . . . 81226
CYP2C9 . . . . . . . . . . . . . . . . . . . . . . . . . . . 81227
Cytogenomic Constitutional Microarray
Analysis . . . . . . . . . . . . . . . . . . . . . 81228-81229
F2 . . . . . . . . . . . . . . . . . . . . . . . . . . . . . . . 81240
F5 . . . . . . . . . . . . . . . . . . . . . . . . . . . . . . . 81241
FANCC . . . . . . . . . . . . . . . . . . . . . . . . . . . 81242
FLT3 . . . . . . . . . . . . . . . . . . . . . . . . . . . . . 81245
FMR1 . . . . . . . . . . . . . . . . . . . . . . . . . 81243-81244
G6PC . . . . . . . . . . . . . . . . . . . . . . . . . . . . 81250
GBA . . . . . . . . . . . . . . . . . . . . . . . . . . . . . 81251
HBA1/HBA2 . . . . . . . . . . . . . . . . . . . . . . . 81257
HEXA . . . . . . . . . . . . . . . . . . . . . . . . . . . . 81255
HFE . . . . . . . . . . . . . . . . . . . . . . . . . . . . . 81256
HLA Class I and II Typing, Low
Resolution . . . . . . . . . . . . . . . . . . . 81370-81371
HLA Class I Typing, Low
Resolution . . . . . . . . . . . . . . . . . . . 81372-81374
HLA Class II Typing, Low
Resolution . . . . . . . . . . . . . . . . . . . 81375-81377
HLA Class I and II Typing,
High Resolution . . . . . . . . . . . . . . . . . . 81378
HLA Class I Typing, High
Resolution . . . . . . . . . . . . . . . . . . . 81379-81381
HLA Class II Typing, High
Resolution . . . . . . . . . . . . . . . . . . . 81382-81383
IGH@ (Immunoglobulin Heavy Chain
Locus) . . . . . . . . . . . . . . . . . . . . . . 81261-81263
IGK@ . . . . . . . . . . . . . . . . . . . . . . . . . . . . 81264
IKBKAP . . . . . . . . . . . . . . . . . . . . . . . . . . 81260
JAK2 . . . . . . . . . . . . . . . . . . . . . . . . . . . . 81270
KRAS . . . . . . . . . . . . . . . . . . . . . . . . . . . . 81275
Long QT Syndrome Gene
Analyses . . . . . . . . . . . . . . . . . . . . 81280-81282
MCOLN1 . . . . . . . . . . . . . . . . . . . . . . . . . . 81290
MECP2 . . . . . . . . . . . . . . . . . . . . . . . 81302-81304
Microsatellite Instability Analysis . . . . . . . . 81301
MTHFR . . . . . . . . . . . . . . . . . . . . . . . . . . . 81291
MLH1 . . . . . . . . . . . . . . . . . . . . . . . . 81292-81294
MSH2 . . . . . . . . . . . . . . . . . . . . . . . . 81295-81297
MSH6 . . . . . . . . . . . . . . . . . . . . . . . . 81298-81300
NPM1 . . . . . . . . . . . . . . . . . . . . . . . . . . . . 81310
PML/RARalpha . . . . . . . . . . . . . . . . . 81315-81316
PMS2 . . . . . . . . . . . . . . . . . . . . . . . . 81317-81319
SERPINA1 . . . . . . . . . . . . . . . . . . . . . . . . 81332
SMPD1 . . . . . . . . . . . . . . . . . . . . . . . . . . . 81330
SNRPN/UBE3A . . . . . . . . . . . . . . . . . . . . . 81331
TRB@ . . . . . . . . . . . . . . . . . . . . . . . 81340-81341
TRG@ . . . . . . . . . . . . . . . . . . . . . . . . . . . . 81342
UGT1A1 . . . . . . . . . . . . . . . . . . . . . . . . . . 81350
VKORC1 . . . . . . . . . . . . . . . . . . . . . . . . . . 81355

**Gene Product**
*See* Protein

**Genioplasty** . . . . . . . . . . . . . . 21120-21123
Augmentation . . . . . . . . . . . . . . . 21120, 21123
Osteotomy . . . . . . . . . . . . . . . . . 21121-21123

**Genitourinary Sphincter, Artificial**
*See* Prosthesis, Urethral Sphincter

**Genotype Analysis**
by Nucleic Acid
Hepatitis C Virus . . . . . . . . . . . . . . . . . 87902

HIV-1 . . . . . . . . . . . . . . . . . . . . . . . . . . . . 87906
Protease/Reverse Transcriptase
Regions . . . . . . . . . . . . . . . . . . . . 87901
Vancomycin Resistance . . . . . . . . . . . 87500

**Gentamicin** . . . . . . . . . . . . . . . . . 80170
Assay . . . . . . . . . . . . . . . . . . . . . . . . . . . . 80170

**Gentamycin Level**
*See* Gentamicin

**Gentiobiase**
*See* Beta Glucosidase

**Genus: Human Cytomegalovirus Group**
*See* Cytomegalovirus

**GERD**
*See* Gastroesophageal Reflux Test

**German Measles**
*See* Rubella

**Gestational Trophoblastic Tumor**
*See* Hydatidiform Mole

**GGT**
*See* Gamma Glutamyl Transferase

**GI Tract**
*See* Gastrointestinal Tract

**Giardia**
Antigen Detection
Enzyme Immunoassay . . . . . . . . . . . . . 87329
Immunofluorescence . . . . . . . . . . . . . . 87269

**Giardia Lamblia**
Antibody . . . . . . . . . . . . . . . . . . . . . . . . . 86674

**Gibbons Stent** . . . . . . . . . . . . . . . 52332

**GIF**
*See* Somatostatin

**GIFT**
*See* Gamete Intrafallopian Transfer

**Gill Operation** . . . . . . . . . . . . . . . 63012

**Gillies Approach**
Fracture
Zygomatic Arch . . . . . . . . . . . . . . . . . 21356

**Gingiva**
*See* Gums

**Gingiva, Abscess**
*See* Abscess
Fracture
*See* Abscess, Gums;Gums
Zygomatic Arch
*See* Abscess, Gums; Gums, Abscess

**Gingivectomy** . . . . . . . . . . . . . . . 41820

**Gingivoplasty** . . . . . . . . . . . . . . . 41872

**Girdlestone Laminectomy**
*See* Laminectomy

**Girdlestone Procedure**
*See* Acetabulum, Reconstruction

**Gla Protein (Bone)**
*See* Osteocalcin

**Gland**
*See* Specific Gland

**Gland, Adrenal**
*See* Adrenal Gland

**Gland, Bartholin's**
*See* Bartholin's Gland

**Gland, Bulbourethral**
*See* Bulbourethral Gland

**Gland, Lacrimal**
*See* Lacrimal Gland

**Gland, Mammary**
*See* Breast

**Gland, Parathyroid**
*See* Parathyroid Gland

**Gland, Parotid**
*See* Parotid Gland

**Gland, Pituitary**
*See* Pituitary Gland

**Gland, Salivary**
*See* Salivary Glands

**Gland, Sublingual**
*See* Sublingual Gland

**Gland, Sweat**
*See* Sweat Glands

**Gland, Thymus**
*See* Thymus Gland

**Gland, Thyroid**
*See* Thyroid Gland

**Glasses**
*See* Spectacle Services

**Glaucoma**
Cryotherapy . . . . . . . . . . . . . . . . . . . . . . 66720
Cyclophotocoagulation . . . . . . . . . . 66710-66711
Diathermy . . . . . . . . . . . . . . . . . . . . . . . 66700
Fistulization of Sclera . . . . . . . . . . . . . . 66150
Provocative Test . . . . . . . . . . . . . . . . . . 92140

**Glaucoma Drainage Implant**
*See* Aqueous Shunt

**Glenn Procedure** . . . . . . . . . 33766-33767

**Glenohumeral Joint**
Arthrotomy . . . . . . . . . . . . . . . . . . . . . . 23040
with Biopsy . . . . . . . . . . . . . . . . . . . . 23100
with Synovectomy . . . . . . . . . . . . . . . 23105
Exploration . . . . . . . . . . . . . . . . . . . . . . 23107
Removal
Foreign or Loose Body . . . . . . . . . . . . 23107

**Glenoid Fossa**
Reconstruction . . . . . . . . . . . . . . . . . . . 21255

**GLN**
*See* Glutamine

**Globulin**
Antihuman . . . . . . . . . . . . . . . . . . 86880-86886
Immune . . . . . . . . . . . . . . . . . . . . 90281-90399
Sex Hormone Binding . . . . . . . . . . . . . . 84270

**Globulin, Corticosteroid-Binding**
*See* Transcortin

**Globulin, Rh Immune**
*See* Immune Globulins, Rho (D)

**Globulin, Thyroxine-Binding**
See Thyroxine Binding Globulin

**Glomerular Procoagulant Activity**
See Thromboplastin

**Glomus Caroticum**
See Carotid Body

**Glossectomies**
See Excision, Tongue

**Glossopexy**
See Tongue, Fixation

**Glossorrhaphy**
See Suture, Tongue

**Glucagon**............................82943
Tolerance Panel ................. 80422-80424
Tolerance Test .......................... 82946

**Glucose** ........ 80422-80424, 80430-80435,
                                    95250-95251
Blood Test.............. 82947-82950, 82962
Body Fluid............................. 82945
Interstitial Fluid
   Continuous Monitoring ........ 95250-95251
Tolerance Test ................. 82951-82952
   with Tolbutamide................... 82953

**Glucose Phosphate Isomerase**
See Phosphohexose Isomerase

**Glucose Phosphate Isomerase Measurement**
See Phosphohexose Isomerase

**Glucose-6-Phosphate**
Dehydrogenase ................. 82955-82960

**Glucosidase** ....................82963

**Glucuronide Androstanediol** ...82154

**Glue**
Cornea Wound....................... 65286
Sclera Wound........................ 65286

**Glukagon**
See Glucagon

**Glutamate Dehydrogenase**
Blood................................82965

**Glutamate Pyruvate Transaminase**
See Transaminase, Glutamic Pyruvic

**Glutamic Alanine Transaminase**
See Transaminase, Glutamic Pyruvic

**Glutamic Aspartic Transaminase**
See Transaminase, Glutamic Oxaloacetic

**Glutamic Dehydrogenase**
See Glutamate Dehydrogenase

**Glutamine**....................82975

**Glutamyltransferase, Gamma**....................82977

**Glutathione**....................82978

**Glutathione Reductase**....82979

**Glutethimide**....................82980

**Glycanhydrolase, N-Acetylmuramide**
See Lysozyme

**Glycated Hemoglobins**
See Glycohemoglobin

**Glycated Protein** ..............82985

**Glycerol Phosphoglycerides**
See Phosphatidylglycerol

**Glycerol, Phosphatidyl**
See Phosphatidylglycerol

**Glycerophosphatase**
See Alkaline Phosphatase

**Glycinate, Theophylline Sodium**
See Theophylline

**Glycocholic Acid**
See Cholylglycine

**Glycohemoglobin** ..............83036

**Glycol, Ethylene**
See Ethylene Glycol

**Glycols, Ethylene**
See Ethylene Glycol

**Glycosaminoglycan**
See Mucopolysaccharides

**GMP**
See Guanosine Monophosphate

**GMP, Cyclic**
See Cyclic GMP

**Goeckerman Treatment** ... 96910-96913

**Gol-Vernet Operation**
See Pyelotomy, Exploration

**Gold**
Assay ............................. 80172

**Goldwaite Procedure** ..........27422

**Golfer's Elbow**
See Tennis Elbow

**Gonadectomy, Female**
See Oophorectomy

**Gonadectomy, Male**
See Excision, Testis

**Gonadotropin**
Chorionic...................... 84702-84704
FSH ............................... 83001
ICSH .............................. 83002
LH ................................ 83002

**Gonadotropin Panel**..........80426

**Gonioscopy** ..................92020

**Goniotomy** ..................65820

**Gonococcus**
See Neisseria Gonorrhoeae

**Goodenough Harris Drawing Test**..................... 96101-96103

**GOTT**
See Transaminase, Glutamic Oxaloacetic

**GPUT**
See Galactose-1-Phosphate, Uridyl Transferase

**Graft**
See Bone Graft; Bypass Graft
Anal.............................. 46753
Aorta.............. 33840-33851, 33860-33877
Artery
   Coronary.................. 33503-33505
Bone
   See Bone Marrow, Transplantation
   Harvesting ................. 20900-20902
   Microvascular/Anastomosis .... 20955-20962
   Osteocutaneous Flap with
   MicrovascularAnastomosis ..... 20969-20973
   Vascular Pedicle................. 25430
   Vertebra ........................ 0222T
      Cervical....................... 0219T
      Lumbar....................... 0221T
      Thoracic...................... 0220T
Bone and Skin ............... 20969-20973
Cartilage
   Costochondral ................. 20910
   Ear to Face .................... 21235
   Harvesting ................. 20910-20912
      See Cartilage Graft
   Rib to Face .................... 21230
Conjunctiva....................... 65782
   Harvesting ..................... 68371
Cornea
   with Lesion Excision ........... 65426
Cornea Transplant
   Allograft Preparation.....0289T-0290T, 65757
   Endothelial..................... 65756
   in Aphakia ..................... 65750
   in Pseudophakia................. 65755
   Lamellar
      Anterior..................... 65710
      Penetrating.................. 65730
Dura
   Spinal Cord.................... 63710
Endovascular ..................... 34900
Eye
   Amniotic Membrane .......... 65778-65780
   Conjunctiva ................... 65782
   Stem Cell ...................... 65781
Facial Nerve Paralysis .......... 15840-15845
Fascia
   Cheek........................ 15840
Fascia Lata
   Harvesting ................. 20920-20922
Gum Mucosa ..................... 41870
Heart
   See Heart, Transplantation
Heart Lung
   See Transplantation, Heart-Lung
Kidney
   See Kidney, Transplantation
Liver
   See Liver, Transplantation
Lung
   See Lung, Transplantation
Muscle
   Cheek........................ 15841-15845
Nail Bed
   Reconstruction.................. 11762
Nerve ...................... 64885-64907
Oral Mucosa...................... 40818
Organ
   See Transplantation
Pancreas
   See Pancreas, Transplantation

Skin
　Biological
　　*See* Allograft, Skin
　Blood Flow Check, Graft . . . . . . . . . . . 15860
　　*See* Skin Graft and Flap
　Harvesting
　　for Tissue Culture . . . . . . . . . . . . . . . 15040
　Vascular Flow Check, Graft . . . . . . . . . . 15860
Tendon
　Finger . . . . . . . . . . . . . . . . . . . . . . . 26392
　Hand . . . . . . . . . . . . . . . . . . . . . . . . 26392
　Harvesting . . . . . . . . . . . . . . . . . . . . 20924
Tissue
　Harvesting . . . . . . . . . . . . . . . . . . . . 20926
Vein
　Cross-Over . . . . . . . . . . . . . . . . . . . . 34520

**Grain Alcohol**
*See* Alcohol, Ethyl

**Granulation Tissue**
Cauterization, Chemical . . . . . . . . . . . . . 17250

**Gravi, Myasthenia**
*See* Myasthenia Gravis

**Gravities, Specific**
*See* Specific Gravity

**Great Toe**
Free Osteocutaneous Flap with
Microvascular Anastomosis . . . . . . . . . . . 20973

**Great Vessels**
Shunt
　Aorta to Pulmonary Artery
　　Ascending . . . . . . . . . . . . . . . . . . . 33755
　　Descending . . . . . . . . . . . . . . . . . . 33762
　Central . . . . . . . . . . . . . . . . . . . . . . 33764
　Subclavian to Pulmonary Artery . . . . . . 33750
　Vena Cava to Pulmonary
　Artery . . . . . . . . . . . . . . 33766-33767
Unlisted Services and Procedures . . . . . . 33999

**Great Vessels Transposition**
*See* Transposition, Great Arteries

**Greater Tuberosity Fracture**
with Shoulder Dislocation
　Closed Treatment . . . . . . . . . . . . . . . 23665
　Open Treatment . . . . . . . . . . . . . . . . 23670

**Greater Vestibular Gland**
*See* Bartholin's Gland

**Green Operation**
*See* Scapulopexy

**Grippe, Balkan**
*See* Q Fever

**Gritti Operation**
*See* Amputation, Leg, Upper; Radical Resection;
Replantation

**Groin Area**
Repair
　Hernia . . . . . . . . . . . . . . . 49550-49557

**Group Health Education** . . . . . . . . . . 98961-98962, 99078

**Grouping, Blood**
*See* Blood Typing

**Growth Factors, Insulin-Like**
*See* Somatomedin

**Growth Hormone** . . . . . . . . . . . . . . . 83003
Human . . . . . . . . . . . 80418, 80428-80430, 86277

**Growth Hormone Release Inhibiting Factor**
*See* Somatostatin

**GTT**
*See* Hydatidiform Mole

**Guaiac Test**
*See* Blood, Feces

**Guanosine Monophosphate** . . . . 83008

**Guanosine Monophosphate, Cyclic**
*See* Cyclic GMP

**Guanylic Acids**
*See* Guanosine Monophosphate

**Guard Stain** . . . . . . . . . . . . . . . . . . . 88313

**Gullet**
*See* Esophagus

**Gums**
Abscess
　Incision and Drainage . . . . . . . . . . . . 41800
Alveolus
　Excision . . . . . . . . . . . . . . . . . . . . . 41830
Cyst
　Incision and Drainage . . . . . . . . . . . . 41800
Excision
　Gingiva . . . . . . . . . . . . . . . . . . . . . 41820
　Operculum . . . . . . . . . . . . . . . . . . . 41821
Graft
　Mucosa . . . . . . . . . . . . . . . . . . . . . 41870
Hematoma
　Incision and Drainage . . . . . . . . . . . . 41800
Lesion
　Destruction . . . . . . . . . . . . . . . . . . . 41850
　Excision . . . . . . . . . . . . . . 41822-41828
Mucosa
　Excision . . . . . . . . . . . . . . . . . . . . . 41828
Reconstruction
　Alveolus . . . . . . . . . . . . . . . . . . . . . 41874
　Gingiva . . . . . . . . . . . . . . . . . . . . . 41872
Removal
　Foreign Body . . . . . . . . . . . . . . . . . 41805
Tumor
　Excision . . . . . . . . . . . . . . 41825-41827
Unlisted Services and Procedures . . . . . . 41899

**Gunning-Lieben Test**
*See* Acetone, Blood or Urine

**Guthrie Test** . . . . . . . . . . . . . . . . . . . 84030

# H

**H Flu**
*See* Hemophilus Influenza

**H1N1**
Immunization
　*See* Vaccines

**H-Reflex Study** . . . . . . . . . . 95934-95936

**HAA (Hepatitis Associated Antigen)**
*See* Hepatitis Antigen, B Surface

**HAAb**
*See* Antibody, Hepatitis

**Haemoglobin F**
*See* Fetal Hemoglobin

**Haemorrhage**
*See* Hemorrhage

**Haemorrhage Rectum**
*See* Hemorrhage, Rectum

**Hageman Factor** . . . . . . . . . . . . . . . 85280

**HAI Test**
*See* Hemagglutination Inhibition Test

**Hair**
Electrolysis . . . . . . . . . . . . . . . . . . . . 17380
KOH Examination . . . . . . . . . . . . . . . . 87220
Microscopic Evaluation . . . . . . . . . . . . 96902
Transplant
　Punch Graft . . . . . . . . . . . . 15775-15776
　Strip Graft . . . . . . . . . . . . . 15220-15221

**Hair Removal**
*See* Removal, Hair

**Hallux**
*See* Great Toe

**Halo**
Body Cast . . . . . . . . . . . . . . . . . . . . . 29000
Cranial . . . . . . . . . . . . . . . . . . . . . . . 20661
　for Thin Skull Osteology . . . . . . . . . . 20664
Femur . . . . . . . . . . . . . . . . . . . . . . . 20663
Maxillofacial . . . . . . . . . . . . . . . . . . . 21100
Pelvic . . . . . . . . . . . . . . . . . . . . . . . . 20662
Removal . . . . . . . . . . . . . . . . . . . . . . 20665

**Haloperidol**
Assay . . . . . . . . . . . . . . . . . . . . . . . . 80173

**Halstead-Reitan Neuropsychological Battery** . . . 96118

**Halsted Mastectomy**
*See* Mastectomy, Radical

**Halsted Repair**
*See* Hernia, Repair, Inguinal

**Ham Test**
*See* Hemolysins

**Hammertoe Repair** . . . . . . . . 28285-28286

**Hamster Penetration Test** . . . . . . 89329

**Hand**
*See* Carpometacarpal Joint; Intercarpal Joint
Amputation
　at Metacarpal . . . . . . . . . . . . . . . . . 25927
　at Wrist . . . . . . . . . . . . . . . . . . . . . 25920
　　Revision . . . . . . . . . . . . . . . . . . . 25922
　Revision . . . . . . . . . . . 25924, 25929-25931
Arthrodesis
　Carpometacarpal Joint . . . . . . . . 26843-26844
　Intercarpal Joint . . . . . . . . . . . 25820-25825
Bone
　Incision and Drainage . . . . . . . . . . . . 26034
Cast . . . . . . . . . . . . . . . . . . . . . . . . . 29085
Decompression . . . . . . . . . . . . . . 26035-26037

Fracture
  Carpometacarpal . . . . . . . . . . . . 26641-26650
  Interphalangeal . . . . . . . . . . . . . 26740-26746
  Metacarpal. . . . . . . . . . . . . . . . 26600-26615
  Metacarpophalangeal . . . . . . . . 26740-26746
  Phalangeal . . . . . . .26720-26735, 26750-26765
Insertion
  Tendon Graft . . . . . . . . . . . . . . . . . . . . 26392
Magnetic Resonance Imaging
(MRI) . . . . . . . . . . . . . . . . . . . . . . . 73218-73223
Reconstruction
  Tendon Pulley. . . . . . . . . . . . . . 26500-26502
Removal
  Implantation. . . . . . . . . . . . . . . . . . . . . 26320
  Tube/Rod . . . . . . . . . . 26390-26392, 26416
Repair
  Blood Vessel. . . . . . . . . . . . . . . . . . . . . 35207
  Cleft Hand . . . . . . . . . . . . . . . . . . . . . . 26580
  Muscle. . . . . . . . . . . . . . . . . . . . . 26591-26593
  Tendon
    Extensor . . . . . . . . . . . . . . . . 26410-26416,
            26426-26428, 26433-26437
    Flexor . . . . . . . . . . . . . 26350-26358, 26440
    Profundus . . . . . . . . . . . . . . . 26370-26373
Replantation. . . . . . . . . . . . . . . . . . . . . . . 20808
Strapping . . . . . . . . . . . . . . . . . . . . . . . . . 29280
Tendon
  Excision . . . . . . . . . . . . . . . . . . . . . . . . 26390
  Extensor . . . . . . . . . . . . . . . . . . . . . . . 26415
Tenotomy . . . . . . . . . . . . . . . . . . 26450, 26460
Tumor
  Excision . . . . . . . . . . . . . . . . . . 26115-26116
  Radical Resection . . . . . . 26117-26118, 26250
Unlisted Services and Procedures . . . . . . . . 26989
X-ray . . . . . . . . . . . . . . . . . . . . . . . . 73120-73130

**Hand Abscess**
See Abscess, Hand

**Hand Phalange**
See Finger, Bone

**Hand(s) Dupuytrens Contracture(s)**
See Dupuytren's Contracture

**Handling**
Device. . . . . . . . . . . . . . . . . . . . . . . . . . . . 99002
Radioelement. . . . . . . . . . . . . . . . . . . . . . 77790
Specimen . . . . . . . . . . . . . . . . . . . 99000-99001

**Hanganutziu Deicher Antibodies**
See Antibody, Heterophile

**Haptoglobin**. . . . . . . . . . . . . . . 83010-83012

**Hard Palate**
See Palate

**Harelip Operation**
See Cleft Lip, Repair

**Harii Procedure** . . . . . . . . . . . . . . .25430

**Harrington Rod**
Insertion . . . . . . . . . . . . . . . . . . . . . . . . . 22840
Removal . . . . . . . . . . . . . . . . . . . . . . . . . 22850

**Hartmann Procedure**
Laparoscopic . . . . . . . . . . . . . . . . . . . . . . 44206
Open . . . . . . . . . . . . . . . . . . . . . . . . . . . . 44143

**Harvest of Upper Extremity Artery
for Coronary Artery Bypass** . . . . .35600

**Harvesting**
Bone Graft . . . . . . . . . . . . . . . . . . 20900-20902

Bone Marrow
  Allogeneic . . . . . . . . . . . . . . . . . . . . . . 38230
  Autologous. . . . . . . . . . . . . . . . . . . . . . 38232
Cartilage Graft . . . . . . . . . . . . . . . 20910-20912
Conjunctival Graft . . . . . . . . . . . . . . . . . 68371
Eggs
  In Vitro Fertilization . . . . . . . . . . . . . . . 58970
Endoscopic
  Vein for Bypass Graft. . . . . . . . . . . . . . 33508
Fascia Lata Graft . . . . . . . . . . . . . . 20920-20922
Intestines . . . . . . . . . . . . . . . . . . . 44132-44133
Kidney . . . . . . . . . . . . 50300-50320, 50547
Liver . . . . . . . . . . . . . . . . 47133, 47140-47142
Lower Extremity Vein
  for Vascular Reconstruction. . . . . . . . . 35572
Skin
  for Tissue Culture. . . . . . . . . . . . . . . . . 15040
Stem Cell . . . . . . . . . . . . . . . . . . 38205-38206
Tendon Graft. . . . . . . . . . . . . . . . . . . . . . 20924
Tissue Grafts . . . . . . . . . . . . . . . . . . . . . 20926
Upper Extremity Artery
  for Coronary Artery Bypass Graft. . . . . . 35600
Upper Extremity Vein
  for Bypass Graft . . . . . . . . . . . . . . . . . . 35500

**Hauser Procedure**. . . . . . . . . . . .27420

**Hayem's Elementary Corpuscle**
See Blood, Platelet

**Haygroves Procedure**
See Reconstruction, Acetabulum; Revision

**HBA1/HBA2**. . . . . . . . . . . . . . . . . . .81257

**HBcAb**
See Antibody, Hepatitis

**HBeAb**
See Antibody, Hepatitis

**HBeAg**
See Hepatitis Antigen, Be

**HBsAb**
See Antibody, Hepatitis

**HBsAg (Hepatitis B Surface
Antigen)**
See Hepatitis Antigen, B Surface

**HCG**
See Chorionic Gonadotropin

**HCO3**
See Bicarbonate

**HCV Antibodies**
See Antibody, Hepatitis C

**HDL**
See Lipoprotein

**Head**
Angiography. . . . . . . . . . . . . 70496, 70544-70546
CT Scan. . . . . . . . . . . . . . . 70450-70470, 70496
Excision. . . . . . . . . . . . . . . . . . . 21011-21070
Fracture and/or Dislocation. . . . . . . 21310-21497
Incision . . . . . . . . . . . . . . 21010, 61316, 62148
Introduction or Removal . . . . . . . . 21076-21116
Lipectomy, Suction Assisted . . . . . . . . . . 15876
Magnetic Resonance Angiography
(MRA) . . . . . . . . . . . . . . . . . . . . . 70544-70546
Nerve
  Graft. . . . . . . . . . . . . . . . . . . . . 64885-64886
Other Procedures . . . . . . . . . . . . . 21299, 21499

Repair/Revision and/or
Reconstruction. . . . . . . . . . . . . . . . 21120-21296
Ultrasound Exam . . . . . . . . . . . . . . 76506, 76536
Unlisted Services and Procedures . . . . . . . 21499
X-ray . . . . . . . . . . . . . . . . . . . . . . . . . . . 70350

**Head Rings, Stereotactic**
See Stereotactic Frame

**Headbrace**
Application . . . . . . . . . . . . . . . . . . . . . . . 21100
Application/Removal . . . . . . . . . . . . . . . . 20661

**Heaf Test**
See TB Test

**Health Behavior**
See Evaluation and Management, Health Behavior

**Health Risk Assessment Instrument**
See Preventive Medicine

**Hearing Aid**
Bone Conduction
  Implantation. . . . . . . . . . . . . . . . . . . . . 69710
  Removal. . . . . . . . . . . . . . . . . . . . . . . . 69711
  Repair. . . . . . . . . . . . . . . . . . . . . . . . . . 69711
  Replacement . . . . . . . . . . . . . . . . . . . . 69710

**Hearing Aid Check** . . . . . . . 92592-92593

**Hearing Aid Services**
Electroacoustic Test. . . . . . . . . . . . 92594-92595
Examination . . . . . . . . . . . . . . . . . 92590-92591

**Hearing Tests**
See Audiologic Function Tests

**Hearing Therapy**. . . . . . . . . 92507-92508,
                                    92601-92604

**Heart**
Ablation . . . . . . . . . . . . . . . . . . . . 33250-33266
Allograft Preparation . . . . . . . . . . . . . . . . 33933
Acoustic Cardiography with Automated
Analysis . . . . . . . . . . . . . . . . . . . .0223T-0225T
Angiography
  Injection . . . . . . . . . . . . . . . . . . . 93565-93566
    See Cardiac Catheterization; Injection
Aortic Arch
  with Cardiopulmonary Bypass. . . . . . . . 33853
  without Cardiopulmonary Bypass . . . . . 33852
Aortic Valve
  Implantation
    Endovascular Approach . . . . . . . . . . . 0256T
    Open Thoracic Approach . . . . . . . . . . 0257T
  Repair
    Left Ventricle . . . . . . . . . . . . . . . . . . 33414
  Replacement . . . . . . . . . . . . . . . 33405-33413
    with Cardiopulmonary
    Bypass . . . . . . . .0259T, 33405-33406, 33410
    without Cardiopulmonary Bypass . . . . 0258T
Arrhythmogenic Focus
  Catheter Ablation. . . . . . . . . . . . . 93650-93652
  Destruction. . . . . . . . . . . 33250-33251, 33261
Atria
  See Atria
Biopsy . . . . . . . . . . . . . . . . . . . . . . . . . . 93505
  Imaging Guidance . . . . . . . . . . . . . . . . 76932
  Ultrasound
    Imaging Guidance. . . . . . . . . . . . . . . 76932
Blood Vessel
  Repair. . . . . . . . . . . . . . . . . . . . . 33320-33322
Cardiac Output Measurements. . . . . . . 93451,
                                    93561-93562
Cardiac Rehabilitation. . . . . . . . . . . 93797-93798
Cardioassist . . . . . . . . . . . . . . . . . 92970-92971

Tricuspid Valve
   *See* Tricuspid Valve
Tumor
     Excision . . . . . . . . . . . . . . . . . . 33120-33130
Unlisted Services and Procedures . . . . . . . . 33999
Ventricular Assist Device (VAD)
     Interrogation and Programming. . . . . . . . 93750
Ventriculography
   *See* Ventriculography
Ventriculomyectomy . . . . . . . . . . . . . . . . . . 33416
Wound
     Repair. . . . . . . . . . . . . . . . . . . . . 33300-33305

## Heart Sounds
Acoustic Cardiography with Automated
Analysis . . . . . . . . . . . . . . . . . . . . . . . .0223T-0225T
Acoustic Recording
     with Computer Analysis. . . . . . . . . . . . . 93799

## Heart Vessels
Angioplasty
     Percutaneous . . . . . . . . . . . . . . . 92982-92984
     *See* Angioplasty; Percutaneous Transluminal
       Angioplasty
Insertion
     Graft. . . . . . . . . . . . . . . . . . . . . 33330-33335
Thrombolysis . . . . . . . . . . . . . . . . . . 92975-92977
Valvuloplasty
   *See* Valvuloplasty
     Percutaneous . . . . . . . . . . . . . . . 92986-92990

## Heat Unstable Haemoglobin
*See* Hemoglobin, Thermolabile

## Heavy Lipoproteins
*See* Lipoprotein

## Heavy Metal . . . . . . . . . . . . . . 83015-83018

## Heel
*See* Calcaneus
Collection of Blood. . . . . . . . . . . . . . 36415-36416
X-ray . . . . . . . . . . . . . . . . . . . . . . . . . . . . 73650

## Heel Bone
*See* Calcaneus

## Heel Fracture
*See* Calcaneus, Fracture

## Heel Spur
Excision. . . . . . . . . . . . . . . . . . . . . . . . . . 28119

## Heine-Medin Disease
*See* Polio

## Heinz Bodies . . . . . . . . . . . . . 85441-85445

## Helicobacter Pylori
Antibody. . . . . . . . . . . . . . . . . . . . . . . . . . 86677
Antigen Detection
     Enzyme Immunoassay . . . . . . . . . 87338-87339
Blood Test. . . . . . . . . . . . . . . . . . . . . . . . . 83009
Breath Test . . . . . . . . 78267-78268, 83013-83014
Stool . . . . . . . . . . . . . . . . . . . . . . . . . . . . 87338
Urease Activity. . . . . . . . . . 83009, 83013-83014

## Heller Operation
*See* Esophagomyotomy

## Heller Procedure . . . . . . . . 32665, 43279,
                          43330-43331

## Helminth
Antibody. . . . . . . . . . . . . . . . . . . . . . . . . . 86682

## Hemagglutination Inhibition
## Test . . . . . . . . . . . . . . . . . . . . . . . . . . . .86280

## Hemangioma
*See* Lesion, Skin; Tumor

## Hemapheresis
*See* Apheresis

## Hematochezia
*See* Blood, Feces

## Hematologic Test
*See* Blood Tests

## Hematology
Unlisted Services and Procedures . . . . . . . . 85999

## Hematoma
Ankle. . . . . . . . . . . . . . . . . . . . . . . . . . . . 27603
Arm, Lower. . . . . . . . . . . . . . . . . . . . . . . . 25028
Arm, Upper
     Incision and Drainage . . . . . . . . . . . . . 23930
Brain
     Drainage. . . . . . . . . . . . . . . . . . 61154-61156
     Evacuation . . . . . . . . . . . . . . . . 61312-61315
     Incision and Drainage . . . . . . . . 61312-61315
Drain. . . . . . . . . . . . . . . . . . . . . . . . . . . . 61108
Ear, External
     Complicated. . . . . . . . . . . . . . . . . . . . . 69005
     Simple . . . . . . . . . . . . . . . . . . . . . . . . 69000
Elbow
     Incision and Drainage . . . . . . . . . . . . . 23930
Epididymis
     Incision and Drainage . . . . . . . . . . . . . 54700
Gums
     Incision and Drainage . . . . . . . . . . . . . 41800
Hip. . . . . . . . . . . . . . . . . . . . . . . . . . . . . 26990
Incision and Drainage
     Neck. . . . . . . . . . . . . . . . . . . . 21501-21502
     Skin . . . . . . . . . . . . . . . . . . . . . . . . . 10140
     Thorax . . . . . . . . . . . . . . . . . . 21501-21502
Knee . . . . . . . . . . . . . . . . . . . . . . . . . . . . 27301
Leg, Lower . . . . . . . . . . . . . . . . . . . . . . . . 27603
Leg, Upper . . . . . . . . . . . . . . . . . . . . . . . . 27301
Mouth . . . . . . . . . . .41005-41009, 41015-41018
     Incision and Drainage . . . . . . . . 40800-40801
Nasal Septum
     Incision and Drainage . . . . . . . . . . . . . 30020
Nose
     Incision and Drainage . . . . . . . . 30000-30020
Pelvis. . . . . . . . . . . . . . . . . . . . . . . . . . . . 26990
Scrotum
     Incision and Drainage . . . . . . . . . . . . . 54700
Shoulder
     Drainage. . . . . . . . . . . . . . . . . . . . . . . 23030
Skin
     Incision and Drainage . . . . . . . . . . . . . 10140
     Puncture Aspiration . . . . . . . . . . . . . . . 10160
Subdural . . . . . . . . . . . . . . . . . . . . . . . . . 61108
Subungual
     Evacuation . . . . . . . . . . . . . . . . . . . . . 11740
Testis
     Incision and Drainage . . . . . . . . . . . . . 54700
Tongue . . . . . . . . . . . . . . 41000-41006, 41015
Vagina
     Incision and Drainage . . . . . . . . 57022-57023
Wrist. . . . . . . . . . . . . . . . . . . . . . . . . . . . 25028

## Hematopoietic Stem Cell
## Transplantation
*See* Stem Cell, Transplantation

## Hematopoietin
*See* Erythropoietin

## Hematuria
*See* Blood, Urine

## Hemic System
Unlisted Procedure. . . . . . . . . . . . . . . . . . . 38999

## Hemiepiphyseal Arrest
Elbow . . . . . . . . . . . . . . . . . . . . . . . . . . . 24470

## Hemifacial Microsomia
Reconstruction
     Mandibular Condyle. . . . . . . . . . . . . . . . 21247

## Hemilaminectomy . . . . . . . . . 63020-63044

## Hemilaryngectomy . . . . . . . 31370-31382

## Hemipelvectomies
*See* Amputation, Interpelviabdominal

## Hemiphalangectomy
Toe . . . . . . . . . . . . . . . . . . . . . . . . . . . . . 28160

## Hemispherectomy
Partial . . . . . . . . . . . . . . . . . . . . . . . . . . . 61543
Total . . . . . . . . . . . . . . . . . . . . . . . . . . . . 61542

## Hemocytoblast
*See* Stem Cell

## Hemodialyses
*See* Hemodialysis

## Hemodialysis . . . . . . . . . . . 90935-90937
Blood Flow Study. . . . . . . . . . . . . . . . . . . . 90940
Duplex Scan of Access . . . . . . . . . . . . . . . 93990
Kt/V Level. . . . . . . . . . . . . . . . . . . . . 3082F-3084F
Plan of Care Documented . . . . . . . . . . . . . 0505F
via Catheter . . . . . . . . . . . . . . . . . . . . . . . 4054F
via Functioning Arteriovenous Fistula . . . . . 4052F
via Functioning Arteriovenous Graft. . . . . . . 4053F

## Hemofiltration . . . . . . . . . . . 90945-90947

## Hemoglobin
A1c (HbA1c) Level . . . . . . . . . . . . . . 3044F-3045F
Analysis
     O2 Affinity . . . . . . . . . . . . . . . . . . . . . 82820
Carboxyhemoglobin . . . . . . . . 82375-82376, 88740
Chromatography. . . . . . . . . . . . . . . . . . . . 83021
Concentration. . . . . . . . . . . . . . . . . . . . . . 85046
Electrophoresis. . . . . . . . . . . . . . . . . . . . . 83020
Fetal . . . . . . . . . . . .83030-83033, 85460-85461
Fractionation and Quantitation. . . . . . . . . . 83020
Glycosylated (A1C). . . . . . . . . . . . . . 83036-83037
Hgb
     Transcutaneous Testing . . . . . . . . . . . . 88738
Methemoglobin . . . . . . . . . . . . . . . . 83045-83050
     Transcutaneous . . . . . . . . . . . . . . . . . . 88741
Non-Automated . . . . . . . . . . . . . . . . . . . . 83026
Plasma . . . . . . . . . . . . . . . . . . . . . . . . . . 83051
Sulfhemoglobin . . . . . . . . . . . . . . . . 83055-83060
Thermolabile . . . . . . . . . . . . . . . . . . 83065-83068
Transcutaneous . . . . . . . . . . . . . . . . . . . . 88740
Urine . . . . . . . . . . . . . . . . . . . . . . . . . . . . 83069

## Hemoglobin F
Fetal
     Chemical . . . . . . . . . . . . . . . . . . . . . . 83030
     Qualitative . . . . . . . . . . . . . . . . . . . . . 83033

## Hemoglobin, Glycosylated
*See* Glycohemoglobin

## Hemogram
Added Indices. . . . . . . . . . . . . . . . 85025-85027
Automated . . . . . . . . . . . . . . . . . . 85025-85027
Manual . . . . . . . . . . . . . . . . 85014-85018, 85032

## Hemolysins . . . . . . . . . . . . . . . . . . .85475
with Agglutinins. . . . . . . . . . . . . . . . 86940-86941

## HIV-1
Antigen Detection
  Enzyme Immunoassay .............. 87390

## HIV-2
Antigen Detection
  Enzyme Immunoassay .............. 87391

## HK3 Kallikrein
*See* Antigen, Prostate Specific

## HLA
Crossmatch .................... 86825, 86826
Molecular Pathology ............ 81370-81383
Typing .................... 86812-86822

## HMRK
*See* Fitzgerald Factor

## HMW Kininogen
*See* Fitzgerald Factor

## Hoffman Apparatus ............. 20690

## Hofmeister Operation
*See* Gastrectomy, Total

## Holotranscobalamin ............ 0103T

## Holten Test
*See* Creatinine, Urine, Clearance

## Home Services
Activities of Daily Living ............... 99509
Anticoagulant Management ....... 99363-99364
Apnea Monitoring ............... 94774-94777
Catheter Care ...................... 99507
Enema Administration ................. 99511
Established Patient .............. 99347-99350
Hemodialysis ....................... 99512
Home Infusion Procedures ........ 99601-99602
Individual or Family Counseling .......... 99510
Intramuscular Injections ............... 99506
Mechanical Ventilation ................ 99504
New Patient ..................... 99341-99345
Newborn Care ...................... 99502
Postnatal Assessment ................. 99501
Prenatal Monitoring .................. 99500
Respiratory Therapy .................. 99503
Sleep Studies ................... 95805-95811
  Actigraphy Testing ................. 95803
Stoma Care ........................ 99505
Unlisted Services and Procedures ........ 99600
Ventilation Assist .................... 94005

## Home Visit
*See* House Calls

## Homocyst(e)ine ................ 83090
Urine ............................. 82615

## Homogenization, Tissue ....... 87176

## Homologous Grafts
*See* Graft

## Homologous Transplantation
*See* Homograft

## Homovanillic Acid
Urine ............................. 83150

## Hormone Assay
ACTH ............................. 82024
Aldosterone
  Blood or Urine ..................... 82088
Androstenedione
  Blood or Urine ..................... 82157

Androsterone
  Blood or Urine ..................... 82160
Angiotensin II ...................... 82163
Corticosterone ..................... 82528
Cortisol
  Total ............................ 82533
Dehydroepiandrosterone ............. 82626
Dihydroelestosterone ............... 82651
Dihydrotestosterone ................ 82651
Epiandrosterone .................... 82666
Estradiol .......................... 82670
Estriol ............................ 82677
Estrogen .................... 82671-82672
Estrone ........................... 82679
Follicle Stimulating Hormone .......... 83001
Growth Hormone .................... 83003
Hydroxyprogesterone ........... 83498-83499
Luteinizing Hormone ................. 83002
Somatotropin ...................... 83003
Testosterone ....................... 84403
Vasopressin ........................ 84588

## Hormone Pellet Implantation ... 11980

## Hormone, Adrenocorticotrophic
*See* Adrenocorticotropic Hormone (ACTH)

## Hormone, Corticotropin-Releasing
*See* Corticotropic Releasing Hormone (CRH)

## Hormone, Growth
*See* Growth Hormone

## Hormone, Human Growth
*See* Growth Hormone, Human

## Hormone, Interstitial Cell-Stimulating
*See* Luteinizing Hormone (LH)

## Hormone, Parathyroid
*See* Parathormone

## Hormone, Pituitary Lactogenic
*See* Prolactin

## Hormone, Placental Lactogen
*See* Lactogen, Human Placental

## Hormone, Somatotropin Release-Inhibiting
*See* Somatostatin

## Hormone, Thyroid-Stimulating
*See* Thyroid Stimulating Hormone (TSH)

## Hormone-Binding Globulin, Sex
*See* Globulin, Sex Hormone Binding

## Hormones, Adrenal Cortex
*See* Corticosteroids

## Hormones, Antidiuretic
*See* Antidiuretic Hormone

## Hospital Discharge Services
*See* Discharge Services, Hospital

## Hospital Services
Inpatient Services ............... 99238-99239
  Discharge Services .......... 99238-99239,
                                   1110F-1111F
  Initial Care
    New or Established Patient ... 99221-99233
  Initial Hospital Care .......... 99221-99223
  Newborn ............. 99460-99462, 99477
  Prolonged Services .......... 99356-99357
  Subsequent Hospital Care ...... 99231-99233

Observation
  Discharge Services .......... 99234-99236
  Initial Care ................. 99218-99220
Same Day Admission
  Discharge Services .......... 99234-99236
Subsequent Newborn Care ............ 99462

## Hot Pack Treatment ............ 97010
*See* Physical Medicine and Rehabilitation

## House Calls ............... 99341-99350

## HPL
*See* Lactogen, Human Placental

## HTLV I
Antibody
  Confirmatory Test ................. 86689
  Detection ........................ 86687

## HTLV II
Antibody ........................... 86688

## HTLV III
*See* HIV

## HTLV III Antibodies
*See* Antibody, HIV

## HTLV IV
*See* HIV-2

## Hubbard Tank Therapy .......... 97036
*See* Physical Medicine/Therapy/Occupational Therapy

## Hue Test ......................... 92283

## Huggin Operation
*See* Orchiectomy, Simple

## Huhner Test ............... 89300, 89320

## Human Chorionic Gonadotropin
*See* Chorionic Gonadotropin

## Human Chorionic Somatomammotropin
*See* Lactogen, Human Placental

## Human Cytomegalovirus Group
*See* Cytomegalovirus

## Human Epididymis Protein ..... 86305

## Human Growth Hormone (HGH) ............. 80418, 80428-80430

## Human Herpes Virus 4
*See* Epstein-Barr Virus

## Human Immunodeficiency Virus
*See* HIV

## Human Immunodeficiency Virus 1
*See* HIV-1

## Human Immunodeficiency Virus 2
*See* HIV-2

## Human Papillomavirus
*See* Vaccine

## Human Papillomavirus Detection .................. 87620-87622

## Human Placental Lactogen
*See* Lactogen, Human Placental

## Human T Cell Leukemia Virus I
*See* HTLV I

## Human T Cell Leukemia Virus I Antibodies
*See* Antibody, HTLV I

## Human T Cell Leukemia Virus II
*See* HTLV II

## Human T Cell Leukemia Virus II Antibodies
*See* Antibody, HTLV II

## Humeral Epicondylitides, Lateral
*See* Tennis Elbow

## Humeral Fracture
*See* Fracture, Humerus

## Humerus
*See* Arm, Upper; Shoulder
Abscess
　Incision and Drainage . . . . . . . . . . . . . . 23935
Craterization. . . . . . . . . . . . . . . . . . . . 23184, 24140
Cyst
　Excision . . . . . . . . . . . . . . . . . . . 23150, 24110
　　with Allograft . . . . . . . . . . . . . . 23156, 24116
　　with Autograft . . . . . . . . . . . . . 23155, 24115
Diaphysectomy. . . . . . . . . . . . . . . . . . . 23184, 24140
Excision. . . . . . . . . . . . . . . 23174, 23184, 23195,
　　　　　　　　　　　　　　24134, 24140, 24150
Fracture
　Closed Treatment . . . . . . . . . . . . . 24500-24505
　　with Manipulation . . . . . . . . . . . . . . . . 23605
　　without Manipulation. . . . . . . . . . . . 23600
　Condyle
　　Closed Treatment . . . . . . . . . . 24576-24577
　　Open Treatment . . . . . . . . . . . . . . . . . 24579
　　Percutaneous Fixation . . . . . . . . . . . . 24582
　Epicondyle
　　Closed Treatment . . . . . . . . . . 24560-24565
　　Open Treatment . . . . . . . . . . . . . . . . . 24575
　　Skeletal Fixation
　　　Percutaneous . . . . . . . . . . . . . . . . . . 24566
　Greater Tuberosity Fracture
　　Closed Treatment with
　　　Manipulation . . . . . . . . . . . . . . . . . . 23625
　　Closed Treatment without
　　　Manipulation . . . . . . . . . . . . . . . . . . 23620
　　Open Treatment . . . . . . . . . . . . . . . . . 23630
　Open Treatment . . . . . . . . . 23615-23616
　Shaft. . . . . . . . . . . . . . . 24500-24505, 24516
　　Open Treatment . . . . . . . . . . . . . . . . . 24515
　Supracondylar
　　Closed Treatment . . . . . . . . . . 24530-24535
　　Open Treatment . . . . . . . . . . 24545-24546
　　Percutaneous Fixation . . . . . . . . . . . . 24538
　Transcondylar
　　Closed Treatment . . . . . . . . . . 24530-24535
　　Open Treatment . . . . . . . . . . 24545-24546
　　Percutaneous Fixation . . . . . . . . . . . . 24538
　　with Dislocation. . . . . . . . . . . . . 23665-23670
Osteomyelitis . . . . . . . . . . . . . . . . . . . . . . 24134
Pinning, Wiring. . . . . . . . . . . . . 23491, 24498
Prophylactic Treatment . . . . . . . . . . 23491, 24498
Radical Resection . . . . . . . . 23220, 24150, 24152
Repair . . . . . . . . . . . . . . . . . . . . . . . . . . . 24430
　Nonunion, Malunion . . . . . . . . 24430-24435
　Osteoplasty . . . . . . . . . . . . . . . . . . . . 24420
　Osteotomy . . . . . . . . . . . . . . 24400-24410
　　with Graft. . . . . . . . . . . . . . . . . . . . . 24435
Resection Head . . . . . . . . . . . . . . . . . . . 23195
Saucerization . . . . . . . . . . . . . . 23184, 24140
Sequestrectomy . . . . . . . . . . . . . 23174, 24134
Tumor

Excision . . . . . . . . . . . . . . . . . . 23150, 23220,
　　　　　　　　　　24071-24076, 24110
　with Allograft . . . . . . . . . . . . . 23156, 24116
　with Autograft . . . . . . . . . . . . 23155, 24115
X-ray . . . . . . . . . . . . . . . . . . . . . . . . . . . 73060

## Hummelshein Operation
*See* Strabismus, Repair

## Humor Shunt, Aqueous
*See* Aqueous Shunt

## HVA
*See* Homovanillic Acid

## Hybridization Probes, DNA
*See* Nucleic Acid Probe

## Hydatid Disease
*See* Echinococcosis

## Hydatid Mole
*See* Hydatidiform Mole

## Hydatidiform Mole
Evacuation and Curettage . . . . . . . . . . . . . 59870
Excision. . . . . . . . . . . . . . . . . . . . . . . . . 59100

## Hydration . . . . . . . . . . . . . . . 96360-96361
Rehydration Oral Solution . . . . . . . . . . . . 4056F
Status . . . . . . . . . . . . . . . . . . . . . . 2030F-2031F

## Hydrocarbons, Chlorinated
*See* Chlorinated Hydrocarbons

## Hydrocele
Aspiration . . . . . . . . . . . . . . . . . . . . . . . . 55000
Excision
　Bilateral
　　Tunica Vaginalis . . . . . . . . . . . . . . 55041
　Unilateral
　　Spermatic Cord. . . . . . . . . . . . . . . 55500
　　Tunica Vaginalis . . . . . . . . . . . . . . 55040
Repair . . . . . . . . . . . . . . . . . . . . . . . . . . 55060

## Hydrochloric Acid, Gastric
*See* Acid, Gastric

## Hydrochloride, Vancomycin
*See* Vancomycin

## Hydrocodon
*See* Dihydrocodeinone

## Hydrogen Ion Concentration
*See* Blood Gases, pH

## Hydrolase, Acetylcholine
*See* Acetylcholinesterase

## Hydrolase, Triacylglycerol
*See* Lipase

## Hydrolases, Phosphoric Monoester
*See* Phosphatase

## Hydrotherapy (Hubbard Tank) . . . . . . . . . . . . . . . . . . . . . . 97036
*See* Physical Medicine/Therapy/Occupational Therapy

## Hydrotubation . . . . . . . . . . . . . . . 58350

## Hydroxyacetanilide
*See* Acetaminophen

## Hydroxycorticosteroid . . . . . . . . 83491

## Hydroxyindolacetic Acid . . . . . . . 83497
Urine . . . . . . . . . . . . . . . . . . . . . . . . . . . 83497

## Hydroxypregnenolone . . . .80406, 84143

## Hydroxyprogesterone . . . . 80402-80406, 83498-83499

## Hydroxyproline . . . . . . . . . . . 83500-83505

## Hydroxytyramine
*See* Dopamine

## Hygroma
Cystic
　Axillary/Cervical
　　Excision. . . . . . . . . . . . . . . . . 38550-38555

## Hymen
Excision. . . . . . . . . . . . . . . . . . . . . . . . . 56700
Incision . . . . . . . . . . . . . . . . . . . . . . . . . 56442

## Hymenal Ring
Revision . . . . . . . . . . . . . . . . . . . . . . . . . 56700

## Hymenectomy . . . . . . . . . . . . . . . .56700

## Hymenotomy . . . . . . . . . . . . . . . . .56442

## Hyoid
Bone
　Fracture
　　Open Treatment . . . . . . . . . . . . . . 21495
Muscle
　Incision and Suspension . . . . . . . . . . . . 21685

## Hyperbaric Oxygen Pressurization . . . . . . . . . . . . . . . . 99183

## Hypercycloidal X-ray . . . . . 76101-76102

## Hyperdactylies
*See* Supernumerary Digit

## Hyperglycemic Glycogenolytic Factor
*See* Glucagon

## Hyperhidrosis . . . . . . . . . . . . 64650-64653

## Hypertelorism of Orbit
*See* Orbital Hypertelorism

## Hyperthermia Therapy
*See* Thermotherapy

## Hyperthermia Treatment . . . . . . . . . . . . . . . . . 77600-77620

## Hypnotherapy . . . . . . . . . . . . . . . . .90880

## Hypodermis
*See* Subcutaneous Tissue

## Hypogastric Plexus
Destruction. . . . . . . . . . . . . . . . . . . . . . . 64681
Injection
　Anesthetic . . . . . . . . . . . . . . . . . . . . . 64517
　Neurolytic. . . . . . . . . . . . . . . . . . . . . 64681

## Hypoglossal Nerve
Anastomosis
　to Facial Nerve. . . . . . . . . . . . . . . . . . 64868

## Hypoglossal-Facial Anastomosis
*See* Anastomosis, Nerve, Facial to Hypoglossal

## Hypopharynges
*See* Hypopharynx

## Hypopharynx
Biopsy . . . . . . . . . . . . . . . . . . . . . . . . . . 42802

**IMT**
*See* Intima-Media Thickness Study

## In Situ Hybridization
*See* Nucleic Acid Probe, Cytogenetic Studies, Morphometric Analysis

## In Vitro Fertilization ....... 58321-58322

## In Vivo Laboratory Procedures
Unlisted Service...................... 88749

## In Vivo NMR Spectroscopy
*See* Magnetic Resonance Spectroscopy

## Incision
*See* Incision and Drainage
Abdomen ........................... 49000
  Exploration....................... 58960
Abscess
  Soft Tissue
    Subfascial..................... 20005
Accessory Nerve ..................... 63191
Anal
  Fistula.................... 46270, 46280
  Septum........................ 46070
  Sphincter..................... 46080
Ankle............................ 27607
  Tendon ................. 27605-27606
Anus
  *See* Anus, Incision
Aortic Valve
  for Stenosis ...................... 33415
Artery
  Nose...................... 30915-30920
Atrial Septum.................. 33735-33737
Bile Duct
  Sphincter ............... 43262, 47460
Bladder
  Catheterization.................... 51045
  with Destruction .......... 51020-51030
  with Radiotracer ............... 51020
Bladder Diverticulum.................. 52305
Brachial Artery
  Exposure....................... 34834
Brain
  Amygdalohippocampectomy ......... 61566
  Subpial........................ 61567
Breast
  Capsules....................... 19370
Burn Scab.................. 16035-16036
Buttock .................. 27027, 27057
Cataract
  Secondary
    Laser Surgery ................. 66821
    Stab Incision Technique ........... 66820
Chest
  Biopsy.................. 32096-32098
  with Therapeutic Wedge
    Resection ............... 32505-32506
Colon
  Exploration....................... 44025
  Stoma
    Creation ............... 44320-44322
    Revision ............... 44340-44346
Cornea
  for Astigmatism.................... 65772
  Laser
    for Keratoplasty .......... 0289T-0290T
Corpus Callosum .................... 61541
Cricothyroid Membrane................ 31605
Dentate Ligament ............. 63180-63182
Duodenum ......................... 44010

Ear, Inner
  Labyrinth
    Transcanal ................. 69801
Elbow .............................. 24000
Esophagus ............... 43020, 43045
  Muscle ....................... 43030
Exploration
  Heart ................. 33310-33315
  Kidney ....................... 50010
Eye
  Adhesions ..................... 65880
    Anterior Segment.......... 65860-65865
    Anterior Synechiae........... 65870
    Corneovitreal ................. 65880
    Posterior ..................... 65875
  Anterior Chamber.............. 65820
  Conjunctiva ................... 0124T
  Trabeculae ................... 65850
Eyelid
  Canthus ..................... 67715
  Sutures....................... 67710
Femoral Artery
  Exposure............... 34812-34813
Fibula ......................... 27607
Finger
  Decompression ................... 26035
  Tendon .......... 26060, 26455-26460
  Tendon Sheath ................. 26055
Foot ............................. 28005
  Capsule ............... 28260-28264
  Fasciotomy.................... 28008
  for Infection ............ 28002-28003
  Tendon ............... 28230, 28234
Frontal Lobe ....................... 61490
Gallbladder........................ 47490
Hand Decompression.......... 26035-26037
  Tendon ............... 26450, 26460
Heart
  Exploration.............. 33310-33315
Hemorrhoids
  External ..................... 46083
Hepatic Ducts
  *See* Hepaticostomy
Hip
  Denervation ................... 27035
  Exploration ................... 27033
  Fasciotomy.................... 27025
  Joint Capsule
    for Flexor Release............. 27036
  Tendon
    Abductor..................... 27006
    Adductor.............. 27000-27003
    Iliopsoas..................... 27005
Hymen
  *See* Hymen, Incision
Hymenotomy ...................... 56442
Hyoid
  Muscle ....................... 21685
Iliac Artery
  Exposure............... 34820, 34833
Intercarpal Joint
  Dislocation.................... 25670
Interphalangeal Joint
  Capsule ..................... 26525
Intestines (Except Rectum)
  *See* Enterotomy
Intestines, Small .................. 44010
  Biopsy....................... 44020
  Creation
    Pouch ..................... 44316
    Stoma ........ 44300-44310, 44314
  Decompression ................ 44021
  Exploration..................... 44020

  Incision........................ 44020
  Removal
    Foreign Body.................. 44020
  Revision
    Stoma..................... 44312
Iris .................. 66500-66505
Kidney.................. 50010, 50045
Knee
  Capsule ..................... 27435
  Exploration.................... 27310
  Fasciotomy................... 27305
  Removal of Foreign Body.......... 27310
Lacrimal Punctum................. 68440
Lacrimal Sac
  *See* Dacryocystotomy
Larynx ............... 31300-31320
Leg, Lower
  Fasciotomy............. 27600-27602
Leg, Upper
  Fasciotomy................... 27305
  Tenotomy ........ 27306-27307, 27390-27392
Lip
  Frenum....................... 40806
Liver
  *See* Hepatotomy
Lung
  Biopsy.................. 32096-32097
  Decortication
    Partial..................... 32225
    Total ...................... 32220
Lymphatic Channels................ 38308
Mastoid
  *See* Mastoidotomy
Medullary Tract .................... 61470
Mesencephalic Tract ................ 61480
Metacarpophalangeal Joint
  Capsule ..................... 26520
Mitral Valve .............. 33420-33422
Muscle
  *See* Myotomy
Nerve .............. 64568, 64575-64580, 64595, 64702-64772
  Foot ....................... 28035
  Root ................. 63185-63190
  Sacral....................... 64581
  Vagus ............... 43640-43641
Nose
  *See* Rhinotomy
Orbit
  *See* Orbitotomy
Palm
  Fasciotomy............. 26040-26045
Pancreas
  Sphincter .................... 43262
Pelvis
  Fasciotomy............. 27027, 27057
Penis
  Prepuce ............... 54000-54001
    Newborn.................... 54000
Pericardium
  with Clot Removal .............. 33020
  with Foreign Body Removal......... 33020
  with Tube .................... 33015
Pharynx
  Stoma....................... 42955
Pleura
  Biopsy....................... 32098
Pleural Cavity
  Empyema ............. 32035-32036
  Pneumothorax ................. 32551
Prostate
  Exposure
    Bilateral Pelvic Lymphadenectomy ... 55865

Insertion Radioactive Substance . . . . . 55860
Lymph Node Biopsy . . . . . . . . . . . . . . 55862
Transurethral . . . . . . . . . . . . . . . . . . . 52450
Pterygomaxillary Fossa . . . . . . . . . . . . . . . . 31040
Pulmonary Valve . . . . . . . . . . . . . 33470-33474
Pyloric Sphincter . . . . . . . . . . . . . . . . . . . . 43520
Retina
Encircling Material . . . . . . . . . . . . . . . . 67115
Sclera
Fistulization
Iridencleisis or Iridotasis . . . . . . . . . . 66165
Sclerectomy with Punch or Scissors
with Iridectomy . . . . . . . . . . . . . . . . 66160
Thermocauterization with Iridectomy . 66155
Trabeculectomy ab Externo in
Absence Previous Surgery . . . . . . . . 66170
Trephination with Iridectomy . . . . . . . 66150
Semicircular Canal
Fenestration . . . . . . . . . . . . . . . . . . . . 69820
Revision . . . . . . . . . . . . . . . . . . . . . . . 69840
Seminal Vesicle . . . . . . . . . . . . . . . 55600-55605
Complicated . . . . . . . . . . . . . . . . . . . . 55605
Shoulder
Bone . . . . . . . . . . . . . . . . . . . . . . . . . . 23035
Capsular Contracture Release . . . . . . . . 23020
Removal
Calcareous Deposits . . . . . . . . . . . . . 23000
Tenomyotomy . . . . . . . . . . . . . . . 23405-23406
Shoulder Joint . . . . . . . . . . . . . . . . 23040-23044
Sinus
Frontal . . . . . . . . . . . . . . . . . . . . 31070-31087
Maxillary . . . . . . . . . . . . . . . . . . 31020-31032
Endoscopic . . . . . . . . . . . . . . . 31256-31267
Multiple . . . . . . . . . . . . . . . . . . . . . . . 31090
Sphenoid
Sinusotomy . . . . . . . . . . . . . . . . 31050-31051
Skin . . . . . . . . . . . . . . . . 10040, 10060-10061,
10080-10081, 10120-10180
Skull . . . . . . . . . . . . . . . . . . . . . 61316, 62148
Suture . . . . . . . . . . . . . . . . . . . . 61550-61552
Spinal Cord . . . . . . . . . . . . . . . . . . . . . . . 63200
Tract . . . . . . . . . . . . . . . 63170, 63194-63199
Stomach
Creation
Stoma . . . . . . . . . . . . . . . . . . . 43830-43832
Exploration . . . . . . . . . . . . . . . . . . . . . 43500
Pyloric Sphincter . . . . . . . . . . . . . . . . 43520
Synovectomy . . . . . . . . . . . . . . . . . . . . . . 26140
Temporomandibular Joint . . . . . . . . . . . . . 21010
Tendon
Arm, Upper . . . . . . . . . . . . . . . . . . . . . 24310
Thigh
Fasciotomy . . . . . . . . . . . . . . . . . . . . . 27025
Thoracoabdominal
Paraesophageal Hiatal Hernia
Repair . . . . . . . . . . . . . . . . . . . 43336-43337
Thorax
Empyema . . . . . . . . . . . . . . . . . 32035-32036
Pneumothorax . . . . . . . . . . . . . . . . . . . 32551
Thyroid Gland
*See* Thyrotomy
Tibia . . . . . . . . . . . . . . . . . . . . . . . . . . . . 27607
Toe
Capsule . . . . . . . . . . . . . . . . . . 28270-28272
Fasciotomy . . . . . . . . . . . . . . . . . . . . . 28008
Tendon . . . . . . . . . . . . . . . . . . . 28232-28234
Tenotomy . . . . . . . . . . . . . . . . . 28010-28011
Tongue
Frenum . . . . . . . . . . . . . . . . . . . . . . . . 41010
Trachea
Emergency . . . . . . . . . . . . . . . . 31603-31605
Planned . . . . . . . . . . . . . . . . . . 31600-31601
with Flaps . . . . . . . . . . . . . . . . . . . . . 31610

Tympanic Membrane . . . . . . . . . . . . . . . . 69420
with Anesthesia . . . . . . . . . . . . . . . . . 69421
Ureter . . . . . . . . . . . . . . . . . . . . . . . . . . . 50600
Ureterocele . . . . . . . . . . . . . . . . . . . . . . . 51535
Urethra . . . . . . . . . . . . . . . . . . . 53000-53010
Meatus . . . . . . . . . . . . . . . . . . . 53020-53025
Uterus
Remove Lesion . . . . . . . . . . . . . . . . . . 59100
Vagina
Exploration . . . . . . . . . . . . . . . . . . . . . 57000
Vas Deferens . . . . . . . . . . . . . . . . . . . . . 55200
for X-ray . . . . . . . . . . . . . . . . . . . . . . . 55300
Vestibule of the Mouth
*See* Mouth, Vestibule of, Incision
Vitreous Strands
Laser Surgery . . . . . . . . . . . . . . . . . . . 67031
Pars Plana Approach . . . . . . . . . . . . . . 67030
Wrist . . . . . . . . . . . . . . . . . . . . . 25100-25105
Capsule . . . . . . . . . . . . . . . . . . . . . . . 25085
Decompression . . . . . . . . . . . . 25020-25025
Tendon Sheath . . . . . . . . . . . . . 25000-25001

# Incision and Drainage

*See* Drainage; Incision
Abdomen
Fluid . . . . . . . . . . . . . . . . . . . . 49082-49083
Pancreatitis . . . . . . . . . . . . . . . . . . . . . 48000
Abscess . . . . . . . . . . . . . . . . . . . . . . . . . 20005
Abdomen . . . . . . . . . . . . . . . . 49020, 49040
Open . . . . . . . . . . . . . . . . . . . . . . . . 49040
Percutaneous . . . . . . . . . . . . . . . . . . 49021
Soft Tissue
Subfascial . . . . . . . . . . . . . . . . . . . 20005
Anal . . . . . . . . . . . . . . . . . . . . . 46045-46050
Ankle . . . . . . . . . . . . . . . . . . . . . . . . . . 27603
Appendix . . . . . . . . . . . . . . . . . . . . . . . 44900
Open . . . . . . . . . . . . . . . . . . . . . . . . 44900
Percutaneous . . . . . . . . . . . . . . . . . . 44901
Arm, Lower . . . . . . . . . . . . . . . . . . . . . . 25028
Arm, Upper . . . . . . . . . . . . . . . . 23930-23931
Auditory Canal, External . . . . . . . . . . . . 69020
Bartholin's Gland . . . . . . . . . . . . . . . . . 56420
Bladder . . . . . . . . . . . . . . . . . . . . . . . . 51080
Brain . . . . . . . . . . . . . . . . . . . . 61320-61321
Breast . . . . . . . . . . . . . . . . . . . . . . . . . 19020
Ear, External
Complicated . . . . . . . . . . . . . . . . . . . 69005
Simple . . . . . . . . . . . . . . . . . . . . . . . 69000
Elbow . . . . . . . . . . . . . . . . . . . . . . . . . 23930
Epididymis . . . . . . . . . . . . . . . . . . . . . . 54700
Eyelid . . . . . . . . . . . . . . . . . . . . . . . . . 67700
Finger . . . . . . . . . . . . . . . . . . . . 26010-26011
Gums . . . . . . . . . . . . . . . . . . . . . . . . . 41800
Hip . . . . . . . . . . . . . . . . . . . . . . . . . . . 26990
Kidney . . . . . . . . . . . . . . . . . . . . . . . . . 50020
Open . . . . . . . . . . . . . . . . . . . . . . . . 50020
Percutaneous . . . . . . . . . . . . . . . . . . 50021
Knee . . . . . . . . . . . . . . . . . . . . . . . . . . 27301
Leg, Lower . . . . . . . . . . . . . . . . . . . . . . 27603
Leg, Upper . . . . . . . . . . . . . . . . . . . . . . 27301
Liver . . . . . . . . . . . . . . . . . . . . . . . . . . 47010
Open . . . . . . . . . . . . . . . . . . . . . . . . 47010
Percutaneous . . . . . . . . . . . . . . . . . . 47011
Lung . . . . . . . . . . . . . . . . . . . . . . . . . . 32200
Percutaneous . . . . . . . . . . . . . . . . . . 32201
Lymph Node . . . . . . . . . . . . . . . 38300-38305
Mouth . . . . . . . . . 40800-40801, 41005-41009,
41015-41018
Nasal Septum . . . . . . . . . . . . . . . . . . . 30020
Neck . . . . . . . . . . . . . . . . . . . . . 21501-21502
Nose . . . . . . . . . . . . . . . . . . . . . 30000-30020
Ovary . . . . . . . . . . . . . . . . . . . . 58820-58822
Abdominal Approach . . . . . . . . . . . . . 58822
Palate . . . . . . . . . . . . . . . . . . . . . . . . . 42000

Paraurethral Gland . . . . . . . . . . . . . . . . . 53060
Parotid Gland . . . . . . . . . . . . . . . 42300-42305
Pelvis . . . . . . . . . . . . . . . . . . . 26990, 45000
Perineum . . . . . . . . . . . . . . . . . . . . . . . 56405
Peritoneum . . . . . . . . . . . . . . . . . . . . . . 49020
Percutaneous . . . . . . . . . . . . . . . . . . 49021
Prostate . . . . . . . . . . . . . . . . . . 55720-55725
Rectum . . . . 45005-45020, 46040, 46050-46060
Retroperitoneal . . . . . . . . . . . . . . . . . . 49060
Open . . . . . . . . . . . . . . . . . . . . . . . . 49060
Salivary Gland . . . . . . . . . . . . . . 42300-42320
Scrotum . . . . . . . . . . . . . . . . . . 54700, 55100
Skene's Gland . . . . . . . . . . . . . . . . . . . 53060
Skin . . . . . . . . . . . . . . . . . . . . . 10060-10061
Subdiaphragmatic
Percutaneous . . . . . . . . . . . . . . 49040-49041
Sublingual Gland . . . . . . . . . . . . 42310-42320
Submaxillary Gland . . . . . . . . . . 42310-42320
Subphrenic
Percutaneous . . . . . . . . . . . . . . 49040-49041
Testis . . . . . . . . . . . . . . . . . . . . . . . . . 54700
Thorax . . . . . . . . . . . . . . . . . . . 21501-21502
Throat . . . . . . . . . . . . . . . . . . . 42700-42725
Tongue . . . . . . . . . . . . 41000-41006, 41015
Tonsil . . . . . . . . . . . . . . . . . . . . . . . . . 42700
Urethra . . . . . . . . . . . . . . . . . . . . . . . . 53040
Uvula . . . . . . . . . . . . . . . . . . . . . . . . . 42000
Vagina . . . . . . . . . . . . . . . . . . . . . . . . . 57010
Vulva . . . . . . . . . . . . . . . . . . . . . . . . . 56405
Wrist . . . . . . . . . . . . . . . . . . . . . . . . . . 25028
Ankle . . . . . . . . . . . . . . . . . . . . . . . . . . . 27610
Bile Duct . . . . . . . . . . . . . . . . . . 47420-47425
Bladder . . . . . . . . . . . . . . . . . . . . . . . . . . 51040
Bulla
Skin
Puncture Aspiration . . . . . . . . . . . . . 10160
Bursa
Ankle . . . . . . . . . . . . . . . . . . . . . . . . . 27604
Arm, Lower . . . . . . . . . . . . . . . . . . . . . 25031
Elbow . . . . . . . . . . . . . . . . . . . . . . . . . 23931
Foot . . . . . . . . . . . . . . . . . . . . . . . . . . 28001
Hip . . . . . . . . . . . . . . . . . . . . . . . . . . . 26991
Knee . . . . . . . . . . . . . . . . . . . . . . . . . . 27301
Leg, Lower . . . . . . . . . . . . . . . . . . . . . . 27604
Leg, Upper . . . . . . . . . . . . . . . . . . . . . . 27301
Palm . . . . . . . . . . . . . . . . . . . . 26025-26030
Pelvis . . . . . . . . . . . . . . . . . . . . . . . . . 26991
Wrist . . . . . . . . . . . . . . . . . . . . . . . . . . 25031
Carbuncle
Skin . . . . . . . . . . . . . . . . . . . . . 10060-10061
Carpals . . . . . . . . . . . . . . . . . . . . 25035, 26034
Comedones
Skin . . . . . . . . . . . . . . . . . . . . . . . . . . 10040
Cyst
Conjunctiva . . . . . . . . . . . . . . . . . . . . . 68020
Gums . . . . . . . . . . . . . . . . . . . . . . . . . 41800
Liver
Open . . . . . . . . . . . . . . . . . . . . . . . . 47010
Percutaneous . . . . . . . . . . . . . . . . . . 47011
Lung . . . . . . . . . . . . . . . . . . . . . . . . . . 32200
Percutaneous . . . . . . . . . . . . . . . . . . 32201
Mouth . . . . . . . . . 40800-40801, 41005-41009,
41015-41018
Ovarian . . . . . . . . . . . . . . . . . . . 58800-58805
Skin . . . . . . . . . . . . . . . 10040, 10060-10061
Pilonidal . . . . . . . . . . . . . . . . . . 10080-10081
Puncture Aspiration . . . . . . . . . . . . . 10160
Spinal Cord . . . . . . . . . . . . . . . . 63172-63173
Thyroid Gland . . . . . . . . . . . . . . . . . . . 60000
Tongue . . . . . . . . 41000-41006, 41015, 60000
Elbow
Abscess . . . . . . . . . . . . . . . . . . . . . . . . 23935
Arthrotomy . . . . . . . . . . . . . . . . . . . . . 24000

## Incisional Hernia Repair
*See* Hernia Repair, Incisional

## Inclusion Bodies

## Incomplete Abortion
*See* Abortion, Incomplete

## Indicator Dilution Studies . . . . . . . . . . . . . . . 93561-93562

## Induced Abortion
*See* Abortion

## Induced Hyperthermia
*See* Thermotherapy

## Induced Hypothermia
*See* Hypothermia

## Induratio Penis Plastica
*See* Peyronie Disease

## Infant, Newborn, Intensive Care
*See* Intensive Care, Neonatal

## Infantile Paralysis
*See* Polio

## Infection

## Infection, Actinomyces
*See* Actinomycosis

## Infection, Bone
*See* Osteomyelitis

## Infection, Filarioidea
*See* Filariasis

## Infection, Postoperative Wound
*See* Postoperative Wound Infection

## Infection, Wound
*See* Wound, Infection

## Infectious Agent

with Direct Optical
    Observation . . . . . . . . . . . . . . 87802-87899
by Nucleic Acid
    Bartonella Henselae . . . . . . . . 87470-87472
    Bartonella Quintana . . . . . . . . . 87470-87472
    Borrelia Burgdorferi . . . . . . . . 87475-87477
    Candida Species. . . . . . . . . . . 87480-87482
    Chlamydia Pneumoniae . . . . . 87485-87487
    Chlamydia Trachomatis . . . . . 87490-87492
    Clostridium Difficile . . . . . . . . . . . . . 87493
    Cytomegalovirus. . . . . . . . . . . 87495-87497
    Enterovirus . . . . . . . . . . . . . . 87498, 87500
    Gardnerella Vaginalis. . . . . . . . 87510-87512
    Gonorrhea. . . . . . . . . . . . . . . . . . . . . 87850
    Hepatitis B Virus. . . . . . . . . . . 87515-87517
    Hepatitis C . . . . . . . . . . . . . . . 87520-87522
    Hepatitis G . . . . . . . . . . . . . . . 87525-87527
    Herpes Simplex Virus . . . . . . . 87528-87530
    Herpes Virus-6 . . . . . . . . . . . 87531-87533
    HIV-1. . . . . . . . . . . . . . . . . . . 87534-87536
    HIV-2. . . . . . . . . . . . . . . . . . . 87537-87539
    Influenza. . . . . . . . . . . . . . . . 87501-87503
    Legionella Pneumophila . . . . . 87540-87542
    Multiple Organisms . . . . . . . . 87800-87801
    Mycobacteria
      Avium-Intracellulare. . . . . . . . 87560-87562
    Mycobacteria Species . . . . . . . 87550-87552
    Mycobacteria Tuberculosis . . . 87555-87557
    Mycoplasma Pneumoniae . . . . 87580-87582
    Neisseria Gonorrhoeae . . . . . . 87590-87592
    Not Otherwise Specified . . . . . 87797-87799
    Papillomavirus, Human. . . . . . . 87620-87622
    Staphylococcus Aureus . . . . . 87640-87641
    Streptococcus, Group A . . . . . 87650-87652
    Streptococcus, Group B . . . . . . . . . . 87653
    Trichomonas Vaginalis . . . . . . . . . . . 87660
    Vancomycin Resistance . . . . . . . . . . 87500
Enzymatic Activity . . . . . . . . . . . . . . . . 87905
Genotype Analysis
  by Nucleic Acid
    Hepatitis C Virus. . . . . . . . . . . . . . . 87902
    HIV-1 Regions. . . . . . . . . . . . . 87901, 87906
Phenotype Analysis
  by Nucleic Acid
    HIV-1 Drug Resistance . . . . . . . 87903-87904
Phenotype Prediction
  by Genetic Database . . . . . . . . . . . . . 87900

## Infectious Mononucleosis Virus
*See* Epstein-Barr Virus

## Inflammatory Process
Localization
  Nuclear Medicine . . . . . . . . . . . 78805-78808

## Inflation
Ear, Middle
  Eustachian Tube
    with Catheterization. . . . . . . . . . . . . 69400
    without Catheterization . . . . . . . . . . 69401
Eustachian Tube
  Myringotomy . . . . . . . . . . . . . . . . . . . 69420
  Anesthesia . . . . . . . . . . . . . . . . . . . . 69424

## Influenza A
Antigen Detection
  Direct Fluorescence . . . . . . . . . . . . . . 87276
  Enzyme Immunoassay . . . . . . . . . . . . 87400

## Influenza B
Antigen Detection
  Enzyme Immunoassay . . . . . . . . . . . . 87400
  Immunofluorescence . . . . . . . . . . . . . 87275

## Influenza Vaccine
*See* Vaccines

## Influenza Virus
Antibody. . . . . . . . . . . . . . . . . . . . . . . 86710
Detection
  by Immunoassay
    with Direct Optical Observation. . . . . 87804
  by Nucleic Acid . . . . . . . . . . . . 87501-87503

## Infraorbital Nerve
Avulsion . . . . . . . . . . . . . . . . . . . . . . . 64734
Incision . . . . . . . . . . . . . . . . . . . . . . . 64734
Transection. . . . . . . . . . . . . . . . . . . . . 64734

## Infrared Light Treatment . . . . . . . 97026
*See* Physical Medicine/Therapy/Occupational
Therapy

## Infratentorial
## Craniectomy . . . . . . . . . . . . . . 61520-61521

## Infusion
Amnion
  Transabdominal . . . . . . . . . . . . . . . . . 59072
Cerebral
  Intravenous
    for Thrombolysis. . . . . . . . . . . . . . . 37195
Intra-Arterial. . . . . . . . . . . . . . . . . . . . 96373
  Unlisted . . . . . . . . . . . . . . . . . . . . . 96379
Intraosseous. . . . . . . . . . . . . . . . . . . . 36680
Intravenous Unlisted . . . . . . . . . . . . . . 96379
  Diagnostic/Prophylactic/
    Therapeutic . . . . . . . . 96365-96368, 96379
  Hydration . . . . . . . . . . . . . . . . 96360-96361
Radioelement. . . . . . . . . . . . . . . . . . . 77750
Subcutaneous. . . . . . . . . . . . . . 96369-96371
Transcatheter Therapy. . . . . . . . 37201-37202

## Infusion Pump
Electronic Analysis
  Spinal Cord. . . . . . . . . . . . . . . 62367-62370
Insertion
  Intra-Arterial . . . . . . . . . . . . . . . . . . . 36260
Intra-Arterial
  Removal . . . . . . . . . . . . . . . . . . . . . 36262
  Revision . . . . . . . . . . . . . . . . . . . . . 36261
Intravenous
  Insertion . . . . . . . . . . . . . . . . . . . . . 36563
  Repair. . . . . . . . . . . . . . . . . . . . . . . 36576
  Replacement . . . . . . . . . . . . . . . . . . 36583
Maintenance . . . . . . . 95990-95991, 96521-96522
  *See* Chemotherapy, Pump Services
Spinal Cord. . . . . . . . . . . . . . . . 62361-62362
Ventricular Catheter. . . . . . . . . . . . . . . 61215

## Infusion Therapy . . . . . . . . 62350-62351,
62360-62362

*See* Injection, Chemotherapy
Arterial Catheterization. . . . . . . . . . . . . 36640
Chemotherapy . . . . . . 96401-96542, 96545, 96549
Home Infusion Procedures . . . . . . . . 99601-99602
Intravenous. . . . . . . . . . . 96365-96368, 96379
Subcutaneous. . . . . . . . . . . 96369-96371, 96379
Transcatheter Therapy. . . . . . . . . . . . . . 75896

## Ingestion Challenge Test . . . . . . 95075
*See* Allergy Tests

## Inguinal Hernia Repair
*See* Hernia, Repair, Inguinal

## INH
*See* Drug Assay

## Inhalation
Pentamidine. . . . . . . . . . . . . . . . . . . . . 94642

## Inhalation Provocation Tests
*See* Bronchial Challenge Test

## Inhalation Treatment . . . . . . . . . . 94640,
94644-94645, 94664, 99503
*See* Pulmonology, Therapeutic

## Inhibin A . . . . . . . . . . . . . . . . . . . . .86336

## Inhibition Test, Hemagglutination
*See* Hemagglutination Inhibition Test

## Inhibition, Fertilization
*See* Contraception

## Inhibitor, Alpha 1-Protease
*See* Alpha-1 Antitrypsin

## Inhibitor, Alpha 2-Plasmin
*See* Alpha-2 Antiplasmin

## Inhibitory Concentration, Minimum
*See* Minimum Inhibitory Concentration

## Initial Inpatient Consultations
*See* Consultation, Initial Inpatient

## Injection
*See* Allergen Immunotherapy; Infusion
Abdomen
  Air. . . . . . . . . . . . . . . . . . . . . . . . . . 49400
  Contrast Material. . . . . . . . . . . . . . . . 49400
Anesthetic Agent
  Sacroiliac Joint . . . . . . . . . . . . . . . . . 27096
  Spine
    Cervical. . . . . . . . 0228T-0229T, 62310, 62318
    Lumbar . . . . . . . 0230T-0231T, 62311, 62319
    Sacral . . . . . . . . . 0230T-0231T, 62311, 62319
    Thoracic . . . . . . . 0228T-0229T, 62310, 62318
Angiography
  Pulmonary . . . . . . . . . . . . . . . . . . . . 75746
Ankle
  Radial. . . . . . . . . . . . . . . . . . . . . . . . 27648
Antibiotic
  *See* Antibiotic Administration
Antigen (Allergen) . . . . . . . . . . . . . 95115-95125
Aorta (Aortography)
  Radiologic . . . . . . . . . . . . . . . . . . . . 93567
Aponeurosis. . . . . . . . . . . . . . . . . . . . 20550
Arthrography
  Sacroiliac Joint . . . . . . . . . . . . . . . . . 27096
Bladder
  Radiologic . . . . . . . . . . . . . . . 51600-51610
Brain Canal. . . . . . . . . . . . . . . . . . . . . 61070
Bronchography
  Segmental . . . . . . . . . . . . . . . . . . . . 31656
Bursa. . . . . . . . . . . . . . . . . . . . 20600-20610
Cardiac Catheterization. . . . . . . . . . 93454-93464,
93563-93568
Carpal Tunnel
  Therapeutic . . . . . . . . . . . . . . . . . . . 20526
Chemotherapy . . . . . . 96401-96542, 96545, 96549
Cistern
  Medication or Other. . . . . . . . . . . . . . 61055
Contrast . . . . . . . . . . . . . . . . . . . . . . . 49465
  via Catheter . . . . . . . . . . . . . . 36598, 49424
Corpora Cavernosa. . . . . . . . . . . . . . . . 54235
Cyst
  Bone. . . . . . . . . . . . . . . . . . . . . . . . . 20615
  Kidney . . . . . . . . . . . . . . . . . . . . . . . 50390
  Pelvis . . . . . . . . . . . . . . . . . . . . . . . . 50390
  Thyroid . . . . . . . . . . . . . . . . . . . . . . . 60300

Aorta . . . . . . . . . . . . . . . . . . . . . . . . . . . 36200
Bile Duct. . . . . . . . . . . . 47525-47530, 75982
 Percutaneous . . . . . . . . . . . . . . . . . . . 47510
Bladder. . . . . . . . . . . . . . 51045, 51701-51703
Brachiocephalic Artery. . . . . . . . . 36215-36218
Brain. . . . . . . . . . . . . . . . . 0169T, 61210, 61770
Breast. . . . . . . . . . . . . . . . . . . . . . . . . . . . 0169T
 for Interstitial Radioelement
 Application . . . . 19296-19298, 20555, 41019
Bronchi. . . . . . . . . . . . . . . . . . . . . . . . . . . 31717
Bronchus
 for Intracavitary Radioelement
 Application . . . . . . . . . . . . . . . . . . . . . 31643
Cardiac
 *See* Catheterization, Cardiac
 Flow Directed . . . . . . . . . . . . . . . . . . . 93503
Ear, Middle. . . . . . . . . . . . . . . . . . . . . . . . 69405
Eustachian Tube. . . . . . . . . . . . . . . . . . . . 69405
Gastrointestinal, Upper . . . . . . . . . . . . . 43241
Jejunum. . . . . . . . . . . . . . . . . . . . . . . . . . 44015
Kidney . . . . . . . . . . . . . . . . . . . . . . . . . . . 50392
Lower Extremity Artery . . . . . . . 36245-36248
Nasotracheal . . . . . . . . . . . . . . . . . . . . . . 31720
Pelvic Artery. . . . . . . . . . . . . . . . . 36245-36248
Pleural Cavity. . . . . . . . . . . . . . . . . . . . . . 32550
Portal Vein . . . . . . . . . . . . . . . . . . . . . . . . 36481
Prostate . . . . . . . . . . . . . . . . . . . . . . . . . . 55875
Pulmonary Artery . . . . . . . . . . . . 36013-36015
Right Heart. . . . . . . . . . . . . . . . . . . . . . . . 36013
Skull . . . . . . . . . . . . . . . . . . . . . . . . . . . . . 61107
Spinal Cord. . . . . . . . . . . . . . . . . 62350-62351
Suprapubic. . . . . . . . . . . . . . . . . . . . . . . . 51010
Thoracic Artery. . . . . . . . . . . . . . 36215-36218
Trachea. . . . . . . . . . . . . . . . . . . . . . . . . . . 31700
Tracheobronchial . . . . . . . . . . . . . . . . . . . 31725
Transthoracic . . . . . . . . . . . . . . . . . . . . . . 33621
Ureter via Kidney. . . . . . . . . . . . . . . . . . . 50393
Urethra. . . . . . . . . . . . . . . . . . 51701-51703
Vena Cava . . . . . . . . . . . . . . . . . . . . . . . . 36010
Venous . . . . . . . . . 36011-36012, 36400-36410,
 36420-36425, 36500-36510,
 36555-36558, 36568-36569
Cecostomy Tube. . . . . . . . . . . . . . . . . . . . . 49442
Cervical Dilation. . . . . . . . . . . . . . . . . . . . . 59200
Cochlear Device. . . . . . . . . . . . . . . . . . . . . 69930
Colonic Tube. . . . . . . . . . . . . . . . . . . . . . . 49442
Distraction Device
 Posterior Spinous Process,
 Lumbar. . . . . . . . . . . . . . . . . . . . . .0171T-0172T
Drug Delivery Implant . . . . . . . . . . . 11981, 11983
Duodenostomy Tube . . . . . . . . . . . . . . . . . 49441
Electrode
 Brain. . . . . . 61531-61533, 61760, 61850-61875
 Heart . . . . . . . . . 33202-33203, 33210-33211,
 33216-33217, 33224-33225, 93620-93622
 Nerve . . . . . . . . . . . . . . . . . . . . . 64553-64581
 Retina. . . . . . . . . . . . . . . . . . . . . . . . . . 0100T
 Sphenoidal. . . . . . . . . . . . . . . . . . . . . . 95830
 Spinal Cord. . . . . . . . . . . . . . . . . 63650-63655
Stomach
 Laparoscopic
 Neurostimulator . . . . . . . . . . . . . . . . 43647
 Stimulation
 Open
 Neurostimulator . . . . . . . . . . . . . . . . 43881
Endotracheal Tube
 Emergency Intubation . . . . . . . . . . . . . . 31500
Filter
 Vena Cava . . . . . . . . . . . . . . . . . . . . . . 37191
Gastrostomy Tube
 Laparoscopic . . . . . . . . . . . . . . . . . . . . 43653
 Percutaneous. . . . . . . . . . . . . . . . . . . . 43246

Graft
 Aorta . . . . . . . . . . . . . . . . . . . . 33330-33335
 Heart Vessel. . . . . . . . . . . . . . . 33330-33335
Guide
 Kidney Pelvis . . . . . . . . . . . . . . . . . . . . 50395
Guide Wire
 Endoscopy . . . . . . . . . . . . . . . . . . . . . . 43248
 Esophagoscopy . . . . . . . . . . . . . . . . . . 43248
 with Dilation. . . . . . . . . . . . . . . . . . . 43226
Heyman Capsule
 Uterus
 for Brachytherapy. . . . . . . . . . . . . . . . 58346
Iliac Artery
 Occlusion Device . . . . . . . . . . . . . . . . . 34808
Implant
 Bone
 for External Speech Processor/
 CochlearStimulator. . . . . . . . . 69714-69718
Infusion Pump
 Intra-Arterial . . . . . . . . . . . . . . . . . . . . 36260
 Intravenous . . . . . . . . . . . . . . . . . . . . . 36563
 Spinal Cord. . . . . . . . . . . . . . . . 62361-62362
Intracatheter/Needle
 Aorta . . . . . . . . . . . . . . . . . . . . . . . . . . 36160
 Arteriovenous Shunt . . . . . . . . . 36147-36148
 Intra-Arterial . . . . . . . . . . . . . . . 36100-36140
 Intravenous . . . . . . . . . . . . . . . . . . . . . 36000
 Kidney . . . . . . . . . . . . . . . . . . . . . . . . . 50392
Intraocular Lens . . . . . . . . . . . . . . . . . . . . . 66983
 Manual or Mechanical
 Technique. . . . . . . . . . . . . . . 66982, 66984
 Not Associated with Concurrent
 Cataract Removal. . . . . . . . . . . . . . . . . 66985
Intrauterine Device (IUD). . . . . . . . . . . . . . 58300
Jejunostomy Tube
 Endoscopy . . . . . . . . . . . . . . . . . . . . . . 44372
 Percutaneous. . . . . . . . . . . . . . . . . . . . 49441
Keel
 Laryngoplasty. . . . . . . . . . . . . . . . . . . . 31580
Laminaria . . . . . . . . . . . . . . . . . . . . . . . . . 59200
Mesh
 Pelvic Floor. . . . . . . . . . . . . . . . . . . . . . 57267
Nasobiliary Tube
 Endoscopy . . . . . . . . . . . . . . . . . . . . . . 43267
Nasopancreatic Tube
 Endoscopy . . . . . . . . . . . . . . . . . . . . . . 43267
Needle
 Bone. . . . . . . . . . . . . . . . . . . . . . . . . . . 36680
 Intraosseous. . . . . . . . . . . . . . . . . . . . . 36680
 Prostate . . . . . . . . . . . . . . . . . . . . . . . . 55875
Needle Wire
 Trachea. . . . . . . . . . . . . . . . . . . . . . . . . 31730
Neurostimulator
 Pulse Generator . . . . . . . . . . . . . . . . . . 64590
 Receiver. . . . . . . . . . . . . . . . . . . . . . . . 64590
Nose
 Septal Prosthesis. . . . . . . . . . . . . . . . . . 30220
Obturator
 Larynx. . . . . . . . . . . . . . . . . . . . . . . . . . 31527
Ocular Implant
 in Scleral Shell. . . . . . . . . . . . . . . . . . . 65130
 Muscles, Attached. . . . . . . . . . . . . . . . 65140
 Muscles, Not Attached . . . . . . . . . . . . 65135
 with Foreign Material . . . . . . . . . . . . . 65155
 with/without Conjunctival Graft . . . . . . 65150
Orbital Transplant . . . . . . . . . . . . . . . . . . . 67550
Oviduct
 Chromotubation. . . . . . . . . . . . . . . . . . 58350
 Hydrotubation . . . . . . . . . . . . . . . . . . . 58350
Ovoid
 Vagina
 for Brachytherapy. . . . . . . . . . . . . . . . 57155

Pacemaker, Heart. . . . . . . . . . . . . . . 33206-33208
 Pulse Generator Only. . . . 33212-33213, 33221
Pacing Cardio-Defibrillator
 Leads . . . . . . . . . . . 33216-33220, 33224-33225,
 33243-33244
 Pulse Generator Only. . . . 33230-33231, 33240
Packing
 Vagina . . . . . . . . . . . . . . . . . . . . . . . . . 57180
Penile Prosthesis, Inflatable
 *See* Penile Prosthesis, Insertion, Inflatable
Pessary
 Vagina . . . . . . . . . . . . . . . . . . . . . . . . . 57160
Pin
 Skeletal Traction . . . . . . . . . . . . . . . . . 20650
Probe
 Brain. . . . . . . . . . . . . . . . . . . . . . . . . . . 61770
Prostaglandin . . . . . . . . . . . . . . . . . . . . . . . 59200
Prostate
 Radioactive Substance . . . . . . . . . . . . . 55860
Prosthesis
 Knee. . . . . . . . . . . . . . . . . . . . 27438, 27445
 Nasal Septal . . . . . . . . . . . . . . . . . . . . 30220
 Palate. . . . . . . . . . . . . . . . . . . . . . . . . . 42281
 Pelvic Floor. . . . . . . . . . . . . . . . . . . . . . 57267
 Penis
 Inflatable . . . . . . . . . . . . . . 54401-54405
 Noninflatable . . . . . . . . . . . . . . . . . . 54400
 Speech. . . . . . . . . . . . . . . . . . . . . . . . . 31611
 Testis . . . . . . . . . . . . . . . . . . . . . . . . . . 54660
 Urethral Sphincter . . . . . . . . . . . 53444-53445
Pulse Generator
 Brain. . . . . . . . . . . . . . . . . . . . . 61885-61886
 Heart . . . . . . . . . . . 33212-33213, 33221
 Spinal Cord. . . . . . . . . . . . . . . . . . . . . . 63685
Radioactive Material
 Bladder. . . . . . . . . . . . . . . . . . . . . . . . . 51020
 Cystourethroscopy . . . . . . . . . . . . . . . . 52250
Radiation Afterloading Apparatus . . . . . . . 57156
 Vagina
 for Brachytherapy. . . . . . . . . . . . . . . . 57156
Receiver
 Brain. . . . . . . . . . . . . . . . . . . . . 61885-61886
 Spinal Cord. . . . . . . . . . . . . . . . . . . . . . 63685
Reservoir
 Brain. . . . . . . . . . . . . . . . . . . . . 61210-61215
 Spinal Cord. . . . . . . . . . . . . . . . . . . . . . 62360
 Subcutaneous . . . . . . . . . . . . . . . . . . . 49419
Shunt. . . . . . . . . . . . . . . . . . . . . . . . . . . . . 36835
 Abdomen
 Vein. . . . . . . . . . . . . . . . . . . . . . . . . . 49425
 Venous . . . . . . . . . . . . . . . . . . . . . . . 49426
 Eye
 to Suprachoroidal Space . . . . . . . . . . . 0253T
 Intrahepatic Portosystemic . . . . . . . . . . 37182
Spinal Instrument. . . . . . . . . . . . . . . . . . . . 22849
 Spinous Process. . . . . . . . .0171T-0172T, 22841
Spinal Instrumentation
 Anterior . . . . . . . . . . . . . . . . . . . . 22845-22847
 Internal Spinal Fixation . . . . . . . . . . . . . 22841
 Pelvic Fixation . . . . . . . . . . . . . . . . . . . 22848
 Posterior Nonsegmental
 Harrington Rod Technique . . . . . . . . . . 22840
 Posterior Segmental . . . . . . . . . . 22842-22844
 Prosthetic Device. . . . . . . . . . . . . . . . . 22851
Stent
 Bile Duct. . . . . . . . . . . . . . . . . 43268, 47801
 Percutaneous . . . . . . . . . . . . . . . . . . 47511
 Bladder. . . . . . . . . . . . . . . . . . . . . . . . . 51045
 Conjunctiva . . . . . . . . . . . . . . . . . . . . . 68750
 Coronary. . . . . . . . . . . . . . . . . . 92980-92981
 Esophagus . . . . . . . . . . . . . . . . . . . . . . 43219
 Gastrointestinal, Upper . . . . . . . . . . . . 43256
 Ileum . . . . . . . . . . . . . . . . . . . . . . . . . . 44383

with Corneoscleral or Corneal
Section . . . . . . . . . . . . . . . . . . . . . . . 66600
with Cyclectomy . . . . . . . . . . . . . . . . 66605
Incision
Iridotomy
Stab . . . . . . . . . . . . . . . . . . . . . . . 66500
with Transfixion as for Iris Bombe . . . . 66505
Lesion
Destruction . . . . . . . . . . . . . . . . . . . . 66770
Repair
with Ciliary Body . . . . . . . . . . . . . . . 66680
Suture . . . . . . . . . . . . . . . . . . . . . . . 66682
Revision
Laser Surgery . . . . . . . . . . . . . . . . . . 66761
Photocoagulation . . . . . . . . . . . . . . . . 66762
Suture
with Ciliary Body . . . . . . . . . . . . . . . 66682

**Iron** . . . . . . . . . . . . . . . . . . . . . . . . . . . .83540

**Iron Binding Capacity** . . . . . . . . . .83550

**Iron Hematoxylin Stain** . . . . . . . .88312

**Iron Stain** . . . . . . . . . . . . . . .85536, 88313

**Irradiation**
Blood Products . . . . . . . . . . . . . . . . . . . . 86945

**Irrigation**
Bladder . . . . . . . . . . . . . . . . . . . . . . . . . 51700
Catheter
Brain . . . . . . . . . . . . . . . . . . . . 62194, 62225
Corpora Cavernosa
Priapism . . . . . . . . . . . . . . . . . . . . . . . 54220
Penis
Priapism . . . . . . . . . . . . . . . . . . . . . . . 54220
Peritoneal
*See* Peritoneal Lavage
Shunt
Spinal Cord . . . . . . . . . . . . . . . . . . . . . 63744
Sinus
Maxillary . . . . . . . . . . . . . . . . . . . . . . 31000
Sphenoid . . . . . . . . . . . . . . . . . . . . . . 31002
Vagina . . . . . . . . . . . . . . . . . . . . . . . . . . 57150
Venous Access Device . . . . . . . . . . . . . . . 96523

**Irving Sterilization**
*See* Ligation, Fallopian Tube, Oviduct

**Ischemic Stroke**
Onset . . . . . . . . . . . . . . . . . . . . . .1065F-1066F
Tissue Plasminogen Activator (tPA)
Documentation That Administration
Was Considered . . . . . . . . . . . . . . . . . 4077F

**Ischial**
Bursa
Excision . . . . . . . . . . . . . . . . . . . . . . 27060
Tumor
Radical Resection . . . . . . . . . . . 27075, 27078

**Ischiectomy** . . . . . . . . . . . . . . . . . . . .15941

**Island Pedicle Flaps** . . . . . . . . . . .15740

**Islands of Langerhans**
*See* Islet Cell

**Islet Cell**
Antibody . . . . . . . . . . . . . . . . . . . . . . . . . 86341

**Isocitrate Dehydrogenase**
*See* Isocitric Dehydrogenase

**Isocitric Dehydrogenase**
Blood . . . . . . . . . . . . . . . . . . . . . . . . . . . 83570

**Isolation**
Sperm . . . . . . . . . . . . . . . . . . . . 89260-89261

**Isomerase, Glucose 6 Phosphate**
*See* Phosphohexose Isomerase

**Isopropanol**
*See* Isopropyl Alcohol

**Isopropyl Alcohol** . . . . . . . . . . . . . .84600

**Isthmusectomy**
Thyroid Gland . . . . . . . . . . . . . . . . 60210-60225

**IUD**
*See* Intrauterine Device (IUD)

**IV**
*See* Injection, Chemotherapy; Intravenous Therapy

**IV Infusion Therapy**
*See* Allergen Immunotherapy; Chemotherapy;
Infusion; Injection, Chemotherapy

**IV Injection**
*See* Injection, Intravenous

**IV, Coagulation Factor**
*See* Calcium

**IVF**
*See* Artificial Insemination; In Vitro Fertilization

**Ivy Bleeding Time** . . . . . . . . . . . . . .85002

**IX Complex, Factor**
*See* Christmas Factor

# J

**Jaboulay Operation**
*See* Gastroduodenostomy

**Jaboulay Operation
Gastroduodenostomy**
*See* Gastroduodenostomy

**JAK2** . . . . . . . . . . . . . . . . . . . . . . . . . . .81270

**Jannetta Procedure**
*See* Decompression, Cranial Nerve; Section

**Japanese Encephalitis Virus**
*See* Vaccine

**Japanese, River Fever**
*See* Scrub Typhus

**Jatene Type** . . . . . . . . . . . . . . . 33770-33781

**Jaw Joint**
*See* Facial Bones; Mandible; Maxilla

**Jaws**
Muscle Reduction . . . . . . . . . . . . . . 21295-21296
X-ray
for Orthodontics . . . . . . . . . . . . . . . . . 70355

**Jejunostomy**
Catheterization . . . . . . . . . . . . . . . . . . . . 44015
Contrast . . . . . . . . . . . . . . . . . . . . . . . . 49465
Insertion
Catheter . . . . . . . . . . . . . . . . . . . . . . 44015
Percutaneous . . . . . . . . . . . . . . . . . . . 49441
Laparoscopic . . . . . . . . . . . . . . . 44186-44187

Non-Tube . . . . . . . . . . . . . . . . . . . . 44187, 44310
Obstructive Material Removal . . . . . . . . . 49460
Replacement . . . . . . . . . . . . . . . . . . . . . 49451
with Pancreatic Drain . . . . . . . . . . . . . . 48001

**Jejunum**
Creation
Stoma
Laparoscopic . . . . . . . . . . . . . . . . . . . . 44186
Transfer
with Microvascular Anastomosis
Free . . . . . . . . . . . . . . . . . . . . . . . . 43496

**Johannsen Procedure** . . . . . . . . .53400

**Joint**
*See* Specific Joint
Acromioclavicular
*See* Acromioclavicular Joint
Arthrocentesis . . . . . . . . . . . . . . 20600-20610
Aspiration . . . . . . . . . . . . . . . . . . 20600-20610
Dislocation
*See* Dislocation
Drainage . . . . . . . . . . . . . . . . . . . 20600-20610
Finger
*See* Intercarpal Joint
Fixation (Surgical)
*See* Arthrodesis
Foot
*See* Foot, Joint
Hip
*See* Hip Joint
Injection . . . . . . . . . . . 0213T-0218T, 20600-20610
Intertarsal
*See* Intertarsal Joint
Knee
*See* Knee Joint
Ligament
*See* Ligament
Metacarpophalangeal
*See* Metacarpophalangeal Joint
Metatarsophalangeal
*See* Metatarsophalangeal Joint
Nuclear Medicine
Imaging . . . . . . . . . . . . . . . . . . 78300, 78315
Radiology
Stress Views . . . . . . . . . . . . . . . . . . . . 77071
Replacement
Vertebral . . . . . . . . . . . . . . . . . . . . . . 0202T
Sacroiliac
*See* Sacroiliac Joint
Shoulder
*See* Glenohumeral Joint
Sternoclavicular
*See* Sternoclavicular Joint
Survey . . . . . . . . . . . . . . . . . . . . . . . . . 77077
Temporomandibular
*See* Temporomandibular Joint (TMJ)
Dislocation Temporomandibular
*See* Dislocation, Temporomandibular Joint
Implant
*See* Prosthesis, Temporomandibular Joint
Wrist
*See* Radiocarpal Joint

**Joint Syndrome,
Temporomandibular**
*See* Temporomandibular Joint (TMJ)

**Jones and Cantarow Test**
*See* Blood Urea Nitrogen; Urea Nitrogen, Clearance

**Jones Procedure** . . . . . . . . . . . . . . .28760

**Joplin Procedure** . . . . . . . . . . . . . . .28294

**Ladd Procedure** . . . . . . . . . . . . . . . .44055

**Lagophthalmos**
Repair . . . . . . . . . . . . . . . . . . . . . . . . .67912

**Laki Lorand Factor**
*See* Fibrin Stabilizing Factor

**Lamblia Intestinalis**
*See* Giardia Lamblia

**Lambrinudi Operation**
*See* Arthrodesis, Foot Joint

**Lamellar Keratoplasties**
*See* Keratoplasty, Lamellar

**Laminaria**
Insertion . . . . . . . . . . . . . . . . . . . . . . .59200

**Laminectomy** . . . . . . . 0202T, 62351, 63001,
63005-63011, 63015-63044, 63180-63200,
63265-63290, 63300-63655
Lumbar . . . . . . . . . . . . . . . . . . . . 22630, 63012
Neural Elements
Decompression . . . . . . . . . . . . . .0274T-0275T
Surgical. . . . . . . . . . . . . . . . . . . . 63170-63172
with Facetectomy. . . . . . . . . .0202T, 63045-63048

**Laminoplasty**
Cervical . . . . . . . . . . . . . . . . . . . . 63050-63051

**Langerhans Islands**
*See* Islet Cell

**Language Evaluation** . . . . . . . . . . .92506

**Language Therapy** . . . . . . . . 92507-92508

**LAP**
*See* Leucine Aminopeptidase

**Laparoscopic Appendectomy**
*See* Appendectomy, Laparoscopic

**Laparoscopic Biopsy of Ovary**
*See* Biopsy, Ovary, Laparoscopic

**Laparoscopy**
Abdominal
Diagnostic . . . . . . . . . . . . . . . . . . .49320
Surgical . . . . . . . . . . . . . . 49321-49327
Unlisted Procedures. . . . . . . . . . . . . .49329
Adrenal Gland
Biopsy. . . . . . . . . . . . . . . . . . . . . .60650
Excision . . . . . . . . . . . . . . . . . . . . .60650
Adrenalectomy. . . . . . . . . . . . . . . . . . .50545
Appendectomy. . . . . . . . . . . . . . . . . . .44970
Aspiration. . . . . . . . . . . . . . . . . . . . . .49322
Biopsy. . . . . . . . . . . . . . . . . . 47561, 49321
Lymph Nodes . . . . . . . . . . . . . . . . . .38570
Bladder
Repair
Sling Operation. . . . . . . . . . . . . . .51992
Urethral Suspension. . . . . . . . . . . .51990
Unlisted . . . . . . . . . . . . . . . . . . . . .51999
Cecostomy . . . . . . . . . . . . . . . . . . . . .44188
Laparoscopic . . . . . . . . . . . . . . . . . .44188
Cholangiography . . . . . . . . . . 47560-47561
Cholecystectomy . . . . . . . . . . 47562-47564
Cholecystenterostomy. . . . . . . . . . . . . .47570
Colectomy
Laparoscopic . . . . . . . . . . . . . . . . . .44213
Partial. . . . . . . . . 44204-44208, 44213
Total . . . . . . . . . . . . . . . . . 44210-44212
Colostomy. . . . . . . . . . . . . . . . . . . . . .44188
Destruction

Lesion. . . . . . . . . . . . . . . . . . . . . . .58662
Drainage
Extraperitoneal Lymphocele . . . . . . . . .49323
Ectopic Pregnancy . . . . . . . . . . . . . . . .59150
with Salpingectomy and/or
Oophorectomy . . . . . . . . . . . . . . .59151
Electrode Implantation
Gastric . . . . . . . . . . . . . . . 43647, 43648
Electrode Removal
Gastric . . . . . . . . . . . . . . . . . . . . .43648
Electrode Replacement
Gastric . . . . . . . . . . . . . . . . . . . . .43647
Electrode Revision
Gastric . . . . . . . . . . . . . . . . . . . . .43648
Enterectomy . . . . . . . . . . . . . . . . . . . .44202
Enterolysis . . . . . . . . . . . . . . . . . . . . .44180
Enterostomy
Closure . . . . . . . . . . . . . . . . . . . . .44227
Esophageal Lengthening . . . . . . . . . . . .43283
Esophagogastric Fundoplasty . . . . . . . . . 43280,
43327-43328
Esophagomyotomy Fundoplasty . . . . . . . .43279
Fimbrioplasty . . . . . . . . . . . . . . . . . . .58672
Gastrectomy
Longitudinal/Sleeve. . . . . . . . . . . . . .43775
Gastric Restrictive Procedures . . . . . 43644-43645,
43770-43775
Gastrostomy
Temporary . . . . . . . . . . . . . . . . . . .43653
Hernia Repair
Epigastric
Incarcerated or Strangulated . . . . . . . .49653
Reducible . . . . . . . . . . . . . . . . . . .49652
Incisional
Incarcerated or Strangulated . . . . . . . .49655
Reducible . . . . . . . . . . . . . . . . . . .49654
Incisional Recurrent
Incarcerated or Strangulated . . . . . . . .49657
Reducible . . . . . . . . . . . . . . . . . . .49656
Inguinal
Initial. . . . . . . . . . . . . . . . . . . . . .49650
Recurrent . . . . . . . . . . . . . . . . . . .49651
Paraesophageal . . . . . . . . . . . 43281-43282
Spigelian
Incarcerated or Strangulated . . . . . . . .49653
Reducible . . . . . . . . . . . . . . . . . . .49652
Umbilical
Incarcerated or Strangulated . . . . . . . .49653
Reducible . . . . . . . . . . . . . . . . . . .49652
Ventral
Incarcerated or Strangulated . . . . . . . .49653
Reducible . . . . . . . . . . . . . . . . . . .49652
Hysterectomy . . . . . . . . . . . . 58541-58544
Radical . . . . . . . . . . . . . . . . . . . . .58548
Total . . . . . . . . . . . . . . . . . 58570-58573
Ileostomy . . . . . . . . . . . . . . . . . . . . . .44187
In Vitro Fertilization . . . . . . . . . . . . . . .58976
Retrieve Oocyte . . . . . . . . . . . . . . . .58970
Transfer Embryo . . . . . . . . . . . . . . . .58974
Transfer Gamete . . . . . . . . . . . . . . . .58976
Incontinence Repair. . . . . . . . . 51990-51992
Jejunostomy. . . . . . . . . . . . . . 44186-44187
Kidney
Ablation . . . . . . . . . . . . . . . 50541-50542
Ligation
Veins, Spermatic . . . . . . . . . . . . . . .55550
Liver
Ablation
Tumor . . . . . . . . . . . . . . . . 47370-47371
Lymphadenectomy . . . . . . . . . . 38571-38572
Lymphatic . . . . . . . . . . . . . . . 38570-38589
Lysis of Adhesions . . . . . . . . . . . . . . . .58660

Lysis of Intestinal Adhesions . . . . . . . . . . .44180
Nephrectomy . . . . . . . . . . . . . 50545-50548
Partial. . . . . . . . . . . . . . . . . . . . . .50543
Omentopexy. . . . . . . . . . . . . . . . . . . .49326
Orchiectomy . . . . . . . . . . . . . . . . . . . .54690
Orchiopexy . . . . . . . . . . . . . . . . . . . . .54692
Oviduct Surgery . . . . . . . . . 58670-58671, 58679
Pelvis. . . . . . . . . . . . . . . . . . . . . . . . .49320
Proctectomy
Complete . . . . . . . . . . . . . . . . . . . .45395
with Creation of Colonic Reservoir . . . .45397
Proctopexy
for Prolapse . . . . . . . . . . . . . 45400-45402
Prostatectomy . . . . . . . . . . . . . . . . . . .55866
Pyeloplasty. . . . . . . . . . . . . . . . . . . . .50544
Rectum
Resection . . . . . . . . . . . . . . . 45395-45397
Unlisted . . . . . . . . . . . . . . . . . . . . .45499
Removal
Fallopian Tube . . . . . . . . . . . . . . . . .58661
Leiomyomata . . . . . . . . . . . . . 58545-58546
Ovaries. . . . . . . . . . . . . . . . . . . . . .58661
Spleen . . . . . . . . . . . . . . . . . . . . . .38120
Testis . . . . . . . . . . . . . . . . . . . . . .54690
Resection
Intestines
with Anastomosis. . . . . . . . . 44202-44203
Rectum . . . . . . . . . . . . . . . 45395-45397
Salpingostomy . . . . . . . . . . . . . . . . . . .58673
Splenectomy. . . . . . . . . . . . . . 38120-38129
Splenic Flexure
Mobilization . . . . . . . . . . . . . . . . . .44213
Stomach . . . . . . . . . . . . . . . 43647-43659
Gastric Bypass . . . . . . . . . . . . 43644-43645
Gastric Restrictive Procedures. . . 43770-43775,
43848, 43886-43888
Gastroenterostomy . . . . . . . . . 43644-43645
Roux-En-Y. . . . . . . . . . . . . . . . . . . .43644
Transplantation
Unlisted Services and Procedures
Abdomen, Peritoneum, and Omentum. . . 49329
Appendix . . . . . . . . . . . . . . . . . . . .44979
Biliary Tract . . . . . . . . . . . . . . . . . . .47579
Bladder. . . . . . . . . . . . . . . . . . . . . .51999
Esophagus . . . . . . . . . . . . . . . . . . .43289
Hernioplasty, Herniorrhaphy,
Herniotomy. . . . . . . . . . . . . . . . . .49659
Intestine. . . . . . . . . . . . . . . . . . . . .44238
Liver . . . . . . . . . . . . . . . . . . . . . . .47379
Lymphatic System . . . . . . . . . . . . . . .38589
Maternity Care and Delivery . . . . 59898-59899
Oviduct, Ovary . . . . . . . . . . . . . . . . .58679
Rectum . . . . . . . . . . . . . . . . . . . . .45499
Renal . . . . . . . . . . . . . . . . . . . . . .50549
Spermatic Cord . . . . . . . . . . . . . . . .55559
Spleen . . . . . . . . . . . . . . . . . . . . . .38129
Stomach. . . . . . . . . . . . . . . . . . . . .43659
Testis . . . . . . . . . . . . . . . . . . . . . .54699
Ureter . . . . . . . . . . . . . . . . . . . . . .50949
Uterus. . . . . . . . . . . . . . . . . 58578-58579
Ureterolithotomy . . . . . . . . . . . . . . . . .50945
Ureteroneocystostomy. . . . . . . . 50947-50948
Urethral Suspension . . . . . . . . . . . . . . .51990
Vaginal Hysterectomy . . . . . . . . 58550-58554
Vaginal Suspension . . . . . . . . . . . . . . . .57425
Vagus Nerves
Transection. . . . . . . . . . . . . . 43651-43652
with X-ray. . . . . . . . . . . . . . . . . . . . . .47560

**Laparotomy**
Electrode Implantation
Gastric . . . . . . . . . . . . . . . . . . . . . . .43881
Electrode Removal

Gastric ........................ 43882
Electrode Replacement
Gastric ........................ 43881
Electrode Revision
Gastric ........................ 43882
Esophagogastric
Fundoplasty ............... 43327-43328
Exploration ....... 47015, 49000-49002
Hiatal Hernia Repair ........... 43332-43333
Hemorrhage Control ............. 49002
Second Look .................... 58960
Staging ................ 49220, 58960
with Biopsy .................... 49000
Stomach .................... 43605

## Laparotomy, Exploratory
See Abdomen, Exploration

## Lapidus Procedure ............ 28297

## Large Bowel
See Anus; Rectum

## Laroyenne Operation
See Vagina, Abscess, Incision and Drainage

## Laryngeal Function Study ...... 92520

## Laryngeal Sensory Testing .................... 92614-92617

## Laryngectomy ............... 31360-31382
Partial ..................... 31367-31382
Subtotal .................... 31367-31368

## Laryngocele
Removal ....................... 31300

## Laryngofissure ................ 31300

## Laryngography ................ 70373
Instillation

## Laryngopharyngectomy
See Excision, Larynx, with Pharynx

## Laryngopharynx
See Hypopharynx

## Laryngoplasty
Burns ......................... 31588
Cricoid Split .................. 31587
Laryngeal Stenosis ............. 31582
Laryngeal Web ................. 31580
Open Reduction of Fracture ...... 31584

## Laryngoscopy
Diagnostic .................... 31505
Direct ..................... 31515-31571
Exploration ....... 31505, 31520-31526, 31575
Fiberoptic ................. 31575-31579
with Stroboscopy .............. 31579
Indirect ................... 31505-31513
Newborn ...................... 31520
Operative .................. 31530-31561

## Laryngotomy ................. 31300
Diagnostic .................... 31320

## Larynx
Aspiration
Endoscopy ................... 31515
Biopsy
Endoscopy ...... 31510, 31535-31536, 31576
Dilation
Endoscopic ................ 31528-31529
Electromyography

Needle ....................... 95865
Endoscopy
Direct ................... 31515-31571
Excision ................. 31545-31546
Exploration ...... 31505, 31520-31526, 31575
Fiberoptic ............... 31575-31579
with Stroboscopy ........... 31579
Indirect ................. 31505-31513
Operative ................ 31530-31561
Excision
Lesion .............. 31512, 31578
Endoscopic .......... 31545-31546
Partial ............... 31367-31382
Total ................. 31360-31365
with Pharynx ......... 31390-31395
Exploration
Endoscopic ..... 31505, 31520-31526, 31575
Fracture ...................... 31584
Insertion
Obturator .................. 31527
Nerve
Destruction ................ 31595
Reconstruction
Burns ..................... 31588
Cricoid Split .............. 31587
Other ..................... 31588
Stenosis .................. 31582
Web ...................... 31580
Removal
Foreign Body
Endoscopic .... 31511, 31530-31531, 31577
Lesion
Endoscopic .... 31512, 31545-31546, 31578
Repair
Reinnervation Neuromuscular Pedicle .. 31590
Stroboscopy ................... 31579
Tumor
Excision ................... 31300
Endoscopic ............. 31540-31541
Unlisted Services and Procedures ........ 31599
Vocal Cord(s)
Injection ............. 31513, 31570-31571
X-ray ........................ 70370
with Contrast ................. 70373

## Laser Surgery
Anus ................... 46614, 46917
Cautery
Esophagus ................. 43227
Hemorrhoids ............... 46930
Lacrimal Punctum ............. 68760
Lens, Posterior ............... 66821
Lesion
Mouth ..................... 40820
Nose .................. 30117-30118
Penis ..................... 54057
Skin ........ 17000-17111, 17260-17286
Myocardium ............. 33140-33141
Prostate ............... 52647-52648
Tumors
Urethra and Bladder ......... 52234
Urethra and Bladder ............. 52214

## Laser Treatment ......... 17000-17286, 96920-96922
See Destruction

## Lateral Epicondylitis
See Tennis Elbow

## Latex Fixation ............ 86403-86406

## LATS
See Thyrotropin Releasing Hormone (TRH)

## Latzko Operation
See Repair, Vagina, Fistula; Revision

## LAV
See HIV

## LAV Antibodies
See Antibody, HIV

## LAV-2
See HIV-2

## Lavage
Colon .......................... 44701
Lung
Bronchial .................... 31624
Total ....................... 32997
Peritoneal .................... 49084
Stomach ...................... 43753

## LCM
See Lymphocytic Choriomeningitis

## LD
See Lactate Dehydrogenase

## LDH ................... 83615-83625

## LDL
See Lipoprotein, LDL

## Lead ......................... 83655

## Leadbetter Procedure ......... 53431

## Lecithin-Sphingomyelin Ratio ....................... 83661

## Lecithinase C
See Tissue, Typing

## Lee and White Test ........... 85345

## LEEP Procedure .............. 57460

## LeFort Procedure
Vagina ........................ 57120

## LeFort I Procedure
Midface Reconstruction ........ 21141-21147, 21155, 21160
Palatal or Maxillary Fracture ...... 21421-21423

## LeFort II Procedure
Midface Reconstruction ......... 21150-21151
Nasomaxillary Complex Fracture ... 21345-21348

## LeFort III Procedure
Craniofacial Separation ......... 21431-21436
Midface Reconstruction ......... 21154-21159

## Left Atrioventricular Valve
See Mitral Valve

## Left Heart Cardiac Catheterization
See Cardiac Catheterization, Left Heart

## Leg
Cast
Rigid Total Contact ............ 29445
Lower
See Ankle; Fibula; Knee; Tibia
Abscess
Incision and Drainage ............ 27603
Amputation ....... 27598, 27880-27882
Revision ................ 27884-27886
Angiography ................... 73706
Artery
Ligation ................... 37618

Finger
  Tendon Sheath . . . . . . . . . . . . . . . . . . . 26160
Foot
  Excision . . . . . . . . . . . . . . . 28080, 28090
Gums
  Destruction . . . . . . . . . . . . . . . . . . . . 41850
  Excision . . . . . . . . . . . . . . 41822-41828
Hand Tendon Sheath . . . . . . . . . . . . . . . 26160
Intestines
  Excision . . . . . . . . . . . . . . . . . . . . . 44110
Intestines, Small
  Destruction . . . . . . . . . . . . . . . . . . . 44369
  Excision . . . . . . . . . . . . . . . . . . . . . 44111
Iris
  Destruction . . . . . . . . . . . . . . . . . . . 66770
Larynx
  Excision . . . . . . . . . . . . . . 31545-31546
Leg, Lower
  Tendon Sheath . . . . . . . . . . . . . . . . . 27630
Lymph Node
  Incision and Drainage . . . . . . . . 38300-38305
Mesentery
  Excision . . . . . . . . . . . . . . . . . . . . . 44820
Mouth
  Destruction . . . . . . . . . . . . . . . . . . . 40820
  Excision . . . . . . . . . . 40810-40816, 41116
  Vestibule
    Destruction . . . . . . . . . . . . . . . . . 40820
    Repair . . . . . . . . . . . . . . . . . . . . . 40830
Nerve
  Excision . . . . . . . . . . . . . . 64774-64792
Nose
  Intranasal
    External Approach . . . . . . . . . . . . . 30118
    Internal Approach . . . . . . . . . . . . . 30117
Orbit
  Excision . . . . . . . . . . . . . . 61333, 67412
Palate
  Destruction . . . . . . . . . . . . . . . . . . . 42160
  Excision . . . . . . . . . . . . . . 42104-42120
Pancreas
  Excision . . . . . . . . . . . . . . . . . . . . . 48120
Pelvis
  Destruction . . . . . . . . . . . . . . . . . . . 58662
Penis
  Destruction
    Cryosurgery . . . . . . . . . . . . . . . . . 54056
    Electrodesiccation . . . . . . . . . . . . . 54055
    Extensive . . . . . . . . . . . . . . . . . . 54065
    Laser Surgery . . . . . . . . . . . . . . . 54057
    Simple . . . . . . . . . . . . . 54050-54060
    Surgical Excision . . . . . . . . . . . . . 54060
  Excision . . . . . . . . . . . . . . . . . . . . . 54060
    Penile Plaque . . . . . . . . . . . 54110-54112
Pharynx
  Destruction . . . . . . . . . . . . . . . . . . . 42808
  Excision . . . . . . . . . . . . . . . . . . . . . 42808
Radiosurgery
  Cranial . . . . . . . . . . . . . . 61796-61800
Rectum
  Excision . . . . . . . . . . . . . . . . . . . . . 45108
Removal
  Larynx . . . . . . . . . . . . . . . 31512, 31578
Resection . . . . . . . . . . . . . . . . . . . . . . 52354
Retina
  Destruction
    Extensive . . . . . . . . . . . 67227-67228
    Localized . . . . . . . . . . . . 67208-67210
    Radiation by Implantation of Source . . . . 67218
Sciatic Nerve
  Excision . . . . . . . . . . . . . . . . . . . . . 64786
Sclera
  Excision . . . . . . . . . . . . . . . . . . . . . 66130

Skin
  Abrasion . . . . . . . . . . . . . . 15786-15787
  Biopsy . . . . . . . . . . . . . . . 11100-11101
  Destruction
    Benign . . . . . . . . . . 17110-17111, 17250
    Malignant . . . . . . . . . . . 17260-17286
    Premalignant . . . . . . . . . . 17000-17004
  Excision
    Benign . . . . . . . . . . . . 11400-11471
    Malignant . . . . . . . . . . . 11600-11646
  Injection . . . . . . . . . . . . . 11900-11901
  Paring or Curettement . . . . . . . . 11055-11057
  Shaving . . . . . . . . . . . . . 11300-11313
Skin Tags
  Removal . . . . . . . . . . . . . 11200-11201
Skull
  Excision . . . . . . . . . . 61500, 61600-61608,
                       61615-61616
Spermatic Cord
  Excision . . . . . . . . . . . . . . . . . . . . . 55520
Spinal Cord
  Destruction . . . . . . . . . . . . 62280-62282
  Excision . . . . . . . . . . . . . . 63265-63273
Stomach
  Excision . . . . . . . . . . . . . . . . . . . . . 43611
Testis
  Excision . . . . . . . . . . . . . . . . . . . . . 54512
Toe
  Excision . . . . . . . . . . . . . . . . . . . . . 28092
Tongue
  Excision . . . . . . . . . . . . . . 41110-41114
Uvula
  Destruction . . . . . . . . . . . . . . . . . . . 42145
  Excision . . . . . . . . . . . . . . 42104-42107
Vagina
  Destruction . . . . . . . . . . . . 57061-57065
Vulva
  Destruction
    Extensive . . . . . . . . . . . . . . . . . 56515
    Simple . . . . . . . . . . . . . . . . . . . 56501
Wrist Tendon
  Excision . . . . . . . . . . . . . . . . . . . . . 25110

**Leu 2 Antigens**
See CD8

**Leucine Aminopeptidase** . . . . . . . 83670

**Leukemia Lymphoma Virus I Antibodies, Human T Cell**
See Antibody, HTLV-I

**Leukemia Lymphoma Virus I, Adult T Cell**
See HTLV I

**Leukemia Lymphoma Virus II Antibodies, Human T Cell**
See Antibody, HTLV-II

**Leukemia Virus II, Hairy Cell Associated, Human T Cell**
See HTLV II

**Leukoagglutinins** . . . . . . . . . . . . . 86021

**Leukocyte**
See White Blood Cell
Alkaline Phosphatase . . . . . . . . . . . . . 85540
Antibody . . . . . . . . . . . . . . . . . . . . 86021
Count . . . . . . . . . . . . 85032, 85048, 89055
Histamine Release Test . . . . . . . . . . . . 86343
Phagocytosis . . . . . . . . . . . . . . . . . . 86344
Transfusion . . . . . . . . . . . . . . . . . . . 86950

**Levarterenol**
See Noradrenalin

**Levator Muscle Repair**
See Blepharoptosis, Repair

**LeVeen Shunt**
Insertion . . . . . . . . . . . . . . . . . . . . 49425
Patency Test . . . . . . . . . . . . . . . . . . 78291
Revision . . . . . . . . . . . . . . . . . . . . . 49426

**Levulose**
See Fructose

**LGV**
See Lymphogranuloma Venereum

**LH**
See Luteinizing Hormone (LH)

**LHR**
See Leukocyte Histamine Release Test

**Lid Suture**
See Blepharoptosis, Repair

**Lidocaine**
Assay . . . . . . . . . . . . . . . . . . . . . . 80176

**Lift, Face**
See Face Lift

**Ligament**
See Specific Site
Collateral
  Repair
    Knee
      with Cruciate Ligament . . . . . . . . . 27409
Dentate
  Section . . . . . . . . . . . . . . 63180-63182
Injection . . . . . . . . . . . . . . . . . . . . . 20550
Release
  Coracoacromial . . . . . . . . . . 23415, 29826
  Transverse Carpal . . . . . . . . . . . . . . 29848
Repair
  Elbow . . . . . . . . . . . . . . . 24343-24346
  Knee Joint . . . . . . . . . . . . . 27405-27409

**Ligation**
Artery
  Abdomen . . . . . . . . . . . . . . . . . . . 37617
  Carotid . . . . . . . . . . . . . . 37600-37606
  Chest . . . . . . . . . . . . . . . . . . . . . 37616
  Coronary . . . . . . . . . . . . . . . . . . . 33502
  Ethmoidal . . . . . . . . . . . . . . . . . . 30915
  Extremity . . . . . . . . . . . . . . . . . . . 37618
  Fistula . . . . . . . . . . . . . . . . . . . . . 37607
  Maxillary . . . . . . . . . . . . . . . . . . . 30920
  Neck . . . . . . . . . . . . . . . . . . . . . 37615
  Temporal . . . . . . . . . . . . . . . . . . . 37609
Esophageal Varices . . . . . . . . . . 43204, 43400
Fallopian Tube
  Oviduct . . . . . . . . . . . 58600-58611, 58670
Gastroesophageal . . . . . . . . . . . . . . . 43405
Hemorrhoids . . . . . . . . . . . . . . 46945-46946
  with Ultrasound . . . . . . . . . . . . . . . 0249T
Oviducts . . . . . . . . . . . . . . . . . . . . 59100
Salivary Duct . . . . . . . . . . . . . . . . . . 42665
Shunt
  Aorta
    Pulmonary . . . . . . . . . . . . . . . . . 33924
  Peritoneal
    Venous . . . . . . . . . . . . . . . . . . . 49428
Thoracic Duct . . . . . . . . . . . . . . . . . 38380
  Abdominal Approach . . . . . . . . . . . . . 38382
  Thoracic Approach . . . . . . . . . . . . . . 38381

Metatarsophalangeal Joint . . . . . . . . . . 28022
Tarsometatarsal Joint . . . . . . . . . . . . . 28020
Toe . . . . . . . . . . . . . . . . . . . . . . . . . . 28022
Wrist . . . . . . . . . . . . . . . . . . . . . . . . . 25101

## Lord Procedure
See Anal Sphincter, Dilation

## Louis Bar Syndrome
See Ataxia Telangiectasia

## Low Birth Weight Intensive Care Services . . . . . . . . . . . . . . . . . . 99478-99480

## Low Density Lipoprotein
See Lipoprotein, LDL

## Low Frequency Ultrasound . . . . . 0183T

## Low Vision Aids
See Spectacle Services
Fitting . . . . . . . . . . . . . . . . . . . . . . . . 92354-92355

## Lower Extremities
See Extremity, Lower

## Lower GI Series
See Barium Enema

## LRH
See Luteinizing Releasing Factor

## LSD
See Lysergic Acid Diethylamide

## LTH
See Prolactin

## Lumbar
See Spine

## Lumbar Plexus
Decompression . . . . . . . . . . . . . . . . . . . 64714
Injection
   Anesthetic . . . . . . . . . . . . . . . . . . . . 64449
Neuroplasty . . . . . . . . . . . . . . . . . . . . . 64714
Release . . . . . . . . . . . . . . . . . . . . . . . . 64714
Repair/Suture . . . . . . . . . . . . . . . . . . . . 64862

## Lumbar Puncture
See Spinal Tap

## Lumbar Spine Fracture
See Fracture, Vertebra, Lumbar

## Lumbar Sympathectomy
See Sympathectomy, Lumbar

## Lumbar Vertebra
See Vertebra, Lumbar

## Lumen Dilation . . . . . . . . . . . . . . . 74360

## Lumpectomy . . . . . . . . . . . . . . 19301-19302

## Lunate
Arthroplasty
   with Implant . . . . . . . . . . . . . . . . . . . 25444
Dislocation
   Closed Treatment . . . . . . . . . . . . . . . 25690
   Open Treatment . . . . . . . . . . . . . . . . 25695

## Lung
Ablation . . . . . . . . . . . . . . . . . . . . . . . 32998
Abscess
   Incision and Drainage
      Open . . . . . . . . . . . . . . . . . . . . . . . 32200
      Percutaneous . . . . . . . . . . . 32200-32201
Aspiration . . . . . . . . . . . . . . . . . . . . . . 32420
Biopsy . . . . . . . . . . . . . . . . . . . . . 32096-32097

Bullae
   Resection-Plication
      Thoracoscopic . . . . . . . . . . . . . . . . . 32655
      Thoracotomy . . . . . . . . . . . . . . . . . . 32141
Cyst
   Incision and Drainage
      Open . . . . . . . . . . . . . . . . . . . . . . . 32200
      Removal . . . . . . . . . . . . . . . . . . . . . 32140
Decortication
   Endoscopic . . . . . . . . . . . . . . . 32651-32652
   Partial . . . . . . . . . . . . . . . . . . . . . . . . 32225
   Total . . . . . . . . . . . . . . . . . . . . . . . . . 32220
   with Parietal Pleurectomy . . . . . . . . . . 32320
Empyema
   Excision . . . . . . . . . . . . . . . . . . . . . . 32540
Excision . . . . . . . . . . . . . . . . . . . 32440-32445
   Bronchus Resection . . . . . . . . . . . . . . 32486
   Completion . . . . . . . . . . . . . . . . . . . . 32488
   Donor
      Heart-Lung . . . . . . . . . . . . . . . . . . . 33930
      Lung . . . . . . . . . . . . . . . . . . . . . . . 32850
   Empyema . . . . . . . . . . . . . . . . . . . . . 32540
   Lobe . . . . . . . . . . . . . . . . . . . . 32480-32482
   Segment . . . . . . . . . . . . . . . . . . . . . . 32484
   Tumor . . . . . . . . . . . . . . . . . . . 32503-32504
Foreign Body
   Removal . . . . . . . . . . . . . . . . . . . . . . 32151
Hemorrhage . . . . . . . . . . . . . . . . . . . . 32110
Insertion
   Bronchial Valve . . . . . . . . . . . . . . . . . 0250T
Lavage
   Bronchial . . . . . . . . . . . . . . . . . . . . . 31624
   Total . . . . . . . . . . . . . . . . . . . . . . . . . 32997
Lysis
   Adhesions . . . . . . . . . . . . . . . . . . . . . 32124
Needle Biopsy . . . . . . . . . . . . . . . . . . . 32405
Nuclear Medicine
   Imaging, Perfusion . . . . . . 78580, 78597, 78598
   Imaging, Ventilation . . . . . 78579, 78582, 78598
   Unlisted Services and Procedures . . . . . . 78599
Placement
   Interstitial Device . . . . . . . . . . . . . . . . 32553
Pneumocentesis . . . . . . . . . . . . . . . . . . 32420
Pneumolysis . . . . . . . . . . . . . . . . . . . . 32940
Pneumothorax . . . . . . . . . . . . . . . . . . . 32960
Puncture . . . . . . . . . . . . . . . . . . . . . . 32420
Removal . . . . . . . . . . . . . . . . . . . 32440-32445
   Bilobectomy
      Thoracoscopic . . . . . . . . . . . . . . . . . 32670
   Bronchial Valve . . . . . . . . . . . . . . . . . 0251T
   Bronchoplasty . . . . . . . . . . . . . . . . . . 32501
   Completion Pneumonectomy . . . . . . . . . 32488
   Extrapleural . . . . . . . . . . . . . . . . . . . . 32445
   Pneumonectomy . . . . . . . . . . . . 32440-32445
      Thoracoscopic . . . . . . . . . . . . . . . . . 32671
   Segmentectomy
      Thoracoscopic . . . . . . . . . . . . . . . . . 32669
   Single Lobe . . . . . . . . . . . . . . . . . . . . 32480
   Single Segment . . . . . . . . . . . . . . . . . 32484
   Sleeve Lobectomy . . . . . . . . . . . . . . . . 32486
   Sleeve Pneumonectomy . . . . . . . . . . . . 32442
   Two Lobes . . . . . . . . . . . . . . . . 32482, 32670
   Volume Reduction . . . . . . . . . . . . . . . . 32491
Repair
   Hernia . . . . . . . . . . . . . . . . . . . . . . . 32800
Resection-Plication
   Emphysematous . . . . . . . . . . . . 32491, 32672
Segmentectomy . . . . . . . . . . . . . 32484, 32669
Tear
   Repair . . . . . . . . . . . . . . . . . . . . . . . 32110
Thoracotomy
   Biopsy . . . . . . . . . . . . . . . . . . . 32096-32097
   Cardiac Massage . . . . . . . . . . . . . . . . 32160

for Post-Op Complications . . . . . . . . . . . 32120
Removal
   Bullae . . . . . . . . . . . . . . . . . . . . . . . 32141
   Cyst . . . . . . . . . . . . . . . . . . . . . . . . . 32140
   Intrapleural Foreign Body . . . . . . . . . . . 32150
   Intrapulmonary Foreign Body . . . . . . . . 32151
   Repair . . . . . . . . . . . . . . . . . . . . . . . 32110
   with Open Intrapleural
      Pneumonolysis . . . . . . . . . . . . . . . . 32124
   with Resection-Plication of Bullae . . . . . 32141
Transplantation . . . . . . . . . . . 32851-32854, 33935
   Allograft Preparation . . . . 32855-32856, 33933
   Donor Pneumonectomy
      Heart-Lung . . . . . . . . . . . . . . . . . . . 33930
      Lung . . . . . . . . . . . . . . . . . . . . . . . 32850
Tumor
   Removal . . . . . . . . . . . . . . . . . 32503-32504
Unlisted Services and Procedures . . . . . . . . 32999

## Lung Function Tests
See Pulmonology, Diagnostic

## Lung Volume Reduction (LVRS)
Emphysematous . . . . . . . . . . . . . . . 32491, 32672

## Lupus Anticoagulant Assay . . . . 85705

## Lupus Band Test
See Immunofluorescent Study

## Luteinizing Hormone (LH) . . . . . . . . . . . . . 80418, 80426, 83002

## Luteinizing Releasing Factor . . . 83727

## Luteotropic Hormone
See Prolactin

## Luteotropin
See Prolactin

## Luteotropin, Placental
See Lactogen, Human Placental

## Lyme Disease . . . . . . . . . . . . . 86617-86618

## Lyme Disease ab
See Antibody, Lyme Disease

## Lyme Disease Vaccine
See Vaccination

## Lymph Duct
Injection . . . . . . . . . . . . . . . . . . . . . . . 38790

## Lymph Nodes
Abscess
   Incision and Drainage . . . . . . . . 38300-38305
Biopsy . . . . . . . . . . 38500, 38510-38530, 38570
   Needle . . . . . . . . . . . . . . . . . . . . . . . 38505
Dissection . . . . . . . . . . . . . . . . . . . . . . 38542
Excision . . . . . . . . . . . . . . . . 38500, 38510-38530
   Abdominal . . . . . . . . . . . . . . . . . . . . 38747
   Inguinofemoral . . . . . . . . . . . . . 38760-38765
   Laparoscopic . . . . . . . . . . . . . . 38571-38572
   Limited, for Staging
      Para-Aortic . . . . . . . . . . . . . . . . . . . 38562
      Pelvic . . . . . . . . . . . . . . . . . . . . . . 38562
      Retroperitoneal . . . . . . . . . . . . . . . . 38564
   Pelvic . . . . . . . . . . . . . . . . . . . . . . . . 38770
   Radical
      Axillary . . . . . . . . . . . . . . . . . 38740-38745
      Cervical . . . . . . . . . . . . . . . . . 38720-38724
      Suprahyoid . . . . . . . . . . . . . . . 38720-38724
      Retroperitoneal Transabdominal . . . . . . 38780
      Thoracic . . . . . . . . . . . . . . . . . . . . . 38746
Exploration . . . . . . . . . . . . . . . . . . . . . 38542

Lumbar . . . . . . . . . . . . . . . . . . . . 72148-72158
   Thoracic . . . . . . . .72146-72147, 72156-72158
Temporomandibular Joint (TMJ). . . . . . . . . 70336
Toe . . . . . . . . . . . . . . . . . . . . . . . . 73721-73723
Unlisted . . . . . . . . . . . . . . . . . . . . . . . . . 76498
Wrist. . . . . . . . . . . . . . . . . . . . . . . . . . . . 73221

## Magnetic Resonance Spectroscopy . . . . . . . . . . . . . . . . . 76390

## Magnetic Stimulation
Transcranial . . . . . . . . . . . . . . . . . . . 90867-90869

## Magnetoencephalography (MEG) . . . . . . . . . . . . . . . 95965-95967

## Magnuson Procedure . . . . . . . . . . 23450

## MAGPI Operation . . . . . . . . . . . . . 54322

## MAGPI Procedure
See Hypospadias, Repair

## Major Vestibular Gland
See Bartholin's Gland

## Malar Area
Augmentation. . . . . . . . . . . . . . . . . . . . . . 21270
Bone Graft . . . . . . . . . . . . . . . . . . . . . . . . 21210
Fracture
   Open Treatment . . . . . . . . . . . . . 21360-21366
   with Bone Graft . . . . . . . . . . . . . . . . . 21366
   with Manipulation . . . . . . . . . . . . . . . . 21355
Reconstruction . . . . . . . . . . . . . . . . . . . . . 21270

## Malar Bone
See Cheekbone

## Malaria Antibody . . . . . . . . . . . . . . 86750

## Malaria Smear . . . . . . . . . . . . . . . . 87207

## Malate Dehydrogenase . . . . . . . . 83775

## Maldescent, Testis
See Testis, Undescended

## Male Circumcision
See Circumcision

## Malformation, Arteriovenous
See Arteriovenous Malformation

## Malic Dehydrogenase
See Malate Dehydrogenase

## Malignant Hyperthermia Susceptibility
Caffeine Halothane Contracture Test
(CHCT). . . . . . . . . . . . . . . . . . . . . . . . . . 89049

## Malleolus
See Ankle; Fibula; Leg, Lower; Tibia; Tibiofibular
Joint

## Mallet Finger Repair . . . . . . . . . . . 26432

## Maltose
Tolerance Test . . . . . . . . . . . . . . . . 82951-82952

## Malunion Repair
Femur
   with Graft. . . . . . . . . . . . . . . . . . . . . . 27472
   without Graft . . . . . . . . . . . . . . . . . . . . 27470
Metatarsal . . . . . . . . . . . . . . . . . . . . . . . . 28322
Tarsal Joint. . . . . . . . . . . . . . . . . . . . . . . . 28320

## Mammalian Oviduct
See Fallopian Tube

## Mammaplasty
See Breast, Reconstruction; Mammoplasty

## Mammary Abscess
See Abscess, Breast

## Mammary Arteries
See Artery, Mammary

## Mammary Duct
X-ray with Contrast . . . . . . . . . . . . . 77053-77054

## Mammary Ductogram
Injection . . . . . . . . . . . . . . . . . . . . . . . . . 19030

## Mammary Stimulating Hormone
See Prolactin

## Mammillaplasty
See Nipples, Reconstruction

## Mammogram
Breast
   Localization Nodule . . . . . . . . . . . . . . . 77032

## Mammography . . . . . . . . . . . 77055-77057
Magnetic Resonance Imaging (MRI)
   with Computer-Aided Detection . . . . . . . 0159T
Screening . . . . . . . . . . . . . . . . . . . . . . . . 77057
with Computer-Aided Detection . . . . 77051-77052

## Mammoplasty
Augmentation. . . . . . . . . . . . . . . . . 19324-19325
Reduction . . . . . . . . . . . . . . . . . . . . . . . . 19318

## Mammotomy
See Incision, Breast; Incision and Drainage, Breast;
Mastotomy

## Mammotropic Hormone, Pituitary
See Prolactin

## Mammotropic Hormone, Placental
See Lactogen, Human Placental

## Mammotropin
See Prolactin

## Mandated Services
On Call Services. . . . . . . . . . . . . . . . . . . 99027

## Mandible
See Facial Bones; Maxilla; Temporomandibular
Joint (TMJ)
Abscess
   Excision . . . . . . . . . . . . . . . . . . . . . . 21025
Bone Graft . . . . . . . . . . . . . . . . . . . . . . . . 21215
Cyst
   Excision . . . . . . . . . . . . 21040, 21046-21047
Fracture
   Closed Treatment
     with Interdental Fixation . . . . . . . . . . 21453
     with Manipulation . . . . . . . . . . . . . . 21451
     without Manipulation. . . . . . . . . . . . . 21450
   Open Treatment . . . . . . . . . . . . . 21454-21470
     External Fixation. . . . . . . . . . . . . . . . 21454
     with Interdental Fixation . . . . . . . . . . 21462
     without Interdental Fixation. . . . . . . . . 21461
   Percutaneous Treatment . . . . . . . . . . . . 21452
Osteotomy . . . . . . . . . . . . . . . . . . 21198-21199
Reconstruction
   with Implant. . . . . . .21244-21246, 21248-21249
Removal
   Foreign Body . . . . . . . . . . . . . . . . . . . 41806
Torus Mandibularis
   Excision . . . . . . . . . . . . . . . . . . . . . . 21031
Tumor
   Excision . . . . . . . . . . . . . . . . . 21040-21047

X-ray . . . . . . . . . . . . . . . . . . . . . . . 70100-70110

## Mandibular Body
Augmentation
   with Bone Graft . . . . . . . . . . . . . . . . . . 21127
   with Prosthesis . . . . . . . . . . . . . . . . . . 21125

## Mandibular Condyle
Fracture
   Open Treatment . . . . . . . . . . . . . . . . . 21465
Reconstruction. . . . . . . . . . . . . . . . . . . . . 21247

## Mandibular Condylectomy
See Condylectomy

## Mandibular Fracture
See Fracture, Mandible

## Mandibular Rami
Reconstruction
   with Bone Graft . . . . . . . . . . . . . . . . . . 21194
   with Internal Rigid Fixation . . . . . . . . . . . 21196
   without Bone Graft . . . . . . . . . . . . . . . . 21193
   without Internal Rigid Fixation . . . . . . . . 21195

## Mandibular Resection Prosthesis . .
21081

## Mandibular Staple Bone Plate
Reconstruction
   Mandible . . . . . . . . . . . . . . . . . . . . . . 21244

## Manganese . . . . . . . . . . . . . . . . . . . 83785

## Manipulation
Chest Wall . . . . . . . . . . . . . . . . . . 94667-94668
Chiropractic . . . . . . . . . . . . . . . . . 98940-98943
Dislocation and/or Fracture. . . . . . . . . . . . 25535
   Acetabulum . . . . . . . . . . . . . . . . . . . . 27222
   Acromioclavicular . . . . . . . . . . . . . . . . 23545
   Ankle . . . . . . . . . . . 27810, 27818, 27860
   Carpometacarpal . . . . . . . . . . . . . 26670-26676
   Clavicular . . . . . . . . . . . . . . . . . . . . . . 23505
   Elbow . . . . . . . . . . . . . . . . . 24300, 24640
   Femoral . . . . . . . 27232, 27502, 27510, 27517
     Peritrochanteric . . . . . . . . . . . . . . . . 27240
   Fibula . . . . . . . . . . . . . . . . . 27781, 27788
   Finger . . . . . . . . . . 26725-26727, 26742, 26755
   Greater Tuberosity
     Humeral . . . . . . . . . . . . . . . . . . . . . 23625
   Hand. . . . . . . . . . . . . . . . . . . 26670-26676
   Heel . . . . . . . . . . . . . . . . . . . 28405-28406
   Hip . . . . . . . . . . . . . . . . . . . . . . . . . . 27257
   Hip Socket . . . . . . . . . . . . . . . . . . . . . 27222
   Humeral . . . . 23605, 24505, 24535, 24577
     Epicondyle . . . . . . . . . . . . . . . . . . . 24565
   Intercarpal . . . . . . . . . . . . . . . . . . . . . 25660
   Interphalangeal Joint. . . . 26340, 26770-26776
   Lunate . . . . . . . . . . . . . . . . . . . . . . . . 25690
   Malar Area. . . . . . . . . . . . . . . . . . . . . 21355
   Mandibular. . . . . . . . . . . . . . . . . . . . . 21451
   Metacarpal. . . . . . . . . . . . . . . . 26605-26607
   Metacarpophalangeal . . . 26700-26706, 26742
   Metacarpophalangeal Joint . . . . . . . . . . 26340
   Metatarsal . . . . . . . . . . . . . . . . 28475-28476
   Nasal Bone. . . . . . . . . . . . . . . . 21315-21320
   Orbit. . . . . . . . . . . . . . . . . . . . . . . . . 21401
   Phalangeal Shaft . . . . . . . . . . . . . . . . . 26727
     Distal, Finger or Thumb . . . . . . . . . . . 26755
     Phalanges, Finger/Thumb. . . . . . . . . . 26725
   Phalanges
     Finger . . . . . . . . 26742, 26755, 26770-26776
     Finger/Thumb. . . . . . . . . . . . . . . . . . 26727
     Great Toe . . . . . . . . . . . . . . . . 28495-28496
     Toes . . . . . . . . . . . . . . . . . . . . . . . . 28515

Radial............... 24655, 25565
Radial Shaft........................ 25505
Radiocarpal....................... 25660
Radioulnar........................ 25675
Scapular.......................... 23575
Shoulder............... 23650-23655
  with Greater Tuberosity.......... 23665
Sternoclavicular................... 23525
  with Neck Fracture.............. 23675
Talus...................... 28435-28436
Tarsal..................... 28455-28456
Thumb..................... 26641-26650
Tibial................. 27532, 27752
Trans-Scaphoperilunar............. 25680
Ulnar............. 24675, 25535, 25565
Vertebral......................... 22315
Wrist........ 25259, 25624, 25635,
    25660, 25675, 25680, 25690
Foreskin.......................... 54450
Globe...................... 92018-92019
Hip............................... 27275
Interphalangeal Joint, Proximal...... 26742
Knee............................. 27570
Osteopathic............... 98925-98929
Shoulder
  Application of Fixation Apparatus..... 23700
Spine
  with Anesthesia.................. 22505
Temporomandibular Joint(s) (TMJ)....... 21073
Tibial, Distal..................... 27762

**Manometric Studies**
Colon............................ 91117
Esophagus........................ 91010
  with Perfusion............. 91013, 0241T
  with Pressure Topography........... 0240T
  with Stimulation........... 91013, 0241T
Gastrointestinal Tract................. 0242T
Kidney
  Pressure....................... 50396
Rectum/Anus...................... 91122
Ureter
  Pressure....................... 50686
Ureterostomy..................... 50686

**Manometry**
Rectum........................... 90911

**Mantoux Test**
*See* TB Test, Skin Test

**Manual Therapy**.............. 97140

**Maquet Procedure**........... 27418

**Marcellation Operation**
*See* Hysterectomy, Vaginal

**Marrow, Bone**
*See* Bone Marrow

**Marshall-Marchetti-Krantz Procedure**.......... 51840-51841, 58152,
    58267, 58293

**Marsupialization**
Bartholin's Gland Cyst.............. 56440
Cyst
  Sublingual Salivary............. 42409
Liver
  Cyst or Abscess................ 47300
Pancreatic Cyst................... 48500
Skin............................. 10040
Urethral Diverticulum.............. 53240

**Mass**
Kidney
  Ablation....................... 50542
    Cryosurgical................. 50250

**Mass Spectrometry and Tandem Mass Spectrometry**
Analyte
  Qualitative.................... 83788
  Quantitative................... 83789

**Massage**
Cardiac.......................... 32160
Therapy.......................... 97124
  *See* PhysicalMedicine/Therapy/Occupational Therapy

**Masseter Muscle/Bone**
Reduction................. 21295-21296

**Mastectomy**
Gynecomastia..................... 19300
Modified Radical.................. 19307
Partial.................. 19301-19302
Radical................. 19303-19306
Simple, Complete................. 19303
Subcutaneous..................... 19304

**Mastectomy, Halsted**
*See* Mastectomy, Radical

**Mastoid**
Excision
  Complete...................... 69502
  Radical....................... 69511
    Modified.................... 69505
    Petrous Apicectomy........... 69530
  Simple........................ 69501
Obliteration...................... 69670
Repair
  by Excision............. 69601-69603
  Fistula....................... 69700
  with Apicectomy................ 69605
  with Tympanoplasty............. 69604

**Mastoid Cavity**
Debridement............. 69220-69222

**Mastoidectomy**
Osseointegrated Implant
  for External Speech Processor/Cochlear
  Stimulator............. 69715, 69718
with Apicectomy................... 69605
with Skull Base Surgery......... 61590, 61597
  Decompression................. 61595
  Facial Nerve................... 61595
with Tympanoplasty....... 69604, 69641-69646
  Cochlear Device Implantation........ 69930
  Complete...................... 69502
    Revision.................... 69601
  Ossicular Chain Reconstruction...... 69605
  Radical....................... 69511
    Modified.................... 69505
    Revision............... 69602-69603
  Simple........................ 69501
  with Labyrinthectomy........... 69910
  with Petrous Apicectomy......... 69530

**Mastoidotomy**............ 69635-69637
with Tympanoplasty................ 69635
  Ossicular Chain Reconstruction...... 69636
    and Synthetic Prosthesis....... 69636

**Mastoids**
Polytomography............. 76101-76102
X-ray.................. 70120-70130

**Mastopexy**...................19316

**Mastotomy**.................19020

**Maternity Care**
*See* Abortion; Cesarean Delivery; Ectopic Pregnancy; Obstetrical Care

**Maternity Care and Delivery**............ 59612-59622, 59898

**Maxilla**
*See* Facial Bones; Mandible
Bone Graft........................ 21210
CT Scan............... 70486-70488
Cyst
  Excision.............. 21048-21049
Excision............ 21030, 21032-21034
Fracture
  Closed Treatment.......... 21345, 21421
  Open Treatment... 21346-21348, 21422-21423
  with Fixation.......... 21345-21347
Osteotomy....................... 21206
Reconstruction
  with Implant... 21245-21246, 21248-21249
Tumor
  Excision.............. 21048-21049

**Maxillary Arteries**
*See* Artery, Maxillary

**Maxillary Sinus**
*See* Sinus/Sinuses, Maxillary

**Maxillary Torus Palatinus**
Tumor Excision.................... 21032

**Maxillectomy**.......... 31225-31230

**Maxillofacial Fixation**
Application
  Halo Type Appliance............. 21100

**Maxillofacial Impressions**
Auricular Prosthesis............... 21086
Definitive Obturator Prosthesis...... 21080
Facial Prosthesis.................. 21088
Interim Obturator Prosthesis........ 21079
Mandibular Resection Prosthesis..... 21081
Nasal Prosthesis.................. 21087
Oral Surgical Splint................ 21085
Orbital Prosthesis................. 21077
Palatal Augmentation Prosthesis..... 21082
Palatal Lift Prosthesis............. 21083
Speech Aid Prosthesis............. 21084
Surgical Obturator Prosthesis........ 21076

**Maxillofacial Procedures**
Unlisted Services and Procedures........ 21299

**Maxillofacial Prosthetics**............ 21076-21089
Unlisted Services and Procedures........ 21089

**Maydl Operation**........ 45563, 50810
*See* Colostomy

**Mayo Hernia Repair**
*See* Hernia, Repair, Umbilicus

**Mayo Procedure**................28292

**Maze Procedure**
  Endoscopic............ 33265-33266
  Open................. 33254-33256

**McBride Procedure**............28292

**McBurney Operation**
See Hernia, Repair, Inguinal

**McCannel Procedure** .......... 66682

**McKissock Surgery**
See Breast, Reduction

**MCOLN1** ...................... 81290

**McVay Operation**
See Hernia, Repair, Inguinal

**Measles Uncomplicated**
See Rubeola

**Measles Vaccine**
See Vaccines

**Measles, German**
See Rubella

**Meat Fibers**
Feces ............................ 89160

**Meatoplasty** ................... 69310

**Meatotomy** ............... 53020-53025
Cystourethroscopy ............... 52281
Infant ........................... 53025
Prostate
  Laser Coagulation .............. 52647
  Laser Vaporization ............. 52648
Transurethral Electrosurgical Resection
  Prostate ....................... 52601
Ureter .......................... 52290
Ureteral
  Cystourethroscopy .......... 52290-52305

**MECP2** ................... 81302-81304

**Meckel's Diverticulum**
Excision ......................... 44800
Unlisted Services and Procedures ........ 44899

**Median Nerve**
Decompression .................... 64721
Neuroplasty ...................... 64721
Release .......................... 64721
Repair/Suture
  Motor Thenar ................... 64835
Transposition .................... 64721

**Median Nerve Compression**
See Carpal Tunnel Syndrome

**Mediastinal Cyst**
See Cyst, Mediastinal; Mediastinum, Cyst

**Mediastinoscopy** ............... 39400

**Mediastinotomy**
Cervical Approach ................. 39000
Transthoracic Approach ............ 39010

**Mediastinum**
See Chest; Thorax
Cyst
  Excision ....................... 32662
  Resection ...................... 39200
Endoscopy
  Biopsy ......................... 39400
  Exploration .................... 39400
Exploration ................. 39000-39010
Incision and Drainage .......... 39000-39010
Needle Biopsy .................... 32405
Removal
  Foreign Body .............. 39000-39010

Thoracoscopy
  Diagnostic ..................... 32601
Tumor
  Excision ....................... 32662
Unlisted Procedures .............. 39499

**Medical Disability Evaluation Services** ............... 99455-99456

**Medical Genetics** ............. 96040
Genetic Counseling ............... 96040

**Medical Team Conference** .............. 99366-99368

**Medical Testimony** ............. 99075

**Medication Therapy Management**
Pharmacist Provided ......... 99605-99607

**Medicine, Preventive**
See Preventive Medicine

**Medicine, Pulmonary**
See Pulmonology

**Medulla**
Tractotomy ....................... 61470

**Medullary Tract**
Incision ......................... 61470
Section .......................... 61470

**Meibomian Cyst**
See Chalazion

**Membrane Oxygenation, Extracorporeal**
See Extracorporeal Membrane Oxygenation

**Membrane, Mucous**
See Mucosa

**Membrane, Tympanic**
See Ear, Drum

**Meninges**
Tumor
  Excision ................. 61512, 61519

**Meningioma**
Excision .................. 61512, 61519
Tumor
  Excision ................. 61512, 61519

**Meningitis, Lymphocytic Benign**
See Lymphocytic Choriomeningitis

**Meningocele Repair** ...... 63700-63702

**Meningococcal**
See Vaccines

**Meningococcal Vaccine**
See Vaccines

**Meningococcus**
See Neisseria Meningitidis

**Meningomyelocele**
See Myelomeningocele

**Meniscectomy**
Knee Joint .................. 27332-27333
Temporomandibular Joint .......... 21060

**Meniscus**
Knee
  Excision ............... 27332-27333
  Repair ......................... 27403

Transplantation ................. 29868

**Mental Nerve**
Avulsion ......................... 64736
Incision ......................... 64736
Transection ...................... 64736

**Meprobamate** .................. 83805

**Mercury** ................ 83015, 83825

**Mesencephalic Tract**
Incision ......................... 61480
Section .......................... 61480

**Mesencephalon**
Tractotomy ....................... 61480

**Mesenteric Arteries**
See Artery, Mesenteric

**Mesentery**
Lesion
  Excision ....................... 44820
Repair ........................... 44850
Suture ........................... 44850
Unlisted Services and Procedures ........ 44899

**Mesh**
Implantation
  Hernia .............. 49568, 49652-49657
Insertion
  Pelvic Floor ................... 57267
Removal
  Abdominal Infected ............. 11008

**Metabisulfite Test**
See Red Blood Cell (RBC), Sickling

**Metabolite** .................... 82520
Thromboxane ...................... 84431

**Metacarpal**
Amputation ....................... 26910
Craterization .................... 26230
Cyst
  Excision ................. 26200-26205
Diaphysectomy .................... 26230
Fracture
  Closed Treatment ............... 26605
    with Fixation ................ 26607
  Open Treatment ................. 26615
  Percutaneous Fixation .......... 26608
  with Manipulation ........ 26605-26607
  without Manipulation ........... 26600
Ostectomy ........................ 26250
Repair
  Lengthening .................... 26568
  Nonunion ....................... 26546
  Osteotomy ...................... 26565
Saucerization .................... 26230
Tumor
  Excision ................. 26200-26205
  Radical Resection .............. 26250

**Metacarpophalangeal Joint**
Arthrodesis ................ 26850-26852
Arthroplasty ............... 26530-26531
Arthroscopy
  Diagnostic ..................... 29900
  Surgical ................. 29901-29902
Arthrotomy ....................... 26075
Biopsy
  Synovium ....................... 26105
Capsule
  Excision ....................... 26520
  Incision ....................... 26520

## Minnesota Multiphasic Personality Inventory
See MMPI

## Miscarriage
Incomplete Abortion . . . . . . . . . . . . . . . . . . . 59812
Missed Abortion
　First Trimester . . . . . . . . . . . . . . . . . . . . 59820
　Second Trimester . . . . . . . . . . . . . . . . . 59821
Septic Abortion . . . . . . . . . . . . . . . . . . . . . . 59830

## Missed Abortion
See Abortion

## Mitchell Procedure . . . . . . . . . . . .28296

## Mitogen Blastogenesis . . . . . . . .86353

## Mitral Valve
Incision . . . . . . . . . . . . . . . . . . . . . 33420-33422
Repair . . . . . . . . . . . . . . . . . . . . . . 33420-33427
　Incision . . . . . . . . . . . . . . . . . . . 33420-33422
Replacement . . . . . . . . . . . . . . . . . . . . . . . 33430

## Mitrofanoff Operation . . . . . . . . . .50845
See Appendico-Vesicostomy

## Miyagawanella
See Chlamydia

## MLC
See Lymphocyte, Culture

## MLH1 . . . . . . . . . . . . . . . . . . . 81292-81294

## MMPI . . . . . . . . . . . . . . . . . . . . 96101-96103
Computer-Assisted . . . . . . . . . . . . . . . . . . 96103

## MMR Shots . . . . . . . . . . . . . . . . .90707
See Vaccines

## Mobilization
Splenic Flexure . . . . . . . . . . . . . . . . . . . . . 44139
　Laparoscopic . . . . . . . . . . . . . . . . . . . . 44213
Stapes . . . . . . . . . . . . . . . . . . . . . . . . . . . 69650

## Moderate Sedation
See Sedation

## Modified Radical Mastectomy
See Mastectomy, Modified Radical

## Mohs Micrographic Surgery . . . . . . . . . . . . . . . . . . 17311-17315

## Molar Pregnancy
See Hydatidiform Mole

## Mold
Culture . . . . . . . . . . . . . . . . . . . . . . . . . . . 87107

## Mole, Carneous
See Abortion

## Mole, Hydatid
See Hydatidiform Mole

## Molecular Cytogenetics . . 88271-88275
Interpretation and Report . . . . . . . . . . . . . 88291

## Molecular Diagnostics . . . 83890-83914
Amplification . . . . . . . . . . . . 83898-83901, 83908
Cell Lysis . . . . . . . . . . . . . . . . . . . . . . . . . 83907
Dot/Slot Production . . . . . . . . . . . . . . . . . 83893
Enzymatic Digestion . . . . . . . . . . . . . . . . 83892
Extraction . . . . . . . . . . . . . . . . . . 83890-83891
Interpretation . . . . . . . . . . . . . . . . . . . . . 83912
Macroscopic Evaluation . . . . . . . . . 88387-88388
Molecular Isolation (Extraction) . . . . . . . . 83890

Mutation Identification . . . . . . . . . . 83904-83906
　Enzymatic Ligation . . . . . . . . . . . . . . . . 83914
Mutation Scanning . . . . . . . . . . . . . . . . . 83903
Nucleic Acid Amplification . . . . . . . . 83900-83901,
　　　　　　　　　　　　　　　　　　　83908
Nucleic Acid Extraction . . . . 83890-83891, 83907
Nucleic Acid Probe . . . . . . . . . . . . . . . . . 83896
Nucleic Acid Transfer . . . . . . . . . . . . . . . . 83897
Polymerase Reaction Chain . . . . . . . . . . . . 83898
Reverse Transcription . . . . . . . . . . . . . . . 83902
RNA Stabilization . . . . . . . . . . . . . . . . . . 83913
Separation . . . . . . . . . . . . . . . . . . . . . . . 83894
Separation and Identification
　High Resolution Technique . . . . . . . . . . 83909

## Molecular Oxygen Saturation
See Oxygen Saturation

## Molecular Pathology . . . . . 81200-81383,
　　　　　　　　　　　　　　81400-81408
See Also Gene Tests

## Molecular Probes . . . . . . . . 88384-88386
Multiple
　Array-Based Evaluation . . . . . . . . 88384-88386

## Molluscum Contagiosum
Destruction . . . . . . . . . 17110-17111, 54050-54065

## Molteno Procedure . . . . . . . . . . . .66180

## Monilia
See Candida

## Monitoring
Blood Pressure, 24 Hour . . . . . . . . . 93784-93790
Cardiovascular Device
　Evaluation and Programming
　　Cardioverter-Defibrillator . . . . . 93282-93284,
　　　　　　　　　　　　93287, 93289-93290, 93292,
　　　　　　　　　　　　93295-93296, 93299
　　Loop Recorder . . . . . . . . . . . 93285, 93291,
　　　　　　　　　　　　93298-93299
　　Pacemaker . . . . . 93279-93281, 93294-93296
Electrocardiogram . . . . . . . . 93268, 93270-93272
　See Electrocardiography
Electroencephalogram . . . . . . . . . . . 95812-95813,
　　　　　　　　　　　　95950-95953, 95956
　with Drug Activation . . . . . . . . . . . . . . . 95954
　with Physical Activation . . . . . . . . . . . . 95954
　with WADA Activation . . . . . . . . . . . . . 95958
Fetal
　During Labor . . . . . . . . . . 59050-59051, 99500
　Interpretation Only . . . . . . . . . . . . . . . . 59051
Glucose
　Interstitial Fluid . . . . . . . . . . . . 95250-95251
Interstitial Fluid Pressure . . . . . . . . . . . . . 20950
Intraocular Pressure . . . . . . . . . . . . . . . . . 0173T
Pediatric Apnea . . . . . . . . . . . . . . . 94774-94777
Seizure . . . . . . . . . . . . . . . . . . . . . 61531, 61760

## Monitoring, Sleep . . . 0244T, 95800-95801
See Polysomnography

## Monoethylene Glycol
See Ethylene Glycol

## Mononuclear Cell Antigen . . . . .86356

## Mononucleosis Virus, Infectious
See Epstein-Barr Virus

## Monophosphate, Adenosine
See Adenosine Monophosphate (AMP)

## Monophosphate, Adenosine Cyclic
See Cyclic AMP

## Monophosphate, Guanosine
See Guanosine Monophosphate

## Monophosphate, Guanosine Cyclic
See Cyclic GMP

## Monospot Test
See Rapid Test for Infection

## Monoxide, Carbon
See Carbon Monoxide

## Monteggia Fracture . . . . . . . 24620-24635

## Monticelli Procedure
See Application, Bone Fixation Device

## Morbilli
See Rubeola

## Morphine Methyl Ether
See Codeine

## Morphometric Analysis
Nerve . . . . . . . . . . . . . . . . . . . . . . . . . . . 88356
Skeletal Muscle . . . . . . . . . . . . . . . . . . . . 88355
Tumor . . . . . . . . . . . . 88358-88361, 88367-88368
Urinary Tract Specimen . . . . . . . . . . 88120-88121

## Morton's Neuroma
See Neuroma, Foot
Excision . . . . . . . . . . . . . . . . . . . . . . . . . 28080

## Mosaicplasty . . . . . . . . . . . . . . . . .27416

## Mosenthal Test
See Urinalysis, Routine

## Mother Cell
See Stem Cell

## Motility Study
Colon . . . . . . . . . . . . . . . . . . . . . . . . . . . 91117
Duodenal . . . . . . . . . . . . . . . . . . . . . . . . 91022
Esophagus . . . . . . . . . . . . . . . . . . . . . . . 91010
　with Perfusion . . . . . . . . . . . . . . 91013, 0241T
　with Pressure Topography . . . . . . 0240T-0241T
　with Stimulation . . . . . . . . . . . . 91013, 0241T
　Imaging . . . . . . . . . . . . . . . . . . . . . . . . 78258
Sperm . . . . . . . . . . . . . . . . . . . . . . . . . . 89300

## Motion Analysis
by Video and 3-D Kinematics . . . . . . 96000, 96004
Computer-based . . . . . . . . . . . . . . . 96000, 96004

## Mouth
Abscess
　Incision and Drainage . . . . . . . . 40800-40801,
　　　　　　　　　　　41005-41009, 41015-41018
Biopsy . . . . . . . . . . . . . . . . . . . . . 40808, 41108
Cyst
　Incision and Drainage . . . . . . . . 40800-40801,
　　　　　　　　　　　41005-41009, 41015-41018
Excision
　Frenum . . . . . . . . . . . . . . . . . . . . . . . . 40819
Hematoma
　Incision and Drainage . . . . . . . . 40800-40801,
　　　　　　　　　　　41005-41009, 41015-41018
Lesion
　Destruction . . . . . . . . . . . . . . . . . . . . . 40820
　Excision . . . . . . . . . . . . . 40810-40816, 41116
　Vestibule
　　Destruction . . . . . . . . . . . . . . . . . . . 40820
　　Repair . . . . . . . . . . . . . . . . . . . . . . . 40830
Mucosa
　Excision . . . . . . . . . . . . . . . . . . . . . . . 40818
Reconstruction . . . . . . . . . . . . . . . . 40840-40845

## Myelin Basic Protein
Cerebrospinal Fluid . . . . . . . . . . . . . . . . . . . 83873

## Myelography
Brain . . . . . . . . . . . . . . . . . . . . . . . . . . . . 70010
Spine
   Cervical . . . . . . . . . . . . . . . . . . . . . . 72240
   Lumbosacral. . . . . . . . . . . . . . . . . . . . 72265
   Thoracic . . . . . . . . . . . . . . . . . . . . . . . 72255
   Total . . . . . . . . . . . . . . . . . . . . . . . . . 72270

## Myelomeningocele
Repair . . . . . . . . . . . . . . . . . . . . . 63704-63706

## Myeloperoxidase (MPO) . . . . . . .83876

## Myelotomy . . . . . . . . . . . . . . . . . . .63170

## Myocardial
Perfusion Imaging . . . . . . . . . . . . . . 78451-78454
   *See* Nuclear Medicine
Positron Emission Tomography (PET) . . . . . . 78459

## Myocardial Imaging . . . . . . . 78466-78469
Perfusion Study
   Positron Emission Tomography
   (PET) . . . . . . . . . . . . . . . . . . . . . 78491-78492
   Single Photon Emission Computed
   Tomography (SPECT) . . . . . . . . . . 78451-78452
Repair
   Postinfarction. . . . . . . . . . . . . . . . . . . 33542

## Myocutaneous
**Flaps** . . . . . . . . . . . . . 15731-15738, 15756

## Myofascial Pain Dysfunction Syndrome
*See* Temporomandibular Joint (TMJ)

## Myofibroma
*See* Leiomyomata

## Myoglobin . . . . . . . . . . . . . . . . . . . .83874

## Myomectomy
Anorectal . . . . . . . . . . . . . . . . . . . . . . . 45108
Uterus . . . . . . . . . . . . .58140-58146, 58545-58546

## Myoplasty
*See* Muscle, Repair

## Myotomy
Esophagus . . . . . . . . . . . . . . . . . . . . . . 43030
Hyoid. . . . . . . . . . . . . . . . . . . . . . . . . 21685

## Myringoplasty . . . . . . . . . . . . . . . .69620

## Myringostomy
*See* Myringotomy

## Myringotomy . . . . . . . . . . . . . 69420-69421

## Myxoid Cyst
*See* Ganglion

# N

## N. Meningitidis
*See* Neisseria Meningitidis

## Naffziger Operation
*See* Decompression, Orbit; Section

## Nagel Test
*See* Color Vision Examination

## Nail Bed
Reconstruction . . . . . . . . . . . . . . . . . . . 11762
Repair . . . . . . . . . . . . . . . . . . . . . . . . 11760

## Nail Fold
Excision
   Wedge . . . . . . . . . . . . . . . . . . . . . 11765

## Nail Plate Separation
*See* Nails, Avulsion

## Nails
Avulsion . . . . . . . . . . . . . . . . . . . 11730-11732
Biopsy. . . . . . . . . . . . . . . . . . . . . . . . . 11755
Debridement. . . . . . . . . . . . . . . . . 11720-11721
Drainage. . . . . . . . . . . . . . . . . . . 10060-10061
Evacuation
   Hematoma, Subungual . . . . . . . . . . . . 11740
Excision. . . . . . . . . . . . . . . . . . . . 11750-11752
KOH Examination . . . . . . . . . . . . . . . . . 87220
Removal . . . . . . . . . . .11730-11732, 11750-11752
Trimming. . . . . . . . . . . . . . . . . . . . . . . 11719

## Narcosynthesis
Diagnostic and Therapeutic . . . . . . . . . . . . 90865

## Nasal Abscess
*See* Nose, Abscess

## Nasal Area
Bone Graft . . . . . . . . . . . . . . . . . . . . . . 21210

## Nasal Bleeding
*See* Epistaxis

## Nasal Bone
Fracture
   Closed Treatment. . . . . . . . . . . . 21310-21320
   Open Treatment . . . . . . . . . . . . . 21325-21335
   with Manipulation . . . . . . . . . . . 21315-21320
   without Manipulation . . . . . . . . . . . . . 21310
X-ray . . . . . . . . . . . . . . . . . . . . . . . . . 70160

## Nasal Deformity
Repair . . . . . . . . . . . . . . . . . . . . 40700-40761

## Nasal Function Study . . . . . . . . . .92512

## Nasal Polyp
*See* Nose, Polyp

## Nasal Prosthesis
Impression . . . . . . . . . . . . . . . . . . . . . . 21087

## Nasal Septum
Abscess
   Incision and Drainage . . . . . . . . . . . . . 30020
Fracture
   Closed Treatment. . . . . . . . . . . . . . . . 21337
   Open Treatment . . . . . . . . . . . . . . . . . 21336
Hematoma
   Incision and Drainage . . . . . . . . . . . . . 30020
Repair . . . . . . . . . . . . . . . . . . . . . . . . 30630
Submucous Resection . . . . . . . . . . . . . . . 30520

## Nasal Sinuses
*See* Sinus/Sinuses

## Nasal Smear
Eosinophils. . . . . . . . . . . . . . . . . . . . . . 89190

## Nasal Turbinate
Fracture
   Therapeutic . . . . . . . . . . . . . . . . . . . 30930

## Nasoethmoid Complex
Fracture
   Open Treatment . . . . . . . . . . . . . 21338-21339
   Percutaneous Treatment . . . . . . . . . . . 21340
Reconstruction . . . . . . . . . . . . . . . 21182-21184

## Nasogastric Tube
Placement. . . . . . . . . . . . . . . . . . . . . . . 43752

## Nasolacrimal Duct
Exploration . . . . . . . . . . . . . . . . . . . . . . 68810
   with Anesthesia. . . . . . . . . . . . . . . . . 68811
Insertion
   Catheter Dilation . . . . . . . . . . . . . . . . 68816
   Stent. . . . . . . . . . . . . . . . . . . . . . . 68815
X-ray
   with Contrast . . . . . . . . . . . . . . . . . . 70170

## Nasomaxillary
Fracture
   Closed Treatment. . . . . . . . . . . . . . . . 21345
   Open Treatment . . . . . . . . . . . . . 21346-21348
   with Bone Grafting. . . . . . . . . . . . . . . . 21348

## Nasopharynges
*See* Nasopharynx

## Nasopharyngoscopy . . . . . . . . . . . .92511

## Nasopharynx
*See* Pharynx
Biopsy. . . . . . . . . . . . . . . . . . . . 42804-42806
Hemorrhage . . . . . . . . . . . . . . . . 42970-42972
Unlisted Services and Procedures . . . . . . . . 42999

## Natriuretic Peptide . . . . . . . . . . . . .83880

## Natural Killer (NK) Cells
Count. . . . . . . . . . . . . . . . . . . . . . . . . 86357

## Natural Ostium
Sinus
   Maxillary . . . . . . . . . . . . . . . . . . . . 31000
   Sphenoid . . . . . . . . . . . . . . . . . . . . 31002

## Navicular
Arthroplasty
   with Implant. . . . . . . . . . . . . . . . . . . 25443
Fracture
   Closed Treatment. . . . . . . . . . . . . . . . 25622
   Open Treatment . . . . . . . . . . . . . . . . . 25628
   with Manipulation . . . . . . . . . . . . . . . 25624
Repair . . . . . . . . . . . . . . . . . . . . . . . . 25440

## Navigation
   Computer Assisted. . . . . . . . . . . 0054T-0055T,
                20985, 31627, 61781-61783

## Neck
Angiography. . . . . . . . . . . . . 70498, 70547-70549
Artery
   Ligation . . . . . . . . . . . . . . . . . . . . . 37615
Biopsy. . . . . . . . . . . . . . . . . . . . . . . . . 21550
Bypass Graft. . . . . . . . . . . . . . . . . . . . . 35901
CT Scan. . . . . . . . . . . . 70490-70492, 70498
Dissection, Radical
   *See* Radical Neck Dissection
Exploration
   Blood Vessel. . . . . . . . . . . . . . . . . . . 35800
   Lymph Nodes . . . . . . . . . . . . . . . . . . 38542
Incision and Drainage
   Abscess . . . . . . . . . . . . . . . . 21501-21502
   Hematoma . . . . . . . . . . . . . . . 21501-21502
Lipectomy, Suction Assisted . . . . . . . . . . . 15876
Magnetic Resonance Angiography
(MRA) . . . . . . . . . . . . . . . . . . . . 70547-70549

## Nerves

Anastomosis
- Facial to Hypoglossal . . . . . . . . . . . . . . . 64868
- Facial to Phrenic . . . . . . . . . . . . . . . . . . . 64870
- Facial to Spinal Accessory . . . . . . . . . . 64866

Avulsion . . . . . . . . . . . . . . . . . . . . . . 64732-64772

Biopsy . . . . . . . . . . . . . . . . . . . . . . . . . . . . . . 64795

Cervical
- Neurostimulator Implant . . . . . . . .0282T-0283T

Decompression . . . . . . . . . . . . . . . . 64702-64727
- Laminotomy/Laminectomy . . . . . . .0274T-0275T

Destruction . . . . . . . . . . . . . . . . . . . 64600-64681
- Laryngeal, Recurrent . . . . . . . . . . . . . . . 31595

Foot
- Excision . . . . . . . . . . . . . . . . . . . . . . . . . . 28055
- Incision . . . . . . . . . . . . . . . . . . . . . . . . . . 28035

Graft . . . . . . . . . . . . . . . . . . . . . . . . 64885-64907

Implantation
- Electrode Array . . . 0282T-0283T, 64553-64581
- to Bone . . . . . . . . . . . . . . . . . . . . . . . . . . 64787
- to Muscle . . . . . . . . . . . . . . . . . . . . . . . . 64787

Incision . . . . . . . . . . .43640-43641, 64732-64772

Injection
- Anesthetic . . . . . . .01991-01992, 64400-64530
- Neurolytic Agent . . . . . . . . . . . . . 64600-64681

Insertion
- Electrode Array . . . . . . . . . . . . . . 64553-64581

Lesion
- Excision . . . . . . . . . . . . . . . . . . . . 64774-64792

Lumbar
- Neurostimulator Implant . . . . . . . .0282T-0283T

Neurofibroma
- Excision . . . . . . . . . . . . . . . . . . . . 64788-64792

Neurolemmoma
- Excision . . . . . . . . . . . . . . . . . . . . 64788-64792

Neurolytic
- Internal . . . . . . . . . . . . . . . . . . . . . . . . . . 64727

Neuroma
- Destruction . . . . . . . . . . . . . . . . . . . . . . . 64632
- Excision . . . . . . . . . . . . . . . . . . . . 64774-64786
- Injection . . . . . . . . . . . . . . . . . . . . . . . . . 64455

Neuroplasty . . . . . . . . . . . . . . . . . . 64702-64721

Removal
- Electrode Array . . . . . . . . . . . . . . . . . . . 64585

Repair
- Graft . . . . . . . . . . . . . . . . . . . . . . . 64885-64911
- Microdissection . . . . . . . . . . . . . . . . . . . 69990
- Suture . . . . . . . . . . . . . . . . . . . . . . 64831-64876

Revision
- Electrode Array . . . . . . . . . . . . . . . . . . . 64585

Spinal Accessory
- Incision . . . . . . . . . . . . . . . . . . . . . . . . . . 63191
- Section . . . . . . . . . . . . . . . . . . . . . . . . . . 63191

Suture . . . . . . . . . . . . . . . . . . . . . . . 64831-64876

Sympathectomy
- Excision . . . . . . . . . . . . . . . . . . . . 64802-64818

Thoracic
- Neurostimulator Implant . . . . . . . .0282T-0283T

Transection . . . . . . . . . .43640-43641, 64732-64772

Transposition . . . . . . . . . . . . . . . . . 64718-64721

Unlisted Services and Procedures . . . . . . . . 64999

## Nervous System

Nuclear Medicine
- Unlisted Services and Procedures . . . . . . 78699

## Nesidioblast
*See* Islet Cell

## Neural Conduction
*See* Nerve Conduction

## Neural Ganglion
*See* Ganglion

## Neurectomy

Foot . . . . . . . . . . . . . . . . . . . . . . . . . . . . . . . . 28055
Gastrocnemius . . . . . . . . . . . . . . . . . . . . . . . 27326
Hamstring Muscle . . . . . . . . . . . . . . . . . . . . . 27325
Leg, Lower . . . . . . . . . . . . . . . . . . . . . . . . . . 27326
Leg, Upper . . . . . . . . . . . . . . . . . . . . . . . . . . 27325
Popliteal . . . . . . . . . . . . . . . . . . . . . . . . . . . . 27326
Tympanic . . . . . . . . . . . . . . . . . . . . . . . . . . . 69676

## Neuroendoscopy

Intracranial . . . . . . . . . . . . . . . . . . . 62160-62165

## Neurofibroma

Cutaneous Nerve
- Excision . . . . . . . . . . . . . . . . . . . . . . . . . 64788

Extensive
- Excision . . . . . . . . . . . . . . . . . . . . . . . . . 64792

Peripheral Nerve
- Excision . . . . . . . . . . . . . . . . . . . . . . . . . 64790

## Neurolemmoma

Cutaneous Nerve
- Excision . . . . . . . . . . . . . . . . . . . . . . . . . 64788

Extensive
- Excision . . . . . . . . . . . . . . . . . . . . . . . . . 64792

Peripheral Nerve
- Excision . . . . . . . . . . . . . . . . . . . . . . . . . 64790

## Neurologic System
*See* Nervous System

## Neurology

Brain Cortex Magnetic
- Stimulation . . . . . . . . . . . . . . . . . . 90867-90869
Brain Mapping . . . . . . . . . . . . . . . . 96020, 90867
Brain Surface Electrode
- Stimulation . . . . . . . . . . . . . . . . . . 95961-95962
Central Motor
- Transcranial Motor
  - Stimulation . . . . . . . . . . . . . . . . 95928-95929
Cognitive Performance . . . . . . . . . . . . . . . . . 96125
Diagnostic
- Anal Sphincter . . . . . . . . . . . . . . . . . . . . . 51785
- Autonomic Nervous Function
  - Heart Rate Response . . . . . . . . 95921-95923
  - Pseudomotor Response . . . . . . 95921-95923
  - Sympathetic Function . . . . . . . . 95921-95923
Electrocorticogram
- Intraoperative . . . . . . . . . . . . . . . . . . . . . 95829
Electroencephalogram (EEG) . . . . . . 95812-95827,
95955
- Brain Death . . . . . . . . . . . . . . . . . . . . . . . 95824
- Electrode Placement . . . . . . . . . . . . . . . 95830
- Intraoperative . . . . . . . . . . . . . . . . . . . . . 95955
- Monitoring . . . . . . . . . . . . . . . . .95812-95813,
95950-95953, 95956
- Physical or Drug Activation . . . . . . . . . . 95954
- Sleep . . . . . . . . . . 95800-95801, 95822, 95827
- Standard . . . . . . . . . . . . . . . . . . . . . . . . . 95819
- WADA Activation . . . . . . . . . . . . . . . . . . . 95958
Electroencephalography (EEG)
- Digital Analysis . . . . . . . . . . . . . . . . . . . . 95957
Electromyography
- Fine Wire
  - Dynamic . . . . . . . . . . . . . . . . . . . . . . . 96004
- Ischemic Limb Exercise Test . . . . . . . . . 95875
- Needle . . . . . . . . . . . . . . 51785, 95860-95872
- Surface
  - Dynamic . . . . . . . . . . . . . . . . . . 96002-96004
Higher Cerebral Function
- Aphasia Test . . . . . . . . . . . . . . . . . . . . . . 96105
- Cognitive Function Tests . . . . . . . . . . . . . 96116
- Developmental Tests . . . . . . . . . 96110-96111
- Neurobehavioral Status . . . . . . . . . . . . . 96116
- Neuropsychological Testing . . . . . 96118-96120

Neuropsychological Testing,
- Computer-Assisted . . . . . . . . . . . . . . . . . 96120
Magnetoencephalography (MEG) . . . 95965-95967
Motion Analysis
- by Accelerometer and Gyroscope . . . . . . 0199T
- by Video and 3-D Kinematics . . . 96000, 96004
- Computer-based . . . . . . . . . . . . . 96000, 96004
Muscle Testing
- Manual . . . . . . . . . . . . . . . . . . . . . 95831-95834
Nerve Conduction
- Motor Nerve . . . . . . . . . . . . . . . . . 95900-95903
- Motor and Sensory Nerve . . . . . . . . . . . 95905
- Sensory Nerve . . . . . . . . . . . . . . . . . . . . 95904
Neurofunctional Testing . . . . . . . . . . . . . . . 96020
Neuromuscular Junction Tests . . . . . . . . . . 95937
Neurophysiological Testing
- Intraoperative . . . . . . . . . . . . . . . 95915-95920
Neuropsychological Testing . . . . . . . 96118-96120
- Cognitive Performance . . . . . . . . . . . . . . 96125
- Computer-Assisted . . . . . . . . . . . . . . . . . 96120
Plantar Pressure Measurements
- Dynamic . . . . . . . . . . . . . . . . . . . 96001, 96004
Polysomnography . . . . . . . . . . . . . . . 95808-95811
Range of Motion . . . . . . . . . . . . . . . 95851-95852
Reflex
- Blink Reflex . . . . . . . . . . . . . . . . . . . . . . . 95933
- H-Reflex . . . . . . . . . . . . . . . . . . . . 95933-95934
Sleep Study . . . . . . . . 95800-95801, 95805-95811
- Actigraphy Testing . . . . . . . . . . . . . . . . . 95803
Somatosensory Testing . . . . . . . . . . 95925-95927,
95938-95939
Cholinesterase Inhibitor Challenge Test . . . . 95857
Therapeutic
- Magnetic Stimulation
  - Transcranial . . . . . . . . . . . . . . . 90867-90869
Unlisted Services and Procedures . . . . . . . . 95999
Urethral Sphincter . . . . . . . . . . . . . . . . . . . . 51785
Visual Evoked Potential, CNS . . . . . . . . . . . 95930

## Neurolysis

Nerve . . . . . . . . . . . . . . . . . . . . . . . . 64704, 64708
- Internal . . . . . . . . . . . . . . . . . . . . . . . . . . 64727

## Neuroma

Acoustic
*See* Brain, Tumor, Excision
Excision
- Cutaneous Nerve . . . . . . . . . . . . . . . . . . 64774
- Digital Nerve . . . . . . . . . . . . . . . 64776-64778
- Foot . . . . . . . . . . . . . . . . . . . . . . . . . . . . 28080
  - Destruction . . . . . . . . . . . . . . . . . . . . . 64632
  - Injection . . . . . . . . . . . . . . . . . . . . . . . 64455
- Foot Nerve . . . . . . . . . . . . . . . . . 64782-64783
- Hand Nerve . . . . . . . . . . . . . . . . . 64782-64783
- Peripheral Nerve . . . . . . . . . . . . . . . . . . 64784
- Sciatic Nerve . . . . . . . . . . . . . . . . . . . . . 64786
Interdigital
*See* Morton‚Äôs Neuroma; Neuroma, Excision,
Foot

## Neuromuscular Junction
Tests . . . . . . . . . . . . . . . . . . . . . . . . . . . . .95937

## Neuromuscular Pedicle
Reinnervation
- Larynx . . . . . . . . . . . . . . . . . . . . . . . . . . . 31590

## Neuromuscular Reeducation . . .97112
*See* Physical Medicine/Therapy/Occupational
Therapy

## Neurophysiologic Testing
Autonomic Nervous Function
- Heart Rate Response . . . . . . . . . . 95921-95923
- Pseudomotor Response . . . . . . . . 95921-95923

Repair
    Adhesions . . . . . . . . . . . . . . . . . . . . . . 30560
    Cleft Lip . . . . . . . . . . . . . . . . . 40700-40761
    Fistula. . . . . . . . . . . . . 30580-30600, 42260
    Rhinophyma . . . . . . . . . . . . . . . . . . . . 30120
    Septum. . . . . . . . . . 30540-30545, 30630
    Synechia. . . . . . . . . . . . . . . . . . . . . . . 30560
    Vestibular Stenosis . . . . . . . . . . . . . . 30465
Skin
    Excision . . . . . . . . . . . . . . . . . . . . . . . 30120
    Surgical Planing . . . . . . . . . . . . . . . . . 30120
Submucous Resection Turbinate
    Excision . . . . . . . . . . . . . . . . . . . . . . . 30140
Turbinate
    Excision . . . . . . . . . . . . . . . 30130-30140
    Fracture . . . . . . . . . . . . . . . . . . . . . . . 30930
    Injection . . . . . . . . . . . . . . . . . . . . . . . 30200
Turbinate Mucosa
    Cauterization . . . . . . . . . . . 30801-30802
Unlisted Services and Procedures . . . . . . . . 30999

**Nose Bleed** . . . . . . . . . . . . . . 30901-30906
*See* Hemorrhage, Nasal

**NPM1** . . . . . . . . . . . . . . . . . . . . . . . 81310

**NTD** . . . . . . . . . . . . . . . . . . . . . . . . 86384
*See* Nitroblue Tetrazolium Dye Test

**Nuclear Antigen**
Antibody . . . . . . . . . . . . . . . . . . . . . . . . 86235

**Nuclear Imaging**
*See* Nuclear Medicine

**Nuclear Magnetic Resonance Imaging**
*See* Magnetic Resonance Imaging (MRI)

**Nuclear Magnetic Resonance Spectroscopy**
*See* Magnetic Resonance Spectroscopy

**Nuclear Matrix Protein 22** . . . . . 86386

**Nuclear Medicine**
Adrenal Gland Imaging . . . . . . . . . . . . . . 78075
Bile Duct
    Imaging . . . . . . . . . . . . . . . 78226-78227
Bladder
    Residual Study . . . . . . . . . . . . . . . . . . 78730
Blood
    Bone
        Density Study . . . . . . . . . . . . 78350-78351
        Imaging. . . . . . . . . . . . . . 78300-78320
        SPECT . . . . . . . . . . . . . . . . . . . . . . 78320
        Ultrasound . . . . . . . . . . . . . . . . . . 76977
        Unlisted Services and Procedures . . . . 78399
    Flow Imaging . . . . . . . . . . . . . . . . . . 78445
    Iron
        Red Cells. . . . . . . . . . . . . . . . . . . . 78140
    Platelet Survival. . . . . . . . . . 78190-78191
    Red Cell Survival . . . . . . . . . . . 78130-78135
    Red Cells . . . . . . . . . . . . . . . 78120-78121
    Unlisted Services and Procedures . . . . . . 78199
    Whole Blood Volume . . . . . . . . . . . . . 78122
Bone Marrow
    Imaging . . . . . . . . . . . . . . . 78102-78104
Brain
    Blood Flow . . . . . . . . . . . . . . . . . . . . 78610
    Cerebrospinal Fluid . . . . . . . . . . . 78630-78650
    Imaging . . . . . . . . . . . . . . . 78600-78609
        Vascular Flow . . . . . . . . . . . . . . . . 78610
Endocrine System
    Unlisted Services and Procedures . . . . . . 78099

Esophagus
    Imaging (Motility) . . . . . . . . . . . . . . . 78258
    Reflux Study. . . . . . . . . . . . . . . . . . . 78262
Gallbladder
    Imaging . . . . . . . . . . . . . . . 78226-78227
Gastric Mucosa
    Imaging . . . . . . . . . . . . . . . . . . . . . . 78261
Gastrointestinal
    Blood Loss Study . . . . . . . . . . . . . . . 78278
    Protein Loss Study . . . . . . . . . . . . . . 78282
    Shunt Testing . . . . . . . . . . . . . . . . . . 78291
    Unlisted Services and Procedures . . . . . 78299
Genitourinary System
    Unlisted Services and Procedures . . . . . 78799
Heart
    Blood Flow . . . . . . . . . . . . . . . . . . . . 78414
    Blood Pool Imaging . . . . . . . . . . 78472-78473,
                  78481-78483, 78494-78496
    Myocardial Imaging . . . . . 78459, 78466-78469
    Myocardial Perfusion . . . . . . . . . 78451-78454
    Shunt Detection . . . . . . . . . . . . . . . . 78428
    Unlisted Services and Procedures . . . . . 78499
Hepatic Duct
    Imaging . . . . . . . . . . . . . . . 78226-78227
Inflammatory Process . . . . . . . . . . 78805-78807
    Injection Procedure . . . . . . . . . . . . . . 78808
Intestines
    Imaging . . . . . . . . . . . . . . . . . . . . . . 78290
Kidney
    Function Study . . . . . . . . . . . . . . . . . 78725
    Imaging . . . . . . . . 78700-78707, 78710
    Vascular Flow. . . . . . . . . . . . 78701-78709
Lacrimal Gland Tear Flow . . . . . . . . . . . . . 78660
Liver
    Imaging . . . . . . . . . . . . . . . 78201-78216
    Vascular Flow. . . . . . . . . . . . . . . . . . 78206
Lung
    Imaging, Perfusion . . . . . . 78580, 78597, 78598
    Imaging, Ventilation . . . 78579, 78582, 78598
    Unlisted Services and Procedures . . . . . 78599
Lymph Nodes . . . . . . . . . . . . . . . . . . . . 78195
Lymphatics . . . . . . . . . . . . . . . . . . . . . . 78195
    Unlisted Services and Procedures . . . . . 78199
Musculoskeletal System
    Unlisted Services and Procedures . . . . . 78399
Nervous System
    Unlisted Services and Procedures . . . . . 78699
Parathyroid Gland Imaging . . . . . . . . . . . . 78070
Pulmonary Perfusion . . . . . . 78580, 78597-78598
Pulmonary Ventilation . . . . . . 78579, 78582, 78598
Salivary Gland Function Study . . . . . . . . . . 78232
    Imaging . . . . . . . . . . . . . . . 78230-78231
Spleen
    Imaging . . . . . . . . . . 78185, 78215-78216
    Unlisted Services and Procedures . . . . . 78199
Stomach
    Blood Loss Study . . . . . . . . . . . . . . . 78278
    Emptying Study . . . . . . . . . . . . . . . . 78264
    Protein Loss Study . . . . . . . . . . . . . . 78282
    Reflux Study. . . . . . . . . . . . . . . . . . . 78262
    Vitamin B-12 Absorption . . . . . . . 78270-78272
Testes
    Imaging . . . . . . . . . . . . . . . . . . . . . . 78761
Therapeutic
    Interstitial. . . . . . . . . . . . . . . . . . . . . 79300
    Intra-Arterial . . . . . . . . . . . . . . . . . . 79445
    Intra-Articular. . . . . . . . . . . . . . . . . . 79440
    Intracavitary . . . . . . . . . . . . . . . . . . . 79200
    Intravenous . . . . . . . . . . . . . . . . . . . 79101
    Intravenous Infusion . . . . . . . . . . . . . 79403
    Oral. . . . . . . . . . . . . . . . . . . . . . . . . 79005
    Thyroid . . . . . . . . . . . . . . . 79200-79300
    Unlisted Services and Procedures . . . . . 79999

Thyroid
    Imaging . . . . . . . . . . . . . . . . . . . . . . 78010
    Imaging for Metastases. . . . . . . 78015-78018
    Imaging with Flow . . . . . . . . . . . . . . 78011
    Imaging with Uptake . . . . . . . . . . . . . 78006
    Metastases Uptake . . . . . . . . . . . . . . 78020
    Uptake . . . . . . . . . . . . . . . . 78000-78003
Tumor Imaging
    Positron Emission
        Tomography . . . . . . . . . . . . . 78811-78816
        with Computed
        Tomography . . . . . . . . . . . . . 78814-78816
Tumor Localization . . . . . . . . . . . . . 78800-78804
Unlisted Services and Procedures . . . . . . . . 78999
Urea Breath Test . . . . . . . . . . . . 78267-78268
Ureter
    Reflux Study. . . . . . . . . . . . . . . . . . . 78740
Vein
    Thrombosis Imaging. . . . . . . . . . 78456-78458

**Nucleases, DNA**
*See* DNAse

**Nucleic Acid Probe** . . . . . . . . . . . 83896
Amplified Probe Detection
    Infectious Agent
        Bartonella Henselae. . . . . . . . . . . . . 87471
        Bartonella Quintana . . . . . . . . . . . . . 87471
        Borrelia Burgdorferi . . . . . . . . . . . . . 87476
        Candida Species. . . . . . . . . . . . . . . . 87481
        Chlamydia Pneumoniae . . . . . . . . . . 87486
        Chlamydia Trachomatis . . . . . . . . . . 87491
        Cytomegalovirus. . . . . . . . . . . . . . . . 87496
        Enterovirus . . . . . . . . . . . . . . 87498, 87500
        Gardnerella Vaginalis . . . . . . . . . . . . 87511
        Hepatitis B Virus. . . . . . . . . . . . . . . . 87516
        Hepatitis C . . . . . . . . . . . . . . . . . . . 87521
        Hepatitis G . . . . . . . . . . . . . . . . . . . 87526
        Herpes Simplex Virus . . . . . . . . . . . . 87529
        Herpes Virus-6 . . . . . . . . . . . . . . . . 87532
        HIV-1 . . . . . . . . . . . . . . . . . . . . . . . 87535
        HIV-2 . . . . . . . . . . . . . . . . . . . . . . . 87538
        Legionella Pneumophila . . . . . . . . . . . 87541
        Multiple Organisms . . . . . . . . . . . . . 87801
        Mycobacteria Avium-Intracellulare . . . 87561
        Mycobacteria Species . . . . . . . . . . . . 87551
        Mycobacteria Tuberculosis . . . . . . . . 87556
        Mycoplasma Pneumoniae . . . . . . . . . 87581
        Neisseria Gonorrheae . . . . . . . . . . . . 87591
        Not Otherwise Specified . . . . . 87798, 87801
        Papillomavirus, Human. . . . . . . . . . . 87621
        Staphylococcus Aureus . . . . . 87640-87641
        Streptococcus, Group A . . . . . . . . . . 87651
        Streptococcus, Group B . . . . . . . . . . 87653
Direct Probe Detection
    Infectious Agent
        Bartonella Henselae. . . . . . . . . . . . . 87470
        Bartonella Quintana . . . . . . . . . . . . . 87470
        Borrelia Burgdorferi . . . . . . . . . . . . . 87475
        Candida Species. . . . . . . . . . . . . . . . 87480
        Chlamydia Pneumoniae . . . . . . . . . . 87485
        Chlamydia Trachomatis . . . . . . . . . . 87490
        Clostridium Difficile . . . . . . . . . . . . . 87493
        Cytomegalovirus. . . . . . . . . . . . . . . . 87495
        Gardnerella Vaginalis . . . . . . . . . . . . 87510
        Hepatitis B Virus. . . . . . . . . . . . . . . . 87515
        Hepatitis C . . . . . . . . . . . . . . . . . . . 87520
        Hepatitis G . . . . . . . . . . . . . . . . . . . 87525
        Herpes Simplex Virus . . . . . . . . . . . . 87528
        Herpes Virus-6 . . . . . . . . . . . . . . . . 87531
        HIV-1 . . . . . . . . . . . . . . . . . . . . . . . 87534
        HIV-2 . . . . . . . . . . . . . . . . . . . . . . . 87537
        Legionella Pneumophila . . . . . . . . . . . 87540
        Multiple Organisms . . . . . . . . . . . . . 87800

Mycobacteria Avium-Intracellulare ... 87560
Mycobacteria Species ............. 87550
Mycobacteria Tuberculosis ......... 87555
Mycoplasma Pneumoniae ......... 87580
Neisseria Gonorrheae ............. 87590
Not Otherwise Specified .......... 87797
Papillomavirus, Human............. 87620
Streptococcus, Group A ........... 87650
Trichomonas Vaginalis ............ 87660
Genotype Analysis
  Infectious Agent
    Hepatitis C Virus................. 87902
    HIV-1 Regions............. 87901, 87906
In Situ Hybridization............. 88120-88121,
                                  88365-88368
Phenotype Analysis
  Infectious Agent
    HIV-1 Drug Resistance ....... 87903-87904
Quantification
  Infectious Agent
    Bartonella Henselae............... 87472
    Bartonella Quintana .............. 87472
    Borrelia Burgdorferi .............. 87477
    Candida Species.................. 87482
    Chlamydia Pneumoniae ........... 87487
    Chlamydia Trachomatis ........... 87492
    Cytomegalovirus................. 87497
    Gardnerella Vaginalis............. 87512
    Hepatitis B Virus................. 87517
    Hepatitis C ..................... 87522
    Hepatitis G ..................... 87527
    Herpes Simplex Virus............. 87530
    Herpes Virus-6 .................. 87533
    HIV-1.......................... 87536
    HIV-2.......................... 87539
    Legionella Pneumophila ........... 87542
    Mycobacteria Avium-Intracellulare ... 87562
    Mycobacteria Species ............. 87552
    Mycobacteria Tuberculosis ......... 87557
    Mycoplasma Pneumoniae ......... 87582
    Neisseria Gonorrheae ............. 87592
    Not Otherwise Specified .......... 87799
    Papillomavirus, Human............. 87622
    Streptococcus, Group A ........... 87652

**Nucleolysis, Intervertebral Disc**
*See* Chemonucleolysis

**Nucleotidase** .................83915

**Nursemaid Elbow** .............24640

**Nursing Facility Discharge Services**
*See* Discharge Services, Nursing Facility

**Nursing Facility Services**
Annual Assessment.................... 99318
Care Plan Oversight Services ...... 99379-99380
Comprehensive Assessments
Discharge Services ... 99315-99316, 1110F-1111F
Initial Care ..................... 99304-99306
Subsequent Care ............... 99307-99310

**Nuss Procedure**
with Thoracoscopy.....................21743
without Thoracoscopy...................21742

**Nutrition Therapy**
Group ........................... 97804
Home Infusion ................. 99601-99602
Initial Assessment..................... 97802
Reassessment ...................... 97803

**Nystagmus Tests**
*See* Vestibular Function Tests
Optokinetic.................. 92534, 92544
Positional ................... 92532, 92542
Spontaneous ................. 92531, 92541

# O

**O2 Saturation**
*See* Oxygen Saturation

**Ober-Yount Procedure** .........27025
*See* Fasciotomy, Hip

**Obliteration**
Mastoid ........................... 69670
Vagina
  Total .................... 57110-57112
  Vault ........................ 57120

**Oblongata, Medulla**
*See* Medulla

**Observation** .... 99217-99220, 99224-99226,
99234-99236
*See* Evaluation and Management; Hospital Services

**Obstetrical Care**
Abortion
  Induced
    by Amniocentesis Injection ... 59850-59852
      *See* Abortion; Cesarean Delivery; Ectopic Pregnancy
    by Dilation and Curettage .......... 59840
    by Dilation and Evaluation .......... 59841
  Missed
    First Trimester.................... 59820
    Second Trimester ................ 59821
  Spontaneous ..................... 59812
  Therapeutic .............. 59840-59852
Antepartum Care ............... 59425-59426
Cesarean Delivery ............. 59618-59622
  Only ........................ 59514
  Postpartum Care ............... 59515
  Routine....................... 59510
  with Hysterectomy................ 59525
Curettage
  Hydatidiform Mole................ 59870
Evacuation
  Hydatidiform Mole................ 59870
External Cephalic Version .............. 59412
Miscarriage
  Surgical Completion.......... 59812-59821
Placenta Delivery..................... 59414
Postpartum Care ............... 59430, 59514
Septic Abortion ..................... 59830
Total (Global) .......... 59400, 59610, 59618
Unlisted Services and
Procedures ................... 59898-59899
Vaginal
  after Cesarean ............... 59610-59614
Vaginal Delivery................ 59409-59410
  Delivery after Cesarean ........ 59610-59614

**Obstruction**
*See* Occlusion

**Obstruction Clearance**
Venous Access Device........... 36595-36596

**Obstruction Colon**
*See* Colon, Obstruction

**Obturator Nerve**
Avulsion ................... 64763-64766
Incision..................... 64763-64766
Transection.................. 64763-64766

**Obturator Prosthesis** ..........21076
Definitive ...................... 21080
Insertion
  Larynx......................... 31527
Interim ......................... 21079

**Occipital Nerve, Greater**
Avulsion ........................... 64744
Incision .......................... 64744
Injection
  Anesthetic ..................... 64405
Transection....................... 64744

**Occlusion**
Bronchi
  Balloon......................... 31634
Extracranial
  Intracranial..................... 61623
Fallopian Tube
  Oviduct .............. 58565, 58615
Penis
  Vein .......................... 37790
Umbilical Cord ..................... 59072

**Occlusive Disease of Artery**
*See* Repair, Artery; Revision

**Occult Blood**............. 82270-82272
by Hemoglobin Immunoassay........... 82274

**Occupational Therapy**
Evaluation..................... 97003-97004

**Ocular Implant**
*See* Orbital Implant
Insertion
  Drainage Device.........0191T-0192T, 0253T
  in Scleral Shell................. 65130
  Muscles, Attached................. 65140
  Muscles, Not Attached ............ 65135
Modification...................... 65125
Reinsertion....................... 65150
  with Foreign Material .............. 65155
Removal ......................... 65175

**Ocular Muscle**
*See* Eye Muscles

**Ocular Orbit**
*See* Orbit

**Ocular Photoscreening** ........99174

**Ocular Prostheses**
*See* Prosthesis, Ocular

**Oculomotor Muscle**
*See* Eye Muscles

**Oddi Sphincter**
*See* Sphincter of Oddi

**Odontoid Dislocation**
Open Treatment/Reduction............22318
  with Grafting .................... 22319

**Odontoid Fracture**
Open Treatment/Reduction.............22318
  with Grafting .................... 22319

## Odontoid Process
Excision............................22548

## Oesophageal Neoplasm
*See* Tumor, Esophagus

## Oesophageal Varices
*See* Esophageal Varices

## Oesophagus
*See* Esophagus

## Oestradiol
*See* Estradiol

## Office and/or Other Outpatient Services
*See* History and Physical Consultation
Established Patient ..............99211-99215
New Patient....................99201-99205
Normal Newborn.....................99432
Office Visit
   Established Patient ........99211-99215
   New Patient................99201-99205
Outpatient Visit
   Established Patient ........99211-99215
   New Patient................99201-99205
   Prolonged Services ..........99354-99355

## Office Medical Services
After Hours..........................99050
Emergency Care.......................99058
Extended Hours ......................99051

## Office or Other Outpatient Consultations
*See* Consultation, Office and/or Other Outpatient

## Olecranon
*See* Elbow; Humerus; Radius; Ulna
Bursa
   Arthrocentesis....................20605
Cyst
   Excision ....................24125-24126
Tumor
   Cyst ...........................24120
   Excision ...................24125-24126

## Olecranon Process
Craterization........................24147
Diaphysectomy.......................24147
Excision.............................24147
   Abscess.........................24138
Fracture
   *See* Elbow; Humerus; Radius
   Closed Treatment.............24670-24675
   Open Treatment.....................24685
Osteomyelitis...................24138, 24147
Saucerization........................24147
Sequestrectomy......................24138

## Oligoclonal Immunoglobulins...............83916

## Omentectomy.......49255, 58950-58958
Laparotomy..........................58960
Oophorectomy .......................58943
Resection Ovarian Malignancy.....58950-58952
Resection Peritoneal Malignancy...58950-58958
Resection Tubal Malignancy.......58950-58958

## Omentum
Excision..............49255, 58950-58958
Flap ........................49904-49905
Free
   with Microvascular Anastomosis.....49906

Omentopexy .......................49326
Unlisted Services and Procedures ........49999

## Omphalectomy .................49250

## Omphalocele
Repair .....................49600-49611

## Omphalomesenteric Duct
Excision.........................44800

## Omphalomesenteric Duct, Persistent
*See* Diverticulum, Meckel's

## Oncoprotein
Des-gamma-carboxyprothrombin (DCP) ....83951
HER-2/neu .........................83950

## Online Internet Assessment and Management
Nonphysician ......................98969
Physician..........................99444

## One Stage Prothrombin Time .....................85610-85611
*See* Prothrombin Time

## Onychectomy
*See* Excision, Nails

## Onychia
Drainage..................10060-10061

## Oocyte
Assisted Fertilization
   Microtechnique ..............89280-89281
Biopsy.......................89290-89291
Culture
   Extended .......................89272
   Less than 4 Days ...............89250
   with Co-Culture .................89251
Identification
   Follicular Fluid ..................89254
Insemination.......................89268
Retrieval
   for In Vitro Fertilization ...........58970
Storage ...........................89346
Thawing ...........................89356

## Oophorectomy ..........58262-58263,
58291-58292, 58552, 58554,
58661, 58940-58943
Ectopic Pregnancy
   Laparoscopic Treatment............59120
   Surgical Treatment................59120

## Oophorectomy, Partial
*See* Excision, Ovary, Partial

## Oophorocystectomy
*See* Cystectomy, Ovarian

## Open Biopsy, Adrenal Gland
*See* Adrenal Gland, Biopsy

## Operating Microscope .........69990

## Operation
Blalock-Hanlon
   *See* Septostomy, Atrial
Blalock-Taussig Subclavian-Pulmonary Anastomosis
   *See* Pulmonary Artery, Shunt, Subclavian
Dunn
   *See* Arthrodesis, Foot Joint
Duvries
   *See* Tenoplasty

Estes
   *See* Ovary, Transposition
Foley Pyeloplasty
   *See* Pyeloplasty
Fontan
   *See* Repair, Heart, Anomaly
Green
   *See* Scapulopexy
Harelip
   *See* Cleft Lip, Repair
Heller
   *See* Esophagomyotomy
Iris, Inclusion
   *See* Iridencleisis
Jaboulay Gastroduodenostomy
   *See* Gastroduodenostomy
Keller
   *See* Keller Procedure
Mumford
   *See* Claviculectomy, Partial
Nissen
   *See* Fundoplasty, Esophagogastric
Ramstedt
   *See* Pyloromyotomy
Richardson Hysterectomy
   *See* Hysterectomy, Abdominal, Total
Schanz
   *See* Femur, Osteotomy
Schlatter Total Gastrectomy
   *See* Excision, Stomach, Total
Winiwarter Cholecystoenterostomy
   *See* Anastomosis, Gallbladder to Intestines

## Operation Microscopes
*See* Operating Microscope

## Operculectomy .................41821

## Operculum
*See* Gums

## Ophthalmic Mucous Membrane Test...............................95060
*See* Allergy Tests

## Ophthalmology
Unlisted Services and Procedures ........92499
   *See* Ophthalmology, Diagnostic

## Ophthalmology, Diagnostic
Color Vision Exam .....................92283
Computerized Scanning
   Anterior .......................92132
   Posterior..................92133-92134
Computerized Screening ..........99172, 99174
Dark Adaptation.......................92284
Electro-oculography....................92270
Electromyography, Needle ..............92265
Electroretinography....................92275
Endoscopy...........................66990
Eye Exam
   Established Patient ..........92012-92014
   New Patient................92002-92004
   with Anesthesia...........92018-92019
Glaucoma Provocative Test..............92140
Gonioscopy..........................92020
Ocular Photography
   External .......................92285
   Internal...................92286-92287
Ophthalmoscopy .................92225-92226
   with Dynamometry...............92260
   with Fluorescein Angiography ......92235
   with Fluorescein Angioscopy........92230
   with Fundus Photography ..........92250

Reconstruction
  Ossicular Chain
    Tympanoplasty with Antrotomy
    or Mastoidotomy . . . . . . . . . . . 69636-69637
    Tympanoplasty with
    Mastoidectomy . . . . . . 69642, 69644, 69646
    Tympanoplasty without
    Mastoidectomy . . . . . . . . . . . . 69632-69633
Release
  Stapes . . . . . . . . . . . . . . . . . . . . . . . . 69650
Replacement
  with Prosthesis . . . . . . . . . . . . 69633, 69637

## Ostectomy
Metacarpal . . . . . . . . . . . . . . . . . . . . . . . . . 26250
Metatarsal . . . . . . . . . . . . . . . . . . . . . . . . . 28288
Phalanges
  Finger . . . . . . . . . . . . . . . . . . . . 26260-26262
Pressure Ulcer
  Ischial . . . . . . . . . . . . . . . . . 15941, 15945
  Sacral . . . . . . . . . . . . . 15933, 15935, 15937
  Trochanteric . . . . . . . . 15951, 15953, 15958
Scapula . . . . . . . . . . . . . . . . . . . . . . . . . . 23190
Sternum . . . . . . . . . . . . . . . . . . . . . . . . . . 21620

## Osteocalcin . . . . . . . . . . . . . . . . . . . . .83937

## Osteocartilaginous Exostoses
*See* Exostosis

## Osteochondroma
*See* Exostosis

## Osteocutaneous Flap
with Microvascular Anastomosis . . . 20969-20973

## Osteoma
Sinusotomy
  Frontal . . . . . . . . . . . . . . . . . . . . . . . . 31075

## Osteomyelitis . . . . . . . . . . . . . . . . .20005
Elbow
  Incision and Drainage . . . . . . . . . . . . . 23935
Excision
  Clavicle . . . . . . . . . . . . . . . . . . . . . . 23180
  Facial . . . . . . . . . . . . . . . . . . . . . . . 21026
  Humerus, Proximal . . . . . . . . . . . . . . 23184
  Mandible . . . . . . . . . . . . . . . . . . . . . 21025
  Scapula . . . . . . . . . . . . . . . . . . . . . . 23182
Femur/Knee
  Incision and Drainage . . . . . . . . . . . . . 27303
Finger
  Incision . . . . . . . . . . . . . . . . . . . . . . 26034
Hand Incision . . . . . . . . . . . . . . . . . . . . . 26034
Hip
  Incision, Deep . . . . . . . . . . . . . . . . . . 26992
Humerus . . . . . . . . . . . . . . . . . . . . . . . . . 24134
  Incision and Drainage . . . . . . . . . . . . . 23935
Incision
  Foot . . . . . . . . . . . . . . . . . . . . . . . . . 28005
  Shoulder . . . . . . . . . . . . . . . . . . . . . 23035
  Thorax . . . . . . . . . . . . . . . . . . . . . . . 21510
Olecranon Process . . . . . . . . . . 24138, 24147
Pelvis
  Incision, Deep . . . . . . . . . . . . . . . . . . 26992
Radius . . . . . . . . . . . . . . . . . . . . 24136, 24145
Sequestrectomy
  Clavicle . . . . . . . . . . . . . . . . . . . . . . 23170
  Humeral Head . . . . . . . . . . . . . . . . . 23174
  Scapula . . . . . . . . . . . . . . . . . . . . . . 23172
  Skull . . . . . . . . . . . . . . . . . . . . . . . . 61501

## Osteopathic Manipulation . . . . . . . . . . . . 98925-98929

## Osteoplasty
Carpal Bone . . . . . . . . . . . . . . . . . . . . . . 25394
Facial Bones
  Augmentation . . . . . . . . . . . . . . . . . 21208
  Reduction . . . . . . . . . . . . . . . . . . . . . 21209
Femoral Neck . . . . . . . . . . . . . . . . . . . . . 27179
Femur . . . . . . . . . . . . . . . . . . . . . . . . . . 27179
  Lengthening . . . . . . . . . . . . . . 27466-27468
  Shortening . . . . . . . . . . . . . . . 27465, 27468
Fibula
  Lengthening . . . . . . . . . . . . . . . . . . . 27715
Humerus . . . . . . . . . . . . . . . . . . . . . . . . . 24420
Metacarpal . . . . . . . . . . . . . . . . . . . . . . . 26568
Phalanges, Finger . . . . . . . . . . . . . . . . . . 26568
Radius . . . . . . . . . . . . . . . . . . . . 25390-25393
Tibia
  Lengthening . . . . . . . . . . . . . . . . . . . 27715
Ulna . . . . . . . . . . . . . . . . . . . . . 25390-25393
Vertebra
  Lumbar . . . . . . . . . . . . . . . . . 22521-22522
  Radiological Supervision . . . . . . 72291, 72292
  Thoracic . . . . . . . . . . . . . . . . 22520-22522

## Osteotomy
Calcaneus . . . . . . . . . . . . . . . . . . . . . . . . 28300
Chin . . . . . . . . . . . . . . . . . . . . . 21121-21123
Clavicle . . . . . . . . . . . . . . . . . . 23480-23485
Femur . . . . . . . . . . . . . . . . . . . . 27140, 27151
  Femoral Neck . . . . . . . . . . . . . . . . . . 27161
  for Slipped Epiphysis . . . . . . . . . . . . . 27181
  with Fixation . . . . . . . . . . . . . . . . . . . 27165
  with Open Reduction of Hip . . . . . . . . . 27156
  with Realignment . . . . . . . . . . . . . . . . 27454
  without Fixation . . . . . . . . . . . . 27448-27450
Fibula . . . . . . . . . . . . . . . . . . . 27707-27712
Hip . . . . . . . . . . . . . . . . . . . . . 27146-27151
  Femoral
    with Open Reduction . . . . . . . . . . . . 27156
    Femur . . . . . . . . . . . . . . . . . . . . . . 27151
Humerus . . . . . . . . . . . . . . . . . . 24400-24410
Mandible . . . . . . . . . . . . . . . . . 21198-21199
  Extra-Oral . . . . . . . . . . . . . . . . . . . . 21047
  Intra-Oral . . . . . . . . . . . . . . . . . . . . . 21046
Maxilla . . . . . . . . . . . . . . . . . . . . . . . . . 21206
  Extra-Oral . . . . . . . . . . . . . . . . . . . . 21049
  Intra-Oral . . . . . . . . . . . . . . . . . . . . . 21048
Metacarpal . . . . . . . . . . . . . . . . . . . . . . . 26565
Metatarsal . . . . . . . . . . . . . . . . 28306-28309
Orbit Reconstruction . . . . . . . . . . . . . . . . 21256
Pelvis . . . . . . . . . . . . . . . . . . . . . . . . . . 27158
Periorbital
  Orbital Hypertelorism . . . . . . . . . 21260-21263
  Osteotomy with Graft . . . . . . . . . 21267-21268
Phalanges
  Finger . . . . . . . . . . . . . . . . . . . . . . . 26567
  Toe . . . . . . . . . . . . . . . 28299, 28310-28312
Radius
  and Ulna . . . . . . . . . . . . . . . . 25365, 25375
  Distal Third . . . . . . . . . . . . . . . . . . . 25350
  Middle or Proximal Third . . . . . . . . . . 25355
  Multiple . . . . . . . . . . . . . . . . . . . . . . 25370
Skull Base . . . . . . . . . . . . . . 61582-61585, 61592
Spine
  Anterior . . . . . . . . . . . . . . . . . 22220-22226
  Posterior
    Posterolateral . . . . . . . . . . . . . 22210-22214
  Posterior or Posterolateral
    Three-Column . . . . . . . . . . . . . 22206-22208
Talus . . . . . . . . . . . . . . . . . . . . . . . . . . . 28302
Tarsal . . . . . . . . . . . . . . . . . . . 28304-28305
Tibia . . . . . . . . 27455-27457, 27705, 27709-27712

Ulna . . . . . . . . . . . . . . . . . . . . . . . . . . . 25360
  and Radius . . . . . . . . . . . . . . 25365, 25375
  Multiple . . . . . . . . . . . . . . . . . . . . . . 25370
Vertebra
  Additional Segment
    Anterior Approach . . . . . . . . . . . . . 22226
    Posterior/Posterolateral Approach . . . . 22216
  Cervical
    Anterior Approach . . . . . . . . . . . . . 22220
    Posterior/Posterolateral Approach . . . . 22210
  Lumbar
    Anterior Approach . . . . . . . . . . . . . 22224
    Posterior/Posterolateral Approach . . . . 22214
  Thoracic
    Anterior Approach . . . . . . . . . . . . . 22222
    Posterior/Posterolateral Approach . . . . 22212
with Graft
  Reconstruction
    Periorbital Region . . . . . . . . . . 21267-21268

## Otolaryngology
Diagnostic
  Exam Under Anesthesia . . . . . . . . . . . . 92502

## Otomy
*See* Incision

## Otoplasty . . . . . . . . . . . . . . . . . . . . .69300

## Otorhinolaryngology
Unlisted Services and Procedures . . . . . . . . 92700

## Ouchterlony Immunodiffusion . . . . . . . . . . . . . .86331

## Outer Ear
*See* Ear, Outer

## Outpatient Visit
*See* History and Physical; Office and/or Other
Outpatient Services

## Output, Cardiac
*See* Cardiac Output

## Ova
Smear . . . . . . . . . . . . . . . . . . . . . . . . . . 87177

## Oval Window
Repair Fistula . . . . . . . . . . . . . . . . . . . . . 69666

## Oval Window Fistula
*See* Fistula, Oval Window

## Ovarian Cyst
*See* Cyst, Ovarian; Ovary, Cyst

## Ovarian Vein Syndrome
Ureterolysis . . . . . . . . . . . . . . . . . . . . . . 50722

## Ovariectomies
*See* Oophorectomy

## Ovariolysis . . . . . . . . . . . . . . . . . . . .58740

## Ovary
Abscess
  Incision and Drainage . . . . . . . 58820-58822
    Abdominal Approach . . . . . . . . . . . . 58822
Biopsy . . . . . . . . . . . . . . . . . . . . . . . . . 58900
Cyst
  Incision and Drainage . . . . . . . . 58800-58805
Excision . . . . . . . . . . . . . . . . . . 58662, 58720
  Cyst . . . . . . . . . . . . . . . . . . . . . . . . 58925
  Partial
    Oophorectomy . . . . . . . . . . . . 58661, 58940
    Ovarian Malignancy . . . . . . . . . . . . . 58943
    Peritoneal Malignancy . . . . . . . . . . . . 58943

# P

## Pancreas, Endocrine Only
*See* Islet Cell

## Pancreatectomy
Donor . . . . . . . . . . . . . . . . . . . . . . . . . . . . 48550
Partial . . . . . . . 48140-48146, 48150-48154, 48160
Total . . . . . . . . . . . . . . . . . . . . . . . 48155-48160
with Transplantation . . . . . . . . . . . . . . . . 48160

## Pancreatic DNAse
*See* DNAse

## Pancreatic Duct
Destruction
    Calculi (Stone) . . . . . . . . . . . . . . . . . . 43265
Dilation
    Endoscopy . . . . . . . . . . . . . . . . . . . . . 43271
Endoscopy. . . . . . . . . . . . . . . . . . . . . . . . 43273
    Collection
      Specimen . . . . . . . . . . . . . . . . . . . 43260
    Destruction
      Calculi (Stone) . . . . . . . . . . . . . . . 43265
      Tumor . . . . . . . . . . . . . . . . . . . . . 43272
    Dilation. . . . . . . . . . . . . . . . . . . . . . . 43271
    Removal (Endoscopic)
      Calculi (Stone) . . . . . . . . . . . . . . . 43264
      Foreign Body. . . . . . . . . . . . . . . . . 43269
      Stent. . . . . . . . . . . . . . . . . . . . . . . 43269
    Sphincter Pressure. . . . . . . . . . . . . . . 43263
    Sphincterotomy . . . . . . . . . . . . . . . . . 43262
    Tube Placement . . . . . . . . . . . . . 43267-43268
Incision
    Sphincter . . . . . . . . . . . . . . . . . . . . . 43262
Removal
    Calculi (Stone) . . . . . . . . . . . . . . . . . 43264
    Foreign Body . . . . . . . . . . . . . . . . . . 43269
    Stent. . . . . . . . . . . . . . . . . . . . . . . . 43269
Tube Placement
    Nasopancreatic . . . . . . . . . . . . . . . . . 43267
    Stent. . . . . . . . . . . . . . . . . . . . . . . . 43268
Tumor
    Destruction. . . . . . . . . . . . . . . . . . . . 43272
X-ray with Contrast
    Guide Catheter. . . . . . . . . . . . . 74329-74330

## Pancreatic Elastase 1 (PE1) . . . .82656

## Pancreatic Islet Cell AB
*See* Antibody, Islet Cell

## Pancreaticojejunostomy . . . . . . .48548

## Pancreatography
Injection Procedure . . . . . . . . . . . . . . . . . 48400
Intraoperative. . . . . . . . . . . . . . . . . 74300-74301
Postoperative . . . . . . . . . . . . . . . . . . . . . 74305

## Pancreatorrhaphy . . . . . . . . . . . . . .48545

## Pancreatotomy
*See* Incision, Pancreas

## Pancreozymin-Secretin Test . . .82938

## Panel
*See* Blood Tests; Organ or Disease-Oriented Panel

## Panniculectomy
*See* Lipectomy

## Pap Smears . . . . . . . . . . . . . . 88141-88155,
88164-88167, 88174-88175

## Paper, Chromatography
*See* Chromatography, Paper

## Papilla, Interdental
*See* Gums

## Papilloma
Destruction
    Anus . . . . . . . . . . . . . . . . . . . . 46900-46924
    Penis. . . . . . . . . . . . . . . . . . . . 54050-54065

## PAPP D
*See* Lactogen, Human Placental

## Para-Tyrosine
*See* Tyrosine

## Paracentesis
Abdomen . . . . . . . . . . . . . . . . . . 49082-49083
Eye
    with Aqueous Aspiration. . . . . . . . . . . 65800
    with Aqueous Release. . . . . . . . . . . . . 65805
    with Discission of Anterior Hyaloid
    Membrane . . . . . . . . . . . . . . . . . . . . 65810
    with Removal
      Blood. . . . . . . . . . . . . . . . . . . . . . 65815
      Vitreous . . . . . . . . . . . . . . . . . . . 65810
Thorax. . . . . . . . . . . . . . . . . . . 32421-32422

## Paracervical Nerve
Injection
    Anesthetic . . . . . . . . . . . . . . . . . . . . 64435

## Paraffin Bath Therapy . . . . . . . . .97018
*See* Physical Medicine/Therapy/Occupational
Therapy

## Paraganglioma, Medullary
*See* Glucagon, Tolerance Panel; Pheochromocytoma

## Parainfluenza Virus
Antigen Detection
    Immunofluorescence . . . . . . . . . . . . . 87279

## Paralysis, Facial Nerve
*See* Facial Nerve Paralysis

## Paralysis, Infantile
*See* Polio

## Paranasal Sinuses
*See* Sinus/Sinuses

## Parasites
Blood. . . . . . . . . . . . . . . . . . . . 87206-87209
Examination . . . . . . . . . . . . . . . . . . . . . 87169
Smear . . . . . . . . . . . . . . . . . . . . . . . . . 87177
Tissue . . . . . . . . . . . . . . . . . . . . . . . . . 87220

## Parasitic Worms
*See* Antibody; Helminth

## Parathormone . . . . . . . . . . . . . . . .83970

## Parathyrin
*See* Parathormone

## Parathyroid Autotransplantation . . . . . . . . . . .60512

## Parathyroid Gland
Autotransplant . . . . . . . . . . . . . . . . . . . 60512
Excision. . . . . . . . . . . . . . . . . . 60500-60502
Exploration . . . . . . . . . . . . . . . . 60500-60505
Nuclear Medicine
    Imaging . . . . . . . . . . . . . . . . . . . . . 78070

## Parathyroid Hormone . . . . . . . . . .83970

## Parathyroid Transplantation
*See* Parathyroid Gland, Autotransplant;
Transplantation, Parathyroid.

## Parathyroidectomy . . . . . . . . 60500-60505

## Paraurethral Gland
Abscess
    Incision and Drainage . . . . . . . . . . . . . 53060

## Paravertebral Nerve
Destruction. . . . . . . . . . . . . . . . . 64633-64636
Injection
    Anesthetic . . . . . . . . . . . . . . . 64470-64484
    Neurolytic. . . . . . . . . . . . . . . . 64633-64636

## Parietal Cell Vagotomies
*See* Vagotomy, Highly Selective

## Parietal Craniotomy . . . . . . . . . . . . .61556

## Paring
Skin Lesion
    Benign Hyperkeratotic . . . . . . . . . 11055-11057
    2 to 4 Lesions . . . . . . . . . . . . . . . . . 11056
    More than 4 Lesions. . . . . . . . . . . . . . 11057
    Single Lesion . . . . . . . . . . . . . . . . . . 11055

## Paronychia
Incision and Drainage . . . . . . . . . . . 10060-10061

## Parotid Duct
Diversion. . . . . . . . . . . . . . . . . . 42507-42510
Reconstruction . . . . . . . . . . . . . . . 42507-42510

## Parotid Gland
Abscess
    Incision and Drainage . . . . . . . . 42300-42305
Calculi (Stone)
    Excision . . . . . . . . . . . . . . . . 42330, 42340
Excision
    Partial. . . . . . . . . . . . . . . . . . 42410-42415
    Total. . . . . . . . . . . . . . . . . . . 42420-42426
Tumor
    Excision . . . . . . . . . . . . . . . . . 42410-42426

## Parotitides, Epidemic
*See* Mumps

## Pars Abdominalis Aortae
*See* Aorta, Abdominal

## Partial
Colectomy
    *See* Colectomy, Partial
Cystectomy
    *See* Cystectomy, Partial
Esophagectomy
    *See* Esophagectomy, Partial
Gastrectomy
    *See* Excision, Stomach, Partial
Glossectomy
    *See* Excision, Tongue, Partial
Hepatectomy
    *See* Excision, Liver, Partial
Mastectomy
    *See* Breast, Excision, Lesion
Nephrectomy
    *See* Excision, Kidney, Partial
Pancreatectomy
    *See* Pancreatectomy, Partial
Splenectomy
    *See* Splenectomy, Partial
Thromboplastin Time
    *See* Thromboplastin, Partial Time
Ureterectomy
    *See* Ureterectomy, Partial

## Particle Agglutination . . . . 86403-86406

## Parvovirus
Antibody . . . . . . . . . . . . . . . . . . . . . . . .86747

Foreign Body.....................33020
with Tube.....................33015
Incision and Drainage.................33025
Puncture Aspiration............33010-33011
Removal
Clot
Endoscopic....................32658
Foreign Body
Endoscopic....................32658
Tumor
Excision.....................32661
Resection.....................33050

**Peridural Anesthesia**
*See* Anesthesia, Epidural

**Peridural Injection**
*See* Epidural, Injection

**Perineal Prostatectomy**
*See* Prostatectomy, Perineal

**Perineoplasty**....................56810

**Perineorrhaphy**
Repair
Rectocele......................57250

**Perineum**
Abscess
Incision and Drainage..............56405
Colposcopy......................99170
Debridement
Infected...................11004, 11006
Removal
Prosthesis......................53442
Repair.........................56810
X-ray with Contrast..................74775

**Perionychia**
*See* Paronychia

**Periorbital Region**
Reconstruction
Osteotomy with Graft.........21267-21268
Repair-Osteotomy..............21260-21263

**Peripheral Artery Disease (PAD) Rehabilitation**...................93668

**Peripheral Nerve**
Repair/Suture
Major......................64856, 64859

**Periprosthetic Capsulectomy**
Breast...........................19371

**Peristaltic Pumps**
*See* Infusion Pump

**Peritoneal Dialysis**...90945-90947, 4055F
Kt/V Level......................3082F-3084F

**Peritoneal Free Air**
*See* Pneumoperitoneum

**Peritoneal Lavage**..............49084

**Peritoneoscopy**
*See* Peritoneum Endoscopy

**Peritoneum**
Abscess
Incision and Drainage..............49020
Percutaneous...................49021
Chemotherapy Administration..........96446
*See* Chemotherapy

Endoscopy
Biopsy........................47561
Diagnostic......................49320
Drainage
Lymphocele....................49323
X-ray.........................47560
Exchange
Drainage Catheter................49423
Injection
Contrast
via Catheter..................49424
Ligation
Shunt........................49428
Removal
Catheter......................49422
Foreign Body...................49402
Shunt........................49429
Tumor
Resection..................58950-58958
Unlisted Services and Procedures........49999
Venous Shunt
Injection......................49427
X-ray.........................74190

**Persistent Truncus Arteriosus**
*See* Truncus Arteriosus

**Persistent, Omphalomesenteric Duct**
*See* Diverticulum, Meckel's

**Personal Care**
*See* Self Care

**Personality Test**...........96101-96103
Computer-Assisted..................96103

**Pessary**
Insertion........................57160

**Pesticides**
Chlorinated Hydrocarbons.............82441

**PET**
*See* Positron Emission Tomography

**Petrous Temporal**
Excision
Apex.........................69530

**Peyronie Disease**
Injection........................54200
Surgical Exposure..................54205
with Graft...................54110-54112

**pH**
*See* Blood Gases
Exhaled Breath Condensate............83987
Other Fluid.......................83986
Urine..........................83986

**Phacoemulsification**
Removal
Extracapsular Cataract........66982, 66984
Secondary Membranous Cataract......66850

**Phagocytosis**
White Blood Cells..................86344

**Phalangectomy**
Toe...........................28150
Partial........................28160

**Phalanges (Hand)**
*See* Finger, Bone

**Phalanx, Finger**
Craterization..................26235-26236

Cyst
Excision...................26210-26215
Diaphysectomy...............26235-26236
Excision.....................26235-26236
Radical
for Tumor.................26260-26262
Fracture
Articular
Closed Treatment.............26740
Open Treatment..............26746
with Manipulation............26742
Distal....................26755-26756
Closed Treatment.............26750
Open Treatment..............26765
Percutaneous Fixation..........26756
Open Treatment................26735
Distal.....................26765
Shaft.....................26720-26727
Open Treatment..............26735
Incision and Drainage...............26034
Ostectomy
Radical
for Tumor.................26260-26262
Repair
Lengthening.................26568
Nonunion...................26546
Osteotomy..................26567
Saucerization................26235-26236
Thumb
Fracture
Shaft.....................26720-26727
Tumor
Excision...................26210-26215

**Phalanx, Great Toe**
*See* Phalanx, Toe
Fracture.........................28490
Open Treatment................28505
with Manipulation..........28495-28496
Percutaneous Fixation...............28496
without Manipulation................28490

**Phalanx, Toe**
Condyle
Excision......................28126
Craterization.....................28124
Cyst
Excision......................28108
Diaphysectomy...................28124
Excision...........28124, 28150-28160
Fracture
Open Treatment................28525
with Manipulation...............28515
without Manipulation..............28510
Repair
Osteotomy.................28310-28312
Saucerization.....................28124
Tumor
Excision......................28108
Radical Resection.................28175

**Pharmaceutic Preparations**
*See* Drug

**Pharmacotherapies**
*See* Chemotherapy

**Pharyngeal Tonsil**
*See* Adenoids

**Pharyngectomy**
Partial..........................42890

**Pharyngolaryngectomy**...31390-31395

**Pharyngoplasty**.................42950

Iontophoresis . . . . . . . . . . . . . . . . . . . . . 97033
Microwave Therapy . . . . . . . . . . . . . . . 97024
Paraffin Bath . . . . . . . . . . . . . . . . . . . . 97018
Traction . . . . . . . . . . . . . . . . . . . . . . . . . 97012
Ultrasound . . . . . . . . . . . . . . . . . . . . . . . 97035
Ultraviolet Light . . . . . . . . . . . . . . . . . . 97028
Unlisted Services and Procedures . . . . . . 97039
Vasopneumatic Device . . . . . . . . . . . . . 97016
Whirlpool Therapy . . . . . . . . . . . . . . . . 97022
Orthotics Training . . . . . . . . . . . . . . . . . . . . 97760
Osteopathic Manipulation . . . . . . . . 98925-98929
Procedures
Aquatic Therapy . . . . . . . . . . . . . . . . . . 97113
Direct . . . . . . . . . . . . . . . . . . . 97032-97039
Gait Training . . . . . . . . . . . . . . . . . . . . . 97116
Group Therapeutic . . . . . . . . . . . . . . . . 97150
Massage Therapy . . . . . . . . . . . . . . . . . 97124
Neuromuscular Reeducation . . . . . . . . . 97112
Physical Performance Test . . . . . . . . . . 97750
Supervised . . . . . . . . . . . . . . 97010-97028
Therapeutic Exercises . . . . . . . . . . . . . 97110
Traction Therapy . . . . . . . . . . . . . . . . . 97140
Work Hardening . . . . . . . . . . . 97545-97546
Prosthetic Training . . . . . . . . . . . . . . . . . . . 97761
Sensory Integration . . . . . . . . . . . . . . . . . . 97533
Therapeutic Activities . . . . . . . . . . . . . . . . 97530
Unlisted Services and Procedures . . . 97139, 97799
Wheelchair Management . . . . . . . . . . . . . . 97542
Work Reintegration . . . . . . . . . . . . . . . . . . 97537

## Physical Therapy
*See* Physical Medicine/Therapy/Occupational
Therapy

## Physician Services
Care Plan Oversight Services . . . . . . 99339-99340,
99374-99380
Domiciliary Facility . . . . . . . . . . 99339-99340
Home Health Agency Care . . . . . . . . . . 99374
Home or Rest Home Care . . . . . . 99339-99340
Hospice . . . . . . . . . . . . . . . . . . . 99377-99378
Nursing Facility . . . . . . . . . . . . . . 99379-99380
Case Management Services . . . . . . . 99366-99368
Direction, Advanced Life Support . . . . . . . . 99288
Online . . . . . . . . . . . . . . . . . . . . . . . . . . . . . 99444
Prolonged
with Direct Patient Contact . . . . . 99354-99357
Inpatient . . . . . . . . . . . . . . . . . 99356-99357
Outpatient/Office . . . . . . . . . . . 99354-99355
without Direct Patient Contact . . 99358-99359
Standby . . . . . . . . . . . . . . . . . . . . . . . . . . . . 99360
Supervision, Care Plan Oversight
Services . . . . . . . . . . 99339-99340, 99374-99380
Team Conference . . . . . . . . . . . . . . . . . . . . 99367
Telephone . . . . . . . . . . . . . . . . . 99441-99443

## Piercing of Ear Lobe . . . . . . . . . . . . 69090

## Piles
*See* Hemorrhoids

## Pilonidal Cyst
Excision . . . . . . . . . . . . . . . . . . . . 11770-11772
Incision and Drainage . . . . . . . . . . . 10080-10081

## Pin
*See* Wire
Insertion/Removal
Skeletal Traction . . . . . . . . . . . . . . . . . 20650
Prophylactic Treatment
Femur . . . . . . . . . . . . . . . . . . . . . . . . . . 27187
Humerus . . . . . . . . . . . . . . . . . . . . . . . . 24498
Shoulder . . . . . . . . . . . . . . . . . . . 23490-23491

## Pinch Graft . . . . . . . . . . . . . . . . . . 15050

## Pinna
*See* Ear, External

## Pinworms
Examination . . . . . . . . . . . . . . . . . . . . . . . . 87172

## Pirogoff Procedure . . . . . . . . . . . . 27888

## Pituitary Epidermoid Tumor
*See* Craniopharyngioma

## Pituitary Gland
Excision . . . . . . . . . . . . . . . . . . . . . 61546-61548
Tumor
Excision . . . . . . . . . . . . . . 61546-61548, 62165

## Pituitary Growth Hormone
*See* Growth Hormone

## Pituitary Lactogenic Hormone
*See* Prolactin

## Pituitectomy
*See* Excision, Pituitary Gland

## PKU
*See* Phenylalanine

## Placement
Adjustable Gastric Restrictive Device . . . . . 43770
Broncheal Stent . . . . . . . . . . . . . . . 31636-31637
Cardiac Stent . . . . . . . . . . . . . . . . . . . . . . 33621
Catheter
Aneurysm Sac
Pressure Sensor . . . . . . . . . . . . . . . 34806
Complete Study . . . . . . . . . . . . . . . 93982
Brain
for Chemotherapy . . . . . . . . . . . . . . . . 0169T
Breast
for Interstitial Radioelement
Application . . . . 19296-19298, 20555, 41019
Bronchus
for Intracavitary Radioelement
Application . . . . . . . . . . . . . . . . . . . . . 31643
*See* Catheterization
Head
Interstitial Radioelement
Application . . . . . . . . . . . . . . . . . . . . 41019
Neck
Interstitial Radioelement
Application . . . . . . . . . . . . . . . . . . . . 41019
Pelvic Organs
Interstitial Radioelement
Application . . . . . . . . . . . . . . . . . . . . 55920
Prostate . . . . . . . . . . . . . . . . . . . . . . . . 55875
Renal Artery
Selective . . . . . . . . . . . . . . . . . 36251-36252
Superselective . . . . . . . . . . . . . 36253-36254
Catheter, Cardiac . . . . . . . . . . . . . . . . . . . 93503
*See* Catheterization, Cardiac
Cecostomy Tube . . . . . . . . . . . . . . 44300, 49442
Colonic Stent . . . . . . 44397, 45327, 45345, 45387
Dosimeter
Prostate . . . . . . . . . . . . . . . . . . . . . . . . 55876
Drainage
Pancreas . . . . . . . . . . . . . . . . . . . . . . . . 48001
Duodenostomy Tube . . . . . . . . . . . . . . . . . 49441
Endovascular Prosthesis
Aorta . . . . . . . . . . . . . . . . . . . . 33883-33886
Enterostomy Tube . . . . . . . . . . . . . . . . . . . 44300
Fiducial Markers
Bronchus . . . . . . . . . . . . . . . . . . . . . . . 31626
Prostate . . . . . . . . . . . . . . . . . . . . . . . . 55876
Gastostomy Tube . . . . . . . . . . . . . 43246, 49440

Guidance
Catheter
Abscess . . . . . . . . . . . . . . . . . . . . . . . 75989
Bile . . . . . . . . . . . . . . . . . . . . . . . . . . . 75982
Specimen . . . . . . . . . . . . . . . . . . . . . . 75989
Prosthesis
Thoracic Aorta . . . . . . . . . . . . 75958-75959
Implant
Vertebra
Intrafacet . . . . . . . . . . . . . . . . 0219T-0222T
Interstitial Device
Abdomen . . . . . . . . . . . . . . . . . 49411-49412
Lungs . . . . . . . . . . . . . . . . . . . . . . . . . 32553
Omentum . . . . . . . . . . . . . . . . . 49411-49412
Pelvis . . . . . . . . . . . . . . . . . . . . 49411-49412
Pleura . . . . . . . . . . . . . . . . . . . . . . . . . 32553
Peritoneum . . . . . . . . . . . . . . . . 49411-49412
Prostate . . . . . . . . . . . . . . . . . . . . . . . . 55876
Retroperitoneum . . . . . . . . . . . . 49411-49412
Intravascular Stent
Coronary . . . . . . . . . . . . . . . . . 92980-92981
Intracranial . . . . . . . . . . . . . . . . . . . . . 61635
Jejunostomy Tube
Endoscopic . . . . . . . . . . . . . . . . . . . . . 44372
Percutaneous . . . . . . . . . . . . . . . . . . . 49441
Metallic Localization Clip
Breast . . . . . . . . . . . . . . . . . . . . . . . . . 19295
Nasogastric Tube . . . . . . . . . . . . . . . . . . . 43752
Needle
Bone . . . . . . . . . . . . . . . . . . . . . . . . . . 36680
Interstitial Radioelement Application
Genitalia . . . . . . . . . . . . . . . . . . . . . . 55920
Head . . . . . . . . . . . . . . . . . . . . . . . . . 41019
Muscle . . . . . . . . . . . . . . . . . . . . . . . 20555
Neck . . . . . . . . . . . . . . . . . . . . . . . . . 41019
Pelvic Organs . . . . . . . . . . . . . . . . . . 55920
Soft Tissue . . . . . . . . . . . . . . . . . . . . 20555
Prostate . . . . . . . . . . . . . . . . . . . . . . . 55875
Needle Wire
Breast . . . . . . . . . . . . . . . . . . . 19290-19291
Orogastric Tube . . . . . . . . . . . . . . . . . . . . 43752
Osteopromotive Material . . . . . . . . . . . . . . 20930
Pressure Sensor . . . . . . . . . . . . . . . . . . . . 34806
Radiation Delivery Device
Intracoronary Artery . . . . . . . . . . . . . . . 92974
Pleural Cavity . . . . . . . . . . . . . . . . . . . . 32553
Sensor, Wireless
Endovascular Repair . . . . . . . . . . . . . . 34806
Seton
Anal . . . . . . . . . . . . . . . . . . . . . . . . . . . 46020
Subconjunctival Retinal Prosthesis . . . . . . . 0100T
Synthetic Device
Vertebra . . . . . . . . . . . . . . . . . . 0220T-0222T
Tracheal Stent . . . . . . . . . . . . . . . . . . . . . 31631
Transcatheter
Pressure Sensor . . . . . . . . . . . . . . . . . 34806
Ureteral Stent . . . . . . . . . . . . . . . . . . . . . . 50947

## Placenta
Delivery . . . . . . . . . . . . . . . . . . . . . . . . . . . 59414

## Placenta Alpha
## Microglobulin-1 . . . . . . . . . . . . . . 84412

## Placental Lactogen
*See* Lactogen, Human Placental

## Placental Villi
*See* Chorionic Villus

## Plagiocephaly . . . . . . . . . . . . . . . . 21175

## Plague Vaccine . . . . . . . . . . . . . . . 90727

Spirometry . . . . . . . . . . . . . . . . 94010-94070
 Evaluation . . . . . . . . . . . . . . 94010-94070
 Patient Initiated with
  Bronchospasm . . . . . . . . . . . 94014-94016
Sputum Mobilization with Inhalants . . . . 94664
Stress Test . . . . . . . . . . . . . . . . . 94621
Stress Test, Pulmonary . . . . . . . . . . . 94620
Therapeutic
 Expired Gas Analysis . . . . . . . . . . . . 94250
 Inhalation
  Pentamidine . . . . . . . . . . . . . . . 94642
 Inhalation Treatment . . . . 94640, 94644-94645,
                        94664, 99503
 Intrapulmonary Surfactant
  Administration . . . . . . . . . . . . . . 94610
 Manipulation of Chest Wall . . . . 94667-94668
 Pressure Ventilation
  Negative CNPB . . . . . . . . . . . . . . 94662
  Positive CPAP . . . . . . . . . . . . . . 94660
 Unlisted Services and Procedures . . . . . 94799
 Ventilation Assist . . . . . . 94002-94005, 99504
Unlisted Services and Procedures . . . . . . 94799

**Pulse Generator**
Electronic Analysis . . . . . . . . .0285T, 95970-95982
Heart
 Insertion . . . . . . . . . . . . 33212-33213, 33221
Neurostimulator
 Electronic Analysis . . . . . . . . . . 95970-95982
Peripheral Field Stimulation
 Electronic Analysis . . . . . . . . . . . . . 0285T
Revision/Removal . . . . . . . . . . . . . . . . 0284T

**Pulse Rate Increased**
*See* Tachycardia

**Pump**
*See* Chemotherapy, Pump Services; Infusion Pump

**Pump Services**
Oxygenator/Heat Exchanger . . . . . . . 99190-99192

**Pump, Infusion**
*See* Infusion Pump

**Punch Graft** . . . . . . . . . . . . . . 15775-15776

**Puncture**
Artery . . . . . . . . . . . . . . . . . . . . . 36600
Chest
 Drainage . . . . . . . . . . . . . . 32421-32422
Cisternal
 *See* Cisternal Puncture
Lumbar
 *See* Spinal Tap
Lung . . . . . . . . . . . . . . . . . . . . . . 32420
Pericardium . . . . . . . . . . . . . . . 33010-33011
Pleural Cavity
 Drainage . . . . . . . . . . . . . . 32421-32422
Skull
 Drain Fluid . . . . . . . . . . . . . 61000-61020
  Cistern . . . . . . . . . . . . . . . . . 61050
 Inject Cistern . . . . . . . . . . . . . . 61055
 Inject Ventricle . . . . . . . . . . . . . 61026
 Shunt
  Drain Fluid . . . . . . . . . . . . . . . 61070
  Injection . . . . . . . . . . . . . . . . 61070
Spinal Cord
 Diagnostic . . . . . . . . . . . . . . . . 62270
 Drain Fluid . . . . . . . . . . . . . . . . 62272
 Lumbar . . . . . . . . . . . . . . . . . . 62270
Tracheal
 Aspiration and/or Injection . . . . . . . . 31612

**Puncture Aspiration**
Abscess
 Skin . . . . . . . . . . . . . . . . . . . . 10160
Bulla . . . . . . . . . . . . . . . . . . . . . 10160
Cyst
 Breast . . . . . . . . . . . . . . . 19000-19001
 Skin . . . . . . . . . . . . . . . . . . . . 10160
Hematoma . . . . . . . . . . . . . . . . . . 10160

**Puncturing**
*See* Puncture

**Pure-Tone Audiometry**
*See* Audiometry, Pure Tone

**Pustules**
Removal . . . . . . . . . . . . . . . . . . . 10040

**Putti-Platt Procedure** . . . . . . . . . 23450

**PUVA**
*See* Dermatology; Photochemotherapy; Ultraviolet
Light Therapy

**Pyelogram**
*See* Urography, Intravenous; Urography, Retrograde

**Pyelography** . . . . . . . . . . . . .74400, 74425
Injection . . . . . . . . . . . . . . . . . . . 50394

**Pyelolithotomy** . . . . . . . . . . . . . 50130
Anatrophic . . . . . . . . . . . . . . . . . . 50075
Coagulum . . . . . . . . . . . . . . . . . . 50130

**Pyeloplasty** . . . . . . . . 50400-50405, 50544
Repair
 Horseshoe Kidney . . . . . . . . . . . . 50540
Secondary . . . . . . . . . . . . . . . . . . 50405

**Pyeloscopy**
with Cystourethroscopy . . . . . . . . . . . 52351
 Biopsy . . . . . . . . . . . . . . . . . . 52354
 Destruction . . . . . . . . . . . . . . . . 52354
 Lithotripsy . . . . . . . . . . . . . . . . 52353
 Removal
  Calculus . . . . . . . . . . . . . . . . 52352
 Tumor Excision . . . . . . . . . . . . . . 52355

**Pyelostogram** . . . . . . . . . . . . . . 50394

**Pyelostolithotomy**
Percutaneous . . . . . . . . . . . . . . 50080-50081

**Pyelostomy** . . . . . . . . 50125, 50400-50405
Change Tube . . . . . . . . . . . . . . . . . 50398

**Pyelotomy**
Complicated . . . . . . . . . . . . . . . . . 50135
Endoscopic . . . . . . . . . . . . . . . . . 50570
Exploration . . . . . . . . . . . . . . . . . 50120
with Drainage . . . . . . . . . . . . . . . . 50125
with Removal Calculus . . . . . . . . . . . . 50130

**Pyeloureterogram**
Antegrade . . . . . . . . . . . . . . . . . . 50394

**Pyeloureteroplasty**
*See* Pyeloplasty

**Pyloric Sphincter**
Incision . . . . . . . . . . . . . . . . . . . 43520
Reconstruction . . . . . . . . . . . . . . . 43800

**Pyloromyotomy** . . . . . . . . . . . . . 43520

**Pyloroplasty** . . . . . . . . . . . . . . 43800
with Vagotomy . . . . . . . . . . . . . . . . 43640

**Pyothorax**
*See* Abscess, Thorax

**Pyridoxal Phosphate** . . . . . . . . . .84207

**Pyrophosphate, Adenosine**
*See* Adenosine Diphosphate

**Pyrophosphorylase, Udp Galactose**
*See* Galactose-1-Phosphate, Uridyl Transferase

**Pyruvate** . . . . . . . . . . . . . . 84210-84220

**Q Fever** . . . . . . . . . . . . . . . .86000, 86638

**Q Fever ab**
*See* Antibody, Coxiella Burnetii

**QST**
*See* Quantitative Sensory Testing

**Quadrantectomy** . . . . . . . . . . .19301-19302

**Quadriceps Repair** . . . . . . . . . . .27430

**Quantitative Sensory Testing (QST)**
Cooling Stimuli . . . . . . . . . . . . . . . . 0108T
Heat-Pain Stimuli . . . . . . . . . . . . . . . 0109T
Other Stimuli . . . . . . . . . . . . . . . . . 0110T
Touch Pressure Stimuli . . . . . . . . . . . . 0106T
Vibration Stimuli . . . . . . . . . . . . . . . 0107T

**Quick Test**
*See* Prothrombin Time

**Quinidine**
Assay . . . . . . . . . . . . . . . . . . . . 80194

**Quinine** . . . . . . . . . . . . . . . . . .84228

**Rabies Vaccine**
*See* Vaccines

**Rachicentesis**
*See* Spinal Tap

**Radial Artery**
*See* Artery, Radial

**Radial Head, Subluxation**
*See* Nursemaid Elbow

**Radial Keratotomy** . . . . . . . . . . . .65771

**Radiation**
*See* Irradiation

**Radiation Physics**
Consultation . . . . . . . . . . . . . . 77336-77370
Unlisted Services and Procedures . . . . . . 77399

**Radiation Therapy** . . . . . . . . 77280-77295
Consultation
 Radiation Physics . . . . . . . . . . . 77336-77370

**Radiation, X**
*See* X-ray

**Radical Excision of Lymph Nodes**
*See* Excision, Lymph Nodes, Radical

**Radical Mastectomies, Modified**
*See* Mastectomy, Modified Radical

**Radical Neck Dissection**

**Radical Resection**

**Radical Vaginal Hysterectomy**
*See* Hysterectomy, Vaginal, Radical

**Radical Vulvectomy**
*See* Vulvectomy, Radical

**Radio-Cobalt B-12 Schilling Test**
*See* Vitamin, B-12, Absorption Study

**Radioactive Colloid Therapy** . . . 79300

**Radioactive Substance**

**Radiocarpal Joint**

**Radiocinematographies**
*See* Cineradiography

**Radioelement**

**Radioelement Substance**

**Radiography**
*See* Radiology, Diagnostic; X-ray

**Radioimmunosorbent Test**
*See* Gammaglobulin, Blood

**Radioisotope Brachytherapy**
*See* Brachytherapy

**Radioisotope Scan**
*See* Nuclear Medicine

**Radiological Marker**

**Radiology**

**Radionuclide CT Scan**
*See* Emission Computerized Tomography

**Radionuclide Imaging**
*See* Nuclear Medicine

**Radionuclide Therapy**
*See* Radiopharmaceutical Therapy

**Radionuclide Tomography,
Single-Photon Emission-Computed**
*See* SPECT

**Radiopharmaceutical Localization**

**Radiopharmaceutical Therapy**

**Radiotherapeutic**
*See* Radiation Therapy

**Radiotherapies**
*See* Irradiation

**Radiotherapy, Surface**
*See* Application, Radioelement, Surface

**Radioulnar Joint**

Open Treatment . . . . . . . . . . . . . . . . . . . 25676
Percutaneous Fixation . . . . . . . . . . . . . 25671

## Radius
*See* Arm, Lower; Elbow; Ulna
Arthroplasty . . . . . . . . . . . . . . . . . . . . . . . 24365
  with Implant. . . . . . . . . . . . . . . 24366, 25441
Craterization. . . . . . . . . . . . . . . . . . 24145, 25151
Cyst
    Excision . . . . . . . . 24125-24126, 25120-25126
Diaphysectomy. . . . . . . . . . . . . . . . . 24145, 25151
Dislocation
    Partial. . . . . . . . . . . . . . . . . . . . . . . . . 24640
    Subluxate . . . . . . . . . . . . . . . . . . . . . . 24640
    with Fracture
      Closed Treatment . . . . . . . . . . . . . 24620
      Open Treatment . . . . . . . . . . . . . . 24635
Excision. . . . . . . . . . . . . . . 24130, 24136, 24145
    Epiphyseal Bar . . . . . . . . . . . . . . . . . . 20150
    Partial. . . . . . . . . . . . . . . . . . . . . . . . . 25145
    Styloid Process. . . . . . . . . . . . . . . . . . 25230
Fracture . . . . . . . . . . . . . . . . . . . . . . . . . . 25605
    Closed Treatment . . . . . . . . . . . 25500-25505,
                25520, 25600-25605
      with Manipulation . . . . . . . . . . . . . 25605
      without Manipulation. . . . . . . . . . . 25600
    Colles . . . . . . . . . . . . . . . . . . . . . . . . . 25600
    Distal . . . . . . . . . . . . . . . . . . . . 25600-25609
      Closed Treatment . . . . . . . . . 25600-25605
      Open Treatment . . . . . . . . . . 25607-25609
    Head/Neck
      Closed Treatment . . . . . . . . . . 24650-24655
      Open Treatment . . . . . . . . . . . 24665-24666
    Open Treatment . . . . . . . 25515, 25525-25526,
                       25574
    Percutaneous Fixation . . . . . . . . . . . . . 25606
    Shaft. . . . . . . . . . . . . . . . . . . . . 25500-25526
      Open Treatment . . . . . . 25515, 25574-25575
    Smith . . . . . . . . . . . . . . . . . . . . . . . . . 25600
    with Ulna . . . . . . . . . . . . . . . . 25560-25565
      Open Treatment . . . . . . . . . . . . . . 25575
Implant
    Removal. . . . . . . . . . . . . . . . . . . . . . . 24164
Incision and Drainage . . . . . . . . . . . . . . . 25035
Osteomyelitis . . . . . . . . . . . . . . . . 24136, 24145
Osteoplasty . . . . . . . . . . . . . . . . . 25390-25393
Prophylactic Treatment . . . . . . . . . 25490, 25492
Repair
    Epiphyseal Arrest. . . . . . . . . . . 25450-25455
    Epiphyseal Separation
      Closed. . . . . . . . . . . . . . . . . . . . . . 25600
      Closed with Manipulation . . . . . . . . . 25605
      Open Treatment . . . . . . . . . 25607-25609
      Percutaneous Fixation . . . . . . . . . . . 25606
    Malunion or Nonunion. . . . . . . . 25400, 25415
    Osteotomy . . . 25350-25355, 25370-25375
      and Ulna . . . . . . . . . . . . . . . . . . . . 25365
    with Graft. . . . . . . . . . 25405, 25420-25426
Saucerization . . . . . . . . . . . . . . . . 24145, 25151
Sequestrectomy . . . . . . . . . . . . . . 24136, 25145
Tumor
    Cyst . . . . . . . . . . . . . . . . . . . . . . . . . 24120
    Excision . . 24125-24126, 25120-25126, 25170
    Radical Resection . . . . . . . . . . . . . . . . 24152

## Ramstedt Operation
*See* Pyloromyotomy

## Ramus Anterior, Nervus Thoracicus
*See* Intercostal Nerve

## Range of Motion Test
Extremities or Trunk. . . . . . . . . . . . . . . . . 95851
Eye . . . . . . . . . . . . . . . . . . . . . . 92018-92019
Hand . . . . . . . . . . . . . . . . . . . . . . . . . . . 95852

## Rapid Heart Rate
*See* Tachycardia

## Rapid Plasma Reagin Test . . . . . . . . . . . . . . . . . . . . . 86592-86593

## Rapid Test for Infection . . . . . . . . . 86308, 86403-86406
Monospot Test . . . . . . . . . . . . . . . . . . . . 86308

## Rapoport Test . . . . . . . . . . . . . . . . . . . 52005

## Raskind Procedure . . . . . . . 33735-33737

## Rat Typhus
*See* Murine Typhus

## Rathke Pouch Tumor
*See* Craniopharyngioma

## Rays, Roentgen
*See* X-ray

## Raz Procedure . . . . . . . . . . . . . . . . . 51845
*See* Repair, Bladder, Neck

## RBC
*See* Red Blood Cell (RBC)

## RBC ab
*See* Antibody, Red Blood Cell

## Reaction
Lip
    without Reconstruction . . . . . . . . . . . . 40530

## Reaction, Polymerase Chain
*See* Polymerase Chain Reaction

## Realignment
Femur
    with Osteotomy . . . . . . . . . . . . . . . . . 27454
Knee
    Extensor . . . . . . . . . . . . . . . . . . . . . . 27422

## Receptor
*See* CD4; Estrogen, Receptor; FC Receptor;
Progesterone Receptors

## Receptor Assay
Hormone. . . . . . . . . . . . . . . . . . . 84233-84235
Non Hormone. . . . . . . . . . . . . . . . . . . . 84238

## Recession
Gastrocnemius
    Leg, Lower . . . . . . . . . . . . . . . . . . . . 27687

## Reconstruction
*See* Revision
Abdominal Wall
    Omental Flap . . . . . . . . . . . . . . . . . . . 49905
Acetabulum . . . . . . . . . . . . . . . . 27120-27122
Anal
    Congenital Absence. . . . . . . . . . 46730-46740
    Fistula. . . . . . . . . . . . . . . . . . . . . . . . 46742
    Graft. . . . . . . . . . . . . . . . . . . . . . . . . 46753
    Sphincter . . . . . . . . 46750-46751, 46760-46762
    with Implant. . . . . . . . . . . . . . . . . . . . 46762
Ankle. . . . . . . . . . . . . . . . . . . . . 27700-27703
Apical-Aortic Conduit . . . . . . . . . . . . . . . 33404
Atrial . . . . . . . . . . . . . . . . . . . . . 33257-33259
    Endoscopic . . . . . . . . . . . . . . . 33265-33266
    Open . . . . . . . . . . . . . . . . . . . 33254-33259
Auditory Canal, External . . . . . . . . . 69310-69320
Bile Duct
    Anastomosis . . . . . . . . . . . . . . . . . . . 47800

Bladder
    and Urethra . . . . . . . . . . . . . . . 51800-51820
      Radiofrequency Micro-Remodeling . . . 53860
    from Colon . . . . . . . . . . . . . . . . . . . . . 50810
    from Intestines. . . . . . . . . . . . 50820, 51960
Breast . . . . . . . . . . . . . . . . . . . . 19357-19369
    Augmentation . . . . . . . . . . . . . 19324-19325
    Mammoplasty . . . . . . . . . . . . . 19318-19325
    Nipple. . . . . . . . . . . . . . . . . . 19350-19355
    Revision . . . . . . . . . . . . . . . . . . . . . . 19380
    Transverse Rectus Abdominis
    Myocutaneous Flap . . . . . . . . . . 19367-19369
      with Free Flap . . . . . . . . . . . . . . . 19364
      with Latissimus Dorsi Flap. . . . . . . . 19361
      with Other Techniques. . . . . . . . . . 19366
      with Tissue Expander. . . . . . . . . . . 19357
Bronchi . . . . . . . . . . . . . . . . . . . . . . . . . 32501
    Graft Repair . . . . . . . . . . . . . . . . . . . 31770
    Stenosis . . . . . . . . . . . . . . . . . . . . . . 31775
Canthus. . . . . . . . . . . . . . . . . . . . . . . . . 67950
Carpal . . . . . . . . . . . . . . . . . . . . . . . . . . 25443
Carpal Bone . . . . . . . . . . . . . . . . 25394, 25430
Cheekbone . . . . . . . . . . . . . . . . . . . . . . 21270
Chest Wall . . . . . . . . . . . . . . . . . . . . . . 32504
    Omental Flap . . . . . . . . . . . . . . . . . . . 49904
    Trauma . . . . . . . . . . . . . . . . . . . . . . . 32820
Cleft Palate. . . . . . . . . . . . . . . . . 42200-42225
Conduit
    Apical-Aortic . . . . . . . . . . . . . . . . . . . 33404
Conjunctiva. . . . . . . . . . . . . . . . . 68320-68335
    with Flap
      Bridge or Partial . . . . . . . . . . . . . . 68360
      Total . . . . . . . . . . . . . . . . . . . . . . 68362
Cranial Bone
    Extracranial . . . . . . . . . . . . . . . 21181-21184
Ear, Middle
    Tympanoplasty with Antrotomy or
    Mastoidotomy
      with Ossicular Chain
      Reconstruction . . . . . . . . . . . 69636-69637
    Tympanoplasty with Mastoidectomy. . . . 69641
      Radical or Complete. . . . . . . . 69644-69645
      with Intact or Reconstructed
      Wall . . . . . . . . . . . . . . . . . . 69643-69644
      with Ossicular Chain
      Reconstruction . . . . . . . . . . . . . . . 69642
    Tympanoplasty without
    Mastoidectomy . . . . . . . . . . . . . . . . . 69631
      with Ossicular Chain
      Reconstruction . . . . . . . . . . . 69632-69633
Elbow . . . . . . . . . . . . . . . . . . . . . . . . . . 24360
    Total Replacement. . . . . . . . . . . . . . . . 24363
    with Implant. . . . . . . . . . . . . . 24361-24362
Esophagus . . . . . . . . . . . . 43300, 43310, 43313
    Creation
      Stoma . . . . . . . . . . . . . . . . . 43350-43352
    Esophagostomy . . . . . . . . . . . . . . . . . 43350
    Fistula. . . . . . . . . . . . . 43305, 43312, 43314
    Gastrointestinal . . . . . . . . . . . . 43360-43361
Eye
    Graft
      Conjunctiva. . . . . . . . . . . . . . . . . . 65782
      Stem Cell . . . . . . . . . . . . . . . . . . 65781
    Transplantation
      Amniotic Membrane. . . . . . . 65778-65780
Eyelid
    Canthus. . . . . . . . . . . . . . . . . . . . . . . 67950
    Second Stage. . . . . . . . . . . . . . . . . . . 67975
    Total . . . . . . . . . . . . . . . . . . . 67973-67975
    Total Eyelid
      Lower, One Stage. . . . . . . . . . . . . . 67973
      Upper, One Stage . . . . . . . . . . . . . 67974

**Rectal Bleeding**
*See* Hemorrhage, Rectum

**Rectal Prolapse**
*See* Procidentia, Rectum

**Rectal Sphincter**

**Rectocele**

**Rectopexy**
*See* Proctopexy

**Rectoplasty**
*See* Proctoplasty

**Rectorrhaphy**
*See* Rectum, Suture

**Rectovaginal Fistula**
*See* Fistula, Rectovaginal

**Rectovaginal Hernia**
*See* Rectocele

## Rectum

*See* Anus

Abscess
  Incision and Drainage . . . . . . . . 45005-45020,
    46040, 46060
Biopsy . . . . . . . . . . . . . . . . . . . . . . . . . . . . 45100
Dilation
  Endoscopy . . . . . . . . . . . . . . . . . . . . . . 45303
Endoscopy
  Destruction
    Tumor . . . . . . . . . . . . . . . . . . . . . . . 45320
  Dilation . . . . . . . . . . . . . . . . . . . . . . . . 45303
  Exploration . . . . . . . . . . . . . . . . . . . . . 45300
  Hemorrhage . . . . . . . . . . . . . . . . . . . . . 45317
  Removal
    Foreign Body . . . . . . . . . . . . . . . . . . 45307
    Polyp . . . . . . . . . . . . . . . . . . . 45308-45315
    Tumor . . . . . . . . . . . . . . . . . . . 45308-45315
  Volvulus . . . . . . . . . . . . . . . . . . . . . . . 45321
Excision
  Partial . . . . . . . . 45111, 45113-45116, 45123
  Total . . . . . . . . 45110, 45112, 45119-45120
  with Colon . . . . . . . . . . . . . . . . . . . . . 45121
Exploration
  Endoscopic . . . . . . . . . . . . . . . . . . . . . 45300
  Surgical . . . . . . . . . . . . . . . . . . . . . . . 45990
Hemorrhage
  Endoscopic . . . . . . . . . . . . . . . . . . . . . 45317
Injection
  Sclerosing Solution . . . . . . . . . . . . . . . 45520
Laparoscopy . . . . . . . . . . . . . . . . . . . . . . 45499
Lesion
  Excision . . . . . . . . . . . . . . . . . . . . . . . 45108
Manometry . . . . . . . . . . . . . . . . . . . . . . . 91122
Prolapse
  Excision . . . . . . . . . . . . . . . . . 45130-45135
Removal
  Fecal Impaction . . . . . . . . . . . . . . . . . 45915
  Foreign Body . . . . . . . . . . . . . 45307, 45915
Repair
  Fistula . . . . . . . . . . . . . . . . . . . 45800-45825
  Injury . . . . . . . . . . . . . . . . . . . 45562-45563
  Prolapse . . . . . . . . . 45505-45541, 45900
  Rectocele . . . . . . . . . . . . . . . . . . . . . . 45560
  Stenosis . . . . . . . . . . . . . . . . . . . . . . . 45500
  with Sigmoid Excision . . . . . . . . . . . . . 45550
Sensation, Tone, and Compliance Test . . . . 91120
Stricture
  Excision . . . . . . . . . . . . . . . . . . . . . . . 45150
Suture
  Fistula . . . . . . . . . . . . . . . . . . . 45800-45825
  Prolapse . . . . . . . . . . . . . . . . . 45540-45541
Tumor
  Destruction . . . . . . . . . . . . . . . . 45190, 45320
  Excision . . . . . . . . . . . . . . . . . 45160-45172
    Transanal Endoscopic . . . . . . . . . . 0184T
Unlisted Services and Procedures . . . . . . . . 45999

## Red Blood Cell (RBC)

Antibody . . . . . . . . . . . . . . . . . . . 86850-86870
  Pretreatment . . . . . . . . . . . . . . 86970-86972
Count . . . . . . . . . . . . . . . . . . . . . 85032-85041
Fragility
  Mechanical . . . . . . . . . . . . . . . . . . . . . 85547
  Osmotic . . . . . . . . . . . . . . . . . 85555-85557
Hematocrit . . . . . . . . . . . . . . . . . . . . . . . 85014
Morphology . . . . . . . . . . . . . . . . . . . . . . 85007
Platelet Estimation . . . . . . . . . . . . . . . . . 85007
Sedimentation Rate
  Automated . . . . . . . . . . . . . . . . . . . . . 85652
  Manual . . . . . . . . . . . . . . . . . . . . . . . . 85651
Sequestration . . . . . . . . . . . . . . . . . . . . . 78140
Sickling . . . . . . . . . . . . . . . . . . . . . . . . . 85660

Survival Test . . . . . . . . . . . . . . . . 78130-78135
Volume Determination . . . . . . . . . . 78120-78121

## Red Blood Cell ab

*See* Antibody, Red Blood Cell

## Reductase, Glutathione

*See* Glutathione Reductase

## Reductase, Lactic Cytochrome

*See* Lactic Dehydrogenase

## Reduction

Forehead . . . . . . . . . . . . . . . . . . 21137-21139
Lung Volume . . . . . . . . . . . . . . . . . . . . . 32491
Mammoplasty . . . . . . . . . . . . . . . . . . . . 19318
Masseter Muscle/Bone . . . . . . . . . . 21295-21296
Osteoplasty
  Facial Bones . . . . . . . . . . . . . . . . . . . 21209
Pregnancy
  Multifetal . . . . . . . . . . . . . . . . . . . . . 59866
Skull
  Craniomegalic . . . . . . . . . . . . . . 62115-62117
Ventricular Septum
  Non-Surgical . . . . . . . . . . . . . . . . . . 93733

## Reflex Test

Blink Reflex . . . . . . . . . . . . . . . . . . . . . . 95933
H-Reflex . . . . . . . . . . . . . . . . . . 95934-95936

## Reflux Study . . . . . . . . . . . . . . . . . . . . 78262

Gastroesophageal . . . . . . . . . . . . 91034-91038

## Refraction . . . . . . . . . . . . . . . . . . . . . . 92015

## Rehabilitation

Artery
  Occlusive Disease . . . . . . . . . . . . . . . 93668
Auditory
  Post-Lingual Hearing Loss . . . . . . . . . . 92633
  Pre-Lingual Hearing Loss . . . . . . . . . . . 92630
  Status Evaluation . . . . . . . . . . 92626-92627
Cardiac . . . . . . . . . . . . . . . . . . . 93797-93798
Services Considered
  Documentation . . . . . . . . . . . . . . . . . 4079F

## Rehabilitation Facility

Discharge Services . . . . . . . . . . . . . . 1110F-1111F

## Rehabilitative

*See* Rehabilitation

## Reimplantation

Arteries
  Aorta
    Prosthesis . . . . . . . . . . . . . . . . . . . 35697
  Carotid . . . . . . . . . . . . 35691, 35694-35695
  Subclavian . . . . . . . . . . . . . . . 35693-35695
  Vertebral . . . . . . . . . . . . . . . . . 35691-35693
  Visceral . . . . . . . . . . . . . . . . . . . . . . 35697
Kidney . . . . . . . . . . . . . . . . . . . . . . . . . 50380
Ovary . . . . . . . . . . . . . . . . . . . . . . . . . . 58825
Pulmonary Artery . . . . . . . . . . . . . . . . . . 33788
Ureter, to Bladder . . . . . . . . . . . . 50780-50785
Ureters . . . . . . . . . . . . . . . . . . . . . . . . . 51565

## Reinnervation

Larynx
  Neuromuscular Pedicle . . . . . . . . . . . . 31590

## Reinsch Test . . . . . . . . . . . . . . . . . . . . 83015

## Reinsertion

Drug Delivery Implant . . . . . . . . . . . . . . . 11983
Spinal Fixation Device . . . . . . . . . . . . . . . 22849

## Relative Density

*See* Specific Gravity

## Release

Carpal Tunnel . . . . . . . . . . . . . . . . . . . . 64721
Elbow Contracture
  with Radical Release of Capsule . . . . . . . 24149
Flexor Muscles
  Hip . . . . . . . . . . . . . . . . . . . . . . . . . . 27036
Muscle
  Knee . . . . . . . . . . . . . . . . . . . . . . . . . 27422
Nerve . . . . . . . . . . . . . . . . . . . . 64702-64726
  Neurolytic . . . . . . . . . . . . . . . . . . . . . 64727
Retina
  Encircling Material . . . . . . . . . . . . . . . 67115
Spinal Cord . . . . . . . . . . . . . . . . . . . . . . 63200
Stapes . . . . . . . . . . . . . . . . . . . . . . . . . 69650
Tarsal Tunnel . . . . . . . . . . . . . . . . . . . . . 28035
Tendon . . . . . . . . . . . . . . . . . . . 24332, 25295

## Release-Inhibiting Hormone, Somatotropin

*See* Somatostatin

## Removal

Adjustable Gastric Restrictive
  Device . . . . . . . . . . . . . . . . . . . 43772-43774
Allograft
  Intestinal . . . . . . . . . . . . . . . . . . . . . . 44137
Artificial Intervertebral Disc
  Cervical Interspace . . . . . . . . . . 0095T, 22864
  Lumbar Interspace . . . . . . . . . . 0164T, 22865
Balloon
  Intra-Aortic . . . . . . . . . . . . . . . . . . . . 33974
Balloon Assist Device
  Intra-Aortic . . . . . . . . . . . . . . . 33968, 33971
Baroreflex Activation Device . . . . . . . 0269T-0271T
Blood Clot
  Eye . . . . . . . . . . . . . . . . . . . . . . . . . . 65930
Blood Component
  Apheresis . . . . . . . . . . . . . . . . 36511-36516
Breast
  Capsules . . . . . . . . . . . . . . . . . . . . . . 19371
  Implants . . . . . . . . . . . . . . . . . 19328-19330
  Modified Radical . . . . . . . . . . . . . . . . . 19307
  Partial . . . . . . . . . . . . . . . . . . . 19300-19302
  Radical . . . . . . . . . . . . . . . . . . 19305-19306
  Simple, Complete . . . . . . . . . . . . . . . . 19303
  Subcutaneous . . . . . . . . . . . . . . . . . . 19304
Bronchial Valve . . . . . . . . . . . . . . . 0251T-0252T
Calcareous Deposits
  Subdeltoid . . . . . . . . . . . . . . . . . . . . . 23000
Calculi (Stone)
  Bile Duct . . . . . . . . . . . . . 43264, 47420-47425
    Percutaneous . . . . . . . . . . . . 47554, 47630
  Bladder . . . . . . . . 51050, 52310-52318, 52352
  Gallbladder . . . . . . . . . . . . . . . . . . . . 47480
  Hepatic Duct . . . . . . . . . . . . . . . . . . . 47400
  Kidney . . . . . . . . . . . . . 50060-50081, 50130,
    50561, 50580, 52352
  Pancreas . . . . . . . . . . . . . . . . . . . . . . 48020
  Pancreatic Duct . . . . . . . . . . . . . . . . . 43264
  Salivary Gland . . . . . . . . . . . . 42330-42340
  Ureter . . . . . 50610-50630, 50961, 50980,
    51060-51065, 52320-52330, 52352
  Urethra . . . . . . . . . . . . . 52310-52315, 52352
Cardiac Event Recorder . . . . . . . . . . . . . . 33284
Cast . . . . . . . . . . . . . . . . . . . . . 29700-29715
Cataract
  Dilated Fundus Evaluation . . . . . . . . . . 2021F
  with Replacement
    Extracapsular . . . . . . . . . . . 66982, 66984
    Intracapsular . . . . . . . . . . . . . . . . . 66983
    Not Associated with Concurrent . . . . . 66983
Catheter
  Central Venous . . . . . . . . . . . . . . . . . 36589
  Fractured . . . . . . . . . . . . . . . . . . . . . . 75961

Nails . . . . . . . . . . . . .11730-11732, 11750-11752
Neurostimulators
    Pulse Generator . . . . . . . . . . . . . . . . . . . 64595
    Receiver . . . . . . . . . . . . . . . . . . . . . . . . . . 64595
Ocular Implant . . . . . . . . . . . . . . 65175, 65920
Orbital Implant . . . . . . . . . . . . . . . . . . . . . . 67560
Ovary
    Laparoscopy . . . . . . . . . . . . . . . . . . . . . . 58661
    with Hysterectomy . . . . 58542, 58544, 58548
Pacemaker System
    Electrodes
      by Thoracotomy . . . . . . . . . . . . . . . . 33236
    Pulse Generator Only . . . . . . . . . . . . . . . 33233
Pacing Cardioverter-Defibrillator System
    Electrodes . . . . . . . . . . . 33243-33244
      via Thoracotomy . . . . . . . . . . . . . . . . 33243
    Pulse Generator Only . . . . . . . . . . . . . . . 33241
Patella, Complete . . . . . . . . . . . . . . . . . . . 27424
Plate
    Skull . . . . . . . . . . . . . . . . . . . . . . . . . . . . 62142
Polyp
    Anal . . . . . . . . . . . . . . . . . . 46610, 46612
    Antrochoanal . . . . . . . . . . . . . . . . . . . . . 31032
    Colon . . . . . . . . . . . . . . . . 44392, 45385
    Colon-Sigmoid . . . . . . . . . . . . . . . . . . . . 45333
    Endoscopy . . . . . . . 44364-44365, 44394
    Esophagus . . . . . . . . . . . . . . 43217, 43250
    Gastrointestinal, Upper . . . . . . . 43250-43251
    Rectum . . . . . . . . . . . . . . . . . . . . . . . . . 45315
    Sphenoid Sinus . . . . . . . . . . . . . . . . . . . 31051
Prosthesis
    Abdomen . . . . . . . . . . . . . . . . . . . . . . . . 49606
    Abdominal Wall . . . . . . . . . . . . . . . . . . 11008
    Hip . . . . . . . . . . . . . . . . . . . . . 27090-27091
    Knee . . . . . . . . . . . . . . . . . . . . . . . . . . . 27488
    Penis . . . . . . . . . . . . 54406, 54410-54417
    Perineum . . . . . . . . . . . . . . . . . . . . . . . . 53442
    Skull . . . . . . . . . . . . . . . . . . . . . . . . . . . 62142
    Urethral Sphincter . . . . . . . . . . . 53446-53447
    Wrist . . . . . . . . . . . . . . . . . . . 25250-25251
Pulse Generator . . . . . . . . . . . . . . . . . . . . 0284T
    Brain . . . . . . . . . . . . . . . . . . . . . . . . . . . 61888
    Spinal Cord . . . . . . . . . . . . . . . . . . . . . . 63688
Pustules . . . . . . . . . . . . . . . . . . . . . . . . . . 10040
Receiver
    Brain . . . . . . . . . . . . . . . . . . . . . . . . . . . 61888
    Spinal Cord . . . . . . . . . . . . . . . . . . . . . . 63688
Reservoir
    Spinal Cord . . . . . . . . . . . . . . . . . . . . . . 62365
Seton
    Anal . . . . . . . . . . . . . . . . . . . . . . . . . . . 46030
Shoulder Joint
    Foreign or Loose Body . . . . . . . . . . . . . . 23107
Shunt
    Brain . . . . . . . . . . . . . . . . . . 62256-62258
    Heart . . . . . . . . . . . . . . . . . . . . . . . . . . 33924
    Peritoneum . . . . . . . . . . . . . . . . . . . . . . 49429
    Spinal Cord . . . . . . . . . . . . . . . . . . . . . . 63746
Skin Tags . . . . . . . . . . . . . . . . . . 11200-11201
Sling
    Urethra . . . . . . . . . . . . . . . . . . . . . . . . . 53442
    Vagina . . . . . . . . . . . . . . . . . . . . . . . . . 57287
Spinal Instrumentation
    Anterior . . . . . . . . . . . . . . . . . . . . . . . . 22855
    Posterior Nonsegmental
      Harrington Rod . . . . . . . . . . . . . . . . 22850
    Posterior Segmental . . . . . . . . . . . . . . . 22852
Stent
    Bile Duct . . . . . . . . . . . . . . . . . . . . . . . . 43269
    Pancreatic Duct . . . . . . . . . . . . . . . . . . . 43269
    Ureteral . . . . . . . . . . . . . . . . . . 50382-50387

Subcutaneous Port
    for Gastric Restrictive
      Procedure . . . . . . . . . . . . . . . 43887-43888
Suture
    Anal . . . . . . . . . . . . . . . . . . . . . . . . . . . 46754
    Anesthesia . . . . . . . . . . . . . . . 15850-15851
Thrombus
    *See* Thrombectomy
Tissue Expanders
    Skin . . . . . . . . . . . . . . . . . . . . . . . . . . . 11971
Transplant
    Intestines . . . . . . . . . . . . . . . . . . . . . . . 44137
    Kidney . . . . . . . . . . . . . . . . . . . . . . . . . 50370
Tube
    Ear, Middle . . . . . . . . . . . . . . . . . . . . . . 69424
    Finger . . . . . . . . . . . . . . . . . . 26392, 26416
    Hand . . . . . . . . . . . . . . . . . . 26392, 26416
    Nephrostomy . . . . . . . . . . . . . . . . . . . . . 50389
Tumor
    Temporal Bone . . . . . . . . . . . . . . . . . . . 69970
Ureter
    Ligature . . . . . . . . . . . . . . . . . . . . . . . . 50940
Urethral Stent
    Bladder . . . . . . . . . . . . . . . . . . 52310-52315
    Urethra . . . . . . . . . . . . . . . . . . 52310-52315
Uterus
    Laparoscopy . . . . . . . . . . . 58541, 58543, 58548
Vein
    Clusters . . . . . . . . . . . . . . . . . . . . . . . . 37785
    Perforation . . . . . . . . . . . . . . . . 37760-37761
    Saphenous . . . . . . . . . 37718-37735, 37780
    Varicose . . . . . . . . . . . . . . . . . 37765-37766
Venous Access Device . . . . . . . . . . . . . . . . 36590
    Obstruction . . . . . . . . . . . . . . . 75901-75902
Ventilating Tube
    Ear, Middle . . . . . . . . . . . . . . . . . . . . . . 69424
Ventricular Assist Device . . . . . . . . 33977-33978
    Extracorporeal . . . . . . . . . . . . . . . . . . . . 0050T
    Intracorporeal . . . . . . . . . . . . . . . . . . . . 33980
Vitreous
    Anterior Approach . . . . . . . . . . . 67005-67010
Wire
    Anal . . . . . . . . . . . . . . . . . . . . . . . . . . . 46754

## Renal Abscess
*See* Abscess, Kidney

## Renal Arteries
*See* Artery, Renal

## Renal Autotransplantation
*See* Autotransplantation, Renal

## Renal Calculus
*See* Calculus, Removal, Kidney

## Renal Cyst
*See* Cyst, Kidney

## Renal Dialyses
*See* Hemodialysis

## Renal Disease Services
*See* Dialysis

## Renal Transplantation
*See* Kidney, Transplantation

## Renin . . . . . . . . . . . . .80408, 80416, 84244
Peripheral Vein . . . . . . . . . . . . . . . . . . . . . 80417

## Renin-Converting Enzyme . . . .82164

## Reoperation
Carotid
    Thromboendarterectomy . . . . . . . . . . . 35390

Coronary Artery Bypass
    Valve Procedure . . . . . . . . . . . . . . . . . . 33530
Distal Vessel Bypass . . . . . . . . . . . . . . . . 35700

## Repair
*See* Revision
Abdomen . . . . . . . . . . . . . . . . . . . . . . . . 49900
    Hernia . . . . . . . . . . . . . 49491-49525, 49565,
                   49570, 49582-49590
    Omphalocele . . . . . . . . . . . . . . 49600-49611
    Suture . . . . . . . . . . . . . . . . . . . . . . . . . 49900
Abdominal Wall . . . . . . . . . . . . . . 15830, 15847
Anal
    Anomaly . . . . . . . . . . . . . . . . . 46744-46748
    Fistula . . . . . . . . . 46288, 46706, 46715-46716
    Stricture . . . . . . . . . . . . . . . . . 46700-46705
Aneurysm
    Aorta
      Abdominal . . . . . . . . . . . . . . . 0078T-0081T
      Infrarenal . . . . . .34800-34805, 34825-34832
        Imaging . . . . . . . . . . . . . . . 75952-75953
      Thoracic . . . . . . . . . . . . . . . 33877-33886
    Iliac Artery . . . . . . . . . . . . . . . . . . . . . . 75954
    Intracranial Artery . . . . . . . . . . . 61697-61708
Ankle
    Ligament . . . . . . . . . . . . . . . . . 27695-27698
    Tendon . . . . 27612, 27650-27654, 27680-27687
Aorta . . . . . . . . . .33320-33322, 33802-33803
    Coarctation . . . . . . . . . . . . . . . 33840-33851
    Graft . . . . . . . . . . . . . . . . . . . . 33860-33877
    Sinus of Valsalva . . . . . . . . . . . 33702-33720
    Thoracic . . . . . . . . . . . . . . . . . 75956-75959
      Endovascular . . . . . . . . . . . . . 33880-33891
Anorectum
    Fistula . . . . . . . . . . . . . . . . . . . . . . . . . 46707
Aortic Arch
    with Cardiopulmonary Bypass . . . . . . . . . 33853
    without Cardiopulmonary Bypass . . . . . . 33852
Aortic Valve . . . . . . . . 0256T-0257T, 33400-33403
    Obstruction
      Outflow Tract . . . . . . . . . . . . . . . . . . 33414
      Septic Hypertrophy . . . . . . . . . . . . . . 33416
      Stenosis . . . . . . . . . . . . . . . . . . . . . 33415
Arm
    Lower . . . . . . . . . . . . . . 25260-25263, 25270
      Fasciotomy . . . . . . . . . . . . . . . . . . . 24495
      Secondary . . . . . . . . . . 25265, 25272-25274
      Tendon . . . . . . . . . . . . . . . . . . . . . . 25290
      Tendon Sheath . . . . . . . . . . . . . . . . . 25275
      Muscle . . . . . . . . . . . . . . . . . . . . . . 24341
      Tendon . . . . . . . . . . . . 24332, 24341, 25280,
              25295, 25310-25316
    Upper
      Muscle Revision . . . . . . . . . . . 24330-24331
      Muscle Transfer . . . . . . . . . . . 24301, 24320
      Tendon Lengthening . . . . . . . . . . . . . . 24305
      Tendon Revision . . . . . . . . . . . . . . . . 24320
      Tendon Transfer . . . . . . . . . . . . . . . . 24301
      Tenotomy . . . . . . . . . . . . . . . . . . . . 24310
Arteriovenous Fistula
    Abdomen . . . . . . . . . . . . . . . . . . . . . . . 35182
      Acquired or Traumatic . . . . . . . . . . . . 35189
    Head . . . . . . . . . . . . . . . . . . . . . . . . . . 35180
      Acquired or Traumatic . . . . . . . . . . . . 35188
    Lower Extremity . . . . . . . . . . . . . . . . . . 35184
      Acquired or Traumatic . . . . . . . . . . . . 35190
    Neck . . . . . . . . . . . . . . . . . . . . . . . . . . 35180
      Acquired or Traumatic . . . . . . . . . . . . 35188
    Thorax . . . . . . . . . . . . . . . . . . . . . . . . . 35182
      Acquired or Traumatic . . . . . . . . . . . . 35189
    Upper Extremity . . . . . . . . . . . . . . . . . . 35184
      Acquired or Traumatic . . . . . . . . . . . . 35190

## Retinopathy
Destruction
    Cryotherapy, Diathermy . . . . . . . . . . . . . 67227
Treatment
    Photocoagulation, Cryotherapy. . . 67228-67229

## Retraction, Clot
*See* Clot Retraction

## Retrieval
Filter
    Vena Cava . . . . . . . . . . . . . . . . . . . . . . 37193
Transcatheter Foreign Body. . . . . . . . . . . . . 37203

## Retrocaval Ureter
Ureterolysis . . . . . . . . . . . . . . . . . . . . . . . 50725

## Retrograde Cholangiopancreatographies, Endoscopic
*See* Cholangiopancreatography

## Retrograde Cystourethrogram
*See* Urethrocystography, Retrograde

## Retrograde Pyelogram
*See* Urography, Retrograde

## Retroperitoneal Area
Abscess
    Incision and Drainage
       Open . . . . . . . . . . . . . . . . . . . . . . . 49060
       Percutaneous . . . . . . . . . . . . . . . . . . 49061
Biopsy . . . . . . . . . . . . . . . . . . . . . . . . . . . 49010
Cyst
    Destruction/Excision . . . . . . . . . 49203-49205
Endometriomas
    Destruction/Excision . . . . . . . . . 49203-49205
Exploration . . . . . . . . . . . . . . . . . . . . . . . . 49010
Needle Biopsy
    Mass . . . . . . . . . . . . . . . . . . . . . . . . . 49180
Tumor
    Destruction/Excision . . . . . . . . . 49203-49205

## Retroperitoneal Fibrosis
Ureterolysis . . . . . . . . . . . . . . . . . . . . . . . 50715

## Retropubic Prostatectomies
*See* Prostatectomy, Retropubic

## Revascularization
Artery
    Femoral/Popliteal. . . . . . . . . . . . 37224-37227
    Iliac. . . . . . . . . . . . . . . . . . . . . 37220-37223
    Tibial/Peroneal. . . . . . . . . . . . . . 37228-37235
Distal Upper Extremity
    with Interval Ligation. . . . . . . . . . . . . . 36838
Interval Ligation
    Distal Upper Extremity. . . . . . . . . . . . . 36838
Penis . . . . . . . . . . . . . . . . . . . . . . . . . . . . 37788
Transmyocardial. . . . . . . . . . . . . . . . 33140-33141

## Reversal, Vasectomy
*See* Vasovasorrhaphy

## Reverse T3
*See* Triiodothyronine, Reverse

## Reverse Triiodothyronine
*See* Triiodothyronine, Reverse

## Revision
*See* Reconstruction
Abdomen
    Intraperitoneal Catheter . . . . . . . . . . . 49325
Adjustable Gastric Restrictive Device . . . . . 43771
Aorta . . . . . . . . . . . . . . . . . . . . . . . . . . . . 33404

Baroreflex Activation Device. . . . . . . .0269T-0271T
Blepharoplasty . . . . . . . . . . . . . . . . . 15820-15823
Broncheal Stent . . . . . . . . . . . . . . . . . . . . 31638
Bronchus. . . . . . . . . . . . . . . . . . . . . . . . . 32501
Bypass Graft
    Vein Patch . . . . . . . . . . . . . . . . . . . . 35685
Cervicoplasty . . . . . . . . . . . . . . . . . . . . . . 15819
Colostomy
    *See* Colostomy, Revision
Cornea
    Prosthesis. . . . . . . . . . . . . . . . . . . . . 65770
    Reshaping
       Epikeratoplasty. . . . . . . . . . . . . . . 65767
       Keratomileusis . . . . . . . . . . . . . . . 65760
       Keratophakia . . . . . . . . . . . . . . . . 65765
Defibrillator Site
    Chest . . . . . . . . . . . . . . . . . . . . . . . . 33223
Ear, Middle . . . . . . . . . . . . . . . . . . . . . . . 69662
External Fixation System. . . . . . . . . . . . . . 20693
Eye
    Aqueous Shunt. . . . . . . . . . . . . . . . . . 66185
Gastric Restrictive Procedure
    Other than Adjustable Gastric Restrictive
    Device . . . . . . . . . . . . . . . . . . . . . . . 43848
Gastrostomy Tube . . . . . . . . . . . . . . . . . . 44373
Hip Replacement
    *See* Replacement, Hip, Revision
Hymenal Ring. . . . . . . . . . . . . . . . . . . . . . 56700
Ileostomy
    *See* Ileostomy, Revision
Infusion Pump
    Intraarterial . . . . . . . . . . . . . . . . . . . 36261
    Intravenous . . . . . . .36576-36578, 36582-36583
Iris
    Iridoplasty . . . . . . . . . . . . . . . . . . . . 66762
    Iridotomy . . . . . . . . . . . . . . . . . . . . . 66761
Jejunostomy Tube . . . . . . . . . . . . . . . . . . 44373
Lower Extremity Arterial Bypass. . . . 35879-35881
Pacemaker Site
    Chest . . . . . . . . . . . . . . . . . . . . . . . . 33222
Pulse Generator . . . . . . . . . . . . . . . . . . . . 0284T
Rhytidectomy . . . . . . . . . . . . . . . . 15824-15829
Semicircular Canal
    Fenestration. . . . . . . . . . . . . . . . . . . . 69840
Shunt
    Intrahepatic Portosystemic . . . . . . . . . . 37183
Sling . . . . . . . . . . . . . . . . . . . . . . . . . . . . 53442
Stapedectomy
    *See* Stapedectomy, Revision
Stomach
    for Obesity . . . . . . . . . . . . . . . . . . . . 43848
Subcutaneous Port
    for Gastric Restrictive Procedure. . . . . . . 43886
Tracheostomy
    Scar . . . . . . . . . . . . . . . . . . . . . . . . . 31830
Urinary-Cutaneous Anastomosis . . . 50727-50728
Vagina
    Prosthetic Graft . . . . . . . . 57295-57296, 57426
    Sling
       Stress Incontinence . . . . . . . . . . . . . 57287
Venous Access Device. . . . . . . . . . . .36576-36578,
                36582-36583, 36585
Ventricle
    Ventriculomyectomy . . . . . . . . . . . . . . 33416
    Ventriculomyotomy . . . . . . . . . . . . . . . 33416

## Rh (D)
*See* Blood Typing

## Rh Immune Globulin
*See* Immune Globulins, Rho (D)

## Rheumatoid Factor . . . . . . . . 86430-86431

## Rhinectomy
Partial . . . . . . . . . . . . . . . . . . . . . . . . . . 30150
Total . . . . . . . . . . . . . . . . . . . . . . . . . . . 30160

## Rhinomanometry . . . . . . . . . . . . . 92512

## Rhinopharynx
*See* Nasopharynx

## Rhinophyma
Repair . . . . . . . . . . . . . . . . . . . . . . . . . . 30120

## Rhinoplasty
Cleft Lip/Cleft Palate . . . . . . . . . . . 30460-30462
Primary . . . . . . . . . . . . . . . . . . . . 30400-30420
Secondary. . . . . . . . . . . . . . . . . . . 30430-30450

## Rhinoscopy
*See* Endoscopy, Nose

## Rhinotomy
Lateral. . . . . . . . . . . . . . . . . . . . 30118, 30320

## Rhizotomy . . . . . . . . . . . . . . . 63185-63190

## Rho Variant Du. . . . . . . . . . . . . . . . 86905

## Rhytidectomy . . . . . . . . . . . . 15824-15829

## Rhytidoplasties
*See* Face Lift

## Rib
Antibody. . . . . . . . . . . . . . . . . . . . . . . . . 86756
Antigen Detection
    by Immunoassay
       with Direct Optical Observation
       Direct Fluorescense . . . . . . . . . . . . . 87280
       Enzyme Immunoassay . . . . . . . . . . . 87420
Excision. . . . . . . . . . . . . . . 21600-21616, 32900
Fracture
    Closed Treatment. . . . . . . . . . . . . . . . 21800
    External Fixation . . . . . . . . . . . . . . . . 21810
       Internal Fixation . . . . . . . . . . .0245T-0248T
    Open Treatment . . . . . . . . .0245T-0248T, 21805
Graft
    to Face . . . . . . . . . . . . . . . . . . . . . . . 21230
Resection . . . . . . . . . . . . . 19260-19272, 32900
X-ray . . . . . . . . . . . . . . . . . . . . 71100-71111

## Riboflavin . . . . . . . . . . . . . . . . . . . 84252

## Richardson Operation Hysterectomy
*See* Hysterectomy, Abdominal, Total

## Richardson Procedure . . . . . . . . 53460

## Rickettsia
Antibody. . . . . . . . . . . . . . . . . . . . . . . . . 86757

## Ridell Operation
*See* Sinusotomy, Frontal

## Ridge, Alveolar
*See* Alveolar Ridge

## Right Atrioventricular Valve
*See* Tricuspid Valve

## Right Heart Cardiac Catheterization
*See* Cardiac Catheterization, Right Heart

## Ripstein Operation
*See* Proctopexy

## Risk Factor Reduction Intervention
*See* Performance Measures, Preventive Medicine

**Scalp Blood Sampling** . . . . . . . . .59030

**Scan**
See Specific Site, Nuclear Medicine
Abdomen
    See Abdomen, CT Scan
CT
    See CT Scan
MRI
    See Magnetic Resonance Imaging
PET
    See Positron Emission Tomography
Radionuclide
    See Emission Computerized Tomography

**Scanning, Radioisotope**
See Nuclear Medicine

**Scanogram** . . . . . . . . . . . . . . . . . . . . .77073

**Scaphoid**
Fracture
    Closed Treatment . . . . . . . . . . . . . . . .25622
    Open Treatment . . . . . . . . . . . . . . . . .25628
    with Manipulation . . . . . . . . . . . . . . . .25624

**Scapula**
Craterization . . . . . . . . . . . . . . . . . . . .23182
Cyst
    Excision . . . . . . . . . . . . . . . . . . . . . . .23140
        with Allograft . . . . . . . . . . . . . . . . .23146
        with Autograft . . . . . . . . . . . . . . . .23145
Diaphysectomy . . . . . . . . . . . . . . . . . .23182
Excision . . . . . . . . . . . . . . . . . .23172, 23190
    Partial . . . . . . . . . . . . . . . . . . . . . . .23182
Fracture
    Closed Treatment
        with Manipulation . . . . . . . . . . . . . .23575
        without Manipulation . . . . . . . . . . . .23570
    Open Treatment . . . . . . . . . . . . . . . . .23585
Ostectomy . . . . . . . . . . . . . . . . . . . . .23190
Repair
    Fixation . . . . . . . . . . . . . . . . . . . . . . .23400
    Scapulopexy . . . . . . . . . . . . . . . . . . .23400
Saucerization . . . . . . . . . . . . . . . . . . .23182
Sequestrectomy . . . . . . . . . . . . . . . . .23172
Tumor
    Excision . . . . . . . . . . . . . . . . .23140, 23210
        with Allograft . . . . . . . . . . . . . . . . .23146
        with Autograft . . . . . . . . . . . . . . . .23145
    Radical Resection . . . . . . . . . . . . . . . .23210
X-ray . . . . . . . . . . . . . . . . . . . . . . . . .73010

**Scapulopexy** . . . . . . . . . . . . . . . . .23400

**Scarification**
Pleural . . . . . . . . . . . . . . . . . . . . . . . .32215

**Scarification of Pleura**
See Pleurodesis

**Schanz Operation**
See Femur, Osteotomy

**Schauta Operation**
See Hysterectomy, Vaginal, Radical

**Schede Procedure** . . . . . . . .32905-32906

**Scheie Procedure**
See Iridectomy

**Schilling Test** . . . . . . . . . . . . . . . . .78270
See Vitamin B-12 Absorption Study

**Schlatter Operation Total
Gastrectomy**
See Excision, Stomach, Total

**Schlicter Test** . . . . . . . . . . . . . . . . .87197
See Bactericidal Titer, Serum

**Schocket Procedure** . . . . . . . . . . .66180
See Aqueous Shunt

**Schuchard Procedure**
Osteotomy
    Maxilla . . . . . . . . . . . . . . . . . . . . . . .21206

**Schwannoma, Acoustic**
See Brain, Tumor, Excision

**Sciatic Nerve**
Decompression . . . . . . . . . . . . . . . . . 64712
Injection
    Anesthetic . . . . . . . . . . . . . . .64445-64446
Lesion
    Excision . . . . . . . . . . . . . . . . . . . . . 64786
Neuroma
    Excision . . . . . . . . . . . . . . . . . . . . . 64786
Neuroplasty . . . . . . . . . . . . . . . . . . . 64712
Release . . . . . . . . . . . . . . . . . . . . . . 64712
Repair/Suture . . . . . . . . . . . . . . . . . . 64858

**Scintigraphy**
See Nuclear Medicine
Computed Tomographic
    See Emission Computerized Tomography

**Scissoring**
Skin Tags . . . . . . . . . . . . . . . . . .11200-11201

**Sclera**
Excision
    Sclerectomy with Punch or Scissors . . . . 66160
Fistulization
    for Glaucoma . . . . . . . . . . . . . . . . . .0123T
    Iridencleisis or Iridotasis . . . . . . . . . . . 66165
    Sclerectomy with Punch or Scissors
      with Iridectomy . . . . . . . . . . . . . . . . 66160
    Thermocauterization with Iridectomy . . . 66155
    Trabeculectomy ab Externo in Absence
    of Previous Surgery . . . . . . . . . . . . . . . 66170
    Trephination with Iridectomy . . . . . . . . . 66150
Incision
    Fistulization
      Iridencleisis or Iridotasis . . . . . . . . . 66165
      Sclerectomy with Punch or Scissors
      with Iridectomy . . . . . . . . . . . . . . . . 66160
      Thermocauterization with Iridectomy . 66155
      Trabeculectomy ab Externo in Absence
      of Previous Surgery . . . . . . . . . . . . . 66170
      Trephination with Iridectomy . . . . . . . 66150
Lesion
    Excision . . . . . . . . . . . . . . . . . . . . . 66130
Repair
    Reinforcement
      with Graft . . . . . . . . . . . . . . . . . . . 67255
      without Graft . . . . . . . . . . . . . . . . . 67250
    Staphyloma
      with Graft . . . . . . . . . . . . . . . . . . . 66225
      without Graft . . . . . . . . . . . . . . . . . 66220
    with Glue . . . . . . . . . . . . . . . . . . . . . 65286
    Wound
      Operative . . . . . . . . . . . . . . . . . . . 66250
      Tissue Glue . . . . . . . . . . . . . . . . . . 65286

**Scleral Buckling Operation**
See Retina, Repair, Detachment

**Scleral Ectasia**
See Staphyloma, Sclera

**Sclerectomy** . . . . . . . . . . . . . . . . . .66160

**Sclerotherapy**
Venous . . . . . . . . . . . . . . . .36468-36471

**Sclerotomy**
See Incision, Sclera

**Screening, Drug**
See Drug Screen
Alcohol and/or Substance Abuse . . . 99408-99409

**Scribner Cannulization** . . . . . . . . .36810

**Scrotal Varices**
See Varicocele

**Scrotoplasty** . . . . . . . . . . . . . .55175-55180

**Scrotum**
Abscess
    Incision and Drainage . . . . . . . . 54700, 55100
Excision . . . . . . . . . . . . . . . . . . . . . . .55150
Exploration . . . . . . . . . . . . . . . . . . . . .55110
Hematoma
    Incision and Drainage . . . . . . . . . . . . .54700
Removal
    Foreign Body . . . . . . . . . . . . . . . . . .55120
Repair . . . . . . . . . . . . . . . . . .55175-55180
Ultrasound . . . . . . . . . . . . . . . . . . . . .76870
Unlisted Services and Procedures . . . . . . . .55899

**Scrub Typhus** . . . . . . . . . . . . . . . . .86000

**Second Look Surgery**
See Reoperation

**Section**
See Decompression
Cesarean
    See Cesarean Delivery
Cranial Nerve . . . . . . . . . . . . . . . . . . 61460
    Spinal Access . . . . . . . . . . . . . . . . . 63191
Dentate Ligament . . . . . . . . . . . . .63180-63182
Gasserian Ganglion
    Sensory Root . . . . . . . . . . . . . . . . . 61450
Medullary Tract . . . . . . . . . . . . . . . . . 61470
Mesencephalic Tract . . . . . . . . . . . . . . 61480
Nerve Root . . . . . . . . . . . . . . .63185-63190
Spinal Accessory Nerve . . . . . . . . . . . . 63191
Spinal Cord Tract . . . . . . . . . . .63194-63199
Tentorium Cerebelli . . . . . . . . . . . . . . . 61440
Vestibular Nerve
    Transcranial Approach . . . . . . . . . . . . 69950
    Translabyrinthine Approach . . . . . . . . . 69915

**Sedation**
Moderate . . . . . . . . . . . . . . . . .99143-99150
    with Independent Observation . . . 99143-99145

**Seddon-Brookes Procedure** . . . .24320

**Sedimentation Rate**
Blood Cell
    Automated . . . . . . . . . . . . . . . . . . . 85652
    Manual . . . . . . . . . . . . . . . . . . . . . . 85651

**Segmentectomy**
Breast . . . . . . . . . . . . . . . . . . . .19301-19302
Lung . . . . . . . . . . . . . . . . . . . . . . . . .32484
    Thoracoscopic . . . . . . . . . . . . . . . . . 32669

**Seidlitz Powder Test**
See X-ray, with Contrast

Arthrography
  Injection
    Radiologic......................23350
Arthroscopy
  Diagnostic .....................29805
  Surgical ...............29806-29828
    Biceps Tenodesis ..............29828
Arthrotomy
  with Removal Loose or Foreign Body ...23107
Biopsy
  Deep..........................23066
  Soft Tissue....................23065
Blade
  *See* Scapula
Bone
  Excision
    Acromion ....................23130
    Clavicle...............23120-23125
    Incision......................23035
  Tumor
    Excision...............23140-23146
Bursa
  Drainage......................23031
Capsular Contracture Release ...........23020
Cast
  Figure Eight ..................29049
  Removal ......................29710
  Spica ........................29055
  Velpeau ......................29058
Disarticulation ...............23920-23921
Dislocation
  Closed Treatment
    with Manipulation .........23650-23655
Exploration ....................23107
Hematoma
  Drainage......................23030
Manipulation
  Application of Fixation Apparatus......23700
Prophylactic Treatment ...........23490-23491
Removal
  Calcareous Deposits ..............23000
  Cast .........................29710
  Foreign Body
    Complicated ..................23332
    Deep........................23331
    Subcutaneous..................23330
  Foreign or Loose Body ............23107
Repair
  Capsule ...............23450-23466
  Ligament Release ...............23415
  Muscle Transfer...........23395-23397
  Rotator Cuff .............23410-23420
  Tendon .........23410-23412, 23430-23440
  Tenomyotomy...............23405-23406
Strapping .....................29240
Surgery
  Unlisted Services and Procedures......23929
Tumor
  Excision ...............23071-23076
  Radical Resection ...........23077-23078
Unlisted Services and Procedures ........23929
X-ray.....................73020-73030
X-ray with Contrast ...............73040

**Shoulder Joint**
*See* Clavicle; Scapula
Arthroplasty
  with Implant..............23470-23472
Arthrotomy
  with Biopsy ..............23100-23101
  with Synovectomy ...........23105-23106
Dislocation
  Open Treatment ..................23660

with Greater Tuberosity Fracture
  Closed Treatment ..............23665
  Open Treatment ...............23670
with Surgical or Anatomical Neck Fracture
  Closed Treatment with
    Manipulation ..................23675
  Open Treatment ...............23680
Excision
  Torn Cartilage...................23101
Exploration ..............23040-23044
Incision and Drainage ..........23040-23044
Removal
  Foreign Body ............23040-23044
X-ray .........................73050

**Shunt(s)**
Aqueous
  to Extraocular Reservoir............66180
  Revision ......................66185
Arteriovenous
  *See* Arteriovenous Shunt
Brain
  Creation ..............62180-62223
  Removal ..............62256-62258
  Replacement .............62160, 62194,
     62225-62230, 62258
  Reprogramming ..................62252
Cerebrospinal Fluid
  *See* Cerebrospinal Fluid Shunt
Creation
  Arteriovenous
    Direct ......................36821
    ECMO ......................36822
    Thomas Shunt..................36835
    Transposition .........36818-36820
    with Bypass Graft..............35686
    with Graft .............36825-36830
  Cerebrospinal Fluid ...............62200
  Thomas Shunt ..................36835
Fetal .........................59076
Great Vessel
  Aorta
    Pulmonary....................33924
  Aorta to Pulmonary Artery
    Ascending....................33755
    Descending...................33762
  Central .......................33764
  Subclavian Pulmonary Artery.........33750
  Vena Cava to Pulmonary
    Artery ...............33766-33768
Intra-Atrial .............33735-33737
LeVeen
  *See* LeVeen Shunt
Nonvascular
  X-ray .........................75809
Peritoneal
  Venous
    Injection ......................49427
    Ligation......................49428
    Removal .....................49429
    X-ray.......................75809
Pulmonary Artery
  *See* Pulmonary Artery, Shunt
Revision
  Arteriovenous.................36832
Spinal Cord
  Creation ...............63740-63741
  Irrigation......................63744
  Removal .....................63746
  Replacement ..................63744
Superior Mesenteric-Caval
  *See* Anastomosis, Caval to Mesenteric
Ureter to Colon..................50815

Ventriculocisternal with Valve
  *See* Ventriculocisternostomy

**Shuntogram**....................75809

**Sialic Acid**....................84275

**Sialodochoplasty**.........42500-42505

**Sialogram**
*See* Sialography

**Sialography**....................70390

**Sickling**
Electrophoresis....................83020

**Siderocytes**....................85536

**Siderophilin**
*See* Transferrin

**Sigmoid**
*See* Colon-Sigmoid

**Sigmoid Bladder**
Cystectomy....................51590

**Sigmoidoscopy**
Ablation
  Polyp........................45339
  Tumor .......................45339
Biopsy........................45331
Collection
  Specimen ....................45331
Exploration .............45330, 45335
Hemorrhage Control ............45334
Injection
  Submucosal ...................45335
Needle Biopsy ..................45342
Placement
  Stent........................45345
Removal
  Foreign Body .................45332
  Polyp.............45333, 45338
  Tumor .............45333, 45338
Repair
  Volvulus .....................45337
Ultrasound ..............45341-45342

**Signal-Averaged Electrocardiography**
*See* Electrocardiogram

**Silica**....................84285

**Silicon Dioxide**
*See* Silica

**Silicone**
Contouring Injections............11950-11954

**Silver Operation**
*See* Keller Procedure

**Silver Procedure**....................28290

**Simple Mastectomies**
*See* Mastectomy

**Single Photon Absorptiometry**
*See* Absorptiometry, Single Photon

**Single Photon Emission Computed Tomography**
*See* SPECT

**Sinu, Sphenoid**
*See* Sinus/Sinuses, Sphenoid

**Free Skin Graft**
Full Thickness . . . . . . . . . . . . . . . 15200-15261
Island Pedicle Flap . . . . . . . . . . . . . . . . . . . . 15740
Muscle . . . . . . . . . . . . . . . 15731-15738, 15842
   Free . . . . . . . . . . . . . . . . . . . . . . . . . . . . 15756
Myocutaneous . . . . . . . . . . . 15731-15738, 15756
Pedicle Flap
   Formation . . . . . . . . . . . . . . . . . . 15570-15576
   Island . . . . . . . . . . . . . . . . . . . . . . . . . . . 15740
   Neurovascular . . . . . . . . . . . . . . . . . . . . . 15750
   Transfer . . . . . . . . . . . . . . . . . . . . . . . . . 15650
Pinch Graft . . . . . . . . . . . . . . . . . . . . . . . . . 15050
Platysmal . . . . . . . . . . . . . . . . . . . . . . . . . . 15825
Punch Graft . . . . . . . . . . . . . . . . . . 15775-15776
Punch Graft for Hair Transplant . . . . . 15775-15776
Recipient Site Preparation . . . . . . . . 15002-15005
Skin
   Free . . . . . . . . . . . . . . . . . . . . . . . . . . . . 15757
Skin Substitute Graft . . . . . . . . . . . . . 15271-15278
Split Graft . . . . . . . . . . . 15100-15101, 15120-15121
Superficial Musculoaponeurotic System . . . 15829
Tissue Transfer . . . . . . . . . . . . . . . . 14000-14350
Tissue-Cultured . . . . . . . . . . 15040, 15150-15157
Transfer . . . . . . . . . . . . . . . . . . . . . . . . . . 15650
Vascular Flow Check . . . . . . . . . . . . . . . . . . 15860

## Skull
Burr Hole
   Biopsy Brain . . . . . . . . . . . . . . . . . . . . . . 61140
   Drainage
      Abscess . . . . . . . . . . . . . . . 61150-61151
      Cyst . . . . . . . . . . . . . . . . . . 61150-61151
      Hematoma . . . . . . . . . . . . . . 61154-61156
   Exploration
      Infratentorial . . . . . . . . . . . . . . . . . . . 61253
      Supratentorial . . . . . . . . . . . . . . . . . . 61250
   Insertion
      Catheter . . . . . . . . . . . . . . . . . . . . . . 61210
      EEG Electrode . . . . . . . . . . . . . . . . . . 61210
      Reservoir . . . . . . . . . . . . . . . . . . . . . 61210
   Intracranial
      Biopsy . . . . . . . . . . . . . . . . . . . . . . . 61140
      with Injection . . . . . . . . . . . . . . . . . . 61120
   Decompression . . . . . . . 61322-61323, 61340-61345
   Orbit . . . . . . . . . . . . . . . . . . . . . . . . . . . 61330
Drill Hole
   Catheter . . . . . . . . . . . . . . . . . . . . . . . . 61107
   Drainage Hematoma . . . . . . . . . . . . . . . . 61108
   Exploration . . . . . . . . . . . . . . . . . . . . . . 61105
Excision . . . . . . . . . . . . . . . . . . . . . . . . . . 61501
Exploration
   Drill Hole . . . . . . . . . . . . . . . . . . . . . . . 61105
Fracture . . . . . . . . . . . . . . . . . . . . . 62000-62010
Hematoma
   Drainage . . . . . . . . . . . . . . . . . . . . . . . . 61108
Incision
   Suture . . . . . . . . . . . . . . . . . . . . . 61550-61552
Insertion
   Catheter . . . . . . . . . . . . . . . . . . . . . . . . 61107
Lesion
   Excision . . . 61500, 61600-61608, 61615-61616
Orbit
   Biopsy . . . . . . . . . . . . . . . . . . . . . . . . . 61332
   Excision
      Lesion . . . . . . . . . . . . . . . . . . . . . . . 61333
   Exploration . . . . . . . . . . . . . . . . . 61332-61334
   Removal Foreign Body . . . . . . . . . . . . . . . 61334
Puncture
   Cervical . . . . . . . . . . . . . . . . . . . . . . . . 61050
   Cisternal . . . . . . . . . . . . . . . . . . . . . . . . 61050
   Drain Fluid . . . . . . . . . . . . . . . . . . . . . . 61070
   Injection . . . . . . . . . . . . . . . . . . . . . . . . 61070
   Subdural . . . . . . . . . . . . . . . . . . . 61000-61001
   Ventricular Fluid . . . . . . . . . . . . . . . . . . . 61020

Reconstruction . . . . . . . . . . . . . . . 21172-21180
   Defect . . . . . . . . . . . . . . . 62140-62141, 62145
Reduction
   Craniomegalic . . . . . . . . . . . . . . . 62115-62117
Removal
   Plate . . . . . . . . . . . . . . . . . . . . . . . . . . 62142
   Prosthesis . . . . . . . . . . . . . . . . . . . . . . 62142
Repair
   Cerebrospinal Fluid Leak . . . . . . . . . . . . 62100
   Encephalocele . . . . . . . . . . . . . . . . . . . 62120
Replacement
   Plate . . . . . . . . . . . . . . . . . . . . . . . . . . 62143
   Prosthesis . . . . . . . . . . . . . . . . . . . . . . 62143
Tumor
   Excision . . . . . . . . . . . . . . . . . . . . . . . . 61500
X-ray . . . . . . . . . . . . . . . . . . . . . . . 70250-70260

## Skull Base Surgery
Anterior Cranial Fossa
   Bicoronal Approach . . . . . . . . . . . . . . . . 61586
   Craniofacial Approach . . . . . . . . . 61580-61583
   Extradural . . . . . . . . . . . . . . . . . 61600-61601
   LeFort I Osteotomy Approach . . . . . . . 61586
   Orbitocranial Approach . . . . . . . . 61584-61585
   Transzygomatic Approach . . . . . . . . . . 61586
Carotid Aneurysm . . . . . . . . . . . . . . . . . . 61613
Carotid Artery . . . . . . . . . . . . . . . . . . . . . 61610
   Transection/Ligation . . . . . . . . . 61609-61612
Craniotomy . . . . . . . . . . . . . . . . . . . . . . . 62121
Dura
   Repair of Cerebrospinal Fluid
      Leak . . . . . . . . . . . . . . . . . . . 61618-61619
Middle Cranial Fossa
   Extradural . . . . . . . . . . . . . . . . . 61605, 61607
   Infratemporal Approach . . . . . . . . 61590-61591
   Intradural . . . . . . . . . . . . . . . . . 61606, 61608
Orbitocranial Zygomatic Approach . . . . . . . 61592
Posterior Cranial Fossa
   Extradural . . . . . . . . . . . . . . . . . . . . . . 61615
   Intradural . . . . . . . . . . . . . . . . . . . . . . 61616
   Transcondylar Approach . . . . . . . 61596-61597
   Transpetrosal Approach . . . . . . . . . . . . 61598
   Transtemporal Approach . . . . . . . . . . . . 61595

**Sleep Study** . . . . . . . . 0244T, 95800-95801, 95806-95807
Actigraphy . . . . . . . . . . . . . . . . . . . . . . . . 95803

## Sliding Inlay Graft, Tibia
*See* Ankle; Tibia, Repair

## Sling Operation
Incontinence . . . . . . . . . . . . . . . . . . . . . . 53440
   Removal . . . . . . . . . . . . . . . . . . . . . . . 53442
Stress Incontinence . . . . . . . . . . . . . 51992, 57287
Vagina . . . . . . . . . . . . . . . . . . . . 57287-57288

## Small Bowel
*See* Intestines, Small
Neoplasm
   *See* Tumor, Intestines, Small

**SMAS Flap** . . . . . . . . . . . . . . . . . . . . . 15829

## Smear
Cervical
   *See* Cervical Smears
Papanicolaou
   *See* Pap Smears

## Smear and Stain
*See* Cytopathology, Smears
Cornea . . . . . . . . . . . . . . . . . . . . . . . . . 65430
Fluorescent . . . . . . . . . . . . . . . . . . . . . . 87206
Gram or Giesma . . . . . . . . . . . . . . . . . . . 87205
Ova/Parasites . . . . . . . . . . . . . . . . 87177, 87209

Parasites . . . . . . . . . . . . . . . . . . . 87207-87209
Wet Mount . . . . . . . . . . . . . . . . . . . . . . . 87210

**Smith Fracture** . . . . . . . . . . . . 25600-25605

## Smith-Robinson Operation
*See* Arthrodesis, Vertebra

**SMPD1** . . . . . . . . . . . . . . . . . . . . . . . . 81330

## Smoking and Tobacco Use Cessation
Counseling . . . . . . . . . . . . . . . . . 99406-99407

**SNRPN/UBE3A** . . . . . . . . . . . . . . . . 81331

## SO4
*See* Sulfate

**Soave Procedure** . . . . . . . . . . . . . . . 45120

**Sodium** . . . . . . . . . . . . . . . . 84295, 84302
Urine . . . . . . . . . . . . . . . . . . . . . . . . . . . 84300

## Sodium Glycinate, Theophylline
*See* Theophylline

## Sofield Procedure
. . . . . . . . . . . . . . . . . . . . . . . . . . . . . . 24410

## Soft Tissue
*See* Tissue, Soft

## Solar Plexus
*See* Celiac Plexus

## Solitary Cyst
*See* Bone, Cyst

## Somatomammotropin, Chorionic
. . . . . . . . . . . . . . . . . . . . . . . . . . . . . . 83632

**Somatomedin** . . . . . . . . . . . . . . . . . . 84305

## Somatosensory Testing
Lower Limbs . . . . . . . . . . . 95926, 95938-95939
Trunk or Head . . . . . . . . . . . . . . . . . . . . 95927
Upper Limbs . . . . . . . . . . . 95925, 95938-95939

**Somatostatin** . . . . . . . . . . . . . . . . . . 84307

**Somatotropin** . . . . . . . . . . . . . . . . . . 83003

## Somatotropin Release Inhibiting Hormone
*See* Somatostatin

## Somatropin
*See* Growth Hormone, Human

## Somnographies
*See* Polysomnography

## Somophyllin T
*See* Theophylline

## Sonography
*See* Echography

**Sonohysterography** . . . . . . . . . . . . 76831
Saline Infusion
   Injection Procedure . . . . . . . . . . . . . . . 58340

## Sore, Bed
*See* Pressure Ulcer (Decubitus)

## Spasm Eyelid
*See* Blepharospasm

Neoplasm
    Excision . . . . . . . . . . . . . . . . . 63275-63290
Puncture (Tap)
    Diagnostic . . . . . . . . . . . . . . . . . . . . 62270
    Drain Fluid . . . . . . . . . . . . . . . . . . . . 62272
    Lumbar . . . . . . . . . . . . . . . . . . . . . . 62270
Radiosurgery
    Stereotactic . . . . . . . . . . . . . . 63620-63621
Reconstruction
    Dorsal Spine Elements . . . . . . . . . . . . . 63295
Release . . . . . . . . . . . . . . . . . . . . . . . . . 63200
Removal
    Catheter . . . . . . . . . . . . . . . . . . . . . . 62355
    Electrode . . . . . . . . . . . . . . . . 63661-63664
    Pulse Generator . . . . . . . . . . . . . . . . . 63688
    Pump . . . . . . . . . . . . . . . . . . . . . . . . 62365
    Receiver . . . . . . . . . . . . . . . . . . . . . . 63688
    Reservoir . . . . . . . . . . . . . . . . . . . . . 62365
Repair
    Cerebrospinal Fluid Leak . . . . . . . 63707-63709
    Meningocele . . . . . . . . . . . . . . 63700-63702
    Myelomeningocele . . . . . . . . . . 63704-63706
Section
    Dentate Ligament . . . . . . . . . . . 63180-63182
    Tract . . . . . . . . . . . . . . . . . . . . 63194-63199
Shunt
    Create . . . . . . . . . . . . . . . . . . . 63740-63741
    Irrigation . . . . . . . . . . . . . . . . . . . . . . 63744
    Removal . . . . . . . . . . . . . . . . . . . . . . 63746
    Replacement . . . . . . . . . . . . . . . . . . . 63744
Stereotaxis
    Aspiration . . . . . . . . . . . . . . . . . . . . . 63615
    Biopsy . . . . . . . . . . . . . . . . . . . . . . . 63615
    Computer-Assisted Procedure . . . . . . . . 61783
    Creation Lesion . . . . . . . . . . . . . . . . . 63600
    Excision Lesion . . . . . . . . . . . . . . . . . 63615
    Stimulation . . . . . . . . . . . . . . . . . . . . 63610
Syrinx
    Aspiration . . . . . . . . . . . . . . . . . . . . . 62268
Tumor
    Excision . . . . . . . . . . . . . . . . 63275-63290

## Spinal Cord Neoplasms
*See* Spinal Cord
Tumor
    *See* Spinal Cord, Tumor; Tumor
    Excision
        *See* Spinal Cord, Tumor; Tumor, Spinal Cord

## Spinal Fluid
*See* Cerebrospinal Fluid

## Spinal Fracture
*See* Fracture, Vertebra

## Spinal Instrumentation
Anterior . . . . . . . . . . . . . . . . . . . 22845-22847
    Removal . . . . . . . . . . . . . . . . . . . . . . 22855
Internal Fixation . . . . . . . . . . . . . . . . . . . 22841
Pelvic Fixation . . . . . . . . . . . . . . . . . . . . 22848
Posterior Nonsegmental . . . . . . . . . . . . . 22840
    Harrington Rod Technique
        Removal . . . . . . . . . . . . . . . . . . . 22850
Posterior Segmental . . . . . . . . . . 22842-22844
    Removal . . . . . . . . . . . . . . . . . . . . . . 22852
Prosthetic Device . . . . . . . . . . . . . . . . . . 22851
Reinsertion of Spinal Fixation Device . . . . . . 22849

## Spinal Manipulation
*See* Manipulation, Chiropractic

## Spinal Nerve
Avulsion . . . . . . . . . . . . . . . . . . . . . . . 64772
Transection . . . . . . . . . . . . . . . . . . . . . 64772

## Spinal Tap
*See* Cervical Puncture; Cisternal Puncture; Subdural
Tap; Ventricular Puncture
Drainage Fluid . . . . . . . . . . . . . . . . . . . 62272
Lumbar . . . . . . . . . . . . . . . . . . . . . . . . 62270

## Spine
*See* Intervertebral Disc; Spinal Cord; Vertebra;
Vertebral Body; Vertebral Process
Allograft
    Morselized . . . . . . . . . . . . . . . . . . . . 20930
    Structural . . . . . . . . . . . . . . . . . . . . . 20931
Arthroplasty
    Lumbar . . . . . . . . . . . . . . . . . 22856-22865
Aspiration . . . . . . . . . . . . . . . . . . . . . . 62267
Augmentation
    Lumbar Vertebra . . . . . . . . . . . . 22524-22525
    Thoracic Vertebra . . . . . . . . . . . 22523, 22525
Autograft
    Local . . . . . . . . . . . . . . . . . . . . . . . . 20936
    Morselized . . . . . . . . . . . . . . . . . . . . 20937
    Structural . . . . . . . . . . . . . . . . . . . . . 20938
Biopsy . . . . . . . . . . . . . . 20250-20251, 22520-22522
CT Scan
    Cervical . . . . . . . . . . . . . . . . . 72125-72127
    Lumbar . . . . . . . . . . . . . . . . . . 72131-72133
    Thoracic . . . . . . . . . . . . . . . . . 72128-72130
Decompression . . . . . . . . . . . . . . . . . . . 62287
Fixation . . . . . . . . . . . . . . . . . . . . . . . . 22842
Foraminotomy . . . . . . . . . . . . . . . . . . . 0202T
Fusion
    Anterior . . . . . . . . . . . . . . . . . 22808-22812
    Anterior Approach . . . . . 22548-22585, 22812
    Exploration . . . . . . . . . . . . . . . . . . . . 22830
    Lateral Extracavitary . . . . . . . . . 22532-22534
    Posterior Approach . . . . . . . . . . 22590-22802
Incision and Drainage
    Abscess . . . . . . . . . . . . . . . . . 22010-22015
Injection
    Cervical . . . . . . . . 0228T-0229T, 62310, 62318
    Lumbar . . . . . . . . . 0230T-0231T, 62311, 62319
    Sacral . . . . . . . . . . 0230T-0231T, 62311, 62319
    Thoracic . . . . . . . . 0228T-0229T, 62310, 62318
Insertion
    Instrumentation . . . . . . . 22840-22848, 22851
Kyphectomy . . . . . . . . . . . . . . . . 22818-22819
Magnetic Resonance Angiography . . . . . . . 72159
Magnetic Resonance Imaging
    Cervical . . . . . . . . 72141-72142, 72156-72158
    Lumbar . . . . . . . . . . . . . . . . . . 72148-72158
    Thoracic . . . . . . . . 72146-72147, 72156-72158
Manipulation
    with Anesthesia . . . . . . . . . . . . . . . . . 22505
Myelography
    Cervical . . . . . . . . . . . . . . . . . . . . . . 72240
    Lumbosacral . . . . . . . . . . . . . . . . . . . 72265
    Thoracic . . . . . . . . . . . . . . . . . . . . . . 72255
    Total . . . . . . . . . . . . . . . . . . . . . . . . 72270
Placement of Osteopromotive Material . . . . 20930
Radiosurgery
    Stereotactic . . . . . . . . . . . . . . 63620-63621
    Computer Assisted (Navigational) . . . . 61783
Reconstruction
    Dorsal Spine Elements . . . . . . . . . . . . . 63295
Reinsertion
    Instrumentation . . . . . . . . . . . . . . . . . 22849
Removal
    Instrumentation . . . . . . . 22850, 22852-22855
Repair, Osteotomy
    Anterior . . . . . . . . . . . . . . . . . 22220-22226
    Posterior . . . . . . . . . . . . . . . . 22210-22214
        Cervical Laminoplasty . . . . . . . 63050-63051
        Posterolateral . . . . . . . . . . . . . . . . 22216

Ultrasound . . . . . . . . . . . . . . . . . . . . . . 76800
Unlisted Services and Procedures,
Surgery . . . . . . . . . . . . . . . . . . . . . . . . 22899
X-ray . . . . . . . . . . . . . . . . . . . 72020, 72090
    Absorptiometry . . . . . . . . . . . . 77080-77082
    Cervical . . . . . . . . . . . . . . . . . 72040-72052
    Lumbosacral . . . . . . . . . . . . . . 72100-72120
    Standing . . . . . . . . . . . . . . . . . . . . . . 72069
    Thoracic . . . . . . . . . . . . . . . . . 72070-72074
    Thoracolumbar . . . . . . . . . . . . . . . . . 72080
    Total . . . . . . . . . . . . . . . . . . . . . . . . 72010
    with Contrast
        Cervical . . . . . . . . . . . . . . . . . . . 72240
        Lumbosacral . . . . . . . . . . . . . . . . 72265
        Thoracic . . . . . . . . . . . . . . . . . . . 72255
        Total . . . . . . . . . . . . . . . . . . . . . 72270

## Spine Chemotherapy
Administration . . . . . . . . . . . . . . . . . . . 96450
    *See* Chemotherapy

## Spirometry . . . . . . . . . . . . . . . . 94010-94070
*See* Pulmonology, Diagnostic
Patient Initiated . . . . . . . . . . . . . . 94014-94016

## Splanchnicectomy
*See* Nerves, Sympathectomy, Excision

## Spleen
Excision . . . . . . . . . . . . . . . . . . 38100-38102
    Laparoscopic . . . . . . . . . . . . . . . . . . 38120
Injection
    Radiologic . . . . . . . . . . . . . . . . . . . . 38200
Nuclear Medicine
    Imaging . . . . . . . . . . 78185, 78215-78216
Repair . . . . . . . . . . . . . . . . . . . . . . . . . 38115

## Splenectomy
Laparoscopic . . . . . . . . . . . . . . . . . . . . 38120
Partial . . . . . . . . . . . . . . . . . . . . . . . . . 38101
Partial with Repair, Ruptured Spleen . . . . . . 38115
Total . . . . . . . . . . . . . . . . . . . . . . . . . 38100
    En bloc . . . . . . . . . . . . . . . . . . . . . . 38102

## Splenoplasty
*See* Repair, Spleen

## Splenoportography . . . . . . . . . . . . . . 75810
Injection Procedures . . . . . . . . . . . . . . . . 38200

## Splenorrhaphy . . . . . . . . . . . . . . . . . 38115

## Splint
*See* Casting; Strapping
Arm
    Long . . . . . . . . . . . . . . . . . . . . . . . . 29105
    Short . . . . . . . . . . . . . . . . . . . 29125-29126
Finger . . . . . . . . . . . . . . . . . . . 29130-29131
Foot . . . . . . . . . . . . . . . . . . . . . . . . . 29590
Leg
    Long . . . . . . . . . . . . . . . . . . . . . . . . 29505
    Short . . . . . . . . . . . . . . . . . . . . . . . . 29515
Oral Surgical . . . . . . . . . . . . . . . . . . . . . 21085
Ureteral
    *See* Ureteral Splinting

## Split Grafts . . . . . 15100-15101, 15120-15121

## Split Renal Function Test
*See* Cystourethroscopy, Catheterization, Ureteral

## Splitting
Blood Products . . . . . . . . . . . . . . . . . . . 86985

## Spontaneous Abortion
*See* Abortion

## Sprengel's Deformity . . . . . . . . . . . 23400

## Sternum
Debridement...................21627
Excision.............21620, 21630-21632
Fracture
    Closed Treatment...............21820
    Open Treatment.................21825
Ostectomy......................21620
Radical Resection.......21630-21632
Reconstruction.........21740-21742, 21750
   with Thoracoscopy.............21743
X-ray.....................71120-71130

## Steroid-Binding Protein, Sex
See Globulin, Sex Hormone Binding

## Steroids
Anabolic
  See Androstenedione
Injection
    Foot Neuroma...........64455, 64632
    Urethral Stricture..............52283
Ketogenic
    Urine.......................83582

## STH (Somatotropic Hormone)
See Growth Hormone

## Stimulating Antibody, Thyroid
See Immunoglobulin, Thyroid Stimulating

## Stimulation
Electric
  See ElectricalStimulation
Lymphocyte
  See Blastogenesis
Spinal Cord
    Stereotaxis...................63610
Transcutaneous Electric
  See Application, Neurostimulation

## Stimulator, Long-Acting Thyroid
See Thyrotropin Releasing Hormone (TRH)

## Stimulators, Cardiac
See Heart, Pacemaker

## Stimulus Evoked Response....51792

## Stoffel Operation
See Rhizotomy

## Stoma
Creation
    Bladder......................51980
    Kidney..................50551-50561
    Stomach
      Neonatal...................43831
      Temporary............43830-43831
    Ureter.......................50860
Ureter
    Endoscopy via..........50951-50961

## Stomach
Anastomosis
    with Duodenum.......43810, 43850-43855
    with Jejunum.....43820-43825, 43860-43865
Biopsy........................43605
Creation
    Stoma
      Temporary.............43830-43831
    Temporary Stoma
      Laparoscopic..............43653
Electrode
    Removal.....................43882
Electrogastrography...........91132-91133

Excision
    Partial.............43631-43635, 43845
    Total...................43620-43622
Exploration....................43500
Gastric Bypass.........43644-43645, 43846
    Revision.....................43848
Gastric Restrictive Procedures.....43770-43775,
                43848, 43886-43888
Implantation
    Electrodes...........43647, 43881
Incision...................43830-43832
    Exploration..................43500
    Pyloric Sphincter.............43520
    Removal
      Foreign Body..............43500
Laparoscopy...............43647-43648
Nuclear Medicine
    Blood Loss Study..............78278
    Emptying Study...............78264
    Imaging......................78261
    Protein Loss Study............78282
    Reflux Study.................78262
    Vitamin B-12Absorption......78270-78272
Reconstruction
    for Obesity......43644-43645, 43842-43847
    Roux-En-Y...........43644, 43846
Removal
    Foreign Body.................43500
Repair........................48547
    Fistula......................43880
    Fundoplasty.........43325, 43327-43328
      Laparoscopic...........43280-43282
    Laceration............43501-43502
    Stoma.......................43870
    Ulcer........................43501
Replacement
    Electrodes...........43647, 43881
Specimen Collection..........43754-43755
Stimulation of Secretion.........43755
Suture
    Fistula......................43880
    for Obesity...........43842-43843
    Stoma.......................43870
    Ulcer.......................43840
    Wound.......................43840
Tumor
    Excision.............43610-43611
Ulcer
    Excision....................43610
Unlisted Services and Procedures...43659, 43999

## Stomatoplasty
See Mouth, Repair

## Stone, Kidney
See Calculus, Removal, Kidney

## Stookey-Scarff Procedure
See Ventriculocisternostomy

## Stool Blood
See Blood, Feces

## Storage
Embryo........................89342
Oocyte........................89346
Reproductive Tissue............89344
Sperm.........................89343

## Strabismus
Chemodenervation..............67345
Repair
    Adjustable Sutures............67335
    Extraocular Muscles...........67340
    One Horizontal Muscle.........67311

    One Vertical Muscle...........67314
    Posterior Fixation Suture
      Technique.............67334-67335
    Previous Surgery, Not Involving
      Extraocular Muscles........67331
    Release Extensive Scar Tissue..67343
    Superior Oblique Muscle.......67318
    Transposition................67320
    Two Horizontal Muscles........67312
    Two or More Vertical Muscles....67316

## Strapping
See Cast; Splint
Ankle.........................29540
    Compression...........29581-29582
Arm
    Compression...........29583-29584
Chest.........................29200
Elbow.........................29260
Finger........................29280
    Compression.................29584
Foot..................29540, 29590
    Compression...........29581-29582
Hand..........................29280
    Compression.................29584
Hip...........................29520
Knee..........................29530
Leg
    Compression...........29581-29582
Shoulder......................29240
Thorax........................29200
Toes..........................29550
Unlisted Services and Procedures.....29799
Unna Boot.....................29580
Wrist.........................29260

## Strassman Procedure.........58540

## Strayer Procedure
Leg, Lower....................27687

## Streptococcus pneumoniae Vaccine
See Vaccines

## Streptococcus, Group A
Antigen Detection
    Enzyme Immunoassay...........87430
    Nucleic Acid.........87650-87652
Direct Optical Observation.........87880

## Streptococcus, Group B
by Immunoassay
    with Direct Optical Observation.......87802

## Streptokinase, Antibody.......86590

## Stress Tests
Cardiovascular.............93015-93024
Multiple Gated Acquisition
(MUGA).....................78472-78473
Myocardial Perfusion Imaging.....78451-78454
Pulmonary..................94620-94621
    See Pulmonology, Diagnostic

## Stricture
Repair
    Urethra...............53400-53405
Urethra
    See Urethral Stenosis

## Stricturoplasty
Intestines.....................44615

## Stroboscopy
Larynx........................31579

## Suspension

Aorta . . . . . . . . . . . . . . . . . . . . . . . . . . . . 33800
Kidney
　*See* Nephropexy
Muscle
　Hyoid . . . . . . . . . . . . . . . . . . . . . . . . . 21685
　Tongue Base . . . . . . . . . . . . . . . . . . . . 41512
Vagina
　*See* Colpopexy

## Suture

*See* Repair
Abdomen . . . . . . . . . . . . . . . . . . . . . . . . . 49900
Aorta . . . . . . . . . . . . . . . . . . . . . 33320-33322
Bile Duct
　Wound . . . . . . . . . . . . . . . . . . . . . . . . 47900
Bladder
　Fistulization . . . . . 44660-44661, 45800-45805,
　　　　　　　　　　　　　　　　51880-51925
　　Vesicouterine . . . . . . . . . . . . . . 51920-51925
　　Vesicovaginal . . . . . . . . . . . . . . . . . 51900
　Wound . . . . . . . . . . . . . . . . . . 51860-51865
Cervix . . . . . . . . . . . . . . . . . . . . . . . . . . . 57720
Colon
　Diverticula . . . . . . . . . . . . . . 44604-44605
　Fistula . . . . . . . . . . . . . . . . . . 44650-44661
　Plication . . . . . . . . . . . . . . . . . . . . . . 44680
　Stoma . . . . . . . . . . . . . . . . . . 44620-44625
　Ulcer . . . . . . . . . . . . . . . . . . . 44604-44605
　Wound . . . . . . . . . . . . . . . . . 44604-44605
Esophagus
　Wound . . . . . . . . . . . . . . . . . 43410-43415
Eyelid . . . . . . . . . . . . . . . . . . . . . . . . . . . 67880
　Closure of . . . . . . . . . . . . . . . . . . . . . 67875
　with Transposition of Tarsal Plate . . . . . . 67882
　Wound
　　Full Thickness . . . . . . . . . . . . . . . . 67935
　　Partial Thickness . . . . . . . . . . . . . . . 67930
Facial Nerve
　Intratemporal
　　Lateral to Geniculate Ganglion . . . . . . 69740
　　Medial to Geniculate Ganglion . . . . . . 69745
Foot
　Tendon . . . . . . . . . . . . . . . . . 28200-28210
Gastroesophageal . . . . . . . . . . . . . . . . . . 43405
Great Vessel . . . . . . . . . . . . . . . . . . 33320-33322
Hemorrhoids . . . . . . . . . . . . . . . . . 46945-46946
Hepatic Duct
　*See* Hepatic Duct, Repair
Intestine
　Large
　　Diverticula . . . . . . . . . . . . . . . . . . 44605
　　Ulcer . . . . . . . . . . . . . . . . . . . . . . . 44605
　　Wound . . . . . . . . . . . . . . . . . . . . . 44605
Intestines
　Large
　　Diverticula . . . . . . . . . . . . . . . . . . 44604
　　Ulcer . . . . . . . . . . . . . . . . . . . . . . . 44604
　　Wound . . . . . . . . . . . . . . . . . . . . . 44604
　Small
　　Diverticula . . . . . . . . . . . . . 44602-44603
　　Fistula . . . . . . . . . . . . . . . . . 44640-44661
　　Plication . . . . . . . . . . . . . . . . . . . . 44680
　　Ulcer . . . . . . . . . . . . . . . . . . 44602-44603
　　Wound . . . . . . . . . . . . . . . . 44602-44603
　　Stoma . . . . . . . . . . . . . . . . . 44620-44625
Iris
　with Ciliary Body . . . . . . . . . . . . . . . . 66682
Kidney
　Fistula . . . . . . . . . . . . . . . . . . 50520-50526
　Horseshoe . . . . . . . . . . . . . . . . . . . . . 50540
　Wound . . . . . . . . . . . . . . . . . . . . . . . 50500

Leg, Lower
　Tendon . . . . . . . . . . . . . . . . . 27658-27665
Leg, Upper
　Muscle . . . . . . . . . . . . . . . . . 27385-27386
Liver
　Wound . . . . . . . . . . . . . . . . . 47350-47361
Mesentery . . . . . . . . . . . . . . . . . . . . . . . 44850
Nerve . . . . . . . . . . . . . . . . . . . . 64831-64876
Pancreas . . . . . . . . . . . . . . . . . . . . . . . . 48545
Pharynx
　Wound . . . . . . . . . . . . . . . . . . . . . . . 42900
Rectum
　Fistula . . . . . . . . . . . . . . . . . . 45800-45825
　Prolapse . . . . . . . . . . . . . . . . . 45540-45541
Removal
　Anesthesia . . . . . . . . . . . . . . . 15850-15851
Spleen
　*See* Splenorrhaphy
Stomach
　Fistula . . . . . . . . . . . . . . . . . . . . . . . . 43880
　Laceration . . . . . . . . . . . . . . . 43501-43502
　Stoma . . . . . . . . . . . . . . . . . . . . . . . . 43870
　Ulcer . . . . . . . . . . . . . . . . . . 43501, 43840
　Wound . . . . . . . . . . . . . . . . . . . . . . . 43840
Tendon
　Foot . . . . . . . . . . . . . . . . . . . . 28200-28210
　Knee . . . . . . . . . . . . . . . . . . . 27380-27381
Testis
　Injury . . . . . . . . . . . . . . . . . . . . . . . . 54670
　Suspension . . . . . . . . . . . . . . . 54620-54640
Thoracic Duct
　Abdominal Approach . . . . . . . . . . . . . . 38382
　Cervical Approach . . . . . . . . . . . . . . . . 38380
　Thoracic Approach . . . . . . . . . . . . . . . 38381
Throat
　Wound . . . . . . . . . . . . . . . . . . . . . . . 42900
Tongue
　Base Suspension . . . . . . . . . . . . . . . . 41512
　to Lip . . . . . . . . . . . . . . . . . . . . . . . . 41510
Trachea
　Fistula
　　with Plastic Repair . . . . . . . . . . . . . . 31825
　　without Plastic Repair . . . . . . . . . . . . 31820
　Stoma
　　with Plastic Repair . . . . . . . . . . . . . . 31825
　　without Plastic Repair . . . . . . . . . . . . 31820
　Wound
　　Cervical . . . . . . . . . . . . . . . . . . . . . 31800
　　Intrathoracic . . . . . . . . . . . . . . . . . . 31805
Ulcer . . . . . . . . . . . . . . . . . . . . . 44604-44605
Ureter . . . . . . . . . . . . . . . . . . . . . . . . . . 50900
　Deligation . . . . . . . . . . . . . . . . . . . . . 50940
　Fistula . . . . . . . . . . . . . . . . . . 50920-50930
Urethra
　Fistula . . . . . . . . . . . . . 45820-45825, 53520
　Stoma . . . . . . . . . . . . . . . . . . . . . . . . 53520
　to Bladder . . . . . . . . . . . . . . . . 51840-51841
　Wound . . . . . . . . . . . . . . . . . . 53502-53515
Uterus
　Fistula . . . . . . . . . . . . . . . . . . 51920-51925
　Rupture . . . . . . . . . . . . . . . . . 58520, 59350
　Suspension . . . . . . . . . . . . . . . 58400-58410
Vagina
　Cystocele . . . . . . . . . . . . . . . . 57240, 57260
　Enterocele . . . . . . . . . . . . . . . . . . . . . 57265
　Fistula
　　Rectovaginal . . . . . . . . . . . . . 57300-57307
　　Transvesical and Vaginal Approach . . . 57330
　　Urethrovaginal . . . . . . . . . . . 57310-57311
　　Vesicovaginal . . . . . . . 51900, 57320-57330
　Rectocele . . . . . . . . . . . . . . . . 57250-57260
　Suspension . . . . . . . . . . . . . . 57280, 57283
　Wound . . . . . . . . . . . . . . . . . 57200-57210

Vas Deferens . . . . . . . . . . . . . . . . . . . . . 55400
Vein
　Femoral . . . . . . . . . . . . . . . . . . . . . . . 37650
　Iliac . . . . . . . . . . . . . . . . . . . . . . . . . . 37660
Wound . . . . . . . . . . . . . . . . . . . 44604-44605

## Swallowing

Evaluation . . . . . . . 92610-92613, 92616-92617
Imaging . . . . . . . . . . . . . . . . . . . . . . . . . 74230
Treatment . . . . . . . . . . . . . . . . . . . . . . . 92526

## Swanson Procedure . . . . . . . . . . .28309

## Sweat Collection

Iontophoresis . . . . . . . . . . . . . . . . . . . . . 89230

## Sweat Glands

Excision
　Axillary . . . . . . . . . . . . . . . . . 11450-11451
　Inguinal . . . . . . . . . . . . . . . . . 11462-11463
　Perianal . . . . . . . . . . . . . . . . . 11470-11471
　Perineal . . . . . . . . . . . . . . . . . 11470-11471
　Umbilical . . . . . . . . . . . . . . . . 11470-11471

## Sweat Test . . . . . . . . . . . . . . . . . . . .82435

*See* Chloride, Blood

## Swenson Procedure . . . . . . . . . .45120

## Syme Procedure . . . . . . . . . . . . . .27888

## Sympathectomy

Artery
　Digital . . . . . . . . . . . . . . . . . . . . . . . . 64820
　Radial . . . . . . . . . . . . . . . . . . . . . . . . 64821
　Superficial Palmar Arch . . . . . . . . . . . . 64823
　Ulnar . . . . . . . . . . . . . . . . . . . . . . . . . 64822
Cervical . . . . . . . . . . . . . . . . . . . . . . . . . 64802
Cervicothoracic . . . . . . . . . . . . . . . . . . . 64804
Digital Artery
　with Magnification . . . . . . . . . . . . . . . 64820
Lumbar . . . . . . . . . . . . . . . . . . . . . . . . . 64818
Presacral . . . . . . . . . . . . . . . . . . . . . . . . 58410
Thoracic . . . . . . . . . . . . . . . . . . . . . . . . 32664
Thoracolumbar . . . . . . . . . . . . . . . . . . . 64809
with Rib Excision . . . . . . . . . . . . . . . . . 21616

## Sympathetic Nerve

Excision . . . . . . . . . . . . . . . . . . 64802-64818
Injection
　Anesthetic . . . . . . . . . . 64508, 64520-64530

## Sympathins

*See* Catecholamines

## Symphysiotomy

Horseshoe Kidney . . . . . . . . . . . . . . . . . 50540

## Symphysis, Pubic

*See* Pubic Symphysis

## Syncytial Virus, Respiratory

*See* Respiratory Syncytial Virus

## Syndactylism, Toes

*See* Webbed, Toe

## Syndactyly

Repair . . . . . . . . . . . . . . . . . . . . 26560-26562

## Syndesmotomy

*See* Ligament, Release

## Syndrome

Adrenogenital
　*See* Adrenogenital Syndrome
Ataxia-Telangiectasia
　*See* Ataxia Telangiectasia

Bloom
See Bloom Syndrome
Carpal Tunnel
See Carpal Tunnel Syndrome
Costen's
See Temporomandibular Joint (TMJ)
Erb -Goldflam
See Myasthenia Gravis
Ovarian Vein
See Ovarian Vein Syndrome
Synechiae, Intrauterine
See Adhesions, Intrauterine
Treacher Collins
See Treacher-Collins Syndrome
Urethral
See Urethral Syndrome

**Syngesterone**
See Progesterone

**Synostosis (Cranial)**
See Craniosynostosis

**Synovectomy**
Arthrotomy with
Glenohumeral Joint . . . . . . . . . . . . . . . . . 23105
Sternoclavicular Joint . . . . . . . . . . . . . . 23106
Elbow . . . . . . . . . . . . . . . . . . . . . . . . . . . . . . 24102
Excision
Carpometacarpal Joint . . . . . . . . . . . . . 26130
Finger Joint . . . . . . . . . . . . . . . . 26135-26140
Hip Joint . . . . . . . . . . . . . . . . . . . . . . . . . 27054
Interphalangeal Joint. . . . . . . . . . . . . . . . 26140
Knee Joint . . . . . . . . . . . . . . . . 27334-27335
Metacarpophalangeal Joint . . . . . . . . . 26135
Palm . . . . . . . . . . . . . . . . . . . . . . . . . . . . . 26145
Wrist . . . . . . . . . . . . . . . 25105, 25118-25119
Radical . . . . . . . . . . . . . . . . . . . . . 25115-25116

**Synovial**
Bursa
See Bursa
Cyst
See Ganglion
Membrane
See Synovium
Popliteal Space
See Baker's Cyst

**Synovium**
Biopsy
Carpometacarpal Joint . . . . . . . . . . . . . 26100
Interphalangeal Joint. . . . . . . . . . . . . . . . 26110
Knee Joint . . . . . . . . . . . . . . . . . . . . . . . . 27330
Metacarpophalangeal Joint
with Synovial Biopsy . . . . . . . . . . . . . 26105
Excision
Carpometacarpal Joint . . . . . . . . . . . . . 26130
Finger Joint . . . . . . . . . . . . . . . . 26135-26140
Hip Joint. . . . . . . . . . . . . . . . . . . . . . . . . . 27054
Interphalangeal Joint. . . . . . . . . . . . . . . . 26140
Knee Joint . . . . . . . . . . . . . . . . 27334-27335

**Syphilis ab**
See Antibody, Treponema Pallidum

**Syphilis Test** . . . . . . . . . . . . . . . 86592-86593

**Syrinx**
Spinal Cord
Aspiration. . . . . . . . . . . . . . . . . . . . . . . . . 62268

**System**
Endocrine
See Endocrine System

Hemic
See Hemic System
Lymphatic
See Lymphatic System
Musculoskeletal
See MusculoskeletalSystem
Nervous
See Nervous System

# T

**T Cell Leukemia Virus I Antibodies, Adult**
See Antibody, HTLV-I

**T Cell Leukemia Virus I, Human**
See HTLV I

**T Cell Leukemia Virus II Antibodies, Human**
See Antibody, HTLV-II

**T Cell Leukemia Virus II, Human**
See HTLV II

**T-Cells**
CD4
Absolute. . . . . . . . . . . . . . . . . . . . . . . . . . 86361
Count. . . . . . . . . . . . . . . . . . . . . . . . . . . . . 86359
Gene Rearrangement. . . . . . . . . . . . 81340-81342
Ratio . . . . . . . . . . . . . . . . . . . . . . . . . . . . . 86360

**T Lymphotropic Virus Type III Antibodies, Human**
See Antibody, HIV

**T-3**
See Triiodothyronine

**T3 Free**
See Triiodothyronine, Free

**T-4** . . . . . . . . . . . . . . . 84436-84439, 86360

**T4 Molecule**
See CD4

**T4 Total**
See Thyroxine, Total

**T-7 Index**
See Thyroxine, Total

**T-8**
See CD8; T-Cells, Ratio

**T-Cell T8 Antigens**
See CD8

**T-Phyl**
See Theophylline

**Taarnhoj Procedure**
See Decompression, Gasserian Ganglion, Sensory Root; Section

**Tachycardia**
Heart
Recording. . . . . . . . . . . . . . . . . . . . . . . . . 93609

**Tacrolimus**
Drug Assay. . . . . . . . . . . . . . . . . . . . . . . . . . 80197

**Tag, Skin**
See Skin, Tags

**Tail Bone**
Excision. . . . . . . . . . . . . . . . . . . . . . . . . . . . 27080
Fracture. . . . . . . . . . . . . . . . . . . . . 27200-27202

**Takeuchi Procedure** . . . . . . . . . . . . .33505

**Talectomy**
See Astragalectomy

**Talotarsal Joint**
Dislocation . . . . . . . . . . . . . . 28570-28575, 28585
Percutaneous Fixation . . . . . . . . . . . . . 28576

**Talus**
Arthrodesis
Pantalar . . . . . . . . . . . . . . . . . . . . . . . . . 28705
Subtalar . . . . . . . . . . . . . . . . . . . . . . . . . 28725
Triple . . . . . . . . . . . . . . . . . . . . . . . . . . . 28715
Arthroscopy
Surgical . . . . . . . . . . . . . . . . . 29891-29892
Subtalar . . . . . . . 29904-29907, 29915-29916
Autograft, Osteochondral . . . . . . . . . . . . 28446
Craterization. . . . . . . . . . . . . . . . . . . . . . . . 28120
Cyst
Excision . . . . . . . . . . . . . . . 28100-28103
Diaphysectomy. . . . . . . . . . . . . . . . . . . . . 28120
Excision. . . . . . . . . . . . . . . . . . . . 28120, 28130
Fracture
Open Treatment . . . . . . . . . . . . . . . . . . . 28445
Percutaneous Fixation . . . . . . . . . . . . . 28436
with Manipulation . . . . . . . . . . . 28435-28436
without Manipulation . . . . . . . . . . . . . 28430
Repair
Osteochondritis Dissecans . . . . . . . . . 29892
Osteotomy . . . . . . . . . . . . . . . . . . . . . . . 28302
Saucerization . . . . . . . . . . . . . . . . . . . . . . 28120
Tumor
Excision . . . . . . . . . . . . . . . 28100-28103
Radical Resection . . . . . . . . . . . . . . . . 27647

**Tap**
Cisternal
See Cisternal Puncture
Lumbar Diagnostic
See Spinal Tap

**Tarsal**
Fracture
Percutaneous Fixation . . . . . . . . . . . . . 28456

**Tarsal Bone**
See Ankle Bone

**Tarsal Joint**
See Foot
Arthrodesis. . . . . . . . . . . . . 28730-28735, 28740
with Advancement. . . . . . . . . . . . . . . . . 28737
with Lengthening. . . . . . . . . . . . . . . . . . 28737
Craterization. . . . . . . . . . . . . . . . . . . . . . . . 28122
Cyst
Excision . . . . . . . . . . . . . . . . 28104-28107
Diaphysectomy. . . . . . . . . . . . . . . . . . . . . 28122
Dislocation . . . . . . . . . . . . . . 28540-28545, 28555
Percutaneous Fixation . . . . . . . . 28545-28546
Excision. . . . . . . . . . . . . . . . . . . . 28116, 28122
Fracture
Open Treatment . . . . . . . . . . . . . . . . . . . 28465
with Manipulation . . . . . . . . . . . 28455-28456
without Manipulation . . . . . . . . . . . . . 28450
Fusion . . . . . . . . . . . 28730-28735, 28740
with Advancement. . . . . . . . . . . . . . . . . 28737
with Lengthening. . . . . . . . . . . . . . . . . . 28737

Oocytes .......................... 89356
Reproductive Tissue................ 89354
Sperm............................ 89353
Previously Frozen Cells .......... 38208-38209

## Thawing and Expansion
of Frozen Cell ........................ 88241

## THBR
*See* Thyroid Hormone Binding Ratio

## Theleplasty
*See* Nipples, Reconstruction

## Theophylline
Assay ................................ 80198

## Therapeutic
Abortion
    *See* Abortion, Therapeutic
Apheresis
    *See* Apheresis, Therapeutic
Drug Assay
    *See* Drug Assay
Mobilization
    *See* Mobilization
Photopheresis
    *See* Photopheresis
Radiology
    *See* Radiology, Therapeutic

## Therapies
Cold
    *See* Cryotherapy
Exercise
    *See* Exercise Therapy
Family
    *See* Psychotherapy, Family
Language
    *See* Language Therapy
Milieu
    *See* Environmental Intervention
Occupational
    *See* Occupational Therapy
Photodynamic
    *See* Photochemotherapy
Photoradiation
    *See* Actinotherapy
Physical
    *See* Physical Medicine/Therapy/Occupational
    Therapy
Speech
    *See* Speech Therapy
Tocolytic
    *See* Tocolysis
Ultraviolet
    *See* Actinotherapy

## Therapy
ACE Inhibitor Therapy
    *See* Performance Measures
Beta Blocker Therapy
    *See* Performance Measures
Desensitization
    *See* Allergen Immunotherapy
Hemodialysis
    *See* Hemodialysis
Hot Pack
    *See* Hot Pack Treatment
Pharmacologic; for Cessation of Tobacco Use
    *See* Performance Measures
Radiation
    Brachytherapy ...................... 0182T
    *See* Irradiation

Speech
    *See* Speech Therapy
Statin Therapy, Prescribed
    *See* Performance Measures

## Thermocauterization
Ectropion
    Repair....................... 67922
Lesion
    Cornea ...................... 65450

## Thermocoagulation
*See* Electrocautery

## Thermotherapy
Prostate ................. 53850-53852
    Microwave................. 53850
    Radiofrequency ........... 53852

## Thiamine ................84425

## Thiersch Operation............15050
*See* Pinch Graft

## Thiersch Procedure ............46753

## Thigh
Fasciotomy ...................... 27025
    *See* Femur; Leg, Upper

## Thin Layer Chromatographies
*See* Chromatography, Thin-Layer

## Thiocyanate ................84430

## Third Disease
*See* Rubella

## Thompson Procedure ..........27430

## Thoracectomy
*See* Thoracoplasty

## Thoracentesis ............32421-32422

## Thoracic
Anterior Ramus
    *See* Intercostal Nerve
Arteries
    *See* Artery, Thoracic
Cavity
    *See* Chest Cavity
Duct
    *See* Lymphatics
    Cannulation ...................... 38794
    Ligation ...................... 38380
        Abdominal Approach .............. 38382
        Thoracic Approach ................ 38381
    Suture
        Abdominal Approach .............. 38382
        Cervical Approach ............... 38380
        Thoracic Approach ............... 38381
Empyema
    *See* Abscess, Thorax
Exposure
    Transthoracic ................ 0258T-0259T
Surgery
    Video-Assisted
        *See* Thoracoscopy
Vertebra
    *See* Vertebra, Thoracic
Wall
    *See* Chest Wall

## Thoracocentesis
*See* Thoracentesis

## Thoracoplasty ..................32905
with Closure Bronchopleural Fistula....... 32906

## Thoracoscopy
Diagnostic
    with Biopsy ..... 32604, 32606, 32607-32609
    without Biopsy..................... 32601
Surgical ...................... 32650-32674
    with Control Traumatic Hemorrhage .... 32654
    with Creation Pericardial Window ..... 32659
    with Diagnostic Wedge Resection ..... 32668
    with Esophagomyotomy............. 32665
    with Excision Mediastinal Cyst, Tumor
    and/or Mass...................... 32662
    with Excision Pericardial Cyst, Tumor
    and/or Mass...................... 32661
    with Lobectomy ................... 32663
    with Mediastinal Lymphadenectomy ... 32674
    with Parietal Pleurectomy ........... 32656
    with Partial Pulmonary Decortication ... 32651
    with Pleurodesis .................. 32650
    with Regional Lymphadenectomy ...... 32674
    with Removal Intrapleural Foreign
    Body........................... 32653
    with Removal of Clot/Foreign Body..... 32658
    with Resection of Thymus ........... 32673
    with Resection-Plication of Bullae ... 32655
    with Sternum Reconstruction ........ 21743
    with Therapeutic Wedge
    Resection.................. 32666, 32667
    with Thoracic Sympathectomy ........ 32664
    with Total Pulmonary Decortication ....32652

## Thoracostomy
Empyema ..................... 32035-32036
Tube, with/without Water Seal .......... 32551

## Thoracotomy
Cardiac Massage..................... 32160
Lymphadenectomy
    Thoracic ...................... 38746
for Post-Op Complications.............. 32120
Hemorrhage ...................... 32110
Removal
    Bullae.......................... 32141
    Cyst........................... 32140
    Defibrillator .................... 33243
    Electrodes ..................... 33238
    Foreign Body
        Intrapleural ................. 32150
        Intrapulmonary ............... 32151
    Pacemaker ................. 33236-33237
Repair
    Paraesophageal Hiatal Hernia... 43334-43335
Resection
    Diagnostic Wedge ................ 32507
    Therapeutic Wedge ........... 32505-32506
Revascularization................. 33140-33141
Transmyocardial Laser
    With Biopsy .............. 32096-32097
    With Lung Repair .............. 32110
    With Open Intrapleural Pneumolysis .. 32124
    With Resection-Plication of Bullae ... 32141

## Thorax
*See* Chest; Chest Cavity; Mediastinum
Angiography......................... 71275
Biopsy............................. 21550
CT Scan...................... 71250-71275
Exposure
    Transthoracic Cardiac ......... 0258T-0259T
Incision
    Empyema ................. 32035-32036

**Thyroid Hormone Uptake** ...... .84479

**Thyroid Stimulating Hormone (TSH)** .......... 80418, 80438-80440, 84443

**Thyroid Stimulating Hormone Receptor ab**
See Thyrotropin Releasing Hormone (TRH)

**Thyroid Stimulating Immune Globulins** ....................... .84445

**Thyroid Stimulator, Long Acting**
See Thyrotropin Releasing Hormone (TRH)

**Thyroid Suppression Test**
See Nuclear Medicine, Thyroid, Uptake

**Thyroidectomy**
Partial ..................... 60210-60225
Secondary ........................ 60260
Total ................... 60240, 60271
Cervical Approach ................ 60271
for Malignancy
Limited Neck Dissection ........ 60252
Radical Neck Dissection ........ 60254
Removal All Thyroid Tissue ...... 60260
Sternal Split/Transthoracic Approach .. 60270

**Thyrolingual Cyst**
See Cyst, Thyroglossal Duct

**Thyrotomy** ..................... .31300

**Thyrotropin Receptor Ab**
See Thyrotropin Releasing Hormone (TRH)

**Thyrotropin Releasing Hormone (TRH)** ............. 80438-80439

**Thyroxine**
Free ......................... 84439
Neonatal ....................... 84437
Total ......................... 84436
True ......................... 84436

**Thyroxine Binding Globulin** ... .84442

**Tibia**
See Ankle
Arthroscopy Surgical ........... 29891-29892
Craterization ................. 27360, 27640
Cyst
Excision ................. 27635-27638
Diaphysectomy ............... 27360, 27640
Excision ................. 27360, 27640
Epiphyseal Bar ................ 20150
Fracture
Arthroscopic Treatment ....... 29855-29856
Plafond ..................... 29892
Closed Treatment .......... 27824-27825
Distal ................. 27824-27825
Intercondylar ............ 27538-27540
Malleolus ... 27760-27766, 27808-27814
Open Treatment ...... 27535-27536,
27758-27759, 27826-27828
Plateau .................. 29855-29856
Closed Treatment ........ 27530-27536
Shaft ................ 27752-27759
with Manipulation ............ 27825
without Manipulation ......... 27824
Incision .................... 27607
Neurostimulation
Posterior .................... 64566
Osteoplasty
Lengthening .................. 27715
Prophylactic Treatment ........... 27745

Reconstruction ............... 27418
at Knee ......... 27440-27443, 27446
Repair ................. 27720-27725
Epiphysis ...... 27477-27485, 27730-27742
Osteochondritis Dissecans
Arthroscopy ............... 29892
Osteotomy ......... 27455-27457, 27705,
27709-27712
Pseudoarthrosis .............. 27727
Saucerization ........... 27360, 27640
Tumor
Excision ............. 27635-27638
Radical Resection .......... 27645
X-ray ..................... 73590

**Tibial**
Arteries
See Artery, Tibial
Nerve
Repair/Suture
Posterior .................. 64840

**Tibiofibular Joint**
Arthrodesis .................. 27871
Dislocation .............. 27830-27832
Disruption
Open Treatment .............. 27829
Fusion ..................... 27871

**TIG**
See Immune Globulins, Tetanus

**Time**
Bleeding
See Bleeding Time
Prothrombin
See Prothrombin Time
Reptilase
See Thrombin Time

**Tinnitus**
Assessment ................. 92625

**Tissue**
Crystal Identification ............ 89060
Culture
Chromosome Analysis ........ 88230-88239
Homogenization .............. 87176
Non-neoplastic Disorder ..... 88230, 88237
Skin Grafts ...... 15100-15101, 15120-15121
Harvesting ................ 15040
Solid Tumor ................ 88239
Toxin/Antitoxin ............. 87230
Virus ................. 87252-87253
Dissection, Macroscopic ......... 88387-88388
Examination, Macroscopic ....... 88387-88388
Enzyme Activity ............... 82657
Examination for Ectoparasites ...... 87220
Examination for Fungi ........... 87220
Expander
Breast Reconstruction with ......... 19357
Insertion
Skin ...................... 11960
Removal
Skin ...................... 11971
Replacement
Skin ...................... 11970
Grafts
Harvesting .................. 20926
Granulation
See Granulation Tissue
Homogenization .............. 87176
Hybridization In Situ ......... 88365-88368
Mucosal
See Mucosa

Preparation
Drug Analysis ................ 80103
Macroscopic ............. 88387-88388
Previously Diagnosed/Archived
Retrieved/Selected for Examination .... 88363
Skin Harvest for Culture ......... 15040
Soft
Abscess ................... 20005
Tumor
See Tumor, Excision
See Tumor, Radical Resection
Transfer
Adjacent
Eyelids ................ 67961
Skin ............... 14000-14350
Facial Muscles ............. 15845
Finger Flap .............. 14350
Toe Flap ............... 14350
Typing
Culture .............. 87140-87158
Human Leukocyte Antigen (HLA)
Antibodies ......... 86812-86817
Crossmatch ......... 86825-86826
Lymphocyte Culture ...... 86821-86822

**Tissue Culture**
from Skin Harvest ............... 15040
Skin Grafts ............... 15150-15157

**Tissue Factor**
See Thromboplastin

**TLC**
See Chromatography, Thin-Layer
Screen ..................... 84375

**TMJ**
See Temporomandibular Joint (TMJ)
Manipulation, Therapeutic
See Manipulation, Temporomandibular Joint
Prostheses
See Prosthesis, Temporomandibular Joint

**Tobacco**
See Performance Measures

**Tobramycin**
Assay ..................... 80200

**Tocolysis** ..................... .59412

**Tocopherol** ................... .84446

**Toe**
See Interphalangeal Joint, Toe;
Metatarsophalangeal Joint; Phalanx
Amputation ............... 28810-28825
Capsulotomy ............. 28270-28272
Fasciotomy ................. 28008
Fracture
See Fracture, Phalanges, Toe
Lesion
Excision ................. 28092
Reconstruction
Angle Deformity ............ 28313
Extra Toes ................ 28344
Hammertoe .............. 28285-28286
Macrodactyly ........... 28340-28341
Syndactyly ............... 28345
Webbed Toe .............. 28345
Repair
Bunion ............... 28290-28299
Muscle ................ 28240
Tendon .......... 28232-28234, 28240
Webbed ................ 28280
Webbed Toe ............... 28345

Tumor
  Excision
    Cervical .......................... 31785
    Thoracic ......................... 31786
  Unlisted Services and Procedures
    Bronchi .......................... 31899
  Wound
    Suture
      Cervical ....................... 31800
      Intrathoracic .................. 31805

## Tracheal
Stent
  Placement ......................... 31631
Tubes
  *See* Endotracheal Tube

## Trachelectomy ................. 57530
Radical .............................. 57531

## Tracheloplasty
*See* Cervicoplasty

## Trachelorrhaphy ............... 57720

## Tracheo-Esophageal Fistula
*See* Fistula, Tracheoesophageal

## Tracheobronchoscopy
through Tracheostomy ................ 31615

## Tracheoplasty
Cervical ............................. 31750
Intrathoracic ........................ 31760
Tracheopharyngeal Fistulization ......... 31755

## Tracheostoma
Revision ...................... 31613-31614

## Tracheostomy
Emergency .................... 31603-31605
Planned ...................... 31600-31601
Revision
  Scar .............................. 31830
Surgical Closure
  with Plastic Repair ................. 31825
  without Plastic Repair .............. 31820
Tracheobronchoscopy through ........... 31615
with Flaps ........................... 31610

## Tracheotomy
Tube Change ......................... 31502

## Tracking Tests (Ocular) ........ 92545
*See* Ear, Nose, and Throat

## Tract, Urinary
*See* Urinary Tract

## Traction Therapy
*See* Physical Medicine/Therapy/Occupational
Therapy
Manual .............................. 97140
Mechanical .......................... 97012

## Tractotomy
Medulla ............................. 61470
Mesencephalon ...................... 61480

## Training
Activities of Daily Living .......... 97535, 99509
Biofeedback ................... 90901-90911
Cognitive Skills ...................... 97532
Community/Work Reintegration .......... 97537
Home Management .............. 97535, 99509
Orthoptic/Pleoptic ................... 92065
Orthotics ............................ 97760
Prosthetics .......................... 97761

Self Care .......... 97535, 98960-98962, 99509
Sensory Integration ................... 97533
Walking (Physical Therapy) ............. 97116
Wheelchair Management ............... 97542

## TRAM Flap
Breast Reconstruction ........... 19367-19369

## Trans-Scaphoperilunar
Fracture/Dislocation
  Closed Treatment ................. 25680
  Open Treatment .................. 25685

## Transaminase
Glutamic Oxaloacetic ................. 84450
Glutamic Pyruvic ..................... 84460

## Transanal Endoscopic Microsurgery (TEMS)
*See* Rectum, Tumor, Excision, Transanal Endoscopic

## Transcatheter
Biopsy .............................. 37200
Closure
  Percutaneous
    Heart .................. 93580-93581
    Transmyocardial
Embolization
  Percutaneous ..................... 37204
  Cranial ...................... 61624-61626
Occlusion
  Percutaneous ..................... 37204
  Cranial ...................... 61624-61626
Placement
  Intravascular Stents .......... 0075T-0076T,
      37205-37208, 37215-37216,
      75960, 92980-92981
  Sensor, Aneurysmal Sac ............. 34806
Therapy
  Embolization ...................... 75894
  Infusion ........... 37201-37202, 75896-75898
  Perfusion
    Cranial .................. 61624-61626
  Retrieval ......................... 75961

## Transcatheter Foreign Body
Retrieval ............................ 37203

## Transcortin ...................... 84449

## Transcranial
Doppler Study (TCP) ............. 93886-93893
Stimulation, Magnetic ............ 90867-90869
Stimulation, Motor ............... 95928-95929
Methemoglobin ...................... 88741

## Transcutaneous Electrical Modulation Pain Reprocessing ................... 0278T

## Transcutaneous Electric Nerve Stimulation
*See* Application, Neurostimulation

## Transcutaneous Testing
Bilirubin ............................ 88720
Carboxyhemoglobin ................... 88740
Hemoglobin (Hgb) .................... 88738
Unlisted In Vivo Procedure ............. 88749

## Transdermal Electrostimulation
*See* Application, Neurostimulation

## Transection
Artery
  Carotid .................. 61610, 61612
Blood Vessel
  Kidney ........................... 50100
Brain
  Subpial ........................... 61567
Carotid
  with Skull Base Surgery ............. 61609
Nerve ...................... 64732-64772
  Vagus .................... 43640-43641
Pulmonary Artery ..................... 33922

## Transesophageal
Doppler Echocardiography ........ 93312-93318

## Transfer
Blastocyst
  *See* Embryo Transfer
Gamete Intrafallopian
  *See* GIFT
Jejunum
  with Microvascular Anastomosis
    Free ............................ 43496
Preparation
  Embryo ........................... 89255
    Cryopreserved .................. 89352
Surgical
  *See* Transposition
Tendon
  *See* Tendon, Transfer
Toe to Hand ................... 26551-26556

## Transferase
Aspartate Amino ...................... 84450
Glutamic Oxaloacetic ................. 84450

## Transferrin ...................... 84466

## Transformation
Lymphocyte .......................... 86353

## Transfusion
Blood ............................... 36430
  Exchange ................... 36450-36455
  Fetal ............................. 36460
  Push
    Infant ......................... 36440
Blood Parts
  Exchange ................... 36511-36516
Unlisted Services and Procedures ........ 86999
White Blood Cells .................... 86950

## Transfusion of, Blood, Autologous
*See* Autotransfusion

## Transluminal
Angioplasty
  Arterial
    Radiological Supervision ..... 75962-75968
Atherectomies
  *See* Artery, Atherectomy
Coronary Balloon Dilatation
  *See* Percutaneous Transluminal Angioplasty
Stent Placement
  *See* Stent, Transluminal Placement

## Transmyocardial Laser Revascularization ......... 33140-33141

## Transosteal Bone Plate
Reconstruction
  Mandible .......................... 21244

## Transpeptidase, Gamma-Glutamyl
*See* Gamma Glutamyl Transferase

**Trigger Point**
Injection
    One or Two Muscles . . . . . . . . . . . . . . . 20552
    Two or More Muscles . . . . . . . . . . . . . . 20553

**Triglyceridase**
See Lipase

**Triglyceride Lipase**
See Lipase

**Triglycerides** . . . . . . . . . . . . . . . . . . . 84478

**Trigonocephaly** . . . . . . . . . . . . . . . . . 21175

**Triiodothyronine**
Free . . . . . . . . . . . . . . . . . . . . . . . . . . . . . 84481
Reverse . . . . . . . . . . . . . . . . . . . . . . . . . . 84482
Total . . . . . . . . . . . . . . . . . . . . . . . . . . . . 84480
True . . . . . . . . . . . . . . . . . . . . . . . . . . . . 84480

**Triolean Hydrolase**
See Lipase

**Trioxopurine**
See Uric Acid

**Tripcellim**
See Trypsin

**Trisegmentectomy** . . . . . . . . . . . . . . 47122

**Trocar Biopsy**
Bone Marrow . . . . . . . . . . . . . . . . . . . . . . 38221

**Trochanteric Femur Fracture**
See Femur, Fracture, Trochanteric

**Trophoblastic Tumor GTT**
See Hydatidiform Mole

**Troponin** . . . . . . . . . . . . . . . . . . . . . . . 84484
Qualitative . . . . . . . . . . . . . . . . . . . . . . . . 84512
Quantitative . . . . . . . . . . . . . . . . . . . . . . . 84484

**Truncal Vagotomies**
See Vagotomy, Truncal

**Truncus Arteriosus**
Repair . . . . . . . . . . . . . . . . . . . . . . . . . . . 33786

**Truncus Brachiocephalicus**
See Artery, Brachiocephalic

**Trunk, Brachiocephalic**
See Artery, Brachiocephalic

**Trypanosomiases**
See Trypanosomiasis

**Trypanosomiasis** . . . . . . . . . 86171, 86280

**Trypsin**
Duodenum . . . . . . . . . . . . . . . . . . . . . . . 84485
Feces . . . . . . . . . . . . . . . . . . . . . . . 84488-84490

**Trypsin Inhibitor, Alpha
1-Antitrypsin**
See Alpha-1 Antitrypsin

**Trypure**
See Trypsin

**Tsalicylate Intoxication**
See Salicylate

**TSH**
See Thyroid Stimulating Hormone

**TSI**
See Thyroid Stimulating Immunoglobulin

**Tsutsugamushi Disease**
See Scrub Typhus

**TT**
See Thrombin Time

**TT-3**
See Triiodothyronine, True

**TT-4**
See Thyroxine, True

**Tuba Auditoria (Auditiva)**
See Eustachian Tube

**Tubal Embryo Stage Transfer**
See Embryo Transfer

**Tubal Ligation** . . . . . . . . . . . . . . . . . 58600
Laparoscopic . . . . . . . . . . . . . . . . . . . . . 58670
with Cesarean Delivery . . . . . . . . . . . . . . 58611

**Tubal Occlusion**
See Fallopian Tube, Occlusion; Occlusion
Create Lesion

**Tubal Pregnancy** . . . . . . . . . . . . . . . 59121
with Salpingectomy and/or
Oophorectomy . . . . . . . . . . . . . . . . . . . . 59120

**Tube Change**
Colonic . . . . . . . . . . . . . . . . . . . . . . . . . 49450
Duodenostomy . . . . . . . . . . . . . . . . . . . . 49451
Gastro-Jejunostomy . . . . . . . . . . . . . . . . 49452
Gastrostomy . . . . . . . . . . . . . . . . 43760, 49446
Jejunostomy . . . . . . . . . . . . . . . . . . . . . . 49451
Tracheostomy . . . . . . . . . . . . . . . . . . . . . 31502

**Tube Placement**
Cecostomy Tube . . . . . . . . . . . . . 44300, 49442
Duodenostomy Tube . . . . . . . . . . . . . . . . 49441
Endoscopic
    Bile Duct, Pancreatic Duct . . . . . . . . . . 43268
    Jejunostomy Tube
        Percutaneous . . . . . . . . . . . . . . . . . 49441
    Nasobiliary, Nasopancreatic
        for Drainage . . . . . . . . . . . . . . . . . . 43267
Enterostomy Tube . . . . . . . . . . . . . . . . . 44300
Gastrostomy Tube . . . . . . . . . . . . 43246, 49440
Nasogastric Tube . . . . . . . . . . . . . . . . . . 43752
Orogastric Tube . . . . . . . . . . . . . . . . . . . 43752

**Tube, Fallopian**
See Fallopian Tube

**Tubectomy**
See Excision, Fallopian Tube

**Tubed Pedicle Flap**
Formation . . . . . . . . . . . . . . . . . . . 15570-15576

**Tubercle Bacilli**
Culture . . . . . . . . . . . . . . . . . . . . . . . . . . 87116

**Tubercleplasty**
Tibia
    Anterior . . . . . . . . . . . . . . . . . . . . . . . 27418

**Tuberculin Test**
See Skin, Tests, Tuberculosis

**Tuberculosis**
Antigen Response Test . . . . . . . . . . 86480-86481
Culture . . . . . . . . . . . . . . . . . . . . . . . . . . 87116
Skin Test . . . . . . . . . . . . . . . . . . . . . . . . 86580

**Tuberculosis Vaccine
(BCG)** . . . . . . . . . . . . . . . . . . . . 90585-90586

**Tubes**
Colonic
    See Colon
Duodenostomy
    See Duodenostomy
Endotracheal
    See Endotracheal Tube
Gastrostomy
    See Gastrostomy Tube
Jejunostomy
    See Jejunostomy

**Tudor 'Rabbit Ear'**
See Urethra, Repair

**Tuffier Vaginal Hysterectomy**
See Hysterectomy, Vaginal

**Tumor**
See Craniopharyngioma
Abdomen
    Destruction/Excision . . . . . . . . . 49203-49205
Abdominal Wall
    Excision . . . . . . . . . . . . . . . . . . 22900-22903
    Radical Resection . . . . . . . . . . . 22904, 22905
Acetabulum
    Excision . . . . . . . . . . . . . . . . . . . . . . . 27076
Ankle
    Excision . . . . . . . . . 27618-27619, 27632-27634
    Radical Resection . . . . . . . . . . . 27615-27616
Arm, Lower
    Excision . . . . . . . . . . . . . . . . . . 25071-25076
    Radical Resection . . . . . . . . . . . 25077-25078
Arm, Upper
    Excision . . . . . . . . . . . . . . . . . . 24071-24076
    Radical Resection . . . . . . . . . . . 24077, 24079
Back/Flank
    Excision . . . . . . . . . . . . . . . . . . 21930-21933
    Radical Resection . . . . . . . . . . . 21935, 21936
Bile Duct
    Destruction . . . . . . . . . . . . . . . . . . . . . 43272
    Extrahepatic . . . . . . . . . . . . . . . . . . . . 47711
    Intrahepatic . . . . . . . . . . . . . . . . . . . . 47712
Bladder . . . . . . . . . . . . . . . . . . . . 52234-52240
    Excision . . . . . . . . . . . . . . . . . . 51530, 52355
Bone
    Ablation . . . . . . . . . . . . . . . . . . . . . . . 20982
Brain . . . . . . . . . . . . . . . . . . . . . . . . . . . 61510
    Excision . . . . . . . . . . . . 61518, 61520-61521,
        61526-61530, 61545, 62164
Breast
    Excision . . . . . . . . . . . . . . . . . . 19120-19126
Bronchi
    Excision . . . . . . . . . . . . . . . . . . . . . . . 31640
Calcaneus
    Excision . . . . . . . . . . . . . . . . . . 28100-28103
    Radical Resection . . . . . . . . . . . . . . . . 27647
Carpal . . . . . . . . . . . . . . . . . . . . . 25130-25136
Cheekbone . . . . . . . . . . . . . . . . . 21030, 21034
Chest Wall
    Excision . . . . . . . . . . . . . . . . . . 19260-19272
Clavicle
    Excision . . . . . . . . . . . . . . . . . . 23140, 23200
    with Allograft . . . . . . . . . . . . . . . . . . . 23146
    with Autograft . . . . . . . . . . . . . . . . . . . 23145
Coccyx . . . . . . . . . . . . . . . . . . . . . . . . . . 49215
Colon
    Destruction . . . . . . . . . . . . . . . . 44393, 45383
Cranial Bone
    Reconstruction . . . . . . . . . . . . . 21181-21184
Destruction
    Chemosurgery . . . . . . . . . . . . . . 17311-17315
    Urethra . . . . . . . . . . . . . . . . . . . . . . . . 53220

Lumbar . . . . . . . . . . . . . . . . . . . . . . . 22102
Thoracic
    Excision. . . . . . . . . . . . . . . . . . . . . . 22101
Wrist . . . . . . . . . . . . . 25071-25076, 25130-25136
    Radical Resection . . . . . . . . . . . 25077, 25078

## Tunica Vaginalis
Hydrocele
    Aspiration. . . . . . . . . . . . . . . . . . . . . 55000
    Excision . . . . . . . . . . . 55040-55041
    Repair . . . . . . . . . . . . . . . . . . . . . . . . 55060

## Turbinate
Excision. . . . . . . . . . . . . . . . . . 30130-30140
Fracture
    Therapeutic . . . . . . . . . . . . . . . . . . 30930
Injection . . . . . . . . . . . . . . . . . . . . . . . . 30200
Submucous Resection
    Nose Excision. . . . . . . . . . . . . . . . . . 30140

## Turbinate Mucosa
Cauterization . . . . . . . . . . . . . . . . . . 30801-30802

## Turcica, Sella
*See* Sella Turcica

## Turnbuckle Jacket . . . . . . . 29020-29025
Removal . . . . . . . . . . . . . . . . . . . . . . . . 29715

## TURP
*See* Prostatectomy, Transurethral

## Tylectomy
*See* Breast, Excision, Lesion

## Tylenol
Urine . . . . . . . . . . . . . . . . . . . . . . . . . . 82003

## Tympanic Membrane
Create Stoma . . . . . . . . . . . . . . . . 69433-69436
Incision . . . . . . . . . . . . . . . . . . . . 69420-69421
Reconstruction . . . . . . . . . . . . . . . . . . . . 69620
Repair . . . . . . . . . . . . . . . . . . 69450, 69610

## Tympanic Nerve
Excision. . . . . . . . . . . . . . . . . . . . . . . . 69676

## Tympanolysis . . . . . . . . . . . . . . . . .69450

## Tympanomastoidectomy
*See* Tympanoplasty

## Tympanometry . . . . . . .92550, 92567, 92570
*See* Audiologic Function Tests

## Tympanoplasty
*See* Myringoplasty
Radical or Complete. . . . . . . . . . . . . . . 69645
    with Ossicular Chain Reconstruction. . . . 69646
with Antrotomy or Mastoidotomy. . . . . . . 69635
    with Ossicular Chain Reconstruction. . . . 69636
      and Synthetic Prosthesis . . . . . . . . . . 69637
with Mastoidectomy . . . . . . . . . . . . . . . 69641
    with Intact or Reconstructed Wall. . . . . . 69643
      and Ossicular Chain Reconstruction . . . 69644
    with Ossicular Chain Reconstruction. . . . 69642
without Mastoidectomy . . . . . . . . . . . . . . 69631
    with Ossicular Chain Reconstruction. . . . 69632
      and Synthetic Prosthesis . . . . . . . . . . 69633

## Tympanostomy . . . . . . . . . . . . 69433-69436

## Tympanotomy
*See* Myringotomy

## Typhoid Vaccine . . . . . . . . . . 90690-90693
AKD . . . . . . . . . . . . . . . . . . . . . . . . . . 90693
H-P . . . . . . . . . . . . . . . . . . . . . . . . . . 90692

Oral . . . . . . . . . . . . . . . . . . . . . . . . . . 90690
Polysaccharide . . . . . . . . . . . . . . . . . . . . 90691

## Typhus
Endemic
    *See* Murine Typhus
Mite-Borne
    *See* Scrub Typhus
Sao Paulo
    *See* Rocky Mountain Spotted Fever
Tropical
    *See* Scrub Typhus

## Typing, Blood
*See* Blood Typing

## Typing, HLA
*See* HLA Typing

## Typing, Tissue
*See* Tissue, Typing

## Tyrosine . . . . . . . . . . . . . . . . . . . .84510

## Tzank Smear . . . . . . . . . . . . . 88160-88161

# U

## UDP Galactose Pyrophosphorylase
*See* Galactose-1-Phosphate, Uridyl Transferase

## UFR
*See* Uroflowmetry

## UGT1A1 . . . . . . . . . . . . . . . . . . . . . .81350

## Ulcer
Anal
    *See* Anus, Fissure
Decubitus
    *See* Debridement; Pressure Ulcer (Decubitus);
    Skin Graft and Flap
Pinch Graft . . . . . . . . . . . . . . . . . . . . . 15050
Pressure . . . . . . . . . . . . . . . . . . 15920-15999
Stomach
    Excision . . . . . . . . . . . . . . . . . . . . . 43610

## Ulcerative, Cystitis
*See* Cystitis, Interstitial

## Ulna
*See* Arm, Lower; Elbow; Humerus; Radius
Arthrodesis
    Radioulnar Joint
      with Resection . . . . . . . . . . . . . . . . . 25830
Arthroplasty
    with Implant. . . . . . . . . . . . . . . . . . . 25442
Centralization or Wrist . . . . . . . . . . . . . . 25335
Craterization. . . . . . . . . . . . 24147, 25150-25151
Cyst
    Excision . . . . . . . .24125-24126, 25120-25126
Diaphysectomy. . . . . . . . . . 24147, 25150-25151
Excision. . . . . . . . . . . . . . . . . . . . . . . 24147
    Abscess . . . . . . . . . . . . . . . . . . . . . 24138
    Complete . . . . . . . . . . . . . . . . . . . . . 25240
    Epiphyseal Bar . . . . . . . . . . . . . . . . . 20150
    Partial. . . . . . . . . . . 25145-25151, 25240
Fracture
    Closed Treatment. . . . . . . . . . . 25530-25535
    Olecranon. . . . . . . . . . . . . . . 24670-24675
    Open Treatment . . . . . . . . . . . 24685, 25545

Shaft. . . . . . . . . . . . . . . . . . 25530-25545
    Open Treatment . . . . . . . . . . . . . . . . . 25574
Styloid
    Closed Treatment . . . . . . . . . . . . . . . . 25650
    Open Treatment . . . . . . . . . . . . . . . . . 25652
    Percutaneous Fixation . . . . . . . . . . . . 25651
    with Dislocation
      Closed Treatment . . . . . . . . . . . . . . . 24620
      Open Treatment . . . . . . . . . . . . . . . . 24635
    with Manipulation . . . . . . . . . . . . . . . 25535
    with Radius . . . . . . . . . . . . . 25560-25565
      Open Treatment . . . . . . . . . . . . . . . . 25575
    without Manipulation . . . . . . . . . . . . . 25530
Incision and Drainage . . . . . . . . . . . . . . . 25035
Osteoplasty . . . . . . . . . . . . . . . 25390-25393
Prophylactic Treatment . . . . . . . . . 25491-25492
Reconstruction
    Radioulnar . . . . . . . . . . . . . . . . . . . . 25337
Repair
    Epiphyseal Arrest. . . . . . . . . . . 25450-25455
    Malunion or Nonunion. . . . . . . 25400, 25415
    Osteotomy . . . . . . . . . . . 25360, 25370-25375
      and Radius . . . . . . . . . . . . . . . . . . . 25365
    with Graft. . . . . . . . . . . 25405, 25420-25426
Saucerization . . . . . . . . . . . . . 24147, 25150-25151
Sequestrectomy . . . . . . . . . . . . . . 24138, 25145
Tumor
    Cyst . . . . . . . . . . . . . . . . . . . . . . . . 24120
    Excision . . .24125-24126, 25120-25126, 25170

## Ulnar Arteries
*See* Artery, Ulnar

## Ulnar Nerve
Decompression. . . . . . . . . . . . . . . . . . . . 64718
Neuroplasty . . . . . . . . . . . . . . . . . 64718-64719
Reconstruction . . . . . . . . . . . . . . 64718-64719
Release . . . . . . . . . . . . . . . . . . . 64718-64719
Repair/Suture
    Motor . . . . . . . . . . . . . . . . . . . . . . . 64836
Transposition . . . . . . . . . . . . . . . . 64718-64719

## Ultrasonic
*See* Ultrasound

## Ultrasonic Cardiography
*See* Echocardiography

## Ultrasonic Procedure . . . . . . . . . .52325

## Ultrasonography
*See* Echography

## Ultrasound
*See* Echocardiography; Echography
3D Rendering . . . . . . . . . . . . . . 76376-76377
Abdomen . . . . . . . . . . . . . . . . . . 76700-76705
Arm
    Complete . . . . . . . . . . . . . . . . . . . . . 76881
    Limited . . . . . . . . . . . . . . . . . . . . . . 76882
Artery
    Intracranial. . . . . . . . . . . . . . 93886-93893
    Middle Cerebral . . . . . . . . . . . . . . . . . 76821
    Umbilical . . . . . . . . . . . . . . . . . . . . . 76820
Bladder . . . . . . . . . . . . . . . . . . . . . . . 51798
Bone Density Study . . . . . . . . . . . . . . . . 76977
Breast . . . . . . . . . . . . . . . . . . . . . . . . 76645
Bronchi
    Endoscopy . . . . . . . . . . . . . . . . . . . . 31620
Chest. . . . . . . . . . . . . . . . . . . . . . . . . 76604
Colon
    Endoscopic . . . . . . . . . . . . . . 45391-45392
Colon-Sigmoid
    Endoscopic. . . . . . . . . . . . . . . 45341-45342

## Ultraviolet Light Therapy

## Umbilectomy . . . . . . . . . . . . . . . . . . .49250

## Umbilical

## Umbilical Cord

## Umbilicus

## Undescended Testicle
See Testis, Undescended

## Unfertilized Egg
See Ova

## Unguis
See Nails

## Unilateral Simple Mastectomy
See Mastectomy

## Unlisted Services and Procedures . . . . . . . . . . . . . . .99499, 99600

Musculoskeletal System . . . . . . . . . . . . 78399
Nervous System. . . . . . . . . . . . . . . . . . . 78699
Therapeutic . . . . . . . . . . . . . . . . . . 79999
Obstetrical Care . . . . . . . . . . . . . . 59898-59899
Omentum . . . . . . . . . . . . . . . . . 49329, 49999
Ophthalmology . . . . . . . . . . . . . . . . . . . . . 92499
Orbit . . . . . . . . . . . . . . . . . . . . . . . . . . . 67599
Otorhinolaryngology . . . . . . . . . . . . . . . . . 92700
Ovary . . . . . . . . . . . . . . . . . . . 58679, 58999
Oviduct . . . . . . . . . . . . . . . . . . 58679, 58999
Palate . . . . . . . . . . . . . . . . . . . . . . . . . 42299
Pancreas Surgery . . . . . . . . . . . . . . . . . . 48999
Pathology . . . . . . . . . . . . . . . . . . . . . . . 89240
Pelvis . . . . . . . . . . . . . . . . . . . . . . . . . 27299
Penis . . . . . . . . . . . . . . . . . . . . . . . . . 55899
Peritoneum . . . . . . . . . . . . . . . 49329, 49999
Pharynx . . . . . . . . . . . . . . . . . . . . . . . . 42999
Physical Therapy . . . . . . . . . 97039, 97139, 97799
Pleura . . . . . . . . . . . . . . . . . . . . . . . . 32999
Pressure Ulcer . . . . . . . . . . . . . . . . . . . 15999
Preventive Medicine . . . . . . . . . . . . . . . . 99429
Prostate . . . . . . . . . . . . . . . . . . . . . . . 55899
Psychiatric . . . . . . . . . . . . . . . . . . . . . . 90899
Pulmonology . . . . . . . . . . . . . . . . . . . . . 94799
Radiation Physics . . . . . . . . . . . . . . . . . . 77399
Radiation Therapy . . . . . . . . . . . . . . . . . 77499
Planning . . . . . . . . . . . . . . . . . . . . . 77299
Radiology, Diagnostic . . . . . . . . . . . . . . . 76499
Radionuclide Therapy . . . . . . . . . . . . . . . 79999
Radiopharmaceutical Therapy . . . . . . . . . . 79999
Rectum . . . . . . . . . . . . . . . . . 45499, 45999
Reproductive Medicine
Laboratory Procedure . . . . . . . . . . . . . . 89398
Salivary Gland . . . . . . . . . . . . . . . . . . . . 42699
Scrotum . . . . . . . . . . . . . . . . . . . . . . . 55899
Seminal Vesicle . . . . . . . . . . . . . . . . . . . 55899
Shoulder Surgery . . . . . . . . . . . . . . . . . . 23929
Sinuses . . . . . . . . . . . . . . . . . . . . . . . 31299
Skin . . . . . . . . . . . . . . . . . . . . . . . . . . 17999
Special Services and Reports . . . . . . . . . . . 99199
Spine . . . . . . . . . . . . . . . . . . . . . . . . . 22899
Stomach . . . . . . . . . . . . . . . . . 43659, 43999
Strapping . . . . . . . . . . . . . . . . . . . . . . 29799
Surgical Pathology . . . . . . . . . . . . . . . . . 88399
Temporal Bone . . . . . . . . . . . . . . . . . . . 69979
Testis . . . . . . . . . . . . . . . . . . 54699, 55899
Throat . . . . . . . . . . . . . . . . . . . . . . . . 42999
Tongue . . . . . . . . . . . . . . . . . . . . . . . . 41599
Tonsil/Adenoid . . . . . . . . . . . . . . . . . . . 42999
Toxoid . . . . . . . . . . . . . . . . . . . . . . . . 90749
Trachea . . . . . . . . . . . . . . . . . . . . . . . 31899
Transfusion . . . . . . . . . . . . . . . . . . . . . 86999
Ultrasound . . . . . . . . . . . . . . . . . . . . . . 76999
Ureter . . . . . . . . . . . . . . . . . . . . . . . . 50949
Urinary System . . . . . . . . . . . . . . . . . . . 53899
Uterus . . . . . . . . . . . . . . . . 58578-58579, 58999
Uvula . . . . . . . . . . . . . . . . . . . . . . . . . 42299
Vaccine . . . . . . . . . . . . . . . . . . . . . . . 90749
Vagina . . . . . . . . . . . . . . . . . . . . . . . . 58999
Vas Deferens . . . . . . . . . . . . . . . . . . . . 55899
Vascular . . . . . . . . . . . . . . . . . . . . . . . 37799
Vascular Endoscopy . . . . . . . . . . . . . . . . 37501
Vascular Injection . . . . . . . . . . . . . . . . . . 36299
Vascular Studies . . . . . . . . . . . . 93799, 93998
Wrist . . . . . . . . . . . . . . . . . . . . . . . . . 25999

**Unna Paste Boot** . . . . . . . . . . . . . . . . . 29580
Removal . . . . . . . . . . . . . . . . . . . . . . . . . 29700

**UPP**
See Urethra Pressure Profile

**Upper**
Digestive System Endoscopy
See Endoscopy, Gastrointestinal, Upper
Extremity
See Arm, Upper; Elbow; Humerus
Gastrointestinal Bleeding
See Gastrointestinal, Upper, Hemorrhage
Gastrointestinal Endoscopy, Biopsy
See Biopsy
Planning
See Biopsy, Gastrointestinal, Upper
Endoscopy; Endoscopy, Gastrointestinal
GI Tract
See Gastrointestinal Tract, Upper

**Urachal Cyst**
See Cyst, Urachal

**Urea Breath Test** . . . . 78267-78268, 83014

**Urea Nitrogen**
See Blood Urea Nitrogen
Clearance . . . . . . . . . . . . . . . . . . . . . . . 84545
Quantitative . . . . . . . . . . . . . . . . . . . . . . 84520
Semiquantitative . . . . . . . . . . . . . . . . . . . 84525
Urine . . . . . . . . . . . . . . . . . . . . . . . . . . 84540

**Urea Nitrogen, Blood**
See Blood Urea Nitrogen

**Urecholine Supersensitivity Test**
See Cystometrogram

**Ureter**
Anastomosis
to Bladder . . . . . . . . . . . . . . . . 50780-50785
to Colon . . . . . . . . . . . . . . . . . 50810-50815
to Intestine . . . . . . . . . . . 50800, 50820-50825
to Kidney . . . . . . . . . . . . . . . . 50740-50750
to Ureter . . . . . . . . . . . . . . . . 50760-50770
Biopsy . . . . . . . 50955-50957, 50974-50976, 52007
Catheterization . . . . . . . . . . . . . . . . . . . . 52005
Continent Diversion . . . . . . . . . . . . . . . . . 50825
Creation
Stoma . . . . . . . . . . . . . . . . . . . . . . . 50860
Destruction
Endoscopic . . . . . . . . . . . . . . . 50957, 50976
Dilation . . . . . . . . . . . . 52341-52342, 52344-52345
Endoscopic . . . . . . 50553, 50572, 50953, 50972
Endoscopy
Biopsy . . . . . . . . . 50955-50957, 50974-50976,
52007, 52354
Catheterization . . . . . . . . 50953, 50972, 52005
Destruction . . . . . . . . . 50957, 50976, 52354
Dilation . . . . . . . . . 52341-52342, 52344-52345
Excision
Tumor . . . . . . . . . . . . . . . . . . . . . . . 52355
Exploration . . . . . . . . . . . . . . . . . . . . . 52351
Injection of Implant Material . . . . . . . . . 52327
Insertion
Stent . . . . 50947, 52282, 52332-52334, 53855
Lithotripsy . . . . . . . . . . . . . . . . . . . . . 52353
Manipulation of Ureteral Calculus . . . . . 52330
Removal
Calculus . . . . . . . . . . . . . 50961, 50980,
52320-52325, 52352
Foreign Body . . . . . . . . . . . . 50961, 50980
Resection . . . . . . . . . . . . . . . . . . . . . . 52355
via Incision . . . . . . . . . . . . . . . 50970-50980
via Stoma . . . . . . . . . . . . . . . . 50951-50961
Exploration . . . . . . . . . . . . . . . . . . . . . . 50600
Incision and Drainage . . . . . . . . . . . . . . . 50600
Injection
Drugs . . . . . . . . . . . . . . . . . . . . . . . . 50391
Radiologic . . . . . . . . . . . . . . . . 50684, 50690

Insertion
Catheter . . . . . . . . . . . . . . . . . . . . . . 50393
Stent . . . . . 50393, 50688, 50947, 52332-52334
Tube . . . . . . . . . . . . . . . . . . . . . . . . 50688
Instillation
Drugs . . . . . . . . . . . . . . . . . . . . . . . . 50391
Lesion
Destruction . . . . . . . . . . . . . . . . . . . . 52354
Lithotripsy . . . . . . . . . . . . . . . . . . . . . . . 52353
Lysis
Adhesions . . . . . . . . . . . . . . . 50715-50725
Manometric Studies
Pressure . . . . . . . . . . . . . . . . . . . . . . 50686
Meatotomy . . . . . . . . . . . . . . . . . . . . . . 52290
Nuclear Medicine
Reflux Study . . . . . . . . . . . . . . . . . . . . 78740
Postcaval
See Retrocaval Ureter
Reconstruction . . . . . . . . . . . . . . . . . . . . 50700
with Intestines . . . . . . . . . . . . . . . . . . 50840
Reflux Study . . . . . . . . . . . . . . . . . . . . . 78740
Reimplantation . . . . . . . . . . . . . . . . . . . . 51565
Removal
Anastomosis . . . . . . . . . . . . . . . . . . . 50830
Calculus . . . . . . . . . . . 50610-50630, 50961,
51060-51065, 52320-52325
Foreign Body . . . . . . . . . . . . . . . . . . . 50961
Stent . . . . . . . . . . . . . . . . . . 50382-50387
Repair . . . . . . . . . . . . . . . . . . . . . . . . . 50900
Anastomosis . . . . . . . . . . . . . . 50740-50825
Continent Diversion . . . . . . . . . . . . . . . 50825
Deligation . . . . . . . . . . . . . . . . . . . . . 50940
Fistula . . . . . . . . . . . . . . . . . . 50920-50930
Lysis Adhesions . . . . . . . . . . . . 50715-50725
Ureterocele . . . . . . . . . . . . . . . . . . . . 51535
Ectopic . . . . . . . . . . . . . . . . . . . . . 52301
Orthotopic . . . . . . . . . . . . . . . . . . . 52300
Urinary Undiversion . . . . . . . . . . . . . . . 50830
Replacement
Stent . . . . . . . . . . . . . . . . . 50382, 50387
with Intestines . . . . . . . . . . . . . . . . . . 50840
Resection . . . . . . . . . . . . . . . . . . . . . . . 52355
Revision
Anastomosis . . . . . . . . . . . . . . 50727-50728
Stent
Change . . . . . . . . . . . . . . . . . . . . . . 50688
Insertion . . . . . . . . . . . . . . . . . . . . . . 50688
Suture . . . . . . . . . . . . . . . . . . . . . . . . . 50900
Deligation . . . . . . . . . . . . . . . . . . . . . 50940
Fistula . . . . . . . . . . . . . . . . . . 50920-50930
Tube
Change . . . . . . . . . . . . . . . . . . . . . . 50688
Insertion . . . . . . . . . . . . . . . . . . . . . . 50688
Tumor Resection . . . . . . . . . . . . . . . . . . . 52355
Unlisted Services and Procedures . . . 50949, 53899
X-ray with Contrast
Guide Catheter . . . . . . . . . . . . . . . . . . 74480
Guide Dilation . . . . . . . . . . . . . . . . . . 74485

**Ureteral**
Catheterization
See Catheterization, Ureter
Guide Wire Insertion . . . . . . . . . . . . . . . . 52334
Meatotomy
See Meatotomy, Ureteral
Splinting . . . . . . . . . . . . . . . . . . 50400-50405
Stent Insertion . . . . . . . . . . . . . . . . . . . . 52332

**Ureterectomy** . . . . . . . . . . . 50650-50660
Partial . . . . . . . . . . . . . . . . . . 50220, 50546
Total . . . . . . . . . . . . . . . . . . . . . . . . . . 50548

**Ureterocalycostomy** . . . . . . . . . . . 50750

# V

## Vaginal Smear
*See* Pap Smears

## Vaginal Suppositories
Induced Abortion . . . . . . . . . . . . . . . . . . . . . . 59855
　　with Dilation and Curettage . . . . . . . . . 59856
　　with Hysterectomy. . . . . . . . . . . . . . . . . 59857

## Vaginectomy
*See* Colpectomy

## Vaginoplasty
Intersex State. . . . . . . . . . . . . . . . . . . . . . . . 57335

## Vaginorrhaphy
*See* Colporrhaphy

## Vaginoscopy
Biopsy. . . . . . . . . . . . . . . . . . . . . . . . . . . . . . 57454
Exploration . . . . . . . . . . . . . . . . . . . . . . . . . 57452

## Vaginotomy
*See* Colpotomy

## Vagotomy
Abdominal . . . . . . . . . . . . . . . . . . . . . . . . . . 64760
Highly Selective . . . . . . . . . . . . . . . . . . . . . . 43641
Parietal Cell . . . . . . . . . . . . . . . . . . . 43641, 64755
Selective. . . . . . . . . . . . . . . . . . . . . . . . . . . 43640
Transthoracic . . . . . . . . . . . . . . . . . . . . . . . 64752
Truncal . . . . . . . . . . . . . . . . . . . . . . . . . . . . 43640
with Gastroduodenostomy Revision,
Reconstruction. . . . . . . . . . . . . . . . . . . . . . . 43855
with Gastrojejunostomy Revision,
Reconstruction. . . . . . . . . . . . . . . . . . . . . . . 43865
with Partial Distal Gastrectomy . . . . . . . . . 43635

## Vagus Nerve
Avulsion
　　Abdominal . . . . . . . . . . . . . . . . . . . . . . 64760
　　Selective . . . . . . . . . . . . . . . . . . . . . . . 64755
　　Thoracic . . . . . . . . . . . . . . . . . . . . . . . . 64752
Incision . . . . . . . . . . . . . . . . . . . . . . 43640-43641
　　Abdominal . . . . . . . . . . . . . . . . . . . . . . 64760
　　Selective . . . . . . . . . . . . . . . . . . . . . . . 64755
　　Thoracic . . . . . . . . . . . . . . . . . . . . . . . . 64752
Injection
　　Anesthetic . . . . . . . . . . . . . . . . . . . . . . 64408
Transection. . . . . . . . . . . . . . . . . . . 43640-43641
　　Abdominal . . . . . . . . . . . . . . . . . . . . . . 64760
　　Selective . . . . . . . . . . . . . . . . . . 43652, 64755
　　Thoracic . . . . . . . . . . . . . . . . . . . . . . . . 64752
　　Truncal . . . . . . . . . . . . . . . . . . . . . . . . . 43651

## Valproic Acid
*See* Dipropylacetic Acid

## Valproic Acid Measurement
*See* Dipropylacetic Acid

## Valsalva Sinus
*See* Sinus of Valsalva

## Valva Atrioventricularis Sinistra (Valva Mitralis)
*See* Mitral Valve

## Valve
Aortic
　*See* Heart, Aortic Valve
Bicuspid
　*See* Mitral Valve
Mitral
　*See* Mitral Valve
Pulmonary
　*See* Pulmonary Valve

Tricuspid
　*See* Tricuspid Valve

## Valve Stenoses, Aortic
*See* Aortic Stenosis

## Valvectomy
Tricuspid Valve . . . . . . . . . . . . . . . . . . . . . . 33460

## Valvotomy
Mitral Valve . . . . . . . . . . . . . . . . . . . 33420-33422
Pulmonary Valve. . . . . . . . . . . . . . . . 33470-33474
Reoperation . . . . . . . . . . . . . . . . . . . . . . . . 33530

## Valvuloplasty
Aortic Valve . . . . . . . . . . . . . . . . . . . 33400-33403
Femoral Vein. . . . . . . . . . . . . . . . . . . . . . . . 34501
Mitral Valve . . . . . . . . . . . . . . . . . . . 33425-33427
Percutaneous Balloon
　　Aortic Valve . . . . . . . . . . . . . . . . . . . . . 92986
　　Mitral Valve . . . . . . . . . . . . . . . . . . . . . 92987
　　Pulmonary Valve. . . . . . . . . . . . . . . . . . 92990
Prosthetic Valve . . . . . . . . . . . . . . . . . . . . . 33496
Reoperation . . . . . . . . . . . . . . . . . . . . . . . . 33530
Tricuspid Valve . . . . . . . . . . . . . . . . . 33463-33465

## Van Den Bergh Test
*See* Bilirubin, Blood

## Vancomycin
Assay . . . . . . . . . . . . . . . . . . . . . . . . . . . . . 80202
Resistance . . . . . . . . . . . . . . . . . . . . . . . . . 87500

## Vanillylmandelic Acid
Urine . . . . . . . . . . . . . . . . . . . . . . . . . . . . . . 84585

## Vanilmandelic Acid
*See* Vanillylmandelic Acid

## Varicella (Chicken Pox)
*See* Vaccines

## Varicella-Zoster
Antibody . . . . . . . . . . . . . . . . . . . . . . . . . . . 86787
Antigen Detection
　　Direct Fluorescence . . . . . . . . . . . . . . . 87290

## Varices Esophageal
*See* Esophageal Varices

## Varicocele
Spermatic Cord
　　Excision . . . . . . . . . . . . . . . . . . . 55530-55540

## Varicose Vein
Ablation . . . . . . . . . . . . . . . . . . . . . 36475-36479
Removal . . . . . . . . . . . . . . . . . . . . . 37765-37785
Secondary Varicosity . . . . . . . . . . . . . . . . . 37785
with Tissue Excision . . . . . . . . . . . . . 37735-37761

## Vas Deferens
Anastomosis
　　to Epididymis . . . . . . . . . . . . . . 54900-54901
Excision. . . . . . . . . . . . . . . . . . . . . . . . . . . 55250
Incision . . . . . . . . . . . . . . . . . . . . . . . . . . . 55200
　　for X-ray . . . . . . . . . . . . . . . . . . . . . . . 55300
Ligation. . . . . . . . . . . . . . . . . . . . . . . . . . . 55450
Repair
　　Suture. . . . . . . . . . . . . . . . . . . . . . . . . 55400
Unlisted Services and Procedures . . . . . . . 55899
Vasography. . . . . . . . . . . . . . . . . . . . . . . . . 74440
X-ray with Contrast . . . . . . . . . . . . . . . . . . 74440

## Vascular Flow Check, Graft . . . 15860

## Vascular Injection
Unlisted Services and Procedures . . . . . . . 36299

## Vascular Lesion
Cranial
　　Excision . . . . . . . . 61600-61608, 61615-61616
Cutaneous
　　Destruction. . . . . . . . . . . . . . . 17106-17108

## Vascular Malformation
Cerebral
　　Repair. . . . . . . . . . . . . . . . . . . . . . . . . 61710
Finger
　　Excision . . . . . . . . . . . . . . . . . 26111-26116
Hand
　　Excision . . . . . . . . . . . . . . . . . 26111-26116

## Vascular Procedures
Angioscopy
　　Non-Coronary Vessels . . . . . . . . . . . . . 35400
Brachytherapy
　　Intracoronary Artery. . . . . . . . . . . . . . . 92974
Digital Visualization
　　Near-Infrared Guidance. . . . . . . . . . . . . 0287T
Endoscopy
　　Surgical . . . . . . . . . . . . . . . . . . . . . . . 37500
Harvest
　　Lower Extremity Vein. . . . . . . . . . . . . . 35572
Intravascular Ultrasound
　　Coronary Vessels . . . . . . . . . . . 92978-92979
　　Non-Coronary Vessels . . . . . . . . 75945-75946
Ligation
　　Vena Cava . . . . . . . . . . . . . . . . . . . . . 37619
Spectroscopy
　　Catheter Based . . . . . . . . . . . . . . . . . . 0205T
Stent
　　Intracoronary . . . . . . . . . . . . . . . 92980-92981
Thrombolysis
　　Coronary Vessels . . . . . . . . . . . 92975-92977
　　Cranial Vessels. . . . . . . . . . . . . . . . . . . 37195

## Vascular Rehabilitation
*See* Peripheral Artery Disease Rehabilitation (PAD)

## Vascular Studies
*See* Doppler Scan, Duplex, Plethysmography
Access and Patency
　　Digital Visualization
　　　　Near-Infrared Guidance . . . . . . . . . . 0287T
Angioscopy
　　Non-Coronary Vessels . . . . . . . . . . . . . 35400
Aorta. . . . . . . . . . . . . . . . . . . . . . . 93978-93979
Arterial Studies (Non-Invasive)
　　Extracranial . . . . . . . . . . . . . . . 93880-93882
　　Extremities. . . . . . . . . . . . . . . . 93922-93924
　　Intracranial. . . . . . . . . . . . . . . . 93886-93890
　　Lower Extremity . . . . . . . . . . . . 93925-93926
　　Middle Cerebral Artery, Fetal . . . . . . . . 76821
　　Umbilical Artery, Fetal . . . . . . . . . . . . . 76820
Artery Studies
　　Upper Extremity . . . . . . . . . . . . 93930-93931
Bioimpedance Cardiovascular Analysis . . . . 93701
Blood Pressure Monitoring,
24 Hour . . . . . . . . . . . . . . . . . . . . . 93784-93790
Cardiac Catheterization
　　Imaging . . . . . . . . . . . . . . . . . . 93452-93461
Hemodialysis Access. . . . . . . . . . . . . . . . . 93990
Kidney
　　Multiple Study
　　　　with Pharmacological Intervention . . . 78709
　　Single Study
　　　　with Pharmacological Intervention . . . 78708
Penile Vessels . . . . . . . . . . . . . . . . 93980-93981
Spectroscopy
　　Catheter Based . . . . . . . . . . . . . . . . . . 0205T
Temperature Gradient . . . . . . . . . . . . . . . . 93740
Unlisted Services and Procedures . . . . . . . 93799

## Vidal Procedure
See Varicocele, Spermatic Cord, Excision

## Video
Esophagus . . . . . . . . . . . . . . . . . . . . . . . 74230
Pharynx. . . . . . . . . . . . . . . . . . . . 70371, 74230
Speech Evaluation . . . . . . . . . . . . . . . . . . 70371
Swallowing Evaluation . . . . . . . . . . . . . . . . 74230

## Video-Assisted Thoracoscopic Surgery
See Thoracoscopy

## Videoradiography
Unlisted Services and Procedures . . . 76120-76125

## VII, Coagulation Factor
See Proconvertin

## VII, Cranial Nerve
See Facial Nerve

## VIII, Coagulation Factor
See Clotting Factor

## Villus, Chorionic
See Chorionic Villus

## Villusectomy
See Synovectomy

## VIP
See Vasoactive Intestinal Peptide

## Viral Antibodies . . . . . . . . . . . . . . . . 86280

## Viral Warts
See Warts

## Virus
AIDS
  See HIV-1
Burkitt Lymphoma
  See Epstein-Barr Virus
Human Immunodeficiency
  See HIV
Influenza
  See Influenza Virus
Respiratory Syncytial
  See Respiratory Syncytial Virus
Salivary Gland
  See Cytomegalovirus

## Virus Identification
Immunofluorescence . . . . . . . . . . . . . . . . . 87254

## Virus Isolation . . . . . . . . . . . . 87250-87255

## Visceral Larval Migrans . . . . . . . 86280

## Viscosities, Blood
See Blood, Viscosity

## Visit, Home
See House Calls

## Visual Acuity Screen . . . . . 99172-99173

## Visual Field Exam . . . . . . . . 92081-92083

## Visual Function Screen . . . 1055F, 99172

## Visual Reinforcement
### Audiometry . . . . . . . . . . . . . . . . . . . . 92579
See Audiologic Function Tests

## Vization
. . . . . . . . . . . . . . . . . . . . . . . . . . . . . 50690

## Vital Capacity Measurement . . . 94150

## Vitamin . . . . . . . . . . . . . . . . . . . . . . . 84591
A . . . . . . . . . . . . . . . . . . . . . . . . . . . . 84590
B Complex
  See B Complex Vitamins
B-1. . . . . . . . . . . . . . . . . . . . . . . . . . . 84425
B-12. . . . . . . . . . . . . . . . . . . . 82607-82608
  Absorption Study . . . . . . . . . . 78270-78272
  Holotranscobalamin . . . . . . . . . . . . . . . 0103T
B-2. . . . . . . . . . . . . . . . . . . . . . . . . . . 84252
B-6. . . . . . . . . . . . . . . . . . . . . . . . . . . 84207
B-6 Measurement
  See Pyridoxal Phosphate
BC
  See Folic Acid
C . . . . . . . . . . . . . . . . . . . . . . . . . . . . 82180
D
  Blood Serum Level
    25 hydroxy . . . . . . . . . . . . . . . . . . 82306
    1, 25 dihydroxy . . . . . . . . . . . . . . . . 82652
    Counseling . . . . . . . . . . . . . . . . . . . 4019F
E . . . . . . . . . . . . . . . . . . . . . . . . . . . . 84446
K . . . . . . . . . . . . . . . . . . . . . . . . . . . . 84597
K Dependent Bone Protein
  See Osteocalcin
K-Dependent Protein S
  See Protein S

## Vitelline Duct
See Omphalomesenteric Duct

## Vitrectomy
Anterior Approach
  Partial. . . . . . . . . . . . . . . . . . . . . . . 67005
for Retinal Detachment . . . . . . . . . . 67112-67113
Monitoring of Intraocular Pressure. . . . . . . 0173T
  by Sampling . . . . . . . . . . . . . . . . . . . 0198T
  Drainage Device. . . . . . . . . . . 0191T, 0192T
Pars Plana Approach . . . . . . . . . . 67036-67043
Subtotal . . . . . . . . . . . . . . . . . . . . . . . 67010
  with Endolaser Panretinal
    Photocoagulation. . . . . . . . . . . . . . . 67040
with Focal Endolaser Photocoagulation . . . . 67039
with Implantation or Replacement
  Drug Delivery System . . . . . . . . . . . . . 67027

## Vitreous
Aspiration. . . . . . . . . . . . . . . . . . . . . . 67015
Excision
  Pars Plana Approach . . . . 67036, 67041-67043
  with Focal Endolaser
    Photocoagulation. . . . . . . . . . . . . . . 67039
Implantation
  Drug Delivery System . . . . . . . . . . . . . 67027
Incision
  Strands. . . . . . . . . . . . . . . . 67030-67031
Injection
  Fluid Substitute . . . . . . . . . . . . . . . . 67025
  Pharmacologic Agent. . . . . . . . . . . . . . 67028
Placement
  Radiation Source . . . . . . . . . . . . . . . . 0190T
Removal
  Anterior Approach . . . . . . . . . . . . . . . 67005
  Subtotal . . . . . . . . . . . . . . . . . . . . . 67010
Replacement
  Drug Delivery System . . . . . . . . . . . . . 67027
Strands
  Discission. . . . . . . . . . . . . . . . . . . . 67030
  Severing. . . . . . . . . . . . . . . . . . . . . 67031
Subtotal . . . . . . . . . . . . . . . . . . . . . . . 67010

## VKORC1 . . . . . . . . . . . . . . . . . . . . . 81355

## VLDL
See Lipoprotein, Blood

## VMA
See Vanillylmandelic Acid

## Vocal Cords
Injection
  Endoscopy . . . . . . . . . . . . . . . . . . . 31513
    Therapeutic. . . . . . . . . . . . . . 31570-31571

## Voice Box
See Larynx

## Voice Button . . . . . . . . . . . . . . . . . 31611

## Voiding Pressure Studies
Abdominal . . . . . . . . . . . . . . . . . . . . . 51797
Bladder . . . . . . . . . . . . . . . . . . . 51728-51729
Rectum . . . . . . . . . . . . . . . . . . . . . . . 51797

## Volatiles . . . . . . . . . . . . . . . . . . . . . 84600

## Volhard's Test
See Water Load Test

## Volkman Contracture. . . . . . 25315-25316

## Volume Reduction
Blood Products. . . . . . . . . . . . . . . . . . . 86960

## Volume Reduction, Lung
See Lung Volume Reduction (LVRS)

## Von Kraske Proctectomy
See Proctectomy, Partial

## VP
See Voiding Pressure Studies

## Vulva
Abscess
  Incision and Drainage . . . . . . . . . . . . . 56405
Colposcopy. . . . . . . . . . . . . . . . . . . . . 56820
  Biopsy. . . . . . . . . . . . . . . . . . . . . . . 56821
Excision
  Complete . . . . . . . . . . . . 56625, 56633-56640
  Partial. . . . . . . . . . . . . . 56620, 56630-56632
  Radical . . . . . . . . . 56630-56631, 56633-56640
    Complete . . . . . . . . . . . . . . . 56633-56640
    Partial . . . . . . . . . . . . . . . . . 56630-56632
  Simple
    Complete . . . . . . . . . . . . . . . . . . 56625
    Partial . . . . . . . . . . . . . . . . . . . . 56620
Lesion
  Destruction. . . . . . . . . . . . . . 56501-56515
Perineum
  Biopsy. . . . . . . . . . . . . . . . . 56605-56606
  Incision and Drainage . . . . . . . . . . . . . 56405
Repair
  Obstetric. . . . . . . . . . . . . . . . . . . . . 59300

## Vulvectomy
Complete . . . . . . . . . . . . . . . 56625, 56633-56640
Partial. . . . . . . . . . . . . . . . . 56620, 56630-56632
Radical . . . . . . . . . . . . 56630-56631, 56633-56640
  Complete
    with Bilateral Inguinofemoral
      Lymphadenectomy . . . . . . . . . . . . . 56637
    with Inguinofemoral, Iliac, and Pelvic
      Lymphadenectomy . . . . . . . . . . . . . 56640
    with Unilateral Inguinofemoral
      Lymphadenectomy . . . . . . . . . . . . . 56634
  Partial
    with Bilateral Inguinofemoral
      Lymphadenectomy . . . . . . . . . . . . . 56632

with Unilateral Inguinofemoral
    Lymphadenectomy . . . . . . . . . . . . . . . 56631
Simple
    Complete . . . . . . . . . . . . . . . . . . . . . . . . 56625
    Partial. . . . . . . . . . . . . . . . . . . . . . . . . . 56620

**VZIG**
*See* Immune Globulins, Varicella-Zoster

# W

**W-Plasty**
*See* Skin, Adjacent Tissue Transfer

**WADA Activation Test** . . . . . . . . . .95958
*See* Electroencephalography

**WAIS** . . . . . . . . . . . . . . . . . . . . . . 96101-96102

**Waldius Procedure** . . . . . . . . . . . .27445

**Wall, Abdominal**
*See* Abdominal Wall

**Walsh Modified Radical
Prostatectomy**
*See* Prostatectomy

**Warts**
Flat
    Destruction. . . . . . . . . . . . . . . . . 17110-17111

**Washing**
Sperm . . . . . . . . . . . . . . . . . . . . . . . . . . . 58323

**Wassmund Procedure**
Osteotomy
    Maxilla. . . . . . . . . . . . . . . . . . . . . . . . 21206

**Water Wart**
*See* Molluscum Contagiosum

**Waterston Procedure** . . . . . . . . . .33755

**Watson-Jones
Procedure**. . . . . . . . . . . . . . . . . 27695-27698

**Wave, Ultrasonic Shock**
*See* Ultrasound

**WBC**
*See* White Blood Cell

**Webbed**
Toe
    Repair. . . . . . . . . . . . . . . . . . . . . . . . . 28280

**Wechsler Memory Scales**
*See* Neuropsychological Testing

**Wedge Excision**
Osteotomy . . . . . . . . . . . . . . . . . . . . . . . 21122

**Wedge Resection**
Ovary. . . . . . . . . . . . . . . . . . . . . . . . . . . . 58920

**Well-Baby Care** . . . . .99381, 99391, 99432

**Wellness Behavior**
*See* Evaluation and Management, Health Behavior

**West Nile Virus**
Antibody. . . . . . . . . . . . . . . . . . . . . 86788-86789

**Westergren Test**
*See* Sedimentation Rate, Blood Cell

**Western Blot**
HIV . . . . . . . . . . . . . . . . . . . . . . . . . . . . 86689
Protein . . . . . . . . . . . . . . . . . . . . 84181-84182
Tissue Analysis . . . . . . . . . . . . . . 88371-88372

**Wheelchair Management**
Training. . . . . . . . . . . . . . . . . . . . . . . . . 97542

**Wheelchair Management/
Propulsion**
*See* Physical Medicine/Therapy/Occupational
Therapy

**Wheeler Procedure**
*See* Blepharoplasty, Entropion
Discission Secondary Membranous
Cataract . . . . . . . . . . . . . . . . . . . . . . . . 66820

**Wheeze Rate**
*See* Acoustic Respiratory Measurements

**Whipple Procedure** . . . . . . . . . . . .48150

**Whirlpool Therapy** . . . . . . . . . . . . .97022
*See* Physical Medicine/Therapy/Occupational
Therapy

**White Blood Cell**
Alkaline Phosphatase . . . . . . . . . . . . . . . 85540
Antibody. . . . . . . . . . . . . . . . . . . . . . . . . 86021
Count. . . . . . . . . . . . . . . . . 85032, 85048, 89055
Differential. . . . . . . . . . . . . . 85004-85007, 85009
Histamine Release Test. . . . . . . . . . . . . . 86343
Phagocytosis . . . . . . . . . . . . . . . . . . . . . 86344
Transfusion
    *See* Leukocyte, Transfusion

**Whitman Astragalectomy**
*See* Talus, Excision

**Whitman Procedure**. . . . . . . . . . . .27120

**Wick Catheter Technique**. . . . . . .20950

**Window**
Oval
    *See* Oval Window
Round
    *See* Round Window

**Window Technic, Pericardial**
*See* Pericardiostomy

**Windpipe**
*See* Trachea

**Winiwarter Operation**
*See* Anastomosis, Gallbladder to Intestines

**Winter Procedure** . . . . . . . . . . . . . .54435

**Wintrobe Test**
*See* Sedimentation Rate, Blood Cell

**Wire**
*See* Pin
Insertion/Removal
    Skeletal Traction . . . . . . . . . . . . . . . 20650
Interdental
    without Fracture. . . . . . . . . . . . . . . . 21497

**Wiring**
Prophylactic Treatment
    Humerus. . . . . . . . . . . . . . . . . . . . . . 24498

**Wirsung Duct**
*See* Pancreatic Duct

**Wisconsin Card Sorting Test**
*See* Neuropsychological Tests

**Witzel Operation** . . . . . . . . 43500, 43520,
43830-43832
*See* Incision, Stomach, Creation, Stoma; Incision
and Drainage

**Womb**
*See* Uterus

**Wood Alcohol**
*See* Methanol

**Work Hardening**. . . . . . . . . . 97545-97546
*See* Physical Medicine/Therapy/Occupational
Therapy

**Work Related Evaluation
Services** . . . . . . . . . . . . . . . . 99455-99456

**Worm**
*See* Helminth

**Wound**
Debridement
    Non-Selective . . . . . . . . . . . . . . . . . . 97602
    Selective . . . . . . . . . . . . . . . . . . 97597-97598
Dehiscence
    Repair. . . . . . . . . . . . . . . 12020-12021, 13160
Exploration
    Penetrating
        Abdomen/Flank/Back. . . . . . . . . . . . 20102
        Chest. . . . . . . . . . . . . . . . . . . . . . . 20101
        Extremity. . . . . . . . . . . . . . . . . . . . 20103
        Neck . . . . . . . . . . . . . . . . . . . . . . . 20100
        Penetrating Trauma . . . . . . . . . . 20100-20103
Infection
    Incision and Drainage
        Postoperative . . . . . . . . . . . . . . . . . 10180
Near-Infrared Spectroscopy
    Lower Extremity. . . . . . . . . . . . . . . . . . 0286T
Negative Pressure Therapy. . . . . . . . 97605-97606
Repair
    Complex. . . . . . . . . . . . . . . . . . . 13100-13160
    Intermediate. . . . . . . . . . . . . . . . 12031-12057
    Simple . . . . . . . . . . . . . . . . . . . 12001-12021
    Urethra. . . . . . . . . . . . . . . . . . . 53502-53515
Strapping
Suture
    Bladder. . . . . . . . . . . . . . . . . . . 51860-51865
    Kidney . . . . . . . . . . . . . . . . . . . . . . . 50500
    Trachea
        Cervical. . . . . . . . . . . . . . . . . . . . . 31800
        Intrathoracic . . . . . . . . . . . . . . . . . 31805
    Urethra. . . . . . . . . . . . . . . . . . . 53502-53515
Vagina
    Repair. . . . . . . . . . . . . . . . . . . 57200-57210

**Wrist**
*See* Arm, Lower; Carpal Bone
Abscess . . . . . . . . . . . . . . . . . . . . . . . . 25028
Arthrocentesis . . . . . . . . . . . . . . . . . . . . 20605
Arthrodesis. . . . . . . . . . . . . . . . . . . . . . . 25800
    with Graft. . . . . . . . . . . . . . . . . . . . . 25810
    with Sliding Graft. . . . . . . . . . . . . . . . 25805
Arthrography . . . . . . . . . . . . . . . . . . . . . 73115
Arthroplasty . . . . . . . . . . . . 25332, 25443, 25447
    Revision . . . . . . . . . . . . . . . . . . . . . . 25449
    Total Replacement. . . . . . . . . . . . . . . 25446
    with Implant. . . . . . .25441-25442, 25444-25445

# X

## X, Coagulation Factor
*See* Stuart-Prower Factor

## X, Cranial Nerve
*See* Vagus Nerve

## X-Linked Ichthyoses
*See* Syphilis Test

## X-ray

Artery
  Abdominal ...................... 75726
  Additional Vessels .............. 75774
  Adrenal................. 75731-75733
  Arm...................... 75710-75716
  Arteriovenous Shunt.............. 75791
  Brachial........................ 75658
  Carotid ................. 75660-75680
  Coronary ....................... 93556
  Coronary Bypass.................. 93556
  Head and Neck................... 75650
  Iliac........................... 75953
  Leg .................... 75710-75716
  Mammary........................ 75756
  Pelvic ......................... 75736
  Pulmonary............... 75741-75746
  Spine........................... 75705
  Transcatheter Therapy ...... 75894-75898
  Vertebral....................... 75685
Bile Duct................. 74300-74320
  Calculus Removal................ 74327
  Catheterization............ 75982-75984
  Drainage................. 75980-75982
  Guide Catheter.......... 74328, 74330
Bladder......... 74430, 74450-74455
Brain................... 70010-70015
Bronchi................. 71040-71060
Central Venous Access Device ....... 36598
Colon
  Barium Enema ........... 74270-74280
Corpora Cavernosa............... 74445
Elbow.......................... 73085
Epididymis ..................... 74440
Gallbladder............... 74290-74291
Gastrointestinal Tract ........ 74246-74249
Hip ........................... 73525
Iliofemoral Artery................ 75630
Intervertebral Disc
  Cervical....................... 72285
  Lumbar ....................... 72295
  Thoracic ...................... 72285
Joint
  Stress Views................... 77071
Kidney
  Cyst.......................... 74470
  Guide Catheter................. 74475
Knee............. 73560-73564, 73580
Lacrimal Duct................... 70170
Larynx......................... 70373
Lymph Vessel
  Abdomen ............... 75805-75807
  Arm................... 75801-75803
  Leg .................. 75801-75803
Mammary Duct ........... 77053-77054
Nasolacrimal Duct................ 70170
  Guide Dilation................. 74485
Oviduct........................ 74740
Pancreas............... 74300-74305
Pancreatic Duct
  Guide Catheter.......... 74329-74330
Perineum ...................... 74775
Peritoneum..................... 74190
Salivary Gland .................. 70390
Seminal Vesicles ................ 74440

Shoulder........................ 73040
Spine
  Cervical....................... 72240
  Lumbosacral ................... 72265
  Thoracic ...................... 72255
  Total ......................... 72270
Temporomandibular Joint
(TMJ) ................... 70328-70332
Ureter
  Guide Catheter................. 74480
  Guide Dilation................. 74485
Urethra................. 74450-74455
Urinary Tract............ 74400-74425
Uterus......................... 74740
Vas Deferens ................... 74440
Vein
  Adrenal................ 75840-75842
  Arm................... 75820-75822
  Hepatic Portal........ 75810, 75885-75887
  Jugular ....................... 75860
  Leg .................. 75820-75822
  Liver ................. 75889-75891
  Neck.......................... 75860
  Orbit ......................... 75880
  Renal................. 75831-75833
  Sampling...................... 75893
  Sinus......................... 75870
  Skull ................. 75870-75872
  Splenic ....................... 75810
  Vena Cava.............. 75825-75827
Wrist .......................... 73115
Wrist...................... 73100-73110

## X-ray Tomography, Computed
See CT Scan

## Xa, Coagulation Factor
See Thrombokinase

## Xenoantibodies
See Antibody, Heterophile

## Xenografts, Skin
See Heterograft, Skin

## Xenotransplantation
See Heterograft

## XI, Coagulation Factor
See Plasma Thromboplastin, Antecedent

## XI, Cranial Nerve
See Accessory Nerve

## XII, Coagulation Factor
See Hageman Factor

## XII, Cranial Nerve
See Hypoglossal Nerve

## XIII, Coagulation Factor
See Fibrin Stabilizing Factor

## Xylose Absorption Test
Blood................................. 84620
Urine................................. 84620

## Yacoub Procedure
See Ascending Aorta Graft

## Yeast
Culture ............................. 87106

## Yellow Fever Vaccine ......... 90717

## Yersinia
Antibody............................ 86793

## YHrium-Aluminum-Garnet (YAG)
## Laser
See Eye, Incision

# Z

## Ziegler Procedure
Discission Secondary Membranous
Cataract ........................... 66820

## Zinc ............................. 84630

## Zinc Manganese Leucine
## Aminopeptidase
See Leucine Aminopeptidase

## Zygoma
See Cheekbone

## Zygomatic Arch
Fracture
  Open Treatment ............ 21356-21366
  with Manipulation.................. 21355

# Notes

# CODING *with* MODIFIERS:

## A Guide to Correct CPT® and HCPCS Level II Modifier Usage, fourth edition

**Modifier changes:**
- **One new**
- **One deleted**
- **Four revised**

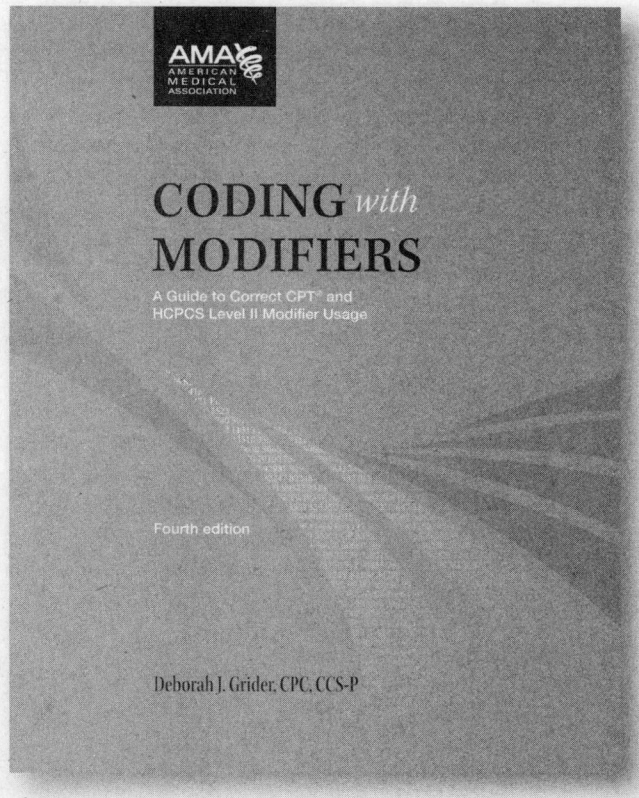

The ultimate modifiers resource—revised. Essential components to the coding process, modifiers help create clear and concise communications between the provider and payer. *Coding with Modifiers* provides guidance on how and when to use modifiers in order to avoid costly payment delays and denials.

Using the 2012 code set, the fourth edition contains new, deleted and revised modifiers, along with updates to Centers for Medicare & Medicaid Services, third-party payer, and AMA-modifier guidelines to assist with coding accuracy.

- **Coding tips**—explain how to use specific modifiers to help clear up confusion surrounding modifier usage

- **Modifiers approved for hospitals and ASCs**—provide information for professional service and hospital reporting requirements

- **Teaching tools**—allow you to create and administer tests using questions and answers developed by the AMA

- **Clinical examples**—guide readers in determining the correct modifier to use with helpful scenarios

- **Test-Your-Knowledge questions**—test your comprehension of the material with more than 190 questions

## Visit amabookstore.com for more information or call (800) 621-8335 to order!

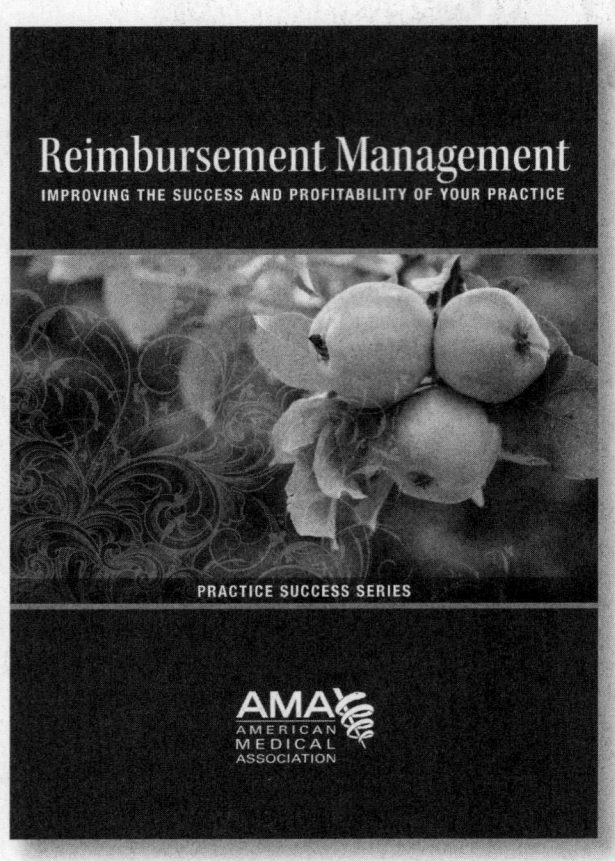

# AMA Coding Online

## Authoritative coding and compliance resources

**Now available!**
**amacodingonline.com**

**NEW!** AMA Coding Online features the American Medical Association's (AMA) best-selling authoritative coding and compliance resources in all-new, web-based formats. These user-friendly online products provide you instant access to the latest coding, billing and compliance changes from the source of CPT®—the AMA.

Monthly updates included!

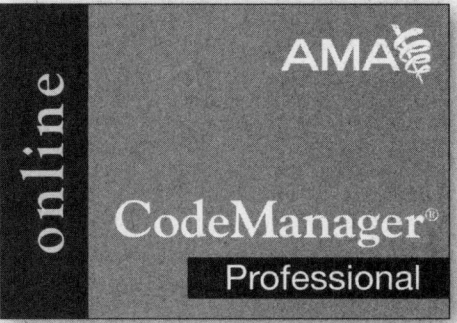

### The authoritative voice of CPT®

Receive a new issue of *CPT® Assistant* every month and rely on instant access to more than 21 years of essential coding articles.

### Built with the coder in mind

Integrated features include:

- The latest edition of *CPT Professional, ICD-9-CM Volumes 1, 2 and 3 and HCPCS Level II*
- Medicare rules and RBRVS calculator
- Date-of-service searching
- Local Coverage Determinations (LCDs)
- And much more!

**Experience *CodeManager Online* today!**

- Sign up for a 14-day free trial of the *Elite* level
- Register for a free monthly webinar hosted by a coding expert
- View a comparison chart of the three *CodeManager Online* levels: Standard, Professional and Elite

### Also available at AMA Coding Online!

Twelve-month subscriptions are available and can be purchased on behalf of an entire office. Discounts are also available for two- and three-year subscriptions and multi-user accounts.

**AMA**
AMERICAN MEDICAL ASSOCIATION

**Visit the new AMA Coding Online site today at *amacodingonline.com* or call (800) 621-8335 to learn more.**